Clinical Management of Infections in Immunocompromised Infants and Children

Clinical Management of Infections in Immunocompromised Infants and Children

Editor

Christian C. Patrick, M.D., Ph.D.

Deputy Chief Medical Officer
Vice President for Medical Services
Member, Departments of Infectious Diseases and Pathology
St. Jude Children's Research Hospital
and
Associate Professor
Department of Pediatrics
University of Tennessee, Memphis
College of Medicine
Memphis, Tennessee

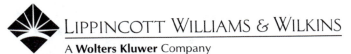

LIPPINCOTT WILLIAMS & WILKINS
A **Wolters Kluwer** Company
Philadelphia · Baltimore · New York · London
Buenos Aires · Hong Kong · Sydney · Tokyo

Acquisitions Editor: Jonathan W. Pine, Jr.
Developmental Editor: Michelle M. LaPlante
Production Editor: John C. Vassiliou
Manufacturing Manager: Benjamin Rivera
Cover Designer: Karen Quigley
Compositor: Lippincott Williams & Wilkins Desktop Division
Printer: Maple-Press

Library of Congress Cataloging-in-Publication Data

Clinical management of infections in immunocompromised infants and children / editor, Christian C. Patrick.
    p. cm.
  Includes bibliographical references and index.
  ISBN 0-7817-1718-3
  1. Immunological deficiency syndromes in children—Complications. 2. Infection in children. I. Patrick, Christian C.
  [DNLM: 1. Infection Control—Child. 2. Immunocompromised Host—Child. WC 195 C641 2000]
RJ387.D42 C56 2000
618.92—dc21
                                                                        00-060888

Care has been taken to confirm the accuracy of the information presented and to describe generally accepted practices. However, the authors, editor, and publisher are not responsible for errors or omissions or for any consequences from application of the information in this book and make no warranty, expressed or implied, with respect to the currency, completeness, or accuracy of the contents of the publication. Application of this information in a particular situation remains the professional responsibility of the practitioner.

The authors, editor, and publisher have exerted every effort to ensure that drug selection and dosage set forth in this text are in accordance with current recommendations and practice at the time of publication. However, in view of ongoing research, changes in government regulations, and the constant flow of information relating to drug therapy and drug reactions, the reader is urged to check the package insert for each drug for any change in indications and dosage and for added warnings and precautions. This is particularly important when the recommended agent is a new or infrequently employed drug.

Some drugs and medical devices presented in this publication have Food and Drug Administration (FDA) clearance for limited use in restricted research settings. It is the responsibility of the health care provider to ascertain the FDA status of each drug or device planned for use in their clinical practice.

10 9 8 7 6 5 4 3 2 1

This book is dedicated to the immunocompromised patients
for whom, hopefully, it will serve.

Contents

III. Infectious Complications as Defined by Anatomic Location

IV. Prevention and Therapy

Contributing Authors

Uma H. Athale, M.D. *Postdoctoral Fellow, Department of Hematology/Oncology, St. Jude Children's Research Hospital, Memphis, Tennessee*

Bettina H. Ault, M.D. *Assistant Professor, Department of Pediatrics, The University of Tennessee Health Science Center, Memphis, Tennessee*

Kenneth M. Boyer, M.D. *Director, Department of Pediatric Infectious Diseases, Rush Children's Hospital; Professor and Associate Chairman, Department of Pediatrics, Rush Medical College, Chicago, Illinois*

R. Clark Brown, M.D., Ph.D. *Fellow, Department of Hematology/Oncology, St. Jude Children's Research Hospital, Memphis, Tennessee*

Stephen A. Chartrand, M.D. *Director, Department of Pediatric Infectious Diseases, Children's Hospital; Professor and Chairman, Department of Pediatrics, Creighton University School of Medicine, Omaha, Nebraska*

P. Joan Chesney, M.D. *Director, Academic Programs Office, St. Jude Children's Research Hospital; Professor, Department of Pediatrics, University of Tennessee, Memphis, Tennessee*

James H. Conway, M.D. *Clinical Assistant Professor, Department of Pediatric Infectious Diseases, James Whitcomb Riley Hospital for Children; Clinical Assistant Professor, Department of Pediatrics, Indiana University Medical School, Indianapolis, Indiana*

Dev M. Desai, M.D., Ph.D. *Chief Resident, Department of Surgery, Stanford University Hospital; Chief Resident, Department of Surgery, Stanford University School of Medicine, Stanford, California*

Patricia M. Flynn, M.D. *Member, Department of Infectious Diseases, St. Jude Children's Research Hospital; Associate Professor, Department of Pediatrics, University of Tennessee, Memphis, Tennessee*

Marc D. Foca, M.D. *Clinical Fellow, Department of Pediatrics, Babies & Children's Hospital; Postdoctoral Clinical Fellow, Department of Pediatrics, Columbia University, New York, New York*

Wayne L. Furman, M.D. *Associate Member, Department of Hematology/Oncology, St. Jude Children's Research Hospital; Associate Professor, Department of Pediatrics, University of Tennessee College of Medicine, Memphis, Tennessee*

Michael Green, M.D., M.P.H. *Attending Physician, Division of Allergy, Immunology, and Infectious Diseases, Children's Hospital of Pittsburgh; Associate Professor, Department of Pediatrics and Surgery, University of Pittsburgh School of Medicine, Pittsburgh, Pennsylvania*

Andreas H. Groll, M.D.   *Senior Clinical Fellow, Immunocompromised Host Section, Pediatric Oncology Branch, National Cancer Institute, National Institutes of Health, Bethesda, Maryland*

William C. Gruber, M.D.   *Vice President, Department of Clinical Research, Wyeth-Lederle Vaccines, Pearl River, New York*

Imelda Celine Hanson, M.D.   *Department of Pediatrics, Texas Children's Hospital; Associate Professor, Department of Pediatrics, Baylor College of Medicine, Houston, Texas*

John P. Heggers, Ph.D., F.A.A.M., C.W.S. (A.A.W.M.)   *Director, Clinical Microbiology and Immunology, Shriners Burns Hospital; Professor, Department of Surgery (Plastic)/Microbiology and Immunology, University of Texas Medical Branch, Galveston, Texas*

Robert W. Hostoffer, D.O. , F.A.C.O.P., F.A.A.P.   *Department of Pediatrics, University Hospital; Clinical Assistant Professor, Department of Pediatrics, Case Western Reserve University, Cleveland, Ohio*

Lisa M. Hunsicker, M.D.   *Resident, Department of Surgery, Shriners Burns Hospital; Resident, Department of Surgery, University of Texas Medical Branch, Galveston, Texas*

Robert S. Irwin, M.D.   *Senior Clinical Fellow, Department of Pediatrics, Madigan Army Medical Center, Tacoma, Washington*

Deborah P. Jones, M.D.   *Director, Dialysis Services, Department of Pediatric Nephrology, LeBonheur Children's Medical Center; Associate Professor, Department of Pediatrics, University of Tennessee, Memphis, Tennessee*

Sheldon L. Kaplan, M.D.   *Chief, Infectious Disease Services, Texas Children's Hospital; Professor and Vice-Chairman for Clinical Affairs, Department of Pediatrics, Baylor College of Medicine, Houston, Texas*

James W. Lee, M.D.   *Medical Director, Department of Oncology, Deaconess Hospital, Evansville, Indiana*

Moise Levy, M.D.   *Chief, Dermatology Division, Texas Children's Hospital; Professor, Departments of Pediatrics and Dermatology, Baylor College of Medicine, Houston, Texas*

Jorge Luján-Zilbermann, M.D.   *Postdoctoral Fellow, Department of Infectious Diseases, St. Jude Children's Research Hospital; Postdoctoral Fellow, Department of Pediatrics, The University of Tennessee Health Science Center, Memphis, Tennessee*

Jonathan A. McCullers, M.D.   *Research Associate, Department of Infectious Diseases, St. Jude Children's Research Hospital, Memphis, Tennessee*

Ross E. McKinney, Jr., M.D.   *Division Chief, Pediatric Infectious Diseases; Associate Professor, Department of Pediatrics, Duke University Medical Center, Durham, North Carolina*

Maria T. Millan, M.D. *Assistant Professor of Surgery, Department of Surgery, Stanford University School of Medicine, Palo Alto, California*

Douglas K. Mitchell, M.D. *Pediatric Infectious Diseases, Children's Hospital of The King's Daughters; Associate Professor, Department of Pediatrics, Eastern Virginia Medical School, Center for Pediatric Research, Norfolk, Virginia*

Janak A. Patel, M.D. *Associate Professor and Division Director, Department of Pediatrics, University of Texas Medical Branch, Galveston, Texas*

Christian C. Patrick, M.D., Ph.D. *Deputy Chief Medical Officer and Vice President for Medical Services, Member, Departments of Infectious Diseases and Pathology, St. Jude Children's Research Hospital; Associate Professor, Department of Pediatrics, University of Tennessee College of Medicine, Memphis, Tennessee*

Larry K. Pickering, M.D., F.A.A.P. *Director, Center for Pediatric Research, Children's Hospital of The King's Daughters; Professor, Department of Pediatrics, Eastern Virginia Medical School, Norfolk, Virginia*

Philip A. Pizzo, M.D. *Physician-in-Chief and Chair, Department of Medicine, Children's Hospital; Thomas Morgan Rotch Professor, Department of Pediatrics, Harvard Medical School, Boston, Massachusetts*

Sujatha Rajan, M.D. *Clinical Instructor, Department of Pediatrics, Columbia University, New York, New York*

Lisa Saiman, M.D., M.P.H. *Associate Attending, Department of Pediatrics, Babies & Children's Hospital; Associate Professor, Department of Pediatrics, Columbia University, New York, New York*

José Ignacio Santos, M.D. *Director, National Child Health Program, Ministry of Health; Professor, Department of Experimental Medicine, Universidad Nacional Autonoma de Mexico, Mexico City, Mexico*

Jerry L. Shenep, M.D. *Associate Member, Department of Infectious Diseases, St. Jude Children's Research Hospital; Professor, Department of Pediatrics, University of Tennessee, Memphis, Tennessee*

Samuel K. S. So, M.D., F.A.C.S. *Associate Professor, Department of Surgery, Stanford University School of Medicine, Palo Alto, California*

Deanna Soloway-Simon, M.D. *Pediatric Resident, Department of Pediatrics, Texas Children's Hospital; Pediatric Resident, Department of Pediatrics, Baylor College of Medicine, Houston, Texas*

Dennis C. Stokes, M.D. *Clinical Director, Department of Pediatric Pulmonary Medicine, Vanderbilt Children's Hospital; Associate Professor, Department of Pediatrics, Vanderbilt University School of Medicine, Nashville, Tennessee*

Russell B. Van Dyke, M.D. *Head, Pediatric Infectious Diseases, Tulane Medical Center; Professor, Department of Pediatrics, Tulane University Health Sciences Center, New Orleans, Louisiana*

Thomas J. Walsh, M.D. *Senior Investigator and Chief, Immunocompromised Host Section, Pediatric Oncology Branch, National Cancer Institute, National Institutes of Health, Bethesda, Maryland*

Winfred C. Wang, M.D. *Member, Department of Hematology/Oncology, St. Jude Children's Research Hospital; Professor, Department of Pediatrics, University of Tennessee, Memphis, Tennessee*

Robert J. Wyatt, M.D. *Professor, Department of Pediatrics, The University of Tennessee Health Science Center, Memphis, Tennessee*

Ram Yogev, M.D. *Director, Section of Pediatric and Maternal HIV Infection, Department of Infectious Diseases/Special ID, Children's Memorial Hospital; Professor, Department of Infectious Diseases, Northwestern University Medical School, Chicago, Illinois*

Foreword

More than a quarter of a century ago, Dr. Waldo E. Nelson asked me to write a review article for the *Journal of Pediatrics* on infections in the compromised host. I asked an eminent immunologist, Dr. William Shearer, to work with me and we coauthored a three-part series of articles concerning this subject. In 38 pages of printed text we were able to encompass what was then known about the predisposing factors, etiology, pathogenesis, clinical diagnosis, and treatment of these disorders. At that time, the management of infections in immunocompromised patients represented a small portion of the consulting practice of a pediatric infectious disease specialist.

Much has changed in the intervening years. The field of immunology has exploded. Cytokines, interferons, interleukins, and many other components of the immunologic response to infection have been described. Therapy with a large variety of agents that can interfere with the normal immune response to infection has been utilized to treat many childhood disorders, thereby creating a population of patients that are predisposed to infection. Our ability to sustain the lives of infants and children in intensive care units has improved markedly. The sustenance of life has required the use of many types of catheters that bypass the normal barriers to infection, predisposing the patient to infection with both common and unusual microorganisms. Many of the organisms themselves have become resistant to commonly used antimicrobial agents.

Dr. Christian C. Patrick has undertaken the task of editing the current body of information concerning infection in immunocompromised infants and children, with particular emphasis placed upon the information most relevant to the clinical management of infections in these patients. Patients with congenital or acquired immunodeficiency, congenital or acquired neutropenias, or those predisposed to infection because the normal barriers to infection have been bypassed now constitute more than 50% of all patients seen by pediatric infectious disease consultants. For this reason, *Clinical Management of Infections in Immunocompromised Infants and Children*, edited by Dr. Patrick, is a needed and welcome addition to the literature.

Dr. Patrick has organized the text logically by dividing it into several sections: i) The Immunocompromised Host, ii) Infections of the Compromised Host, iii) Infectious Complications as Defined by Anatomic Location, and iv) Prevention and Therapy. Individual chapters are devoted to infections following kidney, liver, heart, and stem cell transplantation. Separate chapters are devoted to infections in patients with congenital immunodeficiencies and those with acquired immunodeficiency disease.

A chapter entitled "Immunizations in the Immunocompromised Host" addresses an area of great interest and concern for all physicians who care for children, and particularly for those in general pediatric practice or family medicine.

A chapter devoted to immunomodulation describes the current knowledge in this field, but also gives us a glimpse of the future. The traditional approach to prevention and treatment of infection in children has been to administer aggressive antimicrobial therapy, to immunize them to prevent disease, or both. Recent advances in our basic understanding of the immune system have enabled us to explore methods for manipulation of the immune system as a means of improving the response of the patient to an infectious insult. The use of anticytokine agents (e.g., monoclonal antibodies), colony-stimulating factors, interleukins, interferons, and hematopoietic growth factors that allow treatment or prevention of infection in the immuno-compromised host is in its infancy. The extent to which the efficacy of these agents has been proved is delineated; the ultimate beneficial effects of these agents will require further human trials.

Dr. Patrick and the superbly talented group of authors whom he has chosen are to be complimented for presenting an authoritative, comprehensive, and eminently readable textbook. It should be recommended as required reading for every infectious disease specialist and, in fact, to anyone interested in the care of children.

Ralph D. Feigin, M.D.
President and Chief Executive Officer,
J.S. Abercrombie Professor and Chairman, Department of Pediatrics, and
Distinguished Service Professor, Baylor College of Medicine
Physician-in-Chief, Texas Children's Hospital
Pediatrician-in-Chief, Ben Taub General Hospital
Chief, Pediatric Service, The Methodist Hospital
Houston, Texas

Preface

With the increasing longevity of patients with congenital and acquired immunodeficiencies and the improvement in supportive care concerning cancer and transplant patients allowing increased survival, the care and treatment of infectious diseases in the immunocompromised child is becoming an integral part of pediatric medicine. The spectrum of potential pathogens is diverse, and includes both organisms that are pathogenic in the normal host, and organisms once thought to be nonvirulent that have now been shown to cause life-threatening diseases in the immunocompromised host. The diagnosis and clinical management of such infections is challenging.

The art of caring for an immunocompromised patient was once the purview of the physician specialized in the disciplines associated with immunodeficiency (e.g., the immunologist), the infectious diseases practitioner, the hematologist/oncologist, and the transplant surgeon. These individuals acquired their knowledge and skills in the management of the immunocompromised patient by learning from their mentors and by keeping abreast of new knowledge through conferences and literature review. As the number of immunocompromised patients has increased, so has the number of healthcare providers who are administering care to these patients. This book will hopefully help these individuals to understand the pathobiology of disorders associated with an immunocompromised state and current management.

Clinical Management of Infections in Immunocompromised Infants and Children is an effort to provide information from experts in the field pertinent to the diagnosis and treatment of infections in the immunocompromised patient. The pathogenesis, clinical manifestations, diagnosis, therapy including suppressive care, and prevention of infectious diseases are presented in a manner that will allow the reader to ascertain important points to help manage this increasing patient population.

Clinical Management of Infections in Immunocompromised Infants and Children is structured to afford the reader comprehensive and practical information. It has easy access to up-to-date pertinent information in the management of difficult infectious processes in this unique patient population.

The content is divided into four parts to provide the reader the opportunity to evaluate a particular patient not only in terms of the pathobiology of the immunocompromised host, as delineated in disorders of host defense in Part I, but also as it pertains to the particular compromised host as detailed in Part II, or by anatomical location as depicted in Part III. Part IV affords the opportunity of looking at potential prevention and therapy, through immunizations, particular prevention and therapy, and the use of immunomodulations.

It has been a pleasure to edit this book and to work with this outstanding group of authors. I hope that you, the reader, can obtain as much information from this textbook as I have.

PART I

The Immunocompromised Host

1

Disorders of Host Defense

Robert W. Hostoffer

Department of Pediatrics, Case Western Reserve University, Cleveland, Ohio 44121

The human immune system has developed over millennia into an overlapping network that protects the host from most earthly pathogens. Although it is generally extremely effective, it relies on very intricate molecular mechanisms involving four essential limbs: the humoral, the cellular, the phagocytic, and complement. The first three of these are derived from a pluripotent stem cell (Fig. 1.1). Through various mutations any one of these limbs may become deficient and allow infection to prevail. The loss of even a single limb as a result of a mutation would allow those specific pathogens excluded by that limb to penetrate the host's defenses (Table 1.1). This then may cause infection at a particular time of the host's life, repeated infection, or death.

Careful questioning of the patient should permit the practitioner to ascertain the limb of the immune system that is deficient, which would then allow for the appropriate testing and treatment. Questioning should start with the "immunologist's rule of thumb" (Table 1.2). This table will be used initially as an outline for this chapter. This chapter reviews for the clinical immunologist and infectious disease practitioner those necessary questions that allow determination of the defective limb

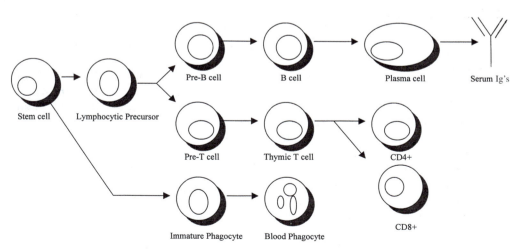

FIG. 1.1. The drawing demonstrates the normal differentiation of both the lymphoid (B- and T-cell) and myeloid limbs from a common stem cell.

TABLE 1.1. *Mutations of the limbs of the immune system causing primary immunodeficiencies*

Disorder	Chromosome	Protein mutation	Peripheral defect
X-linked primary immunodeficiencies			
X-LA	Xq22	Btk	Absent B cells, absent immunoglobulins
X-HIM	Xq26	gp39	Absent IgG and IgA, increased IgM
X-SCID	Xq13	IL-2Rτ	Absent T cells
X-CGD	Xp21	91-kd	Absent superoxide production
WAS	Xp11.2	WASP	Thrombocytopenia, Eczema
Other primary immunodeficiencies			
Omenn's SCID		RAG I/II	T and B cells
Bare lymphocyte SCID	2q12	CIITA	Absent expression of MHC I/II
ZAP70 SCID	16p13	ZAP70	CD8 deficiency
DiGeorge syndrome	22q11.2	6q	T cell, aorta, parathyroid
JAK3 SCID	19p12	JAK3	Absent T cells
AT	11q22.3	AT protein	IgA, ataxia, telangiectasia
Fas defect	10q24.1	Fas protein	Lymphoproliferation
τIFN-τRI/II deficiency	γ	IFN-τ receptor	Recurrent mycobacterial infection

AT, ataxia telangiectasia; CGD, chronic granulomatous disease; HIM, hyperimmunoglobulin M; IFN, interferon; IL, interleukin; SCID, severe combined immunodeficiency; WAS, Wiskott-Aldrich syndrome; X-LA, X-linked agammaglobulinemia.

TABLE 1.2. *Immunologist's rule of thumb for determining immunodeficiency*

Recurrent infections
>10 episodes acute otitis media per year (infant and children)
>2 episodes consolidated pneumonia per year
>2 life-threatening infections per life-time
Unusual organisms
Unusual response to organisms
Recurrent autoimmune phenomena
Dysmorphic features associated with recurrent infection
Infections worsening chronic disorders (asthma or seizure)
Development of vaccine pathogen after vaccination
Family history of immunodeficiencies or recurrent infections

and some of the major described defects within each limb.

RECURRENT INFECTIONS

The most common complaint that should be evaluated for an immunodeficiency is that of recurrent episodes of infection; however, not every patient with this complaint has an immunodeficiency. The differential diagnosis for recurrent infections also includes illnesses such as cystic fibrosis and immotile cilia syndrome, inborn errors of metabolism, and anatomic abnormalities (e.g., deviated septum, narrowed bronchus).

A strict numeric criterion to establish how many infections are too many is difficult to derive, but certain rules of thumb may serve as guidelines. In infants and children, more than one episode of acute otitis media per month warrants an evaluation of the immune system. Such patients present after repeated trips to the family physician, continual use of antibiotics, several days lost from school, and tremendous parental frustrations. Typically patients have already received one or more sets of tympanostomy tubes and/or courses of prophylactic antibiotics, with little improvement in their history of infections.

Sinusitis in children is difficult to diagnose and therefore a difficult parameter to use for recurrent bacterial infections. Often patients present to the immunologist or the infectious disease subspecialist after multiple episodes of yellowish to greenish nasal drainage acutely treated with antibiotics. Substantiation of these past episodes is difficult and may necessitate a period of observation over 4 to 6 months to document the true incidence of infection. Radiographic imaging of the sinuses may also be helpful in the substantiation of sinusitis and in documenting chronic sinus changes.

The number of sinusitis episodes required to indicate an immune workup changes with the age of the patient. As the child becomes an adolescent or adult, more than five episodes per year is incriminating. Inner ear infections become less common as the child becomes an adolescent, so repeated attacks of acute otitis media and/or severe sinusitis with purulent drainage (more than once a year) in an adolescent or adult may warrant an immunologic evaluation.

Recurrent lower respiratory tract infections are also prominently found in the symptom complex of primary immunodeficiency. Typically, more than two consolidated lobar pneumonias per year is suspicious. Some patients may also have continuous low-grade bronchitis. On occasion, chest radiographs may be available to document the pneumonias or bronchitis, but often they are not. A high-resolution, thin-slice computed tomographic (CT) study may be necessary to demonstrate the effects of repeated or chronic lower respiratory tract disease.

Infections in a patient with immunodeficiency may not produce the classic symptom complex experienced by the normal host in response to the pathogen. In fact, the response may be dramatically blunted. Severe end-organ damage may have occurred before diagnosis as a result of this blunting. Therefore, if the patient admits to a chronic cough or shortness of breath (in lieu of repeated antibiotic use for recurrent upper respiratory tract infections), a further evaluation of the pulmonary system (i.e., chest radiograph, pulmonary function tests, and/or CT) should be performed to demonstrate end-organ damage.

UNUSUAL INFECTIONS

Organisms such as *Streptococcus pneumoniae* (the pneumococcus) or *Haemophilus influenzae* routinely occur in a primary care practice and are comfortably treated by the practitioner. The presentation of odd or opportunistic organisms such as *Candida albicans, Klebsiella, Aspergillus* spp., *Pseudomonas aeruginosa/burkholderia,* or *Pneumocystis carinii* that are uncomfortably managed by the practitioner warrant an immunologic evalua-

tion. In other words, organisms causing infection that are typically warded off by a competent immune system may signal an immunologic defect, although there are caveats to this statement.

Some immunodeficiencies allow the host to survive without infection but manifest with an odd organism in an odd place at a random time. Sorenson et al. (1) described an otherwise healthy child with an interleukin-2 (IL-2) deficiency whose only symptom was a cryptococcal osteomyelitis of the scapula. In these patients with relatively minor immunodeficiencies, infection may occur given the right physical circumstances, organisms, and health of the host. These patients should receive an immunodeficiency evaluation. If no defect is determined, they should be referred to a tertiary care institution with basic science laboratories.

Some immunodeficiencies are so specific that the host develops infections with the same odd organism time after time. Ottenhoff et al. (2) described a cohort of patients with defects of the interferon-γ receptor I and II (IFN-γR-I/II) who experienced recurrent episodes of mycobacterial infection.

Some of these odd organisms may also occur in the normal host. For example, *P. carinii* pneumonia has been reported in normal newborns (3). Typically these are one-time events and are not repeated in the host; the patient thrives and has no future infections. An in-depth immunologic evaluation should be performed on these patients. If no abnormalities are identified, the patient should be monitored for several months to years to assess for progressive immunologic deficits such as late-onset adenosine deaminase (ADA) or purine nucleoside phosphorylase (PNP) deficiency.

LIFE-THREATENING INFECTIONS

The immune system is so effective that the normal host is rarely seriously threatened by common microbes. However, life-threatening infections in the normal host do occur. Infants, children, adolescents, and adults may experience at least one life-threatening infection in their lifetime. Newborn sepsis, meningococcus meningitis, or pneumococcus pneumonia with severe respiratory distress are prime examples. The occurrence of two or more life-threatening infections during one's lifetime may signal a breakdown in host defenses and should be investigated.

UNUSUAL RESPONSES TO INFECTION

Infections are typically treated with one course of oral antibiotics. Patients with immunodeficiencies may present with infections that have not been resolved in this manner. Repeated courses of oral or intravenous antibiotics for a single infection may signal an immunodeficiency.

Infections manifest in the normal host with classic symptoms of fever and rigor, among others. Patients with immunodeficiencies may not demonstrate such symptoms. They may present to the office with little symptoms except for a chronic cough, with bronchiectatic changes of the lung found on subsequent CT of the chest.

INFECTIONS COMPLICATING CHRONIC DISORDERS

In some cases patients present with increased difficulty in the management of a pre-existing disease such as asthma or seizure. Further questioning may suggest that the worsening is linked to recurrent infections or fevers. Laboratory evaluation often shows a B-cell defect, in particular hypogammaglobulinemia.

In the case of asthma, sinusitis is followed by exacerbation of asthma symptoms that may require steroid therapy; this may decrease the total serum immunoglobulin level and result in increased susceptibility to infection. The cycle may not resolve until the underlying immunodeficiency is treated.

In the case of seizure disorders, febrility caused by infection may decrease the patient's seizure threshold, thereby increasing the number of seizures. This may complicate the management of the seizure disorder. Defining and treating an immunodeficiency in such patients may help to decrease the number of infections, but it does not alleviate the need for management of the nonfebrile seizures.

TYPES OF ORGANISMS

On occasion an organism may be recovered from the patient with suspected immunodeficiency during an acute infection. The clinician may use this information to determine which limbs of the immune system are involved. Patients with B-cell or complement defects (or both) are most likely to develop infections with polysaccharide-encapsulated organisms such as pneumococcus and *H. influenzae* (4). Because these organisms predominate in the respiratory system, it may be inferred that they are responsible when the signs and symptoms include repeated otitis, sinusitis, bronchitis, and/or pneumonia, especially if accompanied by significant fever. Bacteremia with these organisms is more likely in patients with serious antibody or complement deficiencies, in individuals with impaired splenic function, and in children who have lost their spleens as a result of trauma.

Patients with primary T-cell defects may develop infection with organisms commonly found in patients with human immunodeficiency virus (HIV) infection (i.e., *P. carinii, C. albicans,* and *Mycobacterium avium* complex) (5). In most cases these organisms can be isolated from the lungs and mucus membranes by bronchoscopy or endoscopy, or from the skin.

Patients with phagocytic defects may develop infection with *Staphylococcus aureus, Serratia marcescens, Escherichia coli, Pseudomonas,* or *Aspergillus* species (6). These organisms can be isolated from the lung, lymph nodes, or skin and soft tissue, particularly if an abscess develops that must be incised or drained.

Patients with opsonic complement defects typically experience recurrent episodes of infection with encapsulated organisms and resemble patients with opsonic antibody deficiencies. On the other hand, patients with late complement deficiencies (C5–9) seem to have a unique susceptibility to serious and disseminated infections with *Neisseria* species, including meningitis and gonococcal arthritis (7). The organisms may frequently be isolated from the blood or cerebral spinal fluid and are associated with systemic disease.

TIME OF PRESENTATION

Clinically significant primary immunodeficiencies have specific ages at which the initial infections occur. Although it is not a hard and fast rule, patients with B-cell defects tend to start their infections after 6 months of life. This is primarily a result of the protection provided by transplacental maternal immunoglobulin, the concentration of which diminishes for the first several months of life and is rarely sufficient much beyond 6 months. Babies who fail to produce their own immunoglobulins at this time are unprotected. X-linked agammaglobulinemia (X-LA), immunoglobulin G (IgG) subclass deficiency, and common variable immunodeficiency (CVID) are a few of the B-cell defects that manifest after 6 months of age. Confounding factors such as extreme prematurity or protein-losing syndromes (lymphangiectasia, peritoneal dialysis, respiratory disease such as respiratory distress syndrome, and maternal hypogammaglobulinemia or maternal CVID) often skew the age of presentation downward. Patients presenting before 6 months of age may have immunodeficiencies involving the T-cell, phagocytic, or complement limbs. Although there are exceptions to this rule, it serves as an initial guide to the evaluation and workup.

RESPONSE TO IMMUNIZATION

Vaccinations are used to enhance the host's antibody production against pathogens. They depend on a normal host response for their effectiveness. The development of an infection, after vaccination, with the organism presented in the vaccine may suggest host defense failure, although poorly administered vaccines must be considered as well. For example,

episodes of *H. influenzae* type b after the appropriate administration of the Hib vaccine may suggest a defect in antibody formation. Likewise, the development of a viral infection such as polio after administration of a live polio vaccine may suggest a T-cell defect.

FAMILY HISTORY

A history of recurrent infections or deaths due to infection in family members may assist the clinician in determining the type of immunodeficiency of the proband. For example, deaths occurring only in males on the maternal side suggest X-linked inheritance. One may then choose from the five known X-linked immunodeficiency disorders: X-linked agammaglobulinemia (X-LA), X-linked hyperimmunoglobulin M syndrome (X-HIM), Wiskott-Aldrich syndrome (WAS), X-linked severe combined immunodeficiency (X-SCID), and X-linked chronic granulomatous disease (X-CGD). Recurrent infections or early deaths affecting both men and women suggest an autosomal inheritance pattern. Examples include ADA or PNP deficiency, DiGeorge syndrome, and autosomal CGD.

DYSMORPHIC FEATURES

Many immunodeficiencies are associated with dysmorphic features. Features such as cleft palate, bifid uvula, hypertelorism, and notched pinnae have all been reported with several forms of immunodeficiencies. In addition, many known genetic syndromes such as Down's syndrome, Rubinstein-Taybi syndrome, and DiGeorge syndrome have been shown to be associated with humoral, cellular, phagocytic, and complement deficiencies. Therefore, the finding of isolated dysmorphic features or diagnosis of a genetic syndrome associated with recurrent infections should warrant further evaluation of the patient's immune system.

RECURRENT AUTOIMMUNE PHENOMENA

Recurrent autoimmune disorders (i.e., hemolytic anemia, immune thrombocytopenia, neutropenia) may signal an immune dysregulation. This immune dysregulation may also be large enough to cause recurrent infections.

One type of immune dysregulation may manifest as massive lymphoproliferation secondary to defects in apoptosis or cell defect. Rieux-Laucat et al. (8) described a cohort of patients with a defect of Fas (APO-1, CD95) who experienced recurrent autoimmune disorders, lymphoproliferation in immune organs, and recurrent infections.

MOST COMMON DEFECTS

Defects of the immune system can be ranked from the most common to the uncommon. The least common immunologic defects are those that involve the complement system (2%). The next small group involves the cellular compartment (10%), followed by phagocytic and combined immunodeficiencies (18% and 20%, respectively). The most common immune defects by far involve the B-cell system (50%) (9). It is therefore appropriate for us to start our approach with a review of the B-cell defects.

B-CELL DEFECTS

B-cell defects are a broad set of deficiencies that range from complete absence of B cells to selective absence of antibody responses to specific organisms. Patients with these defects typically present after 6 months of age and may be male or female. These patients are plagued with recurrent upper and lower respiratory tract infections caused by organisms such as pneumococcus and *H. influenzae*, and they may also have chronic and/or recurrent gastrointestinal infections, including giardiasis. B-cell defects manifest with a wide spectrum of clinical consequences, and the severity of chronic endorgan damage (e.g., destructive sinusitis, bronchitis leading to bronchiectasis) is variable depending on the time of or delay in diagnosis. Treatments may range from prophylactic antibiotics to restriction of infectious exposures and/or intravenous immunoglobulin G (IVIgG).

Laboratory Evaluation

If a B-cell defect is suspected, the peripheral B-cell number should be determined with the use of monoclonal antibodies (CD19, CD20) and flow cytometry. The lack of B cells in a male child should suggest X-LA (10). The presence of B cells with lack of serum IgG, IgA, and IgM suggests CVID (11).

Serum immunoglobulins should be quantitated next. Particular attention should be paid to the relative levels of serum IgG, IgA, and IgM, because their distribution may suggest a particular immunologic defect. Complete absence of all isotypes suggests either X-LA or CVID. Low levels of IgG and IgA with increased levels of IgM in a male child may suggest an X-HIM syndrome (12). Isolated defects of individual isotypes, particularly IgA deficiency, are common but may also be associated with ataxia-telangiectasia (AT).

Low to borderline-low IgG levels with or without IgA deficiency may require the evaluation of IgG subclasses. These low levels of IgG may result from equally low IgG1 through IgG3, or they may represent isolated IgG subclass deficiencies. If any single subclass or combination of subclasses, in particular IgG1, IgG2, and IgG4, is completely absent, one may suspect a gene deletion (13). On occasion, abnormal serum IgG subclasses may be found even with normal or increased levels of total IgG (14).

Antibody responses to vaccination may be used to determine the exact nature of the B-cell defect. Serum antibody titers to tetanus and diphtheria (protein) may comment on T-cell–dependent antibody formation, whereas serum antibody titers to pneumococcal or meningococcal polysaccharides may comment on T-cell–independent antibody formation. If no preexisting titers are present, the patient may be challenged with that particular vaccine, with titers drawn 1 month later. Typically, specific antibody response defects accompany abnormal serum immunoglobulins, but on occasion normal serum immunoglobulin levels may be found with abnormal specific antibody responses to either protein or polysaccharide antigens.

X-Linked Agammaglobulinemia

This disorder was first described by Bruton in 1952 (15). A patient with X-LA is male and may or may not have a maternal family history of recurrent infections or early deaths due to infection. This patient usually presents after 6 months of age with recurrent pyogenic infections (pneumococcus and *H. influenzae*) of the upper and lower respiratory tract. Peripheral blood B cells and serum IgG, IgA, IgM, IgE, and IgD are absent (Fig. 1.2). Because B cells make up a large proportion of the cellularity of lymphatic tissue, these patients have a paucity of tonsillar tissue and other lymphatic structures.

Although resistance to viral infection is classically considered to be intact in these patients, there have been reported cases of infections with enteroviruses (i.e., echovirus, coxsackievirus, poliovirus) which have posed particular difficulty in their resolution (16–18). These viruses may become disseminated, possibly leading to meningoencephalitis and complications such as dermatomyositis and hepatitis (17–19).

Opportunistic pathogens are rarely seen in patients with X-LA. Saulsbury (1998) described a patient with *P. carinii* infection (20). This patient's immune system had been compromised for other reasons and may not represent a true association with X-LA.

Researchers have determined that mutations of Bruton's tryosine kinase (Btk), mapping to the long arm of the X chromosome at Xq22, is responsible for the peripheral observations (21). Conley et al. (1998) found various mutations of Btk in 90% to 95% of patients with X-LA (22). Certain mutations of Btk allow for the presence of some serum immunoglobulin although peripheral B cells are still lacking.

In order to characterize Btk mutations and to evaluate carrier states in family members,

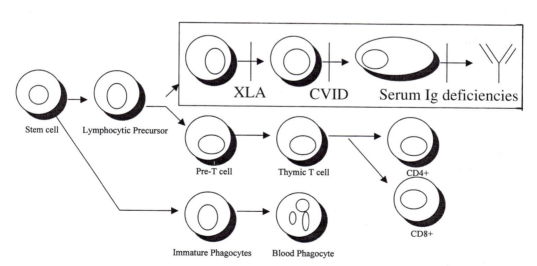

FIG. 1.2. The drawing demonstrates the pathophysiology of B-cell defects. In the bone marrow, pre–B cells develop from stem cells independent of antigen. X-linked agammaglobulinemia occurs when pre–B cells fail to progress to mature peripheral blood B cells, with subsequent lack of antigen-dependent progression to plasma cells. Common variable immunodeficiency occurs when pre–B cells progress to mature B cells but fail to progress to plasma cells. Other antibody formation deficiencies may occur downstream.

B-cell lines are developed from the blood of patients with X-LA. Because of the paucity of B cells in the peripheral blood of these patients, the tests are inherently difficult and time-consuming. Alternatively, monoclonal antibodies against the Btk protein and flow cytometry have been developed and may be used to determine disease and carrier states (23).

Arthritis is often associated with agammaglobulinemia (24). There are three forms: those that resemble rheumatoid arthritis, those that do not (both affecting large joints), and those that are infectious (25). The first two types are rarely helped by the infusion of IVIgG and may develop into a chronic form of arthritis with little destruction of the joint. The third type may be caused by pyogenic organisms or organisms such as *Mycoplasma orale, Mycoplasma hominis,* and *Ureaplasma urealyticum* (26).

Common Variable Immunodeficiency

Although CVID is a disorder that is primarily seen in adulthood, there are forms that manifest in childhood and adolescence (27). In our clinic we have observed two manifestations of CVID in childhood. The first is the development of agammaglobulinemia associated with recurrent autoimmune processes (hemolytic anemia and/or immune thrombocytopenia). Conley et al. (27) described a similar cohort of patients. Additionally, we have observed children with recurrent infections and IgA or IgG subclass deficiencies who slowly lose all ability to form all isotypes of antibodies over a relatively short period of time (28).

CVID does not have a known genetic basis, and care must be taken to differentiate CVID patients from those with X-LA, because 50% of the daughters of X-LA patients are likely to be carriers and the disease may therefore develop in the patient's future male grandchildren. This may be done by the determination of peripheral blood B-cell numbers, which will yield the diagnosis of CVID if they are present.

If B cells are absent, Btk analysis must be done to differentiate between CVID and X-LA.

Despite therapy with antibiotics and/or IVIgG (see later discussion), CVID cases are problematic owing to the presence of concomitant defects in cell-mediated immunity; the propensity to develop autoimmune disorders (29); granulomatous disease (sarcoid) (30); lymphocytic infiltration of the lung, liver, and bowel (31); and chronic intestinal parasitism (*Giardia*) (32). In some cases, immunosuppressive therapy may be required to control autoimmunity and/or the lymphocytic/granulomatous infiltration and save vital organs (33). Splenectomy may be necessary in cases of autoimmune hemolytic anemia or thrombocytopenia and may further compromise the host defenses of patients with CVID.

X-Linked Hyperimmunoglobulin M

Hyperimmunoglobulin M (hyper-IgM) was first described as dysgammaglobulinemia type I (12). It was serologically defined as absent to low IgG and IgA with normal to elevated IgM (12). This particular phenotype may be caused by anticonvulsive drugs (34), but it may also be inherited in either an autosomal (35) or an X-linked pattern (36). For the sake of brevity and scope, only the X-linked inheritance (X-HIM) is discussed here.

Throughout historical descriptions of X-HIM, it has been debated whether its physiologic defect is in the B cell or the T cell. The controversy occurred primarily because these patients develop infections associated with T-cell defects (*P. carinii, Histoplasma capsulatum*), in addition to or instead of those associated with B-cell defects (pneumococcus) (37).

Some investigators initially suggested that a T-cell defect was the cause of the laboratory and clinical profile of X-HIM. In 1986, Mayer et al. (38) reported that a T-cell clone obtained from a patient with Sézary-like syndrome induced B cells from patients with hyper-IgM to secrete IgG and IgA. This suggested that the defect in X-HIM might actually be related to T cells and their ability to interact with and induce class switching in B cells. Evidence supporting a primary T-cell defect was published by Fuleihan et al. (39), who showed that T cells from patients with X-HIM failed to express the normal T-cell surface protein CD40 ligand (CD40L, gp39) for the B-cell receptor CD40, which sends a signal, together with IL-4, for immunoglobulin class switching. It has been shown that the lack of interaction at this receptor level is the primary defect for X-HIM (Fig. 1.3). Several mutations of gp39 have been reported with X-HIM (40).

T cells are schooled through various mechanisms found in the thymus. Thymic nursery, dendritic, and epithelial cells all play their part in educating the T cell. This process is expedited through cell-to-cell contact. Thymic epithelium interacts with the T cell through the CD40-CD40L complex (Fig. 1.4). The lack of CD40L on T cells from patients with X-HIM suggests that these T cells may be skewed inappropriately in the thymus and may function similarly in the periphery.

Because of this defective T-cell phenotype, these patients are at risk for infections of the T-cell defect type. One of our patients with X-HIM syndrome was unable to clear disseminated histoplasmosis and required chronic itraconazole therapy; when the patient discontinued the course of therapy, the infection returned (41). A similar course may be found in patients with HIV infection (Fig. 1.5).

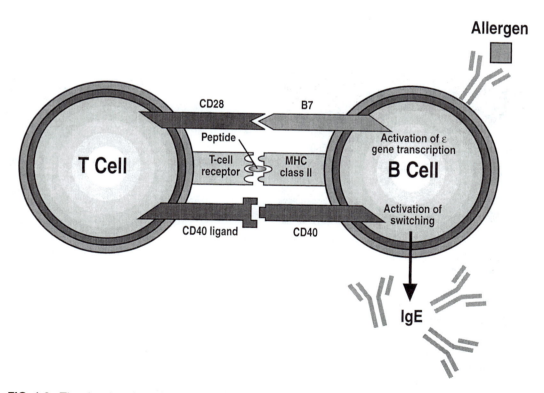

FIG. 1.3. The drawing demonstrates the interaction of T cells with B cells through the CD40/CD40L complex. CD40L on T cells is absent in patients with X-linked hyperimmunoglobulin M.

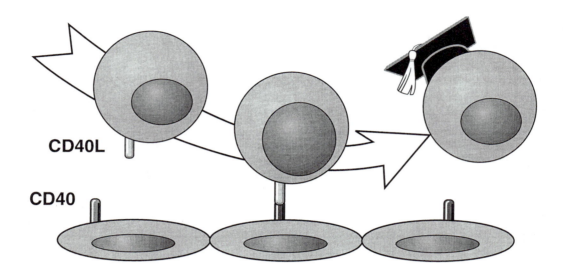

Thymic Epithelium

FIG. 1.4. The drawing demonstrates the interactions between T-cell CD40L and thymic epithelium CD40. The lack of CD40L on T cells of patients with X-linked hyperimmunoglobulin M interferes with T-cell development in the thymus.

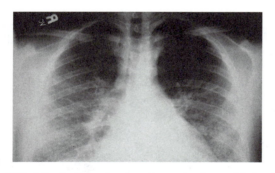
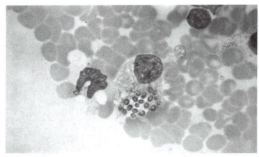

A   B

FIG. 1.5. A: The chest radiograph shows bilateral diffuse interstitial infiltrates in a patient with X-linked hyperimmunoglobulin M. **B:** Light microscopic view of bone marrow aspirate from the same patient shows *Histoplasma capsulatum* (1,000× magnification).

Hyperimmunoglobulin E Syndrome

In most texts hyper-IgE syndrome is listed with phagocytic defects based on the infections and the effects of the increased levels of IgE on chemotaxis of phagocytic cells. For clarity's sake, we have kept this disorder under the heading of B-cell defects.

The syndrome was first reported in 1972 by Buckley et al. (42) and later by others (43,44). It has been known by several names, including Job's syndrome (biblical reference, Job 2:4–9) because of the boils with which the patients are afflicted, Buckley syndrome, Que-Hill syndrome, and hyper-IgE syndrome.

The hallmark of this disorder is extremely high levels of IgE, which may range from 2,150 to 40,000 IU per milliliter, with other immunoglobulin levels remaining normal (42). Pronounced blood and sputum eosinophilia is common (42).

A diverse group of organisms causing infection have been reported with this syndrome, including *S. aureus, C. albicans, H. influenzae,* pneumococcus, and *Aspergillus* spp. (45). The diversity of these organisms does not suggest a primary defect in one particular limb but rather a deficiency in a key modulator of multiple limbs.

Sites of infections are typically skin, lung, and, less often, viscera and blood (46). Classically, the abscesses are described as being "cold" because typical signs of inflammation (e.g., erythema, tenderness) are lacking. The primary defect is unknown, although a polymorphonuclear chemotaxis defect has been described; it may be secondary to other, as yet undefined abnormalities (47). These patients have been reported to have specific IgE antibodies against *S. aureus* and *C. albicans,* which are absent in patients with elevated IgE as a result of allergies and which may contribute to an abnormal inflammatory response (48). Chronic use of antistaphylococcal antibodies may be very helpful to these patients, but formation of pneumatoceles may require surgical intervention. The use of interferon-γ or IVIgG, or both, has been helpful in individual cases (49).

Specific Antipolysaccharide Antibody Deficiency

An intriguing disorder of lacunae antibody deficiencies has been reported involving inadequate responses to polysaccharide antigens in patients with overall normal levels of IgG and its subclasses (50–57). Although precise clinical and laboratory diagnostic criteria are debated, selective antipolysaccharide antibody deficiency (SPAD) is typically defined as absent or diminished antibody response to polysaccharide capsular antigens in polyvalent pneumococcal polysaccharide vaccine, in a patient with normal immunoglobulin and IgG

subclass levels. The pathogenesis of SPAD is unknown, although the nature of the antibody response to polysaccharide antigens is T-cell independent, suggesting a B-cell defect.

The group of patients defined by this clinical history and laboratory data is probably a heterogeneous population in respect to pathogenesis. SPAD has been reported in isolated cases and in association with DiGeorge syndrome (58), Rubinstein-Taybi syndrome (59), and WAS (60).

We have also reported a significant increase in peripheral blood normal CD5+ B cells in patients with SPAD compared with controls (Fig. 1.6), patients with other humoral deficiencies such as CVID and IgG subclass deficiency (61).

Immunoglobulin G Subclass Deficiencies

There are four IgG subclasses. Deficiencies of individual and combined subclasses have been described, although the actual definition of an IgG subclass deficiency has been problematic. For example, patients with very low levels of IgG1 may additionally have low levels of total IgG, a condition that may represent CVID if it is associated with deficiencies of other IgG subclasses and immunoglobulin isotypes.

Other problems have been associated with the definition of IgG subclass deficiency in respect to the variation of normal IgG subclass levels based on age from one reference laboratory to the other. Most researchers agree that IgG subclass deficiency is present when a IgG subclass or multiple subclasses are less than 2 standard deviations below the geometric mean adjusted for age, in association with normal serum IgA and IgM.

Laboratory error also often complicates the diagnosis and definition of IgG subclass deficiency. To determine whether laboratory error has taken place, the practitioner should add all the subclasses together. They should approximately equal the total IgG subclass value given by the reference laboratory. This simple test can help eliminate laboratory error and costly further testing.

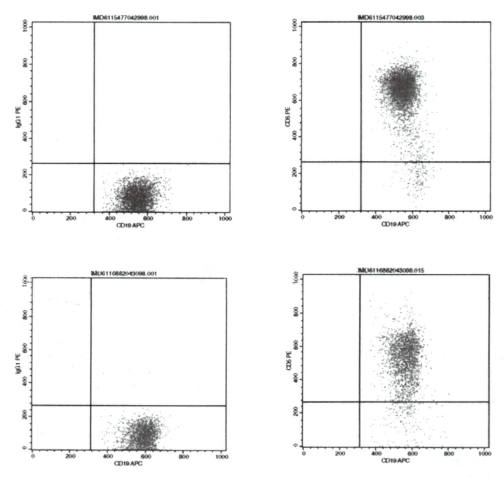

FIG. 1.6. Four-quadrant dot plot of two-color flow cytometry analysis of CD5 versus CD19 expression on peripheral blood B cells of two patients with lack of antibody response to polysaccharide antigens. The panels to the left are the negative controls. The panels to the right show CD5 on the y-axis and CD19 on the x-axis.

Similar clinical observations may be found with all the IgG subclass deficiencies. IgG1 deficiency is often found in association with low total IgG and may be associated with deficiencies of other IgG subclasses, particularly IgG3 (62). Typically, patients with IgG subclass deficiencies have recurrent infections of the upper and lower respiratory system involving pneumococcus and other encapsulated bacteria. IgG2 deficiency may be found as an isolated deficiency, but it may also be associated with IgA and IgG4 deficiency (63). Antibody response defects to polysaccharide antigens have been described in association with selective IgG2 deficiency (64). IgG3 deficiency also may be associated with other IgG subclass deficiencies (65). Recurrent infections of the upper and lower respiratory tract have been reported in association with IgG3 deficiency (66). Isolated IgG4 deficiency and its association with recurrent infections have been controversial, because it is found in a large proportion of normal asymptomatic children (67).

Treatment of Patients with Antibody Production Defects

One of the most frustrating aspects of clinical immunology is the paucity of treatment options. Additionally, the major option that is available (i.e., IVIgG), is overused for nonlabeled indications, resulting in national shortages that have limited its use in labeled indications such as immunodeficiency disorders. IVIgG should be used judiciously, and only in cases in which minimizing infectious disease exposure and prophylactic antibiotics have not been successful (see later discussion).

B-cell defects at the onset may be treated with removal of patients from infectious exposures, prophylactic antibiotics, and/or IVIgG. In cases of transient hypogammaglobulinemia (IgG deficiency with equally low subclasses or isolated IgG subclass deficiency with or without IgA deficiency) that manifests after 6 months with infections that are primarily upper respiratory in nature and with no end-organ damage, elimination of exposures and/or prophylactic antibiotics may be all that is needed. Daily trimethoprim-sulfamethoxazole (TMP/SMX, Bactrim) or amoxicillin (Amoxil) may be used during the entire year or only in the winter months, based on the individual patient's history. The use of prophylactic antibiotics allows the practitioner to sample serum immunoglobulins to repeatedly determine whether the patient has resolved his or her immunodeficiency. Given the rising levels of resistant strains of bacterial pathogens, prophylactic antibiotics should be used thoughtfully and carefully.

In the case of patients with agammaglobulinemia, CVID, or hyper-IgM, the need for IVIgG is unquestioned. Doses of 400 mg per kilogram per dose every 3 to 4 weeks are usually adequate to increase the serum trough IgG levels into the low-normal range. Increasing serum IgG typically is followed by decreasing number of infections. If lung damage in the form of decreased pulmonary function or CT changes (i.e., bronchiectasis) is present (Fig. 1.7), the dose of IVIgG should be in-

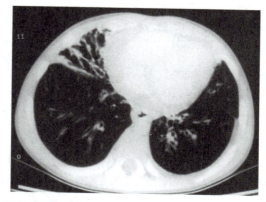

FIG. 1.7. High-resolution thin-sliced computed axial tomogram of a patient with common variable immunodeficiency shows bronchiectatic changes of the lung.

creased to 600 mg per kilogram per dose (68). Patients with borderline-low levels of total IgG, in particular those with only upper respiratory tract infections, may not require IVIgG unless end-organ damage (hearing loss) is determined to be present. In a few cases both prophylactic antibiotics and IVIgG may be useful in preventing recurrent infections.

T-CELL, COMBINED, AND SEVERE COMBINED DEFECTS

A T-cell defect, either isolated or combined with a B-cell defect, may result in profound infectious consequences (Fig. 1.8). Patients with T-cell defects often present before 6 months of age with infections involving organisms such as *P. carinii* (Fig. 1.9), or *C. albicans*. Their diagnosis is established by laboratory evaluation of both T-cell number and function, but the need for this information may complicate reaching the diagnosis in smaller hospitals and in areas where the sophisticated technology required is not available.

The laboratory evaluation of T-cell defects available commercially is limited. The enumeration of T cells using monoclonal antibodies and flow cytometry can be readily obtained (percentages and absolute counts), but

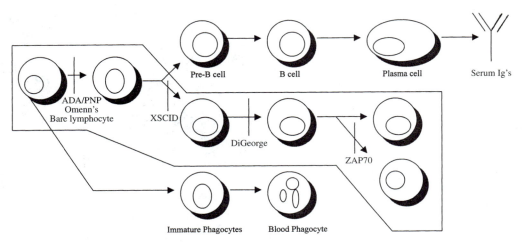

FIG. 1.8. The drawing demonstrates the point at which the defects involved in various T-cell and severe combined immunodeficiency syndromes occurs in normal differentiation.

laboratory error may lead to diagnostic and therapeutic errors (69). Adding up the components of the lymphocyte gait helps to eliminate laboratory error: T cells (CD3+) plus B cells (CD19+) plus natural killer cells (CD16+) equals 100%. Additionally, adding the two T-cell subpopulations together—total T cells (CD3+) equals CD4+ plus CD8+— may check the T-cell compartment. If these two calculations are correct, the T-cell enumerations should be reliable.

The absolute numbers of T cells are on occasion more revealing than the percentages. Even if the T-cell subset percentages are normal, the absolute numbers may be profoundly diminished based on the severity of lymphopenia found on the complete blood count, which must always be submitted simultaneously with flow cytometry for this reason. These numbers must be checked against the laboratory's age-matched control ranges, because the total T and T-cell subset absolute numbers decrease with advancing age. If age-matched control ranges are not taken into account a newborn may be considered to have normal T-cell numbers but in reality have less than 50% of normal for age.

A profound loss of the lymphocyte compartment defines a combined immunodeficiency (i.e., X-SCID, ADA, PNP, bare lymphocyte syndrome, JAK3 deficiency, and ZAP70 deficiency) (70). Typically these patients have less than 10% of the lower limit of normal numbers of T and/or B lymphocytes (70). Low levels of total T cells also may represent diminished subpopulations of CD4+ cells (idiopathic CD4 deficiency), which must be differentiated from HIV infection (71), or CD8+ cells (ZAP70 deficiency) (72). In addition, the application of age-matched controls for the determination of deficiencies is essential in the evaluation of T-cell subsets.

The evaluation of T-cell functions is limited and can be divided into *in vivo* and *in vitro* testing. Delayed hypersensitivity is one *in vivo* method to grossly evaluate T-cell function (73). The intradermal administration of an antigen with appropriate positive and negative controls may determine whether the patient is anergic, suggesting a defective T-cell function. This test may also comment on macrophages and cytokine secretion. The test is not applicable in young infants who have not yet been immunized or exposed to many infectious agents. In these situations, mitogen stimulation must be used (discussed later in this section). Anergy may also be seen in children younger than 2 years of age (74) and in cases of malnutrition (75), illness (76), or technical error and therefore has limited use

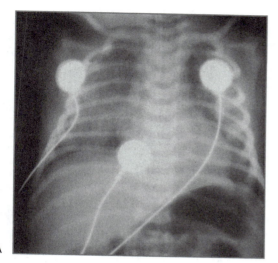

A

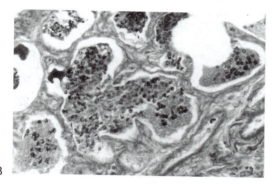

B

FIG. 1.9. A: Chest radiograph of a patient with severe combined immunodeficiency shows diffuse interstitial infiltrates. **B:** Silver stain of a lung biopsy shows *Pneumocystis carinii* (1,000× magnification).

in the evaluation of a hospitalized patient or a busy clinical setting.

In vitro methods of evaluating T-cell function include mitogen and antigen stimulation (76). In this assay, lymphocytes are separated from peripheral blood and suspended in media. Mitogens (phytohemagglutinin [PHA], concanavalin A, pokeweed mitogen) or antigens (tetanus, *C. albicans*) are added to the cell suspensions and then pulsed in 3 to 5 days with radiolabeled thymidine (required for new DNA synthesis). The mitogens or antigens cause the T cells to proliferate, incorporating the radiolabeled thymidine into the cell. Ex-

cess thymidine is washed away. The amount of incorporated thymidine is measured with a gamma counter (counts per minute). This count is an indirect measurement of T-cell proliferation and therefore T-cell function (76). These tests usually are not performed daily at any particular laboratory. Therefore, before drawing the blood the practitioner should find out the exact day on which the tests are performed. A delay in 24 hours between obtaining the blood and starting the culture may alter the response by decreasing the results.

Mitogen and antigen stimulation is particularly useful in the evaluation of DiGeorge syndrome (77), SCID (70), and other T-cell defects. In the case of DiGeorge syndrome, stimulation with the T-cell mitogen PHA serves as a predictive test to determine whether the T-cell counts are likely to return to normal.

DiGeorge Syndrome/ Velocardiofacial Syndrome

In 1965, DiGeorge described the association of recurrent infection, absent thymus/absent thymic shadow (Fig. 1.10), and hypoparathyroidism (78). It was later shown that some of these findings are also associated with a cellular immunodeficiency, congenital heart disease, and abnormal facies (79). The typical facies is elfin in appearance and includes hypognathia, long philtrum, low-set ears, bifid uvula and/or cleft palate, antimongolian slant of the eyes, and hypertelorism (Fig. 1.11). This facies may be difficult to observe in the newborn period if other overt signs are not present.

Most cases of DiGeorge syndrome have been associated with a microdeletion of chromosome 22q11.2 (80), although a new gene locus involving a deletion of chromosome 10p has been found in some patients (81). These deletions are determined by fluorescent *in situ* hybridization (FISH) procedures and cannot be visualized by routine chromosome analysis (Fig. 1.12) (80,81).

These microdeletions have also been found in patients with a broader spectrum of

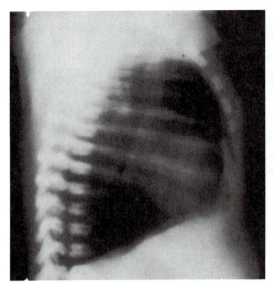

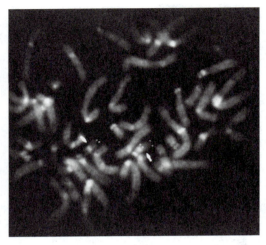

FIG. 1.12. Fluorescent *in situ* hybridization study of a patient with DiGeorge syndrome. Arrows indicate monosomic deletion of 22q11.2.

FIG. 1.10. Lateral chest radiograph of a patient with DiGeorge syndrome shows lack of a thymic shadow in the superior anterior mediastinum.

clinical phenotypes, including velocardiofacial (VCF) anomaly (82) and isolated conotruncal heart defects (83). An acronym has been devised to envelop this spectrum, CATCH 22 (*C*, cardiac defect; *A*, abnormal facies; *T*, hypothymic; *C*, cleft palate; *H*,

hypoparathyroidism) (84). Additionally, the clinician must add developmental delay and central nervous system structural abnormalities (absent or hypoplastic corpus callosum, small cerebellum), because they have become very prominent features (85–87; R. Hostoffer and R. Good, *personal communication*, 1999). The finding of two or more of these observations may warrant evaluation of the chromosomes by FISH and laboratory analysis of T-cell numbers and function. The associations in this spectrum are continually expanding and reported on a monthly basis, although this in my opinion is still one of the most underdiagnosed immunodeficiencies in our clinic, because of its potential subtitles. We have diagnosed patients as old as 15 years of age with DiGeorge/VCF syndrome after observation of recurrent immune cytopenias (88).

Chronic Mucocutaneous Candidiasis

There is a peculiar group of disorders called chronic mucocutaneous candidiasis, initially described by Thorpe and Handely in 1929 (89,90). These patients have persistent candidal infections of the mouth (Fig. 1.13),

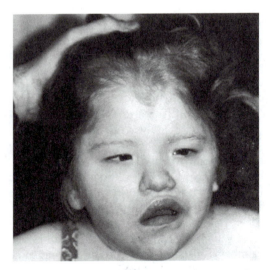

FIG. 1.11. Photograph of a patient with DiGeorge syndrome with the typical facies of the syndrome.

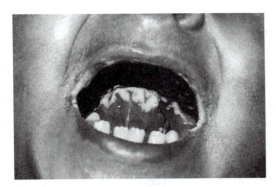

FIG. 1.13. Photograph of thrush in a patient with chronic mucocutaneous candidiasis.

skin, and nails. The infections rarely become systemic (91,92). The patients may also have one or more endocrinologic deficiencies such as hypoparathyroidism, hypoadrenalism, hypothyroidism, or hypogonadism (91). In some cases there is an autosomal dominant or recessive inheritance (92). The primary defect is not known, although cellular (93), humoral (94), and phagocytic (95) defects all have been implicated. Mainstays of therapy include antifungal medication and supportive care.

Combined Immunodeficiency

Wiskott-Aldrich Syndrome

Wiskott first characterized this syndrome in 1937 (96), followed by Aldrich in 1954 (97). It is most notably recognized for the triad of thrombocytopenia, eczema, and recurrent infection (98). The initial presentation for WAS is usually petechiae occurring during the first few months of life. Because of the low number of small platelets, the patients usually first come to the attention of hematologists. These small platelets are pathognomonic for WAS.

The immunologic defect of poor antibody formation, in particular antibodies to polysaccharide antigens in WAS, was described by Krivit, Good, and Cooper (99–101). Low levels of isohemagglutinins; increased IgG, IgA, and IgE; and a low IgM concentration (102) may demonstrate the antibody formation defect. Additional T-cell defects have been pos-

tulated (103). Because of these immunodeficiencies, infections may be prominent. Chronic draining otitis media, pneumonia, and mastoiditis have been reported. The thrombocytopenia may worsen with these infections. The eczematoid rash may vary from isolated crusts behind the ears to severe disfiguring eruptions over large areas of the body and may become superinfected.

The development of malignancies pose a problem in patients with WAS. After the age of 8 years the incidence of malignancy increases dramatically (104). The commonly found malignancies in WAS are lymphoma (105) and reticuloendotheliosis (106) with a predilection for the brain.

The hunt for the pathogenesis of WAS has been pursued by many investigators. Parkman et al. (107) reported that a defect of the platelet surface antigen CD43 was the primary cause of the disease. This was later proved incorrect, because the antigen is encoded on chromosome 16 and not on the X chromosome. Derry and others later showed that mutations of a protein encoded at Xp11.22, now referred to as the WAS protein (WASP), lead to development of the disorder (108,109). The WASP is a 502-amino-acid protein found in the cytoplasm of all hematopoietic cells; it is involved in the cytoskeletal signaling system (110,111). It is not known exactly how mutations in this protein lead to the typical manifestations of WAS.

It has been noted with the localization of the causative gene that WAS, like most immunodeficiencies, may represent a spectrum of clinical observations. On one side of the spectrum are individuals with a certain mutation of the WASP causing isolated X-linked thrombocytopenia without immunodeficiency; at the opposite end, patients with a different mutation have full-blown WAS (111).

Ataxia-Telangiectasia

Initially referred to as Vogt's disease, AT was first reported by Syllaba and Henner in 1926 (112). Later, Boder and Sedgewick in 1957

(113) coined its present-day name, AT. Ataxia, strabismus, athetosis, loss of Purkinje cells in the cerebellum, IgA deficiency, IgG2 subclass deficiency, and recurrent sinopulmonary infections have been described with this devastating disorder.

The ataxia and the telangiectasia have variable onsets. Ataxia may manifest early in infancy, or it may be delayed to as late as 5 years of age (114). The ataxia may be cerebellar at first, progressing to involve generalized muscle weakness and resulting in profound disability. The presentation of the telangiectasia is variably manifest and may occur as early as 1 year of age or as late as 6 (115). The bulbar conjunctiva is typically involved, but telangiectases may also appear on the nose, ears, arms, hands, and feet.

The infections found in patients with AT may involve viral and bacterial pathogens of the sinopulmonary tract, as expected from the IgA and IgG subclass deficiencies. The severity of infections varies from case to case, but chronic lung disease, including bronchiectasis, has been described (116). The predisposition to infections with opportunistic organisms typically is not present.

Chromosomal breakage has been associated with AT. Four common somatic break points have been described involving reciprocal translocations—14q32, 14q12, 7q35, and 7q12 (117–119)—but these may be secondary to underlying enzyme abnormalities in DNA repair. These break points may be detected by routine chromosomal analysis.

Small point germline mutations of the AT gene are responsible for the clinical manifestations of AT. The genes encode for the AT protein (350 kD), which is a key protein kinase (120). This kinase regulates multiple signaling cascades responsible for DNA repair and apoptosis (121).

Severe Combined Immunodeficiency

SCID is a heterogeneous group of disorders having in common deficits in both cellular and humoral immunity. Classically manifesting during early infancy, SCID is characterized by lymphopenia, hypogammaglobuline-

mia, and susceptibility to a broad range of infectious organisms. The presenting features for SCID may include failure to thrive, persistent or unusually severe thrush, or *P. carinii* pneumonia.

X-Linked Severe Combined Immunodeficiency

About 50% of cases of SCID are inherited in an X-linked recessive mode (122). Although it manifests very much like other forms of SCID, X-SCID has a cellular phenotype that is characteristically different. Examination of the lymphocyte compartment of the patient with X-SCID shows absent T cells and low to normal B-cell numbers (123). This phenotype results from a lack of T-cell expansion, caused in part by lack of the IL-2 receptor (IL-2R) γ chain (124) (Fig. 1.14). A similar cellular phenotype of SCID may be seen in female patients who have a deficiency in JAK3, which is a tyrosine kinase downstream of the IL-2R (125).

Adenosine Deaminase/ Purine Nucleoside Deficiency

Giblett et al. (126) described the first immunodeficiency associated with an enzyme deficiency. About 25% of SCID cases are caused by an enzyme deficiency of either ADA or PNP (127). These two enzymes are found in the nucleic acid catabolic pathway. Because of the enzyme deficiency, toxic metabolites such as adenosine diphosphate, guanosine triphosphate, and in particular deoxyadenosine triphosphate begin to accumulate within the lymphocytes. Additionally, deoxyadenosine itself accumulates within the cells. The accumulation of this metabolite affects lymphocyte proliferation, creating a profound lymphopenia involving both T- and B-cell lines (128).

Equilibrium of the metabolites exists between the intracellular space and the plasma, exchanging some of the metabolites, in ADA deficiency. By means of blood transfusion

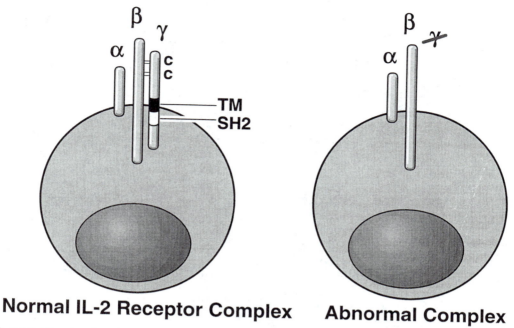

Normal IL-2 Receptor Complex   Abnormal Complex

FIG. 1.14. The drawing shows the pathophysiology of X-linked severe combined immunodeficiency. The figure on the left shows the normal interleukin-2 receptor (IL-2R) heterodimer comprising α, β, and γ chains. The figure on the right shows the absence of the γ chain, which results in X-SCID.

(normal erythrocytes with ADA), the equilibrium may be shifted away from the ADA-deficient lymphocytes, allowing for increased survival of affected cells. However, the necessity of frequent transfusions to treat the defect (every 4 to 6 weeks) obviated its use as a therapy (129). The observation that exogenous enzyme could reduce the intracellular content of toxic metabolites led to the development of bovine-derived ADA coupled (for decreased immunogenicity and increased circulation time) to polyethylene glycol-adeosine deaminase (PEG-ADA, Adagen). This was injected intramuscularly, allowing its activity in the plasma (130). Because of its expense and eventual host antibody response, this therapy has been used only in temporizing settings. Bone marrow transplantation has been the mainstay and definitive treatment if a matched donor is available, but unmatched transplants have not been successful without ablation.

Gene therapy has been performed for the treatment of ADA deficiency (131). Cells are collected from the patient after he or she has received PEG-ADA. These cells are infected with a retrovirus containing the ADA gene. After IL-2 is added to the cell cultures to expand the cells *in vitro,* the cells are washed and given back to the patient (Fig. 1.15). This is by no means a definitive cure, and patients have continued taking PEG-ADA despite having received gene therapy.

Omenn's Syndrome

Omenn first described this syndrome in 1964 (132). It was found in Irish kindred who, since their arrival in the United States, had nomadically traveled the nation. The kindred allowed first cousins to marry, and a matriarch was selected to follow the couple to delivery. At the delivery the matriarch pronounced the child with or without disease. This was based on the presence or absence of a rash now known to be a graft-versus-host reaction caused by maternal transplacentally

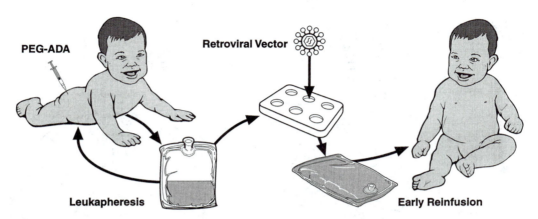

FIG. 1.15. The drawing shows the general procedure used in gene therapy for adenosine deaminase deficiency.

derived T cells. The patients with the rash often have eosinophilia and lymphocytosis. Villa et al. (133) have shown that Omenn's syndrome is associated with a decreased efficiency of V(D)J recombination of antigen receptor loci caused by a missense mutation in the recombinase enzymes, RAGI and RAGII.

Bare Lymphocyte Syndrome

Touraine initially described bare lymphocyte syndrome in 1978 (134). These patients' leukocytes are usually missing the major histocompatibility antigen class II (MHC II) from their cell surface and may or may not have MHC I. Severe functional deficiencies resulting in life-threatening infections have been noted in these patients, who cannot present antigens to T-cell receptors properly (135). The molecular defect in bare lymphocyte syndrome has been shown to be a mutation of the CIITA and RFX5 MHC class II transcriptional regulatory factors (136).

ZAP70 Deficiency

In certain forms of SCID a single T-cell subpopulation is selectively deleted. Such is the case with ZAP70 deficiency. ZAP70 is a tyrosine kinase that is distal to the T-cell receptor. Patients with this deficiency typically have lymphopenia, but more dramatically

they are missing the CD8+ T-cell subcompartment (137). Presentation is similar to that of other forms of SCID, although some patients have survived without transplantation.

Treatment of T-Cell Defects

There are few options in the treatment of T-cell disorders. Initial T-cell and T-cell subset enumerations should be performed. If the total T-cell number is less than 10% of the lower limit of normal, the patient should be evaluated for SCID. Bone marrow transplantation is the standard of care for most forms of SCID (70).

If SCID is not a consideration, as is the case for DiGeorge/VCF syndrome, the CD4 counts should be determined. If the absolute number of CD4+ cells is less than 250 per microliter, *P. carinii* prophylaxis should be initiated. If blood transfusions are required, the blood should be irradiated to prevent graft-versus-host reactions. All blood products should also be cytomegalovirus negative. Live viral vaccination should be avoided, as should persons who recently have received live viral vaccinations. In the case of chicken pox exposure, varicella-zoster immune globulin should be given within 48 hours after exposure. Prophylaxis for respiratory syncytial virus (RSV) should be considered in special cases, which would include the administration of either the polyclonal or monoclonal RSV IgG. A thymic transplantation may be entertained for some patients with DiGeorge/VCF syndrome who have severe deficits of T-cell number and function, but the use of thymic tissue is still controversial (138).

A few T-cell defects may be associated with B-cell functional defects, as found in DiGeorge/VCF syndrome (58). These patients may present with recurrent upper and lower respiratory tract infections. Anticapsular polysaccharide antibody responses to a pneumococcal vaccine may be absent. The use of prophylactic antibiotics and/or IVIgG may be beneficial.

COMPLEMENT DEFECTS

Alper and Rosen (139–141) first described deficiencies of complement components in 1960. Since then, deficiencies of all eleven components have been reported (142). Patients with complement deficiencies typically have one of two manifestations, collagen vascular or infectious. Infections have been associated with deficiencies of C1q, C1r, C1rs, C4, C2, C3, C5–9, and factor D. The most common pathogens are *Neisseria meningitidis* and, less often, pneumococcus. The site of the infection is either blood or meninges.

Deficiencies of plasma control factors have also been associated with recurrent infections. These infections are less common than those just described, but they may involve similar organisms and sites. The factors include factor I, factor H, and properdin.

Most of these deficiencies are inherited. The decreased protein production is a result of the inheritance of two nonfunctioning genes. Inheritance of one nonfunctioning gene results in the heterozygous state, with one half of the normal level. This type of inheritance is called autosomal codominant.

The screening for complement defects is relatively simple. When the patient is well, a CH_{50} test (50% hemolyzing dose of complement, a measurement of the classic pathway function) should be performed. The specimen should be drawn, placed on ice, and delivered immediately to the laboratory. Delay and lack of cooling often result in low levels. If the CH_{50} result is low, an AH_{50} (measurement of the alternative pathway function) should be performed. If this result is low, the defect lies in the common membrane attack complex pathway. Most defects associated with recurrent infections involve members of this portion (143). The clinician may then measure each individual complement component or factor.

Treatment of Complement Defects

Complement defects are extremely rare among all immunodeficiencies (9). There are few treatments available. The use of IVIgG may add additional opsonin to help kill the pathogen. Immunization of the patient and of close household contacts with *H. influenzae, N. meningitidis,* and pneumococcus may also be of assistance. Prophylactic penicillin may be used in endemic areas. The use of fresh-frozen plasma as a source of complement may be added in acute infectious episodes.

PHAGOCYTIC DEFECTS

Phagocytic defects are a diverse group of disorders involving various functional aspects of phagocytosis, adherence, chemotaxis, and killing (Fig. 1.16). These patients present early in infancy and develop infections of the sinopulmonary tract, skin, mucous membranes, liver, and lymph nodes with organisms such as *S. aureus, Aspergillus, Chromobacterium violaceum,* and *Pseudomonas cepacia.*

If a neutrophil defect is suspected, measurement of numbers and function should be performed. The neutrophil count should be scrutinized to determine whether there are adequate numbers for age. Additionally, on the peripheral smear the granules in the neutrophils may be inspected for the absence of specific granules and the presence of abnormally large granules like those found in Chédiak-Higashi syndrome (144).

If a killing defect is suspected, such functional studies as the nitroblue tetrazolium test (145) (Fig. 1.17), chemoluminescence

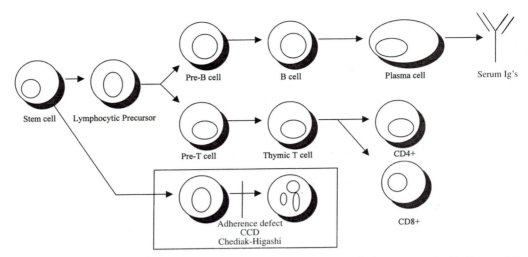

FIG. 1.16. The drawing shows the major defects of the phagocytic limb compared with those of the cellular and humoral limbs.

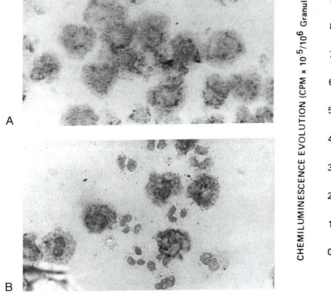

A

B

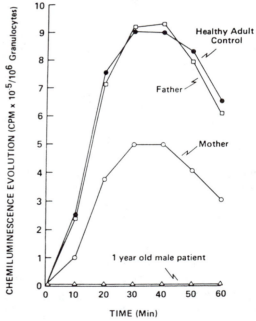

FIG. 1.17. Light microscopic view of polymorpho-nucleocytes (PMNs) after incubation of PMNs with opsonized antigen and nitroblue tetrazolium (NBT). Photograph A shows a normal NBT test. The blue color indirectly demonstrates superoxide production. Photograph B shows the same experiment on a patient who is a carrier for X-linked chronic granulomatous disease. Note that some of the cells have little or no blue color, suggesting lack of superoxide production (1,000× magnification).

FIG. 1.18. The graph shows measurement of chemoluminescence in four individuals. The y-axis measures millivolts and the x-axis measures time. The top two curves represent a normal control subject and the father, suggesting normal superoxide production. The middle curve shows less millivolt production in the mother of a patient with X-linked chronic granulomatous disease, suggesting a carrier state. The bottom curve is from a patient with X-CGD.

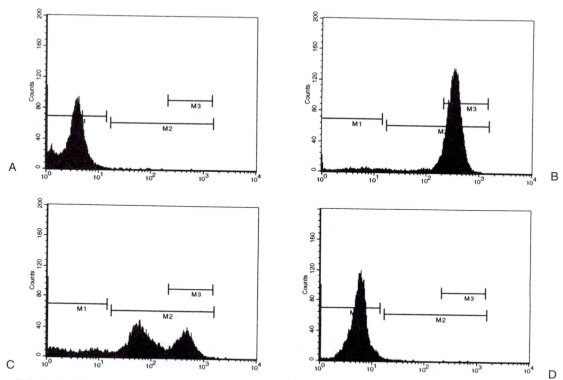

FIG. 1.19. Flow cytometry histogram demonstrates the evaluation of superoxide production. The y-axis shows cell number and the x-axis shows fluorescent intensity in log scale. **A:** This histogram shows the negative control. **B:** This histogram shows a normal superoxide production as measured by flow cytometry. **C:** This histogram shows partial absence of superoxide production, suggesting a carrier state of chronic granulomatous disease. **D:** This histogram shows absent superoxide production by flow cytometry, suggesting CGD.

(Fig. 1.18) (146), or FACS analysis (147) (Fig. 1.19) may be used to determine neutrophil superoxide production indirectly. These tests are readily available in most tertiary institutions.

If an adherence or migrational defect is suspected, the neutrophils may be easily checked by fluorescence-activated cell sorter (FACS) analysis to determine whether the cells have a deficiency of adherence molecules such as CD11a, CD11b, CD11c, or their common CD18 β-receptor (148). Chemotaxis assays may also be performed, but they may not be available commercially.

Chronic Granulomatous Disease

CGD was first described by Janeway et al. in 1954 (149) and later investigated by Good,

Berendes, and Bridges (150,151). These patients have recurrent suppurative infections and hepatosplenomegaly, but, unlike agammaglobulinemics, they actually have hypergammaglobulinemia. Quie et al. (152) determined in 1967 that the defect in this disorder involves intracellular killing. Ingestion of the bacteria by granulocytes was unimpeded, but intracellular killing was impaired due to the lack of superoxide production by those cells. A defect of one of the four structural components of the phagocyte's microbicidal nicotine adenine dinucleotide phosphate (NADPH) oxidase system (plasma membrane cytochrome b_{558}, 91 and 22 kD; cytosolic proteins, 47 and 67 kD) was later determined to be responsible (153). A defect of the 91-kD component results in the most common form,

X-CGD (154), whereas defects of any of the other three components result in the autosomal forms (155).

Infections occur within the first year of life and may be severe. *S. aureus, Aspergillus, C. violaceum,* and *P. cepacia* are typical organisms found in CGD (156). The lung, liver, skin, lymph nodes, and gastrointestinal tract are the most common sites involved in infections (157). Abscess and granulomatous formation is found frequently, but, because of the large inflammatory reaction to relatively few organisms surviving intracellularly, cultures are frequently negative.

Chédiak-Higashi Syndrome

Chédiak-Higashi syndrome is a rare autosomal recessive disorder that is characterized by partial ocular albinism, recurrent infections, neuropathy, and giant granules found in the peripheral leukocytes (144). Infections tend to be less severe than those found in CGD, although these patients do not benefit from IFN-γ. These patients may develop an accelerated phase in response to an infection, involving hepatosplenomegaly, pancytopenia, fever, and jaundice. In some cases this is fatal. Many defects have been found in association with this disorder, including defects of microtubules assembly (158), tubulin tyrosinylation (158), bactericidal activity (159), and natural killer function (160).

Leukocyte Adhesion Defects

In 1987 Anderson and Springer and their colleagues (161) described patients with defects of phagocytic adhesion. These patients fall into two phenotypes, severe and moderate, based on their phagocytic cell surface expression of the glycoprotein heterodimers CD11a/CD18, CD11b/CD18, and CD11c/CD18. The molecular defect involves mutations of the common CD18 subunit. This results in a failure of the units CD11 and CD18 to associate in the endoplasmic reticulum and subsequent absent or decreased expression on the cell surface (162). Patients with this disor-

der develop infections involving *S. aureus,* enterobacteria, *Pseudomonas,* and *C. albicans* (162). The affected organs include the skin, gingiva, bone, sinuses, and lungs. Delayed separation of the umbilical cord (more than 6 weeks) has been reported with this disorder, although in our practice this has not been a reliable observation (163). Leukocytosis during wellness is common owing to the lack of margination. Most patients that live (i.e., with detectable expression of CD11a/CD18, CD11b/CD18, CD11c/CD18) are edentulous because of severe periodontitis. Other defects of adhesion have been described involving absence of CD15 (164); these patients have clinical presentations similar to those of patients with defects of CD11/CD18.

Treatment of Neutrophil Defects

Few modalities exist for the treatment of neutrophil defects. In the homozygous forms of leukocyte adhesion defects, bone marrow transplantation may be indicated (165); the heterozygous forms require symptomatic therapy. Patients with CGD may benefit from IFN-γ therapy, which brings their superoxide production almost to the level of asymptomatic carriers (166). Otherwise, symptomatic care for infectious episodes and complications is the general rule for most phagocytic disorders.

REALITY CHECK

Although historical data is essential for the diagnosis of primary immunodeficiencies, a short warning must be presented to practitioners against those patients and caregivers of patients who receive secondary reward from imaginative and creative recurrent infections. In our clinic this population can be divided into two categories, caregivers (Munchausen syndrome by proxy) and adolescent or adult patients (Munchausen syndrome).

Caregivers typically present unbelievable histories of recurrent infections that are usually accompanied with little objective evidence. The child (infant to early adolescent) appears amazingly well. Depending on previous subspecialist consultations, this patient may have a central venous access line or gastrointestinal tube and may have had several surgical procedures performed; he or she may even have received a trial of IVIgG. The caregiver may be hypervigilant and overdescribe simple episodes. The subspecialist may hear that "no one has been able to help us" or that "we have heard a lot about your clinic and we know you can figure our child out." Careful communication among subspecialists is essential, because the words of one subspecialist may be altered by the caregiver. In reality the detoxification of these parents is very difficult, short of removing the child from the home, because they may simply leave to see another physician. Additionally, even though the patient's issues may be resolved, caregivers may then resume the illness on themselves and involve an entirely new set of adult subspecialists.

Adolescents may present to the recurrent infection clinic with unsubstantiated sinusitis, arthralgias, and fatigue, among other complaints. No previous interventions have made them better. Parents are typically doting or controlling. These patients tend to lack the sophistication to elaborate on their histories during questioning. Gentle movement of these patients to the psychology department assists in the resolution. Serum toxicology may be helpful at the onset to rule out drug abuse. In both cases, the practitioner must rule out pathology first. These will be some of your most difficult patients.

NEW DILEMMAS

With the advent of IVIgG, newer antibiotics, bone marrow transplantation, and better diagnostics, patients with primary immunodeficiencies are living longer, and some of them are at or near childbearing age. The implication of passing on horrific disorders must be addressed, and the patients must be counseled. Additionally, the expanded life expectancy in these patients brings the clinician into uncharted waters in respect to their future

clinical course. Careful observation is clearly required.

IVIgG is a purified blood product. The difficulties inherent in the use of blood products (i.e., contamination) must always be discussed before IVIgG is administered. Although HIV is not transmitted through IVIgG, other viruses have been found in association with its infusion (167). The addition of solvent detergent treatment has reduced if not eliminated the risk of passage of enveloped viruses, stopping hepatitis transmission. Hepatitis C virus, the most recent contaminant (168), was successful in reaching the blood pool partly because of the lack of adequate screening tests for its presence. In several reported cases, patients with immunodeficiencies did develop hepatitis with severe outcome (169,170). At present, risk still exists to the patient receiving IVIgG from viruses that have yet to be identified.

Jakob-Creutzfeldt disease is a progressive, degenerative central nervous system disorder caused by a particle called a prion that is transmitted through transplanted brain tissue or injected brain tissue products (171). These agents are responsible for the "mad cow disease" which has attracted much publicity in the United Kingdom. Although the disease has not been found to be transmitted by blood, many pharmaceutical companies producing IVIgG have voluntarily removed from circulation specific lots of product that were purified from the blood of individuals who later developed Jakob-Creutzfeldt disease. This in turn has decreased the supply of IVIgG to the public and created a panic among recipients of IVIgG based on little scientific evidence and a lot of corporate fears. These types of scenarios in the future will continue to complicate the immunodeficient patient's care and will increasingly require the clinician to provide such patients with accurate information.

Several thousand patients across the United States receive IVIgG monthly as treatment for their primary immunodeficiency. In the past, the demand for the product equaled the supply. More recently, as a result of new federal manufacturing regulations, a shortage has developed. In some areas of the country, patients with primary immunodeficiencies have had to extend their intervals between infusions, use fewer products, switch to a product that was more available, or go without product entirely. This event, although devastating to many, may be short-lived owing to the possible introduction of European products production. It provides a lesson for the clinician, that judicious use of this product is essential.

The mechanisms, diagnostics, and therapeutics of primary immunodeficiency disorders are becoming increasingly intricate and complicated. Behind the grand theories and hypotheses are human beings whose lives are invariably becoming more complicated as well. As practitioners caring for these patients, we must realize their needs and know that depression and loneliness soon follow the discovery and treatment of their defect. Psychosocial interventions will and must play a stronger role in the initial and future care of our patients with primary immunodeficiencies.

CONCLUSION

Primary immunodeficiencies are a diverse group of disorders resulting in recurrent infections in those afflicted. Their diagnosis may be determined through a careful history that includes age at onset, number and type of bacteria causing the infections, seriousness of the infections, response to vaccinations, and family history. From these data, the clinician may order the appropriate testing and treatment.

REFERENCES

1. Sorensen RU, Boehm KD, Kaplan D, et al. Cryptococcal osteomyelitis and cellular immunodeficiency associated with interleukin-2 deficiency. *J Pediatr* 1992; 121:873–879.
2. Ottenhoff THM, Kumararante D, Casanova JL. Novel human immunodeficiencies reveal the essential role of type-1 cytokines in immunity to intracellular bacteria. *Immunol Today* 1998;19:491–494.
3. Stagno S, Pifer LL, Hughes WT, et al. *Pneumocystis carinii* pneumonitis in young immunocompetent infants. *Pediatrics* 1980;66:56–62.
4. Lederman HM, Winkelstein JA. X-linked agammaglobulinemia: an analysis of 96 patients. *Medicine (Baltimore)* 1985;64:145–156.
5. Jose DG, Gatti RA, Good RA. Eosinophilia with *Pneumocystis carinii* pneumonia and immune deficiency syndrome. *J Pediatr* 1971;79:748–754.
6. Malech HL, Gallin JL. Neutrophils in human disease. *N Engl J Med* 1987;317:687–694.
7. Figueroa JE, Densen P. Infectious diseases associated with complement deficiencies. *Clin Microbiol Rev* 1991;4:359–395.
8. Rieux-Laucat F, LeDeist F, Hivroz C, et al. Mutations in Fas associated with human lymphoproliferative syndrome and autoimmunity. *Science* 1995;268: 1347–1349.
9. Ryser O, Morell A, Hitzig WH. Primary immunodeficiencies in Switzerland: first report of the national registry in adults and children. *J Clin Immunol* 1988;8: 478–485.
10. Rosen FS, Cooper MD, Wedgwood RJP. The primary immunodeficiencies. *N Engl J Med* 1984;311:235–242,300–310.
11. Strober W, Eisenstein E, Jaffe JS, et al. New insights into common variable immunodeficiency. *Ann Intern Med* 1993;118:720–730.
12. Notarangelo LD, Duse M, Ugazio AG. Immunodeficiency with hyper IgM (HIM). *Immunodefic Rev* 1992; 3:101–122.
13. Lefranc MP, Hammarstrom L, Smith CIE, et al. Gene deletions in the human immunoglobulin heavy chain constant region locus: molecular and immunologic analysis. *Immunodefic Rev* 1991;2:265–281.
14. Shield JPH, Strobel S, Levinsky RJ, et al. Immunodeficiency presenting as hypergammaglobulinemia with IgG2 subclass deficiency. *Lancet* 1992;340:448–450.
15. Bruton OC. Agammaglobulinemia. *Pediatrics* 1952;9: 722–728.
16. Bardelas JA, Winkelstein JA, Seto DS, et al. Fatal ECHO 24 infection in a patient with hypogammaglobulinemia: relationship to dermatomyositis-like syndrome. *J Pediatr* 1977;90:396–398.
17. Wilfert CM, Buckley RH, Mohanakumar T, et al. Persistent and fatal central-nervous-system ECHO virus infections in patients with agammaglobulinemia. *N Engl J Med* 1977;296:1485–1489.
18. McKinney RE, Katz SL, Wilfert CM. Chronic enteroviral meningoencephalitis in agammaglobulinemia patients. *Rev Infect Dis* 1987;9:334–356.
19. Ziegler JB, Penny R. Fatal ECHO 30 virus infection and amyloidosis in X-linked hypogammaglobulinemia. *Clin Immunol Immunopathol* 1975;3:347–352.
20. Saulsbury FT, Bernstein MTW, Winkelstein JA. *Pneumocystis carinii* pneumonia as the presenting infection in congenital hypogammaglobulinemia. *J Pediatr* 1979;95:559–561.
21. Parolina O, Hejtmancik JF, Allen RC, et al. Linkage analysis and physical mapping near the gene for X-linked agammaglobulinemia at Xp22. *Genomics* 1993; 15:342–349.
22. Conley ME, Mathias D, Treadaway J, et al. Mutations in btk in patients with presumed X-linked agammaglobulinemia. *Am J Hum Genet* 1998;62:1034–1043.
23. Futatani T, Miyawaki T, Tsukada S, et al. Deficient expression of Bruton's tyrosine kinase in monocytes from X-linked agammaglobulinemia evaluated by flow cytometric analysis and its clinical application to carrier detection. *Blood* 1998;91:595–602.
24. Janeway CA, Gitlin D, Craig JM, et al. "Collagen dis-

ease" in patients with congenital agammaglobulinemia. *Trans Assoc Am Physicians* 1956;69:93–97.

25. Good RA, Rotstein J, Mazzitello WF. The simultaneous occurrence of rheumatoid arthritis and agammaglobulinemia. *J Lab Clin Med* 1957;49:343–357.

26. Johnston CLW, Webster ADB, Taylor-Robinson D, et al. Primary late-onset hypogammaglobulinemia associated with inflammatory polyarthritis and septic arthritis due to *Mycoplasma pneumoniae*. *Ann Rheum Dis* 1983;42:108–110.

27. Conley ME, Park CL, Douglas SD. Childhood common variable immunodeficiency with autoimmune disease. *J Pediatr* 1986;108:915–922.

28. Hostoffer RW, Bay CA, Wagner K, et al. Kabuki make-up syndrome associated with acquired hypogammaglobulinemia and anti-IgA antibodies. *Clin Pediatr* 1996;35:273–276.

29. Lee AH, Levinson AI, Schumacher HR Jr. Hypogammaglobulinemia and rheumatic disease. *Semin Arthritis Rheum* 1993;22:252–264.

30. Bronsky D, Dunn YOL. Sarcoidosis with hypogammaglobulinemia. *Am J Med Sci* 1965;250:11–18.

31. Hermans PE, Huizenga KA, Hoffman HN, et al. Dysgammaglobulinemia associated with nodular lymphoid hyperplasia of the small intestine. *Am J Med* 1966;40:78–89.

32. Ament ME, Ochs HD, Davis SD. Structure and function of the gastrointestinal tract in primary immunodeficiency syndromes: a study of 39 patients. *Medicine (Baltimore)* 1973;52:227–248.

33. Fasano MB, Sullivan KE, Sarpon SB, et al. Sarcoidosis and common variable immunodeficiency: report of 8 cases and review of the literature. *Medicine (Baltimore)* 1996;75:251–261.

34. Mitsuya H, Tomino S, Hisamitsu S, et al. Evidence for the failure of IgA specific T helper activity in a patient with immunodeficiency with hyper IgM. *J Clin Lab Immunol* 1979;2:337–342.

35. Brahmi Z, Lazarus KH, Hodes ME, et al. Immunologic studies of three family members with the immunodeficiency with hyper IgM syndrome. *J Clin Immunol* 1983;3:127–134.

36. Notarangelo LD, Parolini O, Albertini A, et al. Analysis of X-chromosome inactivation in X-linked immunodeficiency with hyper IgM (HIGMI): evidence for involvement of different hematopoietic cell lineages. *Hum Genet* 1991;88:103–134.

37. Benkerrou M, Gougeon ML, Griscelli C, et al. Hypogammaglobulinemie G et A avec hypergammaglobulinemie M: propos de 12 observations. *Arch Fr Pediatr* 1990;47:345–349.

38. Mayer L, Kwan SP, Thompson C, et al. Evidence for a defect in "switch" T cells in patients with immunodeficiency and hyperimmunoglobulinemia M. *N Engl J Med* 1986;314:409–418.

39. Fuleihan R, Ramesh N, Loh R, et al. Defective expression of the CD40 ligand in X chromosome-linked immunoglobulin deficiency with normal or elevated IgM. *Proc Natl Acad Sci U S A* 1993;90:2170–2173.

40. Villa A, Notarangelo LD, DiSanto JP, et al. Organization of the human CD40L gene: implications for molecular defects in X chromosome-linked hyper IgM syndrome and prenatal diagnosis. *Proc Natl Acad Sci U S A* 1994;91:2110–2114.

41. Hostoffer RW, Berger M, Clark HT, et al. Dissemi-

nated *Histoplasma capsulatum* in a patient with hyper IgM immunodeficiency. *Pediatrics* 1994;94:234–236.

42. Buckley RH, Wray BB, Belmaker EZ. Extreme hyperimmunoglobulinemia E and undue susceptibility to infection. *Pediatrics* 1972;49:59–70.

43. Hill HR, Quie PG. Raised serum IgE levels and defective neutrophil chemotaxis in three children with eczema and recurrent bacterial infections. *Lancet* 1974;1:183–187.

44. Clark RA, Root RK, Kimball HR, et al. Defective neutrophil chemotaxis and cellular immunity in a child with recurrent infections. *Ann Intern Med* 1973;78:515–519.

45. Donabedian H, Gallin JI. The hyperimmunoglobulinemia E recurrent-infection (Job's) syndrome. *Medicine (Baltimore)* 1983;62:195–208.

46. Merten DF, Buckley RH, Pratt PC, et al. The hyperimmunoglobulinemia E syndrome: radiographic observations. *Radiology* 1979;132:71–78.

47. Hill HR, Quie PG, Pabst HF, et al. Defect in neutrophil granulocyte chemotaxis in Job's syndrome of recurrent "cold" staphylococcus abscesses. *Lancet* 1972;2: 617–619.

48. Berger M, Kirkpatrick CH, Goldsmith PK, et al. IgE antibodies to *Staphylococcus aureus* and *Candida albicans* in patients with the syndrome of hyperimmunoglobulin E and recurrent infections. *J Immunol* 1980;125:2437–2443.

49. King CL, Gallin JI, Malech HL, et al. Regulation of immunoglobulin production in hypergammaglobulin E recurrent infection syndrome by interferon. *Proc Natl Acad Sci USA* 1989;86:10085–10089.

50. Ambrosino DM, Siber GR, Chilmonczyk BA, et al. An immunodeficiency characterized by an impaired antibody response to polysaccharides. *N Engl J Med* 1987; 316:790–793.

51. Herrod HG, Gross S, Insel R. Selective antibody deficiency to *Haemophilus influenzae* type B capsular polysaccharide vaccination in children with recurrent infection. *J Clin Immunol* 1989;9:429–434.

52. Shapiro GG, Virant FS, Furukawa CT, et al. Immunologic defects in patients with refractory sinusitis. *Pediatrics* 1991;87:311–316.

53. Sanders LAM, Rijkers GT, Kluis W, et al. Defective antipneumococcal polysaccharide antibody response in children with recurrent respiratory tract infections. *J Allergy Clin Immunol* 1993;91:110–119.

54. Blecher TE, Soothill JF, Voyve MA, et al. Antibody deficiency syndrome: a case with normal immunoglobulin levels. *Clin Exp Immunol* 1968;3:47–56.

55. Rothbach C, Nagel J, Rabin B, et al. Antibody deficiency with normal immunoglobulins. *J Pediatr* 1979; 94:250–253.

56. Gigliotti F, Herrod HG, Kalwinsky DK, et al. Immunodeficiency associated with recurrent infections and isolated *in vivo* inability to respond to polysaccharides. *Pediatr Infect Dis J* 1988;7:417–420.

57. Germain-Lee EL, Schiffman G, Mules EH, et al. Selective deficiency of antibody responses to polysaccharide antigens in a child mosaic for partial trisomy 1 (46,XX,dir dup(1)(q12-q23)/46,XX). *J Pediatr* 1990; 117:96–97.

58. Rijkers GT, Sanders LAM, Zegers BJM. Anti-capsular polysaccharide antibody deficiency states. *Immunodeficiency* 1993;5:1–21.

59. Lourie EM, Mortimer JC, Cates HL, et al. Rubinstein-

Taybi syndrome associated with cellular and anti-capsular polysaccharide antibody deficiency. *J Allergy Clin Immunol* 1997;99:53.

60. Nahn MH, Blaese RM, Crain MJ, et al. Patients with Wiskott-Alrich syndrome have normal IgG2 levels. *J Immunol* 1986;137:3484–3487.

61. Antall PM, Meyerson H, Kaplan D, et al. Selective anti-polysaccharide antibody deficiency associated with peripheral blood CD5 positive B cell predominance. *J Allergy Clin Immunol* 1999;103:637–641.

62. Schur PH, Borel H, Gelfand EW, et al. Selective gamma-G globulin deficiencies in patients with recurrent pyogenic infections. *N Engl J Med* 1970;283:631–634.

63. Oxelius VA, Laurell AB, Lindquist B, et al. IgG subclasses in selective IgA deficiency: importance of IgG2-IgA deficiency. *N Engl J Med* 1981;304:1476–1477.

64. Geha RS. IgG antibody response to polysaccharides in children with recurrent infections. *Monogr Allergy* 1988;23:97–102.

65. Oxelius VA, Hanson LA, Bjorkander J, et al. IgG3 deficiency: common in obstructive lung disease, hereditary in families with immunodeficiency and autoimmune disease. In: Hanson LA, Soderstrom T, Oxelius VA, eds. *Immunoglobulin subclass deficiencies. Monogr Allergy* 1986;20:106–115.

66. Bjorkander J, Bake B, Oxelius VA, et al. Impaired lung function in patients with IgA deficiency and low levels of IgG2 or IgG3. *N Engl J Med* 1985;313:720–724.

67. Herrod HG. Clinical significance of IgG subclasses. *Curr Opin Pediatr* 1993;5:696–699.

68. Roifman CM, Levison H, Gelfand EW. High dose versus low dose intravenous immunoglobulin in hypogammaglobulinemia and chronic lung disease. *Lancet* 1987;1:1075–1077.

69. Lovett EJ III, Schnitzer B, Keren DF, et al. Application of flow cytometry to diagnostic pathology. *Lab Invest* 1984;50:115.

70. Gelfand EW, Dosch HM. Diagnosis and classification of severe combined immunodeficiency. *Birth Defects* 1983;19:65–72.

71. Edwards KM, Cooper MD, Lawton AR, et al. Severe combined immunodeficiency with absent T4+ helper cells. *J Pediatr* 1984;105:70–72.

72. Elder ME. Severe combined immunodeficiency due to a defect in the tyrosine kinase Zap-70. *Pediatr Res* 1996;39:743–748.

73. Ahmed AR, Blose DA. Delayed-type hypersensitivity skin testing. *Arch Dermatol* 1983;119:934.

74. Gorden EH, Krause A, Kinney JL, et al. Delayed cutaneous hypersensitivity in normals: choice of antigens and comparisons to *in vitro* assays of cell-mediated immunity. *J Allergy Clin Immunol* 1983;72:487–494.

75. Bianco NE. The immunopathology of systemic anergy in infectious diseases: a reappraisal and new perspectives. *Clin Immunol Immunopathol* 1992;62:253–257.

76. Oppenheim JJ, Dougherty S, Chan SP, et al. Use of lymphocyte transformation to assess clinical disorders. In: Vyas GN, Stites DP, Brecher G, eds. *Laboratory diagnosis of immunologic disorder.* New York: Grune & Stratton, 1975:87–109.

77. Bastian J, Law S, Vogler L, et al. Prediction of persistent immunodeficiency in the DiGeorge anomaly. *J Pediatr* 1989;115:391–396.

78. DiGeorge A. A new concept of the cellular basis of immunity [Discussion]. *J Pediar* 1965;67:907–908.

79. Lischner H, DiGeorge A. Role of the thymus in humoral immunity: observations in complete or partial absence of the thymus. *Lancet* 1969;2:1044–1049.

80. Driscoll D, Budarf M, Emanuel B. A genetic etiology for DiGeorge syndrome: consistent deletions and microdeletions of 22q11.2. *Am J Hum Genet* 1992;50:924–933.

81. Daw SCM, Taylor C, Kraman M, et al. A common region of 10p deleted in DiGeorge and velocardiofacial syndromes. *Nat Genet* 1996;13:458–460.

82. Driscoll D, Spinner N, Budarf L, et al. Deletions and microdeletions of 22q11.2 in velo-cardio-facial syndrome. *Am J Hum Genet* 1992;44:261–268.

83. Wilson D, Goodship J, Burn J, et al. Deletions within chromosome 22q11 in familial congenital heart disease. *Lancet* 1992;340:573–575.

84. Hall JG. CATCH 22. *J Med Genet* 1993;30:801–802.

85. Kraynack N, Hostoffer R, Robin N. DiGeorge syndrome associated with agenesis of the corpus callosum. *J Child Neuro* 1999;14:754–756.

86. Ryan AK, Goodship JA, Wilson DI, et al. Spectrum of clinical features associated with interstitial chromosome 22q11 deletions: a European collaborative study. *J Med Genet* 1997;34:798–804.

87. Conley ME, Beckwith JB, Mancer JK, et al. The spectrum of the DiGeorge syndrome. *J Pediatr* 1979;94:883–890.

88. DePiero AD, Lourie EM, Berman BW, et al. Recurrent immune cytopenias in two patients with DiGeorge/velocardiofacial syndrome. *J Pediatr* 1997;131:484–486.

89. Thorpe ES, Handley HE. Chronic tetany and chronic mycelial stomatitis in a child aged four and one half years. *Am J Dis Child* 1929;38:228–338.

90. Craig JM, Schiff LH, Boone JE. Chronic moniliasis associated with Addison's disease. *Am J Dis Child* 1955;89:669–684.

91. Ahonen P, Myllarniemi S, Sipela I, et al. Clinical variation of a autoimmune polyendocrinopathy-candidiasis-ectodermal dystrophy (ADECED) in a series of 68 patients. *N Engl J Med* 1990;322:1829–1836.

92. Blizzard RM, Gibbs JH. Candidiasis: studies pertaining to its association with endocrinopathies and pernicious anemia. *Pediatrics* 1968;42:231–237.

93. Valdimarsson H, Higgs JM, Wells RS, et al. Immune abnormalities associated with chronic mucocutaneous candidiasis. *Cell Immunol* 1973;6:348–361.

94. Bentur L, Nisbet-Brown E, Levinson H, et al. Lung disease associated with IgG subclass deficiency in chronic mucocutaneous candidiasis. *J Pediatr* 1991;118:82–86.

95. Djawari D, Bischoff T, Hornstein OP. Impairment of chemotactic activity of macrophages in chronic mucocutaneous candidosis. *Arch Dermatol Res* 1978;262:247–253.

96. Wiskott A. Familiarer, angeborener Morbus Werihoff? *Wochenschr Kinderheilk* 1937;68:212–216.

97. Aldrich RA, Steinberg AG, Campbell DC. Pedigree demonstrating a sex-linked recessive condition characterized by draining ears, eczematoid dermatitis and bloody diarrhea. *Pediatrics* 1954;13:133–139.

98. Huntley CC, Dees SC. Eczema associated with thrombocytopenia purpura and purulent otitis media: report of five fatal cases. *Pediatrics* 1957;19:351–361.

99. Krivit W, Good RA. Aldrich's syndrome (thrombocytopenia, eczema and infection in infants). *Am J Dis Child* 1959;97:137–153.

100. Cooper MD, Krivit W, Peterson RDA, et al. An immunological defect in Wiskott-Aldrich patients [Abstract]. In: *Transactions American Pediatric Society,* 74th Annual Meeting, Seattle, June 16, 1964.

101. Krivit W, Yunis E, White J. Platelet survival studies in Aldrich syndrome. *Pediatrics* 1966;37:37: 339–341.

102. West CD, Hong R, Holland NH. Immunoglobulin levels from the newborn period to adulthood and in immunological deficiency states. *J Clin Invest* 1962;41: 2054–2064.

103. Blaese RM, Strober W, Brown RS, et al. The Wiskott-Aldrich syndrome: a disorder with a possible defect in antigen processing or recognition. *Lancet* 1968;1: 1056–1061.

104. Brand MM, Marinkovich VA. Primary malignant reticulosis of the brain in Wiskott-Aldrich syndrome. *Arch Dis Child* 1969;44:536–542.

105. Bensel TRW, Stadlan EM, Krivit W. The development of malignancy in the course of the Aldrich syndrome. *J Pediatr* 1966;68:761–767.

106. Sullivan KE, Mullen CA, Blaese RM, et al. A multi-institutional survey of the Wiskott-Aldrich syndrome. *J Pediatr* 1994;125:876–885.

107. Parkman R, Remold-O'Donald E, Cairns L, et al. Immunologic abnormalities in patients lacking a lymphocyte surface glycoprotein. *Clin Immunol Immunopathol* 1984;33:363–370.

108. Derry JMJ, Ochs HD, Francke U. Isolation of a novel gene mutated in Wiskott-Aldrich syndrome. *Cell* 1994;78:635–644.

109. Kolluri R, Shehabeldin A, Peacooke M, et al. Identification of WASP mutations in patients with Wiskott-Aldrich syndrome and isolated thrombocytopenia reveals allelic heterogeneity at the WAS locus. *Hum Mol Genet* 1995;4:1119–1126.

110. Ochs HD. The Wiskott Aldrich syndrome. *Semin Hematol* 1998;35:332–345.

111. Nonoyama S, Ochs H. Characterization of the Wiskott-Aldrich syndrome protein and its role in the disease. *Curr Opin Immunol* 1998;10:407–412.

112. Syllaba L, Henner K. Contribution a l'independence de l'athetose double idiopathique et congenitale: atteinte familiale syndrome dystrophique, signe du reseau vasculaire conjonctival, integrite psychique. *Rev Neurol (Paris)* 1926;1:541–562.

113. Boder E, Sedgwick RP. Ataxia-telangiectasia: a familial syndrome of progressive cerebellar ataxia, oculocutaneous telangiectasia, and frequent pulmonary infection. *Univ South Calif Med Bull* 1957;9:15–27.

114. Boder E, Sedgwick RP. Ataxia-telangiectasia: a review of 101 cases. In: Walsh G, ed. *Cerebellum, Posture and Cerebral Palsy.* Clinics in Developmental Medicine Series No 8. London: The National Spastics Society and Heinemann Medical Books, 1963:110–118.

115. Reed WB, Epstein WL, Boder E, et al. Cutaneous manifestations of ataxia-telangiectasia. *JAMA* 1966; 195:746–753.

116. Ammann AJ, Cain WA, Ishizaka K, et al. Immunoglobulin E deficiency in ataxia-telangiectasia. *N Engl J Med* 1969;281:469–472.

117. McCaw B, Hecht F, Harnden DG, et al. Somatic rearrangement of chromosome 14 in human lymphocytes. *Proc Natl Acad Sci U S A* 1975;72:2071–2075.

118. Aurias A, Dutrillaux B, Buriot D, et al. High frequencies if inversions and translocations of chromosomes 7 and 14 in ataxia-telangiectasia. *Mutat Res* 1980;69:369–374.

119. Kojis TL, Gatti RA, Sparkes RS. The cytogenetics of ataxia-telangiectasia. *Cancer Genet Cytogenet* 1992; 56:143–156.

120. Shiloh Y. Ataxia telengiectasia: ATM and genomic stability—maintaining a delicate balance. Two international workshops on ataxia telengiectasia, related disorders; the ATM protein. *Biochim Biophys Acta* 1998; 1378:R11–R18.

121. Canman CE, Lim DS, Cimprich KA, et al. Activation of the ATM kinase by ionizing radiation and phosphorylation of p53. *Science* 1998;281:1677–1679.

122. Conley ME, Buckley RH, Hong R, et al. X-linked severe combined immunodeficiency: diagnosis in males with sporadic severe combined immunodeficiency and clarification of clinical findings. *J Clin Invest* 1990; 85:1548–1554.

123. Buckley RH, Schiff RI, Schiff SE, et al. Human severe combined immunodeficiency: genetic, phenotypic, and functional diversity in one hundred eight infants. *J Pediatr* 1997;130:378–387.

124. Puck JM, Deschenes SM, Porter JC, et al. The interleukin-2 receptor γ chain maps to Xq13.1 and is mutated in X-linked severe combined immunodeficiency. *Hum Mol Genet* 1993;2:1099–1104.

125. Russell SM, Taybebi N, Nakajima H, et al. Mutation of JAK3 in a patient with SCID: essential role of JAK3 in lymphoid development. *Science* 1995;270:797–802.

126. Giblett ER, Anderson JE, Cohen F, et al. Adenosine deaminase deficiency in two patients with severely impaired cellular immunity. *Lancet* 1972;2:1067–1069.

127. Hirshhorn R. Adenosine deaminase deficiency. *Immunodefic Rev* 1990;2:175–198.

128. Hirschhorn R. Overview of biochemical abnormalities and molecular genetics of adenosine deaminase deficiency. *Pediatr Res* 1993;3[Suppl]:s35–s41.

129. Polmar SH, Stern RC, Schwartz AL, et al. Enzyme replacement therapy for adenosine deaminase deficiency and severe combined immunodeficiency. *N Engl J Med* 1976;295:1337–1343.

130. Hershfield MS, Chaffee S, Sorensen RU. Enzyme replacement therapy with polyethylene glycol-adenosine deaminase in adenosine deaminase deficiency: overview and case reports of three patients, including two now receiving gene therapy. *Pediatr Res* 1993; 3[Suppl]:S42–S48.

131. Blaese RM. Development of gene therapy for immunodeficiency: adenosine deaminase deficiency. *Pediatr Res* 1993;33[Suppl]:S49–S55.

132. Omenn GS. Familial reticuloendotheliosis with eosinophilia. *N Engl J Med* 1965;273:427–432.

133. Villa A, Santagata S, Bozzi F, et al. Partial V(D)J recombination activity leads to Omenn's syndrome. *Cell* 1998;93:885–896.

134. Touraine JL, Betuel H, Gouillet G, et al. Combined immunodeficiency disease associated with absence of cell surface HLA-A and -B antigens. *J Pediatr* 1978; 93:47–51.

135. Touraine JL, Marseglia GL, Betuel LH, et al. The bare lymphocyte syndrome. *Bone Marrow Transplant* 1992; 9[Suppl]:54–56.

136. Steimle V, Reith W, Mach B. Major histocompatibility complex class II deficiency: a disease of gene regulation. *Adv Immunol* 1996;61:327–340.

137. Roifman CM, Hummel D, Martinez-Valdez H, et al. Depletion of CD8+ cells in human thymic medulla results in selective immune deficiency. *J Exp Med* 1989; 170:2177–2182.

138. Mayumi M, Kimata H, Suehiro Y, et al. DiGeorge syndrome with hypogammaglobulinemia: a patient with excess suppressor T cell activity treated with fetal thymus transplantation. *Eur J Pediatr* 1989;148:518–522.

139. Alper CA, Rosen FS. Inherited deficiencies of complement proteins in man. *Springer Semin Immunopathol* 1984;7:251–261.

140. Figueroa JE, Densen P. Infectious disease associated with complement deficiencies. *Clin Microbiol Rev* 1991;4:359–395.

141. Silverstein AM. Essential hypocomplementemia: report of a case. *Blood* 1960;16:1338–1341.

142. Johnston RB Jr. The complement system in host defense and inflammation: the cutting edges of a double-edged sword. *Pediatr Infect Dis J* 1993;12:933–941.

143. Tedesco F, Nurnberger W, Perissutti S. Inherited deficiency of the terminal complement components. *Int Rev Immunol* 1993;10:51–64.

144. Barak Y, Nir E. Chédiak-Higashi syndrome. *Annu J Pediatr Hematol Oncol* 1987;9:42–55.

145. Baehner RL, Nathan DG. Quantitative nitroblue tetrazolium test in chronic granulomatous disease. *N Engl J Med* 1968;287:971–976.

146. Mills EL, Rhool KS, Quie PG. X-linked inheritance in females with chronic granulomatous disease. *J Clin Invest* 1980;66:332–340.

147. Richardson MP, Ayliffe MT, Helbert M, et al. A simple flow cytometry assay using dihydrorhodamine for the measurement of the neutrophil respiratory burst in whole blood: comparison with the quantitative nitrobluetetrazolium test. *J Immunol Method* 1998;219:187–193.

148. Anderson DC, Schmalsteig FC, Finegold MJ, et al. The severe and moderate phenotypes of heritable MAC-1, LFA-1 deficiency: their quantitative definition and relation to leukocyte dysfunction and clinical features. *J Infect Dis* 1985;152:668–689.

149. Janeway C, Craig J, Davidson M, et al. Hypergammaglobulinemia associated with severe recurrent and chronic nonspecific infection. *Am J Dis Child* 1954; 88:388–392.

150. Berendes H, Bridges RA, Good RA. A fatal granulomatous disease of childhood: the clinical study of a new syndrome. *Minn Med* 1957;40:309–312.

151. Bridges RA, Berendes H, Good RA. A fatal granulomatous disease of childhood. *Am J Dis Child* 1959;97: 387–408.

152. Quie PG, White JG, Holmes B, et al. *In vitro* bactericidal capacity of human polymorphonuclear leukocytes: diminished activity in chronic granulomatous disease of childhood. *J Clin Invest* 1967;46:668–679.

153. Segal AW, Jones OTG, Webster D, et al. Absence of a newly described cytochrome b from neutrophils from patients with chronic granulomatous disease. *Lancet* 1978;2:446.

154. Segal AW, Cross AR, Garcia RC, et al. Absence of cytochrome b245 in chronic granulomatous disease: a

155. Nunoi H, Rotrosen D, Gallin JI, et al. Two forms of autosomal chronic granulomatous disease lack distinct neutrophil cytosol factors. *Science* 1988;242: 1298–1301.

156. Gallin JI, Buesher ES, Seligmann BE, et al. Recent advances in chronic granulomatous disease. *Ann Intern Med* 1983;99:657–674.

157. Quie PG. Chronic granulomatous disease of childhood. *Adv Pediatr* 1969;16:287–300.

158. Nath J, Flavin M, Gallin JI. Tubulin tyrosinolation in human polymorphonuclear leukocytes: studies in normal subjects and in patients with the Chédiak-Higashi syndrome. *J Cell Biol* 1982;95:519–526.

159. Root RK, Rosenthal AS, Balestra DJ. Abnormal bactericidal, metabolic and lysosomal functions of Chédiak-Higashi syndrome leukocytes. *J Clin Invest* 1972;51: 649–665.

160. Katz PA, Zaytoun A, Fauce A. Deficiency of active natural killer cells in the Chédiak-Higashi syndrome: localization of the defect using a single cell assay. *J Clin Invest* 1982;69:1231–1238.

161. Marlin SD, Morton CC, Anderson DC, et al. LFA-1 immunodeficiency disease. *J Exp Med* 1986;164: 885–867.

162. Scmalsteig FC. Leukocyte adherence defect. *Pediatr Infect Dis* 1988;7:867–872.

163. Abramson JS, Mills EL, Sawyer MK, et al. Recurrent infections and delayed separation of the umbilical cord in an infant with abnormal phagocytic cell locomotion and oxidative response during particle phagocytosis. *J Pediatr* 1981;99:887–894.

164. Etzioni A, Frydman M, Pollack S, et al. Recurrent severe infections caused by a novel leukocyte adhesion deficiency. *N Engl J Med* 1992;327:1789–1792.

165. LeDiest F, Blanche S, Keable S, et al. Successful HLA nonidentical bone marrow transplantation in three patients with the leukocyte adhesion deficiency. *Blood* 1989;74:512–516.

166. Ezekowitz RAB, Dinauer MC, Jaffe HS, et al. Partial correction of the phagocytic defect in patients with X-linked chronic granulomatous disease by subcutaneous interferon-gamma. *N Engl J Med* 1988;319:146–151.

167. Hitzig WH. Transmission of AIDS by IV Immunoglobulin (Ig) G Prep. Eg. Sandoglobulin (SAGL). In: Petricciani JC, et al. *AIDS: The Safety of Blood and Blood Products.* New York: WHO; Chicester, NY: John Wiley and Sons, 1987:103–116.

168. Centers for Disease Control and Prevention. Outbreak of hepatitis C associated with intravenous gammaglobulin administration—United States. *MMWR Morb Mortal Wkly Rep* 1994;43:505–509.

169. Bresee JS, Mast EE, Coleman PJ, et al. Hepatitis C virus infection associated with administration of intravenous immunoglobulin: a cohort study. *JAMA* 1996; 276:1563–1567.

170. Horowitz B, Prince AM, Hamman J, et al. Viral safety of solvent detergent-treated blood products. *Blood Coagul Fibrinolysis* 1998;5[Suppl 3]:S21–S28, discussion S29–S30.

171. Frantantoni JC. Creutzfeldt-Jakob disease and blood products: FDA policy. *Biologicals* 1999;26:133–134.

PART II

Infections of the Compromised Host

2

Premature Infants

Kenneth M. Boyer

Department of Pediatric Infectious Diseases, Rush Children's Hospital, Chicago, Illinois 60612

Of the almost 4 million babies born in the United States each year, 6.8% have birth weights less than 2,500 g. Approximately 200,000 of these newborn babies have birth weights between 1,500 and 2,500 g. The other 50,000 have birth weights of less than 1,500 g. In the first category, designated low-birth-weight (LBW) infants, the relative risk of neonatal mortality varies with ethnicity but is 3.9- to 7.8-fold higher than in babies with birth weights of more than 2,500 g. Among the 50,000 very-low-birth-weight (VLBW) infants, the relative risk of neonatal mortality is 43.6- to 99.0-fold higher than in babies with birth weights of more than 2,500 g (1). These LBW and VLBW babies, most of whom are premature, constitute the largest population of compromised hosts in pediatric medicine.

The tremendous importance of infectious diseases in these compromised babies is manifested by the administration of empiric antibiotic therapy for suspected infectious disease or of specific antibiotic therapy for documented infectious disease in almost all babies who are admitted to high-risk nursery settings (2). Their enhanced susceptibility to infectious diseases relates not only to immunologic immaturity (described in Chapter 18) but also to the immaturity of many of their natural barriers to infection (integumentary, glottal, and mucosal) and to the transgression of these barriers by the invasive monitoring and therapeutic techniques used in neonatal intensive care.

The majority of infections in premature babies occur during the perinatal period. A substantial minority occur in VLBW premature infants who have survived initial serious problems. During their prolonged hospitalizations, they often experience infections that complicate management of bronchopulmonary dysplasia (BPD), short bowel syndrome, hydrocephalus, cerebrovascular accidents, anoxic/ischemic encephalopathy, and ventilator dependence.

NEONATAL SEPSIS

"Neonatal sepsis" is a much used and often abused term in the nursery setting. The neonatal period, strictly speaking, denotes the first 28 days of life. In the context of infection, however, the term is used generally to include babies younger than 2 months of age and babies older than 2 months of age who remain hospitalized in a neonatal nursery setting. Therefore, the neonatal period for a VLBW baby easily may extend to 4 to 6 months of age (10 to 12 months postconceptional age). *Sepsis* generally implies any life-threatening bacterial infection. *Septicemia* is a more restrictive term that implies bloodstream infection in concert with the pathophysiologic consequences of severe infection, such as circulatory failure, respiratory failure, and disseminated intravascular coagulation (DIC). Although it is useful as a starting point for clinical management of a sick baby, the term "neonatal sepsis" should be used cautiously as a final diagnosis in a patient. The goal of diagnosis in a sick newborn is to identify the specific infecting organism, the source of infection, its portal of entry into the patient, the presence of septicemia, and the extent to which infection has spread to other major organ systems, such as the meninges or skeletal system.

Causative Agents

Many of the pathogens that are responsible for neonatal sepsis are unique to the neonatal period (3). These agents include group B streptococci (GBS), *Escherichia coli,* and *Listeria monocytogenes.* The reasons for their predilection for infecting newborn babies are not clear in all cases but include their propensity to grow in amniotic fluid (GBS), their sialic acid–containing capsules (GBS and *E. coli* serotype K1), and their ability to cross the placenta (*Listeria*). Other common pathogens in neonatal sepsis include the "water bugs," such as *Pseudomonas, Citrobacter, Enterobacter,* and *Klebsiella,* which are capable of persisting in the nursery environment and frequently are associated with nosocomial infection (4). Other categories of organisms frequently associated with invasive neonatal infection are the efficient skin colonizers, such as *Staphylococcus aureus, Staphylococcus epidermidis,* and *Candida albicans.* These organisms also are common isolates in neonatal high-risk nurseries and are particularly associated with lines and catheters that transgress integumentary (skin) barriers (5).

Epidemiology

Although estimates vary, the overall incidence of neonatal sepsis probably is on the order of 5 to 8 per 1,000 births (3). The dominant bacterial isolates in infected babies have varied in the 60 years since good documentation of neonatal sepsis etiology began in the early 1930s (6). From the 1920s through the 1940s, group A streptococcus was the most frequent pathogen isolated. In the 1950s and 1960s, *S. aureus* (particularly bacteriophage type 80/81) was the dominant isolate. In the late 1960s *E. coli* was dominant, and in the 1980s and 1990s GBS was the most frequent isolate. The incidence of infections with nosocomial and device-related pathogens such as *S. epidermidis* and *Candida* is increasing, and they have emerged as the dominant pathogens at the turn of the millennium (7).

Neonatal sepsis is categorized according to age at onset as early-onset or late-onset. Although definitions vary, early-onset infections generally include those occurring in the first week of life. Late-onset infection refers to those occurring after the first week.

The dominant risk factor in early-onset neonatal sepsis is the baby's degree of maturity at delivery (a close correlate of birth weight). Attack rate data derived from retrospective studies of GBS infections have clearly identified a birth weight–specific predisposition to infection (8). In these studies, babies with birth weights between 500 and 1,000 g had an attack rate of 26.6 per 1,000 live births; a stepwise decline in attack rates occurred with increasing birth weight, to a rate of 1.1 per 1,000 live births in babies with birth weights greater than 2,500 g. The 25-fold higher relative risk of infection in the VLBW babies was accompanied by an even more dramatic increase in fatal outcome. Of infected babies weighing less than 1,000 g in this study, 90% died. In contrast, among the infected babies weighing more than 2,500 g, only 1 of 31 (3%) died. Other risk factors predisposing to early-onset GBS sepsis include prolonged membrane rupture (more than 18 hours) and intrapartum maternal fever suggestive of amnionitis.

LBW also is the predominant risk factor for late-onset neonatal sepsis. The other perinatal risk factors do not appear to have a major influence on late-onset disease. Other important risk factors for late-onset disease include surgical procedures, invasive monitoring, mechanical ventilation, hyperalimentation, and prolonged antibiotic treatment. "Devices" that predispose the premature infant to late-onset disease are summarized in Table 2.1 according to the normal protective barriers they compromise.

Pathogenesis

Neonatal sepsis often is fulminant. In the preantibiotic era, the outcome usually was fatal. A unifying scheme of pathogenesis is

TABLE 2.1. *Invasive devices used in the care of premature infants, the protective barriers they bypass, and potential device-related infections*

Invasive device	Protective barriers bypassed	Infections
Scalp electrode	Skin	Neonatal herpes, cellulitis
Intraosseous needle	Skin	Cellulitis
Heelstick blood sampling	Periosteum	Osteomyelitis
Umbilical artery catheter	Skin	Exit site infection
Umbilical vein catheter	Vascular endothelium	Tunnel infection
Peripheral IV (including cutdown)	—	Bacteremia
Percutaneous central venous catheter	—	Septicemia
Cutdown central venous catheter	—	Septic thrombophlebitis–endarteritis
Broviac central venous catheter	—	Septic emboli
Percutaneous arterial catheter	—	Endocarditis
Cutdown arterial catheter	—	Remote hematogenous infection
Peritoneal dialysis catheter	Skin	Exit site infection
Gastrostomy	Peritoneum	Peritonitis
External ventricular drain	Skin	Operative site infection
	Meninges	Ventriculitis
Ventriculoperitoneal shunt	Skin	Operative site infection
	Meninges	Ventriculitis
	Peritoneum	Peritonitis
Chest tube	Skin	Exit site infection
	Pleura	Empyema
Endotracheal tube	Upper respiratory mucosa	Tracheobronchitis
Nasotracheal tube	Skin (tracheostomy)	Pneumonia
Tracheostomy	Glottis	Cellulitis (tracheostomy)
Nasogastric tube	Upper respiratory mucosa	Otitis media
	Eustachean tube, esophagus	Aspiration pneumonia
Urinary catheter	Urethra	Cystitis
Cystostomy	—	Pyelonephritis
Nephrostomy	Urethra, ureteropelvic junction	Pyelonephritis

presented in Fig. 2.1. The major reservoir of causative organisms in early-onset disease is the maternal genital tract. In late-onset disease the major reservoirs are the paraphernalia of neonatal intensive care, including ventilators, incubators, humidification equipment, and vascular access devices. In nosocomial infection, the hands of personnel are the major means by which organisms are transmitted from one patient to another.

The major portals of entry in neonatal sepsis are the baby's respiratory tract, gastrointestinal tract, blood vessels, urinary tract, and skin. In early-onset disease often the proliferation of organisms in amniotic fluid before delivery presents the major inoculum of organisms to the baby's lungs. From the portals of entry the newborn baby's bloodstream is invaded, either by direct entry of pathogens through intact mucous membranes or cutaneous barriers or, more readily, when those barriers have been damaged by physical or anoxic injury. Bloodstream invasions lead to two major consequences: the cascade of pathogenic events in septicemia and the hematogenous infection of distant sites. The pathogenic cascade of septicemia includes endothelial injury, release of inflammatory mediators, stimulation of the release of marrow phagocytic cells, circulatory failure secondary to septic shock and persistent fetal circulation, and the development of DIC with concomitant renal failure (9). This cascade of events can lead to early death. If held in check by host defenses or partially effective therapy, hematogenous infection of distant sites may occur. The most common of these include meningitis, osteomyelitis, endophthalmitis, and endocarditis.

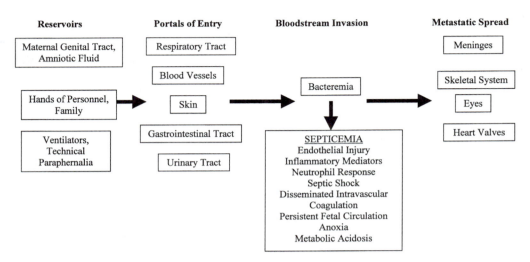

FIG. 2.1. Pathogenetic scheme of neonatal sepsis according to reservoirs of infecting organisms, portals of entry, septicemic cascade, and metastatic spread.

Clinical Manifestations

Depending on the point in the pathogenic scheme, a baby with neonatal sepsis may present with subtle findings or fulminant disease. In a premature infant whose early sepsis was initiated *in utero* during labor and delivery and in whom a well-established amnionitis and prolonged labor and delivery permitted progression of infection, the baby may be desperately ill from the moment of delivery. Such babies typically have poor Apgar scores, require aggressive resuscitation, and are admitted immediately to a special care environment with respiratory and circulatory failure. In other instances a baby may be well at birth and during the first 48 hours of life develop subtle abnormalities, including thermoregulatory problems, poor peripheral perfusion, lethargy, or feeding abnormalities. Failure to recognize and intervene when these abnormalities are present can lead rapidly to the same fulminant septic state seen in the infant infected *in utero*.

Late-onset infection also may vary in severity depending on the pathogenic organism and the mechanism of infection. The most common presentation of sepsis in the VLBW baby who has been hospitalized for a prolonged period and whose infection is nosocomial or device-related is apnea, bradycardia, or deterioration in cardiorespiratory parameters with a resultant need for more aggressive supportive care. The key to recognition of device-related infections is an awareness of the type and location of devices each baby has. Enumeration and evaluation of these devices is an integral part of the physical examination of any hospitalized premature infant.

Diagnosis

Blood culture is the key microbiologic test for diagnosis of neonatal sepsis. When the culture is positive for a recognized neonatal pathogen, and particularly when it is positive after relatively short incubation (24 hours or less) in both bottles of a set, there is little etiologic doubt. Problems arise in interpretation of late-positive results (cultures that turn positive after 48 hours), isolates of uncertain pathogenicity (e.g., viridans streptococci, coagulase-negative staphylococci), multiple isolates in a single specimen, or discordant results (only one of several culture bottles positive) (10). Such results often imply technical errors in collection or inoculation of blood specimens, but occasionally they may be the only tipoff to an occult infection, such as an infected central venous catheter, osteomyelitis, or abscess.

Negative blood cultures do not completely rule out the presence of significant infection. Bacteremia may be masked by prior treatment of the baby or the mother. Bloodstream invasion may be transient, intermittent, confined to a regional circulation (e.g., portal venous), or at a sufficiently low level (e.g., less than one organism per milliliter) that it is missed by the usual limited blood culture volumes obtained from tiny babies. Fastidious organisms (e.g., nutritionally variant streptococci) and slow-growing organisms (e.g., *Malassezia furfur*) may be missed. The concept of the sepsis syndrome (11) is now widely used in adult critical care to describe patients who have multiorgan system compromise that is likely to have an infectious cause, regardless of blood culture status. Although this concept has not been rigorously evaluated in neonates, it is probably valid. Toxin (e.g., endotoxin) or phagocytosed organisms may initiate the syndrome without actual bloodstream invasion by stimulating the release of inflammatory mediators (e.g., tumor necrosis factor [TNF], interleukins, platelet-activating factor) by phagocytic and endothelial cells. Therefore, a broader focus than just the blood culture generally is desirable in diagnosing and managing neonatal sepsis.

The results of complete blood counts, particularly serial studies, are helpful in determining the presence of bacterial infection and therapeutic response. Elevated neutrophil counts or, more impressively, an initial low count followed by a dramatic response after initiation of therapy favors a bacterial etiology (12). A ratio of immature to total neutrophils of 0.2 or more and thrombocytopenia are also helpful hematologic indicators.

Detection of GBS or *E. coli* K1 polysaccharide antigens in urine by latex agglutination is a useful adjunct to blood culture. A positive blood culture with a negative concomitant urine antigen test suggests transient bacteremia. Positive urine antigen tests with negative blood cultures may imply occult in-

fection (e.g., GBS osteomyelitis) or partial treatment by intrapartum therapy. In the majority of instances, however, a positive urine antigen with a negative blood culture implies contamination of the urine sample by "bag" collection (13). In an otherwise healthy baby, this discrepant finding does not justify an extensive diagnostic workup or prolonged treatment.

Evaluation of the baby's mother is another useful diagnostic adjunct, particularly when early-onset neonatal infection is suspected. Pediatricians need to encourage obstetric colleagues to obtain blood cultures from febrile parturients, in addition to other cultures (e.g., urine, lochia, amniotic fluid at cesarean section, placental surfaces), to define maternal infections that imply intrapartum exposure of the neonate. Further, obstetricians must communicate situations in which suspicion of intrapartum infection exists.

Most importantly, an evaluation of the neonate for infection should attempt to identify the extent of spread and the portal of entry. The urinary tract rarely is the portal of entry for bacteremia in a neonate younger than 72 hours (14). In an older baby, however, pretreatment identification of a urinary source for gram-negative sepsis may permit early identification and correction of a structural anomaly. Clean-catch, catheterized, or suprapubic tap urine specimens are superior to bagged urine specimens for culture.

Other potentially helpful bacteriologic information regarding portal of entry often is overlooked. A predominant organism in a Gram-stained gastric aspirate implies significant growth of organisms in amniotic fluid and an infectious challenge to the neonate during labor and delivery. Gram stains and cultures of tracheal aspirates obtained shortly after intubation have a high correlation with etiology in neonatal pneumonia (15). Intravascular catheter tips should always be cultured at the time of removal, using the semiquantitative roll plate technique. The presence of more than 15 colonies on the plate implies a catheter source of bacteremia (16). Stool cultures, if processed to identify predominant aerobic species, may be useful in guiding broad-spectrum therapy in babies with necrotizing enterocolitis (NEC). Cultures of skin lesions, including pustules, intravenous catheter exit sites, surgical wounds, and "weepy" umbilical stumps, may identify the source of bloodstream invasion or focus attention on sites that require removal of hardware, local treatment, or surgical intervention.

Because meningitis is a common site for bacteremic spread in neonatal sepsis, the lumbar puncture is standard in the septic workup. However, because cerebrospinal fluid (CSF) cultures rarely are positive in the absence of bacteremia, there are a few circumstances in which a lumbar puncture may be deferred. For example, lumbar puncture is appropriately deferred in an intubated, asphyxiated, premature newborn whose cardiorespiratory condition is unstable (17) or in an asymptomatic full-term baby in whom blood culture is being performed solely because of maternal prolonged membrane rupture (18). If blood cultures are positive in these situations, subsequent reevaluation should include lumbar puncture. Even if therapy has rendered cultures negative, results of cell counts, chemistries, and antigen detection are likely to identify a baby with meningitis.

Blood culture isolation of certain pathogens often is a clue to particular sites of metastatic spread. An *S. aureus* isolate, for example, implies the possibility of osteomyelitis or endocarditis. *C. albicans* should suggest ocular involvement (chorioretinitis or endophthalmitis) or endocarditis. *Citrobacter diversus* or *Enterobacter sakazakii* should suggest brain abscess.

Treatment

Empiric therapy with combinations of antibiotics is the usual starting point in the management of neonatal sepsis. As a general rule, a decision for workup is a decision for prompt and intensive parenteral treatment, despite the fact that only 5% to 10% of blood cultures are positive. Broad coverage of probable infecting organisms, CSF penetration, safety, and selective pressures for development of drug resistance are the key considerations when choosing regimens. Because actual dosages are tiny, drug costs are not a consideration. Factors that determine probable infecting organisms include the patient's age, birth weight, environment (home or hospital), prior courses of treatment, perinatal or nosocomial exposures to specific pathogens, presence of hardware (e.g., catheters, drains, endotracheal tubes), and identification of specific sites of infection (e.g., pneumonia, meningitis, thrombophlebitis, NEC) (19).

Empiric therapy for early-onset sepsis is predicated on the origin of virtually all infecting organisms in the maternal enteric or genital flora. The usual pathogens include GBS, *E. coli,* enterococci, viridans streptococci, and *L. monocytogenes.* Anaerobes are not uncommon, but positive blood cultures generally clear with or without treatment. Staphylococci, hospital "water bugs," and fungi are rare. The standard regimen for early-onset disease is ampicillin and an aminoglycoside, usually gentamicin or tobramycin. This combination not only provides broad coverage but is synergistic against streptococci and *Listeria.* Cephalosporins, regardless of their generation, are not active against *Listeria* or *Enterococcus* and should not be used without concomitant ampicillin. Moreover, when used with ampicillin they do not offer the advantage of synergism.

Late-onset disease is more heterogeneous in its epidemiology and clinical presentation than early-onset disease and may reflect maternal, family, community, or, most commonly, nosocomial sources for infecting organisms. Consequently, the pathogens involved cover a broad taxonomic spectrum. Bacterial infections in normal infants who have been sent home may include late-onset GBS, *E. coli,* or *Listeria* septicemia; local or disseminated *S. aureus* infections; urosepsis caused by coliforms; or community-acquired *Streptococcus pneumoniae* disease. Most centers now use ampicillin and a third-generation cephalosporin (cefotaxime or ceftriaxone) for empiric treatment of occult infection in older neonates.

The sick premature infant with prolonged hospitalization often has had his or her maternally derived flora eradicated by at least one empiric course of therapy with ampicillin and an aminoglycoside and is particularly prone to nosocomial pneumonia related to prolonged intubation, NEC when feedings are introduced, and intravenous sepsis related to central or peripheral intravascular catheters. Major pathogens include coagulase-negative and coagulase-positive staphylococci, relatively resistant coliforms including *Klebsiella* and *Enterobacter,* and highly resistant opportunists such as *Pseudomonas, Serratia,* and *Candida.*

Selection of empiric regimens for older premature babies is difficult and should be individualized according to the drugs previously used to treat the infant, clinical presentation (e.g., occult infection, suspected NEC, pneumonia, inflamed Broviac tunnel), results of Gram stains and surveillance cultures (e.g., throat, skin, ostomy stomas, catheter exits, endotracheal aspirates), and annual reviews of bacterial isolates from the nursery and their sensitivities. Useful empiric regimens include the combinations of ampicillin, gentamicin, and metronidazole for suspected NEC; vancomycin and ceftazidime for patients with pneumonia, central vascular catheters, or skin breakdown. The known occurrence of methicillin-resistant *S. aureus* (MRSA) infections in a nursery necessitates the use of vancomycin in any situation in which *S. aureus* is a possible cause. Empiric treatment for fungal infection is not advisable. Because of their toxicities, amphotericin B and flucytosine should be reserved for documented invasive fungal infections. Fluconazole is increasingly used for superficial fungal infections.

Empiric antibiotics are a therapeutic first approximation and should be stopped or modified depending on the baby's clinical course and cultures. As a rule, empiric antibiotics should be stopped after 72 hours if cultures, clinical course, and ancillary tests do not support the diagnosis of infection. Even if blood cultures are sterile, however, treatment should be continued in focal infections and in situations in which bacterial infection continues to offer a plausible explanation for a baby's clinical status. Clinical judgment determines the fine line between use and abuse of antibiotics in the nursery.

Specific therapy in septic neonates is determined by whether the infection can be identified as to site and specific infecting organism or organisms. From the available antibiotic alternatives, the list of drugs that can comfortably be recommended for use in the neonatal period is relatively short (Table 2.2) (20,21). A number of once-popular agents have been superseded because of limitations in spectrum, distribution, or toxicity. Among these are carbenicillin, kanamycin, chloramphenicol, moxalactam, and virtually all first- and second-generation cephalosporins. Other recently licensed drugs have not been well studied in newborn infants but are increasingly being used for resistant organisms and apparent clinical failure of conventional agents. Such drugs include piperacillin, aztreonam, imipenem, and metronidazole. The third-generation cephalosporins, cefotaxime, ceftriaxone, and ceftazidime, have been well studied in neonates and have gained a major role in therapy. (Ceftazidime is the only one of the three cephalosporins with reliable activity against *Pseudomonas aeruginosa,* but it is less active against gram-positive organisms.)

Recommended drugs for babies with proven infections by the more common pathogens are summarized in Table 2.3. These recommendations should be considered guidelines. Because most hospital laboratories provide the clinician with susceptibility data on blood culture isolates simultaneously with (or even before) speciation, susceptibilities must be taken into account when modifying an initial empiric regimen.

A number of infecting organisms are best treated with combination therapy. Addition of gentamicin to ampicillin for treatment of listeriosis or enterococcal infection provides synergistic activity and more rapid killing of a large initial inoculum. The same synergism has been documented for GBS, but most clinicians usually stop the aminoglycoside and change to

TABLE 2.2. *Dosage recommendations (mg/kg/d) and intervals of administration for antimicrobial agents commonly used in the treatment of neonatal sepsis and meningitis*

Drug	Routes of administration	Body weight <1,200 g Age <28 d	Body weight <2,000 g Age 0–7 d	Body weight <2,000 g Age >7 d	Body weight >2,000 g Age 0–7 d	Body weight >2,000 g Age >7 d
Amikacin[a]	IV, M	7.5–10 q24h	15 div q12h	22.5 div q8h	20 div q12h	30 div q8h
Amphotericin B[a,b]	IV	0.5–1 q24h	0.5–1 q24h	0.5–1 q24h	0.5–1 q24h	0.5–1 q24h
Ampicillin	IV, IM					
Meningitis		150 div q12h	200 div q12h	300 div q8h	200 div q8h	300 div q6h
Other diseases		50 div q12h	50 div q12h	75 div q8h	75 div q8h	100 div q6h
Aztreonam	IV	60 div q12h	60 div q12h	90 div q8h	90 div q8h	120 div q8h
Cefotaxime	IV, IM	100 div q12h	100 div q12h	150 div q8h	100 div q12h	150–225 div q8h
Ceftazidine	IV, IM	100 div q12h	100 div q12h	150 div q8h	100 div q12h	150 div q8h
Ceftriaxone	IV, IM	NR	50 div q24h	50 div q24h	50 div q24h	80 div q24h
Clindamycin	IV, IM	10 div q12h	10 div q12h	15 div q8h	15 div q8h	20 div q6h
Fluconazole	IV, PO	NR	6 q24h	6 q24h	6 q24h	6 q24h
Flucytosine[a]	PO	NR	100 div q6h	100 div q6h	100 div q6h	100 div q6h
Gentamicin[a]	IV, IM	2.5–3.5 q24h	5 div q12h	7.5 div q8h	5 div q12h	7.5 div q8h
Imipenem	IV, IM	20 div q24h	40 div q12h	40 div q12h	40 div q12h	60 div q8h
Methicillin	IV, IM					
Meningitis		100 div q12h	100 div q12h	150 div q8h	150 div q88	200 div q6h
Other diseases		50 div q12h	50 div q12h	75 div q8h	75 div q8h	100 div q6h
Metronidazole	IV	7.5 q48h	7.5 q12h	15 div q12h	15 div q12h	30 div q12h
Mezlocillin	IV, IM	150 div q12h	150 div q12h	225 div q8h	150 div q12h	225 div q8h
Nafcillin	IV	50 div q12h	50 div q12h	100 div q8h	50 div q8h	150 div q6h
Oxacillin	IV, IM	50 div q12h	50 div q12h	100 div q8h	75 div q8h	150 div q6h
Penicillin G	IV					
Meningitis		150,000 div q12h	300,000 U div q12h	400,000 U div q8h	300,000 U div q8h	400,000 U div q6h
		50,000 div q12h	50,000 U div q12h	750,000 div U q8h	50,000 U div q8h	1000,00 U div q6h
Piperacillin	IV, IM	NR	NR	NR	150 div q8h	200 div q8h
Ticarcillin	IV, IM	150 div q12h	150 div q12h	225 div q8h	225 div q8h	300 div q6h
Tobramycin[a]	IV, IM	2.5–3.5/24h	4 div q12h	6 div q8h	4 div q12h	6 div q8h
Vancomycin[a]	IV	15 q24h	20 div q12h	30 div q8h	20 div q12h	30 div q8h

div, divided; IM, intramuscular; IV, intravenous; NR, no recommendations available; q12h, every 12-hours.

[a]Serum concentration or toxicity monitoring desirable, particularly with birth weights less than 1,200 g, (see Prober CG, Stevenson DR, Benitz NE. The use of antibiotics in neonates weighing less than 1200 grams. *Pediatr Infect Dis J* 1990;9:111).

[b]Gradual dose buildup recommended. Give 0.25 mg/kg first day; 0.50 mg/kg second day; 0.75 mg/kg third day; then 1 mg/kg/d. Dose may be maintained at 0.5 to 0.75 mg/kg/d if flucytosine used concomitantly.

TABLE 2.3. *Recommended specific therapy for selected organisms causing neonatal sepsis*

Organism	Drugs of choice	Alternatives (based on susceptibility)
Bacteroides fragilis	Metronidazole	Clindamycin, imipenem
Candida sp.	Amphotericin B+ flucytosine	Fluconazole
Citrobacter sp.	Cephalosporin[a] + aminoglycoside[b]	Imipenem
Enterobacter sp.	Cephalosporin + aminoglycoside	Imipenem
Enterococcus sp.	Ampicillin + gentamicin	Vancomycin
Escherichia coli	Cephalosporin + aminoglycoside	Ampicillin
Haemophilus influenzae	Cefotaxime	Ampicillin, ceftriaxone
Klebsiella sp.	Cephalosporin + aminoglycoside	Imipenem
Listeria monocytogenes	Ampicillin + gentamicin	
Pseudomonas aeruginosa	Ceftazidime + tobramycin	Ureidopenicillin,[c] aztreonam, imipenem
Salmonella sp.	Cefotaxime	Ceftriaxone, ampicillin
Serratia marcescens	Cephalosporin + aminoglycoside	Imipenem
Staphylococcus aureus	Semisynthetic penicillin[d]	Vancomycin, clindamycin
Staphylococcus sp.	Vancomycin	Semisynthetic penicillin
Streptococcus sp.	Penicillin G	Ampicillin

[a]Cefotaxime, ceftriaxone, or ceftazidime.
[b]Gentamicin, tobramycin, or amikacin.
[c]Ticarcillin, mezlocillin, or piperacillin.
[d]Nafcillin, oxacillin, or methicillin.

"meningitic" doses of penicillin G after initial improvement. Addition of gentamicin to a semisynthetic penicillin dramatically improves bactericidal activity against "tolerant" strains of *S. aureus*. Combination therapy for infections by *Pseudomonas* and *Enterobacter* is important because of the emergence of resistance with single-drug (particularly third-generation cephalosporin) treatment. The addition of flucytosine to amphotericin B for treatment of disseminated candidiasis permits lower dosages of amphotericin (0.5 to 0.75 mg per kilogram per day) to be used.

Duration and route of therapy often are issues, particularly in the current climate of cost efficiency and parent-infant bonding. Isolation of a pathogen from the blood of a sick newborn mandates a minimum 10-day course of parenteral therapy. Longer courses of treatment are necessary for meningitis (2 to 3 weeks) and osteomyelitis (4 to 6 weeks). Clinical judgment determines the duration of treatment in patients with asymptomatic bacteremia, culture-negative sepsis, antigenuria, or focal infection without bacteremia.

A critical decision that usually is necessary for the baby with device-related sepsis is the decision to remove or replace one or more of the baby's monitoring or life support devices. Such decisions are not simple and require judicious weighing of the risk of infection versus the risk of removal of the device in terms of monitoring and treatment capabilities. For devices that are easily removed and replaced, such as endotracheal tubes and urinary catheters, there should be no delay in carrying out these changes of hardware. In patients with line sepsis whose intravascular access is limited by technical considerations or multiple previous lines, treatment with systemic antibiotics alone may be successful in some cases. Antibiotics alone are unlikely to be successful when there is apparent infection of a subcutaneous tunnel or when fungi or gram-negative bacteria are isolated from the blood (5). If a particular intravascular catheter is suspected, antibiotics should be administered through that catheter. If total parenteral nutrition is being administered, it should be re-

duced in nutritional content while the device is accessed for treatment. In patients with multiple-lumen catheters, ports should be rotated for administration of antibiotics. Follow-up blood cultures obtained during treatment usually will identify whether it is successful. If bacteremia persists, the incriminated intravascular device always should be removed.

Other therapeutic considerations in neonatal sepsis include the baby's cardiorespiratory, nutritional, and immunologic status (22,23). Cardiorespiratory monitoring and blood pressure measurements are mandatory in septic newborns. The presence of shock should prompt aggressive volume expansion with fresh-frozen plasma, whole blood, or albumin and may require the use of pressors. DIC should be treated with platelet infusions and fresh-frozen plasma. Persistent fetal circulation, manifested by profound hypoxemia, is a common feature of early-onset GBS infection and usually requires high concentrations of inspired oxygen, mechanical ventilation, and possibly nitric oxide gas mixtures and oscillatory ventilation. Respiratory failure may result from birth asphyxia, neonatal pneumonia, hyaline membrane disease, and "shock lung." Babies with this combination of problems, if they survive, often become long-term residents of neonatal nurseries with BPD. Aggressive early management with surfactant is an important preventive measure.

Nutritional status, particularly in infected premature infants with limited metabolic reserves, is a major consideration during a prolonged course of antimicrobial therapy. Such babies have increased nutritional demands created by thermoregulatory disturbances, cardiopulmonary stress, frequent blood drawing, and surgical procedures. Depending on the site of infection, enteral feedings usually are not introduced or are interrupted during treatment. Delays in starting parenteral nutrition and the often marginal caloric intake provided by "peripheral hyperal" generally lead to weight loss and a negative nitrogen balance at a time when reparative needs are greatest. Despite perceived infection risks, early central hyperalimentation is warranted in many of these babies.

Augmentation of the neonate's marginal supplies of white cells, antibodies, and nonspecific opsonins (e.g., complement, fibronectin) is a logical but unproven adjunct to antimicrobial therapy (24). Fresh-frozen plasma is the preferred volume expander in the nursery because of its content of immunoglobulin G (IgG) and IgM immunoglobulins and nonspecific opsonins. White blood cell transfusions pose difficult logistic problems for the blood bank with only minimal therapeutic benefit. The therapeutic use of intravenous gamma globulin may permit correction of deficiencies in transplacental specific immunoglobulins, enhance localization of infection, and prevent depletion of marrow neutrophil reserves. However, intravenous gamma globulin also is used to block the reticuloendothelial system in the treatment of Kawasaki disease and idiopathic thrombocytopenic purpura. Therapeutic outcome may therefore strike a balance between the benefit of specific opsonins and the risk of nonspecific blockade of phagocytic capacity (25). With the use of hyperimmune globulins and monoclonal antibodies (26), this balance may be shifted in the direction of therapeutic benefit. However, none of these novel approaches has yet proved to be a significant advance in therapy.

Monitoring Therapy

Premature infants with clinical signs of bacterial infection require hospitalization in an intensive care nursery or pediatric unit, not in a normal nursery or at home. In addition to monitoring therapeutic response, monitoring such infants involves recognition of complications and drug toxicity.

Adequate treatment of a septic neonate usually results in a dramatic response within 24 to 48 hours, as manifested by improved activity, respiratory effort, temperature regulation, and peripheral perfusion. White blood cell counts and proportions of segmented neutrophils often rise with treatment, a short-term response that is generally favorable. Babies who do not respond to treatment may have a

resistant organism, an occult focus of infection, or a viral or noninfectious problem. Blood culture should be repeated at the first report of a positive result to document sterilization. Measurement of peak serum bactericidal activity provides a more reliable indication of treatment efficacy than do *in vitro* susceptibility tests (which are based on bacteriostatic activity). Occult bacterial infections associated with slow response or persistence of bacteremia include meningitis, osteomyelitis, abscesses (intraabdominal, renal, brain, subperiosteal), and intravascular infections (suppurative thrombophlebitis, endocarditis). Computed tomography (CT), ultrasonography, echocardiography, and gallium scanning may be helpful in identifying such problems. Disseminated neonatal herpes, in the absence of skin lesions or central nervous system (CNS) abnormalities, can resemble bacterial sepsis. Striking elevation of serum transaminase values is a useful clue to this diagnosis. The patient who does not respond to antibiotics or whose condition deteriorates during therapy may have a noninfectious condition (e.g., hypoplastic left heart syndrome, ductus-dependent cyanotic congenital heart disease, pneumothorax, intraventricular hemorrhage, or intestinal obstruction).

Monitoring serum concentrations of aminoglycosides has become a standard of care in many nurseries, although the occurrence of ototoxicity and nephrotoxicity from these drugs has been difficult to study because of confounding by other conditions such as shock, asphyxia, acidosis, and hyperbilirubinemia. Peak concentrations (at the conclusion of intravenous infusion or 30 minutes after intramuscular injection) and trough concentrations (immediately before the next dose) should be measured in all treated infants. Waiting to measure concentrations until after the third dose of drug is reasonable to ensure equilibration. Target peak and trough antibiotic concentrations in serum are summarized in Table 2.4. Other drugs requiring measurement of serum concentrations during therapy are flucytosine and vancomycin. Vancomycin has been well studied in newborns;

TABLE 2.4. *Suggested target levels of selected antibiotics to optimize efficacy and minimize toxicity*

Drug	Peak (µg/mL)	Trough (µg/mL)
Gentamicin	4–8	<2
Tobramycin	4–8	<2
Netilmicin	4–8	<2
Amikacin	15–25	<6
Vancomycin	15–30	5–10
Flucytosine	50–100	?

experience with flucytosine is anecdotal. Amphotericin B concentrations are difficult to measure and are not well correlated with toxicity. Safe use of amphotericin is best monitored by serial measurements of serum potassium, urea nitrogen, creatinine, and hematologic values and by careful documentation of urine output.

Prevention

The key elements in the prevention of early-onset neonatal sepsis are the prevention of prematurity by appropriate prenatal care and maternal hygiene and the conduct of labor and delivery by the obstetrician aimed at minimizing prolonged membrane rupture and amnionitis. Prevention of late-onset disease can best be accomplished by paying close attention to handwashing; adhering to guidelines for isolation of communicable conditions in mothers, infants, and personnel (27); and minimizing excessive durations of antibiotic treatment.

A substantial proportion of cases of early-onset GBS disease can now be anticipated and prevented by the strategy of selective intrapartum chemoprophylaxis (28). Administration of ampicillin during labor to mothers with prenatal GBS colonization and the obstetric risk factors of premature labor (gestation less than 37 weeks), prolonged membrane rupture (longer than 12 hours), or intrapartum fever (higher than 37.5°C) dramatically reduced neonatal colonization and virtually eliminated early-onset sepsis in one large controlled trial. A number of studies of similar but not identical design have confirmed this observation (29,30).

Based on these studies, the Centers for Disease Control and Prevention (CDC) has now recommended two strategies for intrapartum chemoprophylaxis, which have been widely implemented in the United States (31,32). The "culture-based" strategy involves obtaining prenatal cultures to identify maternal colonization. The "risk-based" strategy is based solely on the presence of obstetric risk factors. Penicillin is recommended as the preferred antibiotic for prophylaxis. A substantial decline in the incidence of GBS early-onset disease has resulted (33).

NECROTIZING ENTEROCOLITIS

NEC is a devastating gastrointestinal condition that principally, but not exclusively, affects premature infants. It affects 1% to 5% of all babies admitted to a special care nursery setting. It is deadly, with case-fatality rates of approximately 40%. After respiratory distress syndrome, it is the most frequent cause of death in babies admitted to a special care nursery environment. The cause is not clearly understood, and treatment has made relatively little progress. The incidence of the disease is increasing as the proportion of VLBW babies who survive increases (34).

Causative Agents

Although the role of infection as the primary event in NEC is argued, there is no question that infection is the usual cause of death. The bacteriology of positive blood cultures, ascitic fluid, and operative or autopsy surgical specimens primarily reflects the bacteria of the gut lumen (35). The list includes common enteric flora such as *E. coli, Klebsiella,* and *Enterobacter.* The common microflora of the intestinal tract, including *Clostridia* and *Bacteroides,* frequently are encountered if cultures are processed anaerobically. Organisms that are likely to populate the gut lumen in patients who have already received antibiotic therapy, such as *S. epidermidis, S. aureus, Pseudomonas, Serratia,* and *Candida,* often are seen in babies with late-onset disease.

Epidemiology

Age at onset of neonatal NEC may range from the first day of life to 90 days of age. The temporal clustering of NEC incidence is much more closely related to the age at initiation of enteral feedings than to actual chronologic age. However, most cases of NEC begin between day 3 and day 10 of life.

The two strongest risk factors associated with NEC are prematurity and feeding. Approximately 90% of all babies with NEC are premature; incidence increases with lower birth weight. In babies with birth weights less than 1,500 g, the incidence was reported to be 12% in one study (36). NEC has been reported in full-term babies. In most instances, such babies have associated clinical problems, such as cyanotic heart disease, polycythemia, or birth asphyxia. However, there are documented cases in previously healthy full-term babies. The other major risk factor for development of NEC is enteral feeding. Ninety percent to 95% of all affected babies have been enterally fed, with either breast milk, formula, or both. An early theory was that the risk of NEC was related to the rapidity of feeding advancement in a premature baby. Recent case-control studies, however, have failed to document this idea. Other purported risk factors for NEC include perinatal asphyxia, polycythemia, respiratory distress syndrome, umbilical catheterization, hypothermia, shock, hypoxia, cyanotic heart disease, and exchange transfusion.

Pathogenesis

Despite three decades of investigation, understanding of the pathogenesis of NEC remains incomplete. Three hypotheses have been proposed: ischemic-hypoxic injury (37), substrate excess (38), and infection (39). Current views are that NEC results from the synergistic impact of all three of these factors.

The ischemic-hypoxic theory relates to the "diving reflex" of aquatic mammals. During prolonged submersion, such mammals prefer-

entially perfuse vital organs, such as the brain and skeletal musculature, with relative ischemia of the kidneys and gastrointestinal tract. This theory could account for the frequent association of NEC with perinatal asphyxia, respiratory distress, shock, and manipulations of the umbilical vessels. In all of these situations there is a relative decrease in mesenteric blood flow with the possibility of hypoxic damage to the enteric mucosa.

The excess substrate theory takes into account the fact that virtually all babies who develop NEC have received enteral feedings. Conversely, the condition rarely manifests in a baby who has been fed exclusively parenterally.

The role of infection as a primary instigator of NEC can be argued. Once the process has begun, however, infection is clearly the dominant process in pathogenesis. Production of gas by invading microorganisms is believed to be the cause of pneumatosis intestinalis.

Septicemic spread, with endotoxemia and release of immunologic mediators, accounts for the cardiovascular collapse and DIC that regularly accompany the disease. Necrotic destruction of the deep submucosal tissues of the intestine leads to perforation and peritonitis. Therefore, the unifying pathogenic theory is that flourishing intestinal bacterial populations, growing in substrate excess, take advantage of intestinal mucosa that is devitalized as a result of ischemic-hypoxic injury. The consequence is the characteristic clinical picture of NEC.

Clinical Manifestations

NEC typically manifests with the combination of abdominal distention and bloody stools. Seen in fewer affected patients are such abnormalities as apnea, bradycardia, abdominal tenderness, retained gastric contents, guaiac-positive stools, a "septic appearance," shock, and bilious emesis. Physical examination findings that are present only in a small number of cases but very specific for NEC are cellulitis of the abdominal wall and the observation of a right lower quadrant mass. The two radiologic hallmarks of NEC are pneumatosis intestinalis (the formation of intramural intestinal gas) and intrahepatic portal venous gas. In most studies these radiographic findings are considered essential for establishing the diagnosis. However, before their occurrence many patients show intestinal distention, ileus, and ascites, which are less specific features. The "persistent bubble sign" is another useful clue in serial radiographs. Advanced disease results in bowel perforation and pneumoperitoneum. In the latter case, free air is best diagnosed with a cross-table lateral abdominal radiograph.

The staging system originally developed by Bell et al. (40) and modified by Walsh and Kleigman (34) is used for most decisions regarding therapy for NEC. This modified Bell's staging criteria scheme is presented in Table 2.5. Stage I disease, suspected NEC, defines the relatively frequent occurrence in the nursery of babies with signs and symptoms suggestive of NEC, which may not ultimately progress. Suspected signs of the disease and absent bowel sounds or pneumatosis intestinalis establish stage II or definite NEC. Mild stage IIA disease has a generally favorable prognosis with medical management. Stage IIB disease frequently progresses to stage III or advanced NEC, which is characterized by signs and symptoms of generalized peritonitis and intestinal perforation and mandates surgical intervention.

TABLE 2.5. *Modified Bell's staging criteria for NEC*

Stage	Systematic signs	Intestinal signs	Radiologic signs	Treatment
IA (suspected NEC)	Temperature instability, apnea, bradycardia, lethargy	Elevated pregavage residuals, mild abdominal distention, emesis, guaiac-positive stool	Normal or intestinal dilation, mild ileus	NPO, antibiotics for 3 d pending culture
IB (suspected NEC)	Same as IA	Bright red blood from rectum	Same as IA	Same as IA
IIA (definite NEC, mildly ill)	Same as IA	Same as IB, plus absent bowel sounds, ± abdominal	Intestinal dilation, ileus, pneumatosis, intestinalis	NPO, antibiotics for 7–10 d if examination is normal in 24–48 h
IIB (definite NEC, moderately ill)	Same as IA, plus mild metabolic acidosis, mild thrombocytopeia	Same as IIA, plus absent bowel sounds, thrombocytopenia, definite abdominal cellulitis or right lower quadrant mass	Same as IIA, plus portal vein gas, ± ascites, ± tenderness	NPO, antibiotics 14 d sodium bicarbonate for acidosis
IIIA (advanced NEC, severely ill, bowel intact)	Same as IIB, plus hypotension, bradycardia, severe apnea, combined respiratory and metabolic acidosis, disseminated intravascular coagulation, neutropenia	Same as IIB, plus signs of generalized peritonitis, marked tenderness and distention of abdomen	Same as IIB plus definite ascites	Same as IIB, plus bolus fluids, inotropic agents, ventilation therapy, paracentesis
IIB (advanced NEC, severely ill, bowel perforated)	Same as IIIA	Same as IIA	Same as IIB, plus pneumoperitoneum	Same as IIIA, plus surgical intervention

NEC, necrotizing enterocolitis; NPO, nothing by mouth.

Diagnosis

The diagnosis of NEC usually is established on the basis of clinical signs and symptoms and radiologic findings and does not depend on culture results. Because hydrogen gas is the dominant component of the intramural accumulations in pneumatosis intestinalis, several investigational approaches have been proposed to detect aberrant gas production. Ultrasound occasionally may reveal portal venous gas before the demonstration of this phenomenon on conventional radiographs (41). Breath hydrogen analysis has been used to demonstrate increased levels of hydrogen gas in babies with NEC. D-Lactate, produced as a byproduct of intestinal fermentation of carbohydrates, has been found in urine samples of babies with NEC; this is consistent with the excessive substrate theory of pathogenesis.

Microbiologic workup of the baby with NEC should include blood cultures and, when appropriate or possible, peritoneal specimens obtained at surgery or by paracentesis (42). The use of stool cultures to define the predominant aerobic flora may be useful in guiding empiric therapy of babies with early disease who do not have proven septicemia or surgical indications.

Hematologic parameters, such as neutropenia and a shifted ratio of immature to total neutrophils, may be helpful in establishing early NEC. Platelet counts are helpful in defining the presence of DIC. Counts lower than 50,000/μL are associated with poor prognosis (43) and with high circulating levels of platelet-activating factor and TNF (44).

Treatment

The key principles in treatment of NEC are bowel decompression, aggressive antimicrobial therapy, nutritional support, and, when indicated, surgical intervention. No studies have clearly established the superiority of one antimicrobial regimen over another in NEC treatment. There is a consensus that treatment should cover a broad spectrum, should be synergistic when possible, and should be administered in high dose. Most centers use a combination of a penicillin, such as ampicillin or ticarcillin, and an aminoglycoside, usually gentamicin or tobramycin. Although studies have not proved its value (45), many centers also use metronidazole or clindamycin for anaerobic coverage. Babies who have had prolonged hospitalizations and are manifesting their NEC late may benefit from treatment with agents that are active against common hospital-acquired flora. In the case of staphylococci (including MRSA) and multiply resistant gram-negative organisms (e.g., *Pseudomonas, Serratia*), these agents include vancomycin and third-generation cephalosporins, respectively.

Nutritional support with parenteral nutrition is essential in the management of advanced disease. Parenteral nutrition usually is administered through a percutaneous central venous catheter or a Broviac permanent line inserted at the time of surgical exploration. Elements of acute surgical management include diversion (jejunostomy, ileostomy, or colostomy), resection of necrotic bowel, and drainage of abscesses (46). Late surgical intervention, up to 2 to 3 months after initial presentation, may be necessary for reanastomosis, lysis of adhesions, repair of intestinal strictures, or drainage of abscesses. Short-bowel syndrome, resulting from extensive resection of necrotic bowel, may result in permanent disability related to malabsorption. Patients for whom resection of the ileocecal valve was necessary and who have less than 25 cm of residual intestine have an ominous prognosis and invariably require prolonged periods of total parenteral nutrition.

Prevention

An effective means of preventing NEC in premature babies is not established. Early studies of the use of oral nonabsorbable antibiotics (such as gentamicin) have not been confirmed, and they are not part of routine care in most nurseries. Early studies demonstrating that rapid feeding progression may be associated with NEC have encouraged most neonatologists to be cautious about feeding progression. This caution, coupled with the increasingly widespread use of total parenteral nutrition, may have some impact on the incidence of NEC in some nurseries—but it also may be compensated by an increased risk of line sepsis. The use of breast milk for feeding had initial enthusiasm but has not been established as a prophylactic approach. In fact, proliferation of bacteria in banked breast milk actually may cause it to have more infection risk than presterilized formulas (47). Oral administration of IgA-enriched immunoglobulin preparations was shown in one unconfirmed study to prevent NEC (48).

NEONATAL MENINGITIS

The highest incidence of meningitis at any age occurs during the newborn period—approximately 1 per 1,000 live births (49). Premature infants have a higher risk than full-term babies, although few birth weight–specific figures are available.

Meningitis connotes bacterial or viral infection of the meninges, but the semantics of CNS infections include a variety of other terms. Aseptic meningitis is a meningitic infectious process in which conventional bacterial cultures are negative. The term implies but is not synonymous with a viral etiology. Ventriculitis is involvement of the third or lateral ventricles by a bacterial process. Encephalitis is an infection of the brain parenchyma itself and implies viral etiology. Cerebritis also is an infection of brain parenchyma, but the term implies a bacterial cause. Brain abscess is a focal infection of brain parenchyma that has undergone liquefaction necrosis and usually represents the further pathogenic evolution of a bacterial cerebritis.

Causative Agents

The two most frequent causes of neonatal bacterial meningitis in the United States are GBS serotype III and *E. coli* K1. Both of these pathogens have a clear predilection for the newborn and a tropism for the meninges. *L. monocytogenes* has a similar pattern but is much less common than GBS III or *E. coli* K1. Most cases of aseptic meningitis are enteroviral (echovirus and coxsackievirus). Congenital infections, such as syphilis, cytomegalovirus (CMV), and toxoplasmosis, and partially treated bacterial meningitis occasionally manifest in a similar fashion.

Coagulase-negative staphylococci and *S. aureus* are the most common causes of device-related infections of the CNS (50). Usually they are opportunists in babies with ventriculoperitoneal shunts, and ventriculitis is the dominant clinical pattern at presentation. Encephalitis is the clinical pattern most strongly associated with herpes simplex viral infection. Species of *Citrobacter, Flavobacterium, Klebsiella,* and *Enterobacter* are rare nosocomial causes of meningitis. When they occur, they often are associated with cerebritis and brain abscess.

Epidemiology

As a component of the early-onset form of neonatal sepsis, meningitis rarely is present in a newborn baby at birth. The peak of incidence for infections by the two most frequent etiologic agents—GBS III and *E. coli* K1—is the latter half of the first week and the second week of life, with gradually declining numbers thereafter The incidence of these infections declines to zero by 6 months of age, with a concomitant increase in attack rates for the usual pathogens of older infants, *Neisseria meningitidis, S. pneumoniae,* and *H. influenzae* type b (all rare pathogens of the neonate).

For unknown reasons the usual perinatal risk factors associated with neonatal sepsis—prematurity, prolonged membrane rupture, and maternal amnionitis—are not as strongly associated with the most common agents of neonatal meningitis as they are with early-onset sepsis. In the majority of instances, meningitis caused by GBS or *E. coli* develops insidiously and affects normal full-term babies, often after hospital discharge. Premature infants are overrepresented in series involving device-related ventriculitis, however, because the most frequent of the conditions predisposing to hydrocephalus—intraventricular hemorrhage and subependymal hemorrhage—are most common in the premature infant. Similarly, the gram-negative pathogens that are the most frequent causes of nosocomial late-onset sepsis often are the causes of neonatal meningitis in premature babies with prolonged hospital stays and complex management.

Pathogenesis

Infection reaches the CNS either hematogenously or by direct extension. Fulminant neonatal sepsis frequently does not involve the meninges, simply because multiorgan circulatory, respiratory, and hematologic failure resulting from sepsis dominates the clinical picture before hematogenous spread to the meninges can occur. When host defenses hold the pathogenic cascade of septic shock in check long enough, meningeal invasion and inflammation can develop.

For meningeal invasion to occur, blood-borne organisms first attach to meningeal capillary endothelial cells, penetrate this barrier by invading the cells or by transiting the junctions between them, and then proliferate rapidly in the CSF. A polymorphonuclear leukocyte inflammatory response follows. Evidence indicates that this is triggered by release of cytokines such as TNF and interleukin-1, which may further mediate inflammation and tissue damage (51). Inflammation is accompanied by alterations in CSF dynamics, the development of superficial cerebral vasculitis, and increasing intracranial pressure due to cerebral edema and acute hydrocephalus. In the absence of intervention, these pathologic processes lead to compression of brain-stem respiratory centers, respiratory arrest, and death (52). Even with intervention, the alterations in CSF dynamics may lead to permanent obstructive or communicating hydrocephalus. Cerebral vasculitis and edema may lead to seizures, localized or generalized cerebral infarction, and ischemic-hypoxic encephalopathy.

Neonatal meningitis that occurs by direct extension most frequently complicates ventricular shunting for hydrocephalus or major congenital defects in the meninges, such as meningomyeloceles or encephaloceles. Depending on the infecting organism, bacteremia and septicemia may not be present unless the process is advanced. Occlusions of shunt hardware frequently are associated with infection; differentiation of infection from a purely mechanical problem may be difficult. The most frequent pathogen in shunt infection, coagulase-negative *Staphylococcus*, usually produces only a modest inflammatory response in the ventricles, without the relentless downhill progression associated with more virulent organisms. More virulent pathogens initiate the same sequence of neurologic dysfunctions as in hematogenous infections, with similar high rates of mortality and long-term morbidity.

Clinical Manifestations

The usual nonspecific presentation of neonatal meningitis makes it difficult to distinguish from neonatal sepsis, as discussed previously. Symptoms and signs that identify a higher probability of CNS involvement as a component of sepsis include focal or generalized seizures, a bulging fontanelle, and the presence of shunt devices or meningeal defects.

Diagnosis

The diagnosis of meningitis is made by laboratory examination of spinal fluid. Unless a clear focal origin of infection can be documented in an otherwise well baby, it is prudent to perform a blood culture study and a CSF examination in any premature infant before initiation of antimicrobial therapy. As discussed previously, there are instances in which lumbar puncture can be deferred, but meningitis can never be ruled out in a baby without a CSF examination. The typical features of the CSF in bacterial meningitis are well known: leukocytosis with polymorphonuclear predominance, low glucose, high protein, and a positive Gram stain; bacteria isolated in culture; and, depending on the organism, a positive antigen detection test. When all of these features are present and coupled with positive results on blood culture and a urinary latex agglutination test for the identical organism, there is no doubt about the diagnosis.

Sometimes the data obtained from a culture survey and CSF examination in a patient do not constitute a coherent whole. Two common examples are prior administration of antibiotics to the baby or the baby's mother during labor, which results in negative cultures, and a CSF specimen that is inadequate due to minimal volume or a bloody tap, which yields uninterpretable cell counts and protein levels. In addition, the range of normal in terms of CSF cell counts, protein, and glucose is substantially wider in a newborn premature infant than in an otherwise healthy older infant and may include values that can be misconstrued as indicating infection (53). Birth trauma, acute or resolving CNS hemorrhagic events, neurosurgical procedures, prior CNS infection, or contamination of specimens by skin flora also may produce abnormalities of the CSF in a premature baby that preclude clearcut interpretation. In all of these situations an element of judgment is required, and infectious disease or neurologic consultation should be sought.

Other diagnostic studies may help to clarify the cause or severity of neonatal meningitis. Detection of the capsular antigens of important pathogens, such as GBS or *E. coli* K1 in CSF or urine, may be helpful. Results may be confounded by contamination of "bagged" urine specimens. Shunt tap rather than lumbar puncture is the preferred approach to examination of spinal fluid in babies with ventriculoperitoneal shunts. Head ultrasound or CT scanning are indicated in all premature babies with meningitis to identify hydrocephalus, brain abscess, and vascular accidents.

Treatment

Central to the treatment of meningitis are the killing of infecting organisms, mainte-nance of cerebral perfusion and oxygenation, and anticipation and treatment of complications. All must be carried out as rapidly as possible after the diagnosis is made or a reasonable suspicion of it is entertained.

Because immunoglobulins and complement are absent in CSF and phagocytosis is relatively ineffectual in the "fluid phase," host defenses seldom hold the relentless progression of a neonatal bacterial meningitis in check. Bactericidal antibiotic therapy is essential. Even if the drugs chosen are bactericidal by the usual laboratory testing procedures, their killing efficacy may be only marginal in clinical situations in which there is a large inoculum (more than 10^5 per milliliter) of infecting organisms—the "inoculum effect" (54). (If any organisms are seen on a Gram stain of CSF, it implies a bacterial count of at least 10^5 per milliliter.) Synergistic combinations of antibiotics—in "meningitic" doses—are the most effective means of rapidly killing organisms and preventing resistance. Combinations of high doses of β-lactam drugs (penicillins and third-generation cephalosporins) with therapeutic doses of aminoglycosides provide the maximum killing power and speed for most neonatal meningeal pathogens, including GBS, *E. coli* K1, *Listeria* (not susceptible to cephalosporins), and most nosocomial gram-negative organisms (55). When third-generation cephalosporins are used against nosocomial gram-negative organisms, concomitant administration of aminoglycosides may impede the emergence of resistant subpopulations during therapy—a particularly troublesome problem with *Enterobacter* and *Pseudomonas* (56).

In shunt-related ventriculitis caused by *S. epidermidis* or *S. aureus,* the increasingly widespread occurrence of methicillin resistance necessitates empiric and therapeutic use of vancomycin. Rifampin or aminoglycosides may be added to achieve more efficient bacterial killing, but there are no comparative studies substantiating their benefit. For methicillin-susceptible organisms, methicillin is believed to penetrate the meninges more effectively than the other semisynthetic penicillins, nafcillin and oxacillin, but no comparative studies are available in terms of therapeutic outcomes.

Duration of treatment in neonatal meningitis usually is longer than in uncomplicated neonatal septicemia or bacterial meningitis in older babies. The usual recommended minimum duration is 14 days for a gram-positive bacterial infection and 21 days for a gram-negative bacterial infection. Longer durations are mandated by slow therapeutic responses, as revealed by follow-up CSF examinations with persistence of positive cultures or by the presence of undrained purulent collections, as in brain abscess or loculated ventriculitis. In device-related ventriculitis, treatment duration should encompass the removal and replacement of hardware and extend beyond it by at least 5 days.

Cerebral perfusion and oxygenation are determined by the dynamic balance (perfusion pressure) between mean arterial blood pressure and intracranial pressure. When meningitis is combined with septic shock, cerebral perfusion may be impaired, even if intracranial pressure is normal. With increased intracranial pressure, normal or even increased mean arterial pressure may be insufficient to maintain local or global perfusion of CNS tissues. Ischemic damage may result from this imbalance. When shock is present, maintenance of normal blood pressure and peripheral perfusion by volume expansion (using colloid solutions) and pressors is a priority. A number of therapeutic adjuncts may be considered in management when increased intracranial pressure due to cerebral edema is present (and clinically manifests as a bulging, firm fontanelle). Most commonly used modalities are moderate fluid restriction, assisted ventilation to maintain the partial pressure of carbon dioxide (P_{CO_2}) in the 25 to 35 mm Hg range, and administration of osmotic agents such as mannitol. The benefits of fluid restriction and hyperventilation are controversial (57,58). However, when septic shock is present, fluid restriction and mannitol are contraindicated until effective intravascular volumes and mean arterial pressures are restored. Steroids (e.g., dexamethasone) have been shown to benefit older infants and children with bacterial (predominantly *H. influenzae* type b) meningitis (59,60). Their benefit may relate to their effects on septic shock or cerebral edema or, most likely, a reduction in cytokine production by inflammatory cells. Controlled trials of their use in neonatal meningitis are in progress.

Respiratory arrest (apnea) commonly accompanies initial presentation of neonatal meningitis. If apnea is sustained or repetitive, intubation and assisted ventilation are mandatory. Ventilator parameters are best chosen to minimize cerebral edema: fractional inspired oxygen (F_{IO_2}) is chosen to maintain oxygen saturation at 95% or greater, and minimal end-expiratory pressure, minimal peak airway pressure, and supraphysiologic rates are chosen to maintain P_{CO_2} in the 25 to 35 mm Hg range.

Inappropriately high production of vasopressin (antidiuretic hormone) is present acutely in most babies with meningitis and persists for several days. Excessive fluid intake in these circumstances can lead rapidly to hyponatremia, enhanced cerebral edema, and increased CNS electrical excitability. Standard practice, unless considerations of shock take precedence, include limiting fluid intake to a fraction of maintenance requirements (usually two thirds) during the first 24 to 48 hours of treatment.

Convulsions commonly complicate management of neonatal meningitis. Although the usual metabolic causes must be ruled out or corrected (i.e., hyponatremia, hypoglycemia, hypocalcemia, and hypomagnesemia), seizures generally are a consequence of irritation of the cortical surface by meningeal inflammation or vasculitis. The usual management agent is phenobarbital. Dosage should be monitored by serum levels of the drug, but toxic levels may be necessary and even beneficial if seizure control is difficult and the patient is maintained with assisted ventilation.

Babies with ventriculitis secondary to ventriculoperitoneal shunt create the difficult management dilemma of the need for shunt removal to achieve eradication of colonized hardware versus the continued need for ventricular drainage to control hydrocephalus. If the system is not obstructed, external ventricular drainage is obligatory, with late replacement of the shunt after sterilization is achieved. If the system is not obstructed but sterilization is not achieved with systemic antimicrobial therapy, then hardware removal also is necessary and may be combined with instillation of antimicrobials directly into the ventricle using an external drain or reservoir (61). The agents that have been used most extensively for this purpose are gentamicin and vancomycin. Preservative-free preparations must be used. Dosages are best based on ventricular volume as estimated by CT scan, ultrasound, or calculations regarding on head circumference and cortical mantle thickness. The therapeutic goal of ventricular injection is to achieve the normal safe levels of drug in ventricular CSF: with vancomycin, 15 to 30 µg per milliliter; with gentamicin, 4 to 8 µg per milliliter. Replacement or internalization of a shunt usually is based on sterilization of CSF for a least 1 week and CSF protein levels of 200 mg per deciliter or less.

Prognosis

The prognosis of neonatal meningitis is guarded at best. As case-fatality rates have improved, the proportion of survivors with residual morbidity is increasing. GBS meningitis now has a case-fatality rate of 21% to 27% (62,63). On long-term follow-up, 30% to 50% of survivors have neurologic impairment ranging from subtle to profound. Outcome figures are equally, if not more, disturbing in neonatal gram-negative meningitis. Three carefully designed and executed clinical trials coordinated by McCracken et al. (64–66) demonstrated overall case-fatality rates of 19% to 32%, with residual neurologic morbidity rates of 33% to 58%. Each of these trials involved what appeared to be a rational alteration in conventional parenteral therapy—including intrathecal gentamicin, intraventricular gentamicin, and the third-generation

cephalosporin, moxalactam. In none of these trials did the study regimen prove superior to conventional parenteral treatment. The trial involving intraventricular gentamicin was terminated early because of a high case-fatality rate in the study regimen group. There is now support for the concept that too rapid killing of infecting organisms, with consequent release of large quantities of endotoxin, may actually do more harm than good. Although the addition of steroids to conventional parenteral regimens is being studied, the major conclusion from previous studies is that the stage of infection at the time treatment is initiated, rather than the specific antimicrobial drug used, determines outcome.

Prevention

In the same manner that early recognition and treatment of neonatal meningitis is associated with improved outcome, early recognition and treatment of neonatal sepsis may prevent the development of meningitis. Selective intrapartum chemoprophylaxis (based on maternal GBS colonization and perinatal risk factors) prevents early-onset neonatal GBS disease in premature infants. It also may have a preventive effect on GBS meningitis, but this is unproven. Immunization of mothers to achieve passive immunization of the fetus and newborn is an appealing approach to preventing GBS diseases (67). The lack of immunogenicity of polysaccharide vaccines and the lower levels of maternally derived specific antibodies in premature infants are important unresolved issues with this approach. Conjugate vaccines with enhanced immunogenicity may soon resolve the problem (65).

Prevention of device-related ventriculitis is related to the technical aspects of shunt insertion. Prophylactic antibiotics during shunt insertion are used by most neurosurgeons, but controlled trials have not shown striking benefits. If prophylactic antibiotics are used, a rational approach is to select them to kill the organisms most likely to colonize the operative sites on the scalp and abdominal skin and to use them preoperatively, intraoperatively, and postoperatively. Vancomycin is the best choice for typical older premature infants who have developed hydrocephalus as the result of a CNS vascular accident. Ampicillin and a third-generation cephalosporin are logical choices for an early shunt in a baby with an open lumbosacral meningomyelocele. If time is available before a procedure, formal documentation of skin flora at the operative sites and their sensitivities affords the greatest chance for a good fit between a prophylactic regimen and the organisms it is designed to interdict.

LATE-ONSET LOWER RESPIRATORY TRACT INFECTIONS

Premature infants are particularly vulnerable to pulmonary infection. Neonatal pneumonia, acquired perinatally, is a frequent component of early-onset sepsis and is discussed in the first section of this chapter. Lower respiratory tract infections manifesting after the first few days of life may be perinatal, nosocomial, or community acquired (69,70). They may be primary, but more often they represent complications of the common noninfectious respiratory conditions of premature infants—hyaline membrane disease and BPD—and their technologic management. In a hospitalized premature baby with marginal respiratory drive and borderline oxygenation-ventilation, these infections are frequently life-threatening. Even long after discharge from the nursery, they are the most important causes of acquired illnesses in premature infants who require hospital readmission.

Causative Agents

The viruses and bacteria that are the most common causes of lower respiratory tract infections may be classified according to their origins and usual age at onset. These are summarized in Fig. 2.2. GBS, herpes simplex,

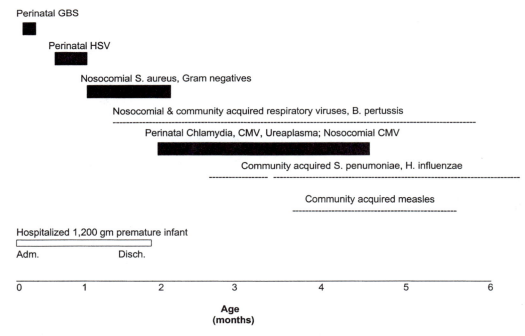

FIG. 2.2. Important causes of perinatal, nosocomial, and community-acquired respiratory tract infections in a hypothetical 1,200-g very-low-birth-weight infant with a 6-week neonatal intensive care unit hospitalization, by age at onset. GBS, group B streptococcus; HSV, herpes simplex virus; CMV, cytomegalovirus; solid bars, usual ages at onset; interrupted bars, possible ages at onset; hatched bar, duration of mechanical ventilation; open bar, remainder of hospitalization.

Chlamydia trachomatis, CMV, and *Ureaplasma urealyticum* usually are acquired perinatally. They manifest at varying ages: GBS exclusively within the first 72 hours of life; herpes simplex usually between the ages of 5 and 14 days; and *Chlamydia,* CMV, and *Ureaplasma* between the ages of 1 and 4 months. *S. aureus,* opportunistic gram-negative rods, CMV, and the common respiratory viruses (respiratory syncytial virus [RSV], parainfluenza viruses 1 to 3, and influenza A and B) may be acquired nosocomially. Nosocomial infections usually manifest after the first week of life, but thereafter may occur any time during the baby's hospitalization and (in the case of *S. aureus* or CMV) up to several months after discharge. After discharge, the same common community-acquired respiratory viruses are the usual causes of lower respiratory tract disease. Pertussis, varicella, and measles can be lethal in an unimmunized premature infant and should not be forgotten.

Epidemiology

The reservoir of infecting organisms in perinatally acquired lower respiratory tract disease is the mother's genital tract or, occasionally, breast milk. The two major reservoirs of infection in nosocomial respiratory tract infection are the hands of personnel and the mechanical devices (ventilators, humidifiers, nebulizers, endotracheal tubes, and tracheostomies) used in treating respiratory failure. The reservoir of most community-acquired respiratory tract infections is other children, particularly siblings in the home or family.

The age at onset for these infections varies with the agent and the mode of acquisition. GBS attacks the lungs as its portal of entry. Because amniotic fluid contamination is the usual mechanism, most affected babies are ill at birth or within a few hours after birth. Herpes simplex attacks the lungs as part of a hematogenous dissemination, usually from a cutaneous or upper respiratory source. Therefore, most affected babies have pneumonia with an overwhelming illness that does not manifest until at least 1 week of age. Perinatal

Chlamydia, CMV, and *Ureaplasma* disease have more prolonged incubation periods.

Nosocomial infections occur during hospitalization or shortly thereafter. Because their access to the lungs usually is via the endotracheal tubes and tracheostomy tubes used for mechanical ventilation, a baby's duration of respiratory failure and intubation determine the major period of vulnerability to bacterial nosocomial pathogens. Viral nosocomial respiratory tract infections can occur at any time during hospitalization. Caretakers with bothersome but relatively mild viral upper respiratory tract infections may inoculate any portion of the baby's respiratory tract, usually by close contact (71). Nosocomial CMV pneumonia is acquired by receiving seropositive unfrozen blood products or banked breast milk (72). As in perinatally acquired CMV, these infections may have a relatively long incubation period.

Community-acquired respiratory illness manifests after hospital discharge in virtually all "premie grads." Most of these infections have strong seasonal patterns, so a baby discharged during the winter is particularly vulnerable to RSV and influenza A and B. Parainfluenza 1 and 2 infections usually occur in the spring and fall. Parainfluenza 3 infections are not seasonal. Loss of maternal humoral immunity at an earlier age than in a full-term baby probably renders premature infants vulnerable to measles and varicella at a younger age than the usual 12 to 15 months, even if the mother's immunity is adequate (73).

The strongest risk factor for serious acquired respiratory tract disease is BPD, the aftermath of aggressive ventilator management of hyaline membrane disease, meconium aspiration, or perinatal pneumonia. Thirty percent to 45% of babies discharged from the hospital with BPD require at least one rehospitalization for respiratory illness, usually triggered by community-acquired viruses, within the first year after discharge. Multiple office and emergency room visits are the norm (74). However, even among VLBW premature infants who have required no mechanical ventilation during their nursery stay, 15%

to 41% require hospitalization within the first year of life for acute respiratory illness (75). Rates of rehospitalization are highest for babies discharged in fall and winter months.

Pathogenesis

Acquired lower respiratory tract infection may develop when pathogens gain direct access to the tracheobronchial tree or alveoli, as in perinatal GBS and nosocomial bacterial infections; when they reach them hematogenously, as in perinatal herpes simplex and nosocomial CMV infections; or when they reach them as part of the invasion of the entire respiratory tract that occurs with perinatal *Chlamydia,* CMV, *Ureaplasma,* and community-acquired respiratory viruses.

The serious consequences of these infections primarily are determined by the anatomic and physiologic severity of preexisting lung compromise. The small caliber and soft consistency of the airways in a premature infant predispose to obstructive phenomena— nasal obstruction, wheezing, or atelectasis— when infection causes inflammatory edema and increased mucus production. Loss of ciliated epithelium and consequent squamous metaplasia in the baby with BPD impairs the lung's usual defense against infection and predisposes to mucus plugging and atelectasis (76). Tracheostomies, subglottic stenosis, or laryngomalacia further impair a baby's ability to clear secretions by coughing.

Marginal oxygenation and ventilation are the usual physiologic hallmarks of BPD and are the result of interstitial fibrosis, coalescence and loss of alveolar units, and ventilation-perfusion mismatching. A respiratory tract infection in a baby with this marginal pulmonary status can easily "tip over" the situation into respiratory failure. Pulmonary hypertension is a physiologic condition associated with enhanced risk of mortality in acquired RSV infection (77), but this association may reflect preexisting pulmonary damage as well as a cardiovascular phenomenon.

The relative immunity of brain-stem respiratory centers and weakness of the diaphragmatic and accessory musculature result in impaired compensatory mechanisms in a baby who develops infection-induced hypoxia, hypercarbia, or obstructive phenomena. These impairments also enhance the risk of respiratory failure and respiratory arrest in the premature infant (78,79).

Clinical Manifestations

The usual signs of respiratory distress— tachypnea, retractions, grunting, rales, wheezing, or cyanosis—are present in most premature babies. Coughing is characteristic of perinatally acquired *Chlamydia,* CMV, and *Ureaplasma* infections (80) and of community-acquired pertussis and measles, but is absent with most other pathogens. Apnea is characteristic of RSV and the other nosocomial or community-acquired respiratory viruses. Wheezing also is most characteristic of viral agents. Fever is an unreliable sign and frequently is absent during a baby's initial hospitalization. In an older premature baby after hospital discharge, fever is a more reliable sign of infection.

In the premature baby with a nosocomial infection, particularly if the child is still intubated and receiving mechanical ventilation, the problem manifests as a deterioration in blood gas status and a need for higher F_{IO_2} and more aggressive ventilator parameters. The usual gradual "weaning" process in an improving baby becomes a "setback." Typically there is an increase in mucus secretions, a need for increased frequency of suctioning, and a change in sputum character from the usual clear and frothy to a more tenacious, purulent appearance.

Diagnosis

Recognition of deterioration in a hospitalized premature baby, or of a significant lower respiratory tract problem in a baby after discharge, usually is not difficult. Differentiation from noninfectious causes, of which there are many, and identification of a specific infectious etiology are problems. These issues have therapeutic implications, however, and are important in management (81).

Chest radiography, blood culture, arterial blood gas determination, and Gram staining or culture of sputum (if available in an incubated patient) are the usual starting points in diagnosis. Comparison with previous chest radiographs is essential in any baby with previous respiratory problems and is the best method for differentiating preexisting scars and lucent areas from newly acquired problems. Elimination of pneumothorax and atelectasis as possible causes can be accomplished quickly. Blood culture usually is a low-yield procedure, but it should be routine. Arterial blood gases determine severity of disease and are essential for initial assessment and documentation of progress. Noninvasive measurement techniques, such as oximetry and transcutaneous monitoring, may substitute for repeated arterial punctures or indwelling lines once a baseline for comparison has been established. Gram stains and cultures of sputum are helpful. Gram staining provides an assessment of the nature of the inflammatory response and the number of bacterial organisms present. A sputum with few polymorphonuclear leukocytes and no visible bacteria is unlikely to represent a nosocomial bacterial process. A dominant polymorphonuclear inflammatory response with visible bacteria (i.e., more than 10^5 per milliliter) is likely to be at least partially bacterial in origin. A single bacterial isolate on culture, particularly if present in significant numbers (i.e., "many" or "moderate"), should guide antibiotic treatment.

Depending on age at onset, season, and severity of the clinical picture, other diagnostic studies may be indicated. Herpes simplex pneumonia, in the context of systemic disseminated disease, is suggested by liver enzyme elevations (usually to "panic" levels) and may be identified rapidly by viral culture of tracheal aspirates or skin lesions. Perinatal *Chlamydia* and *Ureaplasma* infections require specialized culture techniques on tracheal aspirate specimens. Remarkably elevated and stable serum indirect IgG and IgM

immunofluorescence antibody levels also are characteristic of *Chlamydia* pneumonitis, even at the onset of symptoms. A negative serology result rules out this diagnosis. RSV infections (and other respiratory viruses) are most accurately and most quickly identified by direct immunofluorescence staining or enzyme-linked immunosorbent assay (ELISA) of respiratory secretions (tracheal ornasopharyngeal aspirates) (82). Cultures are confirmatory but take longer. Pertussis is best diagnosed by direct immunofluorescent antibody examination of nasopharyngeal swabs smeared on glass slides. Cultivation of *Bordetella pertussis* is difficult and not successful in most hospital clinical microbiology laboratories. Measles is readily confirmed with the use of IgM- and IgG-specific serum antibodies measured by indirect immunofluorescence. IgM is present early; IgG rises during convalescence.

Babies with prolonged intubation and mechanical ventilation create diagnostic difficulties because their lower respiratory tract secretions rarely are sterile. *Pseudomonas* and other opportunistic gram-negative organisms, *S. epidermidis,* and *C. albicans* frequently are encountered. Differentiation of colonization (of the trachea or endotracheal-tracheostomy tube) by these organisms from true infection is difficult (83). The most helpful approach in these situations is to maintain a weekly or twice-weekly surveillance of lower respiratory tract secretion Gram stains and cultures. Abrupt changes in cellular predominance and the appearance of new organisms, coupled with clinical deterioration, should lead to consideration of treatment directed at the newly acquired organisms. Abrupt changes in peripheral white cell count with a left shift further support a bacterial etiology.

Treatment

Because respiratory failure—either blood gas decompensation or apnea—is a frequent presentation of late-onset respiratory tract disease in premature babies, initial treatment efforts involve administration of oxygen, establishment of a secure airway, and mechanical ventilation or increases in ventilator parameters. Accidental problems, such as a dislodged or misplaced endotracheal tube, mucus plugs, and pneumothorax, must be excluded. After the patient has been stabilized, attention can turn to antimicrobial treatment.

Initial empiric treatment usually includes antibiotics, with the choice of regimen depending on Gram stain results, prior infections in the baby, prevalent flora in the nursery, and specific exposures in the community. Third-generation cephalosporins are most frequently used, often combined with vancomycin or an aminoglycoside for the hospitalized baby. Antiviral therapy is imperative for neonatal herpes, although the disease is far advanced if pneumonia is a presenting feature (84). Acyclovir is the drug of choice. For RSV (and probably for other respiratory viruses as well), ribavirin is indicated. A history of prematurity is an indication for treatment, so a fairly aggressive diagnostic effort to document this agent is desirable. There is some controversy regarding the actual benefits of ribavirin, but almost all authorities agree that premature babies with preexisting lung disease are most likely to be helped (85,86). Administration of ribavirin to babies receiving mechanical ventilation requires filtration within the ventilator circuit to prevent crystallization (87). The use of erythromycin for *Chlamydia* and *Ureaplasma* infection is increasingly prevalent, but no controlled studies of efficacy exist in premature infants. Erythromycin also is the drug of choice for pertussis.

Cardiorespiratory monitoring should be routine for any "premie grad" admitted with acute respiratory tract infection because of the risk of apneic spells. The use of bronchodilators has become almost routine in the management of a respiratory illness in which wheezing is a component. Nebulized albuterol is most widely used. Steroids also are frequently used to permit weaning of babies with persistent requirements for mechanical ventilation. Although viral infections, such as CMV or herpes simplex, would be expected to be influenced adversely by steroids, they can be excluded readily before treatment. Other respiratory viral and bacterial illnesses are probably not affected adversely by short-term steroid treatment.

Prevention

Prevention of perinatal GBS disease with intrapartum and postpartum chemoprophylaxis has been discussed previously in this chapter. Prevention of neonatal herpes involves the selective use of cesarean section to interdict vertical transmission and the administration of acyclovir in the weeks before delivery. Erythromycin treatment of colonized pregnant women has been shown to prevent perinatal chlamydial infection (88). There are no data on prevention of perinatal CMV or *Ureaplasma.*

Nosocomial infections in the nursery are best prevented by a thoughtful and enforced set of rules for nursery infection control (27). Careful hand washing between patients, reasonable space allotments for each baby, and appropriate isolation of babies with known communicable diseases are the most effective components of such an approach. Personnel and parents should be aware of their own health. Individuals with upper respiratory tract illnesses should wear masks while working in the nursery or, preferably, should be assigned to desk chores. Individuals with dermatitis of the hands should seek medical attention, which should consist of curative measures, discussions of alternative hand soaps, and use of gloves during direct patient care. Use of ritualistic surgical scrubs on entry to the nursery and of cover gowns may have a psychological rationale, but these measures have no proven benefits (and actually may be harmful).

Certain nosocomial respiratory tract infections have been virtually eliminated from the nursery by the elucidation and elimination of their transmission mechanisms. Acquisition of CMV by susceptible infants through transfusion with CMV-seropositive blood products has been virtually eliminated by blood bank screening or use of frozen deglycerolated red blood cells (89). Nosocomial human immunodeficiency virus (HIV) and hepatitis B infections have been eliminated from the nursery by similar approaches. There appears to be no risk to personnel from any of these agents if "blood precautions" are used during patient care (90).

After hospital discharge, prevention of community-acquired respiratory tract diseases is, to a certain extent, beyond the physician's control. However, parents should be informed about their baby's most likely sources of infection: other children and themselves. Parents who have learned infection control etiquette during their baby's hospitalization should take some elements home with them. This is particularly appropriate for a precarious baby who has had a prolonged hospitalization and is home and receiving supplementary oxygen.

Immunizations are possible against at least some of the pathogens premature babies are exposed to after discharge. There are, however, sparse data on the side effects and serologic responses of premature infants to standard well-baby immunizations. It is usually recommended that premature infants receive pertussis (with diphtheria and tetanus) immunization at the same chronologic (not postconceptional) age as full-term infants (91). However, some delay is not inappropriate for the tiniest hospitalized infants. No specific alterations in immunization schedules for measles and *H. influenzae* type b conjugate vaccines have been made for premature infants. Influenza immunization (with split product vaccine) should be considered for premature infants with chronic respiratory disease who will be discharged during the winter. Repetitive annual vaccination should be carried out routinely in older babies with residual lung damage. Passive immunization with a humanized monoclonal antibody against the fusion glycoprotein of RSV (palivizumab) has a substantial protective effect (92). It is now recommended for all premature infants during the winter respiratory virus seasons (93).

REFERENCES

1. Kleinman JC. Infant mortality among racial/ethnic minority groups, 1983–1984. CDC Surveillance Summaries. *MMWR Morb Mortal Wkly Rep* 1990;39(SS-3):31–52.
2. Lasko SM, Epstein MF, Mitchell AA. Recent patterns of drug use in newborn intensive care. *J Pediatr* 1990;116:985.
3. Klein JO, Marcy SM. Bacterial sepsis and meningitis. In: Remington JS, Kelin JO, eds. *Infectious diseases of the fetus and newborn infant,* 4th ed. Philadelphia: Saunders, 1994:835.
4. Wheeler WE. Waterbugs in the bassinet. *Am J Dis Child* 1961;101:273.
5. Hendeson DK. Bacteremia due to percutaneous intravascular devices. In: Mandell GL, Bennett JE, Dolin R, eds. *Principles and practice of infectious diseases.* New York: Churchill Livingstone, 1995:2987.
6. Freidman RM, Ingram DL, Gross I, et al. A half century of neonatal sepsis at Yale. *Am J Dis Child* 1981;35:140.
7. Gladstone IM, Ehrenkranz RA, Edberg SC, et al. The rise of neonatal sepsis due to skin commensal species. *Pediatr Res* 1990;27:271A.
8. Boyer KM, Gadzala CA, Burd LI, et al. Selective intrapartum chemoprophylaxis of neonatal group B streptococcal early onset disease: I. Epidemiologic rationale. *J Infect Dis* 1983;148:795.
9. Zimmerman JJ, Dietrich KA. Current perspectives on septic shock. *Pediatr Clin North Am* 1987;34:131.
10. Pichichero MD, Todd JK. Detection of neonatal bacteremia. *J Pediatr* 1979;94:958.
11. Bone RC, Fisher CJ Jr, Clemmer TP, et al. Sepsis syndrome: a valid clinical entity. *Crit Care Med* 1990;17:389.
12. Manroe BL, Weinberg AG, Rosenfeld CR, et al. The neonatal blood count in health and disease: I. Reference values for neutrophilic cells. *J Pediatr* 1979;95:89.
13. Sanchez PJ, Siegel JD, Cushion NE, et al. Significance of a positive urine group B streptococcal latex agglutination test in neonates. *J Pediatr* 1990;116:601.
14. Visser VE, Hall RT. Urine culture in the evaluation of suspected neonatal sepsis. *J Pediatr* 1979;94:635.
15. Sherman MP, Goetzman BW, Ahlfors CE, et al. Tracheal aspiration and its clinical correlates in the diagnosis of congenital pneumonia. *Pediatrics* 1980;65:258.
16. Maki DG, Weise CE, Sarafin HW. A semiquantitative method for identifying catheter-related infection. *N Engl J Med* 1977;296:1305.
17. Gleason CA, Martin RJ, Anderson JV, et al. Optimal position for a spinal tap in pre-term infants. *Pediatrics* 1983;71:31.
18. Fielkow S, Reuter S, Gotoff SP. Cerebrospinal fluid examination in symptom-free neonates with risk factors for infections. *J Pediatr* 1991;119:971.
19. Bradley JS. Neonatal infections. *Pediatr Infect Dis* 1985;4:315.
20. McCracken GH Jr, Saez-Llorens X. Clinical pharmacology of antimicrobial agents. In: Remington JS, Klein JO, eds. *Infectious diseases of the fetus and newborn infant,* 4th ed. Philadelphia: Saunders, 1994:1287.
21. Prober CG, Stevenson DR, Benitz NE. The use of antibiotics in neonates weighing less than 1200 grams. *Pediatr Infect Dis J* 1990;9:111.
22. Kaplan SL. Bacteremia and septic shock. In: Feigin RD,

Cherry JD, eds. *Textbook of pediatric infectious diseases,* 4th ed. Philadelphia: Saunders, 1998:807.

23. Mize CE, Squire RH Jr. Starvation. In: Levin DL, Morriss FC, eds. *Essentials of pediatric intensive care,* 2nd ed. St. Louis: Quality Medical, 1997:845.

24. Gonzalez LA, Hill HR. The current status of intravenous gammaglobulin use in neonates. *Pediatr Infect Dis J* 1989;8:315.

25. Weisman LE, Lorenzetti PM. High intravenous doses of human immune globulin suppress neonatal group B streptococcal immunity in rats. *J Pediatr* 1989;115:445.

26. Ziegler EJ, Fisher CJ, Spring CL, et al. HA-1A Sepsis Study Group. Treatment of gram-negative bacteremia and septic shock with HA-1A human monoclonal antibody against endotoxin: a randomized, double-blind, placebo-controlled trial. *N Engl J Med* 1991;324:425.

27. Weinstein RA, Boyer KM, Linn ES. Isolation guidelines for obstetric patients and newborn infants. *Am J Obstet Gynecol* 1983;146:353.

28. Boyer KM, Gotoff SP. Prevention of early onset neonatal group B streptococcal disease with selective intrapartum chemoprophylaxis. *N Engl J Med* 1986;314:1665.

29. Tuppereinen N, Hallman U. Prevention of neonatal group B streptococcal disease: intrapartum detection and prophylaxis of heavily colonized parturients. *Obstet Gynecol* 1989;73:583.

30. Garland SM, Fliejen JR. Group B streptococcus and neonatal infections: the care for intrapartum chemoprophylaxis. *Aust N Z J Obstet Gynecol* 1991;148:915, 1991.

31. Prevention of perinatal group B streptococcal disease: a public health perspective. *MMWR Morb Mortal Wkly Rep* 1996;45(RR-7):1–24.

32. Group B streptococcal infections. In: Peter G, ed. *Report of the committee on infectious diseases,* 24th ed. Elk Grove Village, IL: American Academy of Pediatrics, 1997:494–501.

33. Schreg SJ, Zywicki S, Farley M, et al. Group B streptococcal disease in the era of intrapartum antibiotic prophylaxis. *Clin Infect Dis* 1999;27:972.

34. Walsh MC, Kliegman RM. Necrotizing enterocolitis: treatment based on staging criteria. *Pediatr Clin North Am* 1986;33:179.

35. Kliegman, RM. Models of the pathogenesis of necrotizing enterocolitis. *J Pediatr* 1990;117:S2.

36. Kliegman RM, Pittard WB, Fanaroff AA. Necrotizing enterocolitis in neonates fed human milk. *J Pediatr* 1979;95:450.

37. Nowicki P. Intestinal ischemia and necrotizing enterocolitis. *J Pediatr* 1990;117:S14.

38. Kien CL. Colonic fermentation of carbohydrate in the premature infant: possible relevance to necrotizing enterocolitis. *J Pediatr* 1990;117:552.

39. Kliegman RM. Neonatal necrotizing enterocolitis: implications for an infectious disease. *Pediatr Clin North Am* 1979;26:327.

40. Bell MJ, Ternberg JL, Feigin RD, et al. Neonatal necrotizing enterocolitis: therapeutic decisions based on clinical stating. *Ann Surg* 1978;187:1.

41. Merritt C, Goldsmith J, Sharp M. Sonographic detection of portal venous gas in infants with necrotizing enterocolitis. *Am J Radiol* 1984;143:1059.

42. Koloski AM, Lilly JR. Paracentesis and lavage for diagnosis of intestinal gangrene in neonatal necrotizing enterocolitis. *J Pediatr Surg* 1978;13:315.

43. Hutter JJ Jr, Hathaway WE, Wayne ER. Hematologic abnormalities in severe neonatal necrotizing enterocolitis. *J Pediatr* 1976;88:1026.

44. Caplan MS, Sun XM, Hsueh W, et al. Role of platelet activating factor and tumor necrosis factor–alpha in neonatal necrotizing enterocolitis. *J Pediatr* 1990;116:960.

45. Faix RG, Polley TZ, Grasela TH. A randomized, controlled trial of parenteral clindamycin in neonatal necrotizing enterocolitis. *J Pediatr* 1988;112:271.

46. Walsh MC, Kliegman RM, Hack M. Severity of necrotizing enterocolitis: influence on outcome at 2 years of age. *Pediatrics* 1989;84:808.

47. Botsford KB, Weinstein RA, Boyer KM, et al. Gram-negative bacilli in human milk feedings: quantitation and clinical consequences for premature infants. *J Pediatr* 1986;109:707.

48. Eibl MM, Wolf HM, Furnkranz H, et al. Prevention of necrotizing enterocolitis in low-birth weight infants by IgA-IgG feeding. *N Engl J Med* 1988;319:1.

49. Klein JO, Feigin RD, McCracken JH Jr. Report of the task force on diagnosis and management of meningitis. *Pediatrics* 1986;78[Suppl]:959.

50. Gardner P, Leipzig T, Sadigh M. Infections of mechanical cerebrospinal fluid shunts. In: Remington JS, Swartz MN. *Current clinical topics in infectious disease,* 9th ed. New York: McGraw-Hill, 1988:185.

51. Saez-Llorens X, Ranilo O, Mustafa MM, et al. Molecular pathophysiology of bacterial meningitis: current concepts and therapeutic implications. *J Pediatr* 1990;116:671.

52. Sande ME, Scheld WM, McCracken GH Jr, and the Meningitis Study Group. Pathophysiology of bacterial meningitis: implications for new management strategies. Report of a workshop. *Pediatr Infect Dis* 1987;6:1145.

53. Gyllensward A, Malstrom S. The cerebrospinal fluid in immature infants. *Acta Paediatr Scand* 1962;135 [Suppl]:54.

54. Weeks JL, Mason EO Jr, Baker CJ. Antagonism of ampicillin and chloramphenicol for meningeal isolates of group B streptococci. *Antimicrob Agents Chemother* 1981;20:281.

55. Schweld W, Alliegro GM, Field MR, et al. Synergy between ampicillin and gentamicin in experimental meningitis due to group B streptococci. *J Infect Dis* 1982;146:100.

56. Sanders CC, Sanders WE Jr. Emergence of resistance during therapy with the newer beta-lactam antibiotics: role of inducible beta-lactamases and implications for the future. *Rev Infect Dis* 1983;5:639.

57. Powell KA, Sugarman LI, Eskenazi AE, et al. Normalization of plasma arginine vasopressin concentrations when children with meningitis are given maintenance plus replacement fluid therapy. *J Pediatr* 1990;117:515.

58. Ashwal S, Stringer W, Tomasi L, et al. Cerebral blood flow and carbon dioxide reactivity in children with bacterial meningitis. *J Pediatr* 1990;117:523.

59. Lebel MH, Freij BJ, Syrogiannopoulos GA, et al. Dexamethasone therapy for bacterial meningitis: results of two double-blind, placebo-controlled trials. *N Engl J Med* 1988;319:964.

60. Odio CM, Faingezicht I, Paris M, et al. The beneficial effects of early dexamethasone administration in infants and children with bacterial meningitis. *N Engl J Med* 1991;324:1525.

61. Jackson MA. Cerebrospinal fluid shunt infection. In: Nelson JD, ed. *Current therapy in pediatric infectious disease,* 2nd ed. Toronto: BC Decker, 1988:145.

62. Edwards MS, Rench MA, Haffar AA. Long-term sequelae of group B streptococcal meningitis in infants. *J Pediatr* 1985;106:819.

63. Wald ER, Bergman I, Taylor HG. Long-term outcome of group B streptococcal meningitis. *Pediatrics* 1986; 77:217.

64. McCracken GH Jr, Mize SG. A controlled study of intrathecal antibiotic therapy in gram-negative enteric meningitis in infancy. Report of the Neonatal Cooperative Study Group, *J Pediatr* 1976;89:66.

65. McCracken GH Jr, Mize SG, Threlheld N. Intraventricular gentamicin therapy in gram-negative bacillary meningitis of infancy. Report of the Neonatal Cooperative Study Group. *Lancet* 1980;1:787.

66. McCracken GH Jr, Threlheld N, Mize S, et al. Moxalactam therapy for neonatal meningitis due to gram-negative enteric bacteria. *JAMA* 1984;252:1427.

67. Baker CJ, Rench MA, Kasper DL. Response to type III polysaccharide in women whose infants have had invasive group B streptococcal infection. *N Engl J Med* 1990;322:1857.

68. Lagergard T, Shiloach J, Robbins JB, et al. Synthesis and immunological properties of conjugates composed of group B streptococcus type III capsular polysaccharide covalently bound to tetanus toxoid. *Infect Immun* 1990;58:687.

69. Boyer KM. Nonbacterial pneumonia. In: Feigin RD, Cherry JD, eds. *Textbook of pediatric infectious diseases, 4th ed.* Philadelphia: Saunders, 1998:260.

70. Marks MI, Klein JO. Bacterial infections of respiratory tract. In: Remington JS, Klein JO, eds. *Infectious diseases of the fetus and newborn infant,* 4th ed. Philadelphia: Saunders, 1995:891.

71. Hall CB, Kopelman AE, Douglas RG, et al. Neonatal respiratory syncytial virus infection. *N Engl J Med* 1979;300:393.

72. Yeager AS. Transfusion-acquired cytomegalovirus infection in newborn infants. *Am J Dis Child* 1974;128: 478.

73. Cates KL, Goetz C, Rosenberg N, et al. Longitudinal development of specific and functional antibody in very low birth weight premature infants. *Pediatr Res* 1988; 23:14.

74. Sauve RS, Singhai N. Long-term morbidity of infants with bronchopulmonary dysplasia. *Pediatrics* 1985;76: 725.

75. Cunningham CK, McMillan JA, Gross SJ. Rehospitalization for respiratory illness in infants of less than 32 weeks' gestation. *Pediatrics* 1991;88:527.

76. Naeve C. Tracheal aspirate cytology in neonatal respiratory distress syndrome and bronchopulmonary dysplasia. In: Merritt TA, Northway WH Jr, Boynton BR, eds. *Bronchopulmonary dysplasia.* Boston: Blackwell, 1988:59.

77. McDonald NE, Hall CB, Suffin SC, et al. Respiratory syncytial virus infection in infants with congenital heart disease. *N Engl J Med* 1982;307:397.

78. Bruhn FW, Molcrohisky ST, McIntosch K. Apnea associated with respiratory syncytial virus infection in young infants. *J Pediatr* 1977;90:382.

79. Groothius JR, Gutierrez KM, Lauer BA. Respiratory syncytial virus infection in children with bronchopulmonary dysplasia. *Pediatrics* 1998;82:199.

80. Brasfield DM, Stagno S, Whitley RJ, et al. Infant pneumonitis associated with *Cytomegalovirus, Chlamydia, Pneumocystis,* and *Ureaplasma:* follow-up. *Pediatrics* 1987;79:76.

81. Nickerson BJ. Bronchopulmonary dysplasia, In: Levin DL, Morriss FC, eds. *Essentials of pediatric intensive care,* 2nd ed. St. Louis: Quality Medical, 1997:170.

82. Kellogg IA. Culture vs direct antigen assays for detection of microbial pathogens from lower respiratory tract specimens suspected of containing the respiratory syncytial virus. *Arch Pathol Lab Med* 1991;115:451.

83. Rudermen JW, Morgan MA, Srugo I, et al. Diagnosis of pneumonia in neonates by use of quantitative tracheal aspirates. *Pediatr Res* 1990;27:275A.

84. Whitley R, Arvin AM. Herpes simplex viral infections. In: Remington JS, Klein JO, eds. *Infectious diseases of the fetus and newborn infant,* 4th ed. Philadelphia: Saunders, 1994:354.

85. Groothius JR, Woodin KA, Katz R, et al. Early ribavirin treatment of respiratory syncytial viral infection in high-risk children. *J Pediatr* 1990;117:792.

86. American Academy of Pediatrics Committee on Infectious Diseases. Reassessment of indications of ribavirin therapy. *Pediatrics* 1996;97:137.

87. Smith DW, Frankel LR, Mathers LH, et al. A controlled trial of aerosolized ribavirin in infants receiving mechanical ventilation for severe respiratory syncytial virus infection. *N Engl J Med* 1991;325:24.

88. Schachter J, Sweet RL, Grossman M, et al. Experience with the routine use of erythromycin for chlamydial infections in pregnancy. *N Engl J Med* 1986;314:276.

89. Yeager AS, Grumet FC, Hafleigh EB, et al. Prevention of transfusion-acquired cytomegalovirus infection in newborn infants. *J Pediatr* 1981;98:281.

90. Balfour CL, Balfour HH. Cytomegalovirus is not an occupational risk for nurses in renal transplant and neonatal units. *JAMA* 1986;256:1909.

91. Pertussis. In: Peter G, ed. *Report of the Committee on Infectious Diseases,* 24th ed. Elk Grove Village, IL: American Academy of Pediatrics, 1997:394–407.

92. Meissner HC, Welliver RC, Chartrand SA, et al. Immunoprophylaxis with palivizumab, a humanized respiratory syncytial virus monoclonal antibody, for prevention of respiratory syncytial virus infection in high risk infants: a consensus opinion. *Pediatr Infect Dis J* 1999;18:223.

93. American Academy of Pediatrics Committee on Infectious Diseases. Prevention of respiratory syncytial virus infections: indications for the use of palivizumab and update on the use of RSV-IGIV. *Pediatrics* 1998;102:1211.

3

Pediatric Human Immunodeficiency Virus Infection: Natural History, Perinatal Transmission, and Opportunistic Infections

Russell B. Van Dyke and *Ross E. McKinney, Jr.

*Department of Pediatrics, Tulane University Health Sciences Center, New Orleans, Louisiana 70112;
and *Department of Pediatrics, Duke University Medical Center, Durham, North Carolina 27710*

Pediatric human immunodeficiency virus (HIV) infection is one of the most common causes of severe immune compromise in children. Unlike most conditions affecting the immune system of children, the damage with HIV is progressive, becoming steadily worse with age. In addition, HIV infection produces damage to other organs, such as the central nervous system (CNS), increasing the difficulty in management.

Therapy exists for HIV infection, although it is still only moderately effective. Patients are living longer and better lives, but they are not cured. On the other hand, interventions to prevent mother-to-child HIV transmission can be effective as much as 97% to 98% of the time, making pediatric HIV a relatively preventable disease in countries that can afford to test pregnant women and to offer preventative medications.

BIOLOGY OF HIV DISEASE IN CHILDREN

The time at which HIV is transmitted from mother to infant for most pregnancies can be fairly tightly defined. Transmission can occur before birth (*in utero*), during the delivery process (peripartum), or through breast-feeding after birth. Although infection via breast-feeding is common in much of the world, it is an uncommon means of transmission in developed countries, largely because relatively few HIV-infected women breast-feed. The standard means to determine the timing of an infant's infection is an HIV culture or DNA polymerase chain reaction (PCR) test obtained within the first week of life (1). In the case of an infant infected peripartum (as opposed to *in utero*), the amount of virus present in the first days after infection is small, and as a result HIV cannot be detected by standard PCR or culture techniques. In contrast, if the newborn was infected *in utero*, viral replication has proceeded for a period of time, producing a higher level of peripheral viremia, and virus detection is possible. Investigators have also found integrated proviral DNA in a subset of infected abortuses, suggesting fetal infection (2). Current estimates are that approximately one-third to one-half of HIV-infected infants acquire their virus while *in utero*. Most *in utero* transmissions are thought to occur late in gestation (3).

The known time of infantile infection offers an unusual opportunity to intervene therapeutically. Adult studies have shown that shortly after initiation of an HIV infection the virus disseminates rapidly to multiple organs, particularly lymph nodes (4). A relatively

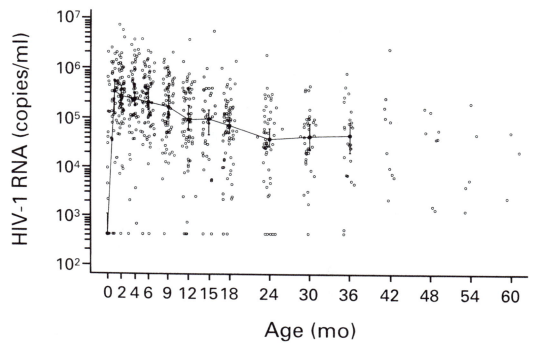

FIG. 3.1. Human immunodeficiency virus RNA concentrations (copy number per milliliter) for 106 HIV-infected children monitored sequentially from birth. The line connects the median value for individual data points; the vertical bars represent the 95% confidence intervals. (From Shearer WT, Quinn TC, LaRussa P, et al. Viral load and disease progression in infants infected with human immunodeficiency virus type 1: Women and Infants Transmission Study Group. *N Engl J Med* 1997;336:1337–1342, with permission.)

high-level viremia follows, as evidenced by detection of large amounts of viral RNA and p24 antigen in serum and plasma (p24 is a protein component of the virus capsid). The adult immune response usually controls this viremia within a matter of weeks, and a period of relatively low viral replication associated with no clinical abnormalities ensues, which may last years (5). Using quantitative RNA PCR, infants have been demonstrated to have higher early virus loads and a slower decline to a plateau level (6) (Fig. 3.1). Evidence is mounting that the immune system of children may not be as effective in controlling virus replication as that of adults, in that few or no cytotoxic T cells may be generated (7) and viral load does not fall to the same degree seen in adults (6,8). Therefore there may be a particular niche for early antiviral therapy in children, as an attempt to limit vi-

ral dissemination while the immune response matures.

EPIDEMIOLOGY

Most pediatric HIV disease has been the result of vertical transmission. There are some pockets of horizontal transmission, such as boys with hemophilia and Romanian children given neonatal blood injections, but they are exceptions to the global rule. Pediatric HIV infection is most prevalent where more women are infected.

As of fall 1999, the United Nations AIDS Program estimated that 34.3 million people were infected with HIV, of whom 15.7 million were women and 1.3 million were children younger than 15 years of age. Infection rates vary tremendously, from a country like Australia where only 550 women and fewer than

100 children are thought to be HIV infected (roughly 0.14%), to KwaZulu Natal Province in South Africa, where almost 30% of pregnant women are HIV infected (9). The highest prevalence rates among women are currently in central and southern Africa, but there are other problem areas (e.g., Southeast Asia) and countries (e.g., India) where the epidemic is growing at an explosive rate.

In addition to variations in the prevalence of HIV infection, there are also variations in vertical transmission rates. These rates reflect many factors, most importantly the availability of antiretroviral therapy to use as perinatal prophylaxis. Transmission rates in Africa are in the range of 25% to 40%, but in the United States and Europe rates as low as 2% to 4% have been reported (Pediatric AIDS Clinical Trials Group Study 247 Team, *personal communication,* 2000). These differences reflect disparities in the ability to identify infected women and in the availability of prophylactic antiviral regimens. Where HIV-infected pregnant women are not identified, targeted prophylaxis does not work as a strategy.

The state of the epidemic among women of child-bearing age is an important predictor of the degree to which vertical transmission of HIV is a problem. In countries like the United States and European nations there is a low prevalence in women, less than 3 per 1,000. However, women have been experiencing a rapid rise in HIV infection rate, especially in areas such as the southeastern United States (10). As a consequence, public policies and attention need to be focused on women in order to reduce the number of infected infants. Interventional efforts have focused on education, improving access to condoms, and attempting to give women social permission to refuse intercourse when condoms are not used. Sexually transmitted disease (STD) prevention and treatment are important, but the same steps that prevent heterosexual HIV transmission also prevent most STDs.

In the developed world, intravenous drug use is also a significant factor in the epidemiology of women and HIV, both because of drug use by women and because many HIV-infected male contacts acquired HIV through shared needles and intravenous drug injection.

NATURAL HISTORY

Pediatric HIV disease is more aggressive than that seen in adults. The median life expectancy of a child born in the United States with vertically acquired HIV infection is about 8 years. Children are more likely to have CNS disease, to have lethal *Pneumocystis carinii* pneumonia (PCP), and to have impaired growth (11).

The rate of progression for pediatric HIV disease has a biphasic distribution (12). Roughly one fourth of children develop acquired immunodeficiency syndrome (AIDS) within the first year of life; the rest have a slower progression, with the median time to AIDS being longer than 5 years, not dissimilar to the interval seen in adults with HIV infection (13). The "rapid progressor" group typically has a high risk for encephalopathy, experiences rapid depletion of CD4+ T lymphocytes, and has more numerous opportunistic infections. The subgroup of children with rapid progression is more likely to have been infected *in utero* (14) and more likely to have a high proviral DNA copy number and a high proportion of CD4+ cells infected, compared with the slow progressor group (14a). The slow progressor group is thought to have been more frequently infected peripartum. The infants infected *in utero* have higher early RNA copy numbers and consequently more rapid disease progression (6). There is, however, considerable overlap in HIV RNA concentrations between children with rapid versus slow progression when early viral loads are evaluated, making viral load a relatively poor prognostic indicator.

The rapid progression seen in some HIV-infected infants may be the result of an inadequate immune response. Katherine Luzuriaga and John Sullivan, while investigating the early T-cell response to HIV, demonstrated that HIV-infected infants have almost no detectable HIV-specific cytolytic T cells (15). In contrast, an adult cytolytic response to HIV is easily demonstrable, particularly early in primary infection (16). Therefore there is a need for interventions that can either contain the virus or boost the child's immune response.

The most typical early manifestations of HIV in infants are oral candidiasis, hepatomegaly, splenomegaly, generalized lymphadenopathy, and a subtle growth delay (17,18). In the typical growth pattern, HIV-infected infants gain weight and length more slowly than do control children (uninfected infants born to HIV-infected women). The HIV effects are seen equally on height and weight, so the infected children are smaller than normal but have normal body proportions, a pattern consistent with growth delay (Fig. 3.2). This is in contrast to the adult wasting syndrome, wherein patients become lean

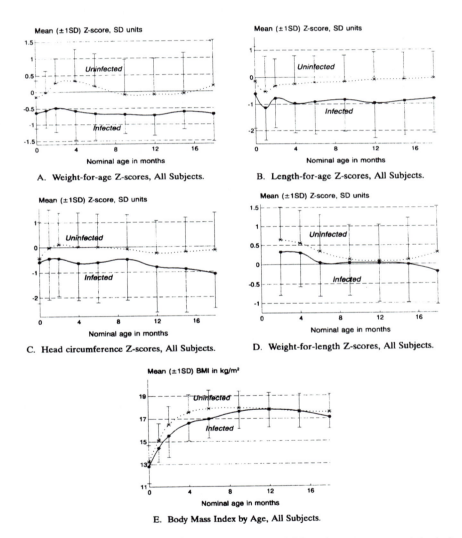

FIG. 3.2. Calculated anthropomorphic measurements on children born to women infected with the human immunodeficiency virus, divided as to whether or not the infant was HIV infected. (From Moye J Jr, Rich KC, Kalish LA, et al. Natural history of somatic growth in infants born to women infected by human immunodeficiency virus. *J Pediatr* 1996;128:58–69, with permission.)

(attain a low weight-for-height). Although some children do become lean late in the course of their disease, loss of lean body mass is a rare early manifestation of HIV disease in children. Growth problems in early HIV disease are almost impossible to diagnose in the individual child and are better seen in aggregate data from groups of children who are infected, compared with those who are simply exposed and not infected.

The most common AIDS-defining opportunistic infection in North America and Europe is *Pneumocystis carinii* pneumonia (PCP) (Fig. 3.3). This infection manifests with fever, tachypnea (usually effortless), hypoxemia, hypocarbia, and sometimes cough. The chest radiograph often shows minimal evidence of disease, with alveolar infiltrates being the most typical abnormality. Compared with adult PCP, the onset is more abrupt, the progression to severe hypoxemia more rapid, and the disease can occur when CD4 counts are still in the normal range. PCP is also more lethal in children. The most effective treatment is prevention, so most HIV-infected children are given trimethoprim-sulfamethoxasole (TMP/SMX) prophylaxis

for their first year of life regardless of their CD4 count (Table 3.1).

Fungal infections are relatively common in HIV-infected children. The most frequent problems are *Candida albicans,* dermatophytes, and histoplasmosis. *Candida* manifests as oral thrush, with white plaques on the tongue and buccal mucosa. Severe oral thrush can affect the gingival mucosa. In some cases, the candidal tongue lesions can appear as glossitis, with hyperemic loss of papillae, rather than as plaques. *Candida* esophagitis is the most common severe form of the disease. The child typically presents with retrosternal pain made worse by swallowing. Some, but not all, cases are associated with oral thrush.

Bacterial infections are frequent in HIV-infected children. The most severe problems are with polysaccharide-encapsulated bacteria (*Streptococcus pneumoniae, Neisseria meningitidis*), and infected children can have unusually frequent bouts of acute otitis media and sinusitis. Invasive bacterial diseases such as meningitis and pneumonia are also more common in HIV-infected children.

Mycobacterial infections can be a profound problem for end-stage HIV patients. The most

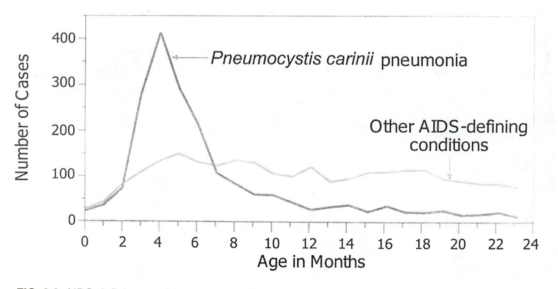

FIG. 3.3 AIDS-defining conditions by age at diagnosis for perinatally-acquired AIDS cases reported through 1997, United States. (Courtesy of the Centers for Disease Control and Prevention.)

TABLE 3.1. *Suggested management for the infant born to an HIV-infected mother*

Age	Management
Birth	CBC
	HIV DNA PCR (peripheral blood, not cord blood)
	Start PO zidovudine (AZT, ZDV), 2 mg/kg/dose q6h or 2.6 mg/kg/dose q8h, within 8–12 h after birth. If can't take PO medications within 24 h, give IV ZDV (1.5 mg/kg/dose IV q6h) until oral medications are tolerated)
2–3 wk	CBC
	HIV DNA PCR (particularly if not done at birth)
6 wk	CBC
	HIV DNA PCR
	Discontinue ZDV (if HIV DNA PCR is negative)
	Start PO TMP/SMX 75 mg/m^2/dose of TMP, b.i.d. on Mondays, Tuesdays, and Wednesdays[a]
4 mo	CBC and lymphocyte subsets
	HIV DNA PCR[b]
12 mo	HIV antibody testing if uninfected or of indeterminate status
18 mo	HIV antibody testing if uninfected or of indeterminate status

CBC, complete blood co~~~~~ an immunodeficiency virus; PCR, polymerase chain reaction; TMP/SMX, trimethoprim-sulfame~~~~

[a]Continue T~~~ age if child is infected or remains of indeterminate status; discontinue if uninfe~~~

~~~mo *and* one at ≥4 mo of age), lymphocyte subsets are normal for ~~~f HIV infection, and child is not breast-feeding, child is considered ~~~d and no further immunologic monitoring is necessary. HIV anti-~~~repeated as necessary to document loss of passive maternal an-tibo~~~

[c]Tw~~~ ~~~oof of HIV infection. The TMP/SMX for PCP prophylaxis should be con~~~ ~~~naged according to the CDC guidelines, based on the child's CD4 T-~~~

common ~~~ than might be expected. Primary infections
terium aviu~ ~~~ith herpes simplex virus (HSV) and varicella-
avium compl~ ~~~ster virus (VZV) are generally well con-
fects children ~ ~~~ed (20). However, recurrent zoster (shin-
phocytes per m~ ~~~is a characteristic disease of children with
manifests with fe~ ~~~ CD4+ cell numbers. Some children
pancytopenia), an~ ~~~d-stage HIV disease develop a chronic
vere enough that p~ ~~~ of VZV disease, with painful, thick,
macrolides (most fre~ lichenified lesions in multiple sites.
warranted once a chil~ ~~~s be- Cryptosporidiosis can be severe in HIV-in-
low 75 to 100 cells per ~~~ fected children. This waterborne parasite pro-

In parts of the world w~ere the bacille Cal-duces profound watery diarrhea that responds
mette-Guérin (BCG) vaccine is used to pre-poorly to therapy. It can last for months, is of-
vent severe tuberculosis, infants with HIV ten associated with wasting, and seems best
and disseminated BCG infection have been controlled by optimizing antiretroviral ther-
reported (19). Knowing a child's HIV status apy. The standard treatment includes paro-
before BCG use would be useful, although in momycin and azithromycin. Efficacy is less
many countries the relative risk of BCG vac-than optimal (21).
cination is believed to be lower than the risk
from exposure to wild-type tuberculosis.

Viral infections controlled by the cell-medi- **PERINATAL TRANSMISSION**
ated immune response are a problem for HIV-
infected children, although to a lesser degree HIV infections among infants and preado-
lescent children result almost exclusively

from transmission from an infected mother to her child. Consequently, in the United States, more than 90% of HIV-infected children have an infected mother. Children can also be infected through the receipt of blood or blood products if blood is not tested for the presence of HIV. However, this has become a rare event with the routine testing of blood. Rarely, children are infected through sexual abuse or close contact with another infected individual, via exchange of blood or bloody secretions.

The mechanism of maternal-child transmission is of considerable interest. Transmission occurs *in utero*, intrapartum by exposure to maternal blood and secretions, and postpartum with breast-feeding (22,23). In the absence of breast-feeding, most transmission probably occurs late in gestation or intrapartum (24). This conclusion is supported by a number of observations. First, infected infants rarely have clinical or laboratory evidence of disease at birth, suggesting that the infection was recently acquired. In addition, at least two thirds of infants who are ultimately shown to be infected do not have detectable HIV in the blood during the first few days of life. These infants develop detectable virus by 4 to 8 weeks of age, suggesting that transmission occurred in the peripartum period. Infection is probably acquired with exposure to blood or bloody secretions in the birth canal; this accounts for the higher transmission rates observed with prolonged rupture of the membranes, with vaginal delivery, and in the firstborn of twins (25–27). Alternatively, small amounts of maternal blood may enter the child's circulation through the placenta during labor. Infants with detectable virus in the peripheral blood in the first 48 hours of life are presumed to have *in utero* acquisition of infection (28).

It has been suggested that some perinatally infected infants spontaneously clear their infection (29). However, when maternal and infant viral sequences have been compared, they are unrelated, suggesting a laboratory error or mixing of blood samples (30). Spontaneous resolution of infection must be an extremely rare event if it occurs at all.

Risk Factors for Maternal-Child Transmission

In the absence of preventive therapy with zidovudine (ZDV), the risk of infection for a non–breast-fed infant born to an infected mother is approximately 25%. However the infection rate varies widely (from 15% to 50%) in different studies and geographic regions (22). Transmission by breast-feeding is well documented, and the additional risk of infection to an infant with breast-feeding is estimated to be 3.2% per year of breast-feeding (31). In developed countries, it is recommended that HIV-infected mothers not breast-feed. However, in developing countries, the risk of breast-feeding needs to be balanced against its established benefit in preventing gastroenteritis and malnutrition in young infants. Therefore, in countries with high infant mortality rates, recommendations regarding breast-feeding must be made locally.

A number of risk factors for maternal-child transmission have been identified (32–36) (Table 3.2). It is likely that variability in these factors accounts for the broad range of transmission rates seen in various studies. Women with advanced HIV infection, as reflected by a high viral load and a low CD4 count, have an increased transmission rate. However, transmission occurs among women with all levels of viral load, and there is no viral load threshold below which transmission does not occur (37). Therefore, in individual cases, the mother's viral load (or CD4 count) has little ability to pre-

TABLE 3.2. *Maternal risk factors for vertical transmission of HIV*

Failure to receive zidovudine preventive therapy
Breast-feeding
Maternal AIDS or advanced HIV infection (decreased CD4+ T-lymphocyte count, high plasma viral load)
Prolonged rupture of membranes
Vaginal delivery
Prematurity or low birth weight
Placental inflammation or chorioamnionitis
Firstborn of twins
Maternal intravenous drug use
Bloody amniotic fluid

AIDS, acquired immune deficiency syndrome; HIV, human immunodeficiency virus.

dict her risk of transmission. Events occurring at delivery, such as prolonged rupture of membranes and preterm delivery, are associated with an increased risk of intrapartum transmission. Likewise, maternal antiretroviral therapy may have a greater protective effect on intrapartum transmission than on *in utero* transmission (38).

Most studies defining risk factors for mother-child transmission of HIV were performed before the routine use of ZDV to prevent transmission. In the presence of preventive therapy, many risk factors lose their importance, including maternal viral load and CD4 count (39). In a study of a non–breast-feeding population in which most women and infants received preventive ZDV, histologic chorioamnionitis was the only independent risk factor for transmission (40).

Prevention of Maternal-Child Transmission

In 1994, the Pediatric AIDS Clinical Trials Group (PACTG) protocol 076 study demonstrated that ZDV can dramatically reduce the rate of maternal-child transmission of HIV. In this placebo-controlled study, ZDV was administered to HIV-infected women during the second and third trimesters of pregnancy, by infusion during labor, and orally to the infant for 6 weeks after birth. This regimen decreased the transmission rate by two thirds, from 22.6% to 7.6% (39,41). As a result of this study, in 1994, the U.S. Public Health Service recommended administration of ZDV to all HIV-infected pregnant women and their infants (42,43). Pregnant women should receive ZDV during the second and third trimester (100 mg orally, five times daily), with an intravenous infusion during active labor until delivery (2 mg per kilogram loading dose over 1 hour, then 1 mg per kilogram per hour until delivery). Their infants should receive 6 weeks of oral therapy (2 mg per kilogram per dose every 6 hours, beginning within 8 to 12 hours after birth) (Table 3.1). If the infant cannot tolerate oral ZDV, the intravenous dose is 1.5 mg per kilogram every 6 hours. Although the PACTG 076 study administered ZDV five times a day to the mother and

four times a day to the infant; many authorities now recommend ZDV 200 mg orally three times a day for the mother and 2.6 to 3 mg per kilogram orally three times a day for the infant. Retrospective data suggest that this strategy still offers some benefit if initiated at the onset of labor or even if administered only to the newborn immediately after delivery (44). Therefore, for women who are not identified as being HIV infected until late in pregnancy or at the time of delivery, it is reasonable to initiate the intervention at that time.

For this intervention to be successful, pregnant women should be offered HIV antibody testing early in pregnancy so that infected women are identified (45). Women who admit to high-risk behavior during pregnancy should be retested during the third trimester even if previously seronegative. Women not previously tested should be tested when they present in labor, because initiation of ZDV therapy at that time may still provide benefit (44).

The PACTG 076 regimen has been well accepted in the United States and Europe. In the United States, it is estimated that 87% of HIV-infected pregnant women are now identified during pregnancy and that more than 65% receive preventive treatment with ZDV (46). This has resulted in a 43% reduction in the number of HIV-infected children born in the United States between 1992 and 1996 (47). The transmission rate in the United States and Europe is currently estimated to be 6% or less. Follow-up of uninfected children in the PACTG 076 study has not shown any long-term adverse effects of *in utero* exposure to ZDV (48).

However, in much of the developing world, the PACTG 076 regimen is impractical because of its high cost and complexity. Many women do not receive prenatal care until late in pregnancy, and they frequently deliver outside of the hospital, making the intrapartum infusion of ZDV impossible. The World Health Organization estimates that 32% of pregnant women in the world receive no prenatal care and 43% deliver unattended (49). In addition, the cost of ZDV in the PACTG 076 regimen (about $800) is prohibitive in many developing countries. In an attempt to define a more practical intervention, short-course modifications of the PACTG 076 regimen have been evaluated. In a study in Thailand, pregnant women received oral ZDV (300 mg twice daily) starting at 36 weeks of gestation, with oral ZDV (300 mg every 3 hours) continued during labor. No ZDV was given to the infants, and the women did not breast-feed. In this placebo-controlled study, there was a 50% reduction in the rate of transmission, from 18.9% to 9.4% (50). In two studies of breast-feeding women in Africa, this strategy was somewhat less effective, with reductions in transmission rate of 38% and 37% (51,52). In one of these studies, women received ZDV for 1 week postpartum in an attempt to prevent transmission through breast-feeding, with no apparent benefit (52). Means to further prevent transmission by breast-feeding are urgently needed and are under study. The regimen used in the Thailand study is likely to become the standard of care in many developing countries, although the need for HIV testing and the cost of ZDV ($50) remain barriers to implementation. The results of these trials support the conclusion that most mother-to-child transmission occurs late in pregnancy or at the time of delivery. Recently, a study in Africa demonstrated that a single dose of nevirapine administered to the mother during labor and to the infant following delivery was effective in substantially reducing the transmission rate (52a). Updated guidelines for preventing mother-to-child transmission of HIV are available (52b).

A number of uncontrolled studies suggest that elective cesarean section, when performed before the onset of active labor, reduces the transmission rate. In a large meta-analysis of 15 prospective cohort studies, elective cesarean section was associated with a lower transmission rate even among women who received antiretroviral therapy; women who received both interventions had a transmission rate of 2% (27). Preliminary results from a randomized, prospective study conducted in Europe suggest a 71% reduction in transmission rate with elective cesarean section (from 10.2% to 3.4%) (53). However, the morbidity of cesarean section in HIV-infected women remains to be adequately defined. In addition, it is not known whether cesarean section provides additional benefit for women who are receiving highly active antiretroviral therapy and who have an extremely low or undetectable HIV viral load, a group at low risk for transmission. The potential benefits and risks of cesarean section should be discussed with HIV-infected pregnant women before delivery.

Interventions at delivery that limit exposure of the infant to maternal blood, such as cleansing of the birth canal, have not been shown to substantially reduce the transmission rate (54). Such simple and inexpensive interventions, if of even limited efficacy, would be very important on a global scale and need further study.

Management of the HIV-Exposed Infant

HIV-infected infants rarely have clinical evidence of disease at birth, and their lymphocyte subset values are usually normal for age. In addition, all infants born to HIV-infected mothers are HIV-seropositive themselves, owing to the presence of maternal transplacental antibody. Therefore, HIV infection in the infant is diagnosed by detecting virus in peripheral blood through culture or DNA PCR testing. HIV DNA PCR is usually the preferred test, because it is readily available, both specific and sensitive, and relatively inexpensive (40). Fewer than one half of infants who are ultimately shown to be infected have detectable HIV in the peripheral blood at birth (55). However, almost all test positive by 3 to 4 months of age. HIV-exposed infants should have testing performed on peripheral blood (not cord blood) before discharge from the nursery, at 1 to 2 months, and at 4 months of age. A positive test should be repeated as soon as possible. HIV infection is confirmed if the child has two positive virologic test results from separate blood draws. A child who is not breast-fed can be considered to be free of infection after two negative virologic test results if one of these was obtained after 1 month of age and the second after 4 months of age. Absence of infection can be confirmed by a negative HIV antibody test, reflecting loss of maternal antibody; this frequently occurs after 12 months of age (40).

Because anemia and neutropenia are the major toxicities seen with ZDV and TMP/SMX, the infant should be evaluated with complete blood counts as suggested in Table 3.1.

All HIV-exposed infants should receive 6 weeks of ZDV therapy according to PACTG 076 regimen described previously. In developed countries, infants of HIV-infected mothers should not breast-feed. In developing countries, the risks and benefits of breast-feeding should be considered locally. At 6 weeks of age, prophylaxis for PCP with TMP/SMX is started; it is discontinued once the child is shown to be noninfected (see later discussion).

DIAGNOSTIC TESTS

The detection of HIV infection in a child (or adult) older than 15 months is a straightforward process, because antibody detection by enzyme-linked immunosorbent assay (ELISA) and Western blot is both sensitive and specific (56). In younger children, however, the presence of transplacentally acquired maternal antibodies complicates the evaluation. Antibody assays can determine whether an infant was exposed to a risk of HIV *in utero*, but it cannot separate the "at risk" infant from the infected one. In most cases the critical determination of infection status is made by one of several strategies: detection of the virus in culture, detection of virus-specific proteins in serum (usually the major capsid protein, p24), or detection of virus-specific genetic sequences through the use PCR assays (or equivalents). These techniques vary in cost, in sensitivity, and in the time it takes to obtain a result (Tables 3.3 and 3.4).

Because infants exposed to HIV *in utero* are antibody positive but have indeterminate HIV infection status, they have been given a specific classification by the Centers for Disease Control and Prevention (CDC), category E (for "exposed") (57). In the previous terminology, children of indeterminate status were placed in category P-0, as opposed to infected children with mild symptoms of HIV disease (P-1) and children with more serious manifestations (P-2).

TABLE 3.3. *Assays to detect HIV*

Assay	Sensitivity (0 to +++)	Cost ($ to $$$)	Time	Advantages	Disadvantages
Antibody detection (ELISA/ Western blot)	+++	$	Hours	Fast, sensitive Inexpensive Suitable for screening	Transplacentally acquired maternal antibodies produce false-positive results in infants
P24 antigen detection	+	$	Hours	Fast Inexpensive Quantitative	Poor sensitivity False-positive results in the first week of life
Immune complex dissociated p24 detection	++	$	Hours	Fast Inexpensive More sensitive than p24 Quantitative	Only moderately sensitive Reproducibility difficult False-positive results in the first week of life
HIV culture	+++	$$$	Weeks	Sensitive Very specific Virus available for genotypic and phenotypic analyses (like antiviral sensitivity)	Requires weeks to complete Requires isolation facility, highly trained personnel Limited availability (mostly research laboratories) Quantitation, although possible, is very difficult and time-consuming
HIV PCR	+++	$$	Days	As sensitive as culture Faster and cheaper than culture Quantitative	False-positive results if not done in a very clean facility No data about virus phenotype Limited information about antiviral sensitivity

ELISA, enzyme-linked immunosorbent assay; HIV, human immunodeficiency virus; PCR, polymerase chain reaction.

TABLE 3.4. *Schema for diagnostic evaluation of children at risk for HIV infection*

Age at initial presentation	Stage of evaluation	Test	Schedule (mo)	Comments
<2 wk	Maternal HIV status unknown	HIV ELISA/Western blot (on mother or infant)	Immediate	If positive, warrants further evaluation per directions below
	Mother HIV infected	HIV PCR and/or culture	Birth, 1–2, 4–6	PCR and culture are roughly equal in sensitivity. Two negative PCRs at 2 mo and at 4–6 mo are good evidence the child is not infected. Start PCP prophylaxis after 6 wk of age pending results. Consider doing two early PCRs (1 and 2 mo) as well as 6 mo.
2 wk to 6 mo	Maternal HIV status unknown	HIV ELISA/Western blot on mother or infant	Immediate	If positive, proceed to next step to determine whether the child is infected in addition to being at risk for HIV.
	Mother HIV infected	HIV PCR and/or culture	Initial visit, 4–6 mo	Consider doing two PCR assays 4 wk apart, then one at >6 mo.
6—15 mo	Maternal HIV status unknown	HIV ELISA/Western blot on mother and infant	Immediate	If ELISA/Western blot on either positive, proceed to next step
	Mother HIV infected	HIV ELISA/Western blot and PCR or culture	ELISA/Western blot and PCR/culture once immediately; repeat ELISA every 3 mo until negative	ELISA assay in children who are going to serorevert to negative will do so at a median of 10 mo of age. Perform PCR or HIV culture initially to determine whether child might need PCP prophylaxis or antiretroviral treatment. If ELISA/Western blot does not serorevert to negative by 15–18 mo, child is HIV infected.
>15 mo	All at risk children	HIV ELISA/Western blot	Once as a screen, twice if confirmation needed	ELISA/Western blot will suffice at >15 mo, because a positive assay means the child is HIV infected. To avoid laboratory errors in a high-risk child, a repeat assay may be worthwhile regardless of first assay's result.

ELISA, enzyme-linked immunosorbent assay; HIV, human immunodeficiency virus; PCP, *Pneumocystis carinii* pneumonia; PCR, polymerase chain reaction.

Antibody Tests

The validity of antibody-based HIV assays depends on the fact that adults and children make specific anti-HIV antibodies only when they are HIV infected. However, immunoglobulin G (IgG) molecules are transferred across the placenta from mother to fetus during pregnancy, so a newborn child has most of the IgG antibody types the mother possessed at the time of delivery. These antibodies can be detected by a variety of techniques. However, it is generally not possible to know whether the antibodies found in an infant younger than 15 months old were endogenously produced in response to infection or were conveyed across the placenta from the mother.

The most widely used antibody detection technique is the ELISA. ELISA assays are very sensitive (greater than 99%), and rarely yield false-positive tests after the first 15 months of life (56). Given the importance of accurately knowing HIV status, in order to ensure that the ELISA is not falsely positive, the results are confirmed using a second category of antibody detection assays, most commonly a Western blot, which identifies antibody to specific viral proteins. A few children have a negative ELISA test and persistently indeterminate Western blot results, with one or more bands that do not meet the diagnostic criteria for positive. If at low risk, these patients are almost certainly not infected (58). If the child has clinical symptoms suggesting HIV infection, an indeterminate Western blot may indicate transition to positive status.

Antigen Detection

HIV antigen detection is relatively inexpensive and rapid, but it is insensitive. The antigen most commonly assayed is p24, one of the structural protein components of the virus capsid. P24 is among the most conserved HIV proteins among strains, varying relatively little from isolate to isolate, which makes it suitable for a diagnostic assay. As HIV replicates, p24 is released from the cells into the surrounding extracellular milieu. The standard detection system is an ELISA assay, which uses anti-p24 antibody adsorbed to a plastic tray. If free p24 antigen is present in the serum, it becomes bound to the antibody and is then detected with the use of another anti-p24 antibody.

Unfortunately, many patients have enough antibody against p24 to complex the protein and limit p24 binding to the antibody in the ELISA tray. In order to improve the rate of detection, techniques have been developed to break up the p24-containing immune complexes (59). The resulting method, called immune complex–dissociated p24 (ICD-p24) detection, is more sensitive than the normal p24 assay, although not the equal of HIV culture or gene detection by PCR. The overall sensitivity of ICD-p24 detection is 81% in children aged 6 weeks to 13 years (59). Because this test is not as sensitive as HIV detection by PCR, it is generally considered to be a second-tier diagnostic assay.

HIV Culture

The "gold standard" for determination of HIV infection status is culture. HIV culture is a very accurate test with an extremely low rate of false-positive results (60). Its sensitivity is excellent, approximating that of PCR. Both tests are unable to detect virus in approximately 50% of infected newborns (younger than 7 days old). The sensitivity is low in patients at that age because virus transmission often occurs perinatally and the amount of virus is below the level of detection (61). Beyond the

4 to 6 weeks of life, the largest shortcomings of HIV culture are the need for an expensive isolation facility (for the protection of laboratory staff), the length of time until culture becomes positive (as long as 3 to 4 weeks), and the expense of the technicians and reagents. Its virtues include the abilities to perform quantitative assays, to determine certain *in vitro* properties of the virus that correlate with prognosis, and to obtain large amounts of virus for molecular and antiviral resistance studies.

Polymerase Chain Reaction

PCR assays are a laboratory means to amplify a specific gene. In the context of HIV detection, this allows the use of defined primers to find HIV-specific DNA or RNA sequences. Although both RNA and DNA PCR assays can be used to determine infection status, if the only question is whether an infant is infected, the DNA PCR is more often used. DNA PCR detects proviral DNA within the chromosomes of infected mononuclear cells (62).

The sensitivity of DNA PCR is essentially the same as that of HIV culture and is greater than 95% in children after the first month of life (56). The major concern with PCR is false-positive results, because the assay is so sensitive that even a small amount of contamination can produce a positive test result (61). To protect against this problem, most PCR laboratories go to great lengths to isolate their sample preparation areas, and new methods have been developed that begin by digesting DNA that has been synthesized within the lab. These methods eliminate PCR product as a detectable contaminant.

Strategies for Virus Detection

When an infant younger than 18 months of age is seen for the first time and HIV infection is considered a possibility, the initial task is to determine whether the child is at risk for infection. Performing an HIV ELISA and confirmatory Western blot on the mother or infant can make this determination. If either the child or the mother has a positive antibody test, further evaluations should be performed.

Status of infection cannot be established by an antibody-only approach until the infant is more than 18 months old unless the child has an AIDS-defining clinical event. The latter possibility is too great, and the widespread availability of PCR makes an antibody-based diagnostic approach obsolete.

Although there are no absolute guidelines for diagnostic strategies, most HIV-exposed children should have a PCR or culture performed as soon as possible after birth. A positive assay on a sample obtained within the first 7 days of life is thought to be a poor prognostic sign because it appears to indicate *in utero* infection and perhaps a larger virus inoculum. Some investigators believe infections detected early warrant more aggressive antiretroviral therapy. Given the poor sensitivity of assays in the first weeks of life, a second culture or PCR should be obtained at 2 to 4 weeks of age. Most physicians retest at 2 to 4 months, and if the previous results are negative a final PCR should be obtained at 4 to 5 months or older. Two negative cultures or PCR assays, including at least one at age 4 months or older, is considered adequate evidence that a child is not infected.

For those children who present at age 18 months or older, the only necessary diagnostic test is an HIV ELISA and Western blot. If the child has symptoms consistent with HIV and a negative ELISA result, quantitative immunoglobulin concentrations should be obtained to be certain that the child is not hypogammaglobulinemic and DNA or RNA PCP. In addition, a small proportion of HIV-infected children, particularly those severely affected by the virus, are ELISA positive and Western blot negative (63). In those instances where antibody assays are suspected of being misleading, PCR can be performed.

TREATMENT

Pediatric HIV infection is a difficult condition to manage. The disease is complex, manifests as more than simple immunosuppression, and occurs in a population in which families are often ill-equipped to administer medications according to complex schedules. The best approach for patient care is to use a multidiscipli-nary team that is able to optimize medical management, minimize psychosocial problems, improve nutrition, and monitor developmental progress. The medical issues are the most straightforward aspect of pediatric HIV care; the psychosocial problems, which have enormous effect, are beyond the scope of this text.

Staging the Disease

The CDC developed a staging scheme for HIV disease that includes both clinical and immunologic components (57) (Table 3.5). In addition, many physicians rely on HIV RNA concentrations as an additional element for determining when to start or change antiretroviral regimens.

There are four levels of clinical disease in the CDC's classification scheme for pediatric HIV disease. In advancing level of severity, they are levels N, A, B, and C. The N stands for *nonsymptomatic*, whereas the A, B, and C represent incremental increases in clinical severity, roughly correlated with prognosis.

The CDC's immunologic categories are designed to compensate for the normal decrease of CD4+ cell numbers as children grow. Absolute CD4 counts are normally highest in the first few months of life, then decline gradually (64). The decrease continues in healthy, noninfected children until 5 to 6 years of age. In contrast to the absolute CD4 count, the percentage of CD4+ lymphocytes (as a percentage of all circulating lymphocytes) stabilizes more quickly, between 1 and 2 years old. Either the absolute count or the percentage can be used as a marker of prognosis, and in general as a marker of cumulative immunologic damage. A low CD4 count or percentage is evidence of damage.

The most short-term marker of disease activity is measurement of HIV RNA copy numbers in plasma by PCR technology. Quantitative RNA assays reflect the level of replicative activity of the virus and therefore, indirectly, the rate at which damage is occurring. In general, immediately after infection there is a burst of viral replication that peaks at 100,000 (5 logs) to more than 1,000,000 (6 logs) RNA copies per milliliter. In an HIV-infected adult, the im-

TABLE 3.5. *Centers for Disease Control and Prevention 1994 revised classification system for human immunodeficiency virus infection in children younger than 13 years of age*

Immunologic category (evidence of suppression)	CD4+ T lymphocytes based on age		Clinical category (signs/symptoms)[a]			
	cells/μL	%	N (none)	A (mild)	B (moderate)	C (severe)
1 (none)			N1	A1	B1	C1
<12 mo	≥1,500	≥25				
1–5 y	≥1,000	≥25				
6–12 y	≥500	≥25				
2 (moderate)			N2	A2	B2	C2
<12 mo	750–1,499	15–24				
1–5 y	500–999	15–24				
6–12 y	200–499	15–24				
3 (severe)			N3	A3	B3	C3
<12 mo	<750	<15				
1–5 y	<500	<15				
6–12 y	<200	<15				

[a]Category N (not symptomatic).

Category A (mildly symptomatic) = Two or more of the following conditions, but none from Category B: lymphadenopathy, hepatomegaly, splenomegaly, dermatitis, parotitis, recurrent or persistent upper respiratory infections or otitis media.

Category B (moderately symptomatic) = Moderate symptoms attributed to HIV: anemia, neutropenia, thrombocytopenia; bacterial disease—single episode (meningitis, sepsis, pneumonia); persistent candidiasis; cardiomyopathy; CMV infection (onset before 1 mo of age); diarrhea (recurrent or chronic); hepatitis; herpes simplex stomatitis; herpes simplex disease before 1 mo of age (bronchitis, pneumonitis, esophagitis); herpes zoster; leiomyosarcoma; lymphocytic interstitial pneumonitis; nephropathy; nocardiosis; persistent fever; toxoplasmosis (onset before 1 mo of age); disseminated varicella.

Category C (severely symptomatic) = Severe illnesses attributed to HIV: multiple serious bacterial infections; esophageal or pulmonary candidiasis; disseminated cryptococcosis; disseminated coccidioidomycosis; cryptosporidiosis; Isosporiasis; CMV disease (onset after 1 mo of age); encephalopathy; persistent or severe herpes simplex infection; histoplasmosis; Kaposi's sarcoma; lymphoma; extrapulmonary tuberculosis; disseminated nontuberculous mycobacterial infection; *Pneumocystis carinii* pneumonia; progressive multifocal leukoencephalopathy; recurrent *Salmonella* septicemia; toxoplasmosis of the brain; wasting syndrome.

From the Centers for Disease Control and Prevention. 1994 Revised classification system for human immunodeficiency virus (HIV) infection in children less than 13 years of age. *MMWR Morb Mortal Wkly Rep* 1994;(RR-12):1–10, with permission.

mune response rapidly trims replication, and the RNA copy number (viral load) declines to a lower plateau. The general dogma is that this plateau, once achieved, establishes an equilibrium that can last for years (65). The higher the plateau, the sooner the patient will go on to symptomatic disease or AIDS. In children infected at birth, there is much less early virus containment, so high levels of plasma RNA are maintained longer than in adults. The differences in RNA concentration between infants with rapid progression rates and those with slower progression are statistically significant but hard to separate clinically (6).

Both CD4 count and viral load contribute prognostic information (66). In basic terms, the CD4 count is a marker of cumulative progression, and the RNA copy number an indicator of progression rate at a single point in time. The RNA copy number can change rapidly in response to therapy, and there are many nuances in its interpretation (67). Interpreting the extremes is relatively easy: patients with RNA values higher than 100,000 have a high risk of disease progression, particularly if they also have a low CD4 count; patients with viral loads lower than 1,000 copies per milliliter have very little likelihood of serious new clinical events, unless they have an extremely low CD4 count (68).

When patients are treated with highly active antiretroviral therapy (often referred to as "HAART" or "triple therapy," given the most common pattern—two nucleoside reverse transcriptase inhibitors and one protease inhibitor), their viral load may drop below the level of detectability. Depending on the assay used, this limit may be 400, 50, 20, or even fewer copies per milliliter. For patients receiving HAART, the lower the RNA value, the more durable the viral suppression.

Controversy remains regarding the use of RNA in management with antiretroviral drugs. If HAART is started and the child's virus load reaches undetectable levels, an issue arises if and when the virus becomes detectable again. Should the patient's therapeutic regimen be switched immediately? As discussed later, with the currently available drugs, any given patient probably has only two effective therapeutic strategies. After that, the odds of long-term virus suppression become extremely small. Therefore, the decision to switch from the first antiretroviral regimen to a second should not be made lightly. Clinical trials have not yet resolved whether it is better to make the change while the patient's virus load is still low but detectable (which gives a higher probability of reachieving undetectable status), or to wait until the old drug regimen no longer has clear therapeutic effect (i.e., a viral load greater than 50,000 RNA copies per milliliter, a falling CD4 count, or clinical progression). At this point, the options should be discussed with the patient and the patient's parents, because the data regarding antiviral strategy options are very limited.

Antiretroviral Therapy

No ideal antiretroviral drug has yet been developed. An ideal drug would be curative without side effects, and a drug that could control the virus without toxicities would be acceptable. Currently licensed drugs decrease the virus burden only moderately and have significant side effects. In the long term, optimization of therapy involves combinations of antiretroviral drugs, either attacking multiple sites in the virus life cycle or convergently inhibiting a single step. The range of drugs available for children is smaller than that for adults. In some cases the compounds are difficult to prepare as liquids or in other formulations that can be titered by size. In other cases, toxicities make it difficult to use the compounds. For example, it is very difficult to diagnose either peripheral neuropathy or the early symptoms of pancreatitis in a preverbal child, and both of these are known adverse events with some antiretroviral drugs.

Reverse Transcriptase Inhibitors

Reverse transcriptase inhibitors can be divided into two broad categories, nucleoside (NRTIs) and non-nucleoside (NNRTIs). The NRTIs are modified nucleosides that take advantage of a relatively high affinity of the virus reverse transcriptase for certain types of nucleotide modifications. Two of the commonly used NRTIs are derived from thymidine, ZDV, and stavudine (D4T). One or the other is used as a foundation for most therapeutic regimens. Because ZDV inhibits stavudine phosphorylation and thus its activation, the drugs should not be used simultaneously.

Both ZDV and D4T are available in liquid and solid preparations, and clinical trials support their use in children (69,70). They are comparable in their virologic effect, typically lowering viral load by 0.5 to 1.0 $\log_{10}$ RNA copies as monotherapy (67). The most common adverse events with ZDV in children are anemia and neutropenia. Rarely a child has a ZDV-related myopathy (71), and some children appear to develop a drug-related attention deficit problem. Nausea, headaches, and fatigue are symptoms often described in the period after initiation of ZDV, although most improve with time.

D4T is well tolerated by most children (67). There are rare instances of peripheral neuropathy, but this seems to be less common than in adults. Pancreatitis can also occur rarely.

In a pattern similar to that of the thymidine analogs, nonthymidine NRTIs, such as didanosine (ddI), lamivudine (3TC), and zalcitabine (ddC), usually are not given in combination with each other. They are, however, typically combined with ZDV or d4T.

3TC is available as a liquid or tablet. Although 3TC is a moderately potent monotherapy, resistance develops with a single point mutation at codon 184 (72). When combined with ZDV, 3TC has shown positive clinical effects on growth and prevention of disease progression end points (73). 3TC is generally well tolerated, with few adverse events. Despite early reports, pancreatitis has not proved to be a significant problem.

ddI, also known as dideoxyinosine, is acid labile and therefore must be given in combination with antacids. It may also be somewhat better absorbed on an empty stomach, although the marginal increase in absorption should be weighed against the effect on compliance of avoiding mealtimes. The pediatric suspension is usually dissolved in a liquid antacid such as Maalox, although tablets that can be dissolved in water are also available. The suspension must be kept refrigerated, and the shelf life is relatively short (approximately 4 weeks).

ddI has proved to be a potent nucleoside. Several studies have shown virologic and clinical effects that were comparable to those of combination nucleosides (e.g., PACTG study protocol 152) (74). ddI is generally well tolerated, although adverse events such as peripheral neuropathy and pancreatitis can occur. The pancreatitis is typically symptomatic, with elevations in both serum amylase and lipase. It should be noted that many HIV-infected children also have elevated serum amylase concentrations related to salivary gland inflammation, so that increased amylase concentrations should be further evaluated with a fractionated amylase assay (to separate pancreatic and salivary isoenzymes) or by confirming the abnormality with a lipase. Salivary inflammation does not generally lead to an increased serum lipase concentration, but pancreatic inflammation does.

ddC is commercially available only in capsules. Its virologic effects are similar to those of ddI, and there is a high degree of cross-resistance between the two compounds. ddC monotherapy in antiretroviral-experienced children led to improved weight gain (75). ddC has also been studied in combination with ZDV, and where it produced a mild positive effect on CD4 counts (76). The most common adverse events are peripheral neuropathy and oral ulcers.

A sixth NRTI, abacavir (ABC), has been approved and is available in both liquid and solid forms. It appears to have excellent activity when used as a first-line agent, but it may have more limited efficacy when used after other NRTIs have lost their effect. Serious hypersensitivity reactions to abacavir can occur.

Non-Nucleoside Reverse Transcriptase Inhibitors

The NNRTIs inhibit the initiation of virus transcription. Nevirapine (NVP) and efavirenz (EFZ) are licensed for pediatric use. A liquid preparation is available for NVP. NNRTI resistance develops very quickly when the drugs are used as monotherapy (77), so they are almost always used in combinations. In addition, resistance to the currently licensed NNRTIs appears to be across the category, so that switching from one NNRTI to another is of little use if the reason for the switch is clinical progression or disease (rather than side effects or compliance issues).

NVP has been evaluated in combination with NRTIs in children (78,79). It shows beneficial effects, although it probably has less potency than protease inhibitors do. Because of its long half-life, NVP is being evaluated as part of a regimen for perinatal prophylaxis in PACTG protocol 316. One dose administered orally to the pregnant woman while in labor, followed by one dose given to the infant, is an effective supplement to routine prophylactic treatment (52a). NVP will also be evaluated as a potential two-dose monotherapy in countries where a full course of ZDV prophylaxis is untenable. The two major problems with NVP are rash and hepatitis. Patients who develop a macular rash, often associated with fever, should have their NVP stopped. This early rash can progress into a life-threatening Stevens-Johnson syndrome. The incidence of rash appears to be similar to that in adults. Hepatitis occurs most frequently early during NVP administration, but it can occur at any point.

Clinical experience with EFZ in children is relatively limited. However, it appears to be an effective alternative to protease inhibitors, and it has been used effectively in combination with them (80). The drug has a very long half-life and can be administered once daily. The major side effect of EFZ has been rash, which is probably more common in children than adults. Unlike the situation with NVP, in most cases the rash with EFZ fades if the drug is continued. The other common adverse event seen with EFZ is CNS disturbance, which can include sleep problems and behavioral changes. In most patients the CNS effects are limited in time.

Protease Inhibitors

Development of protease inhibitors has been slower in children than in adults. Protease inhibitors are technically difficult to formulate into palatable liquid preparations, and their pharmacokinetics in children appears to be disadvantageous when compared with adult pharmacology with larger doses required. The capsule forms of several agents are large soft gel preparations that exceed the size (and dose) a child can swallow.

The most widely used protease inhibitor in children is nelfinavir (NLV). NLV is available as capsules and as a granular powder. The latter formulation allows size-titered dosing in children. The initial pharmacokinetic studies of NLV suggested a dosage range of 25 to 30 mg per kilogram per dose, given every 8 hours. However, more recent studies indicated that a higher dose should be used, especially in young children, and some physicians are using doses in the range of 55 mg per kilogram per dose, given every 12 hours.

Combinations including NLV are able to reduce the viral load to undetectable levels, although success rates are below those in the adult experience, probably related to compliance issues, pharmacology, and the higher viral loads with which most children begin (81). The major side effect of NLV is diarrhea, which usually is manageable through the use of symptomatic therapy with antidiarrheal agents. The powder formulation is somewhat difficult to use, and many children dislike its gritty, granular character and a large volume is often required.

Ritonavir (RTV) is approved for children in the United States and has proved to be clinically effective (82). However, it is a difficult drug to use, with a vile-tasting liquid preparation and numerous side effects. The liquid is 43% ethanol, which by itself makes the drug difficult for children to tolerate. Side effects include nausea, liver transaminase elevations, increased serum lipid concentrations, perioral paresthesias, and numerous drug interactions. RTV is one of the most potent cytochrome P450 inhibitors known, so the metabolism of many drugs is dramatically changed. Many commonly used drugs are contraindicated in the face of RTV: meperidine (Demerol), cisapride (Propulsid), astemizole (Hismanal), ergotamine, flurazepam (Dalmane), propoxyphene (Darvon), midazolam (Versed), and many others. The company provides small wallet cards to help the patient and physician recall which drugs are and are not allowed.

Indinavir is difficult to use in children because there is no liquid preparation. Older children can be treated with capsules, although it appears that clearance of the drug may be more rapid in children than in adults. The side effect profile is similar to that in adults: nephrolithiasis, elevated liver function tests, occasional hyperbilirubinemia, and numerous drug interactions. It may be possible to sprinkle capsules on applesauce (studies are pending).

There is little experience with saquinavir in children since the introduction of the relatively large and better absorbed soft-gel capsules. Saquinavir has a resistance pattern that is different from those of other protease inhibitors, so it may have a niche as part of a therapeutic regimen when initial treatment fails or as one element in a combination protease inhibitor approach.

Antiretroviral Treatment Strategies in Children

Considerable controversy exists about when to start antiretroviral drugs in children (83), although consensus guidelines have been published (84). Most of the controlled data comes from adult studies that must be extrapolated with reservation to pediatric patients. There are several important differences between pediatric and adult HIV disease that make the translation a tenuous one. First, children are more likely to have CNS involvement. Second, the virus has different effects on a growing immune system than on a mature one. Third, perinatally transmitted pediatric disease appears to be more aggressive than adult HIV disease. Children who are infected perinatally do not limit viral replication as effectively as adults do during their primary infection (15), and more children have a rapidly progressive course, including AIDS or death within 2 years after the time of infection (85). Therefore, there may be a special niche for treatment to limit early viral replication so that the child's immune responses can have time to mature.

Adult data have demonstrated that treatment during the "primary infection"—the time immediately after HIV inoculation—offers therapeutic benefits (16). However, adults are rarely aware of their disease in time for early therapy. In contrast, infants infected with HIV are always within months after their time of infection (which happens either *in utero* or at birth) and so may be treated at a time when virus dissemination is less well established. Consequently, many specialists believe that antiviral therapy should be started in all infected infants as soon as they are identified. Although this hypothesis has not yet been clinically verified, there are supporting data from animal models. The difficulty comes in trying to persuade a family to treat their well-appearing infant with a complex and rigid regimen including several poorly tolerated medications. As discussed later, absolute compliance is critical for success in combination antiretroviral regimens.

Two approaches are most often used in making the decision whether to treat an HIV-infected child with antiretroviral therapy. If the child is known to be HIV infected in the first few months of life, early treatment is justified. The infected child is at high risk for progression, laboratory tests are of little prognostic value (because all HIV-infected newborns have a high viral load), and dissemination and the development of genetic diversity

is still early. If the child is older than 3 to 6 months of age, there are no data on which to base a recommendation about when to start treatment. However, all children should be treated before they reach the threshold at which PCP prophylaxis is warranted, and most pediatric infectious disease specialists begin treatment as soon as the CDC immunologic category reaches 2 or worse, or the CDC clinical category reaches B or C (57,84).

When treatment is started, combinations of antiretroviral drugs are more appropriate than monotherapy. Although there are only limited data, as a nucleoside base for a regimen, ZDV/ddI appears to be similar to ZDV/ddC. ZDV/3TC is probably equal to ZDV/ddI (73), and combinations of either ddI or 3TC with D4T are probably comparable to ZDV-containing regimens, although the side effect profiles are different. Most physicians begin with three-drug regimens containing two NRTIs and either a protease inhibitor or an NNRTI. Some practitioners believe that a four-drug regimen is more effective, particularly in young infants with their high initial viral loads. However, compliance is a serious problem for most families, especially those with infants. If the family is noncompliant with a four-drug regimen and viral resistance develops, future therapeutic options will be severely limited. Therefore, the selection of which families should be prescribed a complex regimen is an important decision, one that often involves a multidisciplinary team.

Supportive Therapies

Anemia and neutropenia are commonly observed in children infected with HIV. These hematologic findings may be produced by the HIV infection itself, as a toxicity of the most commonly used drugs, or as a consequence of superinfections such as parvovirus B19 or MAC. Although chronic anemia can be treated with transfusions, this form of therapy is expensive and carries the risk of blood-borne infections such as hepatitis B and C. Given the short half-life of polymorphonuclear leukocytes, there is essentially no role for leukocyte transfusions in HIV. Fortunately there are other therapeutic alternatives.

Chronic anemia can be treated with recombinant erythropoietin. The cost is expensive, 25% to 50% of patients still require periodic transfusions, and erythropoietin must be given subcutaneously several days each week. It is, however, a reasonable option for patients with chronic anemia, particularly those who have difficulty tolerating marrow suppression related to ZDV. The treatment of ZDV-related anemia may also require adjustments in ZDV dose, typically through downward increments of 30%, the choice of PCP prophylaxis (to a drug other than TMP/SMX or dapsone), or treatment of superinfections (parvovirus with intravenous immunoglobulin (IVIG), MAC with a combination of antimycobacterial drugs).

Neutropenia also is a common problem in HIV-infected children. Granulocyte colony stimulating factor (G-CSF) can be effective treatment for this condition. The usual dose is 1 to 20 µg per kilogram per day as a single subcutaneous injection. The dose should start at the low end of the dosage range and advance as needed. The cost is quite high, and attempts should always be made to adjust ZDV or TMP/SMX dosing to determine whether these drugs may be the cause of the neutropenia.

Nutrition

HIV-infected children do not grow at a normal rate (18). HIV produces a growth delay that affects both height and weight within a few months after birth. However, because the effect is comparable for both height and weight, the children are generally appropriate in their weight-for-height. Only in the late stages of HIV disease do children become lean (develop a low weight-for-height). Early on, a reasonable emphasis on appropriate, balanced nutrition is important. There is no point in constructing rigid dietary plans, because children are unlikely to comply. The issue of dietary supplements is unresolved. Although there are advocates for 24-calorie formulas (instead of the standard 20 calories per ounce), no evidence yet exists for its benefit being studied.

Children in late disease are often given nutritional supplements such as Ensure and Sustacal. Although these can provide a balanced diet, their main advantage is the ease with which they can be swallowed. Some children are fed via a nasogastric or gastrostomy tube, but this type of drastic step has its cost, particularly in quality of life for the child. Intravenous nutrition is most useful to support a child with an acute gastrointestinal problem. Chronic total parenteral nutrition is expensive and requires placement of a central venous access line, making it a generally unsatisfactory therapy. Appetite stimulants such as megestrol (Megace) and cyproheptadine (Periactin) may increase oral intake and produce some growth. However, in late HIV disease almost all interventions produce more fat than increase in lean body mass, making their utility marginal. Effective antiretroviral therapy and aggressive treatment of opportunistic infections are probably the most important determinants of optimal growth. In the future, recombinant growth hormone may prove to have a role; preliminary studies in adults have shown improved lean body mass and few side effects. Because the growth pattern in HIV-infected children appears to be a growth delay, growth hormone may be a particularly useful in small, HIV-infected children.

Cardiomyopathy

Cardiomyopathy is a moderately frequent complication of HIV in children; it often manifests as an acute deterioration in cardiac function. Although some children ultimately recover to normal, most are left with some residual cardiac dysfunction. No single therapeutic strategy can be used to treat the condition, but most patients respond to a combination of digoxin, an afterload-reducing medication such as enalapril, and diuretics.

OPPORTUNISTIC INFECTIONS IN HIV-INFECTED CHILDREN

AIDS was first recognized in 1981 when an unusual clustering of cases of PCP occurred among young gay men in Southern California. Subsequently, other opportunistic infections were identified in this population, including disseminated mycobacterial infections, toxoplasmosis, and cytomegalovirus (CMV) retinitis. Soon thereafter, these same opportunistic infections were identified in children. Indeed, the occurrence of opportunistic infections remains central to the case definition of AIDS. The recognition that HIV-infected individuals are at increased risk for certain specific opportunistic pathogens has stimulated the development of strategies to prevent these infections.

In both children and adults, PCP remains the most commonly reported AIDS-defining diagnosis (86) (Table 3.6). Other common opportunistic infections in children include chronic and recurrent mucosal and esophageal candidiasis, CMV infections, nontuberculous mycobacteria (principally MAC), *Cryptosporidium* enteritis, herpes zoster, and mucocutaneous HSV. HIV-infected children also have an increased incidence of common childhood infections such as otitis media, sinusitis, viral respiratory infections, bacterial pneumonia, bacteremia, and meningitis.

TABLE 3.6. *Pediatric AIDS-defining diseases in the United States, 1997 (N = 473)*

Disease	% of Cases
Pneumocystis carinii pneumonia	25
HIV encephalopathy	23
Multiple/recurrent bacterial infections	18
Lymphoid interstitial pneumonitis	17
Failure to thrive	15
Candidiasis, esophageal or pulmonary	13
Cytomegalovirus	9
Nontuberculous mycobacteria	7
Herpes simplex virus infection	3
Cryptosporidiosis	2
Tuberculosis, disseminated	1
CNS toxoplasmosis	1
Lymphoma	1

AIDS, acquired immune deficiency syndrome; CNS, central nervous system; HIV, human immunodeficiency virus.

From the Centers for Disease Control and Prevention. *HIV/AIDS Surveillance Report* 1997;9:18, with permission.

The advent of potent combination antiretroviral therapy (HAART) has resulted in a dramatic decrease in the incidence of opportunistic infections in HIV-infected adults and children. This in turn has produced a dramatic decrease in mortality from AIDS in the United States (87). Therefore, the most effective means of preventing opportunistic infections is to aggressively treat the underlying HIV infection. However, it is anticipated that, with failure of HAART, the incidence of opportunistic infections may once again increase in the future. In addition, infections that occur in children with higher CD4 counts, such as bacterial infections and herpes zoster, are likely to remain common problems despite HAART.

Comprehensive guidelines for the prevention of opportunistic infections in children and adults have been published as have guidelines for the treatment of opportunistic infections in children (88,89).

Pneumocystis carinii Pneumonia

PCP remains the most common opportunistic infection in HIV-infected children. In children, PCP manifests at a much younger age than do other opportunistic infections; the incidence peaks at 4 to 5 months of age. Among children with perinatally acquired AIDS diagnosed within in the first year of life, 61% presented with PCP (90). In contrast, only 19% of older children with an AIDS diagnosis had PCP. Among all HIV-infected infants, without prophylaxis, the risk of PCP in the first year of life is 7% to 20%.

PCP can progress rapidly in young infants, resulting in a mortality rate as high as 50%. The aggressive nature of the infection presumably reflects an impaired cellular immune response at this age. In contrast to the situation in adults, PCP in infancy results from a primary infection with *Pneumocystis*, and the lack of prior immunity to the organism probably contributes to the aggressive nature of the infection.

Children with PCP typically present acutely with tachypnea, hypoxia, fever, and bilateral diffuse alveolar infiltrates on chest radiograph. The differential diagnosis includes lymphoid interstitial pneumonitis (LIP), MAC, and viral pneumonia (including CMV, Epstein-Barr virus, and the respiratory viruses). Children with LIP are distinguished from children with PCP by being older, without fever, and less acutely ill and having prominent hilar and peripheral lymphadenopathy and higher CD4 counts.

Diagnosis

Definitive diagnosis of PCP requires histologic demonstration of the organism in lung tissue or secretions obtained from the lower respiratory tract. An open lung biopsy or transbronchial biopsy is the most reliable means of identifying PCP and also serves to diagnose LIP. Frequently, the organism can be recovered from materials obtained by bronchoalveolar lavage or from tracheal secretions obtained from an endotracheal tube. The organism may even be identified in the induced sputum of an older child or adult. The cyst of the organism is readily visualized with the Grocott-Gomori methenamine silver stain, but this may take up to 24 hours to prepare. A Giemsa stain can be performed much more rapidly, and an experienced observer can identify the trophozoite and sporozoite forms of the organism. Immunofluorescent monoclonal antibody stains are now commercially available and are extremely sensitive.

Treatment

The drug of choice for the treatment of PCP is TMP/SMX (TMP 15 to 20 mg per kilogram per day intravenously in three to four divided doses over 1 hour). With clinical improvement, treatment can be completed with oral therapy (TMP 20 mg per kilogram per day orally in three to four divided doses to complete 2 to 3 weeks of therapy). Children who are intolerant to TMP/SMX and those who fail to improve after 5 to 7 days of intravenous TMP/SMX are often treated with intravenous pentamidine (4 mg per kilogram per day intravenously as a single infusion over 2 hours). Pentamidine has efficacy similar to that of TMP/SMX but has greater toxicity, including hypoglycemia, hy-

potension, hypocalcemia, and hepatic, pancreatic, renal, and hematologic toxicity. Atovaquone has been shown to a useful agent for the treatment of PCP in adults (91). Although it is somewhat less effective than TMP/SMX, it has minimal toxicity. Atovaquone is an option for children with mild-to-moderate PCP who cannot tolerate TMP/SMX. Once therapy for PCP is completed, the child should be given long-term secondary prophylaxis.

The early use of corticosteroids reduces morbidity in adults with PCP (92,93). Although anecdotal reports suggest a similar benefit in children, a definitive pediatric trial has not been performed (94). However, many authorities recommend early initiation of corticosteroids for children with PCP. The recommended regimen is methylprednisolone for 5 days at 2 mg per kilogram per day divided every 6 hours, followed by 3 days at 1 mg per kilogram per day divided every 12 hours, then 2 days at 0.5 mg per kilogram per day as a single dose.

Prevention

Antibiotic prophylaxis is effective in preventing PCP. Because the principal risk factor for PCP is advanced immunosuppression, guidelines for initiating prophylaxis in adults and older children are based on the CD4 count. There are several considerations when developing criteria for prophylaxis in infants. First, normal CD4 counts are higher in infants than in older children, with values decreasing over the first few years of life. Therefore, guidelines for the initiation of PCP prophylaxis in HIV-infected children are based on age-adjusted CD4 values (95) (Table 3.7). In addition, the CD4 count of HIV-infected infants can fall rapidly in the first year of life with rapid progression of disease. In infancy, PCP is frequently the presenting sign of HIV infection, occurring before the child is known to be HIV infected. In many cases, the child's mother is not known to be HIV infected (90). For these reasons, it is recommended that PCP prophylaxis be initiated in all infants at risk (i.e., those born to HIV-infected moth-

TABLE 3.7. *Indications for PCP prophylaxis in children*

PCP prophylaxis should be initiated for any of the following indications:
  After an episode of PCP
  At any age: CDC category C or 3, or rapidly falling CD4+ T-lymphocyte count
  Age <1 y: Start prophylaxis at 4–6 wk of age in all exposed infants and stop if child is proven to be not HIV
    infected (two negative cultures and/or PCR results, with one at ≥4 mo of age)
  Age-adjusted CD4 count thresholds:
    Age 1–5 y: CD4 count <500 cells/μL or <15%
    Age 6–12 y: CD4 count <200 cells/μL or <15%

PCP, *Pneumocystis carinii* pneumonia.
  Adapted from the Centers for Disease Control and Prevention. 1995 Revised guidelines for prophylaxis against *Pneumocystis carinii* pneumonia in children infected with or perinatally exposed to human immunodeficiency virus. *MMWR Morb Mortal Wkly Rep* 1995;44(RR-4):1–11, with permission.

ers). Because PCP rarely occurs before the age of 3 months, prophylaxis can be safely initiated at 6 to 8 weeks of age. Once a child is shown to be noninfected with HIV, prophylaxis can be stopped. Indications for prophylaxis in children older than 1 year of age are based on the CD4 values (Table 3.7). The decision to continue prophylaxis in an infected child who is older than 1 year of age and who no longer meets criteria for prophylaxis should be made on an individual basis.

The drug of choice for PCP prophylaxis is TMP/SMX (Table 3.8). As many as 15% of children are intolerant to TMP/SMX; adverse reactions include rash, fever, neutropenia, anemia, and the Stevens-Johnson syndrome. Neutropenia is particularly troublesome in children receiving both TMP/SMX and ZDV. If the adverse reaction is mild, rechallenge with TMP/SMX may be successful; gradually increasing the dose over 8 to 14 days im-

proves tolerance. Oral desensitization has been reported to be successful in adults and may be successful in children as well (96). For children who are infected with *Toxoplasma gondii,* PCP prophylaxis with TMP/SMX also appears to be effective in preventing *Toxoplasma* reactivation.

Alternatives for prophylaxis in young children who cannot tolerate TMP/SMX include oral dapsone atovaquone and intravenous pentamidine (97). Older children (generally older than 5 years of age) can be taught to receive aerosol pentamidine, although efficacy data is lacking in children (98). Delivery of pentamidine by the aerosol route to infants as young as 8 months has been reported (99). Potential advantages of atovaquone include a long half-life, low toxicity, and the ability to kill *Pneumocystis* in an animal model in which pentamidine and TMP/SMX only suppress the organism.

TABLE 3.8. *PCP prophylaxis in children*

Agent of choice: TMP/SMX, 150/750 mg/m^2/d in two divided doses, PO b.i.d. for three consecutive days per
  week.
Other acceptable dosage schedules:
  Single dose three times per week on consecutive days
  Two divided doses every day
  Two divided doses PO three times per week on alternate days
Alternatives:
  Dapsone, 2 mg/kg PO once daily or 4 mg/kg once weekly (max 100 mg)/(max 200 mg)
  Aerosol pentamidine (age >5 y), 300 mg by Respirgard II inhaler once monthly
  Atovaquone (age 1–3 mo and >24 mo: 30 mg/kg PO q.d.; age 4–24 mo: 45mg/kg PO q.d.)
  Parenteral (IV) pentamidine, 4 mg/kg/dose every 2–4 wk

PCP, *Pneumocystis carinii* pneumonia; TMP/SMX, trimethoprim-sulfamethoxazole.
  From the Centers for Disease Control and Prevention. 1999 USPHS/IDSA guidelines for the prevention of opportunistic infections in persons infected with human immunodeficiency virus. *MMWR Morb Mortal Wkly Rep* 1999;48(RR-10):1–66, with permission.

A limited number of adults who have responded to HAART with an increase in their CD4 count to more than 200 cells per microliter have been able to safely stop PCP prophylaxis (100). These patients usually have not had a prior episode of PCP, their CD4 counts have been increased for at least 6 months, and their HIV viral load is low or undetectable. The safety of discontinuing PCP prophylaxis in children has not been established.

Invasive Bacterial Infections

HIV-infected children are at increased risk for common childhood infections such as otitis media and sinusitis. Recurrent sinusitis can be problematic in some children. In addition, children have more frequent invasive bacterial infections, including pneumonia, bacteremia, and meningitis. The organisms causing these infections are generally the same as those in normal children, with *S. pneumoniae* the predominant pathogen (101,102). Diagnosis and management of these infections is similar to that for the normal child. The choice of antibiotics should reflect the increasing prevalence of penicillin-resistant pneumococci worldwide. This is an even greater problem in the HIV-infected population, where chronic antibiotic usage for PCP prophylaxis is common. Therefore, a third-generation cephalosporin or vancomycin should be included in the initial therapy.

All HIV-infected children should be vaccinated with the conjugate *Haemophilus influenzae* type b vaccine according to the routine schedule. In addition, all should receive the conjugate pneumococcal vaccine at 24 months of age and the influenza vaccine each year (88).

The use of TMP/SMX for PCP prophylaxis results in fewer bacterial infections; there may be an advantage to using daily dosing (150 mg TMP and 750 mg SMX per square meter per day in two divided doses) in children with recurrent infections. TMP/SMX prophylaxis does not prevent all pneumococcal infections, because the majority of penicillin-resistant strains are also resistant to TMP/SMX. Other antibiotics may be considered for prophylaxis in individual cases, recognizing the risk of promoting drug resistance.

Infusions of IVIG (400 mg per kilogram per dose, given once a month) have been shown to be effective in preventing recurrent bacterial infections in selected children (101,102). This is rational because HIV-infected children have functional hypogammaglobulinemia, even though immunoglobulin levels are commonly elevated. Because of the cost, risk of complications, and discomfort associated with IVIG infusions, its use is generally limited to children with the following indications (89):

1. Children who experience recurrent bacterial infections despite appropriate antimicrobial prophylaxis and therapy. In children with hypogammaglobulinemia, it may be reasonable to initial IVIG infusions without attempting antimicrobial prophylaxis. IVIG may not provide additional benefit to children receiving daily TMP/SMX prophylaxis (102).
2. Children living in a region with a high prevalence of measles who are without detectable antibody to measles despite receiving two measles immunizations.
3. Children who have HIV-associated thrombocytopenia (platelet count, lower than 20,000 cells per microliter) while receiving antiretroviral therapy.
4. HIV-infected children with chronic bronchiectasis who fail to respond to antibiotics and pulmonary care may respond to high-dose IVIG (600 mg per kilogram per month).

Candidiasis

Oral candidiasis is the most common mucocutaneous disease of HIV-infected children. Chronic and recurrent infections of skin and mucous membranes are frequently the presenting infection in HIV-infected children. These infections usually respond to topical or oral therapy but may promptly recur once therapy is discontinued. Oral candidiasis may be confused with oral hairy leukoplakia, but this disease is rare in children. If there is no response to initial therapy, a culture and scraping or biopsy of the lesion should be performed to confirm the presence of *Candida* and rule out coinfection with CMV or HSV. Esophageal candidiasis, characterized by dysphagia and retrosternal pain on swallowing, should be considered in a child who is eating poorly. Endoscopy is necessary to confirm the diagnosis of esophageal candidiasis and to rule out other causes of esophagitis such as HSV, CMV, and MAC. Acute airway obstruction with stridor has been reported in children with *Candida* epiglottitis and supraglottitis (103,104). Disseminated candidiasis is uncommon in HIV-infected children in the absence of an indwelling central venous catheter.

Oral candidiasis often responds to topical therapy with nystatin suspension, clotrimazole troches or cream, or oral amphotericin B suspension (105). Refractory cases require treatment with an oral azole (fluconazole, 3 to 6 mg per kilogram per day in one to two doses, or ketoconazole, 5 to 10 mg per kilogram per day in one to two doses). Hepatotoxicity is uncommon in children treated with the azoles. Long-term suppressive therapy with an oral azole may be required for frequently recurrent disease, but it should be limited because of the risk of development of resistance. Esophageal candidiasis requires systemic therapy with fluconazole, ketoconazole, or amphotericin B. Some isolates of *Candida krusei* and *Torulopsis glabrata* are resistant to fluconazole and require amphotericin B therapy.

Cytomegalovirus

CMV infection is common in HIV-infected children. However, infection is often asymptomatic, and it is difficult to determine the extent to which CMV is contributing to disease (106). In young children, CMV infection often represents a primary infection rather than reactivation of a prior infection, the more common situation in adults. Although most HIV-infected women are also CMV-infected, infants born to dually infected mothers do not have an increased risk of CMV infection (107). However, CMV coinfection is likely to accelerate the course of HIV disease (108).

Clinical manifestations of CMV disease in children with advanced HIV infection include chorioretinitis, enteritis, CNS infection, interstitial pneumonitis, hepatitis, neutropenia, and thrombocytopenia (106). Retinitis is the most important disease; it can progress rapidly to permanent loss of vision in the involved eye (109). Perivascular exudates with hemorrhage are seen on funduscopic examination. Diagnosis is based on the funduscopic findings, because viral cultures of blood and urine are not uniformly positive.

CMV enteritis is characterized by ulceration of the gastrointestinal mucosa. The colon is the most commonly involved site, but lesions may involve the small intestine and esophagus. Massive hemorrhage and obstruction have been described as complications of enteric disease (110). The differential diagnosis of enteric ulcers includes HSV, *Candida,* and MAC.

Infection of the CNS with CMV is described (111). However, encephalopathy in HIV-infected children is generally caused by HIV infection of the brain, and the relative contribution of CMV to encephalopathy is uncertain. A brain biopsy is required to make a definitive diagnosis of CMV encephalitis, but it is rarely performed. Ganglioneuronitis of intestinal ganglion cells has been described in infants (112).

CMV may cause a chronic interstitial pneumonitis in HIV-infected children. However, CMV is commonly isolated from bronchoalveolar lavage specimens or lung biopsy material, and its clinical significance is often unclear. Frequently, another pathogen such as *P. carinii* is also identified (113,114). Coinfection with CMV has not been shown to increase the severity of PCP (114). Genital skin ulcers caused by CMV have been described in adults. A diaper dermatitis caused by CMV has been reported in an HIV-infected child with disseminated CMV (115).

Diagnosis

The diagnosis of active CMV disease is complicated by the fact that excretion of CMV in urine and respiratory secretions is common in children with asymptomatic CMV infection. In addition, many features of CMV infection can be caused by HIV or by other opportunistic infections. However, the detection of CMV in blood or tissues by virus isolation or PCR is strongly suggestive of active CMV disease. The shell-vial system allows for early identification of a positive CMV culture. Histopathologic evidence of viral cytopathology is required for confirmation of specific organ involvement. Biopsy materials can be stained for viral antigens with the use of immunoperoxidase techniques. Reagents that allow for the rapid detection of viral antigens in peripheral blood polymorphonuclear leukocytes are commercially available (116). The presence of detectable antigen correlates well with active clinical disease, and this appears to be an important advance in the diagnosis of CMV disease.

Treatment

Treatment of CMV retinitis and gastrointestinal disease results in clinical improvement. Ganciclovir is the drug of choice for treating CMV disease in children. The pediatric dose is 10 mg per kilogram per day intravenously, divided in two daily doses for 14 to 21 days. The principal toxicity of ganciclovir is bone marrow suppression, which develops in up to 50% of patients. Bone marrow toxicity is potentiated by the combination of ganciclovir and ZDV. Ganciclovir-resistant strains of CMV have been isolated from patients receiving chronic suppressive therapy, and patients who fail to respond to ganciclovir should be treated with foscarnet (180 mg per kilogram per day intravenously, given in three divided doses). Foscarnet is effective in treating ganciclovir-resistant CMV retinitis in adults (117). The principal side effect of foscarnet is nephrotoxicity. Other options when therapy fails include the combination of ganciclovir and foscarnet, intraocular injections of ganciclovir, and intravenous cidofovir (118).

Without immunologic reconstitution, relapse is common after treatment of acute CMV retinitis, and long-term suppressive therapy is required (119). Intravenous infusions of ganciclovir (5 mg per kilogram, 5 days a week) and foscarnet (90 to 120 mg per kilogram daily) are effective in reducing the risk of recurrence. Alternatives for suppression include intraocular ganciclovir implants (which do not prevent disease in the contralateral eye or other organs) and oral ganciclovir. The combination of an implant in the affected eye plus oral ganciclovir is an appealing strategy for many patients. Reports suggest that some patients whose CD4 counts increase after HAART therapy may be able to safely discontinue CMV prophylaxis. However, criteria for discontinuing prophylaxis remain to be defined, and further experience is required before this therapy can be recommended for children.

Prevention

HIV-infected children who are CMV seronegative and require transfusion should receive CMV-seronegative or leukocyte-depleted blood products. CMV-seropositive children with advanced HIV infection should be evaluated by an experienced ophthalmologist on a regular basis in order to detect early retinitis. Children should be taught to recognize "floaters" and changes in visual acuity that could represent retinitis. Prophylaxis with oral ganciclovir may be considered in CMV-infected children who are severely immunosuppressed (120). Factors to consider include cost, the toxicity of oral ganciclovir (anemia and neutropenia), limited efficacy, and the risk of developing resistant virus. A liquid preparation of ganciclovir for use in children can be prepared from the parenteral preparation. The dose is 30 mg per kilogram per dose, given orally three times a day.

Nontuberculous Mycobacterial Infections

Disseminated infections with nontuberculous environmental mycobacteria are common in advanced AIDS, representing 7% of pediatric AIDS-defining diagnoses in the United States (Table 3.6). More than 85% of these infections are caused by MAC. An excellent review of this group of organisms has been published (121).

Without prophylaxis, between 10% and 18% of children with AIDS develop MAC infection (122,123). MAC is rare in the first year of life but becomes more common with increasing age and a falling CD4 count. Among cases reported to the CDC, the mean age of MAC diagnosis was 3.3 years for children with perinatal HIV and 8.7 years for children infected by transfusion (124). The median CD4 count in children with MAC is 17 cells per microliter, with 70% of children having fewer than 50 cells per microliter. However, among children younger than 24 months of age, MAC occurs at substantially higher CD4 counts than in older children (125).

Features of disseminated MAC include fever, night sweats, anorexia, failure to thrive, weight loss, abdominal pain, and diarrhea (122). Anemia and neutropenia are common laboratory findings. It may be difficult to differentiate symptoms of MAC from those of advanced HIV disease. Because MAC infections occur in children with advanced HIV disease, the reported survival time is brief; in one series, the median survival time after a diagnosis of MAC was only 5 months (124). However, with the restoration of immune function resulting from HAART, the prognosis has greatly improved, and cure of MAC infection has been reported (126).

Diagnosis

The child with suspected MAC should have at least two mycobacterial blood cultures obtained. Sustained bacteremia is common with disseminated infection, and the degree of bacteremia is usually high enough that blood cultures for mycobacteria are positive. An organism isolated from the blood should be identified to species by the laboratory.

The isolation of MAC from stool or respiratory secretions, in the absence of a positive blood culture, probably represents colonization rather than disseminated infection and should not necessarily prompt therapy. Surveillance cultures of stool have not proved to be useful and are not recommended. The identification of mycobacteria in internal organs confirms the presence of a disseminated infection. Acid-fast organisms can be identified on histologic examination of biopsy materials. However, tissues should be cultured to confirm the presence of the organism and identify the species, ruling out *Mycobacterium tuberculosis*. The clinical value of sensitivity testing remains controversial (127).

Treatment

Treatment of established MAC infection in patients with AIDS is challenging. Because of a poor clinical response to monotherapy, coupled with the rapid development of resistance, therapy with multiple drugs is recommended (128). Clinical responses to combination therapy include resolution of fever and night sweats, weight gain, and an improved sense of well-being. Frequently there is an elimination or reduction in the number of organisms present in quantitative blood cultures.

The macrolide antibiotic clarithromycin has assumed a key role in the treatment of MAC (129). This agent has excellent killing activity against MAC and is able to penetrate macrophages to reach intracellular organisms. In a controlled trial, clarithromycin was superior to azithromycin when combined with ethambutol (130). Therapy should include the combination of clarithromycin (15 mg per kilogram per day in two divided doses; maximum dose, 500 mg) and ethambutol (15 to 20 mg per kilogram per day as a single dose; maximum dose, 1,600 mg). Because optic neuritis is a complication of ethambutol, regular ophthalmologic evaluations are recommended. The addition of rifabutin (5 to 10 mg per kilogram per day, given once daily; maximum dose, 300 mg) as a third drug may reduce the likelihood of drug resistance but is associated with greater toxicity, including iritis, and the potential for multiple drug interactions (131). In addition, improved efficacy with the addition of rifabutin has not been demonstrated. A liquid formulation of rifabutin for use in children is not available. The clinician should be familiar with the toxicities and frequent drug interactions that occur with these drugs (121). After a clinical response to treatment, therapy should be continued for the long term. Immune reconstitution associated with HAART may allow discontinuation of therapy if the child is able to maintain an adequate CD4 count (126). An inflammatory lymphadenitis due to MAC has been reported in patients with a subclinical MAC infection after initiation of HAART (132).

Prevention

Prophylaxis of disseminated MAC is recommended for individuals with advanced HIV disease. Studies of adults have demonstrated the efficacy of rifabutin, clarithromycin, and azithromycin (133–135). MAC prophylaxis in children is currently being studied. However, based on adult studies, prophylaxis is recommended with clarithromycin (7.5 mg per kilogram per dose, maximum 500 mg, given orally twice a day) or azithromycin (20 mg per kilogram per dose, maximum 1,200 mg, given once weekly) for children with advanced immunosuppression (88). The criteria for initiating prophylaxis are based on the CD4 count, as noted in Table 3.9. A MAC blood culture should be obtained before prophylaxis is

TABLE 3.9. *Criteria for initiating MAC prophylaxis in children*

Age (y)	CD4+ T-lymphocyte count (cells/μL)
≥6	<50
2–6	<75
1–2	<500
<1	<750

MAC, *Mycobacterium avium* complex.
From the Centers for Disease Control and Prevention. 1999 USPHS/IDSA guidelines for the prevention of opportunistic infections in persons infected with human immunodeficiency virus. *MMWR Morb Mortal Wkly Rep* 1999;48(RR-10):1–66, with permission.

started. The safety of discontinuing MAC prophylaxis with immunologic reconstitution from HAART is currently under study.

Cryptosporidium Infection

Cryptosporidium, a protozoan, is a common cause of self-limited watery diarrhea in normal infants and children. Transmission is by fecal-oral spread, and outbreaks of *Cryptosporidium* infection are frequent in the day care setting (136). Large outbreaks in metropolitan areas have resulted from contaminated drinking water, and several outbreaks have been associated with public swimming pools. Other sources of infection include lake and river water, contaminated foods, and young household pets. In children with advanced HIV infection, *Cryptosporidium* causes severe and protracted diarrhea with abdominal pain and anorexia. The infection may result in substantial weight loss and even death. The stools are watery in consistency and may contain mucus but lack blood and inflammatory cells. Patients with advanced immunosuppression have protracted infections that rarely clear (137). *Cryptosporidium* has been implicated as a cause of sclerosing cholangitis (138).

The diagnosis of *Cryptosporidium* can be made by examination of a fresh stool sample. The oocyst of the organism stains with the modified Kinyoun acid-fast stain; this differentiates it from yeast cells, which are of similar size and shape. Frequently, the number of oocysts present in the stool is high and concentration of the stool is not necessary to visualize the organism. The organism may also be identified on histologic examination of a biopsy of enteric mucosa. Reagents are commercially available that allow the identification of the organism by indirect immunofluorescence.

Children with severe immunodeficiency should avoid exposure to the sources of *Cryptosporidium* noted previously. Families may choose to avoid having their child drink tap water; boiling water for 1 minute reduces the risk of infection. Use of bottled water and a submicron personal-use water filter may also reduce the risk of infection; effective filtering of bottled water should be confirmed. Clarithromycin and rifabutin, when used for MAC prophylaxis, may prevent the development of cryptosporidiosis (139). This benefit is not seen with azithromycin. Protease inhibitors may also have a direct effect in preventing cryptosporidiosis.

The treatment of chronic diarrhea due to cryptosporidiosis requires careful attention to fluid and electrolyte balance and caloric intake. Antidiarrheal agents such as loperamide may be helpful if they are used with caution. Persistent watery diarrhea that is unresponsive to other modalities may respond to treatment with somatostatin (octreotide acetate) (140). A variety of antimicrobial agents have been used to treat *Cryptosporidium,* but none has proved uniformly successful. These agents include nitazoxanide, paromomycin, azithromycin, spiramycin, oral IVIG, and oral hyperimmune bovine colostrum (141,142). Paromomycin, an aminoglycoside that is not absorbed when taken orally, has been reported to produce a clinical response in some patients and is currently the recommended treatment (30 to 40 mg per kilogram per day, divided in three to four doses, for at least 14 days; maximum dose, 1,000 mg) (143,144). A liquid preparation of paromomycin is not available.

The most effective treatment of cryptosporidiosis is HAART. Symptoms frequently resolve with an increase in the CD4 count (145). However, if the CD4 count should subsequently decline, symptomatic disease may recur.

CHILDHOOD IMMUNIZATIONS

HIV-infected and HIV-exposed children should be immunized according to the Immunization Schedule for HIV-Infected Children included in the 1999 *U.S. Public Health Service IDSA Guidelines for the Prevention of Opportunistic Infections in Persons Infected with Human Immunodeficiency Virus* (88). As now recommended for all children, the inactivated polio vaccine should be ad-

ministered rather than the live polio vaccine. The live attenuated measles-mumps-rubella (MMR) vaccine should be administered to all HIV-infected children except those with severe immunodeficiency (CDC immunologic category 3). The second dose of the MMR vaccine may be given as early as 1 month after the first dose, recognizing that the younger, less immunosuppressed child is more likely to respond to the vaccine. The influenza vaccine should be administered annually beginning at 6 months of age. The live attenuated varicella vaccine has been shown to be immunogenic and safe in HIV-infected children with normal lymphocyte subsets and is now recommended for children of CDC class N1 and A1; it is contraindicated for all other HIV-infected children (88). A 7-valent pneumococcal conjugate vaccine (PCV7) has been approved for use in children and is recommended for all HIV-infected and exposed children (145a). Infants should receive 4 doses of the PCV7 in the first 15 months of life, followed by a dose of the 23-valent pneumococcal polysaccharide vaccine (23PS) at 24 months of age. A second dose of the 23PS is administered 3–5 years after the first dose. Older children should have "catch-up" immunization with the PCV7 and 23PS vaccine as described in the American Academy of Pediatrics recommendations. The live attenuated varicella vaccine has been shown to be immunogenic and safe in HIV-infected children with normal lymphocyte subsets and is recommended for children in CDC classes N1 and A1; it is contraindicated for other HIV-infected children (88,146).

Suboptimal responses to both live and killed vaccines have been demonstrated in HIV-infected children, particularly those with advanced immunosuppression (147,148). However, serologic testing after receipt of any of the childhood vaccines is not recommended (149). In regions experiencing a measles outbreak, serologic testing for measles immunity may be considered to identify susceptible children who would benefit from immunoglobulin prophylaxis.

REFERENCES

1. Bryson YJ, Luzuriaga K, Sullivan JL, et al. Proposed definitions for *in utero* versus intrapartum transmission of HIV-1. *N Engl J Med* 1992;327:1246–1247.
2. Soeiro R, Rubinstein A, Rashbaum WK, et al. Maternofetal transmission of AIDS: frequency of human immunodeficiency virus type 1 nucleic acid sequences in human fetal DNA. *J Infect Dis* 1992;166:699–703.
3. Kalish LA, Pitt J, Lew J, et al. Defining the time of fetal or perinatal acquisition of human immunodeficiency virus type 1 infection on the basis of age at first positive culture. *J Infect Dis* 1997;175:712–715.
4. Fauci AS. Multifactorial nature of human immunodeficiency virus disease: implications for therapy. *Science* 1993;262:1011–1018.
5. Daar ES, Moudgil T, Meyer RD, et al. Transient high levels of viremia in patients with primary human immunodeficiency virus type 1 infection. *N Engl J Med* 1991;324:961–964.
6. Shearer WT, Quinn TC, LaRussa P, et al. Viral load and disease progression in infants infected with human immunodeficiency virus type 1. *N Engl J Med* 1997;336:1337–1342.
7. Luzuriaga K, McQuilken P, Alimenti A, et al. Early viremia and immune responses in vertical human immunodeficiency virus type 1 infection. *J Infect Dis* 1993;167:1008–1013.
8. Palumbo PE, Kwok S, Waters S, et al. Viral measurement by polymerase chain reaction-based assays in human immunodeficiency virus-infected infants. *J Pediatr* 1995;126:592–595.
9. United Nations AIDS Program. *Report on the Global HIV/AIDS epidemic—June 2000.* Available at: http://www.unaids.org/epidemic update/report/Epi report.htm glob.
10. Centers for Disease Control and Prevention. Update: AIDS among women—United States, 1994. *MMWR Morb Mortal Wkly Rep* 1995;44:81–84.
11. Oxtoby MJ. Vertically acquired HIV infection in the United States. In: Pizzo PA, Wilfert CM, eds. *Pediatric AIDS: the challenge of HIV infection in infants, children, and adolescents,* 2nd ed. Baltimore: Williams & Wilkins, 1994:3–20.
12. Auger I, Thomas P, DeGruttola V, et al. Incubation periods for paediatric AIDS patients. *Nature* 1988;336:575–577.
13. European Collaborative Study. Children born to women with HIV-1 infection: natural history and risk of transmission. *Lancet* 1991;337:253–260.
14. Bryson Y, Chen I, Miles S, et al. A prospective evaluation of HIV co-culture for early diagnosis of perinatal HIV infection. Abstract W.B.2014. In: *Proceedings and Abstracts, VII International Conference on AIDS (Florence).* June 16–21, 1991:185.
14a. Dickover RE, Dillon M, Gillette SG, et al. Rapid increases in load of human immunodeficiency virus correlate with early disease progression and loss of CD4 cells in vertically infected infants. *J Infect Dis* 1994;170:1279–1284.
15. Pikora CA, Sullivan JL, Panicali D, et al. Early HIV-1 envelope-specific cytotoxic T lymphocyte responses in vertically infected infants. *J Exp Med* 1997;185:1153–1161.
16. Rosenberg ES, Billingsley JM, Caliendo AM, et al. Vigorous HIV-1-specific CD4+ T cell responses associated with control of viremia. *Science* 1997;278:1447–1450.
17. McKinney RE, Robertson JWR, Duke Pediatric AIDS Clinical Trials Unit. The effect of human immunodeficiency virus infection on the growth of young children. *J Pediatr* 1993;123:579–582.
18. Moye J Jr, Rich KC, Kalish LA, et al. Natural history of somatic growth in infants born to women infected by human immunodeficiency virus. *J Pediatr* 1996;128:58–69.
19. Raton JA, Pocheville I, Vicente JM, et al. Disseminated bacillus Calmette-Guérin infection in an HIV-infected child: a case with cutaneous lesions. *Pediatr Dermatol* 1997;14:365–368.
20. Gershon AA, Mervish N, LaRussa P, et al. Varicella-zoster virus infection in children with underlying human immunodeficiency virus infection. *J Infect Dis* 1997;176:1496–1500.
21. Griffiths JK. Human cryptosporidiosis: epidemiology, transmission, clinical disease. *Adv Parasitol* 1998;40:37–85.
22. Bryson YJ. Perinatal HIV-1 transmission: recent advances and therapeutic interventions. *AIDS* 1996;10 [Suppl 3]:S33–S42.
23. Van De Perre P, Simonon A, Msellati P, et al. Postnatal transmission of human immunodeficiency virus type 1 from mother to infant: a prospective cohort study in Kigali, Rwanda. *N Engl J Med* 1991;325:593–598.
24. Bertolli J, St. Louis ME, Simonds RJ, et al. Estimating the timing of mother-to-child transmission of human immunodeficiency virus in the breast-feeding population in Kinshasa, Zaire. *J Infect Dis* 1996;174:722–726.
25. Landesman SH, Kalish LA, Burns DN, et al. Obstetrical factors and the transmission of human immunodeficiency virus type 1 from mother to child. *N Engl J Med* 1996;334:1617–1623.
26. Duliege A-M, Amos CI, Felton S, et al. Birth order, delivery route, and concordance in the transmission of human immunodeficiency virus type 1 from mothers to twins. *J Pediatr* 1995;126:625–632.
27. The International Perinatal HIV Group. Mode of delivery and vertical transmission of HIV-1: a meta-analysis from fifteen prospective cohort studies. *N Engl J Med* 1999;340:977–987.
28. Bryson YJ, Luzuriaga K, Sullivan JL, et al. Proposed definitions for *in utero* versus intrapartum transmission of HIV-1. *N Engl J Med* 1992;327:1246–1247.
29. Bryson YJ, Pang S, Wei LS, et al. Clearance of HIV infection in a perinatally infected infant. *N Engl J Med* 1995;332:833–838.
30. Frenkel LM, Mullins JI, Learn GH, et al. Genetic evaluation of suspected cases of transient HIV-1 infection of infants. *Science* 1998;280:1073–1077.
31. Leroy V, Newell ML, Dabis F, et al. International multicentre pooled analysis of late postnatal mother-to-child transmission of HIV-1 infection. *Lancet* 1998;352:597–600.
32. Gabiano C, Tovo PA, deMartino M, et al. Mother to child transmission of human immunodeficiency virus type 1: risk of infection and correlates of transmission. *Pediatrics* 1992;90:369–374.
33. Dickover RE, Garratty EM, Herman SA, et al. Identification of levels of maternal HIV-1 RNA associated with risk of perinatal transmission: effect of maternal

zidovudine treatment on viral load. *JAMA* 1996;275: 599–605.

34. Mandelbrot L, Mayaux M-J, Bongain A, et al. Obstetric factors and mother-to-child transmission of human immunodeficiency virus type 1: the French perinatal cohorts. *Am J Obstet Gynecol* 1996;175:661–667.

35. St. Louis ME, Kamenga M, Brown C, et al. Risk for perinatal HIV-1 transmission according to maternal immunologic, virologic and placental factors. *JAMA* 1993;269:2853–2859.

36. Pitt J, Brambilla D, Reichelderfer P, et al. Maternal immunologic and virologic risk factors for infant human immunodeficiency virus type 1 infection: findings from the Women and Infants Transmission Study. *J Infect Dis* 1997;175:567–575.

37. Cao Y, Krogstad P, Korber BT, et al. Maternal HIV-1 viral load and vertical transmission. *Nat Med* 1997;3: 549–552.

38. Kuhn L, Steketee RW, Weedon J, et al. Distinct risk factors for intrauterine and intrapartum human immunodeficiency virus transmission and consequences for disease progression in infected children. *J Infect Dis* 1999;179:52–58.

39. Sperling RS, Shapiro DE, Coombs RW, et al. Maternal viral load, zidovudine treatment, and the risk of transmission of human immunodeficiency virus type 1 from mother to infant. *N Engl J Med* 1996;335: 1621–1629.

40. Van Dyke RB, Korber BT, Popek E, et al. The Ariel Project: a prospective cohort study of risk factors for maternal-child transmission of human immunodeficiency virus type 1 in the era of maternal antiretroviral therapy. *J Infect Dis* 1999;179:319–328.

41. Connor EM, Sperling RS, Gelber R, et al. Reduction of maternal-infant transmission of human immunodeficiency virus type 1 with zidovudine treatment: results of AIDS clinical trials group protocol 076. *N Engl J Med* 1994;331:1173–1180.

42. Centers for Disease Control and Prevention. Zidovudine for the prevention of HIV transmission from mother to infant. *MMWR Morb Mortal Wkly Rep* 1994;43:285–287.

43. Centers for Disease Control and Prevention. Recommendations of the U.S. Public Health Service Task Force on the use of zidovudine to reduce perinatal transmission of human immunodeficiency virus. *MMWR Morb Mortal Wkly Rep* 1994;43(RR-11):1–20.

44. Wade NA, Birkhead GS, Warren BL, et al. Abbreviated regimens of zidovudine prophylaxis and perinatal transmission of the human immunodeficiency virus. *N Engl J Med* 1998;339:1409–1414.

45. Stoto MA, Almario DA, McCornick MC, eds. *Reducing the odds: preventing perinatal transmission of HIV in the United States*. Washington DC: National Academy Press, 1998. Available at: http://books.nap.edu/books/0309062861/html/index.html.

46. Centers for Disease Control and Prevention. Success in implementing public health service guidelines to reduce perinatal transmission of HIV. *MMWR Morb Mortal Wkly Rep* 1998;47:688–691.

47. Centers for Disease Control and Prevention. Update: perinatally acquired HIV/AIDS—United States, 1997. *MMWR Morb Mortal Wkly Rep* 1997;46: 1086–1092.

48. Culnane M, Fowler M, Lee SS, et al. Lack of long-term effects of *in utero* exposure to zidovudine among uninfected children born to HIV-infected women. *JAMA* 1999;281:151–157.

49. World Health Organization. *Coverage of maternal care: a listing of available information,* 4th ed. Geneva: WHO, 1997.

50. Shaffer N, Chuachoowong R, Mock PA, et al. Short-course zidovudine for perinatal HIV-1 transmission in Bangkok, Thailand: a randomized controlled trial. *Lancet* 1999;353:773–780.

51. Wiktor SZ, Ekpini E, Karon JM, et al. Short-course oral zidovudine for prevention of mother-to-child transmission of HIV-1 in Abidjan, Côte d'Ivoire: a randomized trial. *Lancet* 1999;353:781–785.

52. Dabis F, Mselli P, Meda N, et al. 6-month efficacy, tolerance, and acceptability of a short regimen of oral zidovudine to reduce vertical transmission of HIV in breastfed children in Côte d'Ivoire and Burkina Faso: a double-blind placebo-controlled multicentre trial. *Lancet* 1999;353:786–792.

52a. Guay LA, Musoke P, Fleming T, et al. Intrapartum and neonatal nevirapine compared with zidovudine for prevention of mother-to-child transmission of HIV-1 in Kampala, Uganda: HIVNET 012 randomized trial. *Lancet* 1999;354:795.

52b. Centers for Disease Control and Prevention. U.S. public health service task force recommendations for the use of antiretroviral drugs in pregnant women infected with HIV-1 for maternal health and for reducing perinatal HIV-1 transmission in the United States. *MMWR Morb Mortal Wkly Rep* 1998;47(RR-2):1–29. Available in an updated version at: http://www.hivatis.org/trtgdlns.html.

53. The European Mode of Delivery Collaboration. Elective caesarean-section versus vaginal delivery in prevention of vertical HIV-1 transmission: a randomised clinical trial. *Lancet* 1999;353:1035–1039.

54. Bigger RJ, Miotti PG, Taha TE, et al. Perinatal intervention trial in Africa: effect of a birth canal cleansing intervention to prevent HIV transmission. *Lancet* 1996;347:1647–1650.

55. Bremer JW, Lew JF, Cooper E, et al. Diagnosis of infection with human immunodeficiency virus type 1 by a DNA polymerase chain reaction assay among infants enrolled in the Women and Infants' Transmission Study. *J Pediatr* 1996;129:198–207.

56. Rogers MF, Schochetman G, Hoff R. Advances in diagnosis of HIV infection in infants. In: Pizzo PA, Wilfert CM, eds. *Pediatric AIDS: the challenge of HIV infection in infants, children, and adolescents,* 2nd ed. Baltimore: Williams & Wilkins, 1994:219.

57. Centers for Disease Control. CDC 1994 revised classification system for HIV-infection in children less than 13 years of age. *MMWR Morb Mortal Wkly Rep* 1994; 43(RR-12):1–10.

58. Jackson JB, MacDonald KL, Caldwell J, et al. Absence of HIV infection in blood donors with indeterminate Western blot tests for antibody to HIV-1. *N Engl J Med* 1990;322:217.

59. Miles SA, Balden E, Magpantay L, et al. Rapid serologic testing with immune-complex-dissociated HIV p24 antigen for early detection of HIV infection in neonates. *N Engl J Med* 1993;328:297.

60. Frenkel LM, Mullins JI, Learn GH, et al. Genetic eval-

uation of suspected cases of transient HIV-1 infection of infants. *Science* 1998 15;280:1073–1077.

61. Borkowsky W, Krasinski K, Pollack H, et al. Early diagnosis of human immunodeficiency virus infection in children <6 months of age: comparison of polymerase chain reaction, culture, and plasma antigen capture techniques. *J Infect Dis* 1992;166:616–619.

62. Rogers MF, Ou C-Y, Rayfield M, et al. Use of the polymerase chain reaction for early detection of the proviral sequences of human immunodeficiency virus in infants born to seropositive mothers. *N Engl J Med* 1989;320:1649.

63. Walter EB, McKinney RE, Lane BA, et al. Interpretation of Western blots in HIV-1 infected children: implications for prognosis and diagnosis. *J Pediatr* 1990;117:255.

64. The European Collaborative Study. Age-related standards for T-lymphocyte subsets based on uninfected children born to human immunodeficiency virus 1-infected mothers. *Pediatr Infect Dis J* 1999;11: 1018–1026.

65. Mellors JW, Rinaldo CR, Gupta P, et al. Prognosis in HIV-1 infection predicted by the quantity of virus in plasma. *Science* 1996;272:1167–1170.

66. Mofenson LM, Korelitz J, Meyer WA, et al. The relationship between serum human immunodeficiency virus type 1 (HIV-1) RNA level, CD4 lymphocyte percent, and long-term mortality risk in HIV-1 infected children. *J Infect Dis* 1997;175:1029–1038.

67. McKinney RE. Antiretroviral therapy: evaluating the new era in HIV treatment. *Adv Pediatr Infect Dis* 1996:12:297–323.

68. Valentine ME, Jackson CR, Vavro C, et al. Evaluation of surrogate markers and clinical outcomes in two-year follow-up of 86 HIV-infected pediatric patients. *Pediatr Infect Dis J* 1998;17:18–23.

69. McKinney RE Jr, Maha MA, Connor EM, et al. A multicenter trial of oral zidovudine in children with advanced human immunodeficiency virus disease. *N Engl J Med* 1991;324:1018–1025.

70. Kline MW, Van Dyke RB, Lindsey JC, et al. A randomized comparative trial of stavudine (d4T) versus zidovudine (ZDV, AZT) in children with human immunodeficiency virus infection. *Pediatrics* 1998;101:214–220.

71. Morgello S, Wolfe D, Godfrey E, et al. Mitochondrial abnormalities in human immunodeficiency virus-associated myopathy. *Acta Neuropathol* 1995;90:366–374.

72. Kuritzkes DR, Quinn JB, Benoit SL, et al. Drug resistance and virologic response in NUCA 3001, a randomized trial of lamivudine (3TC) versus zidovudine (ZDV) versus ZDV plus 3TC in previously untreated patients. *AIDS* 1996;10:975–981.

73. McKinney RE Jr, Johnson GM, Stanley K, et al., Pediatric AIDS Clinical Trials Group Protocol 300 Study Team. A randomized study of combined zidovudine-lamivudine versus didanosine monotherapy in children with symptomatic therapy-naïve HIV-1 infection. *J Pediatr* 1998;133:500–508.

74. Englund JA, Baker CJ, Raskino C, et al. Zidovudine, didanosine, or both as the initial treatment for symptomatic HIV-infected children. *N Engl J Med* 1997; 336:1704–1712.

75. Spector SA, Blanchard S, Wara DW, et al. Comparative trial of two dosages of zalcitabine in zidovudine-experienced children with advanced human immuno-

76. Bakshi SS, Britto P, Capparelli E, et al. Evaluation of pharmacokinetics, safety, tolerance, and activity of combination of zalcitabine and zidovudine in stable, zidovudine-treated pediatric patients with human immunodeficiency virus infection. *J Infect Dis* 1997;175: 1039–1050.

77. Richman DD, Havlir D, Corbeil J, et al. Nevirapine resistance mutations of human immunodeficiency virus type 1 selected during therapy. *J Virol* 1994;68: 1660–1666.

78. Luzuriaga K, Bryson Y, McSherry G, et al. Pharmacokinetics, safety, and activity of nevirapine in human immunodeficiency virus type 1-infected children. *J Infect Dis* 1996;174:713–721.

79. Luzuriaga K, Bryson Y, Krogstad P, et al. Combination treatment with zidovudine, didanosine, and nevirapine in infants with human immunodeficiency virus type 1 infection. *N Engl J Med* 1997;336:1343–1349.

80. Kahn J, Mayers D, Riddler S, et al. Durable clinical anti-HIV-1 activity (60 weeks) and tolerability for efavirenz (DMP 266) in combination with indinavir (IDV) suppression to "less than 1 copy/mL" (OD=background) by Amplicor as a predictor of virologic treatment response [DMP 266-003, cohort IV] [Abstract 692]. In: *Program and Abstracts of the 5th Conference on Retroviruses and Opportunistic Infections,* Chicago, February 1–5. 1998:208.

81. Martel L, Valentine M, Ferguson L, et al. Virologic and CD4 response to treatment with nelfinavir in therapy experienced but protease inhibitor naïve HIV-infected children [Abstract 233]. In: *Program and Abstracts of the 5th Conference on Retroviruses and Opportunistic Infections,* Chicago, February 1–5. 1998:123.

82. Mueller BU, Nelson RP Jr, Sleasman J, et al. A phase I/II study of the protease inhibitor ritonavir in children with human immunodeficiency virus infection. *Pediatrics* 1998;101:335–343.

83. McKinney RE Jr. Use of antiretroviral therapy in children and pregnant women [Review]. *Adv Exper Med Biol* 1996;394:345–354.

84. Centers for Disease Control and Prevention. Guidelines for the use of antiretroviral agents in pediatric HIV infection. *MMWR Morb Mortal Wkly Rep* 1998; 47(RR-4):1–43. Available in an updated version at: http://www.hivatis.org/trtgdlns.html.

85. Scott GB, Hutto C, Makuch RW, et al. Survival in children with perinatally acquired human immunodeficiency virus type 1 infection. *N Engl J Med* 1989;321: 1791.

86. Centers for Disease Control and Prevention. *HIV/AIDS Surveillance Report* 1997;9:18.

87. Palella FJ, Delaney KM, Moorman AC, et al. Declining morbidity and mortality among patients with advanced human immunodeficiency virus infection. *N Engl J Med* 1998;338:853–861.

88. Centers for Disease Control and Prevention. 1999 USPHS/IDSA guidelines for the prevention of opportunistic infections in persons infected with human immunodeficiency virus. *MMWR Morb Mortal Wkly Rep* 1999;48(RR–10):1–66.

89. Working Group on Antiretroviral Therapy and Medical Management of Infants, Children, and Adolescents With HIV Infection. Antiretroviral therapy and med-

ical management of pediatric HIV infection. *Pediatrics* 1998;102:1005–1062.

90. Simonds RJ, Oxtoby MJ, Caldwell MB, et al. *Pneumocystis carinii* pneumonia among US children with perinatally acquired HIV infection. *JAMA* 1993;270: 470–473.

91. Hughes WT, Leoung G, Kramer F, et al. Comparison of atovaquone and trimethoprim-sulfamethoxazole to treat *P. carinii* pneumonia in patients with AIDS. *N Engl J Med* 1993;328:1521–1527.

92. Bozzette SA, Sattler FR, Chiu J, et al. A controlled trial of early adjunctive treatment with corticosteroids for *Pneumocystis carinii* pneumonia in the acquired immunodeficiency syndrome. *N Engl J Med* 1990; 323:1451–1457.

93. National Institutes of Health–University of California Expert Panel for Corticosteroids as Adjunctive Therapy for *Pneumocystis* Pneumonia. Consensus statement on the use of corticosteroids as adjunctive therapy for *Pneumocystis* pneumonia in the acquired immunodeficiency syndrome. *N Engl J Med* 1990; 323:1500–1504.

94. Sleasman JW, Hemenway C, Klein AS, et al. Corticosteroids improve survival of children with AIDS and *Pneumocystis carinii* pneumonia. *Am J Dis Child* 1993;147:30–34.

95. Centers for Disease Control and Prevention. 1995 revised guidelines for prophylaxis against *Pneumocystis carinii* pneumonia in children infected with or perinatally exposed to human immunodeficiency virus. *MMWR Morb Mortal Wkly Rep* 1995;44(RR-4):1–11.

96. Gluckstein D, Ruskin J. Rapid oral desensitization to trimethoprim-sulfamethoxazole (TMP-SMX): use in prophylaxis for *Pneumocystis carinii* pneumonia in patients with AIDS who were previously intolerant to TMP-SMZ. *Clin Infect Dis* 1995;20:849–853.

97. Stavola JJ, Noel GJ. Efficacy and safety of dapsone prophylaxis against *Pneumocystis carinii* pneumonia in human immunodeficiency virus-infected children. *Pediatr Infect Dis J* 1993;12:644–647.

98. Hand IL, Wiznia AA, Porricolo M, et al. Aerosolized pentamidine for prophylaxis of *Pneumocystis carinii* pneumonia in infants with human immunodeficiency virus infection. *Pediatr Infect Dis J* 1994;13: 100–104.

99. Katz BZ, Rosen C. Aerosolized pentamidine in young children. *Pediatr Infect Dis J* 1991;12:958.

100. Schneider MME, Borleffs JCC, Stolk RP, et al. Discontinuation of prophylaxis for *Pneumocystis carinii* pneumonia in HIV-1-infected patients treated with highly active antiretroviral therapy. *Lancet* 1999;353: 201–203.

101. NICHD IVIG Study Group. Intravenous immune globulin for the prevention of bacterial infection in children with symptomatic human immunodeficiency virus infection. *N Engl J Med* 1991;325:73–80.

102. Spector SA, Gelber RD, McGrath N, et al. A controlled trial of intravenous immune globulin for the prevention of serious bacterial infections in children receiving zidovudine for advanced human immunodeficiency virus infection. *N Engl J Med* 1994;331:1181–1187.

103. Bye MR, Palomba A, Bernstein L, et al. Clinical *Candida* supraglottitis in an infant with AIDS-related complex. *Pediatr Pulmonol* 1987;3:280–281.

104. Balsam D, Sorrano D, Barax C. *Candida* epiglottitis presenting as stridor in a child with HIV infection. *Pediatr Radiol* 1992;22:235–236.

105. Alban J, Groel JT. Amphotericin B oral suspension in the treatment of thrush. *Curr Ther Res Clin Exp* 1970; 12:479–484.

106. Frenkel LD, Gaur S, Tsolia M, et al. Cytomegalovirus infection in children with AIDS. *Rev Infect Dis* 1990;12[Suppl 7]:S820–S826.

107. Mussi-Pinhata MM, Yamamoto Y, Figueiredo LTM, et al. Congenital and perinatal cytomegalovirus infection in infants born to mothers infected with human immunodeficiency virus. *J Pediatr* 1998;132:285–290.

108. Nigro G, Krzystofiak A, Gattinara G, et al. Rapid progression of HIV diseases in children with CMV DNAemia. *AIDS* 1996;10:1127–1133.

109. Dennehy PJ, Warman R, Flynn JT, et al. Ocular manifestations in pediatric patients with acquired immunodeficiency syndrome. *Arch Ophthalmol* 1989;107: 978–982.

110. Dolgin SE, Larsen JG, Shah KD, et al. CMV enteritis causing hemorrhage and obstruction in an infant with AIDS. *J Pediatr Surg* 1990;25:696–698.

111. Belec L, Tayot J, Tron P, et al. Cytomegalovirus encephalopathy in an infant with congenital acquired immuno-deficiency syndrome. *Neuropediatrics* 1990;21: 124–129.

112. Anderson VM, Greco MA, Recalde AL, et al. Intestinal cytomegalovirus ganglioneuronitis in children with human immunodeficiency virus infection. *Pediatr Pathol* 1990;10:167–174.

113. Cohen-Abbo A, Wright PF. Complex etiology of pneumonia in infants perinatally infected with human immunodeficiency virus 1. *Pediatr Infect Dis J* 1991;10: 545–547.

114. Glaser JH, Schuval S, Burstein O, et al. Cytomegalovirus and *Pneumocystis carinii* pneumonia in children with acquired immunodeficiency syndrome. *J Pediatr* 1992;120:929–931.

115. Thiboutot DM, Beckford A, Mart CR, et al. Cytomegalovirus diaper dermatitis. *Arch Dermatol* 1991; 127:396–398.

116. Landry ML, Ferguson D. Comparison of quantitative cytomegalovirus antigenemia assay with culture methods and correlation with clinical disease. *J Clin Microbiol* 1993;31:2851–2856.

117. Studies of Ocular Complications of AIDS Research Group, in Collaboration with the AIDS Clinical Trials Group. Mortality in patients with the acquired immunodeficiency syndrome treated with either foscarnet or ganciclovir for cytomegalovirus retinitis. *N Engl J Med* 1992;326:213–220.

118. The Studies of Ocular Complications of AIDS Research Group in collaboration with the AIDS Clinical Trials Group. Combination foscarnet and ganciclovir therapy vs. monotherapy for the treatment of relapsed cytomegalovirus retinitis in patients with AIDS. *Arch Ophthalmol* 1996;114:23–33.

119. Jacobson MA, O'Donnell JJ, Brodie HR, et al. Randomized prospective trial of ganciclovir maintenance therapy for cytomegalovirus retinitis. *J Med Virol* 1988;25:436–440.

120. Spector SA, McKinley GF, Lalezari JP, et al. Oral ganciclovir for the prevention of cytomegalovirus diseae in persons with AIDS. *N Engl J Med* 1996;334: 1491–1497.

121. Inderlied CB, Kemper CA, Bermudez LEM. The *Mycobacterium avium* complex. *Clin Microbiol Rev* 1993;6:266–310.

122. Hoyt L, Oleske J, Holland B, et al. Nontuberculous mycobacteria in children with acquired immunodeficiency syndrome. *Pediatr Infect Dis J* 1992;11: 354–360.

123. Rutstein RM, Cobb P, McGowan KL, et al. *Mycobacterium avium intracellulare* complex infection in HIV-infected children. *AIDS* 1993;7:507–512.

124. Horsburgh CR Jr, Caldwell MB, Simons RJ. Epidemiology of disseminated nontuberculous mycobacterial disease in children with acquired immunodeficiency syndrome. *Pediatr Infect Dis J* 1993;12:219–222.

125. Lindegren ML, Hanson C, Saletan S, et al. *Mycobacterium avium* complex (MAC) in children with AIDS, United States: need for specific prophylaxis guidelines for children less than 6-years-old [abstract We.B.420]. *XI International Conference on AIDS,* Vancouver, Canada, July 7–12, 1996;11:27.

126. Aberg JA, Yajko DM, Jacobson MA. Eradication of AIDS-related disseminated *Mycobacterium avium* complex infection after 12 months of antimycobacterial therapy combined with highly active antiretroviral therapy. *J Infect Dis* 1998;178:1446–1449.

127. Shafran SD, Talbot JA, Chomyc S, et al. Does *in vitro* susceptibility to rifabutin and ethambutol predict the response to treatment of *Mycobacterium avium* complex bacteremia with rifabutin, ethambutol, and clarithromycin? *Clin Infect Dis* 1998;27:1401–1405.

128. Hoy J, Mijch A, Sandland M, et al. Quadruple-drug therapy for *Mycobacterium avium-intracellulare* bacteremia in AIDS patients. *J Infect Dis* 1990;161: 801–805.

129. Chaisson RE, Benson CA, Dube MP, et al. Clarithromycin therapy for bacteremic *Mycobacterium avium* complex disease: a randomized, double-blind, dose-ranging study in patients with AIDS. *Ann Intern Med* 1994;121:905–911.

130. Ward TT, Rimland D, Kauffman C, et al. Randomized, open-label trial of azithromycin plus ethambutol vs. clarithromycin plus ethambutol as therapy for *Mycobacterium avium* complex bacteremia in patients with human immunodeficiency virus infection. *Clin Infect Dis* 1998;27:1278–1285.

131. Benson CA. Treatment of disseminated disease due to the *Mycobacterium avium* complex in patients with AIDS. *Clin Infect Dis* 1994;18[Suppl 3]:S237–S242.

132. Race EM, Adelson-Mitty J, Kriegel G, et al. Focal mycobacterial lymphadenitis following initiation of protease-inhibitor therapy in patients with advanced HIV-1 disease. *Lancet* 1998;351:252–255.

133. Nightingale SD, Camaron DW, Gordin FM, et al. Two controlled trials of rifabutin prophylaxis against *Mycobacterium avium* complex infection in AIDS. *N Engl J Med* 1993;329:828–833.

134. Pierce M, Crampton S, Henry D, et al. A randomized trial of clarithromycin as prophylaxis against disseminated *Mycobacterium avium* complex infection in patients with advanced acquired immunodeficiency syndrome. *N Engl J Med* 1996;335:384–391.

135. Havlir DV, Dube MP, Sattler FR, et al. Prophylaxis against disseminated *Mycobacterium avium* complex with weekly azithromycin, daily rifabutin, or both. *N Engl J Med* 1996;335:392–398.

136. Cordell RL, Addiss DG. Cryptosporidiosis in child care settings: a review of the literature and recommendations for prevention and control. *Pediatr Infect Dis J* 1994;13:310–317.

137. Flanigan T, Whalen C, Turner J, et al. Cryptosporidium infection and CD4 counts. *Ann Intern Med* 1992;116: 840–842.

138. Cello JP. Acquired immunodeficiency syndrome cholangiopathy: spectrum of disease. *Am J Med* 1989; 86:539–546.

139. Holmberg SD, Moorman AC, Von Bargen JC, et al. Possible effectiveness of clarithromycin and rifabutin for cryptosporidiosis chemoprophylaxis in HIV disease. *JAMA* 1998;279:384–386.

140. Cook DJ, Kelton JG, Stannosis AM, et al. Somatostatin treatment of cryptosporidial diarrhea in a patient with the acquired immunodeficiency syndrome. *Ann Intern Med* 1988;108:708–709.

141. Tzipori S, Roberton D, Chapman D. Remission of diarrhea due to cryptosporidiosis in an immunodeficient child treated with hyperimmune bovine colostrum. *BMJ* 1986;293:1276–1277.

142. Borowitz SM, Saulsbury FT. Treatment of chronic cryptosporidial infection with orally administered human serum immune globulin. *J Pediatr* 1991;119: 593–595.

143. Scaglia M, Atzori C, Marchetti G, et al. Effectiveness of aminosidine (paromomycin) sulfate in chronic *Cryptosporidium* diarrhea in AIDS patients: an open, uncontrolled, prospective clinical trial. *J Infect Dis* 1994;170:1349–1350.

144. White AC, Chappell CL, Hayat CS, et al. Paromomycin for cryptosporidiosis in AIDS: a prospective, double blind trial. *J Infect Dis* 1994;170:419–424.

145. Carr A, Marriott D, Field A, et al. Treatment of HIV-1 associated microsporidiosis and cryptosporidiosis with combination antiretroviral therapy. *Lancet* 1998; 351:256–261.

145a. American Academy of Pediatrics, Committee on Infectious Diseases. Policy statement: recommendations for the prevention of pneumococcal infections, including the use of pneumococcal conjugate vaccine (Prevnar), pneumococcal polysaccharide vaccine, and antibiotic prophylaxis. *Pediatrics* 2000;106: 362–366.

146. Levin M, Gershon A, Weinberg A, et al. Administration of varicella vaccine to HIV-infected children [Abstract 440]. *Sixth Conference on Retroviruses and Opportunistic Infections,* Chicago, January 31–February 4, 1999:150.

147. Arpadi SM, Markowitz LE, Baughman AL, et al. Measles antibody in vaccinated human immunodeficiency virus type 1-infected children. *Pediatrics* 1996;97:653–657.

148. Peters VB, Diamant EP, Hodes DS, et al. Impaired immunity to pneumococcal polysaccharide antigens in children with human immunodeficiency virus infection immunized with pneumococcal vaccine. *Pediatr Infect Dis J* 1994;13:933–934.

149. Centers for Disease Control and Prevention. Update: vaccine side effects, adverse reactions, contraindications, and precautions. Recommendations of the Advisory Committee on Immunization Practices (ACIP). *MMWR Morb Mortal Wkly Rep* 1996;45(RR-12):1–32.

4

Congenital Immunodeficiencies

Imelda Celine Hanson

Department of Pediatrics, Baylor College of Medicine, Houston, Texas 77030

Technologic advances in molecular genetics have enabled clinicians to identify a growing number of the congenital (primary) immune deficiencies by prenatal or immediate postnatal testing (1–3). However, most primary immune deficiencies continue to be identified by clinical presentation with unusual infections or infections with microorganisms of low pathogenicity in the immune-competent host. In this review, congenital immunodeficiencies (B-lymphocyte defects, T-lymphocyte defects, combined B- and T-lymphocyte syndromes, granulocyte defects, and complement deficiencies) and their presenting infectious complications are reviewed.

B-CELL DEFICIENCIES

B-lymphocyte cells produce five immunoglobulin classes, and primary deficiencies have been described in all (IgM, IgA, IgG, IgD, and IgE). Specific antibody production plays an important role in affording protection against invading organisms. Specific immunoglobulin synthesis and secretion occurs after exposure of antigen to B lymphocytes presented by antigen-presenting cells of the immune system (e.g., monocytes, macrophages). Immunoglobulin linked with antigen can initiate antigen elimination through Fc receptor interactions with phagocytes producing ingestion and killing, through activation of antibody-dependent cytotoxicity

of T lymphocytes or natural killer (NK) cells, and through lysis of invading antigens (microorganisms) by activation of the classic complement cascade (4). All classes of immunoglobulin exist in circulating peripheral blood. IgA plays a prominent role in mucosal immunity by protecting against invading agents at gastrointestinal, respiratory, and genitourinary surfaces.

Antibody deficiency makes up about 50% of all congenital immunodeficiencies. Their incidences in the general population are reported as frequent to rare. IgA deficiency has been reported in as many as 1 in every 200 individuals. In contrast, X-linked hypogammaglobulinemia is reported in 1 of every 100,000 live births (5). This chapter reviews common infectious complications of the following B-lymphocyte defects: X-linked agammaglobulinemia (X-LA, Bruton's agammaglobulinemia), common variable immune deficiency (CVID), selective IgA deficiency, and IgG subclass deficiencies.

X-Linked Agammaglobulinemia

X-LA is an X-linked disease affecting male patients. The molecular defect is a lack of cytoplasmic Bruton's tyrosine kinase (Btk), which results in arrest of maturation of B lymphocytes and absence of circulating and tissue CD19+ and CD20+ B lymphocytes (6). T-lymphocyte function is preserved in these young infants. Clinical illness usually begins at 4 to 6 months of life, when passively acquired (transplacental) circulating maternal antibodies wane. For a subset of patients, presenting clinical illness may be accompanied by neutropenia (1 week in duration); associated pathogens include *Staphylococcus aureus* and *Pseudomonas* sp. (7). Presentations include serious bacterial infections such as sinopulmonary disease, meningitis, septicemia, diarrheal illnesses, and septic arthritis (8). Sinopulmonary disease has been described with as many as 1.0 pneumonias per treatment year in a small cohort of X-LA patients with 12.5 years of follow up; predictors of improved pulmonary outcome included early diagnosis and compliance with gamma globulin replacement and oral antibiotic therapy. Respiratory pathogens isolated from bronchoalveolar lavage and biopsies in asymptomatic X-LA infants were more likely to be bacterial (*Haemophilus influenzae* predominated) rather than viral (9). Other pathogens implicated in clinical disease include *Streptococcus pneumoniae* and *Mycoplasma* (10).

Gastrointestinal illnesses in X-LA include the pathogens *Giardia lamblia, Salmonella* spp., and rotavirus (11). Viral infections in X-LA are primarily linked with central nervous system (CNS) disease but have also been described as causes of exudative enteropathy and arthritis. Enteroviruses have been identified with greater incidence in hypogammaglobulinemic patients, specifically vaccine-associated poliomyelitis and chronic enteroviral meningoencephalitis (12,13). The impact of the latter infection can be devastating, with persistent encephalopathy and identification of virus isolation from spinal fluid despite aggressive therapy including antiviral therapy and intraventricular immunoglobulin. Aggressive and early antimicrobial treatment of infections in patients with X-LA, combined with monthly administration of intravenous immunoglobulin (IVIG)—400 to 600 mg per kilogram per month to sustain serum IgG levels higher than 500 mg/dL—are the mainstay of current therapy and are effective in reducing bacter-

ial infections and pulmonary insufficiency (14). Past use of IVIG has been associated with some iatrogenic infections, specifically hepatitis C virus (HCV) infection (15). Careful attention to IVIG preparation has diminished the likelihood that further HCV or other known viral infections will be transmitted through aggressive IVIG therapy. As in all patients with antibody deficiencies, aggressive search for infection is necessary and relies heavily on the actual detection of the pathogen and not on serologic responses (enzyme immunoassays and IgG, IgA, or IgM tests). Tissue- or blood-specific microbial staining, culture, or polymerase chain reaction (PCR) assay is imperative to identify pathogens in these patients.

Avoidance of live viral vaccines is important in this antibody disorder, because neutralizing antibody plays an important role in prevention of some viral illnesses. This is particularly true of poliovirus. Risk for vaccine-associated paralytic poliovirus is 20,000 times greater in X-LA patients than in the general population. The shift in the childhood vaccine schedule to inactivated poliovirus vaccine delivery should diminish the likelihood that paralytic polio will continue to affect patients with X-LA.

Common Variable Immunodeficiency

The term CVID is applied to a group of disorders that probably represent varied alterations to B-cell development. Findings suggest that upregulation of interleukin-12 (IL-12) production leads to dysregulation of the IL-12/interferon-γ (IFN-γ) circuit, which may be responsible for downregulation of antibody production (16). Other studies suggest that a subset of CVID patients have impaired B-cell protein tyrosine phosphorylation representing a signal transduction defect (17). This disorder is more commonly reported in the second or third decade of life, although patients younger than 5 years old have been described (18). For some CVID patients, Epstein-Barr virus (EBV) has been implicated as the heralding event that triggers development of the immune deficiency (19). Immunologically, these individuals lack evidence of circulating antibody, specifically IgG, IgA, and IgM. In contrast to patients with X-LA, these male and female patients have evidence of circulating mature B lymphocytes (normal numbers and/or percentages of CD19+ and CD20+ lymphocytes). Those patients with the lowest circulating B-cell numbers and serum immunoglobulin levels appear to have the worst clinical prognosis. T-cell function is variably affected (approximately 40% of patients affected). All patients have recurrent sinopulmonary disease (bronchitis, sinusitis, otitis, pneumonia). Chronic sinusitis in these patients is often refractory to traditional oral antimicrobial therapy, and linkage with aggressive surgical intervention is necessary (20). Common sinopulmonary pathogens include *H. influenzae, S. pneumoniae,* and anaerobes. Pathogens associated with bronchiectasis in CVID include adenovirus, CMV, and rhinoviruses (9). Noninfectious causes of pulmonary disease include lymphoid interstitial pneumonitis, which is responsive to antiinflammatory therapy.

Other clinical presentations include autoimmune phenomena (arthritis, inflammatory bowel disease, granulomatous skin or gastrointestinal changes), meningitis, infectious arthritis, and exudative enteropathy. CNS disease (i.e., meningoencephalitis) has already been described for X-LA patients. Bowel disease includes infectious causes, namely *G. lamblia, Salmonella* spp., and viral causes. In addition, celiac sprue has been described in patients with CVID (21). Infectious arthritis has been associated with *Mycoplasma* and *Ureaplasma* infections in CVID patients, representing more than 40% of all identified pathogens in joints (22). Fungal (*Penicillium marneffei*) erosive arthritis was described in one child with CVID (23).

Treatment for CVID mirrors that previously outlined for X-LA. However, because CVID patients may have abnormalities of T-cell function, additional coverage for *Pneumocystis carinii* pneumonia (PCP) with trimethoprim-sulfamethoxazole (TMP/SMX)

prophylaxis is often offered at 5 mg per kilogram per dose, given twice daily for three consecutive days or on alternating days (24). Additionally, the use of prophylactic antibiotics for pulmonary disease, specifically chronic bronchiectasis, is not uncommon. Therapy is usually offered based on sensitivities of cultured pathogens from the lower respiratory tract obtained through bronchoscopy or induced sputum production.

Selective Immunoglobulin A Deficiency

Selective IgA deficiency is the most common of primary immune deficiencies. Immune definition of selective IgA deficiency is a serum IgA level of less than 10 mg/dL and no evidence of any accompanying immune defects (T-lymphocyte, B-lymphocyte, complement, or phagocytic disorders). Sporadic and familial cases are reported in the literature; progression of selective IgA deficiency to CVID has been described (25). The specific defect in patients with selective IgA deficiency is unknown. However, studies have shown that addition of IL-4 and IL-10 to IgA-deficient B cells can restore IgA levels to normal *in vitro* (26). Acquired IgA deficiency has been described with the use of certain drugs, specifically anticonvulsants. Many individuals with selective IgA deficiency are asymptomatic; symptomatic individuals have a clinical disease presentation consistent with deficient mucosal immunity: absent IgA at mucosal surfaces (27). Sinopulmonary disease is the hallmark of symptomatic presentation (28). Common pathogens include *S. pneumoniae, H. influenzae,* and *Moraxella catarrhalis.* Other less frequent bacterial species include group A streptococcus, group C streptococcus, viridans streptococci, *Peptostreptococcus* sp., other *Moraxella* species and *Eikenella corrodens.* Anaerobic infection is not common, but fungal infections, specifically sinusitis, may be found. Treatment for selective IgA deficiency includes aggressive antimicrobial therapy for identified pathogens. Unlike the patient with X-LA or CVID, the patient with selective IgA deficiency can mount an IgG and IgM response to pathogens; for this reason, serology and culture or PCR results are helpful in diagnosis. Replacement of IgA with exogenous pooled human IgA is limited by its short half-life and its relatively low distribution in peripheral blood compared with IgG.

Noninfectious complications of selective IgA deficiency include autoimmune disease (celiac disease, hypothyroidism, systemic lupus erythematosus (SLE), Sjögren's syndrome, immune thrombocytopenia). The incidence of selective IgA deficiency in celiac disease has been reported to be almost 2% (29). Vasculitis has also been described either in association with known autoimmune diseases (rheumatoid arthritis or SLE) or as a selective finding (30). Defective mucosal immunity predisposes patients with selective IgA deficiency to some increased incidence of food intolerances and allergic rhinitis. Absent IgA deficiency has been associated with transfusion reactions but is a rare event, occurring 1 in 20,000 to 47,000 transfusions (31). No clear predictor of transfusion reaction has been identified. All IgA-deficient patients and their health care providers should be aware of the potential risk of anaphylaxis with transfusions.

Immunoglobulin G Subclass Deficiency Syndrome

IgG subclass deficiency syndrome has been described in isolation and in association with IgA depression (10% of IgA deficiencies). IgG as distributed in peripheral blood is divided into four subcategories: IgG1, IgG2, IgG3, and IgG4. The clinical significance of these deficiencies continues to be controversial. IgG1 deficiency is most often associated with additional immune defects, such as CVID. IgG2 has been demonstrated as an isolated event and in association with IgG4 deficiency. IgG3 deficiency is relatively rare but has been associated with viral lung disease. IgG4 deficiency may represent a variant of the normal population (approximately 10%) or may be associated with pulmonary illness.

Associated clinical diseases include sinopulmonary diseases (otitis, sinusitis, and pneumonia). Severity of clinical presentation has been associated with poor antibody response to encapsulated organism challenge, specifically pneumococcal and *H. influenzae* antibody production (32). Treatment has included the use of antimicrobial agents targeting specific microorganisms (TMP/SMX, ampicillin, or amoxicillin clavulanate). Replacement therapy with IVIG has been suggested for patients with both abnormalities of IgG subclass levels and evidence of functional hypogammaglobulinemia, specifically for responses to polysaccharide antigens. Subclass abnormalities have been suspected in association with childhood asthma. Two European studies were unable to identify a significant association of IgG subclass deficiency in infants with asthma or persistent wheezing (33,34).

CELLULAR DEFECTS

In general, T-lymphocyte defects are associated with very poor prognosis without transplantation intervention. Stem cells traverse through the thymus and commit to T-lymphocyte lineages. T lymphocytes work alone or in concert with B lymphocytes to eradicate foreign antigens and pathogens. Their byproducts, interleukins and chemokines, are responsible for and integral to the development and proliferation of the immune repertoire. Great strides in the molecular genetics of primary T-cell defects have been made in the past decade. Primary deficiencies discussed here include DiGeorge syndrome, severe combined immunodeficiency (SCID), ataxia-telangiectasia (AT), and Wiskott-Aldrich syndrome (WAS). Patients with these disorders are afflicted not only with overwhelming infections but also with transfusion risks of graft-versus-host disease and malignancy, because normal T-cell protection is aberrant.

DiGeorge Syndrome

The DiGeorge syndrome is considered the prototypical T-lymphocyte defect, because associated B-cell defects are exceedingly rare. In this congenital disorder, the heart, parathyroid glands, and thymus are affected. Thymic hypoplasia/aplasia leads to absent response of circulating T lymphocytes to mitogen (phytohemagglutin A) and antigen stimulation, which persists without transplant intervention (35). Deletions in the chromosome region of 22q11 have been identified with the DiGeorge syndrome as well as with velocardiofacial syndrome and conotruncal anomaly face syndrome (36). Clinical presentation of DiGeorge syndrome is early in life (days after birth) and is usually not related to infectious complications but rather to congenital heart disease (e.g., murmur, cyanosis) or to hypocalcemia, including frank seizures, from parathyroid dysfunction. Infectious complications include recurrent pneumonia complicated by congenital heart disease. Pulmonary pathogens have included *P. carinii,* bacteria (*H. influenzae, Streptococcus* sp., *Mycobacteria tuberculosis*) and fungi (*Aspergillus, Candida*), as well as significant viral illnesses (37). Resultant pulmonary complications include bronchiolitis obliterans and lymphoid interstitial pneumonia. Almost all tissues (gastrointestinal, genitourinary, lung, bone marrow) have been affected by viral infections in DiGeorge syndrome. The infectious agents include rotavirus, astrovirus, cytomegalovirus (CMV), adenovirus, EBV (especially in association with malignancies), and human herpes viruses (38,39).

Management of the patient with DiGeorge syndrome includes correction of parathyroid abnormalities to prevent seizures, therapy for congenital heart disease to maximize cardiac output and decrease congestive heart failure (including both medical and surgical interventions), and augmentation of the immune system. Transplantation with stem cells and thymus tissue in the complete syndrome has been successful in restoring immune function. Success in immunorestoration is best predicted when transplantation occurs early in the clinical course, before development of serious sequelae of infectious processes (40). Prevention strategies to reduce infectious complications of DiGeorge syndrome and other cellular deficiencies include provision of PCP prophylaxis and delivery of passive immunization with specific immunoglobulin (e.g., hepatitis, measles, CMV, varicella) when exposures are identified in a timely fashion. Other prevention strategies include delivery of blood products that are irradiated, CMV negative, and/or leukocyte reduced (to reduce the risk graft-versus-host reactions) and avoidance of live viral vaccines.

Severe Combined Immunodeficiency

SCID now describes more than 10 genetic defects manifesting in a similar clinical fashion. Patterns of inheritance include X-linked recessive defects of the IL-2 receptor γ chain, autosomal recessive disorders, and sporadic mutations (41,42). Boys are more often affected than girls, and the incidence is reported to be 1 in 200,000 live births. Variants of SCID have been associated with other disorders, including α_1-antitrypsin deficiency, red and white blood cell enzymatic defects (purine nucleoside phosphorylase deficiency, adenosine deaminase [ADA] deficiency), short-limbed dwarfism, and reticuloendothelial defects (Letterer-Siwe disease, Ommen's syndrome) (43).

The clinical manifestation of SCID is in early infancy and is most often associated with infectious complications and wasting. Pathogens include fungi (*Candida albicans*), viruses (adenovirus, CMV, EBV, rotavirus, and enteroviruses), and *P. carinii* (Table 4.1). Bacterial infections are not uncommon but usually manifest later, because passively acquired maternal antibodies provide some protection in early infancy. Nosocomial bacterial infections plague the hospitalized SCID patient, causing significant morbidity (e.g., central line sepsis, genitourinary infection). A typical clinical course for SCID includes oral thrush nonresponsive to traditional therapy (oral fungicides), progressive wasting, indolent cough, and diarrhea. For survivors, complications of infections can produce significant morbidity including bronchiolitis obliterans (PCP, CMV), blindness (CMV retinitis), and sensorineural hearing defects (44).

TABLE 4.1. *Common infections in severe combined immunodeficiency and other cell-mediated primary immunodeficiencies*

Bacterial
  Staphylococcus epidermidis
  Listeria monocytogenes
  Serratia sp.
  Pseudomonas sp.
Fungal
  Candida sp.
  Aspergillus sp.
Viral
  Cytomegalovirus
  Epstein-Barr virus
  Adenovirus
  Rotavirus
  Herpes viruses
Protozoa
  Pneumocystis carinii
  Toxoplasmosis gondii

Immunologic presentation is most often associated with lymphopenia and hypogammaglobulinemia. In infants with PCP as their presenting clinical illness, peripheral eosinophilia can confound early SCID diagnosis, with wasted infants believed to have an allergy to cow's milk until hypoxia is noted. Serum immunoglobulins are usually markedly depressed and show either no or limited response to antigen challenge (diphtheria, tetanus, blood group antigens). *In vitro* lymphoproliferative responses of T lymphocytes to mitogens (phytohemagglutunin, concanavalin A, pokeweed mitogen) or to specific antigens (e.g., *Candida,* tetanus) are markedly depressed or absent. Peripheral blood cell analysis for phenotyping differs by defect. For example, JAK3 deficiency is defined by low circulating CD8+ T lymphocytes. However, all patients have marked depression of circulating mature T lymphocytes (CD3+, CD2+). NK cells may be increased in some SCID patients; B-cell markers may show compensatory increase. Phenotypic differences have been reported to predict transplantation outcome; B cell–positive SCID infants fare better than B cell–negative SCID infants, with successful engraftment in 60% versus 35%, respectively (45).

In SCID, identification of infectious pathogens is made difficult because the anti-body response is usually absent, so serologic evidence for acute or past infection is often not helpful. In addition, most patients are immediately given replacement IVIG, and this confounds the use of diagnostic serologic tests. An aggressive search for infections includes evaluation of affected tissue (biopsy, bronchoscopy, endoscopy/colonoscopy) with staining (e.g., Gram, Geimsa, silver), culture, or PCR. This is necessary because empiric therapy is often unhelpful and may lead to significant sequelae (e.g., deafness, renal disease). Prevention strategies for infectious complications are not dissimilar to those described for the DiGeorge syndrome and include (a) TMP/SMX for PCP prophylaxis, (b) avoidance of live viral vaccines, (c) avoidance of direct contact with ill person, (d) fungal prophylaxis (e.g., nystatin for oral thrush), and (e) monthly IVIG (400 to 600 mg per kilogram per dose) until immune reconstitution is realized. The last treatment may be replaced by hyperimmuneglobulin for CMV when exposure is noted (i.e., CMV-seropositive bone marrow donor or mother). Length of therapy for CMV-specific immunoglobulin differs among centers. CMV pp65 antigenemia monitoring has been a helpful and cost-effective strategy for prevention of CMV disease (46). Other preventive strategies include use of irradiated, leukocyte-reduced, and/or CMV-negative blood products to reduce the risks of both graft-versus-host disease and CMV. Early treatment of CMV antigenemia in transplanted patients is recommended, although efficacy in prevention of fatal CMV disease is not clearly established (47).

Without medical intervention, death from infectious complications is likely in the first year of life for SCID infants. Therapeutic options include hematopoietic stem cell transplantation (histocompatible bone marrow transplantation [BMT], haploidentical BMT, matched unrelated donor marrow transplantation, fetal tissue transplantation, or umbilical cord blood transplantation) and gene therapy (48–50). Immune dysfunction in the subset of patients with ADA deficiency can be corrected with glycol-modified adenosine deaminase (PEG-ADA) even without transplantation or gene therapy interventions (51).

Wiskott-Aldrich Syndrome

WAS, first described in 1937, is an X-linked recessive disorder (chromosome Xp11.22) that manifests in infancy with eczema, microthrombocytopenia (bleeding), and recurrent infections (52). Immune dysfunction includes both T-lymphocyte abnormalities and B-lymphocyte defects and is linked with actin cytoskeleton abnormalities. Disorders of the WAS protein (WASP), which is responsible for signal transduction from the cell membrane to the actin cytoskeleton, translate into defects of cell motility and function. Specific immune abnormalities in this disorder include lymphopenia; lymphocyte depletion in the thymus, lymph nodes and marginal zone of the spleen; defective delayed hypersensitivity reactions; poor antibody responses to polysaccharide antigens; and abnormal serum IgA and IgG levels (marked elevation and depression, respectively) (53,54).

In a review of 301 cases, infection-related morbidity was reported in 59% of patients, followed by bleeding (27%) and malignancy (12%) (55). Infectious morbidity is related to recurrent pneumonias with and without sepsis. Implicated pathogens include CMV, *P. carinii*, varicella, herpesviruses, enteroviruses, and EBV. Skin infections are particularly bothersome, and commonly include *S. aureus, S. pneumoniae,* and molluscum contagiosum. Persistent sinusitis and otitis are common findings. Autoimmune manifestations have included hemolytic anemia, arthritis/arthralgias, colitis, and leukocytoclastic vasculitis.

Treatment options include provision of antibiotic and IVIG prophylaxis. Splenectomy may be useful in reducing the morbidity of microthrombocytopenia but has no effect on eczema or T- and B-lymphocyte function (56). Stem cell transplantation can correct immune defects and should be considered in younger patients with histocompatible donors. In a retrospective review of WAS patients (n = 26) who underwent BMT, excellent outcome of hu-

man leukocyte antigen (HLA)–matched BMT was shown (57). In children with severe sequelae of WAS (i.e., bleeding, sepsis, vasculitis), haploidentical BMT resulted in engraftment but long-term survivors were relatively few. Complications of the process included viral infections (CMV, EBV) and EBV-induced lymphoproliferative disorders. Untreated patients with WAS are at risk for malignancy, especially lymphomas (Hodgkin's and non-Hodgkin's).

Ataxia-Telangiectasia

AT is an autosomal recessive complex that includes cerebellar ataxia, telangiectases, variable combined-lymphocyte and cellular defects, radiosensitivity, and cancer predisposition (58). Identification of the ataxia-telangiectasia mutated (ATM) gene mutation on chromosome 11q22-23 for AT has provided great insight into cancer risk, specifically the breast cancer risk for heterozygotes. The ATM gene is thought to play a crucial role in signal transduction processes that regulate genetic recombination, apoptosis, and other cellular responses to DNA damage. Immunologic dysfunction is characterized by a defective IgG antibody response to polysaccharide antigens; the response to protein moieties often is normal (59). Serum IgA levels are usually depressed, and IgG2, IgG3, or both may also be diminished. Serum IgE may be absent. Thymic architecture in AT is markedly abnormal and resembles that of a fetal thymus. It is postulated that, in addition to elevated serum α-fetoprotein levels, thymic abnormalities reflect a defect in thymic tissue maturation.

The disorder manifests in the first years of life with ataxia and oculocutaneous abnormalities. Recurrent infections with sinusitis, pneumonia, and bronchiectasis occur later in childhood. These infections often are related to progressive neurologic dysfunction, including oropharyngeal dysphagia and aspiration (60). Common pathogens include *H. influenzae, S. pneumoniae, Enterococcus, Pseudomonas* spp., and anaerobes. In contrast to patients with other primary immunodeficiencies, AT patients rarely succumb to opportunistic infections. Mortality occurs primarily as progression of neurologic disease, with aspiration pneumonia and progressive pulmonary failure or occurrence of malignancy. In mouse AT models, ATM mutations show a marked apoptosis defect induced by genomic stress (i.e., ATM functions to dispose of neurons with excessive genomic damage). ATM mutations may be responsible for CNS abnormalities or ionizing sensitivity after irradiation (61). AT patients often present with poorly differentiated oncologic processes that respond poorly to conventional therapy. Reported malignancies include non-Hodgkin's lymphoma (CNS, thorax, bone), poorly differentiated Hodgkin's lymphoma, and T-cell acute lymphoid leukemia (62). B-cell tumors are rare in AT patients. Treatment is supportive and includes aggressive and often prolonged use of antimicrobials for identified infections. IVIG may be used for prophylaxis in patients with functional hypogammaglobulinemia, but this therapy does not affect the morbidity from progressive neurologic dysfunction.

PHAGOCYTIC DEFECTS

Circulating phagocytic cells include polymorphonuclear leukocytes, macrophages, monocytes, and eosinophils. The polymorphonuclear leukocyte (PMN) is the most abundant in the circulation and also the best characterized phagocyte. Like T and B lymphocytes, PMNs originate from stem cells that commit to myeloid lineage. PMN functions include chemotaxis, adhesion, aggregation, phagocytosis, respiratory burst activity, and bacterial killing. Several disorders of PMN function are outlined, including chronic granulomatous disease (CGD), leukocyte adhesion deficiency (LAD), and Chédiak-Higashi syndrome. Molecular defects associated with these disorders have been identified and, as with other primary immunodeficiencies, new technology has allowed for early detection.

Chronic Granulomatous Disease

CGD is an inherited immunodeficiency syndrome caused by a defect in nicotine adenine dinucleotide phosphate (NADPH) oxidase system that makes PMNs incapable of appropriate production of reactive oxygen metabolites. This renders the host susceptible to recurrent bacterial and fungal infections. The enzyme NADPH oxidase comprises membrane components (gp91phox and p22phox) and cytosolic components (p47phox, p67phox, and p40phox). GP91phox is encoded on the X chromosome, and 60% to 65% of all CGD patients have this NADPH subunit defect; p22phox, p47phox, and p67phox are all on different autosomal chromosomes (63).

Affected children have multisystem infections with sinopulmonary, gastrointestinal, lymphatic, skin, and genitourinary diseases, in order of prevalence. For example, sinopulmonary infections comprise almost 80% of all CGD infections and are the most likely to be associated with mortality. Pulmonary manifestations include bronchopneumonia, empyema, suppuration of hilar lymph nodes, and lung abscesses. Chronic sinusitis is a common finding. Hepatic and perihepatic abscesses, although less frequently encountered (50% of all CGD patients) than pulmonary disease in CGD, are identified far more frequently in CGD than in the general population (64). Clinical presentation of hepatic abscesses includes prolonged fever and malaise. Aggressive evaluation with abdominal cavity imaging (i.e., ultrasound), nuclear imaging (computed tomography, magnetic resonance imaging) and plain films may be helpful in identifying abscesses in the almost universal absence of symptoms of abdominal pain.

Osteomyelitis occurs in more than 33% of all CGD patients. Unlike bony infections of the immunocompetent host, osteomyelitis in CGD patients involves small bones of the hands and feet. Other infectious complications of CGD include periodontal disease, urinary tract infections, and skin disease (furuncles, erthyroderma, and rectal abscesses).

Noninfectious complications of CGD include granuloma formation causing obstruction of hollow lumens (gastrointestinal obstruction with gastric outlet lesions, pulmonary obstructive lesions with laryngeal or bronchial lesions, genitourinary obstructive lesions), which can lead to secondary infectious complications. Chorioretinal lesions have also been described in CGD patients, although visual disturbance is not always associated with these lesions (65). Patients with CGD may have associated McLeod syndrome, absence of a red-blood-cell Kell antigen, and should be screened before transfusion (66). The locus for the McLeod syndrome defect has been mapped to a region between the loci for muscular dystrophy and CGD, Xp21. Sensitization by repeated transfusion of Kell-negative individuals can cause a profound hemolytic anemia.

Catalase-positive organisms are the predominate cause of infectious complications in CGD (Table 4.2). Catalase-negative organisms (e.g., *S. pneumoniae*) are less likely to cause disease, owing to their inability to clear endogenous bacterial oxygen metabolites. *S. aureus* is the most prevalent infectious pathogen in CGD, and antimicrobial prophylaxis is directed toward this pathogen. TMP/SMX, dicloxacillin, and rifampin have all been used as antimicrobial prophylactic agents for children with CGD or other white blood cell disorders. Staphylococcal disease has been reported in all organ systems (i.e., skin, gastrointestinal tract, genitourinary tract, and respiratory tract).

TABLE 4.2. *Common pathogens in chronic granulomatous disease*

Bacteria
  Aerobes
    Staphylococcus aureus
    Pseudomonas cepacia
    Klebsiella sp.
    Escherichia coli
    Serratia marcescens
    Salmonella sp.
    Listeria sp.
    Mycobacteria sp.
  Anaerobes
    Chromobacterium sp.
    Clostridium sp.
Fungal
  Aspergillus fumigatus
  Aspergillus spp.
  Candida spp.
Viral
  Varicella-zoster virus
  Herpes simplex virus
  Picornavirus

Treatment for staphylococcal disease is the same as in the immunocompetent host, with provision of antibiotics that are least expensive, most palatable, with the least serious sequelae but the greatest sensitivity to the identified pathogen. In closed-space diseases such as sinusitis or abscesses/empyemas, surgical intervention with drainage, excision, or both is an adjunctive and important curative measure. In a review of 10 patients with CGD, the average number surgical interventions for infectious complications was 2.9 procedures per child (67). The appropriate and early use of radiographic interventions to exclude bony involvement is prudent in this cohort. Cutaneous staphylococcal disease is often refractory to standard intervals of oral antimicrobial therapy. Length of therapy in CGD patients is predicted by documented downward changes in markers of inflammation (C-reactive protein, erythrocyte sedimentation rate) and diminished tissue involvement. Cutaneous lesions may be superinfected with fungal pathogens. The addition of scrapings for fungal pathogens can assist with clearance of cutaneous lesions. Aggressive wound care with or without debridement is helpful for cutaneous lesions, especially perirectal abscesses. Often stool softeners are necessary, not only to minimize pain but also to assist with more rapid cutaneous healing.

Other bacterial causes of infection in CGD include gram-negative organisms such as *Serratia marcescens, Escherichia coli, Salmonella* sp., *Legionella* sp., *Mycobacteria* sp., *Burkholderia gladioli,* and *Klebsiella* sp. Disseminated tuberculosis has been documented after bacille Calmette-Guérin immunization in CGD patients (68). *Pseudomonas cepacia,* but not *Pseudomonas aeroginosa,* can cause disease in CGD patients. This is a curious finding, because both organisms are catalase positive. Studies of *Pseudomonas* species killing by CGD PMNs indicate that *P. cepacia* is resistant to neutrophil-mediated nonoxidative bactericidal effects of the PMNs and therefore produces significant disease (69) *P. cepacia* is often a devastating illness in CGD patients because it may not be covered by the broad-spectrum antibiotics used for traditional gram-negative disease (i.e., ticarcillin, gentamicin, amikacin).

Anaerobes are increasingly documented in patients with CGD and include *Chromobacterium* and *Clostridium* species. Nocardiosis and actinomycoses are particularly problematic for CGD patients, because their identification can be significantly delayed and ongoing local inflammatory responses may lead to necrotizing destruction of affected tissue. Resistant strains of *Nocardia* may cause particularly destructive pulmonary disease (70).

Fungal infections of CGD include *Aspergillus* spp., *Candida* spp., and *Scedosporium apiospermum* (71). Much like *Nocardia,* fungal infections can present significant therapeutic challenges, because even in the face of optimal antifungal coverage suppurative infection may progress with necrosis of affected tissue and/or drug toxicity may impede successful completion of therapy. *Aspergillus* pulmonary infection has been associated with significant recurrence in this population (e.g., 89% in children younger than 10 years of age). Standardized antifungal therapy includes amphoterocin B at standard doses but with extension of length of therapy by weeks. Length of therapy for fungal or bacterial infections is often empiric in CGD patients, balancing drug toxicity risk with that of pathogen recurrence. Liposomal amphoterocin B therapy is clearly indicated in the CGD patient with fungal disease and renal toxicity. *Candida* species are not common pathogens in CGD but have been reported to cause sepsis, hepatic abscesses, and meningitis.

Viral infections are not common in CGD patients. However, recurrent varicella-zoster has been described, but not with fatal outcome. Other phagocytic defects appear to have greater morbity from viral infection than CGD.

Prophylaxis for CGD patients, as mentioned earlier, includes long-term TMP/SMX use. This therapy has decreased the incidence of nonfungal infections from 7.1 to 2.4 per 100 patient-months in patients with autosomal CGD and from 15.8 to 6.9 per 100 patient-months for patients with X-linked CGD (72). Itraconazole prophylaxis for fungal infections has been proven to have efficacy in neutropenic or hematologic transplantation patients but is not routinely used in CGD with the exception of secondary prophylaxis (i.e., for patients with already documented systemic fungal disease) (73,74). Concerns in the CGD cohort center on breakthrough invasive fungal disease with low trough itraconazole levels, as described by Glasmacher in neutropenic patients receiving itraconazole prophylaxis (75).

Recombinant human interferon-γ (rIFNg) has been shown to reconstitute defective neutrophil function in CGD and to decrease morbidity from common pathogens (76). In an uncontrolled, open-label study of 28 patients, the use of rIFNg at a dose of 0.5 mg per square meter resulted in an increase in median infection-free time to 993 days (77). Leukocyte transfusions have been used in selected clinical situations with reported efficacy (78). These situations are usually when evidence of antimicrobial or antifungal treatment failure is suggested. Management of noninfectious granulomas in CGD includes use of antiinflammatory agents: corticosteroids for gastric outlet obstruction, sulfasalazine and cyclosporine for large bowel disease, and cholestyramine for gallbladder dysfunction (79).

Correction of CGD has been attempted with BMT in humans and with gene therapy in CGD mouse knockouts, with varying degrees of success (80,81). Best results in human BMT are with HLA-identical siblings.

Leukocyte Adhesion Deficiency

LAD, previously described as MAC-1 deficiency, involves a defect in the CD11/CD18 integrins, a series of related heterodimers involved in cell-matrix and cell-cell adhesion functions. These protein markers are present on progenitors of all myeloid and red blood cells (82). LAD is associated with an inability of neutrophils to bind to ligands on endothelium, which normally allows PMNs to leave the circulation and assist with tissue infection. Two types of LAD are described: LAD type I, with complete absence of CD11a/CD18 β_2-integrins, and LAD type II, which results from a generalized defect in fucose metabolism (83,84). In patients with complete absence of integrins, clinical severity is suggested to be worse and risk for fatality the highest. Exceptions to this association of clinical severity and integrin expression have been described.

Infectious sites are nonpurulent in LAD and eventually become necrotic because of poor wound healing. The disorder is characterized by markedly elevated circulating PMNs (more than 20,000 cells per microliter). Sites of infection include the abdominal wall (omphalitis in newborns), long skeletal muscles with nonpurulent cellulitis, gastrointestinal infections, cutaneous infections, and sepsis.

Pathogens include bacterial, fungal, and viral organisms. Recurrent varicella-zoster and herpes simplex viral infections have been associated with fatality in LAD type I. Correction of LAD has been described with BMT, with both HLA-identical sibling cord blood and unrelated matched donor blood, but successful engraftment is described in only small numbers of patients with LAD type I (85,86).

Chédiak-Higashi Syndrome

Chédiak-Higashi syndrome is an autosomal disorder characterized by variable degrees of oculocutaneous albinism, bleeding (platelet dense bodies), recurrent infections with neutropenia, impaired chemotaxis, and impaired NK cell function. The presence of cytoplasmic granules in circulating granulocytes is unique to this syndrome. In the mouse model for Chédiak-Higashi syndrome, a lyst gene has been identified that may have connection to the human LYST gene on chromosome 1q42; approximately 86% sequence homology has been determined for these genes (87). Clinical infections occur early in life and include impetigo, pyoderma, cellulitis, bronchitis, bronchopneumonia, recurrent sinusitis, and otitis media.

Noninfectious complications include neurologic abnormalities (peripheral neuropathy), platelet defects with bleeding, and exaggerated lymphoproliferative responses.

Pyogenic infections are the hallmark of Chédiak-Higashi syndrome, with more than 60% of all affected patients reporting febrile infections. *S. aureus* is a prominent pathogen in affected individuals. Other pathogens include group A β-hemolytic streptococcus, *H. influenzae, Shigella flexneri,* and *Klebsiella, Pseudomonas, Proteus, Aspergillus,* and *Candida* species. EBV infection has been linked with an accelerated lymphoma-like phase (88). Management of infections is supportive, with standardized therapeutic intervention for immunocompetent individuals applied. Chemoprophylaxis has no proven efficacy in Chédiak-Higashi syndrome.

Hyperimmunoglobulin E Syndrome

Hyperimmunoglobulin E syndrome (HIES), or Job's syndrome, is an autosomal dominant disorder with variable penetrance and clinical presentation of recurrent skin abscesses, pneumonia, bony and dental abnormalities, and elevated serum IgE concentrations. HIES has been linked to chromosome 4, specifically the proximal 4q region (89). Immune dysfunction in this disorder includes defective production of IFN-γ, which results in defective PMN chemotaxis and increased levels of IgE (90). This is postulated to be caused by lack of appropriate negative feedback in IL-4 production. In addition, inappropriate response of HIES B lymphocytes to IL-12 may result in specific anergy to antigens such as *S. aureus*.

In a study of 30 patients with HIES, nonimmunologic features of the disorder could be identified in all patients older than 8 years of age (91). Common findings included recurrent fractures (57% of HIES patients), hyperextensible joints (68%), and scoliosis (76% over 16 years). In this review, delayed shedding of primary teeth was identified in 72% of patients. The classic findings of cutaneous infections, pneumonia, and immunologic abnormalities occurred in 77% of those older than 8 years of age. Of 27 relatives at risk for HIES expression, only 10 had classic HIES; 6 had combinations of dental, bony, or immunologic abnormalities, and 11 were completely unaffected.

Pulmonary infections are the primary cause of significant morbidity and mortality in HIES. Common radiographic changes include bronchiectasis, empyema, blebs, and chronic perihilar infiltrates. Deep-seated infections (organ and skin abscesses, bacteremia, CNS infections, osteomyelitis, and endocarditis) are infrequently reported (92,93). In fact, soft tissue infections predominate, and bony involvement is rarely reported (94). Eczematous lesions may be prominent in HIES, and superinfection is a common occurrence. The soft tissue abscesses of HIES are often termed "cold abscesses" because of their lack of erythema or localized warmth (95). Other cutaneous findings include exaggerated wheal and flare responses after trauma, which are not related to infection. Lymphoma has been reported in HIES; persistent lymph node enlargement should prompt evaluation for oncologic processes.

Buckley (1972) described the universal presence of *S. aureus* infection in patients with HIES (96). Other described pathogens include *C. albicans, H. influenzae, Streptococcus* sp., *Aspergillus* spp., and miscellaneous gram-negative organisms. Impaired immune response, as outlined earlier (impaired chemotaxis and defective IL-12 production), predicts poor response to polysaccharides and clinical disease with these pathogens.

Clinical management of HIES has included prophylaxis for cutaneous infections and pneumonia with either TMP/SMX or dicloxacillin. Elucidation of immunologic defects in HIES has prompted study of IVIG prophylaxis for recurrent bacterial infections. It is likely that the *in vitro* finding of correction of IFN-γ production with recombinant IL-12 may prompt further evaluation of the role of IL-12 therapy in HIES.

COMPLEMENT DEFECTS

Protection against invading organisms depends on interactions of the various arms of the immune system: cell-mediated immunity, specific immunoglobulin synthesis, phagocytic functions, and an intact complement system. The complement system is often divided into an alternate pathway and a classic pathway, with both composed of proenzymes and molecules responsible for organism elimination. The classic pathway is activated by antigen-antibody complexes and uses the molecules of C1 through C9. The pathway for interaction includes recognition of the Fc receptor of immunoglobulins (IgG and IgM) on antigen-antibody complexes by C1q (one of three molecules—C1q, C1r, and C1s—that comprise C1). Binding of C1q to the antigen-antibody complex results in activation of the C1 complex and subsequent activation by C1s of C4 and C2, the next components in the activation cascade. Activated C4 and C2 fragments combine to form a C4b2b complex (C3 convertase), with resultant activation of the C3 molecule. Cleavage of C3 produces C3b, which fixes to the antigen-antibody complex through the antigen membrane and to C4b2b. This binding greatly enhances phagocytosis and enhances PMN clearance of antigen-antibody complexes. C5 is activated by the C3b and C4b2b complexes and fragments into C5a and C5b. C5a serves to promote recruitment of PMNs to the antigen-antibody complex site, increase tissue permeability, and enhance local edema. C5b binds with C6 and C7 to form a complex that binds to the antigenic membrane. This complex serves as a recruiter for C8 and C9 and the lytic C5–9 complex (membrane attack complex) is formed; this complex is responsible for antigen lysis via rapid influx of water and ions. This represents activation of the classic pathway of complement.

The classic pathway is dependent on antibody complexing. In the alternative pathway, C3 fixation occurs without antibody. Molecules involved in C3 fixation include factor B, factor I, and properidin. Polysaccharide antigens are potent stimulators of the alternative pathway. Defects of all molecules in the classic and alternative pathways have been described. This review focuses on complement deficiencies associated with serious infectious sequelae, namely C3 deficiency, lytic component (C5–9) deficiency, and factor I deficiency.

C3 deficiency has been reported in multiple ethnic groups and geographic areas in the world (97). Multiple mutations in C3 have been identified, including defects in C3 secretion and proenzyme defects (98). C3 deficiency is associated with membranoproliferative glomerulonephritis and with collagen vascular disease, but more commonly the patient presents clinically with recurrent pyogenic infections. Infections are usually severe and include meningococcal, gonococcal, and pneumococcal disease (pneumonia, bacteremia). Lytic complex (C5–9) deficiencies are associated with recurrent *Neisseria* infections. Unlike the more heterogenous presentation of C3 deficiency, C6 deficiency has been reported at highest incidence in blacks in the Southeastern United States, with the frequency approaching 1 in 1,600 in this population (99). Factor I deficiency is also known to be associated with pyogenic infections, including otitis, sinusitis, bronchopneumonia, meningitis, and bacteremia (100,101). Factor I deficiency has been linked to glomerulonephritis but not to collagen vascular disease.

Clinical management of the primary complement deficiencies is supportive. *Neisseria meningitidis* strains causing disease in complement deficiencies have not been proven to differ from those causing disease in the general population (102). Protection against meningococcal disease in complement-deficient patients may be afforded by vaccination with the tetravalent meningococcal capsular polysaccharide vaccine; revaccination should be offered every 3 years (103). The role of prophylactic antibiotics (penicillin) in prevention of recurrent neisserial disease is controversial.

In summary, the clinical management of infections in primary immunodeficiencies is not dissimilar within groupings of disorders, namely, B-lymphocyte defects, T-lymphocyte defects, phagocytic defects, and complement deficiencies. Great strides in molecular genetics have led to options for interventions, such as transplantation and gene therapy, that may provide total or incomplete correction of the underlying immune defect, thus eliminating the need to chronically manage infectious sequelae. Earlier detection of disease, especially prenatal diagnosis, offers great hope for curative intervention in these congenital disorders.

REFERENCES

1. Wengler GS, Parolini O, Fiorini M, et al. A PCR-based non-radioactive X-chromosome inactivation assay for genetic counseling in X-linked primary immunodeficiencies. *Life Sci* 1997;61:1405–1411.
2. Davidson A, Khandelwal M, Punnett HH. Prenatal diagnosis of the 22q11 deletion syndrome. *Prenat Diagn* 1997;17:380–383.
3. Touraine JL, Raudrant D, Laplace S, et al. Stem cell transplants *in utero* for genetic diseases: treatment and a model for induction of immunologic tolerance. *Transplant Proc* 1999;31:681–682.
4. Burton DR, Woof JM. Human antibody effector function. *Adv Immunol* 1992;51:1–84.
5. Lederman HM, Winkelstein JA. X-linked hypogammaglobulinemia. *J Infect* 1989;18:175–177.
6. Vihenen M, Vetrie D, Maniar HS, et al. Structural basis for chromosome X-linked agammaglobulinemia: a tyrosine kinase disease. *Proc Natl Acad Sci U S A* 1994;91:12803–12807.
7. Farrar JE, Rohrere J, Conley ME. Neutropenia in X-linked agammaglobulinemia. *Clin Immunol Immunopathol* 1996;81:271–276.
8. Sweinberg SK, Wodell RA, Grodofsky MP, et al. Retrospective analysis of the incidence of pulmonary disease in hypogammaglobulinemia. *J Allergy Clin Immunol* 1991;88:96–104.
9. Kainulainen L, Nikoskelainen J, Vuroinen T, et al. Viruses and bacteria in bronchial samples from patients with primary hypogammaglobulinemia. *Am J Respir Crit Care Med* 1999;159:1199–1204.
10. Roifman CM, Rao CP, Lederman HM, et al. Increased susceptibility to *Mycoplasma* infection in patients with hypogammaglobulinemia. *Am J Med* 1986;80:590–594.
11. LoGalbo PR, Sampson HA, Buckley RH. Symptomatic giardiasis in three patients with X-linked agammaglobulinemia. *J Pediatr* 1982;101:78–80.
12. Paralytic poliomyelitis—United States, 1980–1994. *MMWR Morb Mortal Wkly Rep* 1997;31:79–83.
13. Mishah SA, Spickett GP, Ryba PC, et al. Chronic enteroviral meningoencephalitis in agammaglobulinemia: a case report and literature review. *J Clin Immunol* 1992;12:266–270.
14. Quartier P, Debre M, DeBlic J, et al. Early and prolonged intravenous immunoglobulin replacement therapy in childhood agammaglobulinemia: a retrospective survey of 31 patients. *J Pediatr* 1999;134:589–596.
15. Quiti I, Pandolfi F, Pagnelli R, et al. HCV infection in patients with primary defects of immunoglobulin production. *Clin Exp Immunol* 1995;102:11–16.

16. Cambronero R, Sewell WA, North ME, et al. Up-regulation of IL-12 in monocytes: a fundamental defect in common variable immunodeficiency. *J Immunol* 2000; 164:488–494.

17. Schwartz R, Porat YB, Handzel Z, et al. Identification of a subset of common variable immunodeficiency patients with impaired B-cell tyrosine phosphorylation. *Clin Diagn Lab Immunol* 1999;6:856–860.

18. Cunningham-Rundles C, Bodian C. Common variable immunodeficiency: clinical and immunological features of 248 patients. *Clin Immunol* 1999;92:34–48.

19. Zucarro G, Della Bella S, Polizzi B, et al. Common variable immunodeficiency following Epstein-Barr virus infection. *J Clin Lab Immunol* 1997;49:41–45.

20. Buehring I, Friedrich B, Schaaf J, et al. Chronic sinusitis refractory to standard management in patients with humoral immunodeficiencies. *Clin Exp Immunol* 1997;109:468–472.

21. Heneghan MA, Stevens FM, Cryan EM, et al. Celiac sprue and immunodeficiency states: a 25-year review. *J Clin Gastroenterol* 1997;25:421–425.

22. Bonilla HF, Chenoweth CE, Tully JG, et al. *Mycoplasma felis* septic arthritis in a patient with hypogammaglobulinemia. *Clin Infect Dis* 1997;24:222–225.

23. Lin WC, Dai YS, Tsai MJ, et al. Systemic *Penicillium marneffei* infection in a child with common variable immunodeficiency. *J Formos Med Assoc* 1998;97: 780–783.

24. Hughes WT. *Pneumocystis* in infants and children. *N Engl J Med* 1995;333:320–321.

25. Vorechovsky I, Blennow E, Nordenskjold M, et al. A putative susceptibility locus on chromosome 18 is not a major contributor to human selective IgA deficiency: evidence from meiotic mapping of 83 multiple-case families. *J Immunol* 1999;163:2236–2240.

26. Marconi M, Plebani A, Avanzini MA, et al. IL-10 and IL-4 co-operate to normalize *in vitro* IgA production in IgA-deficient (IgAD) patients. *Clin Exp Immunol* 1998;112:528–532.

27. Lamm ME. Interaction of antigens and antibodies at mucosal surfaces. *Annu Rev Microbiol* 1997;51: 311–340.

28. Dacle JJ. Chronic sinusitis in children. *Acta Otorhinolaryngol Belg* 1997;51:285–304.

29. Cataldo F, Marino V, Bottaro G, et al. Celiac disease and selective immunoglobulin A deficiency. *J Pediatr* 1997;131:306–308.

30. Liu MF, Li JS, Tsao CJ, et al. Selective IgA deficiency with recurrent vasculitis of the central nervous system. *Clin Exp Rheumatol* 1998;16:77–79.

31. Sandler SG, Mallory D, Malamut D, et al. IgA anaphylactic transfusion reactions. *Transfus Med Rev* 1995;9:1–8.

32. French MA, Denis KA, Dawkins R, et al. Severity of infections in IgA deficiency: correlation with decreased serum antibodies to pneumococcal polysaccharides and decreased serum IgG2 and/or IgG4. *Clin Exp Immunol* 1995;100:47–53.

33. Hegel PH, Nigerian B, Header G. Age related IgG subclass concentrations in asthma. *Arch Dis Child* 1994;70:179–182.

34. Karma O, Eggs A, Uzuner N. Immunoglobulin G subclasses in wheezing infants. *Acta Paediatr Jpn* 1998; 40:564–566.

35. Markert ML, Hummell DS, Rosenblatt HM, et al. Complete DiGeorge syndrome: persistence of profound immunodeficiency. *J Pediatr* 1998;132:15–21.

36. Sergi C, Serpi M, Muller-Navia J, et al. Catch 22 syndrome: report of 7 infants with follow-up data and review of the recent advancements in the genetic knowledge of the locus 22q11. *Pathologica* 1999;91:166–172.

37. Deerojanawong J, Chang AV, Eng PA, et al. Pulmonary diseases in children with severe combined immunodeficiency and DiGeorge syndrome. *Pediatr Pulmonol* 1997;24:324–330.

38. Wood DJ, David TJ, Chrystie IL, et al. Chronic enteric virus infection in two T-cell immunodeficient children. *J Med Virol* 1988;24:435–444.

39. Ramos JT, Lopez-Laso E, Ruiz-Contreras J, et al. B cell non-Hodgkin's lymphoma in a girl with the DiGeorge anomaly. *Arch Dis Child* 1999;81:444–445.

40. Markert ML, Boech A, Hale LP, et al. Transplantation of thymus tissue in complete DiGeorge syndrome. *N Engl J Med* 1999;14:1180–1189.

41. Fugmann SD, Muller S, Friedrich W, et al. Mutations in the gene for the common gamma chain (gammac) in X-linked severe combined immunodeficiency. *Hum Genet* 1998;103:730–731.

42. Schumacher RF, Mella P, Lalatta F, et al. Prenatal diagnosis of JAK3 deficient SCID. *Prenat Diagn* 1999; 19:653–656.

43. Ommen GS. Familial reticuleoendotheliosis with eosinophilia. *N Engl J Med* 1963;273:427.

44. Baumal CR, Levin AV, Read SE. Cytomegalovirus retinitis in immunosuppressed children. *Am J Opthalmol* 1999;127:550–558.

45. Bertrand Y, Landais P, Friedrich W, et al. Influence of severe combined immunodeficiency phenotype on the outcome of HLA non-identical, T-cell-depleted bone marrow transplantation: a retrospective European survey from the European Group for Bone Marrow Transplantation and the European Society for Immunodeficiency. *J Pediatr* 1999;134:740–748.

46. Kusne S, Grossi P, Irish W, et al. Cytomegalovirus PP65 antigenemia monitoring as a guide for preemptive therapy: a cost effective strategy for prevention of cytomegalovirus disease in adult liver transplant recipients. *Transplantation* 1999;68:1125–1131.

47. Shimokawa T, Morishima Y, Kitaori K, et al. Early treatment of CMV antigenemia with ganciclovir for prevention of fatal CMV disease in patients receiving marrow from HLA-matched unrelated donors. *Int J Hematol* 1999;70:119–126.

48. Knutsen AP, Wall DA. Kinetics of T-cell development of umbilical cord blood transplantation in severe T-cell immunodeficiency disorders. *J Allergy Clin Immunol* 1999;103:823–832.

49. Buckley RH, Schiff SE, Schiff RL, et al. Hematopoietic stem-cell transplantation for the treatment of severe combined-immunodeficiency. *N Engl J Med* 1999;340:508–516.

50. Ondonera M, Nelson DM, Sakiyama Y, et al. Gene therapy for severe combined immunodeficiency caused by adenosine deaminase deficiency: improved retroviral vectors for clinical trials. *Acta Haematol* 1999;101:89–96.

51. Herschfield MS, Arredondo-Vega FX, Santisteban I. Clinical expression, genetics and therapy of adenosine deaminase (ADA) deficiency. *J Inherit Metab Dis* 1997;20:179–185.

52. Thrasher AJ, Burns S. Wiskott-Aldrich syndrome: a disorder of haematopoietic cytoskeletal regulation. *Microsc Res Tech* 1999;15:107–113.

53. Ochs HD. The Wiskott-Aldrich syndrome. *Semin Hematol* 1998;35:332–345.

54. Vermi W, Blanzuoli L, Kraus MD, et al. The spleen in the Wiskott-Aldrich syndrome: histopathologic abnormalities of the white pulp correlate with the clinical phenotype of the disease. *Am J Surg Pathol* 1999;23:182–191.

55. Perry GS, Spector BD, Schuman LM. The Wiskott-Aldrich syndrome in the United States and Canada (1892–1979). *J Pediatr* 1980;97:72.

56. Litzman J, Jones A, Hann I, et al. Intravenous immunoglobulin, splenectomy, and antibiotic prophylaxis in Wiskott-Aldrich syndrome. *Arch Dis Child* 1996;75:436–439.

57. Ozsahin H, LeDeist F, Benkerrou M, et al. Bone marrow transplantation in 26 patients with Wiskott-Aldrich syndrome from a single center. *J Pediatr* 1996;129:238–244.

58. Satisvsky K, Barr-Shira A, Gilad S, et al. A single ataxia telangiectasia gene with a product similar to PI-3 kinase. *Science* 1995;268:1749–1753.

59. Sanal O, Ersoy F, Yel J, et al. Impaired IgG antibody production to pneumococcal polysaccharides in patients with ataxia-telangiectasia. *J Clin Immunol* 1999;19:326–334.

60. Lefton-Grief MA, Crawford TO, Winkelstein JA, et al. Oropharyngeal dysphagia and aspiration in patients with ataxia-telangiectasia. *J Pediatr* 2000;135:225–231.

61. Chong MJ, Murray MR, Gosink EC, et al. Atm and bax cooperate in ionizing radiation-induced apoptosis in the central nervous system. *Proc Natl Acad Sci U S A* 2000;97:889–894.

62. Taylor AM, Metcalfe JA, Thick J, et al. Leukemia and lymphoma in ataxia telangiectasia. *Blood* 1996;87:423–428.

63. Meischl C, Roos D. The molecular basis of chronic granulomatous disease. *Springer Semin Immunopathol* 1998;19:417–434.

64. Anderson D. Infectious complications resulting from phagocytic cell dysfunction. In: Feigin RD, Cherry JD, eds. *Textbook of pediatric infectious diseases.* Philadelphia: Saunders, 1990:63–78.

65. Goldblatt D, Butcher J, Thrasher AJ, et al. Chorioretinal lesions in patients and carriers of chronic granulomatous disease. *J Pediatr* 1999;134:780–783.

66. Ho MF, Monaco AP, Blonden LA, et al. Fine mapping of the McLeod locus (XK) to a 150–380-kb region in Xp21. *Am J Hum Genet* 1992;50:317–320.

67. Eckert JW, Abramson SL, Starke J, et al. The surgical implications of chronic granulomatous disease. *Am J Surg* 1995;169:320–323.

68. Gonzalez B, Morena S, Curdach R. Clinical presentation of bacillus Calmette-Guérin infections in patients with immunodeficiency disorders. *Pediatr Infect Dis J* 1989;8:210.

69. Speert DP, Bond M, Woodman RC, et al. Infection with *Pseudomonas cepacia* in chronic granulomatous disease: role of nonoxidative killing by neutrophils in host defense. *J Infect Dis* 1994;170:1524–1531.

70. Shetty AK, Arvin AM, Gutierrez KM. *Nocardia farcinica* pneumonia in chronic granulomatous disease. *Pediatrics* 1999;104:961–964.

71. Jabado N, Casanova HL, Haddad E, et al. Invasive pulmonary infection due to *Scedosporium apiospermum* in two children with chronic granulomatous disease. *Clin Infect Dis* 1998;27:1437–1441.

72. Margolis DM, Melnick DA, Allikng DW, et al. Trimethoprim-sulfamethoxazole prophylaxis in the management of chronic granulomatous disease. *J Infect Dis* 1990;162:723–726.

73. Foot AB, Veys PA, Gibson BE. Itraconazole oral solution as antifungal prophylaxis in children undergoing stem cell transplantation or intensive chemotherapy for haematological disorders. *Bone Marrow Transplant* 1999;24:1089–1093.

74. Nucci M, Biasoli I, Akiti T, et al. A double-blind, randomized, placebo-controlled trial for itraconazole capsules as antifungal prophylaxis for neutropenic patients. *Clin Infect Dis* 2000;30:300–305.

75. Glasmacher A, Hahn C, Leutner C, et al. Breakthrough invasive fungal infections in neutropenic patients after prophylaxis with itraconazole. *Mycoses* 1999;42:443–451.

76. Sechler JM, Malech HL, White CJ, et al. Recombinant human interferon-gamma reconstitutes defective phagocyte function in patients with chronic granulomatous disease of childhood. *Proc Natl Acad Sci U S A* 1988;85:4874–4878.

77. Weening RS, Leitz GJ, Seger RA. Recombinant human interferon-gamma in patients with chronic granulomatous disease—European follow up study. *Eur J Pediatr* 1995;154:295–298.

78. Buckley RH. Immunodeficiency. *J Allergy Clin Immunol* 1983;72:627–631.

79. Barton LL, Moussa SL, Villar RG, et al. Gastrointestinal complications of chronic granulomatous disease: case report and literature review. *Clin Pediatr* 1998;37:231–236.

80. Malech HL. Progress in gene therapy for chronic granulomatous disease. *J Infect Dis* 1999;179:S318–325.

81. Leung T, Chik K, Li C, et al. Bone marrow transplantation for chronic granulomatous disease: long-term follow-up and review of literature. *Bone Marrow Transplant* 1999;24:567–570.

82. Mazzone A, Ricevuti G. Leukocyte CD11/CD18 integrins: biological and clinical relevance. *Haematologica* 1995;80:161–175.

83. Marquardt T, Brune T, Luhn K, et al. Leukocyte adhesion deficiency II syndrome, a generalized defect in fucose metabolism. *J Pediatr* 1999;134:681–688.

84. Hogg N, Stewart MP, Scarth SL, et al. A novel leukocyte adhesion deficiency caused by expressed but nonfunctional beta2 integrins Mac-1 and LFA-1. *J Clin Invest* 1999;103:97–106.

85. Mancias C, Infante AJ, Kamani NR. Matched unrelated donor bone marrow transplantation in leukocyte adhesion deficiency. *Bone Marrow Transplant* 1999;24:1261–1263.

86. Stary J, Bartunkova J, Kobylka P, et al. Successful HLA-identical sibling cord blood transplantation in a 6-year-old boy with leukocyte adhesion deficiency syndrome. *Bone Marrow Transplant* 1996;18:249–252.

87. Introne W, Boissy RE, Gahl WA. Clinical, molecular, and cell biological aspects of Chédiak-Higashi syndrome. *Mol Genet Metab* 1999;68:283–303.

88. Blume RS, Wolff SM. The Chédiak-Higashi syndrome studies in 4 patients and a review of the literature. *Medicine (Baltimore)* 1972;51:247–250.

89. Grimbacher B, Schaffer AA, Holland SM, et al. Genetic linkage of hyper-IgE syndrome to chromosome 4. *Am J Hum Genet* 1999;65:735–744.

90. Borges WG, Augustine NH, Hill HR. Defective interleukin-12/interferon-gamma pathway in patients with hyperimmunoglobulinemia E syndrome. *J Pediatr* 2000;136:176–180.

91. Grimbacher B, Holland SM, Gallin JI, et al. Hyper-IgE syndrome with recurrent infections: an autosomal dominant multisystem disorder. *N Engl J Med* 1999; 340:692–702.

92. Garty BZ, Wolach B, Ashkenazi S, et al. Cryptococcal meningitis in a child with hyperimmunoglobulin E syndrome. *Pediatr Allergy Immunol* 1995;6:175–177.

93. Yates AB, Mehrotra D, Moffit JE. *Candida* endocarditis in a child with hyperimmunoglobulinemia E syndrome. *J Allergy Clin Immunol* 1997;99:770–772.

94. Misago N, Tanaka T, Takeuchi M, et al. Necrotizing fasciitis in association with hyperimmunoglobulin E syndrome. *J Dermatol* 1995;22:673–676.

95. Hill HR. The syndrome of hyperimmunoglobulinemia E and recurrent infections. *Am J Dis Child* 1982;136: 767–771.

96. Buckley HR, Wray BB, Belmaker EZ. Extreme hyperimmunoglobulinemia E and undue susceptibility to infection. *Pediatrics* 1972;49:59–64.

97. Singer L, Colten HR, Wetsel RA. Complement C3 deficiency: human, animal, and experimental models. *Pathobiology* 1994;62:14–28.

98. Katz Y, Singer L, Wetsel RA, et al. Inherited complement C3 deficiency: a defect in C3 secretion. *Eur J Immunol* 1994;24:1517–1522.

99. Shu Z, Atkinson TP, Hovanky KT, et al. High prevalence of complement component C6 deficiency among African-Americans in the southeastern USA. *Clin Exp Immunol* 2000;119:305–310.

100. Vyse TJ, Spath PJ, Davies KA, et al. Hereditary complement factor I deficiency. *QJM* 1994;87: 385–401.

101. Sadallah S, Gudat F, Laissue JA, et al. Glomerulonephritis in a patient with complement factor I deficiency. *Am J Kidney Dis* 1999;33:1153–1157.

102. Fijen CA, Kuijper EJ, Dankert J, et al. Characterization of *Neisseria meningitidis* strains causing disease in complement-deficient and complement-sufficient patients. *J Clin Microbiol* 1998;36:2342–2345.

103. Fijen CA, Kuijper EJ, Drogari-Apiranthitou M, et al. Protection against meningococcal serogroup ACYW disease complement-deficient individuals vaccinated with the tetravalent meningococcal capsular polysaccharide vaccine. *Clin Exp Immunol* 1998;114: 362–369.

5

Management of Specific Infectious Complications in Children with Leukemias and Lymphomas

Andreas H. Groll, *Robert S. Irwin, †James W. Lee, ‡Philip A. Pizzo, and Thomas J. Walsh

*Immunocompromised Host Section, Pediatric Oncology Branch, National Cancer Institute, National Institutes of Health, Bethesda, Maryland 20819; *Department of Pediatrics, Madigan Army Medical Center, Tacoma, Washington 98431; †Department of Oncology, Deaconess Hospital, Evansville, Indiana 47713; and ‡Department of Medicine, Children's Hospital, Boston, Massachusetts 02115*

Childhood cancer is second only to accidents as the leading cause of death in children younger than 15 years of age. Of the 6,500 new cases diagnosed each year in the United States, leukemia and lymphoma constitute approximately 50%, followed by central nervous system (CNS) tumors (20%) and cancers of the sympathetic nervous system, soft tissues, kidney, bone, liver, eye, and germ cells. Enormous progress has been achieved in the treatment of these neoplasms, and more than half of these patients are now being cured.

Because childhood neoplasms are characterized by a high growth fraction with a propensity for frequent, early micrometastases, chemotherapy has become the cornerstone of treatment. Many therapeutic regimens are composed of dose-intensive combinations of agents, and few dosage modifications are made for myelosuppression or infection. With a number of childhood cancers, induction therapy is followed by maintenance regimens that may last 1 to 3 years, thus prolonging the period of immunosuppression and continuing the risk for infection.

Accordingly, infections have become expected sequelae after therapy for childhood cancer (1,2). The magnitude of risk for infection varies closely with the depth and duration of granulocytopenia (3). Fewer than 30% of patients whose duration of neutropenia is less than 1 week have fever or evidence of infection, compared with almost 100% of patients who receive more intensive chemotherapy and have neutropenia lasting longer than 1 week (4,5). The extent of the underlying malignancy closely correlates with the intensity and duration of chemotherapy and contributes to the increased rate of infection. For example, children with low-risk acute lymphocytic leukemia (ALL) have a lower incidence of serious infectious complications than those with high-risk ALL, reflecting both the severity of the leukemia and the intensity of chemotherapy used to treat it. However, once remission is achieved, the risk for infection-related morbidity and mortality declines (6).

Fever remains the most important indicator of infection in children with cancer. Fever is a nonspecific sign, however, and can result from both infectious and noninfectious causes. Although it is less commonly observed than in adults, fever can be caused by the child's underlying malignancy. This is especially true for tumors that are associated with tissue necrosis (e.g., Ewing sarcoma), or the production of pyrogens (e.g., certain lymphomas) (7). Nevertheless, most fevers in children with cancer appear to be associated with granulocytopenia and infection. For example, in a prospective analysis of 1,001 episodes of fever in pediatric and young adult cancer patients admitted to the National Cancer Institute (NCI) between 1975 and 1980, almost half developed fever during therapy, and 80% of these cases occurred during periods of granulocytopenia (defined as fewer than 500 polymorphonuclear leukocytes and band forms per cubic millimeter) (8). Almost 75% of those patients with fever and granulocytopenia could eventually be shown to have a clinically or microbiologically documented site of infection; this contrasted sharply with patients who became febrile while they were nongranulocytopenic, of whom fewer than 20% had a defined infectious cause for their fever. This study helped to delineate the association of fever and granulocytopenia with infection in children with cancer and supported the use of empiric antibiotic treatment in the overall management of these cases.

During the 1980s the more rapid employment of empiric antibiotic treatment in febrile granulocytopenic patients limited the ability to define an infectious origin for febrile episodes. In the late 1980s, only 30% to 40% of cases of fever associated with granulocytopenia had a definable infectious cause (9). It is unlikely that these patients actually had fewer infections, especially in view of the continually increasing intensity of treatment. Rather, actual infections were probably being masked by the early use of antibiotics. Other notable changes during the late 1980s and throughout the 1990s were the increased use of indwelling intravenous catheters and an increase in gram-positive bacterial infections together with a decline in those caused by gram-negative organisms, especially *Pseudomonas aeruginosa*. Today, management in neutropenic children initially revolves around the management of fever as a manifestation of infection, as detailed in Chapter 17. Neverthe-

less, there is also a need to understand the management of proven infections, particularly those that may emerge after the initial management of fever and neutropenia. The focus of this chapter is on those pediatric patients with hematologic malignancies in whom an infectious etiology is defined.

FACTORS CONTRIBUTING TO THE RISK OF INFECTION

There are many factors that contribute to diminished host defenses and increase the rate of infection in children and adolescents with cancer. They include abnormalities in mucosal and integumentary physical defense barriers, decreases in phagocyte numbers and functions, profound alterations in cellular and humoral immune defenses, and alterations in innate recognition immunity. Coupled with these changes in the patient's host defense matrix are alterations in the endogenous microbial flora and exposure to new potential pathogens secondary to treatment with cytotoxic and antimicrobial agents, the use of intravascular devices, and hospitalization (10).

The pediatric cancer patient's integumentary and mucosal physical defense barriers can be altered by both chemotherapy and radiation therapy. (For example, high-dose methotrexate can cause mucositis, and radiation treatment to the mediastinum for Hodgkin's disease can cause severe esophagitis.) Oroesophageal and intestinal mucositis is a particularly frequent complication of anticancer treatment and may provide a nidus and portal for systemic infection. Furthermore, the widespread use of implanted intravenous devices, such as Hickman- or Broviac-type catheters or subcutaneously implanted Port-a-Cath systems, offers sites for local and systemic infection. Altered nutrition, a common problem in many cancer patients, contributes to loss of integrity of the integument and mucosal surfaces and to impaired phagocytic capacity, macrophage mobilization, and lymphocyte function (11,12).

The depth and duration of granulocytopenia is directly related to the frequency of serious infections and remains the single most important risk factor associated with infection (3,13). In addition to these well-defined quantitative defects, qualitative abnormalities in neutrophil function have been reported, including defects in chemotaxis, generation of superoxide, phagocytosis, and bactericidal activity *in vitro* (10,14). Glucocorticosteroids given in pharmacologic dosages rapidly and profoundly decrease neutrophil migration, phagocytosis, and intracellular microbicidal activity (15–17). Glucocorticosteroids also alter macrophage function, diminishing host defenses against tissue-invasive fungi and other pathogens, including intracellular bacteria (e.g., *Mycobacterium, Listeria*), protozoans, and viruses (18–22). In addition, a number of antineoplastic agents, including vinca alkaloids, L-asparaginase, 6-mercaptopurine, methotrexate, and anthracyclines, have been shown to significantly decrease phagocytic and bactericidal activity (23).

Children and adolescents undergoing therapy for pediatric cancers show profound quantitative and qualitative defects in cell-mediated immunity (24). The severity and clinical impact of these defects depends on the underlying disease, the chemotherapeutic agents used, and the dose-intensity of antineoplastic chemotherapy (10). Treatment with glucocorticosteroids aggravates these defects, making the patients even more susceptible to infections by viruses (e.g., varicella-zoster virus [VZV], herpes simplex virus [HSV], cytomegalovirus [CMV]) and certain fungal infections (e.g., pneumocystosis, cryptococcosis, histoplasmosis) (20). Although little is known about the indirect effects of chemotherapeutic agents or glucocorticosteroids on the cytokine network, it is conceivable that interferences with this immunoregulatory system may alter responses of either the phagocyte or the lymphocyte arms to infections (10).

Cytotoxic chemotherapy and radiation therapy can also diminish B-cell functions, leading to decreased immunoglobulin concentrations, lowered opsonic activity, inadequate agglutination and lysis of bacteria, and deficient neutralization of bacterial toxins (25–27). Immunoglobulin deficiency is associated with a particular susceptibility to encapsulated bacteria (28), and there exists a markedly increased risk for *Haemophilus influenzae* type b and pneumococcal bloodstream infections in pediatric cancer patients (29). Cytotoxic chemotherapy also depresses the responses to common antiviral and antibacterial vaccines after both primary and booster challenges (10). Depending on the underlying malignancy, the dose-intensity of antineoplastic chemotherapy, and the vaccine used, such defective antibody production can be observed for up to 5 years after completion of anticancer therapy (30,31). The spleen serves as an important organ in host defense because it acts as a phagocytic filter for microorganisms and improves opsonization. It is also important in antibody production, as evidenced by the inferior antibiotic response to polysaccharide capsular vaccines seen in splenectomized children (29). If the spleen is infiltrated by leukemia and lymphoma or removed for diagnostic or therapeutic reasons, the risk of fulminant infection from such encapsulated bacteria as *Streptococcus pneumoniae, H. influenzae,* and *Neisseria meningitidis* is considerably increased (32,33).

At the same time that their host defenses are impaired, patients undergoing treatment for cancer become rapidly colonized after their initial presentation with aerobic gram-negative bacteria (*Escherichia coli, Klebsiella* spp., *P. aeruginosa*) (34). Colonization by *Candida* spp. is also common, in particular in patients receiving broad-spectrum antibiotics (35). This mostly nosocomially acquired endogenous flora provides a point source for systemic invasion through mucosal surfaces that have been denuded as a result of chemotherapy or radiation therapy, or for ingress through indwelling catheters or invasive monitoring devices.

MANAGEMENT OF SPECIFIC INFECTIOUS COMPLICATIONS

Even though most patients do not have a site of proven infection, the prompt use of appropriate antimicrobial therapy is crucial to successful outcome, and delayed or ineffective therapy can result in serious or even fatal sequelae in these patients. In clinical practice, however, once a site of infection becomes apparent, modifications of antimicrobial therapy are often required.

In an NCI study of 550 episodes of fever and granulocytopenia in which patients were randomly assigned to receive either monotherapy with ceftazidime or combination therapy with cephalothin, carbenicillin, and gentamicin, patients who were eventually found to have a clinically or microbiologically documented infection required modifications of their initial therapy in 59% of the episodes, regardless of which initial antibiotic regimen was used (9). Modifications included adding anaerobic coverage for necrotizing gingivitis or perirectal cellulitis and adding vancomycin for gram-positive infections caused by coagulase-negative staphylococci; in patients with prolonged neutropenia, the addition of antifungal therapy was also frequently required. These findings documenting the need for modification of initial antimicrobial therapy for proven or suspected infections were further reflected in a large clinical trial investigating imipenem versus ceftazidime for initial management of fever and neutropenia in pediatric and adult patients (36). Despite their broad spectrum, modification of these regimens was necessary in a considerable proportion of patients. Therefore, the successful management of prolonged neutropenia requires careful follow-up to guide appropriate modification of antimicrobial therapy.

Bloodstream Infections

Between 10% and 20% of febrile and neutropenic cancer patients have a bacteremia. Common sources for bacteremia are the lungs (25%), perioral cellulitis (10%), the gastrointestinal tract (5%), and, with increasing frequency, indwelling intravascular devices. The genitourinary tract is less commonly a source unless urethral catheters are in place. No clinically reliable method has been reported for prospectively distinguishing between those febrile and granulocytopenic patients who have a bacteremia and those who do not (8,35).

It is notable, however, that the pattern of bacterial isolates has changed over recent years, from the previously predominant gram-negative aerobic organisms to gram-positive organisms such as *Staphylococcus aureus,* coagulase-negative staphylococci, *Streptococcus* sp., *Corynebacterium jeikeium,* and *Bacillus* sp. (37). The increasing number of coagulase-negative staphylococcal infections is probably related to the increased use of catheters (38). *C. jeikeium* is a particularly antibiotic-resistant organism that tends to cause bacteremia in patients with prolonged granulocytopenia (39). The streptococci have also evolved into important pathogens, including both the group D streptococci and, in patients who are receiving cytosine arabinoside and who develop oral mucositis, the viridans streptococci (40,41). Furthermore, along with the use of broad-spectrum antibiotics, gram-negative bacilli that are more resistant to antibiotics (e.g., non-*aeruginosa Pseudomonas* spp., *Serratia marcescens, Enterobacter* sp., *Citrobacter* sp.) are more commonly isolated (42).

The expanded use of third-generation cephalosporins has been associated in some institutions with the emergence of organisms expressing high levels of extended-spectrum β-lactamases, including stably derepressed chromosomal AmpC (formerly type 1) β-lactamases (43). These type 1 β-lacatamases hydrolyze ceftazidime and other third-generation cephalosporins. Consequently, patients infected by these organisms may present with septic shock occurring as a breakthrough event after successful resolution of the initial episode of neutropenic fever. *Enterobacter* sp., *Citrobacter freundii, S. marcescens,* and *Morganella morganii* are the most common organisms implicated in these infections; occasionally, *P. aeruginosa* causes this pattern of sepsis. Soon after the recognition of the aforementioned resistant organisms, strains of *Klebsiella pneumoniae* and *E. coli* were also identified as being resistant to the oxyimio-β-lactams, a property which was transmissible by multiresistance plasmids carrying mutations of TEM-1 and SHV-1 that could also hydrolyze third-generation cephalosporins. Imipenem or meropenem is the preferred antimicrobial agent for treatment of these organisms in neutropenic hosts; fluorinated quinolones or trimethoprim-sulfamethoxazole (TMP/SMX) may be effective alternatives in patients who are intolerant of or refractory to the class of penems. More recently, the introduction of cefepime, a fourth-generation cephalosporin, has raised the possibility of using this agent in lieu of ceftazidime for prevention of breakthrough infections by these organisms (43).

Empiric therapy for bacteremia is usually directed at gram-negative organisms, especially *P. aeruginosa,* because of the potentially high morbidity and mortality if these organisms go untreated (44); a relative increase of gram-negative organisms has recently been reported from several oncologic centers (45). In addition to gram-negative bacteria, which are an uncommon cause of breakthrough bacteremias to date, gram-positive organisms, especially coagulase-negative staphylococci, can cause secondary infections. These infections tend to be more indolent than those caused by gram-negative organisms. Among 550 episodes of fever and granulocytopenia, vancomycin was eventually required in 39; in almost all cases, vancomycin was not added until the gram-positive organism had been identified, yet patients survived without excess mortality or morbidity (46). The expanding problem of vancomycin-resistant *Enterococcus* clearly warrants caution in the empiric use of vancomycin (47); its use should be restricted to microbiologically documented or clinically proven infections or specific epidemiologic settings.

The incidence of *S. pneumoniae* and *H. influenzae* bloodstream infections in children with cancer does not appear to be increased in comparison with that in normal children, although 80% of pneumococcal bacteremias occur in association with granulocytopenia (29). The risk of sepsis from these pathogens

is increased, however, in splenectomized children (32,33).

The signs of infection (inflammation, tenderness) may be minimal in granulocytopenic patients, and it is important to evaluate and examine the patient extremely thoroughly for a possible focus for bacteremia, because the identification of such a site could influence therapy. For example, minimal erythema and serous discharge at a catheter exit site may indicate tunnel or exit site infection that requires increased coverage for gram-positive organisms or removal of the catheter. Minimal perirectal erythema may require antianaerobic and possibly antienterococcal coverage, even if blood cultures grow only a gram-negative rod. The absence of specific physical findings does not exclude a life-threatening bacteremia, because more than half of bacteremic patients lack such signs (8).

The treatment for bacteremia begins with the prompt initiation of broad-spectrum empiric antibiotics as soon as fever and granulocytopenia occur. Such empiric therapy may consist of the combination of a broad-spectrum β-lactam (often a semisynthetic penicillin such as ticarcillin or piperacillin) with an aminoglycoside or another β-lactam, or it may involve monotherapy using a third-generation cephalosporin or a carbapenem, which as single agents have broad bactericidal activity (48–50). Table 5.1 provides a list of commonly used antibacterial agents and their pediatric dosing regimens. Of note, no particular combination of antibiotics has been shown to be superior to any another combination or to monotherapy. (For a complete discussion of empiric therapy, see Chapter 17.) Some regimens also include empiric vancomycin because of concern over the rising incidence of gram-positive infections. However, because most of these organisms are relatively avirulent (especially *Staphylococcus epidermidis*) compared with gram-negative aerobes, vancomycin therapy, as discussed previously, can be delayed until the organism has been isolated (46,51). On the other hand, even when a gram-positive bacteremia is identified, broad-spectrum empiric antibiotics

TABLE 5.1. *Common antibacterial agents and their pediatric dosages*

Antimicrobial agent	Daily dosage (mg/kg)	Comment
Azlocillin	200–300 in 4–6 divided doses (max. 21 g)	Broad gram-negative spectrum (particularly, *Pseudomonas aeruginosa*); active against anaerobes, enterococci. In neutropenic patients, use only in combination with an aminoglycoside.
Mezlocillin	200–300 in 4–6 divided doses (max. 21 g)	
Piperacillin	200–300 in 4–6 divided doses (max. 21 g)	
Ceftazidime	60–100 in 3 divided doses (max. 6 g)	Broad gram-negative spectrum, including *P. aeruginosa;* limited gram-positive spectrum; no activity against anaerobes. Combination with an aminoglycoside recommended for gram-negative bacteremia.
Ceftriaxone	75–100 in 1 single dose	Option for empiric therapy in non-neutropenic patients with an indwelling centralvenous catheter; no coverage of *P. aeruginosa.*
Imipenem	50 in 4 divided doses (max. 4 g)	Broad gram-negative and gram-positive spectrum, including *P. aeruginosa;* broad antianaerobic activity. Combination with an aminoglycoside is recommended for treatment of *P. aeruginosa* infections.
Meropenem	60 in 3 divided doses (max. 3 g)	
Aztreonam	100–150 in 4 divided doses (max. 6 g)	Exclusive gram-negative spectrum including many strains of *P. aeruginosa.* Option for combination therapy with vancomycin (± aminoglycoside) in patients with β-lactam allergy.
Vancomycin	40 in 2–4 divided doses (max. 2 g)	Spectrum limited to gram-positive bacteria. Monitoring of serum levels required with vancomycin.
Teicoplanin	10 in 1 single dose[a]	
Gentamicin	5 in 1 or 3 divided doses	Combinatory agent for empiric therapy and for treatment of documented gram-negative infections. Monitoring of serum levels required.
Tobramycin	5 in 1 or 3 divided doses	
Amikacin	15 in 1 or 2–3 divided doses (max. 1.5 g)	
Metronidazole	30 in 4 divided doses (max. 4 g)	Active against anaerobes (abdominal/perirectal processes); first choice for treatment of *Clostridium difficile* infection (PO).
Erythromycin	30–50 in 4 divided doses (max. 4 g)	Therapy for proven/suspected infections by *Chlamydia, Mycoplasma,* and *Legionella.*
Azithromycin	5–10 in 1 single dose (max. 4 g)	
Clarithomycin	15–20 in 2 divided doses	

[a]Not approved in the United States; loading dose, 10 mg/kg q12h for 36 hr.

should not be narrowed in patients who are expected to have prolonged neutropenia (more than 7 days), because almost half of persistently neutropenic patients in whom the antibiotic regimen was narrowed in this way developed a secondary infection with gram-negative aerobes (52). Narrowing the antibiotic regimen when a gram-negative bacteremia occurs may not be advantageous, because it is associated with a greater need for

additions or modifications to the antibiotic regimen (53).

The duration of treatment should be for at least 10 to 14 days, although persistent granulocytopenia and a slowly resolving primary site of infection (especially perianal cellulitis/abscess) may require longer treatment. In patients who had a response but remain neutropenic for longer than 14 days, treatment should not be discontinued before granulocyte counts have recovered, because the likelihood of recurrent fever and infection is up to 30% under these circumstances (54).

Catheter-Associated Bloodstream Infections

The increased use of both transiently placed and permanent central venous catheters has led to an increase in catheter-associated bacteremias, with rates of infections of these catheters ranging from 3% to 60% (55,56) (see Chapter 17). The diagnosis of catheter-associated bacteremia is made by finding positive blood cultures from both a catheter lumen and a peripheral venous site. Quantitative cultures (e.g., using lysis-centrifugation systems) help define a catheter-associated bacteremia more rapidly. It is important to culture all ports of multilumen catheters, since only one may be infected. The risk of catheter-associated bacteremia apparently does not appear to be decreased with the use of subcutaneous catheters (e.g., Port-a-Cath), as demonstrated in a prospective, randomized study comparing Hickman-Broviac and Port-a-Cath systems performed at the NCI (57).

The offending organisms are usually coagulase-negative staphylococci, but other gram-positive bacteria (especially *S. aureus, Streptococcus* sp., *Corynebacterium* sp., and *Bacillus* sp.), gram-negative bacteria (*Acinetobacter* spp., *P. aeruginosa*), and, with increasing frequency, yeast-type fungi (in particular *Candida albicans,* but also non-*albicans Candida* species and previously uncommon pathogens such as *Trichosporon beigelii, Rhodotorula rubra, Hansenula anomala, Malassezia furfur,* and *Cryptococcus laurentii*) cause intraluminal infections as well (58,59). Catheter exit site or tunnel infections due to *Aspergillus* spp. or mycobacteria (especially *Mycobacterium fortuitum* and *Mycobacterium chelonei*) have also been described (60–62). Given the frequency of catheter-associated bloodstream and exit site infections, careful examination and, if appropriate, culture of all ports and exit sites are important in the approach to the patient with an indwelling central venous line.

The treatment of most clinically apparent catheter-associated infections is outlined in Fig. 5.1. This paradigm applies to coagulase-negative staphylococci and most other gram-positive infections, which tend to be indolent and treatable without removal of the catheter. For the most part, only when blood cultures remain positive for more than 24 to 48 hours after antibiotics have been started or when a "tunnel" infection (tenderness or induration along the subcutaneous track of the catheter) exists is catheter removal required (13). Exceptions must be made, however, for organisms such as *Candida* spp., atypical mycobacteria, and *Bacillus* sp., which usually cannot be successfully treated without catheter removal even if the organisms are sensitive to the antimicrobial agents being administered (13,58,63).

Detection of *Candida* spp. and other yeasts in blood cultures of a child with a hematologic malignancy virtually always represents invasive candidiasis and warrants systemic antifungal therapy (58,64,65). Whether it is the primary source of fungemia or a target for attachment of circulating organisms, the intravascular catheter serves as a source for continued seeding of the bloodstream and should be removed whenever feasible. Lecciones et al. (58), in a 10-year retrospective survey of 155 episodes of vascular catheter-associated fungemia among inpatients at the NCI, found that the longer the central venous catheter remained in place, the greater the frequency of persistent fungemia and complications of disseminated candidiasis. Similar conclusions were drawn from two smaller studies in unselected pediatric patients, which found catheter removal to be an important determinant of outcome of fungemia (66,67).

Accompanied by the removal of the intravascular catheter, uncomplicated candidemia can be treated by a 2-week course of amphotericin B at 0.5 mg per kilogram body weight per day (64) (Table 5.2). Fluconazole was equivalent to amphotericin B in the treatment of uncomplicated catheter-associated

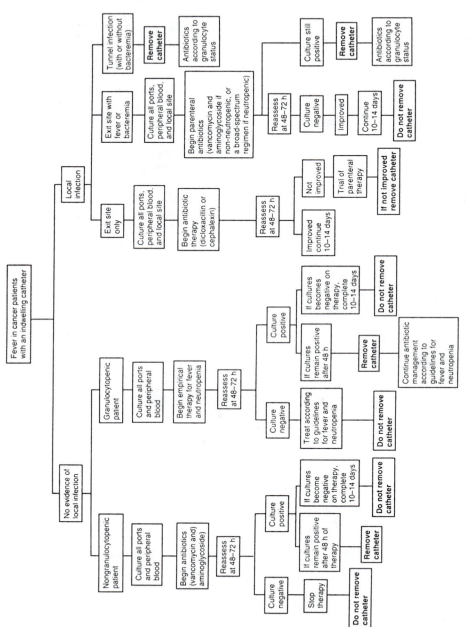

FIG. 5.1. Algorithm for the management of fever in the cancer patient with an indwelling intravenous catheter.

TABLE 5.2. *Common antifungal and antiviral agents and their pediatric dosages*

Antimicrobial agent	Daily dosage (mg/kg)	Comment
Amphotericin B	0.5–0.6 in 1 single dose	Empiric antifungal therapy; invasive *Candida* infections
	0.7–1.0 in 1 single dose	Therapy for infections by *Cryptococcus neoformans*
	0.5–1.0 in 1 single dose	Therapy for infections by *Histoplasma, Blastomyces,* and *Coccidioides*
	1.0 in 1 single dose	Infections by *Candida tropicalis* and *Candida parapsilosis*
	1.0–1.5 in 1 single dose	Infections by *Aspergillus* spp. and other opportunistic molds
ABCD	5 in 1 single dose	Therapy for presumed or proven invasive fungal infections refractory to or intolerant of conventional amphotericin B (all).
ABLC	5 in 1 single dose	Empiric antifungal therapy in neutropenic patients
L-AmB	5 in 1 single dose	(L-AmB only, 3 mg/kg)
5-Fluorocytosine (flucytosine)	100–150 in 3–4 divided doses	In combination with D-AmB for treatment of cryptococcosis, *Candida* meningitis, and endophthalmitis, as well as renal and disseminated candidiasis
Fluconazole	6 in 1 single dose	Prevention of *Candida* infections in patients undergoing myeloablation
	8 in 1 single dose	Maintenance therapy for cryptococcal infections
	6–12 in 1 single dose	Invasive infections by susceptible *Candida* strains in stable patients and therapy for infections by *Trichosporon beigelii* (+ D-AmB in neutropenic patients)
Itraconazole	5 in 1 single dose	Maintenance therapy for invasive *Aspergillus* or cryptococcal infections
Trimethoprim-sulfamethoxazole (TMP/SMX)	5 in 2 divided doses	Prophylaxis of *Pneumocystis carinii* pneumonitis (PCP)
	15–20 in 4 divided doses	Therapy for proven/suspected PCP
Pentamidine	3–4 in 1 single dose (max. 300 mg)	Therapy for proven/suspected PCP in patients intolerant to TMP/SMX
Acyclovir	15 in 3 divided doses	Therapy for *Herpes simplex* mucocutaneous infections
	30–45 in 3 divided doses	Therapy for chickenpox and herpes zoster
Ganciclovir	10 in 2 divided doses	Induction therapy for cytomegalovirus (CMV) disease (day 1–14)
	5 in 1 single dose	Maintenance therapy for CMV disease (day 15 onward)
Foscarnet	80–120 in 2–3 divided doses	Mucocutaneous herpes due to aciclovir-resistant virus
	120–180 in 2–3 divided doses	Herpes zoster due to aciclovir-resistant virus (indication not FDA-approved)
	180 in 3 divided doses	Alternative therapy for CMV infections (indication not FDA-approved)

FDA, U.S. Food and Drug Administration.

fungemia in non-neutropenic adults (68); whether these findings can be extended to granulocytopenic children warrants further study. Given the lower level of susceptibility in these patients, fungemia due to *Candida tropicalis* and *Candida parapsilosis* may require higher doses of amphotericin B (0.75 to 1.0 mg per kilogram per day) and more protracted courses; *Candida lusitaniae, Candida guilliermondii,* and *Candida lipolytica* are frequently resistant to amphotericin B *in vitro* and *in vivo* (64). *Candida krusei* and *Candida glabrata* are considered intrinsically resistant

to fluconazole and may be found as causes of fungemia in neutropenic patients receiving antifungal prophylaxis with fluconazole (69). Depending on the species and susceptibility pattern of the isolate, persistent fungemia may require increasing the dosage of the primary agent, adding flucytosine, or treating with an alternative compound (64). *T. beigelii* is resistant to the fungicidal effects of amphotericin B, but antifungal triazoles such as fluconazole result in significant decline in tissue burden. The current recommendation for candidemia in persistently neutropenic patients is amphotericin B plus fluconazole; in non-neutropenic patients it may be treated with fluconazole alone (64).

The risk for a catheter-associated bacteremia may influence the management of fever in a cancer patient with an indwelling catheter (Fig. 5.1). Even when no local infection is evident in a nongranulocytopenic patient, because of the potential sequelae of an untreated gram-negative infection, we administer a 48- to 78-hour trial of antibiotics while awaiting culture results. In general, a long-acting third-generation cephalosporin (e.g., ceftriaxone), is administered. Alternatively, the combination of vancomycin plus gentamicin can be given. When patients have a double- or triple-lumen catheter in place, it is important to rotate antibiotic administration among the ports or lumens, because infection may be restricted to only one of them. If cultures are negative, antibiotics may be discontinued; if they are positive, a 1- to 14-day course of treatment is given. We have found that even in neutropenic patients with a catheter there is no advantage to including vancomycin in the initial broad-spectrum antibiotic coverage. Therefore, we treat fever and granulocytopenia without empiric vancomycin regardless of whether the patient has a catheter (70).

Upper Respiratory Tract Infections

Otitis

Although the symptoms and signs of ear infection (pain, drainage, fever) may be present in children with cancer, the profoundly granulocytopenic patient may have only minimal tympanic erythema. Unlike the nongranulocytopenic patient, whose most likely pathogens are *S. pneumoniae* or *H. influenzae,* granulocytopenic children are also susceptible to other gram-positive bacteria as well as to gram-negative organisms. Therefore broad-spectrum therapy is initially required for granulocytopenic patients (11).

Increased rates of infection are also observed in patients with anatomic changes secondary to tumor or treatment-induced changes in the outer ear, middle ear, or eustachian tube. Mastoiditis, for example, can occur when a tumor (e.g., rhabdomyosarcoma) erodes the middle ear. Also, *P. aeruginosa* can be the cause of malignant otitis externa (extension of infection through the petrous bone into the brain), for which aggressive antipseudomonal treatment and surgical drainage are required (2).

Sinusitis

In children with cancer, obstruction of the sinuses by tumor (e.g., Burkitt lymphoma, rhabdomyosarcoma) can lead to acute or chronic sinusitis. Again, unlike immunocompetent children, in whom *S. pneumoniae, H. influenzae,* and *Branhamella catarrhalis* constitute the predominant pathogens, the granulocytopenic child or the cancer patient with mechanical obstruction is at risk for infection with gram-negative and gram-positive aerobes as well as anaerobes (71,72). For such patients, appropriate therapy includes agents with antianaerobic activity (73). Therapy is usually begun empirically; but for patients who fail to improve within 72 hours, aspiration or biopsy of the sinus is generally indicated.

For patients who develop sinusitis during an episode of neutropenia, attention must be directed at filamentous fungi, such as *Aspergillus* and *Fusarium* spp., *Pseudallescheria boydii, Bipolaris* spp., and the zygomycetes (74–81). Infections with these organisms can begin with crusting and eschar formation of the anterior nares, the turbinates, or the hard palate, and they can be accompanied by destructive and erosive extension into the orbit, cavernous sinus, and brain (rhinocerebral syndrome). A careful radiographic evaluation including computed tomographic (CT) scans or magnetic resonance imaging (MRI) is needed to assess the anatomic extent of suspected fungal sinusitis and to guide diagnostic biopsies. Fungal sinusitis caused by the aforementioned filamentous molds can be a devastating infection and requires aggressive therapy with high dosages of conventional amphotericin B (1.0 to 1.5 mg per kilogram per day) or one of the lipid formulations of amphotericin B (recommended starting dosage, 5 mg per kilogram per day) (64,82). Itraconazole can be effective in the treatment of sinusitis due to dematiaceous molds, as indicated by a recent case series (83). Surgical interventions during neutropenia should be minimally invasive, but extensive debridement may be required for progressively invasive disease that proves refractory to antifungal chemotherapy (81). Restoration of host defenses, always a prerequisite for successful outcome, includes reversal of granulocytopenia and discontinuation of corticosteroids, if feasible.

Epiglottitis

H. influenzae infection can result in epiglottitis in the child with cancer, as much as in the nonimmunocompromised child, but staphylococcal and *Candida* epiglottitis also must be considered. Infection with any of these organisms can lead to life-threatening airway obstruction. Presenting signs and symptoms may include odynophagia, hoarseness, and stridor. Diagnosis is by laryngoscopy-guided visualization and swabbing of the epiglottis, and therapy consists of airway protection and rapid initiation of antimicrobial therapy (84,85).

Lower Respiratory Tract Infections

Pulmonary infections are the most common site of primary and disseminated infections in cancer patients. Because the lungs are also a site of many noninfectious complications of neoplastic diseases and their treatment (e.g., metastasis or diffuse neoplastic infiltration, graft-versus-host disease [GVHD], pulmonary edema, pulmonary hemorrhage, pulmonary embolization and infarction, chemotherapy- or radiation-induced pneumonitis), the differential diagnosis is complex (Table 5.3) and the management can be complicated (Table 5.4). On an operational management level, pediatric cancer patients with pulmonary infiltrates can generally be divided into four groups depending on the type

---

TABLE 5.3. *Differential diagnosis of pulmonary infiltrates in cancer patients*

Localized infiltrate	Diffuse infiltrate
Non-neutropenic patients	
Bacteria: *Streptococcus pneumoniae, Hemophilus, Mycobacteria, Mycoplasma*	Parasites: *Toxoplasma gondii, Strongyloides*
Fungi: *Cryptococcus, Histoplasma, Coccidioides*	Bacteria: *Mycobacteria, Nocardia, Legionella, Chlamydia, Mycoplasma*
Viruses: RSV, adenovirus	Viruses: HSV, VZV, CMV, measles, influenza, parainfluenza, adenovirus
	Fungi: *Candida, Cryptococcus, Pneumocystis carinii*
Noninfectious causes: drugs, radiation, GVHD, hemorrhage, infarcts, underlying tumor of metastases	Noninfectious causes: radiation pneumonitis, drugs, GVHD, hemorrhage, edema, neoplastic infiltration
Neutropenic patients	
Bacteria: any gram-positive or gram-negative bacteria, mycobacteria, *Nocardia*	Bacteria: any gram-positive or gram-negative bacteria, mycobacteria, *Nocardia, Legionella, Chlamydia*
Fungi: *Aspergillus, Fusarium, Zygomycetes, Cryptococcus, Histoplasma*	Fungi: *Candida, Cryptococcus, Aspergillus, Fusarium, Histoplasma, P. carinii*
Viruses: HZV, VZV, adenovirus, RSV	Parasites: *Toxoplasma gondii, Strongyloides*
Noninfectious causes: drugs, radiation, GVHD, hemorrhage, infarcts, underlying tumor or metastases	Viruses: HSV, VZV, CMV, measles, influenza, parainfluenza, adenovirus, RSV
	Noninfectious causes: radiation, drugs, GVHD, hemorrhage, edema, neoplastic infiltration

CMV, cytomegalovirus; GVHD, graft-versus-host disease; HSV, herpes simplex virus; RSV, respiratory syncytial virus; VZV, varicella-zoster virus.

TABLE 5.4. *Approach to management in the cancer patient who has a pulmonary infiltrate*

Patchy or localized infiltrate		Diffuse or interstitial infiltrate	
Nongranulocytopenic	Granulocytopenic	Nongranulocytopenic	Granulocytopenic
Standard evaluation and therapy according to microbiologic diagnosis	*If not already receiving antibiotics:* Standard evaluation, start empiric broad-spectrum antibiotics Reassess: If improved, continue therapy If not improved, continue diagnostic evaluation, consisting of HRCT and bronchoscopy with lavage or lung biopsy[a]; add empiric antifungal therapy and modify antibacterial therapy according to findings *If already receiving antibiotics:* Continue therapy expectantly if granulocyte count is rising and patient is stable and well If granulocytopenia persists: HRCT and bronchoscopy with lavage or lung biopsy[a] as indicated; add empiric antifungal therapy and modify antibacterial therapy according to findings For patients who cannot tolerate an invasive procedure, add empiric antifungal therapy and broaden antibacterial therapy empirically	Standard evaluation plus bronchoscopy with lavage If diagnostic, treat according to findings If nondiagnostic, start empiric therapy with TMP/SMX and macrolide If bronchoscopy and lavage is not feasible or available, start empiric treatment with TMP/SMX and macrolide Reassess: If improved or stable, continue empiric regimen If patient progressively deteriorates, consider open or percutaneous endoscopic lung biopsy	*If not already receiving antibiotics:* Standard evaluation plus bronchoscopy with lavage, start empiric broad-spectrum antibiotics If lavage is diagnostic, add appropriate therapy If lavage is nondiagnostic, add empiric TMP/SMX and macrolide If bronchoscopy and lavage is not feasible or available, start empiric treatment with broad-spectrum antibiotics, TMP/SMX, and macrolide Reassess; consider empiric antifungal therapy and open or percutaneous endoscopic lung biopsy if patient progressively deteriorates *If already receiving antibiotics:* Standard evaluation plus bronchoscopy with lavage, start empiric antifungal therapy If lavage is diagnostic, add appropriate therapy If lavage is nondiagnostic, add empiric TMP/SMX and macrolide If bronchoscopy and lavage is not feasible or available, modify antibacterial regimen, start empiric antifungal therapy; start empiric therapy with TMP/SMX and macrolide Reassess; consider open or percutaneous endoscopic lung biopsy if patient progressively deteriorates

HRCT, high-resolution computed tomography; TMP/SMX, trimethoprim-sulfamethoxazole.
[a]Transthoracic needle aspiration, open lung biopsy, or percutaneous endoscopic lung biopsy after platelet support in patients with stable plasmatic coagulation.

of infiltrate (patchy versus diffuse) and the neutrophil count at presentation (more than versus fewer than 500 cells per microliter).

Patchy Infiltrates in Non-Neutropenic Children

In non-neutropenic patients presenting with localized infiltrates, the usual community-acquired pathogens predominate. They include common, mostly gram-positive bacteria (e.g., *S. pneumoniae, H. influenzae*); respiratory viruses (e.g., respiratory syncytial virus [RSV], adenoviruses, influenza viruses, parainfluenza viruses, measles in nonimmunized children) (2); *Mycoplasma* (86); and, rarely, *Legionella* and *Chlamydia* spp. (87,88). The diagnosis may be apparent from culture or stains of respiratory specimens, or it may be established by antigen-detecting immunoassays of nasopharyngeal secretions (respiratory viruses, measles, *Legionella, Chlamydia*) or urine (*Legionella pneumophila* serotype I, adenoviruses) or by serologic studies (*Mycoplasma*), although antibody responses may not be adequate. Therapy should be guided by the patient's clinical status and age, community versus hospital acquisition of the organism, prior antimicrobial therapy, and the specific organism found. In patients with pulmonary metastases, obstructive bronchopneumonia may necessitate an interventional bronchoscopy, and antianaerobic antibiotic treatment should be strongly considered.

Mycobacterium tuberculosis has become an increasingly common pathogen in immunocompromised patients who are not neutropenic. This may reflect the changing reservoir of *M. tuberculosis,* in particular in the demographic setting of large urban areas (89,90). The incidence of tuberculosis among cancer patients is significantly increased compared with that in the general population, and both miliary pulmonary infiltrates and extrapulmonary manifestations are more frequent (90–92). The pulmonary infiltrates can easily be confused with other infections or with the underlying malignancy (91,93). Because immunocompromised children usually present with primary tuberculosis and may have disseminated disease (94), the potential mortality is considerable and a high index of suspicion is important. Therapy should always include at least three drugs initially and should be continued for a total of at least 9 months. Prolonged maintenance therapy may be indicated for patients in whom the underlying deficit in host responses has not resolved. Atypical mycobacteria are exceedingly rare pulmonary pathogens in patients with cancer. In contrast to *M. tuberculosis,* the diagnosis usually relies on isolation of the organism from otherwise sterile sites. In potentially contaminated specimens from the lower respiratory tract, repeat recovery of the same species in sufficient amounts and clinical correlation are required (89).

Patchy Infiltrates in Neutropenic Children

The neutropenic patient is prone to develop pneumonia from a wide variety of microorganisms throughout the course of neutropenia. Early in neutropenia, particularly during the first 7 days, bacterial pathogens predominate. These bacterial organisms usually stem from the endogenous flora of the patient, which, in turn, is mostly hospital acquired and includes predominantly gram-negative bacteria (95). Although almost any gram-positive or gram-negative bacterium can cause pneumonia in neutropenic patients, *Klebsiella* sp., other Enterobacteriaceae, and *P. aeruginosa* are the most common (96). Although the diagnosis may be apparent from blood cultures and sometimes from cultures of respiratory specimens, most neutropenic patients, particularly children, are not able expectorate sputum. Sputum induced by aerosolized hypertonic saline may occasionally aid in the diagnosis.

Given the predominance of bacterial pneumonias early in the course of neutropenia, the child with localized or patchy pulmonary infiltrates may initially be treated empirically with broad-spectrum antibiotics. Such empiric therapy may consist of combinations of a β-lactam antibiotic plus an aminoglycoside or monotherapy with a third-generation cephalosporin or a carbapenem, as discussed earlier. If the patient's condition has stabilized or improved after 48 to 72 hours, treatment should be continued for 10 to 14 days.

If clinical or radiographic findings worsen, indicating a pneumonia refractory to initial empiric antibiotic therapy, invasive evaluation may be essential to the identification of other potentially treatable organisms, including *Legionella, Nocardia,* mycobacteria, and especially fungi. Fiberoptic bronchoscopy with bronchoalveolar lavage (BAL) is a rapid procedure and is associated with low morbidity and virtually no mortality in immunocompromised children (97–103). In the absence of cardiovascular instability, coagulopathy, or thrombocytopenia (fewer than 50,000 cells per microliter), bronchoscopy and BAL are feasible in almost any clinical situation. Relative contraindications are severe hypoxia (positive end-expiratory pressure greater than 10 mm Hg or fraction of inspired oxygen [FiO_2] greater than 60% in intubated patients; use of continuous positive airway pressure or greater than 50% FiO_2 for partial pressure of oxygen in arterial blood [PaO_2] greater than 75 mm Hg in nonintubated patients); marked hypercapnia; severe airway obstruction; and pulmonary hypertension (104,105). Although the exact diagnostic yield of BAL in neutropenic children with focal or patchy pulmonary infiltrates is unknown (100,103), microbiologic advances have considerably increased the ability to diagnose infectious causes of pulmonary disease from BAL material (as discussed later in this chapter and in Chapter 18) (106). In comparison to fiberoptic bronchoscopy with BAL, transbronchial biopsy, percutaneous transthoracic needle aspiration, and percutaneous transthoracic needle biopsy are all associated with increased morbidity through pulmonary hemorrhage and air leak (104,107,108), but they may be useful in individual cases. Open lung biopsy remains the diagnostic gold standard if the clinical situation mandates a diagnosis and less invasive procedures were nondiagnostic (109). In conjunction with a comprehensive

conventional microbiologic and histologic laboratory workup, newer immunohistochemical and molecular diagnostic methods hold promise to expand the yield of tissue diagnosis for infectious agents, even in cases with nonspecific morphologic findings (109,110).

For the neutropenic patient with focal or patchy infiltrates not responding to broad-spectrum antibiotic therapy or the patient who presents with new focal or patchy infiltrates late in the course of neutropenia, filamentous fungi are the most common pathogens (111,112). Because of the life-threatening nature of these infections, aggressive diagnostic evaluation, as outlined previously, is indicated. In addition, high-resolution CT of the chest can be very helpful in the early detection and description of pulmonary lesions by filamentous fungi (113) and may identify patients at high risk for pulmonary hemorrhage (114). However, an exact microbiologic diagnosis should always be sought, because it may affect the choice, dose, and duration of antifungal therapy and allow for discontinuation of other potentially toxic empiric treatments. Nevertheless, if the clinical condition of the patient interdicts an invasive procedure, high-dose conventional amphotericin B or one of the lipid formulations of amphotericin B (82) should be added empirically to the antibiotic regimen.

The only exception to this approach is when the granulocytopenic patient develops a new infiltrate while the granulocyte count is rising, in which case the patient usually does well without therapeutic modifications, especially if afebrile and clinically well (112). Presumably, this infiltrate simply represents localization of the now available white blood cells to the previously infected area of the lung.

Legionella *Infection*

Legionella should be considered in the differential diagnosis of both localized or diffuse pulmonary infiltrates refractory to empiric broad-spectrum antibiotic therapy. Fatal pulmonary *Legionella* infections have been reported in patients after bone marrow transplantation (115) and in children with leukemia (88). In addition, autopsy studies indicate a surprisingly high prevalence of the organism in deceased patients with hematologic malignancies (116). The organism is ubiquitous in water and has been isolated from air conditioning cooling towers and hospital showerheads (117). Although legionellosis is a multisystem disease with fever, diarrhea, bradycardia, and neurologic dysfunction as the most frequent presenting signs, the lung is the primary target organ (118). Infiltrates initially are patchy and alveolar and involve a single lobe, usually with consolidation, although diffuse infiltrates can also occur. Diagnosis is best made by direct fluorescent antibody (DFA) testing on respiratory specimens, lung tissue, and urine. However, because the DFA is specific for *L. pneumophila* serotype I, infections by other species or serotypes, which account for approximately 20% of clinical legionellosis cases, are not detected, and a negative DFA result does not rule out disease. Moreover, there is cross-reactivity of the DFA with *Bordetella pertussis*, which may be present in the respiratory tract but has never been reported to cause pneumonitis in pediatric cancer patients. Cultures on charcoal-yeast-extract medium may yield growth of *Legionella* spp. within 2 *to 7 days. The historical standard of therapy for* Legionella infections is erythromycin (30 to 60 mg per kilogram per day in four divided doses for 3 weeks). The addition of rifampin to erythromycin may provide additional benefits for seriously ill patients. Azithromycin, clarithromycin, and the quinolones are newer but less well studied alternatives for treatment of legionellosis (119).

Nocardia *Infection*

Nocardia species (*Nocardia* asteroides and *Nocardia* brasiliensis) can cause severe illness in cancer patients. The respiratory tract is the main portal of entry, and focal pulmonary infections are the main clinical manifestations, although miliary patterns can also occur. Some 30% of patients with *Nocardia* pneumonia have subcutaneous abscesses and brain abscesses as well (120–122). Therefore, the differential diagnosis of a focal pulmonary process and new CNS signs and symptoms in a cancer patient should always include *Nocardia* infection. Diagnosis requires a positive culture or tissue showing invasive organisms. Treatment options include sulfadiazine or TMP/SMX (122) and the combination of either imipenem-cilastatin or amoxicillin-clavulanic acid plus amikacin if the patient is unable to tolerate or does not respond to sulfonamides (123).

Fungal Pneumonias

Fungal pneumonias have long been known to occur in the general population in certain geographic areas of the Americas. These endemic mycoses include infections by *Histoplasma capsulatum, Coccidioides immitis,* and *Blastomyces dermatitidis.* In the normal host, clinical manifestations are most often self-limited and may include transient localized pulmonary infiltrates. In severely immunocompromised cancer patients, the endemic fungal pathogens generally cause invasive and often disseminated diseases that are life-threatening and that require aggressive therapeutic interventions (124). Approaches to antifungal therapy consist of amphotericin B deoxycholate (all mycoses; 0.5 to 1.0 mg per kilogram per day), itraconazole (histoplasmosis and blastomycosis; 5 to 12 mg per kilogram per day) and fluconazole (coccidioidomycosis; 8 to 12 mg per kilogram per day) (125,126).

The most frequent primary respiratory fungal pathogens in cancer patients are the opportunistic molds, in particular *Aspergillus* spp. (127). Yeastlike organisms such as *Candida* spp. and *T. beigelii* are less common and cause pulmonary disease primarily by hematogenous dissemination from a different portal of entry (128). A notable exception is *Cryptococcus neoformans,* for which the lungs are the usual entry site for invasive disease (129).

C. albicans and, with increasing frequency, non-*albicans* Candida species (130,131) are the most common yeastlike pathogens in pediatric cancer patients and can cause primary pneumonia (132). More often, however, the disease process present in the lung reflects disseminated hematogenous disease (127, 128,133). There is no characteristic chest roentgenographic appearance, and false-negative chest films are common (134). High-resolution computed tomography (HRCT) may detect abnormalities when the plain film is negative or shows a questionable finding; nevertheless, no specifically diagnostic HRCT pattern can be ascribed (113). Diagnosis can be elusive because positive cultures in secretions of the lower respiratory tract may reflect oropharyngeal contamination or respiratory colonization and blood cultures can be negative even in the face of widely disseminated infection (128). In the presence of abnormal radiographic findings, isolation of *Candida* from the bloodstream and high colony counts in semiquantitative cultures with microscopic visualization of pseudohyphae in lower respiratory tract secretions are strongly indicative of pulmonary candidiasis (103). However, a definite diagnosis always requires histologic proof of tissue-invasive disease (128). The dilemma is frequently whether to perform an invasive procedure or treat the patient empirically. Because a fungal pneumonia requires protracted therapy, it is preferable to establish the diagnosis. Nevertheless, if a biopsy cannot be performed and the patient is at risk for fungal pneumonia (e.g., new and progressive infiltrates in a neutropenic patient who is already receiving appropriate antibiotics), empiric therapy with amphotericin B (0.5 to 1.0 mg per kilogram per day for suspected *Candida* pneumonia) is always warranted.

Invasive aspergillosis (caused by *Aspergillus fumigatus, Aspergillus flavus,* and, less commonly, *Aspergillus niger, Aspergillus terreus,* and other species) has emerged as an important cause for morbidity and mortality in patients with hematologic malignancies and those undergoing bone marrow transplantation (127,135–138). More recent pediatric series indicate a frequency of 4.5% to 10% in

these settings (139–144). However, considering the low rate of postmortem examination, the generally high proportion of cases detected only at autopsy, and the exclusion of cases of early infection that may resolve with empiric therapy, the true incidence of invasive aspergillosis may be considerably higher than actually reported (127,144).

Because of the airborne route of infection, the lungs are the most commonly affected site (135,127). Initially causing a necrotizing bronchopneumonia, the organisms typically invade blood vessels adjacent to bronchial structures, causing thrombosis and hemorrhagic infarction; hematogenous dissemination, in particular to the CNS, occurs in approximately 30% of patients. If the acute infection is survived, influx of neutrophil granulocytes during bone marrow recovery may result in the erosion of major pulmonary arteries and life-threatening hemoptysis (145,146). In a retrospective analysis of 116 patients with acute leukemia and infections by opportunistic filamentous fungi, major hemoptysis was the cause of death in 10% (147). As in the series of Albelda et al. (145), massive hemoptysis in this series occurred exclusively within 7 days after the granulocyte count exceeded 500 cells per microliter.

Because there is no characteristic radiographic pattern, *Aspergillus* spp. and other opportunistic molds should be considered as the cause of any new infiltrate in a neutropenic patient already receiving antibiotics (148,149). HRCT facilitates early detection and accurate characterization of such infiltrates (149–151). In cancer patients, HRCT findings consistent with invasive pulmonary aspergillosis (IPA), such as the CT halo sign and nodules or masses progressing to air crescent formation or cavitation, have become a widely accepted definition of presumptive IPA (114,149–154). Nevertheless, because other opportunistic molds can cause identical HRCT patterns, and because blood cultures are only exceptionally positive (155), detection of the organism in respiratory secretions or tissues is required for definite diagnosis. However, with conventional microscopic and culture techniques, the organism is detectable by BAL in only one half of histologically confirmed cases (145,156), and even open lung biopsy may be tainted by a considerable number of false-negative findings (109). Regardless of this low sensitivity, detection of septate hyphae or positive cultures in respiratory specimens of a patient with prolonged neutropenia and fever and a progressive infiltrate correlates highly with *Aspergillus* pneumonia and should prompt immediate antifungal treatment (157). Various polymerase chain reaction (PCR) and antigen-based assays are currently under investigation and hold promise to improve recognition and monitoring of IPA.

The current standard of initial medical treatment of IPA consists of high-dose D-AmB (1.0 to 1.5 mg per kilogram per day). The lipid formulations of amphotericin B (ABCD, ABLC, L-AmB) are indicated for patients who have refractory disease or who are intolerant of D-AmB, and itraconazole may be used in stable patients for consolidation or maintenance therapy (Table 5.2) (82). The utility of colony-stimulating factors remains to be established; because neutrophil recovery is the most critical prognostic factor to survival, their use is recommended in persistently neutropenic patients with IPA (64,158). Although surgery can be safely and effectively performed in patients who have localized IPA, even during neutropenia, its exact role and timing in the management of IPA have yet to be defined (144). In a series of 36 patients with hematologic malignancies and proven or probable IPA, surgery combined with medical treatment was successful in 15 of 16 patients. The intervention was performed for diagnostic purposes in 4 cases and for therapy in 12. In eight of the latter cases, surgery was an emergency procedure based on observations by repeat chest CT scans that showed contact of lesions with larger pulmonary arteries; six of these patients were neutropenic. Surgery was uneventful in all cases. Serial CT scans were an important part of this novel approach, and, altogether, 72% of the 36 patients responded to medical or combined medical and surgical treatment (114).

The zygomycetes (the most commonly encountered genuses being *Mucor* and *Rhizo-*

pus) (159,160), *Fusarium* spp. (70,161), *P. boydii* (77), and an ever-expanding array of previously uncommon hyaline or pigmented septated molds (*Acremonium, Paecilomyces,* and *Trichoderma*; and *Bipolaris, Alternaria,* and *Curvularia*, respectively) (81) can all cause primary necrotizing pneumonias with vascular invasion and thrombosis that are clinically and radiographically undistinguishable from IPA. As in IPA, local tissue destruction and hematogenous dissemination are common, and definite diagnosis relies on detection of the organism from the site of infection. However, owing to their production of adventitious conidia-like structures in tissues (162), *Fusarium, Acremonium,* and *Paecilomyces* spp. are among the few opportunistic filamentous fungi that can cause clinically detectable fungemia (81). Approaches to treatment include aggressive antimicrobial therapy with high dosages of amphotericin B (1 to 1.5 mg per kilogram per day) or one of the lipid formulations (5 mg per kilogram or more per day) combined with surgery, as appropriate. Despite neutrophil recovery, many of these opportunistic mold infections are unresponsive to amphotericin B therapy. However, limited experience with itraconazole (83) and recent preclinical work indicate that refractory infections may be amenable to newer antifungal triazoles such as SCH56592163 or voriconazole (164).

Cryptococcosis occurs most commonly in patients with profound impairment of cellular immunity (129). Compared with invasive mold infections, pulmonary cryptococcosis is a rare opportunistic infection in children with hematologic malignancies, but it may manifest as part of a disseminated infection (165). In patients with pediatric sarcomas treated with intensive cytotoxic chemotherapy, pulmonary cryptococcosis may be a differential diagnosis of lung metastasis (166). Initial therapy for pulmonary cryptococcosis is not different from that for cryptococcal meningoencephalitis.

Less common yeastlike opportunistic pathogens, such as *T. beigelii, Saccharomyces cerevisiae, R. rubra, H. anomala,* and *M. fur-*

fur, can also cause serious pneumonia in association with disseminated infection in profound and prolonged neutropenia. Notable among them is *T. beigelii,* which causes white piedra in onimmunocompromised hosts but causes fungemia and infects the lungs, kidney, skin, and eyes of immunocompromised patients (167,168). The pulmonary infiltrates of *Trichosporon* pneumonia consist of either bronchopneumonia after aspiration from an oropharyngeal source or multiple nodular infiltrates from hematogenous dissemination. Diagnosis is aided by the cryptococcal latex agglutination test, which is positive owing to shared antigens with *C. neoformans* (169). *Trichosporon* is resistant to the fungicidal effects of amphotericin B (169–171) and therefore may break through empiric amphotericin B therapy for refractory neutropenic fever (81). Although subjects given conventional amphotericin B or a multilamellar formulation of amphotericin B were not different from untreated controls, therapy with fluconazole resulted in a significant decline in tissue burden in animal models of disseminated trichosporonosis (172). Because neutropenic patients are also at risk for azole-resistant yeast infections and invasive aspergillosis, the current recommendation for treatment in persistently neutropenic patients is amphotericin B plus high-dose fluconazole (8 to 12 mg per kilogram per day); non-neutropenic patients may be treated with fluconazole alone (64).

Diffuse Infiltrates in Neutropenic Children

The pediatric cancer patient who presents with diffuse or interstitial pulmonary infiltrates while neutropenic has an even broader range of possible infectious diseases than a child with patchy infiltrates does (Table 5.3). In addition to the aforementioned fungi, *Legionella, Chlamydia, Mycoplasma,* and gram-positive and gram-negative bacteria—all of which can cause diffuse infiltrates as well as focal ones—as well as *Pneumocystis carinii,* protozoa (*Strongyloides stercoralis, Toxoplasma gondii*), and viruses (especially CMV, but also the common respiratory viruses and

measles) must be considered (2). The management approach is conceptually different than that for patchy infiltrates in that fiberoptic bronchoscopy with BAL should be performed as soon as possible, whenever feasible. If the procedure is nondiagnostic and if the patient's condition deteriorates under empiric therapy (TMP/SMX; a macrolide; broad-spectrum antibacterial therapy), a lung biopsy may be indicated, depending on the overall assessment of the disease status of the patient. If fiberoptic bronchoscopy with BAL is not available or feasible, primary empiric therapy with the aforementioned agents is clearly justified. Again, patients who present late in the course of neutropenia with new, diffuse infiltrates, in particular while receiving antibiotics, are at high risk for an invasive fungal infection, and additional empiric antifungal therapy should be given even if BAL is negative for filamentous fungi.

Specific issues related to *Pneumocystis* and protozoal and viral pneumonias are discussed in the following paragraphs. Diffuse fungal, *Legionella,* and bacterial pneumonias are managed identically to patchy infection patterns caused by the same organisms.

Pneumocystis carinii *and Protozoal Pneumonias*

P. carinii (now recognized as a fungus based on modern molecular phyloanalysis) and the protozoal organisms *T. gondii* and *S. stercoralis* can cause diffuse infiltrates in both neutropenic and non-neutropenic patients. Toxoplasmosis and strongyloidiasis are both rare but should be kept in mind as causes of disseminated disease with pneumonia in those with exposure to the cysts of *T. gondii* (from cats or consumption of raw meat) (173–175) and in those patients from subtropical areas endemic for *S. stercoralis* helminthic infections (176,177).

Children with hematologic malignancies who are receiving dose-intensive antineoplastic chemotherapy are at high risk for development of life-threatening *Pneumocystis carinii* pneumonia (PCP) (178), although its frequency has decreased dramatically with the introduction of prophylactic TMP/SMX (179,180). PCP should be considered in the patient who presents with fever, cough, tachypnea, low Pao$_2$, and a chest roentgenogram showing a hazy bilateral alveolar and/or interstitial infiltrate that typically begins at the hilum and spreads peripherally. The duration of symptoms at presentation may be several weeks, but more often PCP in cancer patients has an acute course measured in a few days (179,181). Fiberoptic bronchoscopy with BAL is the diagnostic standard approach, allowing for the microscopic demonstration of cysts or trophozoites by silver and direct fluorescence stains within a few hours (182,183). The yield of sputum induction in pediatric cancer patients is unknown; a negative result with conventional methods does not rule out PCP and usually necessitates follow-up by bronchoscopy and BAL (184). The treatment of choice consists of TMP/SMX (15 to 20 mg per kilogram per day for 14 to 21 days); secondary alternatives are intravenous pentamidine or atovaquone. In patients with significant hypoxemia (Pao$_2$ less than 70 mm Hg at room air), adjuvant therapy with prednisone is recommended (1 mg per kilogram twice daily for days 1 through 5 of therapy; 0.5 mg per kilogram twice daily on days 6 through 10; and 0.25 mg per kilogram on days 11 through 21) (185,186).

If the BAL result is negative in a patient with diffuse pulmonary infiltrates and the patient has received appropriate prophylaxis with TMP/SMX and was compliant, PCP is unlikely (180). In patients who have received no prophylaxis or prophylactic modalities other than TMP/SMX, it is appropriate to treat empirically with TMP/SMX plus erythromycin and to proceed to open lung biopsy only if there is clinical deterioration and a new result would change the management regimen (187).

Viral Pneumonias

Although the precise role of viruses in causing febrile episodes in children with can-

cer is still unclear, illness caused by common respiratory viruses may occur and may be life-threatening.

Adenoviruses can cause severe invasive infections in immunocompromised patients (188). A frequency as high as 10% was reported among children undergoing bone marrow or liver transplantation, and the crude mortality rate was as high as 70% in patients with pneumonitis (189,190). The organism can be detected from respiratory secretions, urine, stool, buffy coat, and tissues by culture and DFA; because adenoviruses can lead to lifelong persistent infections, their recovery from the respiratory tract of an immunocompromised host requires careful interpretation and clinical correlation (106).

Little is known about measles in immune children with cancer; in nonimmune children, the risk of pneumonitis is greater than 60% and mortality ranges from 36% to 83%. The typical clinical presentation of the disease (exanthema, enanthema) is often absent, especially in cases with complicated course, and serology results and the patient's history of exposure are often noncontributory (191,192).

Children receiving antineoplastic chemotherapy are at maximum risk for complicated infections by RSV. In a prospective study of hospitalized patients, pneumonitis occurred in 100% of cases, even in the older age groups, and the mortality rate was 15%. More than half of the infections were nosocomially acquired (193). The experience reported from adult patients with acute leukemia is similar and underscores the high morbidity and mortality of RSV pneumonitis in patients undergoing dose-intensive chemotherapy (194,195).

Parainfluenza viruses can cause similarly severe infections of the lower respiratory tract in immunocompromised patients. The frequency of documented parainfluenza infections ranges between 2% and 3% in bone marrow transplantation patients, and pneumonitis occurs in approximately 70% of these cases, with an associated mortality of up to 50% (196,197).

The risk for influenza-associated disease is increased in children with cancer (198). The pattern and severity of clinical symptoms do not appear to be different from those observed in immunocompetent patients, although a prolonged clinical course has been noted. Infections are frequently complicated by bacterial superinfections of the respiratory tract, but no increased risk for primary influenza pneumonitis appears to exist (198,199).

Because orthoviruses and paramyxoviruses do not establish persistent infections, the isolation of one of these agents from the respiratory tract is always proof of active disease (106). Diagnosis can be established by shell-vial assay and antigen detection from secretions of the nasopharynx ("nasal wash"), lower respiratory tract, and biopsy specimens. PCR-based methods are also available. The options for specific treatment are limited and may include amantadine, rimantadine, ribavirin, and, for influenza, neuraminidase inhibitors (200).

CMV is found in the urine or saliva of 27% of children with leukemia (201) and can cause gastrointestinal, hepatosplenic, chorioretinal, CNS, pulmonary, and disseminated disease. Pneumonitis is the most common manifestation of CMV disease in the cancer setting. In patients who have undergone allogeneic bone marrow transplantation, its incidence is between 10% and 40%, with an associated mortality rate of up to 50% (202). Risk factors include a positive serostatus and bone marrow transplantation with total body irradiation and development of GVHD (203). The close association of GVHD with CMV pneumonitis underscores the importance of a disordered immune response in the pathogenesis of CMV infection. The typical onset of pneumonia is within 3 months after transplantation, although later cases can occur in association with chronic GVHD (204). Conversely, CMV pneumonitis is relatively infrequent in children who do not have GVHD, including those who have undergone similarly intensive preparative regimens along with autologous rather than allogeneic transplantation.

Results of serology and antigen detection in urine are difficult to interpret. A potentially useful parameter is the quantitative detection of virus or antigen in granulocytes of peripheral blood by PCR or DFA, respectively (205,206). For the diagnosis of pneumonitis, however, centrifugation cultures of BAL material with staining for early CMV antigen possess the highest sensitivity and specificity, and results can be expected within 24 to 48 hours (207). PCR-based assays are still tainted by their high sensitivity (106) and have not been standardized for clinical use.

Treatment has been difficult for CMV pneumonia. Ganciclovir does not appear to improve the outcome of fully developed CMV pneumonia in allogeneic bone marrow transplantation patients (208), although somewhat better responses have been obtained with a combination of ganciclovir and intravenous anti-CMV immunoglobulin (209). The focus has therefore been to prevent CMV pneumonia. Major breakthroughs in reducing the frequency of CMV pneumonitis have been achieved by using only seronegative blood products (210) and by early treatment in patients exhibiting evidence of increased viral replication in serial buffy coat or BAL examinations after transplantation (211,212).

Primary varicella in the child with cancer has a natural mortality rate of 7% to 20% if untreated; visceral varicella infection particularly affects the liver, lungs, and CNS, leading to severe interstitial pneumonitis transaminitis and the syndrome of inappropriate antidiuretic hormone secretion (SIADH) (213). Such dissemination occurs in approximately 32% of patients, with pneumonitis occurring in the majority of cases (213,214). Interstitial pneumonitis has also been noted to occur in association with zoster, although at a low frequency (215). Diagnosis is usually evident from the skin lesions, which generally precede the pneumonia by a few days, although atypical initial presentations without skin involvement have been reported (216). A DFA is available for rapid diagnosis. If skin lesions are not apparent, bronchoscopy or open lung biopsy with DFA and virus culture on BAL material or lung tissue may be required. Therapy must begin promptly with intravenous acyclovir (500 mg per square meter of body area every 8 hours) (Table 5.2). However, acyclovir therapy appeared to be effective even in children with varicella who had already developed pulmonary infiltrates when treatment was initiated (217).

HSV type 1 or 2 can cause viremia and then disseminate to the lungs, liver, or brain. Severe diffuse pulmonary infiltrates occur rarely and require BAL or lung biopsy with DFA and viral culture to secure a diagnosis. Early treatment with acyclovir at the same dose as for varicella is essential to arrest further dissemination (218,219).

Diffuse Infiltrates in Non-Neutropenic Children

A non-neutropenic child with diffuse pulmonary infiltrates is unlikely to have a bacterial or fungal pneumonia. The most commonly encountered pathogen in this setting is *P. carinii,* although viruses, *Legionella, Mycoplasma,* and *Chlamydia* can also cause diffuse infiltrates in these patients (2). The diagnostic and therapeutic algorithm is similar to that described for neutropenic children, with the exception that empiric antibacterial and antifungal therapy usually is not required.

Infections of the Orointestinal Tract

Children with cancer, and especially those with leukemia and lymphoma who are receiving S-phase specific chemotherapeutic agents (e.g., methotrexate, cytosine arabinoside, 5-fluorouracil), frequently develop oral mucositis. Cytotoxic drugs and radiation therapy can provide a nidus that permits the overgrowth of microorganisms constantly present in the gastrointestinal tract, leading to local infections and serving as the major portal of entry for systemic infection (see also Chapter 19).

Oral Mucositis

The mucosal toxicity associated with chemotherapy can sometimes be exceedingly severe, requiring total parenteral nutrition and patient-directed continuous analgesia with morphine derivatives. The periodontium, gingiva, buccal mucosa, and posterior pharynx may be affected (220). Marginal or necrotizing gingivitis, recognizable by an erythematous periapical line, is caused by anaerobes, however, and is an indication for specific antianaerobic drugs (e.g., clindamycin or metronidazole). For uncomplicated mucositis, mouth-cleansing solutions help decrease the discomfort and control superinfection.

Frequently the initial drug-induced mucositis becomes superinfected with *Candida,* HSV, or bacteria (including streptococci), the manifestations of which can be clinically indistinguishable from each other or from simple drug- or radiation-induced mucositis. Swabbing of lesions for direct staining for *Candida,* immunofluorescence testing for HSV, and viral cultures is important for the diagnosis. Treatment of oral candidiasis can be done with oral clotrimazole troches (50 mg five times daily), a short course of either fluconazole (3 to 6 mg per kilogram per day) or cyclodextrin-itraconazole (5 mg per kilogram per day), or intravenous amphotericin B (0.5 mg per kilogram or less per day for 5 days) (125). Oral HSV infection requires treatment with acyclovir orally if the patient can reliably swallow these pills, but intravenous treatment is often necessary if the child has difficulty with oral medications (221).

Esophagitis

Although infectious esophagitis is rare in non-neutropenic patients, in the compromised host with granulocytopenia *Candida,* followed by HSV and bacteria (especially gram-positive species), is a frequent cause of infectious esophagitis; CMV is rather uncommon in this setting (222). Noninfectious esophagitis also occurs secondary to chemotherapy or mediastinal irradiation. Establishing a diagnosis can be difficult, because barium swallow or esophagoscopy cannot reliably distinguish *Candida* from HSV or other causes of esophagitis. Therefore, endoscopic biopsy, culture, and histologic examination are necessary for diagnosis, but this procedure may be risky in a profoundly thrombocytopenic patient, and an experienced operator is essential. Another option is to treat empirically for *Candida* and HSV. This may include fluconazole (3 to 6 mg per kilogram per day), cyclodextrin-itraconazole (5 mg per kilogram per day), or low-dose amphotericin B (0.5 mg per kilogram or less per day) and empiric acyclovir. However, resolution of symptoms does not necessarily signify the eradication of esophageal candidiasis, and a persistently febrile neutropenic patient may still require empiric amphotericin B despite an apparent clinical response (64).

Intraabdominal and Perirectal Infections

The immunosuppressed cancer patient is at increased risk for many abdominal infections, not only from bone marrow suppression but also from the underlying disease itself (e.g., hepatitis secondary to hepatitis B or hepatitis C virus after transfusions, *Clostridium difficile* diarrhea secondary to antibiotics). The clinical presentation can be muted by granulocytopenia, delaying the diagnosis.

Antibiotic-Associated Colitis

Antibiotic-associated colitis is common among cancer patients because of their frequent exposure to broad-spectrum β-lactam antibiotics and clindamycin, as well as antineoplastic agents that can also increase the risk for this disease. Most of these cases are caused by *C. difficile* and its toxin, which produces watery or mucoid diarrhea, often with fever and abdominal pain (223). This presentation can easily be confused with the side effects of chemotherapy or abdominal irradiation. Diagnosis requires a positive stool toxin assay, not just positive cultures (asymptomatic patients can be culture positive but toxin negative). Treatment is usually successful with oral metronidazole; although 10% to 20% of patients have a relapse, they respond to a second course of therapy. Because *C. difficile* can be nosocomially transmitted, affected patients should be treated with enteric precaution measures.

Typhlitis

Unique to granulocytopenic cancer patients is the syndrome of typhlitis, an inflammatory necrotizing cellulitis of the cecum that is associated with a 30% to 50% mortality rate. The patient presents with subacute or acute onset of right lower quadrant abdominal pain that often progresses rapidly to generalized abdominal pain with high fever, diarrhea, and prostration (224). Abdominal ultrasonography may show bowel wall thickening and ascites, supporting the diagnosis (225). The offending agents are mostly gram-negative bacteria, and prompt institution of antibiotic therapy is essential. The differential diagnosis includes appendicitis, and surgical resection is often critical to the patient's survival. This situation is one in which surgery is indicated even in the profoundly neutropenic child (226). In this situation, intensive platelet support is essential for patients who are also thrombocytopenic.

Chronic Disseminated ("Hepatosplenic") Candidiasis

Chronic disseminated candidiasis (CDC) is an uncommon but potentially life-threatening condition in patients with cancer that develops during prolonged granulocytopenia but usually becomes apparent only on recovery from granulocytopenia. It preferentially affects the liver and spleen. The characteristics of CDC include persistent fever despite granulocyte recovery, often coupled with right upper quadrant abdominal pain and increased serum alkaline phosphatase levels (227,228). Ultrasonography, CT scans, or MRI scans performed at this time demonstrate multiple lesions in the liver and spleen, and not infrequently in other organs such as kidneys and lungs, that correspond to large granulomas with a core of necrosis and an outer ring of inflammatory cells and fibrosis (229). Despite the apparently distinct clinical and radiographic presentation, prompt biopsy is important to rule out other infectious, neoplastic, or inflammatory processes and to justify the long-term administration of antifungal agents that may be fraught with significant adverse effects (64). Approaches to the management of hepatosplenic candidiasis include administration of conventional amphotericin B, usually in combination with flucytosine (64,227), or therapy with amphotericin B lipid complex (230), followed by long-term fluconazole for susceptible isolates. Fluconazole has also been used with success in patients who are intolerant of amphotericin B or who have CDC refractory to amphotericin B treatment (231,232). Antifungal therapy is recommended until resolution or calcification of lesions, which may require 6 months to 1 year (64). During therapy for CDC, further antineoplastic chemotherapy can be administered without progression or breakthrough fungemia, provided that the disseminated infection has stabilized or is resolving (233).

Perirectal Cellulitis

Perirectal cellulitis, although less frequently diagnosed than in the early stages of intensive anticancer therapy, can be a problem in children with prolonged, profound granulocytopenia. The risk of this problem increases if perirectal mucositis (secondary to chemotherapy or radiation therapy), hemorrhoids, fissure, or rectal manipulation has occurred. Perianal pain and tenderness often are the first and only indications of infection, because the usual signs of infection (erythema, induration, fluctuance) are delayed. Treatment should begin early with antibiotics to cover aerobic gram-negative bacilli, anaerobes, and group D streptococci, along with sitz baths, stool softeners, and a low-residue diet (234). Surgical incision and drainage can usually be avoided with prompt antibiotic therapy but may be necessary if inflammation or fluctuance persists after granulocyte recovery or if signs of progressive ischiorectal fossa infection occur despite appropriate antibiotic therapy (235).

Genitourinary Infections

Infections of the genitourinary tract are uncommon in children with cancer unless obstruction by tumor, catheterization, neurologic dysfunction (secondary to cord compression or drugs such as vincristine) or changes resulting from local surgery or irradiation have increased the risk. Gram-negative aerobic bacilli and enterococci are the usual pathogens (2). The criterion for treating bacteriuria differs from that in nongranulocytopenic patients, however, in that a colony count of more than 10^3 colony-forming units (CFU) per milliliter of a single organism with symptoms (dysuria, urgency, frequency, fever), or 10^5 CFU/mL even without symptoms, is an indication for therapy. Pyuria may not be seen in the granulocytopenic patient. The indications for treating candiduria may be confusing because colonization without invasion frequently occurs in patients with indwelling urinary catheters and in those receiving broad-spectrum antibiotics. However, persistently positive *Candida* urine cultures (two or more positive fungal cultures of at least 10^3 CFU/mL obtained 24 hours apart by clean catch or catheterization plus fungal elements noted from appropriate stains), in association with fever and worsening azotemia, are highly suggestive of upper urinary tract disease and should prompt appropriate imaging studies and systemic antifungal therapy with amphotericin B plus flucytosine or fluconazole for probable renal candidiasis. In the absence of these signs, candiduria that persists after removal of a catheter or a stent may indicate a superficial bladder infection that can be effectively treated with fluconazole or intravenous amphotericin B, depending on the isolated species and *in vitro* susceptibility (64).

Cutaneous Infections

The pediatric cancer patient is susceptible to cutaneous infections caused by bacteria, fungi, and viruses, not only because of immunosuppression but also because of frequent disruption in this primary defense barrier, as previously mentioned (see also Chapter 21). The skin may also be involved in systemic infections, and careful examination for early lesions with subsequent aspiration or biopsy for culture, Gram stain, potassium hydroxide, methylene blue, or specific viral DFA may permit early diagnosis of generalized infections (236).

Bacterial skin infections include common local gram-positive infections (*S. aureus*, β-hemolytic streptococci), often starting at sites of invasive devices or skin breaks, wounds, radiation, burns, or furuncles (especially in patients receiving glucocorticosteroids). However, gram-negative organisms, in particular *P. aeruginosa*, can cause a fulminant local infection (pyoderma gangrenosum), and embolic- or vasculitic-appearing lesions can be seen with bacteremia caused by *P. aeruginosa*, *Aeromonas hydrophilus*, *Corynebacterium equi*, or *S. marcescens*. Fresh lesions therefore should be aspirated or biopsied, then cultured and Gram stained; treatment should cover both gram-positive and gram-negative bacteria (236).

Fungemia may manifest with embolic skin lesions (especially with *Candida* spp., but also *T. beigelii*, *H. capsulatum*, and *Cryptococcus*, *Fusarium*, *Paecilomyces*, *Acremonium* spp.). Candidemia can sometimes cause nodular, erythematous lesions, notably on the extremities, but cultures are often negative and biopsy may not always reveal organisms unless the lesion is fresh. In any case, a high index of suspicion for fungemia is required in a febrile granulocytopenic patient who is receiving broad-spectrum antibacterial antibiotics and has a new skin lesion (237).

Primary infections of the skin and subcutaneous tissues by *Aspergillus* have been described in association with skin lacerations by armboards, electrodes, and tape (238–243) and at the insertion sites of peripheral (238) or central venous catheters (62,244). With an overall cure rate of approximately 50% after combined medical and surgical therapy, the prognosis of these infections may not be as dismal as that of other forms of invasive aspergillosis (238). Among the filamentous fungi, *Fusarium* has become increasingly recognized as a cause of paronychia in neutropenic patients that may lead to widespread dissemination (80).

Viral cutaneous infections are often seen as a result of HSV or VZV. Fresh vesicles should be unroofed and the base scraped well with a swab, which then should be used to smear a microscope slide for DFA staining. DFA is highly sensitive and specific for both HSV and VZV (245). Wright-Giemsa staining (Tsanck test) for multinucleated giant cells cannot differentiate between HSV and VZV, and viral cultures may take from 2 days (HSV) to 4 weeks (VZV) to turn positive. The diagnosis is important because it determines appropriate management, such as the dose of acyclovir and the need for isolation. The initial therapy of choice for VZV and HSV is intravenous acyclovir, although the dose for zoster (500 mg per square meter every 8 hours) can be halved for uncomplicated mucocutaneous HSV infection. The duration of treatment is usually 7 days, although longer courses may be necessary depending on the response. Hydration should be adequately maintained to prevent renal toxicity. Oral acyclovir is poorly absorbed and therefore cannot be uniformly recommended (217). Novel compounds such as valaciclovir and famciclovir, prodrugs of aciclovir and penciclovir, have improved oral bioavailability and may be used for consolidation therapy in uncomplicated cases (246). The risk of visceral dissemination with VZV is low with therapy, although cutaneous dissemination may occur in 5% to 50% of cases (247). Late complications of VZV include postherpetic neuralgia, secondary bacterial skin infections, and, uncommonly, aseptic meningitis, myelitis, and zoster encephalitis, either by direct VZV infection or as a postinfectious syndrome.

Primary varicella, on the other hand, is the most serious vesicular eruption in children with cancer because of the high rate of visceral dissemination and considerable mortality (213,214,216). The risk of dissemination is higher in patients receiving chemotherapy at the time of infection, especially if the patient is also lymphopenic (fewer than 500 cells per microliter). Prompt initiation, preferably within 48 to 72 hours after exposure, of acyclovir (500 mg per square meter intravenously every 8 hours) is essential to reduce or eliminate dissemination and to reduce the duration of skin lesions and fever (217).

Prevention of primary varicella in pediatric cancer patients is important, given the severity of illness in these children. The most important measure is patient education and avoidance of exposure to individuals with either chickenpox or herpes zoster. If a seronegative patient is exposed to VZV (varicella infection is contagious starting 2 days before the development of skin lesions), immunoprophylaxis with VZV immune globulin should be given intravenously as soon as possible but not later than 72 hours after the exposure (248). Patient and point source should remain separated until the latter is no longer infectious in order to avoid continuous inoculation. The patient should not receive immunosuppressive therapy for approximately 21 days after exposure, and not until scabs heal over if disease develops. If hospitalized, these potentially infected children should be placed in reverse isolation for 21 days after the exposure. Staff members who do not have a history of chickenpox or who are seronegative should refrain from contact with these children. Postexposure chemoprophylaxis, reported for acyclovir as being effective in nonimmunocompromised children (249,250), has not been sufficiently evaluated in the immunocompromised patient population and therefore cannot be recommended.

Central Nervous System Infections

CNS infections are surprisingly infrequent in children (see Chapter 20). When an Ommaya reservoir is present, it can become infected by skin organisms, including staphylococci, *Corynebacterium* spp., *Propionibacterium acnes,* or, rarely, enterococci, gram-negative bacilli, or *Candida* spp. Patients may be asymptomatic, or they may have fever, headache, increased intracranial pressure, and clinical evidence of meningitis. Most shunt infections can be treated by systemic antibiotics, or by antibiotic instillation into the reservoir, without shunt removal

(251). A notable exception is shunt infections caused by *Candida* spp. (252).

Meningitis

In a retrospective review of bacterial and fungal meningitis in pediatric cancer patients from a single institution, most patients (65%) had neurosurgery, a CNS device, or cerebrospinal fluid (CSF) leak. Fever and altered mental status were the most consistent signs at presentation, and *S. aureus* and *S. pneumoniae* were the most common microbiologic isolates (253). Meningitis or meningoencephalitis can also occur secondary to *C. neoformans* or *Listeria monocytogenes* infection, especially in children with decreased cell-mediated immunity.

Cryptococcal meningoencephalitis usually manifests as an indolent process, with symptoms of headache, mental status changes, and low-grade fever; rarely, meningismus, increased intracranial pressure, coma, or focal deficits are present (254). The CSF typically reveals a mild mononuclear pleocytosis, slightly low glucose, and only sometimes (50%) visible organisms on India ink preparation. Diagnosis relies on identification of the organism in blood or CSF; the most reliable and rapid diagnosis is by serum or CSF cryptococcal antigen determination (64). We recommend that treatment of cryptococcal meningoencephalitis be initiated with amphotericin B (0.7 mg per kilogram per day) plus flucytosine (starting dose, 100 mg per kilogram per day) for at least 2 weeks and for 4 to 6 weeks in continuously symptomatic patients; this should be followed by consolidation therapy with fluconazole (8 to 12 mg per kilogram per day) for at least 4 weeks after completion of induction therapy (64,82). For patients who are unable to tolerate conventional amphotericin B, we recommend liposomal amphotericin B at 5 mg per kilogram per day (255); and for those not tolerating antifungal polyenes, the combination of fluconazole and flucytosine.

L. monocytogenes is the most common cause of bacterial meningitis in adult cancer patients (256) and carries an exceedingly high crude mortality rate (257,258). Awareness of the disease is particularly important, because the usual empiric antibiotic regimens used in the febrile cancer patient are not active against *Listeria*. The clinical manifestations of human listeriosis include bacteremia and/or meningitis and encephalitis with a characteristic predilection for the brain stem (259). Diagnosis is usually made by the isolation of the organism from blood or CSF. Standard therapy consists of the administration of ampicillin with or without gentamicin; high-dose TMP/SMX is recommended as a first best alternative (260,261). However, the bactericidal activity of TMP/SMX, its excellent intracellular and intracerebral penetration (261), and limited clinical experience (262,263) suggest that the combination of ampicillin with TMP/SMX, administered for at least 3 weeks, may be the most effective therapy for cerebral listeriosis.

Encephalitis

Encephalitis is generally rare and is usually caused by HSV, VZV, or measles. Patients commonly present with signs of meningeal irritation, mental status changes, and focal neurologic signs or seizures. Diagnosis may be hampered because CSF signs are nonspecific, and CT scans may be negative or unable to help distinguish between infections and neoplastic, toxic, or metabolic causes. Although a brain biopsy is required for definitive diagnosis, it is rarely done. Maximum doses of acyclovir are recommended in clinically suspected cases of viral encephalitis (200).

If one or more enhancing lesions are seen in the brain, *Toxoplasma* should be considered. The diagnosis is based on a typical radiographic appearance on CT scans of the head, results of serologic investigations, isolation of the organism from blood, and demonstration of tachyzoites in tissue or cytologic preparations of body fluids such as BAL material. Brain biopsy is advocated to exclude other disease processes that mimic or coexist with cerebral toxoplasmosis, such as mass lesions

caused by fungi, *Nocardia,* or common gram-positive or gram-negative bacteria (264). Because of the potentially devastating course, therapy with pyrimethamine and sulfadiazine or TMP/SMX may be instituted empirically before establishment of the diagnosis (173). However, brain biopsy should be performed whenever feasible to establish a diagnosis.

CONCLUSIONS

Given the numerous possible causes for the various specific infectious complications in children with cancer, most clinical situations involve starting empiric therapy before a definitive diagnosis is found. Furthermore, as the rate of finding a documented pathogen decreases with early antibiotic therapy, the management of fever in neutropenic patients becomes more empiric. The complex aspects of empiric management and the specific antimicrobial agents available today are discussed in Chapter 19.

REFERENCES

1. Pizzo PA. Infectious complications in the child with cancer: I. Pathophysiology of the compromised host and the initial evaluation and management of the febrile cancer patient. *J Pediatr* 1981;98:341.
2. Pizzo PA. Infectious complications in the child with cancer: II. Management of specific infectious organisms. *J Pediatr* 1981;98:513.
3. Bodey GP, Buckley M, Sathe YS, et al. Quantitative relationships between circulating leukocytes and infection in patients with acute leukemia. *Ann Intern Med* 1966;64:328.
4. Pizzo PA, Robichaud KJ, Edward BK, et al. Oral antibiotic prophylaxis in cancer patients: a double-blind randomized placebo controlled trial. *J Pediatr* 1983; 102:125.
5. Pizzo PA, Commers JR, Cotton DJ, et al. Approaching the controversies in the antibacterial management of cancer patients. *Am J Med* 1984;76:436.
6. Young LS. Management of infections in leukemia and lymphoma. In: Rubin RH, Young LS, eds. *Clinical approaches to the infections in the compromised Host.* New York: Plenum, 1988:439.
7. Browder AA, Hoff JA, Petersdorf RG. The significance of fever in neoplastic disease. *Ann Intern Med* 1961;55:932.
8. Pizzo PA, Robichaud KJ, Wesley R, et al. Fever in the pediatric and young adult patient with cancer: a prospective study of 1001 episodes. *Medicine (Baltimore)* 1982;61:153.
9. Pizzo PA, Hathorn JW, Heimenz JW, et al. A random-

ized trial comparing ceftazidime alone with combination antibiotic therapy in cancer patients with fever and neutropenia. *N Engl J Med* 1986;315:552.

10. Lehrenbecher T, Foster C, Vasquez N, et al. Therapy-induced alterations in host defense in children receiving therapy for cancer. *J Pediatr Hematol Oncol* 1997; 19:399–417.

11. Pizzo PA, Myers J. Infection in the cancer patient. In: Devita VT, Hellman S, Rosenberg SA, eds. *Principles and practice of oncology.* Philadelphia: JB Lippincott, 1989:2008.

12. Keusch GT. Nutrition and infection. In: Remington JS, Swartz NM, eds. *Current clinical topics in infectious disease.* New York: McGraw-Hill, 1984:106.

13. Pizzo PA. Diagnosis and management of infectious disease problems in the child with malignant disease. In: Rubin RH, Young LS, eds. Clinical approaches to the infections in the compromised host. New York: Plenum, 1988:439.

14. Curnette JT, Boxer LA. Clinically significant phagocytic cell defects. In: Remington J, Swartz M, eds. Current clinical topics in infectious diseases. New York: McGraw-Hill, 1985:103.

15. Wiener S, Wiener R, Urivetsky M, et al. The mechanism of action of a single dose of methylprednisolone on acute inflammation *in vivo. J Clin Invest* 1975;56: 679–689.

16. Handin RI, Stossel TP. Effect of corticosteroid therapy on the phagocytosis of antibody-coated platelets by human leukocytes. *Blood* 1978;51:771–779.

17. Nelson DH, Meikle AW, Benowitz B, et al. Cortisol and dexamethasone suppression of superoxide anion production by leukocytes from normal subjects. *Trans Assoc Am Physicians* 1978;91:381–387.

18. Schaffner A, Douglas H, Braude A. Selective protection against conidia by mononuclear and against mycelia by polymorphonuclear phagocytes in resistance to *Aspergillus. J Clin Invest* 1982;69:617.

19. Rinehard J, Sagone A, Balcerzak S, et al. Effects of corticosteroid therapy on human monocyte function. *N Engl J Med* 1975;292:236–241.

20. Dale DC, Petersdorf RG. Corticosteroids and infectious disease. *Med Clin North Am* 1973;57:1277.

21. Cesario TC, Slater L, Poo WJ, et al. The effect of hydrocortisone on the production of gamma-interferon and other lymphokines by human peripheral blood mononuclear cells. *J Interferon Cytokine Res* 1986;6: 337–347.

22. Walsh TJ, Hiemenz J, Pizzo PA. Evolving risk factors for invasive fungal infections: all neutropenic patients are not the same [Editorial]. *Clin Infect Dis* 1994;18: 793–798.

23. Baehner RL, Neiburger RG, Johnson DG, et al. Transient bactericidal defect of peripheral blood phagocytes from children with acute lymphoblastic leukemia receiving craniospinal irradiation. *N Engl J Med* 1973;289:1209.

24. Mackall C, Fleisher T, Brown M, et al. Age, thymopoiesis, and CD4+ T-lymphocyte regeneration after intensive chemotherapy. *N Engl J Med* 1995;332: 143–149.

25. Abrahamsson J, Marky I, Mellander L. Immunoglobulin levels and lymphocyte response to mitogenic stimulation in children with malignant disease during treatment and follow-up. *Acta Paediatr* 1995;84:177–182.

26. Hitzig W, Pluss H, Joller P, et al. Studies on the immune status of children with acute lymphocytic leukemia. *Clin Exp Immunol* 1976;26:414–418.

27. Reid M, Craft A, Todd J. Serial studies of number of circulating T and B lymphocytes in children with acute lymphoblastic leukemia. *Arch Dis Child* 1977;52: 245–247.

28. Rosen F, Cooper M, Wedgewood R. The primary immunodeficiencies: part 2. *N Engl J Med* 1984;311: 300–310.

29. Siber GR. Bacteremias due to *Hemophilus influenzae* and *Streptococcus pneumoniae*: their occurrence and course in children with cancer. *Am J Dis Child* 1980; 134:668.

30. Katz J, Walter BO, Bennetts GA, et al. Abnormal cellular and humoral immunity in childhood acute lymphoblastic leukemia in long-term remission. *West J Med* 1987;146:179–187.

31. Layward K, Levinsky R, Butler M. Long-term abnormalities in T and B lymphocyte function in children following treatment for acute lymphoblastic leukemia. *Br J Hematol* 1981;49:251–258.

32. Donaldson SS, Glatstein E, Vosti K-L. Bacterial infections in pediatric Hodgkin's disease: relationship to radiation, chemotherapy and splenectomy. *Cancer* 1978; 41:1949.

33. Chilcote R, Baehner R, Hammond D. Septicemia and meningitis in children splenectomized for Hodgkin's disease. *N Engl J Med* 1976;295:798–800.

34. Fainstain V, Rodriquez V, Turk M, et al. Patterns of oropharyngeal and fecal flora in patients with leukemia. *J Infect Dis* 1981;144:10.

35. Kramer BK, Pizzo PA, Robichaud KJ, et al. Role of serial microbiological surveillance and clinical evaluation in the management of cancer patients with fever and granulocytopenia. *Am J Med* 1982;72:561.

36. Freifeld AG, Walsh TJ, Marshall D, et al. Monotherapy for fever and neutropenia in cancer patients: a randomized comparison of ceftazidime vs. imipenem. *J Clin Oncol* 1995;13:165–176.

37. Pizzo PA, Ladisch SL, Gill F, et al. Increasing incidence of gram-positive sepsis in cancer patients. *Med Pediatr Oncol* 1978;5:241.

38. Wade JC, Schimpff SC, Newman KA, et al. *Staphylococcus epidermidis: an increasing cause of infection in patients with granulocytopenia.* Ann Intern Med 1982;97:507.

39. Gill VJ, Manning C, Lamson M, et al. Antibiotic-resistant group JK bacteria in hospitals. *J Clin Microbiol* 1982;13:472.

40. Cohen J, Donnelly JP, Worsley Am, et al. Septicemia caused by viridans streptococci in neutropenic patients with leukemia. *Lancet* 1983;2:1452.

41. Bochud PY, Calandra T, Francioli P. Bacteremia due to viridans streptococci in neutropenic patient: a review. *Am J Med* 1994;97:256.

42. Todeschini G, Rubin M, Gill V, et al. Non-*aeruginosa* bacteremias in cancer patients: review of 10 years' experience at the National Cancer Institute. In: *Proceedings of the 27th Interscience Conference on Antimicrobial Agents and Chemotherapy.* Washington, DC: American Society for Microbiology, 1987:265.

43. Jacoby GA. Extended spectrum beta-lactamases and other enzymes providing resistance to oxyimino-beta-lactams. *Infect Dis Clin North Am* 1997;11:875–887.

44. McCabe WR, Jackson GG. Gram-negative bacteremia. *Arch Intern Med* 1982;110:847.

45. Aquino VM, Pappo A, Buchanan GR, et al. The changing epidemiology of bacteremia in neutropenic children with cancer. *Pediatr Infect Dis J* 1995;14:140.

46. Rubin M, Hathorn JW, Marshall D, et al. Gram-positive infections and the use of vancomycin in 550 episodes of fever and neutropenia. *Ann Intern Med* 1988;108:30.

47. Boyce JM. Vancomycin-resistant *Enterococcus. Infect Dis Clin North Am* 1997;11:367–384.

48. Pizzo PA, Thaler M, Hathorn J, et al. New β-lactamase antibiotics in the granulocytopenic patient: new options and new questions. *Am J Med* 1985;79:75.

49. Birnbaum J, Kaham FM, Kropp H, et al. Carbapenems, a new class of beta-lactam antibiotics: discovery and development of imipenem/cilastatin. *Am J Med* 1985;78[Suppl 6A]:3021.

50. Neu H-C. β-Lactam antibiotics: structural relationships affecting *in vitro* activity and pharmacologic properties. *Rev Infect Dis* 1986;8[Suppl 3]:S237.

51. Karp JE, Dick JD, Angelopoulos C, et al. Empiric use of vancomycin during prolonged treatment-induced granulocytopenia: randomized, double blind, placebo-controlled clinical trial in patients with acute leukemia. *Am J Med* 1986;81:237.

52. Pizzo PA, Ladisch SL, Robichaud K. Treatment of gram-positive septicemia in cancer patients. *Cancer* 1980;45:206.

53. Cotton D, Marshall D, Gress J, et al. Pathogen-specific vs broad-spectrum antibiotics for granulocytopenic patients with proven infection. In: *Proceedings of the 24th Interscience Conference on Antimicrobial Agents and Chemotherapy '84.* Washington, DC: American Society for Microbiology, 1984:158.

54. Pizzo PA, Robichaud KJ, Gill FA, et al. Empiric antibiotic and antifungal therapy for cancer patients with prolonged fever and granulocytopenia. *Am J Med* 1984;72:101.

55. Lazarus HM, Lowder JHN, Herzog R-H. Occlusion and infection in Broviac catheters during intensive chemotherapy. *Cancer* 1983;52:2342.

56. Begala JE, Maher K, Cherry J-D. Risk of infection associated with the use of Broviac and Hickman catheters. *Am J Infect Control* 1981;10:17.

57. Mueller BU, Skelton J, Callender DP, et al. A prospective randomized trial comparing the infectious and noninfectious complications of an externalized catheter versus a subcutaneously implanted device in cancer patients. *J Clin Oncol* 1992;10:1943–1948.

58. Lecciones JA, Lee JW, Navarro E, et al. Vascular catheter-associated fungemia in cancer patients: analysis of 155 episodes. *Rev Infect Dis* 1992;14:875–883.

59. Raad II, Bodey GP. Infectious complications of indwelling vascular catheters. *Clin Infect Dis* 1992;15:197–210.

60. Allo MD, Miller J, Townsend T, et al. Primary cutaneous aspergillosis associated with Hickman intravenous catheters. *N Engl J Med* 1987;317:1105.

61. Hoy JF, Rolston KVI, Hopfer RL, et al. *Mycobacterium fortuitum* bacteremia in patients with cancer and long term venous catheters. *Am J Med* 1987;83:213.

62. Burch PA, Karp JE, Merz WG, et al. Favorable outcome of invasive aspergillosis in patients with acute leukemia. *J Clin Oncol* 1987;5:1985–1993.

63. Cotton DJ, Gu V, Heimenz J, et al. *Bacillus* bacteremias in an immunocompromised patient population: clinical features, therapeutic interventions, and relationship to chronic intravascular catheters in sixteen cases. *J Clin Microbiol* 1987;25:672.

64. Walsh TJ, Gonzalez CE, Lyman CA, et al. Invasive fungal infections in children: recent advances in diagnosis and treatment. *Adv Pediatr Infect Dis* 1996;11:187–290.

65. Berenguer J, Buck M, Witebsky F, et al. Lysis-centrifugation blood cultures in the detection of tissue-proven invasive candidiasis: disseminated versus single organ infection. *Diagn Microbiol Infect Dis* 1993;17:103–109.

66. Dato V, Dajani A. Candidemia in children with central venous catheters: role of catheter removal and amphotericin B therapy. *Pediatr Infect Dis J* 1990;9:309–314.

67. Eppes SC, Troutman JL, Gutman LT. Outcome of treatment of candidemia in children whose central catheters were removed or retained. *Pediatr Infect Dis J* 1989;8:99–104.

68. Rex JH, Bennett JE, Sugar AM, et al. A randomized trial comparing fluconazole with amphotericin B for the treatment of candidemia in patients without neutropenia. *N Engl J Med* 1994;331:1325–1330.

69. Wingard JR, Merz WG, Rinaldi MG, et al. Increase in *Candida krusei* infection among patients with bone marrow transplantation and neutropenia treated prophylactically with fluconazole. *N Engl J Med* 1991;325:1274–1277.

70. Rubin M, Todeschini G, Marshall D, et al. Does the presence of an indwelling venous catheter affect the type of infection in neutropenic cancer patients? An analysis of 505 episodes. In: *Proceedings of the 27th Interscience Conference on Antimicrobial Agents and Chemotherapy '87.* Washington, DC: American Society for Microbiology, 1987:264.

71. Wald ER, Milmoe GJ, Bowen AD, et al. Acute maxillary sinusitis in children. *N Engl J Med* 1982;304:749.

72. Caplan ES, Hoyt NJ. Nosocomial sinusitis. *JAMA* 1982;247:639.

73. Frederick J, Braude AI. Anaerobic infection of the paranasal sinuses. *N Engl J Med* 1974;290:135.

74. Berkow RL, Weisman SJ, Provisor AJ, et al. Invasive aspergillosis of paranasal tissues in children with malignancies. *J Pediatr* 1983;103:49–53.

75. Kavanagh KT, Hughes WT, Parham DM, et al. Fungal sinusitis in immunocompromised children with neoplasms. *Ann Otol Rhinol Laryngol* 1991;100:331–336.

76. Choi SS, Milmoe GJ, Dinndorf PA, et al. Invasive *Aspergillus* sinusitis in pediatric bone marrow transplant patients: evaluation and management. *Arch Otolaryngol Head Neck Surg* 1995;121:1188–1192.

77. Travis LB, Roberts GD, Wilson WR. Clinical significance of *Pseudallescheria boydii: a review of 10 years' experience.* Mayo Clin Proc 1985;60:531–537.

78. Antoine GA, Raternik MH. *Bipolaris: a serious new fungal pathogen of the paranasal sinus.* Otolaryngol Head Neck Surg 1989;100:158–162.

79. Kline MW. Mucormycosis in children: review of the literature and report of cases. *Pediatr Infect Dis* 1985;4:672–676.

80. Boutati EI, Anaissie EJ. *Fusarium,* a significant emerging pathogen in patients with hematologic malignancy: ten years' experience at a cancer center and implications for management. *Blood* 1997;90:999–1008.

81. Walsh TJ, Groll AH. Emerging fungal pathogens: evolving challenges to immunocompromised patients for the twenty-first century. *Transplant Infect Dis* 1999;1:247–261.

82. Groll AH, Mueller FM, Piscitelli SC, et al. Lipid formulations of amphotericin B: clinical perspectives for the management of invasive fungal infections in children with cancer. *Klin Padiatr* 1998;210:264–273.

83. Sharkey K, Graybill JR, Rinaldi MG, et al. Itraconazole treatment of phaeohyphomycosis. *J Am Acad Dermatol* 1990;23:577–586.

84. Walsh TJ, Gray W. *Candida* epiglottis in immunocompromised patients. *Chest* 1987;9:482.

85. Hass A, Hyatt AC, Kattan M, et al. Hoarseness in immunocompromised children: association with invasive fungal infection. *J Pediatr* 1987;111:731–733.

86. Weiner LB, Vladimer GM. *Mycoplasma pneumoniae* in a pediatric tumor clinic population. *Pediatr Res* 1974;8:430/156.

87. Gaydos CA, Fowler CL, Gill VJ, et al. Detection of *Chlamydia pneumoniae* by polymerase chain reaction-enzyme immunoassay in an immunocompromised population. *Clin Infect Dis* 1993;17:718–723.

88. Kovatch AL, Jardine DS, Dowling JN, et al. Legionellosis in children with leukemia in relapse. *Pediatrics* 1984;73:811–815.

89. Centers for Disease Control and Prevention. Diagnosis and management of mycobacterial infection and disease in persons with human immunodeficiency virus infection. *Ann Intern Med* 1987;106:254–256.

90. Libshitz HI, Pannu HK, Elting LS, et al. Tuberculosis in cancer patients: an update. *J Thorac Imaging* 1997; 12:41–46.

91. Kaplan MH, Armstrong D, Rosen P. Tuberculosis complicating neoplastic disease: a review of 201 cases. *Cancer* 1974;33:850–858.

92. Scogberg K, Ruutu P, Tukiainen P, et al. Effect of immunosuppressive therapy on the clinical presentation and outcome of tuberculosis. *Clin Infect Dis* 1993;17: 1012–1017.

93. Feld R, Bodey GP, Groschel D. Mycobacteriosis in patients with malignant disease. *Arch Intern Med* 1976; 136:67.

94. Groll AH, Schwabe D, Lerman E, et al. Successfully treated extra-pulmonary tuberculosis in two children with leukemia during intensive chemotherapy. *J Cancer Res Clin Oncol* 1992;118:R34.

95. Schimpff SC, Young VM, Greene WH, et al. Origin of infection in acute nonlymphocytic leukemia: significance of hospital acquisition of potential pathogens. *Ann Intern Med* 1972;77:707–714.

96. Pizzo PA, Robichaud KJ, Gill FA, et al. Empiric antibiotic and antifungal therapy for cancer patients with prolonged fever and granulocytopenia. *Am J Med* 1982;72:101–111.

97. Bye MR, Bernstein L, Shah K, et al. Diagnostic bronchoalveolar lavage in children with AIDS. *Pediatr Pulmonol* 1987;3:425–428.

98. DeBlic J, McKelvie P, Le Burgeois M, et al. Value of bronchoalveolar lavage in the management of severe acute pneumonia and interstitial pneumonitis in the immunocompromised child. *Thorax* 1987;42:759–765.

99. Frankel LR, Smith DW, Lewiston NJ. Bronchoalveolar lavage for diagnosis of pneumonia in the immunocompromised child. *Pediatrics* 1988;81:785–788.

100. McCubbin MM, Trigg ME, Hendricker C, et al. Bronchoscopy with bronchoalveolar lavage in the evaluation of pulmonary complications of bone marrow transplantation in children. *Pediatr Pulmonol* 1992;12: 43–47.

101. Pattishall EN, Noyes BE, Orenstein DM. Use of bronchoalveolar lavage in immunocompromised children with pneumonia. *Pediatr Pulmonol* 1988;5:1–5.

102. Riedler J, Grigg J, Robertson CF. Role of bronchoalveolar lavage in children with lung disease. *Eur Respir J* 1995;8:1725–1730.

103. Stokes DC, Shenep JL, Parham D, et al. Role of flexible bronchoscopy in the diagnosis of pulmonary infiltrates in pediatric patients with cancer. *J Pediatr* 1989; 115:561–567.

104. Levine SJ, Stover DE. Bronchoscopy and related techniques. In: Shelhamer J, Pizzo PA, Parillo JE, et al., eds. *Respiratory disease in the immunosuppressed host.* Philadelphia: JP Lippincott, 1991:73–93.

105. Wood RE, Postma D. Endoscopy of the airway in infants and children. *J Pediatr* 1988;112:1–6.

106. Shelhamer JH, moderator. The laboratory evaluation of opportunistic pulmonary infections. *Ann Intern Med* 1996;124:585–599.

107. Crawford SW, Meyers JD. Respiratory disease in bone marrow transplant patients. In: Shelhamer J, Pizzo PA, Paillo JE, et al. eds. *Respiratory disease in the immunocompromised host.* Philadelphia: JB Lippincott, 1991:595–623.

108. Burt ME, Fly MW, Webbert BL, et al. Prospective evaluation of aspiration needle, cutting needle, transbronchial, and open lung biopsy in patients with pulmonary infiltrates. *Ann Thorac Surg* 1981;32:146.

109. McCabe RE, Brooks RG, Mark JB, et al. Open lung biopsy in patients with acute leukemia. *Am J Med* 1985;78:609–616.

110. Groll AH, Sehrt P, Ahrens P, et al. Diagnostic approach to the pediatric cancer patient with fever and pulmonary infiltrates. *Monatsschr Kinderheilk* 1997;145: 1197–1207.

111. Krick JA, Remington JS. Opportunistic invasive fungal infections in patients with leukemia and lymphoma. *Clin Haematol* 1976;5:249.

112. Commers JC, Robichaud K, Pizzo PA. New pulmonary infiltrates in granulocytopenic patients being treated with antibiotics. *Pediatr Infect Dis* 1984;3:423.

113. Wheeler JH, Fishman EK. Computed tomography in the management of chest infections: current status. *Clin Infect Dis* 1996;23:332–340.

114. Caillot D, Casasnovas O, Bernard A, et al. Improved management of invasive pulmonary aspergillosis in neutropenic patients using early thoracic computed tomography scan and surgery. *J Clin Oncol* 1997;15: 139–147.

115. Schwebke JR, Hackman R, Bowden R. Pneumonia due to *Legionella micdadei* in bone marrow transplant recipients. *Rev Infect Dis* 1990;12:824–828.

116. Schurmann D, Ruf B, Pfannkuch F, et al. Fatal legionellosis in patients with malignant hematologic diseases. *Blut* 1988;56:27–31.

117. Tobin J, Beare J, Dunnill MS, et al. Legionnaires' disease in a transplant unit: isolation of the causative agent from shower baths. *Lancet* 1980;2:118.

118. Kirby BD, Snyder KM, Meyer RD, et al. Legionnaires' disease: report of sixty-five nosocomially acquired

cases and review of the literature. *Medicine (Baltimore)* 1980;59:188.

119. Vergis EN, Yu VL. *Legionella* species. In: Yu VL, Merigan TC, Barriere SL, eds. *Antimicrobial therapy and vaccines.* Baltimore: Williams & Wilkins, 1999: 257–272.

120. Young LS, Armstrong D, Blevins A, et al. *Nocardia asteroides* infection complicating neoplastic disease. *Am J Med* 1971;50:356–367.

121. Smego RA, Gallis HA. The clinical spectrum of *Nocardia brasiliensis* infection in the United States. *Rev Infect Dis* 1984;6:164.

122. Berkey P, Bodey GP. Nocardial infection in patients with neoplastic disease. *Rev Infect Dis* 1989;11: 407–412.

123. McNeill MM, Brown JM. *Nocardia* species. In: Yu VL, Merigan TC, Barriere SL, eds. *Antimicrobial therapy and vaccines.* Baltimore: Williams & Wilkins, 1999:310–323.

124. Kauffman CA, Israel KS, Smith JW, et al. Histoplasmosis in immunocompromised patients. *Am J Med* 1978;64:923.

125. Mueller FM, Groll AH, Walsh TJ. Current approaches to diagnosis and treatment of fungal infections in HIV-infected children. *Eur J Pediatr* 1999;158:187–199.

126. Groll, AH, Piscitelli SC, Walsh TJ. Clinical pharmacology of systemic antifungal agents: a comprehensive review of agents in clinical use, current investigational compounds, and putative targets for antifungal drug development. *Adv Pharmacol* 1998;44:343–500.

127. Groll AH, Shah PM, Mentzel C, et al. Trends in the postmortem epidemiology of invasive fungal infections at a university hospital. *J Infect* 1996;33:23–32.

128. Meunier F. Candidiasis. *Eur J Clin Microbiol Infect Dis* 1989;8:438–447.

129. Perfect JR. Cryptococcosis. *Infect Dis Clin North Am* 1989;3:77–102.

130. Wingard JR. Importance of *Candida* species other than *C. albicans* as pathogens in oncology patients. *Clin Infect Dis* 1995;20:115–125.

131. Nguyen MH, Peacock JE Jr, Morris AJ, et al. The changing face of candidemia: emergence of non-*Candida albicans* species and antifungal resistance. *Am J Med* 1996;100:617–623.

132. Haron E, Vartivarian S, Anaissie E, et al. Primary *Candida* pneumonia: experience at a large cancer center and review. *Medicine (Baltimore)* 1993;72:137–142.

133. Masur H, Rosen PP, Armstrong D. Pulmonary diseases caused by *Candida* species. *Am J Med* 1977;63: 914–925.

134. Edward JE, Lehrer RI, Stiehm ER, et al. Severe candidal infections: clinical perspective, immune defense mechanisms and current concepts of therapy. *Ann Intern Med* 1978;89:91.

135. Meyer RD, Young LS, Armstrong D. Aspergillosis complicating neoplastic disease. *Am J Med* 1973;54: 6–15.

136. Meyers JD. Fungal infections in bone marrow transplant patients. *Semin Oncol* 1990;17[Suppl 6]: S10–S13.

137. Anaissie EJ. Opportunistic mycoses in the immunocompromised host: experience at a cancer center and review. *Clin Infect Dis* 1992;14[Suppl 1]:S43–S53.

138. Wald A, Leichsenring W, van Burik JA, et al. Epidemiology of *Aspergillus* infections in a large cohort of patients undergoing bone marrow transplantation. *J Infect Dis* 1997;175:1459–1466.

139. Boemelburg T, Roos N, Fegeler W, et al. Invasive aspergillosis during chemotherapy in children. *Hematology and Blood Transfusion* 1994;36:778–781.

140. Cole CH, Pritchard S, Rogers PCJ, et al. Intensive conditioning regimen for bone marrow transplantation in children with high-risk hematological malignancies. *Med Pediatr Oncol* 1994;23:464–469.

141. Ritter J, Roos N. Special aspects related to invasive fungal infections in children with cancer. *Baillieres Clin Infect Dis* 1995;2:179–204.

142. Trigg ME, Morgan D, Burns TL, et al. Successful program to prevent *Aspergillus* infections in children undergoing marrow transplantation: use of nasal amphotericin B. *Bone Marrow Transplant* 1997;19: 43–47.

143. Harris RE, Sather HN, Feig SA. High-dose cytosine arabinoside and L-asparaginase in refractory acute lymphoblastic leukemia: the Children's Cancer Group experience. *Med Pediatr Oncol* 1998;30:233–239.

144. Groll AH, Kurz M, Schneider W, et al. Five-year survey of invasive aspergillosis in a pediatric cancer center: incidence, clinical presentation, management, and long-term survival. *Mycoses* 1999;42:431–442.

145. Albelda SM, Talbot GH, Gerson ST, et al. Pulmonary cavitation and massive hemoptysis in invasive pulmonary aspergillosis: influence of bone marrow recovery in patients with acute leukemia. *Am Rev Respir Dis* 1985;131:115–120.

146. Panos R, Barr L, Walsh TJ, et al. Factors associated with fatal hemoptysis in cancer patients. *Chest* 1988; 94:1008.

147. Pagano L, Ricci P, Nosari A, et al. Fatal hemoptysis in pulmonary filamentous mycosis: an underevaluated cause of death in patients with acute leukemia in hematological complete remission. A retrospective study and review of the literature. *Br J Haematol* 1995;89:500–505.

148. Young RC, Bennett JE, Vogel CL, et al. Aspergillosis: the spectrum of the disease in 98 patients. *Medicine (Baltimore)* 1970;49:147.

149. Kuhlman JE, Fishman EK, Siegelman SS. Invasive pulmonary aspergillosis in acute leukemia: characteristic findings on CT, the CT halo sign, and the role of CT in early diagnosis. *Radiology* 1985;157:611–614.

150. Kuhlman JE, Fishman EK, Burch PA, et al. Invasive pulmonary aspergillosis in acute leukemia: the contribution of CT to early diagnosis and aggressive management. *Chest* 1987;92:95–99.

151. von Eiff M, Zuehlsdorf M, Roos N, et al. Pulmonary fungal infections in patients with hematological malignancies: diagnostic approaches. *Ann Hematol* 1995; 70:135–141.

152. Taccone A, Occhi M, Garaventa A, et al. CT of invasive pulmonary aspergillosis in children with cancer. *Pediatr Radiol* 1993;23:177–180.

153. Blum U, Windfuhr M, Buitrago-Tellez C, et al. Invasive pulmonary aspergillosis: MRI, CT and plain radiographic findings and their contribution to early diagnosis. *Chest* 1994;106:1156–1167.

154. Winer-Muram HT, Arheart KL, Jennings SG, et al. Pulmonary complications in children with hematological malignancies: accuracy of diagnosis with chest radiography and CT. *Radiology* 1997;204:643–649.

155. Denning DW. Therapeutic outcome in invasive aspergillosis. *Clin Infect Dis* 1996;23:608–615.
156. Khan FW, Jones JM, England DM. The role of bronchoalveolar lavage in the diagnosis of invasive pulmonary aspergillosis. *Am J Clin Pathol* 1986;86:518–523.
157. Yu VL, Muder RR, Poorsattar A. Significance of isolation of *Aspergillus* from the respiratory tract in diagnosis of invasive pulmonary aspergillosis: results from a three-year prospective study. *Am J Med* 1986;81:249–254.
158. Nemunaitis J. A comparative review of colony-stimulating factors. *Drugs* 1997;54:709–729.
159. Sugar AM. Mucormycosis. *Clin Infect Dis* 1992;14 [Suppl 1]:S126–S129.
160. Irwin RG, Rinaldi MG, Walsh TJ. Zygomycosis of the respiratory tract. In: Sarosi G, Davies S. *Fungal diseases of the lung,* 3rd ed. Philadelphia: Lippincott Williams & Wilkins, 1999.
161. Martino P, Gastaldi R, Raccah R, et al. Clinical patterns of *Fusarium* infections in immunocompromised patients. *J Infect Dis* 1994;[Suppl 1]:7–15.
162. Liu K, Howell DN, Perfect JR, et al. Morphologic criteria for the preliminary identification of *Fusarium, Paecilomyces,* and *Acremonium* species by histopathology. *Am J Clin Pathol* 1998;109:45–54.
163. Lozano-Chiu M, Arikan S, Paetznick VL, et al. Treatment of murine fusariosis with SCH 56592. *Antimicrob Agents Chemother* 1999;43:589–591.
164. McGinnis MR, Pasarell L, Sutton DA, et al. *In vitro* activity of voriconazole against selected fungi. *Med Mycol* 1998;36:239–242.
165. Kaplan MS, Rosen PP, Armstrong D. Cryptococcal meningitis: a study of 111 cases. *Ann Intern Med* 1977;80:176.
166. Allende M, Horowitz M, Pass HI, et al. Pulmonary cryptococcosis presenting as metastases in children with sarcoma. *Pediatr Infect Dis J* 1993;12:240–243.
167. Walsh TJ, Newman KR, Moody M, et al. Trichosporonosis in patients with neoplastic disease. *Medicine (Baltimore)* 1986;65:268.
168. Hoy J, Hsu K, Rolston K, et al. *Trichosporon beigelii* infection: a review. *Rev Infect Dis* 1986;8:959–967.
169. Melcher GA, Reed KD, Rinaldi MG, et al. Demonstration of a cell wall antigen cross-reacting with cryptococcal polysaccharide in experimental disseminated trichosporonosis. *J Clin Microbiol* 1991;29:192–196.
170. Walsh TJ, Melcher G, Rinaldi M, et al. *Trichosporon beigelii: an emerging pathogen resistant to amphotericin B.* J Clin Microbiol 1990;28:1616–1622.
171. Walsh TJ, Melcher GP, Lee JW, et al. Infections due to *Trichosporon* species: new concepts in mycology, pathogenesis, diagnosis, and treatment. *Curr Top Med Mycol* 1993;5:79–113.
172. Walsh TJ, Lee JW, Melcher GP, et al. Experimental disseminated trichosporonosis in persistently granulocytopenic rabbits: implications for pathogenesis, diagnosis, and treatment of an emerging opportunistic infection. *J Infect Dis* 1992;166:121–133.
173. Ruskin J, Remington JS. Toxoplasmosis in the compromised host. *Ann Intern Med* 1976;84:193.
174. Hirsh R, Burke BA, Kersey JH. Toxoplasmosis in bone marrow transplant recipients. *J Pediatr* 1984;105:426–428.
175. Derouin F, Gluckman E, Beauvais B, et al. *Toxoplasma*

176. Daubenton JD, Buys HA, Hartley PS. Disseminated strongyloidiasis in a child with lymphoblastic lymphoma. *J Pediatr Hematol Oncol* 1998;20:260–263.
177. Scowden EB, Schaffner W, Stone WJ. Overwhelming strongyloidiasis: an unappreciated opportunistic infection. *Medicine (Baltimore)* 1978;57:527.
178. Hughes WT, Feldman S, Aur JR, et al. Intensity of immunosuppressive therapy and the incidence of *Pneumocystis carinii* pneumonitis. Cancer 1975;36:2004–2009.
179. Hughes WT. *Pneumocystis carinii* pneumonia. *N Engl J Med* 1977;297:381.
180. Hughes WT, Rivera G, Schell MJ, et al. Successful intermittent chemoprophylaxis for *Pneumocystis carinii* pneumonitis. *N Engl J Med* 1987;316:1627–1632.
181. Kovacs JA, Hiemenz JW, Macher Am, et al. *Pneumocystis carinii* pneumonia: a comparison of clinical features in patients with the acquired immune deficiency syndrome and patients with other immune diseases. *Ann Intern Med* 1984;100:663.
182. Kovacs JA, Ng VL, Masur H, et al. Diagnosis of *Pneumocystis carinii* pneumonia: improved detection in sputum with use of monoclonal antibodies. *N Engl J Med* 1988;318:589–593.
183. Hopewell PC. *Pneumocystis carinii* pneumonia: diagnosis. *J Infect Dis* 1988;157:1115–1119.
184. Ognibene FP, Gill VJ, Pizzo PA, et al. Induced sputum to diagnose *Pneumocystis carinii* pneumonia in immunosuppressed pediatric patients. *J Pediatr* 1989;115:430–433.
185. Freifeld AG, Walsh TJ, Pizzo PA. Infectious complications in the pediatric cancer patient. In: Pizzo PA, Poplack DG, eds. *Principles and practice of pediatric oncology,* 3rd ed. Philadelphia: JP Lippincott, 1996:1069–1114.
186. Masur H. Prevention and treatment of *Pneumocystis* pneumonia. *N Engl J Med* 1992;327:1853–1860.
187. Browne MJ, Potter D, Gress J, et al. A randomized trial of open lung biopsy versus empiric antimicrobial therapy in cancer patients with diffuse pulmonary infiltrates. *J Clin Oncol* 1990;8:222.
188. Flomenberg P, Babbitt J, Drobyski WR, et al. Increasing incidence of adenovirus disease in bone marrow transplant recipients. *J Infect Dis* 1994;169:775–781.
189. Michaels MG, Green M, Wald ER, et al. Adenovirus infection in pediatric liver transplant recipients. *J Infect Dis* 1992;165:170–174.
190. Wasserman R, August C, Plotkin S. Viral infections in pediatric bone marrow transplant patients. *Pediatr Infect Dis J* 1988;7:109–115.
191. Gray MM, Hann IM, Glass S, et al. Mortality and morbidity caused by measles in children with malignant disease attending four major treatment centres: a retrospective review. *Br Med J* 1987;295:19–22.
192. Kernahan J, McQuillin J, Craft AW. Measles in children who have malignant disease. *Br Med J* 1987;295:15–18.
193. Hall CB, Powell KR, McDonald NE, et al. Respiratory syncytial viral infection in children with compromised immune function. *N Engl J Med* 1986;315:77–81.
194. Whimbey E, Couch RB, Englund JA, et al. Respiratory syncytial virus pneumonia in hospitalized adult pa-

infection after human allogeneic bone marrow transplantation: clinical and serological study of 80 patients. *Bone Marrow Transplant* 1986;1:67–73.

tients with leukemia. *Clin Infect Dis* 1995;21: 376–379.

195. Harrinton RD, Hooton TM, Hackman RC, et al. An outbreak of respiratory syncytial virus in a bone marrow transplant center. *J Infect Dis* 1992;165:987–993.

196. Wendt CH, Weisdorf DJ, Jordan MC, et al. Parainfluenza virus respiratory infection after bone marrow transplantation. *N Engl J Med* 1992;326:921–926.

197. Whimbey E, Vartivarian SE, Champlin RE, et al. Parainfluenza virus infection in adult bone marrow transplant recipients. *Eur J Clin Microbiol Infect Dis* 1993;12:699.

198. Kempe A, Hall CB, McDonald ME, et al. Influenza in children with cancer. *J Pediatr* 1989;115:33–39.

199. Feldman S, Webster RG, Sugg M. Influenza in children and young adults with cancer: 20 cases. *Cancer* 1997;39:350–353.

200. Balfour HH. Antiviral drugs. *N Engl J Med* 1999;340: 1255.

201. Henson D, Siegel SE, Fuccillo DA, et al. Cytomegalovirus infection during acute childhood leukemia. *J Infect Dis* 1972;126:469.

202. Sable CA, Donowitz GR. Infections in bone marrow transplant recipients. *Clin Infect Dis* 1994;18: 273–284.

203. Weiner RS, Bortin MM, Gale RP, et al. Interstitial pneumonitis after bone marrow transplantation. *Ann Intern Med* 1986;104:168.

204. Wingard JR, Santos GW, Saral R. Late onset interstitial pneumonia following allogeneic bone marrow transplantation. *Transplantation* 1985;39:21.

205. Boeckh M, Bowden RA, Goodrich JM, et al. Cytomegalovirus antigen detection in peripheral blood leucocytes after allogenic bone marrow transplantation. *Blood* 1992;80:1358–1364.

206. Gerna G, Furione M, Baldanti F, et al. Quantitation of human cytomegalovirus DNA in bone marrow transplant recipients. *Br J Haematol* 1995;91:674–683.

207. Crawford SW, Bowden RA, Hackman RC, et al. Rapid detection of cytomegalovirus pulmonary infection by bronchoalveolar lavage and centrifugation culture. *An Intern Med* 1988;108:180.

208. Balfour HH Jr. Management of cytomegalovirus disease with antiviral drugs. *Rev Infect Dis* 1990;12 [Suppl 7]:S849–S860.

209. Winston DJ, Gale RP. Prevention and treatment of cytomegalovirus infection and disease after bone marrow transplantation in the 1990s. *Bone Marrow Transplant* 1991;8:7–11.

210. Bowden RA, Sayers M, Flournoy N, et al. Cytomegalovirus immune globulin and seronegative blood products to prevent primary cytomegalovirus infection after marrow transplantation. *N Engl J Med* 1986;314:1006.

211. Goodrich J, Zellner S, Bradsher R, et al. Itraconazole treatment of phaeohyphomycosis. *J Am Acad Dermatol* 1990;23:577–586.

212. Schmidt CA, Oettle H, Wilborn F, et al. Demonstration of cytomegalovirus after bone marrow transplantation by polymerase chain reaction, virus culture and antigen detection in buffy coat leukocytes. *Bone Marrow Transplant* 1994;13:71–75.

213. Morgan ET, Smalley LA. Varicella in immunocompromised children: incidence of abdominal pain and organ involvement. *Am J Dis Child* 1983;137:883.

214. Feldman S, Lott L. Varicella in children with cancer: impact of antiviral therapy and prophylaxis. *Pediatrics* 1987;80:465–472.

215. Feldman S, Hughes WT, Kim HY. Herpes zoster in children with cancer. *Am J Dis Child* 1973;126: 178–184.

216. Rowland P, Wald R, Mirro JR, et al. Progressive varicella presenting with pain and minimal skin involvement in children with acute lymphoblastic leukemia. *J Clin Oncol* 1995;13:1697–1703.

217. Prober CG, Kirk LE, Keeney RE. Acyclovir therapy of chicken pox in immunosuppressed children a collaborative study. *J Pediatr* 1982;101:622.

218. Ramsey PG, Fife FH, Hackman RC, et al. Herpes simplex virus pneumonia: clinical, virologic and pathologic features in 20 patients. *Ann Intern Med* 1982;97: 813–820.

219. Hirsch MS, Schooley RT. Treatment of herpes virus infections. *N Engl J Med* 1983;309:963,1034.

220. Peterson DE, Minah GE, Overholser CD, et al. Microbiology of acute peridontal infection in myelosuppressed cancer patients. *J Clin Oncol* 1987;5:1461.

221. Shepp DH, Newton BA, Dandliker PS, et al. Oral acyclovir therapy for mucocutaneous herpes simplex virus infections in immunocompromised marrow transplant recipients. *Ann Intern Med* 1985;102:783.

222. McDonald GB, Sharma P, Hackman RC, et al. Esophageal infections in immunosuppressed patients after marrow transplant. *Gastroenterology* 1985;88: 1111.

223. Bartlett JG, Chang TW, Gurwith M, et al. Antibiotic associated pseudomembranous colitis due to toxin producing clostridia. *N Engl J Med* 1978;298:531.

224. Sloas MM, Flynn PM, Kaste SC, et al. Typhlitis in children with cancer: a 30-year experience. *Clin Infect Dis* 1993;17:484.

225. Gootenberg JE, Abbondanzo SL. Rapid diagnosis of neutropenic entercolitis (typhlitis) by ultrasonography. *Am J Pediatr Hematol Oncol* 1987;9:222.

226. Varki AP, Armitage JO, Feagler JR. Typhlitis in acute leukemia: successful treatment by early surgical intervention. *Cancer* 1979;43:695.

227. Thaler M, Pastakia B, Shawker TH, et al. Hepatic candidiasis in cancer patients: the evolving picture of the syndrome. *Ann Intern Med* 1988;108:88.

228. Haron E, Feld R, Tuffnell P, et al. Hepatic candidiasis: an increasing problem in immunocompromised patients. *Am J Med* 1987;83:17–26.

229. Thaler M, Bacher J, O'Leary T, et al. Evaluation of single-drug and combination antifungal therapy in an experimental model of candidiasis in rabbits with prolonged neutropenia. *J Infect Dis* 1988;158:80–88.

230. Walsh TJ, Whitcomb P, Piscitelli S, et al. Safety, tolerance, and pharmacokinetics of amphotericin B lipid complex in children with hepatosplenic candidiasis. *Antimicrob Agents Chemother* 1997;41:1944–1948.

231. Kauffman CA, Bradley SF, Ross SC, et al. Hepatosplenic candidiasis: successful treatment with fluconazole. *Am J Med* 1991;91:137–141.

232. Anaissie E, Bodey GP, Kantarjian H, et al. Fluconazole therapy for chronic disseminated candidiasis in patients with leukemia and prior amphotericin B therapy. *Am J Med* 1991;91:142–150.

233. Walsh TJ, Whitcomb PO, Revankar SG, et al. Successful treatment of hepatosplenic candidiasis through re-

peated cycles of chemotherapy and neutropenia. *Cancer* 1995;76:2357–2362.

234. Glenn J, Cotton D, Wesley R, et al. Anorectal infections in patients with malignant diseases. *Rev Infect Dis* 1988;10:42.

235. Barnes SG, Sattler FR, Ballard JO. Improved survival after drainage of perirectal infection in patients with acute leukemia. *Ann Intern Med* 1984;100:515.

236. Kinston ME, Mackey D. Skin clues in the diagnosis of life-threatening infections. *Rev Infect Dis* 1986;8:1.

237. Walsh TJ, Pizzo PA. Nosocomial fungal infections: a classification for hospital-acquired fungal infections and mycoses arising from endogenous flora or reactivation. *Annu Rev Microbiol* 1988;42:517.

238. Walmsley S, Devi S, King S, et al. Invasive *Aspergillus* infections in a pediatric hospital: a ten-year review. *Pediatr Infect Dis J* 1993;12:673–682.

239. Prystowski SD, Vogelstein B, Ettinger DS, et al. Invasive aspergillosis. *N Engl J Med* 1976;295:655–658.

240. Grossmann ME, Fithian EC, Behrens C, et al. Primary cutaneous aspergillosis in six leukemic children. *J Am Acad Dermatol* 1985;12:313–318.

241. McCarty JM, Flam MS, Pullen G, et al. Outbreak of primary cutaneous aspergillosis related to intravenous armboards. *J Pediatr* 1986;108:721–724.

242. Barson WJ, Ruymann FB. Palmar aspergillosis in immunocompromised children. *Pediatr Infect Dis J* 1986;5:264–268.

243. Golladay ES, Baker SB. Invasive aspergillosis in children. *J Pediatr Surg* 1987;22:504–505.

244. Allo M, Miller J, Townsend T, et al. Primary cutaneous aspergillosis associated with Hickman intravenous catheters. *N Engl J Med* 1987;317:1105–1113.

245. Drew WL, Mintz L. Rapid diagnosis of varicella-zoster virus infection by direct immunofluorescence. *Am J Clin Pathol* 1980;73:699.

246. Wood MJ. Nucleoside analogues: aciclovir, penciclovir, valaciclovir, and famciclovir. In: Yu VL, Merigan TC, Barriere SL, eds. *Antimicrobial therapy and vaccines.* Baltimore: Williams & Wilkins, 1998; 1434–1441.

247. Locksley RM, Flournoy N, Sullivan KM, et al. Varicella zoster virus infection after marrow transplantation. *J Infect Dis* 1985;152:1172.

248. Centers for Disease Control and Prevention. Prevention of varicella: recommendations of the Advisory Committee on Immunization Practices (ACIP). *MMWR Morb Mortal Wkly Rep* 1996;45:1–36.

249. Asano Y, Yoshikawa T, Suga S, et al. Postexposure prophylaxis of varicella in family contact by acyclovir. *Pediatrics* 1993;92:219–222.

250. Huang YC, Lin TY, Chiu CH. Acyclovir prophylaxis of varicella after household exposure. *Pediatr Infect Dis J* 1995;14:152–154.

251. Browne M, Dinndorf P, Perek D, et al. Infectious complications of intraventricular reservoirs in cancer patients. *Pediatr Infect Dis* 1987;6:182.

252. Chiou CC, Wong TT, Lin HH, et al. Fungal infection of ventriculoperitoneal shunts in children. *Clin Infect Dis* 1994;19:1049–1053.

253. Sommers LM, Hawkins DS. Meningitis in pediatric cancer patients: a review of forty cases from a single institution. *Pediatr Infect Dis J* 1999;18:902–907.

254. Kaplan MH, Rosen PP, Armstrong D. Cryptococcosis in a cancer hospital: clinical and pathological correlates in forty-six patients. *Cancer* 1977;39:2265–2274.

255. Leenders AC, Reiss P, Portegies P, et al. Liposomal amphotericin B both followed by oral fluconazole in the treatment of AIDS-associated cryptococcal meningitis. *AIDS* 1997;11:1463–1471.

256. Nieman RE, Lorber B. Listeriosis in adults: a changing pattern. Report of eight cases and review of the literature. *Rev Infect Dis* 1980;2:207–227.

257. Tim MW, Jackson MA, Shannon K, et al. Non-neonatal infection due to *Listeria monocytogenes. Pediatr Infect Dis* 1984;3:213–217.

258. Skogberg K, Syrjanen J, Jahkola M, et al. Clinical presentation and outcome of listeriosis in patients with and without immunosuppressive therapy. *Clin Infect Dis* 1992;14:815–821.

259. Lorber B. Listeriosis. *Clin Infect Dis* 1997;24:1–9.

260. Jones EM, MacGowan AP. Antimicrobial chemotherapy of human infection due to *Listeria monocytogenes. Eur J Clin Microbiol Infect Dis* 1995;14:165–175.

261. Hof H, Nichterlein T, Kretschmar M. Management of listeriosis. *Clin Microbiol Rev* 1997;10:345–357.

262. Merle-Merlet M, Dossou-Gbete L, Maurer P, et al. Is amoxicillin-cotrimoxazole the most appropriate antibiotic regimen for meningoencephalitis? Review of 22 cases and the literature. *J Infect* 1996;33:79–85.

263. Wacker P, Ozsahin H, Groll AH, et al. Trimethoprime-sulfamethoxazole salvage for refractory listeriosis during maintenance chemotherapy for ALL. *J Pediatr Hematol Oncol* 2000;22:340–343.

264. Khan EA, Correa AG. Toxoplasmosis of the central nervous system in non-human immunodeficiency virus-infected children: case report and review of the literature. *Pediatr Infect Dis J* 1997;16:611–618.

6

Infections Following
Kidney Transplantation in Children

Maria T. Millan, Dev M. Desai, and Samuel K.S. So

Department of Surgery, Stanford University School of Medicine, Palo Alto, California 94304

Optimal therapy for end-stage renal disease in children is renal transplantation. In contrast to hemodialysis and peritoneal dialysis, transplantation provides these children with the best opportunity for normal growth and neuropsychological development and a normal lifestyle (1,2). A successful renal allograft further eliminates the common problems associated with chronic dialysis in the pediatric population. It leads to improvements in nutrition, fluid and electrolyte balance, and renal osteodystrophy. Avoided are problems with dialysis access and potential line and catheter infections. The quality of life is clearly improved as the child is able to attend school and lead a more normal life, unrestricted by a dialysis schedule.

Kidney transplantation can now be done safely in children, with long-term patient survival of more than 90%. With improvements in surgical technique, organ preservation, and immunosuppressive regimens, there has been a steady improvement in renal allograft survival in pediatric recipients over the past 10 years. Up to 80% to 99% of kidneys transplanted into pediatric recipients function at 1 year, and 70% to 85% function at 5 years (3,4). Even small infants, the highest-risk subgroup undergoing kidney transplantation, now experience up to 98% 3-year and 85% 8-year graft survival (5). Acute rejection in the infant and pediatric kidney transplant recipient is often irreversible and has been a major cause of graft loss; a more intense immunosuppressive regimen has been correlated with improved survival in this subgroup (6). However, this approach of intensified immunosuppression also increases the risk for opportunistic and nonopportunistic infections in the pediatric kidney transplant recipient.

MORBIDITY AND MORTALITY OF INFECTION

Despite the enormous success of kidney transplantation in children, infection remains a major cause of morbidity and mortality after transplantation. The North American Pediatric Renal Transplant Cooperative Study (NAPRTCS) found that the primary cause of mortality in children after transplantation was infectious complications, which accounted for 40% of deaths occurring during the first 6 months after transplantation (7). In more recent reports, infection still accounted for 83% of mortality in these patients (1997 annual report, NAPRTCS). Furthermore, of the 50% to 60% of renal transplant recipients who required rehospitalization, approximately 30% were admitted for the treatment of infectious complications (approximately 15% for viral and 13% for bacterial infections) (8,9).

The incidence of posttransplantation bacterial infection varies with age, with younger children being more susceptible. In one center's review of 164 pediatric renal transplant recipients, the incidence of bacterial infection was found to be significantly higher in the younger age groups: 87% in patients younger than 2 years of age, 72% in those 2 to 5 years old, 51% in those 6 to 12 years old, and 40% in those 13 to 17 years old (8). The most common bacterial infection in patients 5 years old or younger was *Clostridium difficile*–associated diarrhea. In those older than 5 years, urinary tract infections (UTIs) were most common. In contrast, the incidence of viral infections did not show any significant propensity for a particular age group.

Posttransplantation infection is the leading cause of mortality among pediatric kidney transplant recipients. Of 2,457 patients in the NAPRTCS 1994 registry who were monitored for 5,481 patient-years, 40% of the deaths were primarily from infection (9,10). Infection accounted for 44% of deaths in kidney transplant recipients younger than 1 year of age and for 36%, 42%, and 40% of the deaths among recipients aged 2 to 5 years, 6 to 12 years, and 13 to 17 years, respectively (7). The risk of death from infection is greatest during the first year after transplantation, and some have reported that up to 50% of infection-related deaths occurred within 6 months after transplantation (11). Polymicrobial infections were associated with increased mortality. In one report, 65% of infectious mortality was caused by cytomegalovirus (CMV) associated with bacterial, fungal, or *Pneumocystis* infections (12).

FEVER AFTER TRANSPLANTATION

Under immunosuppressive therapy, the kidney transplant recipient is predisposed to a variety of opportunistic bacterial, fungal, viral, and protozoal infections, which can occur at unusual sites and can be rapidly lethal if left untreated or inadequately treated. Furthermore, the signs and symptoms of infection can be masked by the use of steroids and antilymphocyte immunosuppressive preparations. A high index of suspicion is imperative in the evaluation of fever in any patient who has undergone transplantation to ensure prompt diagnosis and treatment of the infection.

Fever in the transplant recipient is caused by infection in 74% to 78% of cases (13). Renal allograft rejection can also manifest as fever and accounted for 13% of febrile episodes in one series (14). Viral infection was the most common cause of fever during the first 4 months after transplantation; it was responsible for more than half of the febrile episodes. CMV infection, either alone or in conjunction with rejection or other systemic infections, accounted for 51% of febrile episodes. During the early posttransplantation period, bacterial infection was responsible for 14% and fungal infection for 5% of the febrile episodes. Beyond the first year from transplantation, bacterial infection is the major cause of fever in these patients (13). Other causes of fevers in transplant recipients include drug fever and malignancy (e.g., lymphoma).

In renal transplant recipients who present with fever and a rising creatinine concentration, the diagnosis of urinary tract infection and viral illness should be ruled out, in addition to the workup and treatment for allograft rejection. The first two to three doses of antilymphocyte preparations are frequently associated with fever (38° to 40°C) caused by cytokine release, but fever persisting beyond the third dose or fever occurring late in the course of antilymphocyte treatment is more likely to be related to infection.

Fever in a transplant recipient should lead to a thorough search for common and uncommon bacterial, fungal, viral, and protozoal infections of the ear, throat, nasal sinuses, and urinary, respiratory, gastrointestinal, and central nervous systems occurring either alone or concomitantly. A systematic, thorough approach to the workup of febrile episodes in the pediatric renal transplant recipient is proposed in Fig. 6.1.

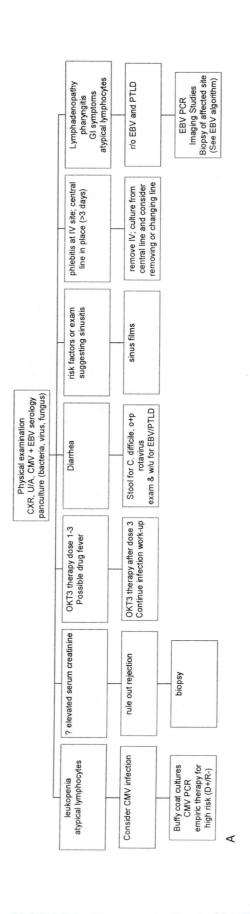

Physical examination
CXR, U/A, CMV + EBV serology
panculture (bacteria, virus, fungus)

leukopenia
atypical lymphocytes

Consider CMV infection

Buffy coat cultures
CMV PCR
empiric therapy for
high risk (D+/R-)

? elevated serum creatinine

rule out rejection

biopsy

OKT3 therapy dose 1-3
Possible drug fever

OKT3 therapy after dose 3
Continue infection work-up

Diarrhea

Stool for C. difficile, o+p
rotavirus
exam & w/u for EBV/PTLD

risk factors or exam
suggesting sinusitis

sinus films

phlebitis at IV site; central
line in place (>3 days)

remove IV; culture from
central line and consider
removing or changing line

Lymphadenopathy
pharyngitis
GI symptoms
atypical lymphocytes

r/o EBV and PTLD

EBV PCR
Imaging Studies
Biopsy of affected site
(See EBV algorithm)

A

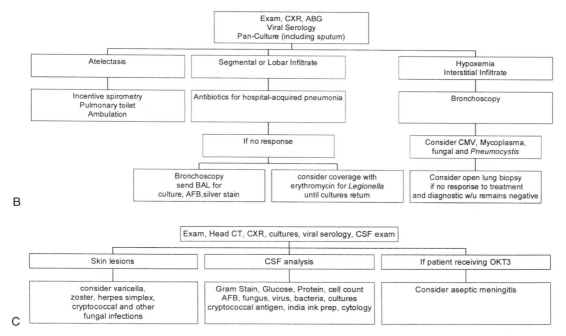

FIG. 6.1. Evaluation of posttransplantation fever in the absence of localizing symptons **(A)**, in the presence of respiratory symptoms **(B)**, and with accompanying headache or neurologic symptoms **(C)**.

TIMING OF INFECTION AFTER TRANSPLANTATION

The propensity of infections to occur within the first few months after transplantation is directly related to the high doses of immunosuppressive agents and the frequent use of monoclonal or polyclonal antilymphocyte preparations early during the posttransplantation period to prevent or treat rejection. The types of infections and their times of peak occurrence after solid organ transplantation follow a pattern, as shown in Fig. 6.2 (15). In the first few weeks after transplantation, infections are mainly bacterial and candidal (16). More than 95% of these infections are the same as those occurring in nonimmunosuppressed patients undergoing similar kinds of surgery. Within the first month after transplantation, three distinct types of infections predominate. The first category includes infections related to contamination of the organ, wound infection, pneumonia, and line sepsis. The second type is that caused by untreated infections that were present in the recipient before transplantation or history of recurrent prior infections. For example, untreated pneumonia in the would-be recipient can have a major impact after transplantation and almost guarantees superinfection with nosocomial gram-negative bacilli, fungi, or both. Children with a history of ear infections are at high risk for recurrent otitis media within the first month after transplantation.

In Chavers' series of 164 pediatric patients transplanted between 1985 and 1993, *C. difficile* colitis was the most common bacterial infection encountered in the first 2 weeks after transplantation. UTI was the second most common bacterial infection, followed by bacteremia and line sepsis. In this cohort, few viral infections occurred within the first 2 weeks (8).

Opportunistic infections (e.g., *Listeria monocytogenes*) and immunomodulating viruses such as CMV and Epstein-Barr virus (EBV) are the most common type of infection seen

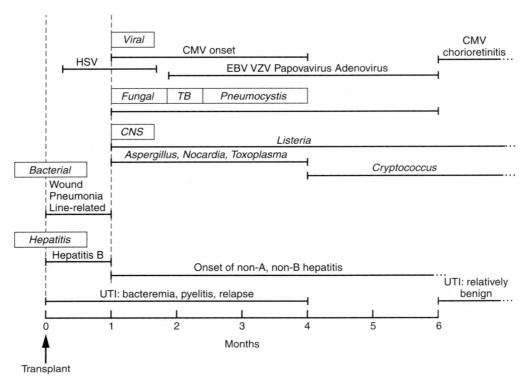

FIG. 6.2. Timetable of infection after organ transplantation. (From Rubin RH, et al. Infection in the renal transplant patient. *Am J Med* 1981;70:405, with permission.)

between 1 and 6 months after transplantation and are related to the individual's net state of immunosuppression. Factors associated with increased risk for opportunistic infections are poor allograft function (17), antirejection therapy, and chronic viral disease (18).

Beyond the first year after transplantation, when maintenance immunosuppression is at the lowest doses, more than 90% of infections are UTIs and chronic infections. However, there is still a potential for lethal infection from hospital-acquired or community-acquired bacteria or, less often, opportunistic infections. Patients at risk for infection during this late phase (1 to 6 years after transplantation) are those who have had repeated rejection episodes or chronic rejection requiring repeated courses of heavy immunosuppression. The most common viral infection beyond the first 6 months after transplantation is

varicella-zoster virus (VZV), which tends to occur more frequently in younger children and can have severe manifestations (8).

BACTERIAL INFECTIONS

The most common form of bacterial infection in the renal transplant recipient in the first 6 months after transplantation occurs in the urinary tract. There is a wide range in incidence, from 6% (19) to as high as 85% (16). In comparison with the nonimmunosuppressed host, infections in these patients are more often associated with pyelonephritis and bacteremia and there is a high rate of relapse when they are treated with a conventional course of antibiotics (17). Renoult found that 7% of UTIs were complicated by sepsis, and recurrence was found in 40% (20). UTIs account for 40% to 60% of episodes of sepsis and 60% of cases of gram-negative bacteremia. *Escherichia coli* is the predominant organism, followed in incidence by gram-positive organisms (*Staphylococcus* sp. and *Enterococcus*) and by *Proteus* and *Klebsiella.* Other organisms include *Enterobacter, Serratia, Acinetobacter, Citrobacter,* and *Pseudomonas.* Bladder catheterization is the main mode of bacterial contamination; the reported bacteremia rate is 5% to 10% per day (21). Early postoperative removal of the bladder catheter is advocated whenever possible, because it is associated with a lower rate of UTIs and no increase in urologic complications (22). Risk factors for the development of posttransplantation UTI include female sex, history of UTI before renal transplantation, polycystic kidneys left unremoved when there is a past history of recurrent upper UTIs, chronic viral infection, diabetes mellitus (a more important factor in adults), and a high cumulative dose of antirejection drugs (23). From this group's experience, pediatric recipients with prune-belly syndrome, those with Eagle-Barrett syndrome (who frequently have other urologic anomalies), those with ileal conduits, and those who require intermittent bladder catheterization for neurogenic bladder have a higher incidence of UTI than other pediatric kidney transplant recipients. Because of this, our practice is to use the native bladder whenever possible and to perform an antireflux ureteral implantation in all cases (24).

Although some have maintained that vesicoureteral reflux does not increase the incidence of UTI or pyelonephritis in the transplant recipient (20), others have reported an incidence of pyelonephritis as high as 84% in patients with reflux and UTI (24–26). In contrast to the normal host, the transplant recipient who develops UTI has a higher predisposition for development of pyelonephritis commonly associated with bacteremia and a significant decline in allograft function. Some advocate routine monitoring of urinary cultures and evaluation for vesicoureteral reflux after transplantation, suggest the use of prophylactic antibiotics with documented reflux, and recommend ureteral reimplantation for those with recurrent UTI due to reflux (26). In our center, we advocate the use of an antireflux procedure from the start, at the time of transplantation, to avoid the potential for reflux, spare the patient frequent radiologic evaluations for reflux, and minimize the risk of posttransplantation UTIs. We preferentially apply the Politano-Leadbetter technique for antireflux ureteral implantation in pediatric kidney transplant recipients (24). In the case of a small, defunctionalized bladder or a "difficult" bladder where this standard implantation cannot be performed, we have applied a technique developed at our center, the so-called "trough" technique for creation of a neosubmucosal antireflux tunnel (27).

Prompt recognition and treatment of posttransplantation UTIs can avert complications including fatal bacterial septicemia. The clinical presentation varies from asymptomatic pyuria to fever, chills, and rigor, which can be associated with tenderness over the bladder or over the native or the transplanted kidney. UTI can also mimic acute rejection when the patient presents with an elevation in serum creatinine with or without fever. Acute pyelonephritis can cause acute renal failure and must be aggressively treated with intravenous antibiotics. Ultrasound studies should be performed to identify any associated hydronephrosis; any obstruction should be relieved acutely, and any significant reflux or obstruction should be definitively repaired after an interval of stabilization.

The prevention of posttransplantation UTI should begin when the patient is first evaluated for a kidney transplantation. The native kidneys should be removed if the patient has a history of frequent UTI associated with either moderate to severe ureteral reflux or polycystic and hydronephrotic kidneys. Any urologic anomalies such as posterior urethral valve should be repaired before transplantation. During the preoperative period, the use of antibiotics, strict aseptic technique during Foley catheter insertion, elimination of the use of external ureteral stents, and early removal of the Foley catheter (within 5 to 7 days) are techniques useful for minimizing the risks of postoperative UTIs. Many groups, including our own, give these patients low-dose antibiotic prophylaxis (trimethoprim-sulfamethoxazole [TMP/SMX]) for the first few months after transplantation; this approach has been shown to decrease the incidence of UTIs (28).

Candidal UTI after kidney transplantation is rare in our experience; when it does occur, it usually is responsive to oral fluconazole. Amphotericin B bladder irrigation is reserved for resistant or persistent candidal infections of the urinary tract.

C. difficile diarrhea was reported to be the leading pathogen in the first 2 weeks after transplantation in one large series of pediatric kidney transplant recipients. Most of those patients responded within 7 days after initiation of oral metronidazole or vancomycin. In the same series, the incidence of bacteremia and line sepsis was found to be more common in recipients younger than 5 years of age (8). This group also found a significant number of positive peritoneal cultures in those patients receiving pretransplantation peritoneal dialysis. Nevertheless, there was no adverse effect on mortality or graft survival, so long as the peritoneal dialysis catheter was removed at the time of transplantation and the patient was given appropriate antibiotics.

Although less common than UTI, bacterial pneumonia is the most frequent cause of infectious disease mortality in the immunosuppressed patient, being responsible for 50% of deaths among renal transplant recipients. This complication is more prevalent in the first month after transplantation. Workup should include clinical examination, chest radiograph, sputum culture, and bronchioalveolar lavage, especially if an opportunistic infection suspected. There is increased risk among patients receiving antilymphocyte preparations for the prevention or treatment of rejection (29).

Vancomycin-resistant enterococcus (VRE) has been associated with a 25% mortality rate in the immunosuppressed patient (30,31). In a retrospective review of 32 organ transplant recipients who were colonized or infected with VRE, risk factors identified were prolonged hospitalization, the presence of invasive lines and catheters or invasive procedures, increased immunosuppression for rejection, and prior antibiotic use, particularly vancomycin (31). In this series, the VRE was susceptible to chloramphenicol (100%), nitrofurantoin (100%), and tetracycline (77%). Cure was achieved in 83%, but 8 of 32 patients who cultured positive for VRE died, with four deaths attributed directly to VRE infection (31).

Prophylactic therapy should consist of perioperative antibiotics to protect against wound infections and possible acquired bacterial infection. As previously noted, we use low-dose antibiotic prophylaxis for urinary tract protection. Because TMP/SMX (Bactrim) therapy has been helpful in the prevention of *Pneumocystis carinii* pneumonia (PCP), we use it for prophylaxis against both UTIs and PCP. In those cases in which Bactrim is not used, inhaled or intravenous pentamidine monthly after transplantation is an alternate form of prophylaxis against PCP (8).

INFLUENCE OF IMMUNOSUPPRESSIVE AGENTS ON THE INCIDENCE OF BACTERIAL INFECTIONS

In a comparison of single- versus triple-drug immunosuppressive regimens, there was no difference in the rate of bacterial infection (32). Further, the number of days of hospitalization due to infectious complications was equal in patients receiving double therapy (azathioprine and prednisone) versus triple therapy (cyclosporine, azathioprine, and prednisone) (33). The Pittsburgh group reported no difference in the rate of bacterial infections between recipients receiving tacrolimus (FK-506) and those receiving cyclosporine preparations (34). Steroids, which are a component of almost every transplant-related immunosuppressive regimen, have clearly been associated with increased risk of bacterial infections (35). In itself, exposure to anti-CD3 monoclonal antibody therapy (OKT3) did not increase the risk of bacterial infection, but repeated courses with higher cumulative dose was associated with increased incidence of infections (36). Development of life-threatening infections after treatment for acute rejection was more frequent among those treated with OKT3 than among those treated with steroids or antithymocyte globulin (ATG) (37).

VIRAL INFECTIONS

Herpesviruses

Cytomegalovirus

Presentation and Diagnosis

CMV infection is the most common opportunistic infection in kidney transplant recipients. It is a major cause of morbidity and mortality in the pediatric renal transplant recipient in the first 3 to 6 months after transplantation. Especially before the era of CMV prophylaxis, the incidence of CMV infection in adult kidney transplant recipients has been reported to be high, as much as 75%. In the pediatric kidney transplant population, the incidence is lower, with a national incidence of 5.6% according to the NAPRTCS registry, but some centers report an incidence of more than 20% (38). The risk for CMV infection is clearly increased with transplantation a CMV-seropositive donor organ and has been correlated with the degree of immunosuppression. CMV infection is particularly common after the use of monoclonal or polyclonal antilymphocyte preparations employed either as induction therapy or for the treatment of acute rejection (37,39,40). Manifestations range from asymptomatic disease to invasive multiorgan involvement to severe infections resulting in death. CMV disease usually manifests 1 to 4 months after kidney transplantation or within 2 to 4 weeks after treatment of acute rejection with monoclonal or polyclonal antilymphocyte preparations. The most common clinical presentation is a CMV syndrome that often begins with prolonged fever associated with malaise, myalgias, arthralgias, and anorexia, frequently with concomitant leukopenia. Thrombocytopenia and liver function

abnormalities can also be found. Unlike infectious mononucleosis associated with EBV, lymphadenopathy and pharyngitis are not associated with the CMV syndrome. The most common serious complication of CMV disease is CMV pneumonitis. The clinical presentation includes fever associated with tachypnea, hypoxemia, and a dry cough. Chest roentgenography may reveal a bilateral interstitial infiltrate. CMV infection of the gastrointestinal tract can cause ulceration in the esophagus, stomach, small bowel, and colon (especially the cecum and right colon), which can manifest as bleeding or perforation. Other manifestations of CMV infection include meningoencephalitis, retinitis, and CMV-associated renal dysfunction presenting as glomerulopathy or nephritis. Mortality rates have varied from 3% to 40%, the wide range possibly resulting from polymicrobial infections complicating some cases (11,41). Additionally, CMV disease has been associated with an increased incidence of renal allograft rejection (42), and improved renal allograft survival among those who develop CMV has been correlated with prior institution of CMV prophylaxis (40). There should be a high index of suspicion when a transplant recipient presents with the aforementioned symptoms, especially if they have been exposed to risk factors for CMV disease. These patients require prompt diagnosis and aggressive therapy to minimize morbidity and mortality of disease.

Diagnostic laboratory studies include detection of a fourfold increase in immunoglobulin G (IgG) or IgM titers, but serologic response may be slow or absent in primary infection, and false-positive reactions may occur. Pathologic evaluations of tissue specimens for the presence of inclusion bodies are helpful, but this finding is present only in advanced infection and with tissue invasion. Immunohistochemical stains to identify CMV antigens in tissue may be a more sensitive test to detect organ involvement. Other diagnostic modalities include shell-vial direct culture of buffy coat, bronchoalveolar fluid, tissue material, urine swab, or throat swab. More recently, the use of polymerase chain reaction

(PCR) assays to detect CMV DNA in peripheral blood leukocytes has afforded a sensitive and highly specific test for detection of disease (43). This assay is being used with more frequency and is available at most transplantation centers. However, some authors caution that PCR may be overly sensitive and may lead to overtreatment when used as a basis for preemptive therapy. This may be especially true in cases of CMV-seropositive patients who have a high rate of reactivation but a low rate of progression to CMV disease (44). On the other hand, PCR is superior to other modalities for the diagnosis of gastrointestinal CMV disease, a situation in which viremia is typically absent. The development of quantitative PCR assays and the accumulation of more experience with these assays will undoubtedly lead to wider application of this technique for the diagnosis of CMV infection.

Treatment of active CMV disease consists of judicious reduction of immunosuppression and a 14-day course of intravenous ganciclovir at a dose of 5 mg per kilogram administered twice daily. In cases of resistant infection, severe CMV hepatitis, or CMV pneumonitis, the addition of CMV-hyperimmune globulin or intravenous pooled gammaglobulin may improve response to ganciclovir. Foscarnet has been used to treat ganciclovir-resistant CMV isolates, but one should be cautious because of the significant nephrotoxicity associated with this drug.

Prophylaxis

To minimize the incidence of CMV disease after renal transplantation, risk stratification based on donor and recipient CMV status should be performed and prophylaxis should be instituted based on those results. Data from the adult renal transplantation experience has demonstrated that CMV-seronegative recipients (R–) who acquire primary CMV infection after receiving a seropositive donor kidney or blood product (D+) have a 60% risk of developing symptomatic primary infection. Reactivation of latent CMV infection in a seropositive recipient (R+) who received a kidney from a seronegative donor (D–) yields a 20% risk of developing symptomatic disease. Secondary infection (caused by reactivation of latent virus, reinfection, or superinfection with new virus) of an R+ patient transplanted with a D+ kidney places the patient at intermediate risk of developing symptomatic disease, between 20% and 60% (45). Because most pediatric patients are CMV-seronegative at time of transplantation and donors are most often CMV-seropositive adults, most pediatric recipients fall into the high- or intermediate-risk categories and require CMV prophylaxis. According to the pediatric transplant registry, more than 75% of patients hospitalized with CMV disease received D+ kidneys; R– patients who received D+ kidneys represented 51% of those hospitalized for CMV disease, whereas the R+/D+ combination accounted for 25% of the group hospitalized for CMV disease. Recipients of a D– kidney, regardless of their CMV exposure status, had a significantly lower incidence of hospitalization for CMV infection (40). This is consistent with the single-center experience from the University of Minnesota, where there was a 10% overall infection rate, and 80% of those who developed CMV infection had received D+ kidneys. In that report, recipients of D+ kidneys had a 40% to 50% incidence of CMV infection (39).

Prophylaxis against CMV has reduced both the incidence of CMV disease and the incidence of organ involvement in those who develop the infection (40). Currently there are at least four antiviral prophylactic modalities for the prevention CMV infection: the antibody preparations, intravenous immunoglobulin G (IVIgG), CMV-hyperimmune globulin, and the antiviral agents, acyclovir and ganciclovir. IVIgG prophylaxis has been shown to decrease the incidence of symptomatic CMV disease from 71% to 17% in the high-risk group of R– children who received D+ allografts (46). The use of CMV-hyperimmune globulin has decreased the attack rate from 60% to 20% and 30% in two different trials (47,48), but the group performing these trials concede that other modalities should be considered because of the cost of IVIgG preparations (49).

Acyclovir acts by competitively inhibiting viral DNA polymerase; it can be administered as an oral agent, is relatively inexpensive, and has minimal toxicity. Despite low *in vitro* activity against CMV, acyclovir has been shown to prevent CMV infection in renal transplant recipients (50). However, when used as prophylaxis for patients receiving induction antirejection therapy with antibody preparations, acyclovir did not decrease the incidence of CMV disease in the D+/R− combinations (51). Therefore, patients receiving antilymphocyte preparations either for induction or as treatment of steroid-resistant rejection, who are at increased susceptibility for CMV infection, need better coverage with either CMV-enriched immunoglobulin therapy or a stronger antiviral agent.

Ganciclovir is another antiviral agent with excellent *in vitro* activity against CMV and all members of the herpes family of viruses. In its active, phosphorylated form, it inhibits DNA polymerase and competes with deoxyguanosine triphosphate to act as a terminator of biosynthesis of the viral strand. This agent has been tested in various trials alone, in combination with acyclovir, and in combination with CMV-enriched immunoglobulin. The results of prophylaxis with ganciclovir as a sole agent are discussed here. When used alone for the high-risk D+/R− combination, short-term (2 to 4 weeks) intravenous ganciclovir has not been effective in reducing CMV infection (52,53). When it was used for prolonged periods (100 days) in liver transplant recipients, there was a reduction in CMV disease even in the high-risk D+R− group (54). Disadvantages with the use of ganciclovir are the less optimal safety profile marked by significant bone marrow and renal toxicity, the need for prolonged intravenous access, the cost of prolonged intravenous administration, and the potential for induction of ganciclovir-resistant strains. With the introduction and availability of an oral form of ganciclovir, many programs, including our own, are evaluating its use for long-term CMV prophylaxis in the high-risk patient. Typically, the patient would receive at least 1 week of intravenous ganciclovir therapy, after which time the drug would be administered in oral form. Pharmacokinetic studies in high CMV-risk pediatric renal transplant recipients in whom a target trough level of 0.91 ± 0.68 µg per milliliter was attained have yielded the following formula for oral ganciclovir dosing: the daily dosage of ganciclovir (milligrams per kilogram per day) is equal to the Schwartz-calculated glomerular filtration rate (GFR) (55). The daily dose is divided into three daily doses unless the GFR is less than 40 mL per minute per 1.73 m^2, in which case only two daily doses are given. Based on these studies, a dosing guideline is proposed (Table 6.1). We and others have incorporated the use of prophylactic oral ganciclovir for pediatric

TABLE 6.1. *Dosing regimen for prophylactic oral ganciclovir*[a]

Condition	Dose	Dosing schedule
Weight >50 kg	1000 mg	t.i.d.
Weight 37.5–50 kg	750 mg	t.i.d.
Weight 24–37.5 kg	500 mg	t.i.d.
GFR <100 mL/min per 1.73 m^2	Dose (mg/kg) per day = GFR	—[b]
GFR ≤50 mL/min per 1.73 m^2	Reduce dose by 50%	—[b]
GFR ≤25 mL/min per 1.73 m^2	Reduce dose by 75%	—[b]

CMV, cytomegalovirus; GFR, glomerular filtration rate.

[a]Based on pharmacokinetic studies in 14 pediatric renal transplant recipients who were CMV-negative and received CMV-positive organs.

[b]The daily dose should be divided into three daily doses unless GFR is <40 mL/min per 1.73 m^2, in which case only two daily doses are given.

From Filler G, et al. Prophylactic oral ganciclovir after renal transplantation: dosing and pharmacokinetics. *Pediatr Nephrol* 1998;12:6–9, with permission.

transplant patients (kidney and liver) who are at high risk of developing CMV infection; although the early results seem promising, interval evaluations should be carried out to assess its efficacy.

There are other agents under investigation for CMV prophylaxis in kidney transplant recipients. The antiviral agent foscarnet is being considered; its major disadvantages are the need for intravenous administration and its nephrotoxic potential. CMV monoclonal antibody is being developed but, because it is likely to be expensive, its use may be limited to high-risk prophylaxis or treatment of CMV disease.

A nucleotide analog, hydroxyphosphoryl methoxypropylcytosine, has the highest anti-CMV activity of any antiviral agent, is effective against ganciclovir-resistant strains, has a favorable dosing schedule of once weekly or even less often, but is also nephrotoxic. Lobucavir (Bristol-Myers Squibb) is an oral anti-CMV agent whose clinical efficacy for prophylaxis is yet to be determined (53).

Although the best prophylactic regimen in pediatric renal transplant patients is still not defined, especially for the highest-risk D+/R– combination, it is clear from the cumulative data that prophylaxis for pediatric patients transplanted with kidneys from CMV-seropositive donors benefit from CMV prophylaxis. Furthermore, patients who receive any form of CMV prophylaxis and ultimately re-

quire hospitalization for CMV disease appear to have a significantly higher graft survival rate and better graft function than those who did not receive CMV prophylaxis (40). Therefore, some form of CMV prophylaxis is warranted for all pediatric renal transplant recipients, or at a minimum for all of those receiving D+ allografts, antibody preparations, or prolonged intensive care unit or hospital stays. A proposed CMV prophylaxis protocol is outlined in Table 6.2.

Epstein-Barr Virus and Posttransplantation Lymphoproliferative Disease

Manifestations of EBV infection in children encompass a wide range of symptoms, including fever, flu-like symptoms, lymphadenopathy, splenomegaly, respiratory symptoms from tonsillar enlargement or airway involvement, and a number of gastrointestinal symptoms. The virus may induce a lymphoproliferative process that can progress to full-blown lymphoma; both of these manifestations are associated with significant mortality. In contrast to what is seen with adults, EBV infections in young children are usually primary because children are usually EBV-seronegative before transplantation. Because primary EBV infections are more likely to result in a lymphoproliferative disorder, children have a greater risk than adults (56). Mortality complicating post-

TABLE 6.2. *Cytomegalovirus prophylaxis based on Stanford Pediatric Kidney Transplant Protocol*[a]

Risk stratification	Indications for risk assignment	Recommended prophylaxis

High	Donor + and recipient –
	Treatment of acute rejection
	    with OKT3 or antithymocyte globulin
	    with pulse steroids (relatively high risk)
	Antibody induction therapy in Donor + and
	    recipient +
	Plasmapheresis
		IV ganciclovir while hospitalized; then
		    oral ganciclovir for total of 100 d

Low-intermediate	Donor – and recipient +
	Donor + and Recipient +
		IV ganciclovir while hospitalized
		    (maximum of 2 wk); then oral
		    acyclovir 40 mg/kg/d divided
		    t.i.d. or q.i.d. for 100 d

Lowest	Donor – and Recipient –	No antiviral prophylaxis except low-dose acyclovir for herpes simplex virus
Unknown serology	Begin prophylaxis and change when serology results are available	IV ganciclovir

[a]The symbols, + and – denote Cytomegalovirus serologic status at time of transplantation.

transplantation lymphoproliferative disease (PTLD) may result from gastrointestinal obstruction and bleeding, respiratory obstruction, or sepsis with shock.

Until recently, most of the experience with EBV and associated PTLD was in pediatric liver transplant recipients. In our institution, we found that 38.5% of pediatric liver transplant recipients with symptomatic EBV infections had diarrhea, gastrointestinal bleeding, or both at the time of presentation. This compelled us to advocate early endoscopy and biopsy for the prompt diagnosis of PTLD (57). The mean time to development of symptomatic EBV infection in our series was 2 years among patients receiving cyclosporine-based therapy and 0.8 years among those receiving tacrolimus. We observed a higher incidence among younger children (under the age of 5 years) (58); with those younger than 2 years of age had a 37% incidence of disease, and those between 2 and 17 years old had an incidence of 23.6% (57). Mortality rates in EBV-associated PTLD have been as high as 36% (59) to 60% (60). The use of antibody preparations (OKT3 and lymphocyte preparations) and of high tacrolimus levels has been associated with an increased incidence of PTLD in pediatric liver transplant recipients (61).

It has been suggested that aggressive prophylaxis and modification of the immunosuppressive regimen in high-risk pediatric liver transplant patients may decrease the incidence of PTLD to as low as 5%. (62). This particular group advocates an aggressive prophylactic regimen in patients with a high risk of PTLD. High-risk recipients—EBV D+R– combinations—were treated by this group with 100 days of intravenous ganciclovir (6 to 10 mg per kilogram per day). Lower-risk patients (D+R+, D–R–, and D–R+) received intravenous ganciclovir during their initial hospitalization, with conversion to oral acyclovir (40 mg per kilogram per day) at the time of discharge. Semiquantitative EBV PCR determinations were made at 1- to 2-month intervals, and those with increasing viral copy number had their tacrolimus levels decreased. When PTLD was diagnosed, tacrolimus was stopped and intravenous ganciclovir was reinstituted. Using this approach, the group reported no cases of PTLD and one case of EBV disease (mononucleosis-like syndrome) in the high-risk group (n = 18; mean age, 14 ± 15 months; mean follow-up, 243 ± 149 days) and two cases of PTLD in the low-risk group (n = 22; mean age, 64 ± 65 months; mean follow-up, 275 ± 130 days). The overall incidence of PTLD had fallen from 10% to 5% at this center among patients treated with primary tacrolimus therapy after liver transplantation (62). In our center, where CMV prophylaxis but not specific EBV prophylaxis is applied, we have also lowered the incidence of PTLD to 5.4% among pediatric liver transplant patients (63) by adopting a regimen that involves lower doses of tacrolimus and prednisone, limiting the use of antibody induction therapy, and adopting an aggressive diagnostic approach when patients present with suspicious symptoms that include the use of PCR to screen for EBV DNA (64). We believe that routine monitoring for EBV in asymptomatic but high-risk patients is helpful for early identification of those at risk for development of EBV-associated disease (65).

In the past, the incidence of PTLD among pediatric kidney transplant patients was 1.2%. More cases were identified with the use of tacrolimus in these patients, and this may have been related to early inexperience with this immunosuppressive agent and overimmunosuppression. The incidence rate of PTLD among tacrolimus recipients (48 of 4,084 patients) reported by the NAPRTCS was 16%, compared with 1.1% among those receiving cyclosporine (46/4,084) (66). In a center experience of 84 pediatric patients receiving renal transplants from 1986 to 1998, a 7% incidence of PTLD was reported among patients who received quadruple immunosuppression with antilymphocyte preparation, methylprednisolone, cyclosporine, and azathioprine or mycophenolate mofetil (MMF) (67). Most of these patients were seronegative for EBV at the time of transplantation, all received viral prophylaxis with intravenous ganciclovir during their transplantation hospitalization, and all continued taking daily oral acyclovir after hospital discharge. These patients were managed by reducing immunosuppression and initiating antiviral therapy; in one case, additional chemotherapy and CMV-hyperimmune globulin were used. All of these patients had resolution of disease, and all were alive with functioning grafts at the time of the report (67). In a comprehensive analysis of children at another center who underwent renal transplantation with tacrolimus-based immunosuppression, the EBV combination R–D+ predicted a high risk for seroconversion and for development of PTLD or lymphoma. Among those with known donor EBV serologies, 15 (79%) of 19 R– patients who received D+ grafts seroconverted at a mean of 6.6 ± 2.6 months after transplantation (68). The authors proposed that EBV viral load should be used to predict the risk for development of PTLD. They monitored EBV viral load by peripheral blood quantitative competitive-PCR. If the initial viral load exceeded 5,000 genome copies per 10^5 peripheral blood leukocytes or rose to 1,000 or more copies per 10^5 peripheral blood leukocytes, intravenous gan-

ciclovir and CMV-hyperimmune globulin were instituted with a modest reduction of immunosuppression. Among those with extranodal involvement (PTLD), these antiviral agents were administered together with a 50% to 100% reduction in tacrolimus dose and discontinuation of prednisone. In this particular series, there was absence of mortality, systemic symptoms resolved within 14 days, and extranodal lesions disappeared within 4 to 8 weeks of initiation of therapy. Maintenance immunosuppression was reintroduced at modified doses within 2 to 3 months (68).

In contrast to the experience with CMV, antiviral prophylaxis has not been clearly demonstrated to reduce the incidence of EBV and associated PTLD (67,68). However, an aggressive diagnostic approach should be applied, especially for high-risk (D+R–) patients who present with even the most subtle symptom. A proposed treatment algorithm is outlined in Fig. 6.3. Response to therapy should be monitored by clinical status, assessing for presence of fever, palpable adenopathy, and organomegaly; monitoring allograft function;

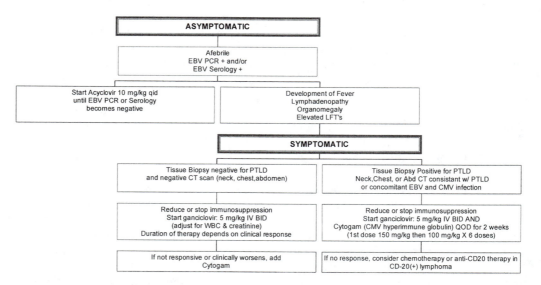

FIG. 6.3. Diagnostic and treatment algorithm for Epstein-Barr virus and posttransplantation lymphoproliferative disease. (Derived from Cao S, et al. Posttransplant lymphoproliferative disorders and gastrointestinal manifestations of Epstein-Barr virus infection in children following liver transplantation. *Transplantation* 1998;66:851–856, with permission.)

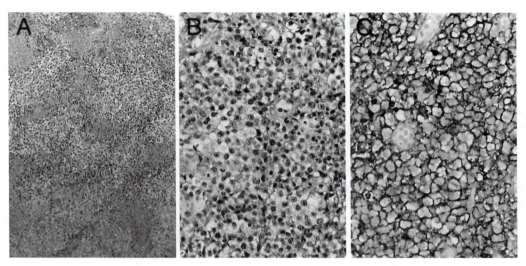

FIG. 6.4. A: Lymph node with diffuse effacement of architecture by an atypical lymphoid infiltrate associated with ulceration and necrosis. **B:** Lymphoid infiltrate comprising pleomorphic large cells with vesicular chromatin and increased mitotic activity. **C:** Immunohistochemical stain for CD20 highlights atypical large cells and confirms B-lineage origin for this diffuse large cell lymphoma. (Courtesy of Dr. Yasodha Natkunam, Department of Pathology, Stanford University Medical Center, Stanford, California; 250× magnification.)

and obtaining serial EBV PCR and follow-up computed tomographic scans to assess extranodal disease and organ involvement. Duration of therapy with antiviral agents can range from 8 to 20 weeks or longer, depending on the clinical response. In our center's experience, chemotherapy was required for one liver transplant recipient with lymphoma, but this patient eventually died from the disease. Two pediatric transplantation patients at our center (one a liver allograft recipient and the other a kidney allograft recipient) with CD20+ monomorphic B-cell lymphomas received monoclonal antibody directed against CD20 (rituximab) in addition to antiviral therapy; both patients had complete response and are alive to date (Fig. 6.4).

Varicella Infections

VZV is a herpesvirus that causes significant morbidity in renal transplant recipients in both its primary (varicella) and reactivation (herpes zoster) forms. In early series, when vaccination was not in wide application, it represented the most common viral infection occurring beyond 6 months after transplantation and was more common in younger recipients (8). In nonimmunosuppressed children, chickenpox is a relatively mild disease. After an incubation period of 10 to 21 days, symptoms appear and consist of fever and malaise followed by development of the classic superficial vesicles, each surrounded by a halo of erythema. The vesicles are most numerous on the trunk but also appear on the face, scalp, mucous membranes, and neck. The lesions change from macules to papules to vesicles and are accompanied by pruritus. In immunocompetent children, new lesions form for an average of 4 days after onset, and 50% of the lesions heal within 1 week. If untreated, the immunosuppressed children could form new vesicles for as long as 2 weeks (69). Those not treated with antiviral medications have a 32% incidence of varicella pneumonitis and a 10% mortality rate (70). The diagnosis of varicella should be sought when the patient presents with the aforementioned lesions and fever, especially if there is a history of exposure to other children with chickenpox. The laboratory diagnosis can be established by culturing the virus from the lesions and by obtaining acute and convalescent serum VZV antibody titers.

Treatment of varicella in the transplant recipient consists of immediate admission to the hospital for intravenous acyclovir therapy and observation for evidence of cutaneous and visceral dissemination. Baseline values for liver enzymes, a coagulation profile, and serum creatinine should be obtained. Early treatment decreases the risk of visceral dissemination, and this risk was found to be greater in children who were not treated until the fifth day of the rash compared with those whose treatment started earlier (71). In a child with normal renal function, intravenous acyclovir should be started at a dose of 10 mg per kilogram of ideal body weight given every 8 hours for 7 to 10 days. The patient should be kept well hydrated during acyclovir therapy to prevent crystallization of the drug in the renal tubules. For all patients with impaired renal function, acyclovir serum levels should be determined and the dose should be adjusted to 5.0 to 7.5 mg per kilogram. To minimize the risk of dissemination, azathioprine and MMF should be withheld at least until all the lesions have crusted and there are no new vesicles. Calcineurin inhibitors (tacrolimus and cyclosporine) and steroids should be continued to protect against graft rejection. It is important to diagnose and treat these infections aggressively because, mortality rates as high as 25% have been reported in pediatric transplant recipients who developed varicella infections (72).

Many children have acquired natural immunity to VZV before transplantation. To promote such immunization for varicella, early exposure to chickenpox should be encouraged in children with renal disease who are destined to develop chronic renal failure. Kidney transplantation should be postponed in circumstances where the would-be recipient has serologic evidence or a history of recent exposure to chickenpox. Susceptible transplant recipients exposed to chickenpox should be given passive immunization with varicella-zoster immune globulin (VZIG) within 98 hours after exposure (73).

Even with the availability of live attenuated virus vaccine, immunization of children with renal failure who are receiving maintenance dialysis is hindered by lower seroconversion rates and the development of lower peak antibody levels to immunization, especially among those patients receiving chronic peritoneal dialysis. To address many of these issues, the Southwest Pediatric Nephrology Study Group (SPNSG) is conducting a study to provide information on the safety and efficacy of varicella vaccine in children with renal insufficiency who are receiving maintenance hemodialysis or peritoneal dialysis. Other studies have demonstrated effective vaccination with the Oka strain in patients with end-stage renal disease and have shown durable titers after transplantation in most of these patients. In a study of 34 pediatric patients, 17 patients with end-stage renal disease being treated with chronic dialysis and 17 renal transplant recipients were inoculated with an attenuated varicella virus. Eighty-five percent of these patients developed titers greater than 1:40, and 76% maintained their antibodies titers at 2 years. Three renal transplant recipients, who initially demonstrated antibody titers of 1:640, developed a mild form of varicella 2 to 4 years after vaccination (74). In a larger series of 704 pediatric patients who underwent transplantation between 1973 to 1994, Broyer et al. (41) examined the effectiveness of varicella immunization before transplantation. The vaccine appeared to induce a strong and lasting immune response, because 62% and 42% of vaccinated patients had antibody titers at 1 and 10 years, respectively. More importantly, there was a significant reduction in the incidence of varicella infection after transplantation in naïve patients who were immunized (26/212, 12%) compared with naïve patients who were not immunized (22/49, 45%). Severity of varicella infection was much less in the former group. Moreover, all of the deaths from varicella infection occurred in the nonimmunized group (3/22, 14%) (41). In another series of 160 pediatric renal transplant recipients who were

VZV-seropositive before transplantation and who received triple immunosuppressive therapy (MMF, cyclosporine A, and prednisone), there was an extremely low incidence of varicella infection (1.9%). These patients had mild disease that was managed with oral acyclovir and had uncomplicated recoveries (75). Based on these reports, VZV vaccination should be administered to all children who have not had chickenpox before transplantation. The immunization guideline should be followed according to the Red Book Schedule in patients with chronic renal failure and in dialysis patients awaiting transplantation, but, because it is a live virus, this vaccine should not be administered within 8 weeks before transplantation or after transplantation (76). Results from the SPNSG will be helpful in guiding any future vaccination practices in these patients.

Herpes zoster, the reactivation form of VZV infection, is estimated to have a 9.5% risk of visceral dissemination in the untreated immunocompromised host (77). Because it is uncertain who will develop cutaneous or visceral dissemination, it is recommended that these children be treated with intravenous acyclovir at 7.5 mg per kilogram of ideal body weight. As with the treatment of primary varicella infection, azathioprine and MMF should be withheld during the treatment of herpes zoster, until all lesions have crusted and no new lesions are forming. Varicella vaccination also appears to have a beneficial effect on herpes zoster outbreaks, because only 7% of vaccinees developed zoster, compared with 38% of naïve patients and 13% of patients with a history of varicella. The widespread employment of varicella vaccination before pediatric renal transplantation should significantly reduce the incidence and the morbidity and mortality from primary varicella infection as well as herpes zoster.

Herpes Simplex Viruses

The development of herpes simplex virus (HSV) oral or genital mucocutaneous lesions is more commonly seen in adult kidney transplant recipients and is usually caused by reactivation of disease in seropositive patients (78). The infection is frequently mild, consisting of a cold sore on the lip or oral mucosa, but in some cases it can produce severe esophagitis. These lesions are predisposed to secondary bacterial and *Candida* infections. Visceral dissemination rarely complicates the disease but could produce severe hepatitis and disseminated intravascular coagulation in extreme cases. Prophylaxis with oral acyclovir at a dose of 5 mg per kilogram twice a day for 3 months after transplantation is recommended. For treatment of severe disease, intravenous acyclovir at a dose of 5 mg per kilogram of ideal weight should be administered every 8 hours for a 7- to 10-day course.

Other Viral Infections

Adenovirus infection in the renal transplant recipient can manifest as acute hemorrhagic cystitis, which has been reported to be self-limited with complete resolution not requiring a reduction in immunosuppression (79). Adenovirus hepatitis, on the other hand, is associated with severe disease leading to fulminant hepatic failure and a high mortality rate. In these cases, a reduction in immunosuppression has been advocated (80). In a pediatric liver transplant recipient with severe respiratory compromise, a positive bronchoalveolar lavage result for adenovirus, and evidence of systemic disease, we had success with intravenous ribavirin therapy. This patient also had concomitant CMV that was treated with ganciclovir and intravenous CMV-enriched immunoglobulin. With therapy, this patient had complete resolution of the pneumonia, was eventually extubated, and is alive, 2 years after the event (81).

Respiratory syncytial virus (RSV) has been reported in 3% of pediatric renal transplant recipients (82). Onset of disease was 1 day to 7 months after transplantation. Symptoms included rhinorrhea, cough, tachypnea, retractions, fever, and abnormal chest radiograph. The course of infection did not differ from that reported in nonimmunosuppressed children, and these patients responded to treatment included bronchodilators, chest physiotherapy, antiviral therapy with ribavirin, and use of a mist tent.

Influenza and parainfluenza viruses produce a spectrum of disease—from mild upper respiratory symptoms to croup, bronchiolitis, pneumonia, and severe infection that may result in death. In contrast to the disease manifestations seen in adults, children are more likely to experience febrile seizures and to have gastrointestinal complaints, pneumonia, and CNS involvement. Influenza B occurs more commonly in children, whereas influenza A is more commonly seen in elderly patients. There are few reports describing parainfluenza and influenza B virus in immunosuppressed children. A combined incidence of 8% was reported from a large center experience (83). The authors observed a difference in incidence according to the type of organ transplanted: 3% of 75 kidney transplant recipients, 29% of 14 small bowel transplant recipients, and 8% of 328 liver transplant recipients had positive cultures for parainfluenza or influenza. They found that the clinical presentations and outcomes were similar regardless of the virus isolated or the type of organ transplanted. Eight of the 42 affected patients died with infection, and half of these patients had coinfection (CMV and bacterial). Poor outcome was observed in those patients younger than 6 months of age, in those treated with supplemental steroids or OKT3 within 1 week of viral isolation, and in those with onset of infection within 1 month after transplantation. Viral isolation was from respiratory specimen–nasopharyngeal swabs or aspirates, throat swabs, endotracheal aspirates, or bronchoalveolar lavage. Duration of viral shedding ranged from 1 to 49 days, and timing of cases of infection coincided with outbreaks in the community. In particular, influenza B infection can present as fever with respiratory illness, gastrointestinal manifestations, or neurologic symptoms, with an interval to onset of disease as long as 54 months. Severe morbidity and mortality have been reported from manifestations such as neurologic complications with uncal herniation,

respiratory failure requiring intubation, development of chronic reactive airway disease, and development of a pericardial effusion (84). Some have a mild form of the disease and require only supportive care, respiratory toilet, and intravenous hydration. Patients who present with suggestive symptomatology should have upper respiratory tract cultures. In addition, bronchoalveolar lavage in some cases has yielded the only positive culture, and it should be pursued if upper respiratory tract cultures are negative. An aggressive workup should be pursued, especially if suspicion is high or if respiratory tract disease manifests during the influenza season.

Ribavirin is the only effective current therapy against influenza B, but is approved by the U.S. Food and Drug Administration (FDA) only for use against RSV. Because specific therapy of influenza is limited, annual immunization of pediatric renal transplant recipients and those with end-stage renal disease who are candidates for transplantation may offer the most effective means of preventing bad outcome from the disease. Only 1% to 11% of children have been immunized against influenza (85), and none of the transplant recipients in a report from the University of Minnesota were immunized (84). The question arises as to the effect of immunosuppressive agents on the efficacy and longevity of the vaccine. Among 20 adult renal transplant recipients who were given the vaccine, only 60% developed protective antibody titers, compared with 100% of 15 normal healthy control subjects (86). However, it has been shown in the elderly population that, despite the achievement of effective antiinfluenza immunization in only 30% to 40% of those immunized, annual immunization in these high-risk patients lessens the severity of disease and prevents hospitalization and death (87). In our own program, we recommend influenza vaccine for children with end-stage renal disease and for pediatric kidney transplant recipients, especially infants, who are at least 6 to 8 months away from transplantation.

Parvovirus B19 has been associated with unexplained anemia in renal transplant recipients symptomatic with fatigue, palpitation, and hematocrits as low as 15%. Diagnosis is confirmed by serology or PCR. Treatment with IVIG has been successful in case reports (88).

Human herpesvirus 6 (HHV-6) is a ubiquitous virus found in more than 80% of the adult population worldwide (89). Little is known about the role of this virus in the transplant recipient, but it is known to lead to transactivation of heterologous viruses such as CMV, which may lead to increased CMV replication (90). In a longitudinal study of organ transplant recipients subjected to HHV-6 serologic screening, manifestations of a positive test were mild to absent unless there was accompanying CMV infection (89). Transmission of another human herpesvirus, HHV-8, has been reported (91) but the implications are not yet well defined. Some caution that this virus may be related to the development of posttransplantation Kaposi's sarcoma, but there is currently no firm evidence for this risk (92).

CONCLUSION

Opportunistic infection is a major cause of morbidity and mortality after renal transplantation in children. The clinical manifestations may be atypical, involve unusual sites, or be caused by unusual bacterial, viral, fungal, and protozoal organisms occurring either alone or in combination. A high index of suspicion is necessary to ensure prompt diagnosis and treatment of these infections. In recent years it has become evident that most posttransplantation infections do not occur at random but follow a more or less predictable timetable after transplantation or after treatment of rejection when the maximum immunosuppressive therapy has been given. Based on this information and an understanding of the pathogenesis of the various infections, useful strategies such as those shown in the proposed algorithms would be useful for prompt diagnosis and early treatment of these opportunistic infections. Future developments in newer and more specific immunosuppressive therapies and the development of more effective antiviral agents and vaccines may further help to decrease the morbidity and mortality associated with opportunistic infections after transplantation.

REFERENCES

1. Fine RN. Renal transplantation for children: the only realistic choice. *Kidney Int* 1985;28:S15.
2. So SKS, Chang PN, Najarian JS, et al. Growth and development in infants after renal transplantation. *J Pediatr* 1987;110:343.
3. Salvatierra O Jr, et al. Superior outcomes in pediatric renal transplantation. *Arch Surg* 1997;132:842–849.
4. Ishitani M, Isaacs R, Norwood V, et al. Predictors of graft survival in living-related kidney transplant recipients. *Transplantation* 2000;70:288–292.
5. Millan MT, et al. 100% 2-year graft survival can be attained in high-risk, < 15 kg infant recipients of kidney allografts. *Arch Surg* 2000 (*in press*).
6. Tejani A, et al. Steady improvement in renal allograft survival among North American children: a five year appraisal by the North American Pediatric Renal Transplant Cooperative Study. *Kidney Int* 1995;48:551–553.
7. Tejani A, et al. Posttransplant deaths and factors that influence the mortality rate in North American children. *Transplantation* 1994;57:547–553.
8. Chavers BM, Gillingham KJ, Matas AJ. Complications by age in primary pediatric renal transplant recipients. *Pediatr Nephrol* 1997;11:399–403.
9. Warady BA, et al. Renal transplantation, chronic dialysis, and chronic renal insufficiency in children and adolescents. The 1995 Annual Report of the North American Pediatric Renal Transplant Cooperative Study. *Pediatr Nephrol* 1997;11:49–64.
10. Kohaut EC, Tejani A. The 1994 report of the North American Pediatric Renal Transplant Cooperative Study. *Pediatr Nephrol* 1996;10:422–434.
11. Harmon WE. Opportunistic infection in children following renal transplantation. J *Pediatr Nephrol* 1991;5:118.
12. Peterson PK, et al. Infectious diseases in hospitalized renal transplant recipients: a prospective study of a complex and evolving problem. *Medicine (Baltimore)* 1982;71:345.
13. Peterson PK, et al. Fever in renal transplant recipients: causes, prognostic significance and changing patterns at the University of Minnesota Hospital. *Am J Med* 1981; 71:345–351.
14. Chang FY, et al. Fever in liver transplant recipients: changing spectrum of etiologic agents. *Clin Infect Dis* 1998;26:59–65.
15. Rubin RH, et al. Infection in the renal transplant patient. *Am J Med* 1981;70:405.
16. Schmaldienst S, Hörl WH, Bacterial infections after renal transplantation. *Nephron* 1997;75:140–153.
17. Rubin RH. Infectious disease complications of renal transplantation. *Kidney Int* 1993;44:221–236.
18. Gray JR, Kasiske BL. Patient and renal allograft survival in the late posttransplant period. *Semin Nephrol* 1992;12:343–352.
19. Dummer JS, et al. Early infections in kidney, heart and liver transplant recipients on cyclosporine. *Transplantation* 1983;36:259–267.
20. Renoult E, et al. Factors influencing early urinary tract infections in kidney transplant recipients. *Transplant Proc* 1994;26:2056–2058.

21. Warren JW, et al. Antibiotic irrigation and catheter-associated urinary tract infections. *N Engl J Med* 1978; 299:570–573.
22. Sealowsky AI, et al. Urologic complications in 505 renal transplants with early catheter removal. *J Urol* 1983; 129:929–932.
23. Grino JM, et al. Antilymphocyte globulin versus OKT3 induction therapy in cadaveric kidney transplantation: a prospective randomized study. *Am J Kidney Dis* 1992; 20:603–610.
24. Salvatierra O Jr. Management of vesico-ureteral reflux in renal allografts transplanted into pediatric recipients [Editorial]. *Pediatr Transplant* 1999;3:171–174.
25. Hanevold CD, et al. Vesicoureteral reflux and urinary tract infection in renal transplant recipients. *Am J Dis Child* 1987;141:982–984.
26. Dunn SP, et al. Pyelonephritis following pediatric renal transplant: increased incidence with vesicoureteral reflux. *J Pediatr Surg* 1987;22:1095–1099.
27. Salvatierra O Jr, et al. A new, unique and simple method for ureteral implantation in kidney recipients with small, defunctionalized bladders. *Transplantation* 1999; 68:731–738.
28. Fox BC, et al. A prospective, randomized, double-blind study of trimethoprim-sulfamethoxazole for prophylaxis of infection in renal transplantation: clinical efficacy, absorption of trimethoprim-sulfamethoxazole, effects on the microflora, and the cost-benefit of prophylaxis. *Am J Med* 1990;89:255–274.
29. Hanto DW, et al. Induction immunosuppression with antilymphocyte globulin or OKT3 in cadaver kidney transplantation. *Transplantation* 1994;57:377–384.
30. Hall LM, Chen HY, Williams RJ. Vancomycin-resistant *Enterococcus durans. Lancet* 1992;340:1105.
31. Sastry V, et al. Vancomycin-resistant enterococci: an emerging pathogen in immunosuppressed transplant recipients. *Transplant Proc* 1995;27:954–955.
32. Tarantino A, et al. A randomized prospective trial comparing cyclosporine monotherapy with triple-drug therapy in renal transplantation. *Transplantation* 1991;52: 53–57.
33. Brinker KR, et al. A randomized trial comparing double-drug and triple-drug therapy in primary cadaveric renal transplants. *Transplantation* 1990;50:43–49.
34. Shapiro R, et al. A prospective randomized trial of FK506-based immunosuppression after renal transplantation. *Transplantation* 1995;59:485–490.
35. Fryer JP, et al. Steroid-related complications in the cyclosporine era. *Clin Transplant* 1994;8:224–229.
36. Mayes JT, et al. Reexposure to OKT3 in renal allograft recipients. *Transplantation* 1988;45:349–353.
37. Oh C-S, et al. Increased infections associated with the use of OKT3 for treatment of steroid-resistant rejection in renal transplantation. *Transplantation* 1988;45: 68–73.
38. Granger DK, et al. Incidence and timing of infections in pediatric renal transplant recipients in the cyclosporine era. *Transplant Proc* 1994;26:64.
39. Burd RS, et al. Diagnosis and treatment of cytomegalovirus disease in pediatric renal transplant recipients. *J Pediatr Surg* 1994;29:1049–1054.
40. Bock GH, et al. Cytomegalovirus infections following renal transplantation—effects of antiviral prophylaxis: a report of the North American Pediatric Renal Transplant Cooperative Study. *Pediatr Nephrol* 1997;11:665–671.
41. Broyer M, et al. Varicella and zoster in children after kidney transplantation: long-term results of vaccinations. *Pediatrics* 1997;99:35–39.
42. Acott PD, et al. Infection concomitant with pediatric renal allograft rejection. *Transplantation* 1996;62: 689–691.
43. Boeckh M, et al. Plasma polymerase chain reaction for cytomegalovirus DNA after allogeneic marrow transplantation. *Transplantation* 1997;64:108–113.
44. Brennan DC, et al. Polymerase chain reaction-triggered preemptive or deferred therapy to control cytomegalovirus-associated morbidity and costs in renal transplant patients. *Transpl Proc* 1997;29:809–811.
45. Davis CL. The prevention of cytomegalovirus disease in renal transplantation. *Am J Kidney Dis* 1990;16: 175–188.
46. Flynn JT, et al. Intravenous immunoglobulin prophylaxis of cytomegalovirus infection in pediatric renal transplant recipients. *Am J Nephrol* 1997;17:146–152.
47. Snydman DR, et al. Use of cytomegalovirus immune globulin to prevent cytomegalovirus disease in renal-transplant recipients. *N Engl J Med* 1987;317: 1049–1054.
48. Snydman DR. Prevention of cytomegalovirus-associated diseases with immunoglobulin. *Transplant Proc* 1991;23[Suppl 3]:131–135.
49. Tsevat J, et al. Which renal transplant patients should receive cytomegalovirus immune globulin? *Transplantation* 1991;52:259–265.
50. Balfour HH, et al. A randomized placebo-controlled trial of oral acyclovir for the prevention of cytomegalovirus disease in recipients of renal allografts. *N Engl J Med* 1989;320:1381.
51. Frey DJ, et al. Sequential therapy: a prospective randomized trial of MALG versus OKT3 for prophylactic immunosuppression in cadaver renal allograft recipients. *Transplantation* 1992;54:50.
52. Rondreau E, et al. Effect of prophylactic ganciclovir on cytomegalovirus infection in renal transplant recipients. *Nephrol Dial Transplant* 1993;8:858.
53. Patel R, et al. Cytomegalovirus prophylaxis in solid organ transplant recipients. *Transplantation* 1996;61: 1279–1289.
54. Winston DJ, et al. Randomized comparison of ganciclovir and high-dose acyclovir for long-term cytomegalovirus prophylaxis in liver transplant patients. *Lancet* 1995;346:43.
55. Filler G, et al. Prophylactic oral ganciclovir after renal transplantation: dosing and pharmacokinetics. *Pediatr Nephrol* 1998;12:6–9.
56. Ho M, et al. The frequency of Epstein-Barr virus infection and associated lymphoproliferative syndrome after transplantation and its manifestation in children. *Transplantation* 1988;45:719–727.
57. Cao S, et al. Posttransplant lymphoproliferative disorders and gastrointestinal manifestations of Epstein-Barr virus infection in children following liver transplantation. *Transplantation* 1998;66:851–856.
58. Cox KL, et al. Increased incidence of Epstein-Barr (EBV) infection and lymphoproliferative disease (LPD) in young children on FK506 after liver transplantation. *Transplantation* 1995;59:524.
59. Cacciarelli TR, et al. Factors affecting survival after orthotopic liver transplantation in infants. *Transplantation* 1997;64:242–247.

60. Newell KA, et al. Posttransplant lymphoproliferative disease in pediatric liver transplantation. *Transplantation* 1996;62:370–375.

61. Sokal EM, et al. Early signs and risk factors for the increased incidence of Epstein-Barr virus-related posttransplant lymphoproliferative disease in pediatric liver transplant recipients treated with tacrolimus. *Transplantation* 1997;64:1438–1442.

62. McDiarmid SV, et al. Prevention and preemptive therapy in posttransplant lymphoproliferative disease in pediatric liver recipients. *Transplantation* 1998;66:1604–1611.

63. Cao S, et al. Strategies in reducing EBV-associated PTLD in pediatric liver recipients [Abstract 1705]. In: *The Transplantation Society XVII World Congress,* Montreal, 1998.

64. Martinez OM, et al. Viral and immunologic aspects of Epstein-Barr virus infection in pediatric liver transplant recipients. *Transplantation* 1995;59:519–523.

65. Krieger NR, et al. The significance of detecting EBV-specific sequences in the peripheral blood of asymptomatic pediatric liver transplant recipients. *Liver Transplant* 2000;6:62–66.

66. Dharnidharka VR, et al. Risk factors for post transplant lympho-proliferative disorder (PTLD): an analysis of the cases in the North American Pediatric Renal Transplant Cooperative Study (NAPRTCS). *Transplantation* 1999;67:S215.

67. Srivastava T, et al. Posttransplant lymphoproliferative disorder in pediatric renal transplantation. *Pediatr Nephrol* 1999;13:748–754.

68. Ellis D, et al. Epstein-Barr virus-related disorders in children undergoing renal transplantation with tacro-limus-based immunosuppression. *Transplantation* 1999;68:997–1003.

69. Balfour HH Jr. Varicella zoster virus infections in immunocompromised hosts a review of the natural history and management. *Am J Med* 1988;85[Suppl 2A]:68.

70. Feldman S, Lott L. Varicella in children with cancer: impact of antiviral therapy and prophylaxis. *Pediatrics* 1987;80:465.

71. Balfour HH Jr. Intravenous acyclovir therapy for varicella in immunocompromised children. *J Pediatr* 1984;104:134.

72. Lynfield R, Herrin JT, Rubin RH. Varicella in pediatric renal transplant recipients. *Pediatrics* 1992;90:216–220.

73. Center for Disease Control and Department of Health and Human Services. Varicella-zoster immune globulin for the prevention of chicken pox: recommendations of the immunization practices advisory committee. *Ann Intern Med* 1984;100:859.

74. Zamora I, et al. Attenuated varicella virus vaccine in children with renal transplant. *Pediatr Nephrol* 1994;8:190–192.

75. Rothwell WS, et al. Disseminated varicella infection in pediatric renal transplant recipients treated with mycophenolate mofetil. *Transplantation* 1999;68:158–161.

76. Fivush BA, Neu AM. Immunization guidelines for pediatric renal disease. *Semin Nephrol* 1998;18:256–263.

77. Balfour HH Jr, et al. Acyclovir halts progression of herpes zoster in immunocompromised patients. *N Engl J Med* 1983;308:1448.

78. Armstrong JA, et al. Viral infections in renal transplant recipients. *Infect Immun* 1976;14:970.

79. Koga S, et al. Acute hemorrhagic cystitis caused by adenovirus following renal transplantation: review of the literature. *J Urol* 1993;149:838–839.

80. Koneru B, et al. Adenoviral infections in pediatric liver transplant recipients. *JAMA* 1987;258:489–492.

81. Shetty AK, et al. Intravenous ribavirin therapy for adenovirus pneumonia. *Pediatr Pulmonol* 2000;29:69–73.

82. Miller RB, Chavers BM. Respiratory syncytial virus infections in pediatric renal transplant recipients. *Pediatr Nephrol* 1996;10:213–215.

83. Apalsch AM, et al. Parainfluenza and influenza virus infections in pediatric organ transplant recipients. *Clin Infect Dis* 1995;20:394–399.

84. Mauch TJ, et al. Influenza B virus infection in pediatric solid organ transplant recipients. *Pediatrics* 1994;94:225–229.

85. Serwint JR, Miller RM, Korsch BM. Influenza type A and B infections in hospitalized pediatric patients. *Am J Dis Child* 1991;145:623–626.

86. Kumar S, Ventura AK, VanderWerf B. Influenza vaccination in renal transplant recipients. *JAMA* 1978;239:840–842.

87. Gardner P, Schaffner W. Immunization of adults. *N Engl J Med* 1993;328:1252–1258.

88. Mathias RS. Chronic anemia as a complication of parvovirus B19 infection in a pediatric kidney transplant patient. *Pediatr Nephrol* 1997;11:355–357.

89. Herbein G, et al. Longitudinal study of human herpesvirus 6 infection in organ transplant recipients. *Clin Infect Dis* 1996;22:171–173.

90. Dockrell DH, Smith TF, Paya CV. Subspecialty clinics: human herpesvirus-6. *Mayo Clin Proc* 1999;74:163–170.

91. Regamey N, et al. Transmission of human herpesvirus 8 infection from renal-transplant donors to recipients. *N Engl J Med* 1998;339:1358–1363.

92. Ho M. Human herpesvirus 8: let the transplantation physician beware. *N Engl J Med* 1998;339:1391–1392.

7

Infectious Complications of Liver Transplantation in Children

Michael Green

Department of Pediatrics and Surgery, University of Pittsburgh School of Medicine,
Pittsburgh, Pennsylvania 15261

Liver transplantation has gained increasing acceptance as treatment for end-stage disease of the liver and may provide a potential cure for some of the metabolic diseases of childhood. Improving surgical techniques and the availability of new and more potent immunosuppressive regimens have led to enhanced short- and long-term survival rates that now approach or exceed 80%. In response to these excellent results, an expanding number of children are being referred to a rapidly growing list of transplantation centers for liver transplantation. To accommodate the increasing number of children on liver transplant waiting lists, newer procedures, including reduced grafts, split liver grafts, and living-related donor liver transplantation have been developed to increase the donor pool.

Infectious complications have been a significant cause of morbidity and mortality in children undergoing liver transplantation since this procedure was widely introduced in the 1980s. However, careful review of the expanding experience of liver transplantation in children along with the increasing availability of new antiinfective agents and diagnostic tools has led not only to the evolution of improved treatment regimens but to the development of many strategies aimed at prevention of infectious complications in these patients. This chapter provides a general approach to the problem of infection after liver transplantation in children.

PREDISPOSING FACTORS

Liver transplantation is associated with a set of technical and medical conditions that predispose to a unique set of infectious complications. The abdomen is the most common site of infection in patients undergoing this procedure (1), almost certainly because of the occurrence of local ischemic injury and bleeding, as well as potential soilage with contaminated material (2). Additional factors predisposing to infection can be divided into those that exist before transplantation and those that occur secondary to intraoperative and posttransplantation activities.

PRETRANSPLANTATION FACTORS

The underlying illnesses leading to transplantation may be associated with intrinsic risk factors for infection. Some disorders may have required palliative surgery that increases the technical difficulty of the transplantation and may result in an enhanced risk for development of posttransplantation infections (3). Some palliative procedures (e.g., Kasai procedure [choledocojejunostomy] as a treatment for biliary atresia) may predispose to recurrent infections before transplantation, increasing the likelihood of colonization with bacteria resistant to multiple antibiotics that can cause infection after liver transplantation. Complications of end-stage liver disease may also predispose to infection after transplantation. For example, a history of one or more episodes of spontaneous bacterial peritonitis before transplantation in patients with ascites has been associated with an increased rate of bacterial infections after liver transplantation (4).

Age, another important pretransplantation factor, is a major determinant of susceptibility to certain agents, severity of expression of infection, and immune maturation. Young children undergoing liver transplantation may experience moderate to severe infection with certain viral organisms (e.g., respiratory syncytial virus [RSV]) or bacterial pathogens (e.g., coagulase-negative staphylococci) that would produce only mild infections in adult recipients. In contrast, certain pathogens, such as *Cryptococcus neoformans,* uncommonly manifest infection before young adulthood (5). Age is also an important factor governing clinical expression of infection with cytomegalovirus (CMV) or Epstein-Barr virus (EBV). There is a high likelihood that young patients undergoing liver transplantation will be seronegative for CMV and EBV and therefore susceptible to primary infections, which are more severe than infections caused by reactivation (6,7).

Another set of pretransplantation factors to consider comprises donor-related issues. Transplant recipients are at risk for acquiring infections that may be active or latent within the donor at the time of organ harvesting. Perhaps the best example of this is CMV, the most frequent and important viral pathogen among transplant recipients (8). Other pathogens established as causing donor-associated infections include EBV (9), human immunodeficiency virus (HIV) (10), and histoplasmosis (11).

INTRAOPERATIVE FACTORS

Operative factors unique to liver transplantation may predispose to infectious complications. For example, patients undergoing roux en Y cholodocoduodenostomy experience more infectious episodes than those who undergo a choledocho-choledochostomy with T-tube drainage (12,13). However, usually only the former option is performed in children undergoing liver transplantation because of the small size of their bile ducts. Prolonged operative time (longer than 12 hours) during the initial transplantation has been associated with an increased risk of infection after transplantation (13,14) and is probably a surrogate marker for the technical difficulty of the surgery. Finally, intraoperative events such as contamination of the operative field clearly predispose to postoperative infections.

POSTTRANSPLANTATION FACTORS

Technical problems, immunosuppression, presence of indwelling cannulas, and nosocomial exposures are major postoperative risk factors for infectious complications. Thrombosis of the hepatic artery is the most serious technical problem and predisposes to areas of necrotic liver and the development of hepatic abscesses and bacteremia (12,15). Bile duct strictures, developing as a sequela of thrombosed hepatic artery and ischemia or caused by technical error, may predispose to cholangitis (12).

Immunosuppression is the critical postoperative factor predisposing to infection in transplant recipients. Immunosuppressive regimens have evolved in an attempt to achieve more specific control of rejection with the least impairment of immunity. This evolution is aimed not only at improved control of rejection but also at decreased morbidity and mortality from infections. The use of cyclosporine-based regimens has resulted in a decreased incidence of infections among renal and cardiac transplant recipients (1,16–17). More recently, the introduction of tacrolimus (FK-506) has allowed management in many patients without the use of steroids (18,19). Although reported rates of infection have been similar in patients treated with tacrolimus and those receiving cyclosporine, an apparent decrease in morbidity and mortality, especially from viral pathogens, has been noted with tacrolimus (18,20). In contrast to these results, some centers have reported an increased rate of EBV-associated posttransplantation lymphoproliferative disease (PTLD) in patients receiving tacrolimus (21). However, data from the University of Pittsburgh suggest that the short- and long-term incidence of EBV-associated PTLD is similar in pediatric liver transplant recipients treated with cyclosporine and those treated with tacrolimus (22).

The treatment of rejection with additional or higher doses of immunosuppressants increases the risk of invasive and potentially fatal infection. Of particular concern is the use of antilymphocyte preparations, especially OKT3, which is often indispensable in the treatment of steroid-refractory rejection (8,13,14).

The prolonged use of an indwelling cannula at any site is an important cause of infection throughout the postoperative course. The presence of a central venous catheter is a cause of bacteremia after transplantation. Similarly, urinary tract infections and bacterial pneumonia are associated with the use of urethral catheters and prolonged nasotracheal or endotracheal intubation, respectively (13,14).

Nosocomial exposures constitute the final group of postoperative risk factors. Transplant recipients, especially children, may be exposed to many common viral pathogens (e.g., rotavirus, RSV, influenza) while in the hospital. In addition, all transplant recipients are at risk of exposure to transfusion-associated pathogens such as hepatitis B virus (HBV), hepatitis C virus (HCV), or HIV. Finally, the presence in the hospital of heavy areas of contamination with pathogenic fungi (e.g., *Aspergillus*) may increase the risk of invasive fungal disease in these patients.

TIMING OF INFECTIONS

The time of onset of infection with various pathogens after transplantation tends to be predictable. The majority of clinically im-

portant infections occur within the first 180 days after transplantation (13,23). The timing of infections can be divided into three intervals: early (0 to 30 days after transplantation), intermediate (30 to 180 days after transplantation) and late (more than 180 days after transplantation). Additionally, some infections may occur throughout the postoperative course. These divisions, although arbitrary, are generally useful in approaching a patient with fever after transplantation and can provide a guide to differential diagnosis. An overview of the infectious complications occurring during each of these time periods is provided in Tables 7.1 through 7.3 and summarized in the following sections.

Early Infections (0 to 30 Days)

Early infections tend to be associated with preexisting conditions and surgical manipulations (Table 7.1). In general, they are caused by either bacteria or yeast. Cholangitis or spontaneous bacterial peritonitis manifesting at or near the time of liver transplantation may lead to intraabdominal infection after the operation. Herpes simplex infection can also reactivate and cause early symptomatic disease (13), although this is uncommon in children. Technical difficulties (e.g., thrombosis of the hepatic artery or portal vein, biliary strictures) predispose to early bacterial infections. Likewise, reexploration of the abdomen is associated with an increased rate of fungal infection (13).

Intermediate Period (31 to 180 Days)

The intermediate period is the typical time of onset for infections associated with donor transmission (either organ or blood products), reactivated viruses, or opportunistic pathogens (Table 7.2). CMV infection peaks in incidence during this time (8,13). This period is also when many patients begin to present with EBV-associated PTLD (7) or *Pneumocystis carinii* pneumonia (PCP) (13).

TABLE 7.1. *Differential diagnosis of infectious complications during the early period (0–30 d) after liver transplantation at Children's Hospital of Pittsburgh*

Clinical syndrome	Associated pathogens
Wound infection (superficial, deep)	*Staphylococcus aureus,* enterococci, Enterobacterciae, *Candida* sp.
Intraabdominal infection (peritonitis, intraabdominal abscess, intrahepatic abscess ± bacteremia)	Enterobacterciae, enterococci, *Candida* sp.
Bloodstream infection, associated with	
Central venous catheterization	Coagulase-negative staphylococci
	Enterococci
	S. aureus
	Candida sp.
Hepatic artery thrombosis	Enterobacterciae
	Enterococci
	Candida sp.
Bacterial cholangitis	Enterobacterciae
	Enterococci
	Candida sp.
Urinary tract infection	Enterobacterciae
	Enterococci
	Candida sp.
Ventilator-associated pneumonia	Enterobacterciae
	Enterococci
	S. aureus
	Candida sp.
Nosocomial acquisition of common community pathogens	Respiratory syncytial virus
	Parainfluenza virus
	Influenza virus
	Rotavirus
Noninfectious causes	Rejection
	Drug fever

TABLE 7.2. *Differential diagnosis of infectious complications during the intermediate period (31–180 d) after liver transplantation at Children's Hospital of Pittsburgh*

Clinical syndrome	Associated pathogens
Viral syndrome (fever, leukopenia, thrombocytopenia ± atypical lymphocytosis)	CMV, EBV
Hepatitis	CMV, EBV, adenovirus, hepatitis B, hepatitis C
Enteritis	CMV, EBV, rotavirus, adenovirus, *Clostridium difficile*
PTLD	EBV
Bacterial cholangitis[a]	Enterobacterciae, enterococci, *Candida* sp.
Pneumonia	*Streptococcus pneumoniae,* CMV, adenovirus, RSV, parainfluenza, influenza, *Pneumocystis carinii, Aspergillus fumigatus*
Adenopathy	EBV/PTLD
Pulmonary nodules	EBV/PTLD, *Aspergillus fumigatus*

CMV, cytomegalovirus; EBV, Epstein-Barr virus; PTLD, posttransplantation lymphoproliferative disease; RSV, respiratory syncytial virus.

[a]Usually associated with the presence of technical complication (e.g., biliary stricture).

TABLE 7.3. *Differential diagnosis of infectious complications during the late period (>180 d) after liver transplantation at Children's Hospital of Pittsburgh*

Clinical syndrome	Associated pathogens
Bacterial cholangitis[a]	Enterobacterciae, enterococci, *Candida* sp.
Posttransplantation lymphoproliferative disease	Epstein-Barr virus
Varicella-zoster	Varicella-zoster virus

[a]Usually associated with the presence of technical complication (e.g., biliary stricture).

Late Infections (More Than 180 Days)

Late infections after liver transplantation are less well characterized than those of other periods because patients usually have been discharged from the transplantation center to their respective homes, often quite far away (Table 7.3). This makes the accurate accumulation of data on these late infections difficult. Problems such as recurrent episodes of bacterial cholangitis (typically associated with underlying problems of the biliary tree) and PTLD (24) occur in this time period and usually require the return of the patient to the transplantation center for definitive diagnosis and management.

Infections Occurring throughout the Postoperative Course

Iatrogenic factors are an important cause of bacterial and fungal infections at all times, but they predominate in the early posttransplantation period. Central venous lines are maintained for a variable time; the risk of infection persists for the entire period that the catheter remains in place. Similarly, the presence of a uretheral catheter or endotracheal tube also increases the risk of infection whenever the device is in place.

Nosocomial acquisition of community viruses, such as RSV, rotavirus, or influenza A or B, can occur at any time after transplantation. These viruses spread easily in hospital environments from personnel or other hospitalized patients to transplant recipients. It is therefore important to modify diagnostic considerations according to local epidemiologic considerations.

BACTERIAL AND FUNGAL INFECTIONS

Bacterial and fungal infections are a frequent and early problem after liver transplantation (12–14,25,26). Rates for bacterial infection of 40% to 70% (12–14,23,24) and for fungal infection of up to 63% (26–28) have been reported from multiple series. Bacteremia is a frequent problem and may be seen in association with a central venous catheter, intraabdominal infection, or no obvious source. Enteric gram-negative organisms account for more than 50% of episodes (6,13,26). Bacterial infections involving the abdomen or wound occur frequently in most series. Infectious complications of the transplanted liver also occur (29). The most important of these is a hepatic abscess associated with hepatic artery or portal vein thrombosis (13), which may be accompanied by refractory bacteremia. Urgent retransplantation in addition to antimicrobial therapy is necessary if the patient is to survive (12,25). Percutaneous drainage of the intrahepatic abscess may allow stabilization of the patient before retransplantation (15).

Another common infection seen after transplantation is ascending cholangitis, usually associated with biliary abnormalities. This diagnosis is typically made on clinical grounds in a patient with fever and biochemical evidence of bile duct disease. Empiric antibiotic treatment is chosen to include enteric gram-negative bacteria and enterococcal species.

Of increasing concern is the importance of antimicrobial resistance among the bacterial pathogens infecting pediatric liver transplant recipients. Outbreaks of colonization and disease due to vancomycin-resistant *Enterococcus faecium* and ceftazidime-resistant *Klebsiella pneumoniae* have been reported (30,31). Spread of these multiply resistant bacteria between patients has been documented, prompting consideration of the imposition of strict infection control procedures. Reports of multiply resistant strains of *Enterobacter cloacae* associated with derepression of a chromosomally located broad-spectrum β-lactamase enzyme have identified this very resistant organism as an important pathogen after liver transplantation in adults (32). Similarly, *E. cloacae* strains demonstrating this broad-spectrum resistance pattern have frequently been recovered from pediatric liver transplant recipients at the University of Pittsburgh. The increasing prevalence of these resistant organisms limits the therapeutic options available for treatment of bacterial infections after liver transplantation and in some instances may result in the unavailability of proven therapeutic agents to treat these complications.

Candida is the most common fungal pathogen after liver transplantation in children; it is usually associated with intraabdominal or catheter-related infections. The availability of newer azole antifungal agents (e.g., fluconazole) increases the number of therapeutic options for the treatment of *Candida* infections. However, acquired or inherent resistance to the azoles is an increasing concern, as are drug-drug interactions between the azoles and both cyclosporine and tacrolimus. Episodes of invasive aspergillosis occur infrequently in pediatric liver transplant recipients (33). Although uncommon, this pathogen is very important because infections with *Aspergillus* are frequently fatal. A suggested approach to the diagnosis and management of fungal infections after liver transplantation in children is summarized in Table 7.4.

TABLE 7.4. *Overview of diagnosis and management of fungal infections after liver transplantation in children*

Parameter	Candida noninvasive (mucositis, dermatitis, and cystitis)	Candida invasive	Aspergillus	Cryptococcus	Others (e.g., Histoplama, Mucor, Fusarium, Blastomycetes, Altenaria)
Frequency	Common (>5%)	Common (>5%)	Uncommon (1%–5%)	Rare (<1%)	Rare (<1%)
Diagnostic tests	Clinical examination Culture Gram stain	Culture Gram stain Histology	Culture Gram stain Histology Radiographic staging[a]	Culture Antigen test India Ink stain Histology CSF examination	Culture Histology Antigen testing (when appropriate)
Treatment Primary Secondary Adjunctive	Nystatin Clotrimazole Topical Amphotericin B[b] Fluconazole[c]	Amphotericin B[d] Fluconazole[c,e] 5-Flucytosine[f] Removal of central lines	Amphotericin B[d] Itraconazole[c,g,h] 5-Flucytosine[6] Surgical resection	Amphotericin B[d] Fluconazole[c,e] 5-Flucytosine[f]	Amphotericin B[d] Azole therapy (for susceptible organisms)[c] Surgical debridement
Duration of therapy	Dependent on rate of clearance	Dependent on the rate of clearance: minimum 14 d	Dependent on the rate of clearance: minimum 4 wk, usually 8–12 wk	Minimum 6–8 wk Many would continue with fluconazole indefinitely	Dependent on rate of clearance
Follow-up	Clinical examination Repeat urine analysis/cultures	Dependent on clinical scenario	Dependent on clinical scenario	Clinical examination Antigen testing Repeat culture of appropriate source (sputum, CSF, urine) Radiographs if relevant	Clinical examination Antigen testing Repeat culture of appropriate source (sputum, CSF, urine) Radiographs if relevant

CSF, cerebrospinal fluid.

[a]Radiographic staging includes computed tomography of head, chest, and abdomen.

[b]Topical amphotericin B for bladder wash for noninvasive candiduria—ultrasound of kidneys is recommended to determine that no invasive disease is present.

[c]Azole use must be accompanied by close follow-up of levels of cyclosporine or tacrolimus. In general tacrolimus dosing should be cut in half when using a standard dose of fluconazole.

[d]Amphotericin B dosed at 0.75–1.0 mg/kg/d; lipid formulations are used if renal failure is present.

[e]Fluconazole is alternative drug for invasive disease if the species is known to be sensitive to fluconazole and the patient is clinically stable. Fluconazole is dosed at 6–12 mg/kg/day based on severity of infection.

[f]5-Flucytosine should not be used alone but is synergistic when used in conjunction with Amphotericin B. Flucytosine is dosed at 100 to 150 mg/kg/d divided every 6 h.

[g]Itraconazole can be used long-term for patients who have been treated for invasive aspergillus but in general is not recommended as first-line therapy.

[h]Itraconazole absorption can be erratic. Accordingly, monitoring of itraconazole levels is recommended. Itraconazole is dosed at 3–5 mg/kg/d as a single dose. Dosing adjustment based on monitoring of levels is recommended. Adjustment of cyclosporine or tacrolimus dosing should be individualized.

VIRAL INFECTIONS

Cytomegalovirus

CMV continues to be the most common and one of the most important viral pathogens after liver transplantation in children. CMV infection can be asymptomatic or symptomatic and may be caused by primary infection (from the donor graft or blood products), reactivation of latent infection, or superinfection with a different CMV strain in a previously seropositive child. Before the use of prophylaxis, the incidence of symptomatic CMV infection was reported to be as high as 22% in adult (13) and 40% in pediatric (8) liver transplant recipients. Use of ganciclovir prophylaxis has resulted in a decreased rate and severity of CMV disease (34).

Primary CMV infection is typically acquired from the donor organ (or passenger donor leukocytes transfused) at the time of transplantation. Primary CMV infection is historically associated with the greatest risk of morbidity, though CMV-associated death has become a rare evident in the era of ganciclovir treatment and prophylaxis (34,35). Reactivation or reinfection occurs frequently in seropositive patients but is generally associated with asymptomatic or mild disease (6). CMV disease appears to be more likely in seropositive recipients of seropositive donor organs than in seropositive recipients of seronegative donors (35). The use of heavy amounts of immunosuppression, especially antilymphocyte preparations, may increase the severity of any episode of CMV, including those occurring in seropositive patients (8,13).

Symptomatic CMV disease typically manifests between 1 and 3 months after transplantation. A characteristic constellation of fever (which may be high-grade, long-lasting, and hectic) and hematologic abnormalities (including leukopenia, atypical lymphocytosis, and thrombocytopenia) occurs frequently in symptomatic patients and has been called the "CMV syndrome." The CMV syndrome occurs in 25% to 50% of patients with symptomatic CMV infection. Invasive CMV disease occurs when involvement of the gastrointesti-

nal tract, liver, and/or lungs is noted. CMV hepatitis appears to be more common among those receiving liver transplants, compared with other types of organ transplants. In contrast to patients with the acquired immunodeficiency syndrome (AIDS), CMV chorioretinitis is rare in organ transplant recipients.

Diagnosis of invasive CMV disease is confirmed by culture and histologic examination of the involved organ. Results of viral cultures of urine or bronchoalveolar lavage specimens alone can be difficult to interpret, because patients frequently shed CMV asymptomatically in these secretions. Review of histopathologic abnormalities to correlate positive cultures with clinical disease is critical. Many centers now use the CMV pp65 antigenemia assay as another tool for diagnosing CMV disease (36). This quantitative assay detects the presence of the CMV pp65 antigen in neutrophils. The finding of the pp65 antigen does not necessarily reflect infection of the neutrophil; rather, it is a marker of active CMV infection anywhere in the body and subsequent phagocytosis of this soluble antigen by the circulating neutrophils. Some centers have also begun to evaluate the usefulness of monitoring CMV viral load, as measured by a polymerase chain reaction (PCR) assay of the peripheral blood. Although quantitative CMV PCR offers great promise and can probably provide information similar to that obtained from the CMV pp65 antigenemia assay, it is also prone to all of the same difficulties in identifying patients who have CMV infections without disease. In addition, less published experience is available with this assay. Accordingly, endorsement of the use of this test can not be given at this time.

Antiviral agents with activity against CMV, such as ganciclovir and foscarnet, have improved the survival of transplant recipients with CMV disease. Fatal, disseminated CMV disease occurred in 19% of infected children (8) and 5% of infected adults undergoing liver transplantation in the preganciclovir era (37). The use of ganciclovir for prevention and treatment of CMV has led to dramatic improvements in the outcome of CMV infection in liver transplant recipients (18,34,35,38). The incidence and outcome of CMV disease among pediatric liver transplant recipients who initially received 2 weeks of intravenous ganciclovir as CMV prophylaxis and ganciclovir as treatment for symptomatic CMV infection has been reviewed (35). Seven (11%) of 59 children, including 4 (28%) of 14 high-risk patients (CMV-seronegative recipient, CMV-seropositive donor) developed symptomatic CMV disease. Invasive disease occurred in 5 (8%) of the 59 children, including 3 (21%) of the 14 high-risk patients. Breakthrough cases of CMV disease (including episodes of invasive disease) were mild and were not associated with mortality or chronic rejection. Recurrent episodes of CMV disease were seen in 2 of the 7 children diagnosed with CMV disease in this series. Similarly, recurrent CMV disease was previously reported in approximately 25% of patients treated with ganciclovir (38). Recurrences occur about 1 month after primary infection and may be associated with invasive disease.

Clinical response to ganciclovir is usually seen 5 to 7 days after initiation of therapy; the course is continued for a total of 14 to 21 days.

In addition to ganciclovir therapy, we also recommend a reduction in immunosuppression for approximately 1 week or until the patient shows a clinical response or has evidence of rejection. Some patients with CMV disease have also received high-titer anti-CMV antibody (CytoGam) as part of their treatment regimen (39). However, clear evidence supporting a benefit for the additional use of this agent is not available. Some centers have begun to use serial measurements of the CMV pp65 early antigen as a marker of clinical response to antiviral therapy. However, very few reports have been published describing the course of CMV pp65 antigenemia in patients treated for symptomatic CMV disease. Accordingly, use of this tool as a marker of response to antiviral therapy must be undertaken with caution. Careful monitoring of the patient's clinical status remains the gold standard for determining clinical response to treatment. Finally, the use of foscarnet should be considered for patients with apparent or proven ganciclovir-resistant CMV. A summary of our suggested approach to the diagnosis and management of CMV infection is provided in Table 7.5.

TABLE 7.5. *Overview of diagnosis and management of viral infections after liver transplantation in children–part 1*

Parameter	Herpes simplex virus	Cytomegalovirus	Epstein-Barr Virus (EBV)	Respiratory syncytial virus (RSV)	Influenza	Parainfluenza
Frequency	Uncommon (1%–5%)	Common (5%)	Common (5%)	Uncommon (1%–5%)	Uncommon (1%–5%)	Uncommon (1%–5%)
Diagnostic tests	Culture Tzank smear	Culture pp65 antigen Histology	EBV PCR Histology Serology	NP aspirate for antigen detection and culture	NP aspirate for antigen detection and culture	NP aspirate for culture
Treatment						
Primary	Acyclovir (5 mg/kg t.i.d.)	Ganciclovir (5 mg/kg b.i.d.)	Decrease IS	Supportive care	Supportive care	Supportive care
Secondary	Foscarnet[a]	Foscarnet	—	Aerosolized ribavirin	Amantadine/ rimantadine	
Adjunctive	Decrease IS	Decrease IS CMV-IVIG	Ganciclovir IVIG	RSV-IVIG Decrease IS	Decrease IS	Decrease IS
Duration of therapy	Site-dependent	Site-dependent	Individualized	Individualized	Individualized	Individualized
Follow-up	Chronic acyclovir prophylaxis	Monitor pp65 antigen	Monitor EBV PCR Repeat imaging studies if positive at outset	None	None	None

CMV, cytomegalovirus; IS, immune suppression; IVIG, intravenous immunoglobulin; NP, nasopharyngeal; PCR, polymerase chain reaction.

[a]Foscarnet used for CMV infection when ganciclovir resistance is suspected or proven. Experience from patients with human immunodeficiency virus infection suggests that a synergistic benefit will be obtained from the combined use of both of these agents when ganciclovir resistance is present.

Epstein-Barr Virus

EBV and PTLD are important problems after liver transplantation (7,40,41). PTLD is more common after primary EBV infection, placing seronegative recipients of organs from seropositive donors at higher risk. Several schemas describing the clinical syndromes of PTLD have been proposed (7,24,25), including three distinguishable presentations: mononucleosis (i.e., exudative tonsillitis, lymphadenopathy, and hepatosplenomegaly), a similar syndrome progressing to disseminated lymphoproliferation, and isolated extranodal lymphoma (7). Onset of the first and second syndromes is typically within the first year, whereas extranodal lymphoma tends to occur later.

It has become apparent that EBV is also responsible for additional clinical syndromes, including a febrile illness similar to the CMV syndrome, enteritis, and hepatitis. Like mononucleosis and the disseminated lymphoproliferative syndromes, these manifestations of EBV typically manifest in the first year after organ transplantation. Although these syndromes are considered hyperplastic and do not meet the classic criteria for EBV-associated PTLD, they are increasingly being recognized as an important cause of morbidity after transplantation and may represent "early" manifestations of EBV, before progression to the more ominous (and perhaps neoplastic) PTLD. Accordingly, it is important to diagnose these EBV-associated syndromes, not only to determine the cause of illness in febrile transplant recipients but also perhaps to intervene before the infection can progress to a neoplastic manifestation.

An EBV-associated syndrome should be considered in patients who present with a febrile illness associated with exudative tonsillitis, peripheral adenopathy, and abnormalities of the complete blood count (including leukopenia, atypical lymphocytosis, and thrombocytopenia). The diagnosis of EBV should also be considered in children with unexplained gastrointestinal symptoms, prolonged diarrhea (particularly if it is associated with gross or microscopic blood), or hepatitis. Diagnostic evaluation of children presenting with one or more of these symptoms should include evaluation for other pathogens (including CMV) and performance of computed tomographic scans of the chest and abdomen to look for occult lesions. Endoscopy should be considered in those children with gastrointestinal manifestations. Whenever possible, tissue samples should be obtained to confirm the diagnosis.

Histologic classification generally describes whether the lesions are polymorphic or monomorphic. Special stains are used to demonstrate the presence of EBV within a lesion. Gene rearrangement studies are used to determine the clonality of PTLD lesions (polyclonal, oligoclonal, or monoclonal). The histology of a lesion is used together with these tests to differentiate between EBV-associated hyperplastic disease and neoplastic disease. This differentiation may be of use in considering therapeutic options for EBV in organ transplant recipients.

The use of an elevated EBV viral load in the peripheral blood, as measured by PCR assay, has been proposed as an additional tool for the diagnosis of symptomatic EBV infection and PTLD (42–44). Each of the reporting groups was able to show a quantitative relation between the amount of EBV in peripheral blood and the presence of PTLD in organ transplant recipients. Although several of the reports of EBV viral load based results on semiquantitative assays (42,43), Rowe has developed a true quantitative assay that accurately and reproducibly determines the EBV viral load in peripheral blood (44). The availability of these assays appears to provide an excellent screening tool for evidence of active EBV disease in symptomatic transplant recipients.

The management of PTLD is controversial; however, initial reduction or withdrawal of immunosuppression is recommended (7,24,25). Although they are widely used, the role of antiviral agents has not been formally studied (45). Withdrawal of immunosuppression in combination with either acyclovir or ganciclovir resulted in resolution of PTLD in 31

(86%) of 36 pediatric liver transplant recipients diagnosed with PTLD under tacrolimus immunosuppression (46). Whether similar results could have been obtained without the use of acyclovir or ganciclovir remains an important question. The role of antiviral therapy, like those of monoclonal antibodies, interferon, and chemotherapy, awaits formal clinical trials to fully determine its impact on PTLD. A summary of our suggested approach and management of EBV/PTLD is provided in Table 7.5.

Other Herpesviruses

Other herpesviruses can also be hazardous after transplantation. Herpes simplex can reactivate early after surgery or after augmentation of immunosuppression. Prophylaxis with acyclovir has been beneficial in these situations. A summary of the suggested approach to the diagnosis and management of HSV is provided in Table 7.5. Varicella in nonimmune transplant recipients can lead to disseminated, fatal disease (47) and should be treated early and aggressively with intravenous acyclovir.

Adenovirus

Adenovirus has been reported to be the third most important virus affecting pediatric liver transplant recipients. It occurred in 10% of our series of 484 children undergoing liver transplantation under cyclosporine-based immunosuppression (48). Symptomatic disease (ranging from self-limited fever, gastroenteritis, or cystitis to devastating illness with necrotizing hepatitis or pneumonia) occurred in more than 60% of infected patients. Infection occurred within the first 3 months after transplantation. The frequency of invasive adenovirus infection after pediatric liver transplantation appears to have decreased markedly with the use of tacrolimus for immunosuppression (49).

It is very difficult to presumptively diagnose infection caused by adenovirus in pediatric liver transplant recipients, because fever, hepatitis, or pneumonia may be caused by a variety of other pathogens. The presence of high-grade fever and symptoms suggestive of adenovirus infection should prompt serial cultures for viruses (including adenovirus) from the buffy coat, stool, throat, and urine. Unexplained elevations in hepatocellular enzymes suggestive of hepatitis should warrant consideration of a liver biopsy. Histologic examination for the presence of adenoviral inclusions, as well as the use of immunohistochemical stains, helps to confirm this diagnosis in most cases.

There is no definitive treatment for adenoviral infection at this time. The most impor-

TABLE 7.6. *Overview of diagnosis and management of viral infections after liver transplantation—part 2*

Parameter	Adenovirus	Enterovirus	Hepatitis B (HBV)	Hepatitis C (HCV)
Frequency	Uncommon (1%–5%)	Uncommon (1%–5%)	Rare (<1%)	Rare (1%)
Diagnostic tests	Viral culture Histology	Viral culture	HBV serologies HBV PCR Histology	HCV serologies HCV viral load
Treatment				
Primary	Decrease IS	Decrease IS	Lamivudine	Interferon
Secondary	IV Ribavirin[a]	Supportive Care	Interferon	IV Ribavirin[b]
Adjunctive	IVIG[a]			
Duration of therapy	Individualized	Individualized	Indefinite	Indefinite
Follow-up	None	None	HBV PCR Serial liver function tests	HCV viral load Serial liver function tests

IS, immune suppression; IVIG, intravenous immunoglobulin; PCR, polymerase chain reaction.
[a]Use of this agent based on anecdotal experience.
[b]Recent data suggest that combined use of IV ribavirin with interferon may be of benefit for HCV infection.

tant component of therapy is supportive care along with a decrease in immunosuppression. The role of antiviral agents is unproven. A small number of case reports describe the use of ribavirin (50–52) or ganciclovir (53) in the treatment of single patients with adenoviral infection after solid-organ or bone marrow transplantation. *In vitro* evidence supports the theoretical role of ribavirin but not that of ganciclovir in the treatment of these infections. In addition to these published reports, an adult lung transplant recipient with disseminated adenovirus type 7 improved after treatment with cidofovir (HPMPC) and pooled, high-titered immunoglobulin against RSV (RespiGam) along with decreased immunosuppression (54). A single case report also raised the possible role of intravenous immunoglobulin as a treatment for adenovirus infection (55). However, no conclusive evidence of the efficacy of these antiviral agents or immunoglobulin therapy can be drawn from these reports. A summary of the suggested approach to diagnosis and management of adenovirus infection is provided in Table 7.6.

Common Community-Acquired Viruses

Although the course of illness has been poorly documented, most children who undergo liver transplantation experience the usual respiratory viruses and gastrointestinal illnesses without significant problems. However infections caused by influenza, parainfluenza, or RSV lead to more severe disease in young children, especially if infection occurs soon after transplantation and during periods of maximal immunosuppression (56, 57). A summary of suggested strategies for the diagnosis and management of these community-acquired viruses can be found in Table 7.5.

Other Viruses

Other viruses, including both pathogens that are nosocomially acquired (e.g., HBV, HCV) and those that are community acquired

(e.g., enterovirus), are relatively uncommon causes of infection after liver transplantation. Suggested approaches to the diagnosis and management of these viral pathogens are provided in Tables 7.5 and 7.6.

OPPORTUNISTIC INFECTIONS

P. carinii is a well-documented cause of pneumonia in immunocompromised patients, including liver transplant recipients. Prophylactic trimethoprim-sulfamethoxazole (TMP/SMX) is safe, inexpensive, and effective (58). The use of this strategy has eliminated PCP in these patients at our center. Alternative prophylactic regimens for the sulfa-allergic patient include aerosolized pentamidine (for patients older than 5 years of age) (59) and dapsone (60).

Tuberculosis (TB) is a particular concern in immunosuppressed hosts, including recipients of liver transplants. Although only limited published information is available describing TB in these patients, transplant recipients known to have a positive purified protein derivative (PPD) test and those who come from areas endemic for TB appear to be at increased risk for symptomatic reactivation after transplantation (61,62). Additional factors predisposing to the development of TB after transplantation include severe hepatic failure at the time of transplantation, aggressive antirejection therapy, and concurrent HIV infection (61,62). Experience among adult renal transplant recipients suggests that although the risk appears greatest in patients who received inadequate or no prior TB therapy (63,64), the disease also can occur in patients who received appropriate anti-TB therapy before transplantation (63–65). Although TB has only rarely been encountered among our pediatric liver transplant recipients, our current practice is to carefully screen for TB by history and PPD testing, along with review of a chest radiograph for lesions consistent with healed TB. Patients with a positive TB history and those with a positive PPD test result receive isoniazid for 6 to 12 months after transplantation, although some experts recommend indefinite continuation while these patients remain on immunosuppression. Attempts at a more definitive diagnosis are indicated for patients from endemic areas who have a negative PPD result but a suspicious chest radiograph. Careful evaluation for evidence of side effects, particularly hepatotoxicity, is maintained, and isoniazid is discontinued when unacceptable toxicity is identified.

Additional potential opportunistic infections include cryptococcosis, coccidioidomycosis, and histoplasmosis, although these pathogens have not been frequently reported among pediatric liver transplant recipients. Prior infection with these pathogens is associated with exposure to geographic areas where they are endemic. Because patients often travel to transplantation centers distant from their homes, it is imperative that transplantation physicians be aware of the local environmental risks for each patient. Experience with coccidioidomycosis in transplant recipients suggests that a minimum of 4 months of antifungal therapy (e.g., fluconazole) should be given to transplant recipients with this history (66). Similarities between coccidioidomycosis and other fungal pathogens suggest that similar strategies may be necessary for patients with a positive history of prior fungal infection with pathogens known to recur after resolution of primary infection.

MANAGEMENT

Pretransplantation Evaluation

A pretransplantation evaluation is helpful in the management of infectious complications in liver transplant recipients (Table 7.7). A complete history and physical examination should be performed, with particular attention to previous infections, immunizations, and drug allergies. An intermediate-strength tuberculin skin test should be performed on all patients.

We recommend obtaining serology results for CMV, EBV, varicella, HSV, hepatitis A virus, HBV, HCV, and HIV on all candidates. Serologic tests on the donor should include

TABLE 7.7. *Pretransplantation evaluation for candidates for pediatric liver transplantation*

Complete history and physical examination
  Emphasis on prior history of infections
  Immunization status
  Drug allergies
Evaluation for tuberculosis
  History of prior infection or potential contact
  Placement of purified protein derivative
Serologic screening
  Cytomegalovirus
  Epstein-Barr virus
  Varicella
  Herpes simplex virus
  Hepatitis A, B, and C
  Human immunodeficiency virus

HIV, HBV, HCV, CMV, and EBV. Donors positive for HIV or HBV should be excluded. The use of organs from HCV-positive donors is controversial. Knowledge of donor and recipient status for these viruses allows one to anticipate infection, identifying patients who might benefit from prophylactic regimens and guiding the diagnostic evaluation of fever.

Prophylactic Regimens

Prophylactic regimens vary among transplantation centers. These strategies have been divided into perioperative and long-term prophylaxis and often evolve to reflect the infectious complications seen at individual institutions.

Perioperative prophylaxis is used to prevent intraoperative sepsis and wound infection. It is based on individual patient characteristics and expected normal flora. If sepsis is suspected in the donor, antibiotics are chosen to cover those organisms identified from the donor and treatment is usually extended to a therapeutic course of 10 to 14 days.

Considerations regarding long-term prophylaxis against infections occurring beyond the perioperative period include the risk and severity of infection and the toxicity, cost, and efficacy of the prophylactic strategy. Nystatin is recommended for all pediatric transplant recipients in an effort to prevent oropharyngeal candidiasis. TMP/SMX is used to prevent PCP. Although some centers recommend using TMP/SMX for only the first 6 months after liver transplantation, anecdotal experience with patients presenting with PCP long after transplantation, as well as the relative safety of this agent, have led us to recommend its use indefinitely after liver transplantation in children.

The frequency and severity of CMV infections in transplant recipients prompts consideration of prophylactic strategies. Although acyclovir was initially used (67), many centers now use ganciclovir, which has greater *in vitro* activity against CMV. Winston et al. (68) demonstrated a decline in CMV disease to 1% among adult liver transplant recipients who received intravenous ganciclovir for the first 100 days after transplantation. More recently, the efficacy of 14 weeks of oral ganciclovir in adult liver transplant recipients was evaluated against that of a placebo (69). The investigators were able to demonstrate a decline in CMV disease from 19% to 5% with oral ganciclovir therapy. Although these results are encouraging, their applicability to pediatric liver transplant recipients may be confounded by the poor absorption of oral ganciclovir in children. Further, it is possible that similar rates of prevention might be obtained with the use of shorter courses of either intravenous or oral ganciclovir. Several centers have also evaluated intravenous immunoglobulin (both high-titer anti-CMV and commercially available products) in the prevention of CMV disease among liver transplant recipients (67,70,71). This strategy has tended to be less effective in preventing CMV disease among high-risk patients with donor-recipient mismatching. Finally, the excellent outcome of children receiving only 2 weeks of intravenous ganciclovir as CMV prophylaxis at our center emphasizes the need for clinical trials to determine the most cost-effective and safest strategies to prevent CMV disease and to identify those children who are likely to benefit from them.

An alternative approach has used the presence of a rise in CMV pp65 antigenemia as a marker for an increased risk of subsequent development of symptoms in patients at risk for CMV disease (36). In these preemptive strategies, intravenous ganciclovir is started when the results of the CMV pp65 antigenemia assay exceed predetermined cutoff values. Despite fairly broad acceptance of this approach, there is little published evidence to confirm its effectiveness or define acceptable cutoff points for treatment in CMV-seronegative and CMV-seropositive transplant recipients. Similarly, the possible role of quantitative CMV PCR as a measure of the CMV viral load may offer an alternative approach to preemptive therapy. As noted earlier, the limited amount of published data describing the use of this test for this purpose prevents any comparison of these two approaches at this time. Additional studies are necessary to delineate the effectiveness of these therapies and to determine the relative superiority of prophylactic versus preemptive strategies.

Finally, the increasing attention paid to the importance of EBV disease and PTLD in pediatric liver transplant recipients has prompted efforts to prevent these problems. The prolonged use of oral acyclovir as chemoprophylaxis against EBV failed to prevent PTLD in pediatric liver transplant recipients (34). As with preemptive strategies against CMV, several sets of investigators have attempted to use rising EBV viral loads, as measured by EBV PCR assays of peripheral blood lymphocytes, to guide preemptive efforts against EBV. However, the complicated nature of EBV infection of B cells limits the likelihood that a direct antiviral therapeutic approach using a nucleoside analog will be effective. However, these investigators have effectively used additional strategies, including decreasing immunosuppression (72) and the use of intravenous immunoglobulin (73), although neither of these approaches has been subject to controlled trials. A third approach of immunoprophylaxis using intravenous immunoglobulin from the time of transplantation is supported by the severe combined immunodeficiency (SCID) mouse model of EBV-associated lymphoma (74) and is now under study among pediatric liver transplant recipients.

SUMMARY

Infections remain an important problem after liver transplantation. Knowledge of the type, timing, and predisposing risk factors for these infectious complications allows for their timely and appropriate diagnosis and management.

REFERENCES

1. Dummer JS, Hardy A, Poorsattar A, et al. Early infections in kidney, heart and liver transplant recipients on cyclosporine. *Transplantation* 1983;36:259–267.
2. Ho M, Dummer JS. Risk factors and approaches to infection in transplant recipients. In: Mandell GL, Douglas RG Jr, Bennett JE, eds. *Principles and practice of infectious diseases,* 3rd ed. New York: Churchill Livingstone, 1990.
3. Cuervas-Mons V, Rimola A, Van Thiel DH, et al. Does previous abdominal surgery alter the outcome of pediatric patients subjected to orthotopic liver transplantation. *Gastroenterology* 1986;90:853–857.
4. Ukah FO, Merhave H, Kramer D. Early outcome of liver transplantation in patients with a history of spontaneous bacterial peritonitis. *Transplant Proc* 1993;25: 1113–1115.
5. Wittner M. Cryptococcosis. In: Feigin RD, Cherry JD, eds. *Textbook of pediatric infectious diseases,* 2nd ed. Philadelphia: Saunders, 1987.
6. Breinig MK, Zitelli B, Starzl TE, et al. Epstein-Barr virus, cytomegalovirus, and other viral infections in children after liver transplantation. *J Infect Dis* 1987; 156:273–279.
7. Ho M, Jaffe R, Miller G, et al. The frequency of Epstein-Barr virus infection and associated lymphoproliferative syndrome after transplantation and its manifestations in children. *Transplantation* 1988;45:719–727.
8. Bowman JS, Green M, Scantlebury VP, et al. OKT3 and viral disease in pediatric liver transplant recipients. *Clin Transplant* 1991;5:294–300.
9. Cen H, Breinig MC, Atchinson RW, et al. Epstein-Barr virus transmission via the donor-organ in solid-organ transplantation: polymerase chain reaction and restriction fragment length polymorphism analogue of IR2, IR3, IR4. *J Virol* 1991;65:976–980.
10. Dummer JS, Siegfried E, Breinig MK, et al. Infection with human immunodeficiency virus in the Pittsburgh transplant population. *Transplantation* 1989;47:134–139.
11. Wong SY, Allen DM. Transmission of histoplasmosis via cadaveric renal transplantation: case report and review of the literature. *Clin Infect Dis* 1992;14:232–234.
12. Schroter GPJ, Hoelscher M, Putnam CW, et al. Infections complicating orthotopic liver transplantation. *Arch Surg* 1976;111:1337–1347.
13. Kusne S, Dummer JS, Singh N, et al. Infection after liver transplantation: an analysis of 101 consecutive cases. *Medicine (Baltimore)* 1988;67:132–143.
14. George DL, Arnow PM, Fox AS, et al. Bacterial infection as a complication of liver transplantation: epidemiology and risk factors. *Rev Infect Dis* 1991;13:387–396.
15. Rollins NK, Andrews WS, Currino G, et al. Infected bile lakes following pediatric liver transplantation: nonsurgical management. *Radiology* 1988;166:169–171.
16. Hofflin JM, Potasman I, Baldwin JC, et al. Infectious complication in heart transplant recipients receiving cyclosporine and corticosteroids. Ann Intern Med. 1987; 106:209–216.
17. Najarian JS, Fryd DS, Strand M, et al. A single institution, randomized, prospective trial of cyclosporine versus azathioprine-antilymphocyte globulin for immunosuppression in renal allograft recipients. *Ann Surg* 1985;201:142–157.
18. Green M, Tzakis A, Reyes J, et al. Infectious complications of pediatric liver transplantation under FK 506. *Transplant Proc* 1991;23:3038–3039.
19. Todo S, Fung JJ, Starzl TE, et al. Liver, kidney, and thoracic organ transplantation under FK 506. *Ann Surg* 1990;212:295–307.
20. Alessiani M, Kusne S, Martin FM, et al. Infections with FK 506 immunosuppression: preliminary results with primary therapy. *Transplant Proc* 1990;22:44–46.
21. Cox KL, Lawrence-Miyasaki LS, Garcia-Kennedy R, et al. An increased incidence of Epstein-Barr virus infection and lymphoproliferative disorder in young children on FK506 after pediatric liver transplantation. *Transplantation* 1995;59:524–529.
22. Cacciarelli TV, Jaffe R, Green M, et al. A decreased incidence of post-transplant lymphoproliferative disorder (PTLD) in pediatric liver transplant recipients under primary tacrolimus (FK506) therapy [Abstract 289]. *Program and Abstracts of the 16th Annual Scientific Committee of the American Society for Transplant Physicians.* 1997:157.
23. Green M, Michaels M. Infectious complications after solid-organ transplantation. *Adv Pediatr Infect Dis* 1992;7:181–204.
24. Malatack JJ, Gartner JC, Urbach AH, et al. Orthotopic liver transplantation, Epstein-Barr virus, cyclosporine and lymphoproliferative syndrome: a growing concern. *J Pediatr* 1991;118:667–675.
25. Zitelli BJ, Gartner JC, Malatach JJ, et al. Pediatric liver transplantation: patient evaluation and selection, infectious complications, and life-style after transplantation. *Transplant Proc* 1987;19:3309–3316.
26. Colonna JO, Winston DJ, Brill JE, et al. Infectious complications in liver transplantation. *Arch Surg* 1988;123: 360–364.
27. Hiatt JR, Ament ME, Berquist ME, et al. Pediatric liver transplantation at UCLA. *Transplant Proc* 1987;19: 3282–3288.
28. Andrews W, Fyock B, Gray S, et al. Pediatric liver transplantation: the Dallas experience. *Transplant Proc* 1987;19:3267–3276.
29. Cienfugos JA, Dominguez RM, Tamelchoff PJ, et al. Surgical complications in the postoperative period of liver transplantation in children. *Transplant Proc* 1984 16:1230–1235.
30. Green M. Vancomycin resistant enterococci: impact and management in pediatrics. *Adv Pediatr Infect Dis* 1998;13:257–277.
31. Green M, Barbadora K. Recovery of ceftazidime-resistant *Klebsiella pneumoniae* from pediatric liver transplant recipients. *Pediatr Transplant* 1998;2:224–230.
32. Chow JW, Fine MJ, Shlaes DM, et al. *Enterobacter* bacteremia: clinical features and emergence of antibiotic

resistance during therapy. *Ann Intern Med* 1991;115: 585–590.

33. Green M, Wald ER, Tzakis A, et al. Aspergillosis of the central nervous system in a pediatric liver transplant recipient and review of the literature. *Rev Infect Dis* 1991;13:653–657.

34. Green M, Kaufmann M, Wilson J, et al. Comparison of intravenous ganciclovir followed by oral acyclovir with intravenous ganciclovir alone for prevention of cytomegalovirus and Epstein-Barr virus disease after liver transplantation in children. *Clin Infect Dis* 1997;25: 1344–1349.

35. Green M, Weinfeld A, Mazariegos G, et al. Short-course intravenous ganciclovir prophylaxis against cytomegalovirus disease following liver transplantation in children. *Pediatr Transplant* 1998;2[Suppl 1]:75.

36. The TH, van der Ploeg M, van der Berg A, et al. Direct detection of cytomegalovirus in peripheral blood leukocytes: a review of the antigenemia assay and polymerase chain reaction. *Transplantation* 1992;54:193–198.

37. Singh N, Dummer S, Kusne S, et al. Infections with cytomegalovirus and other herpesviruses in 121 liver transplant recipients: transmission by donated organ and the effect of OKT3 antibodies. *J Infect Dis* 1988; 155:202–206.

38. Stratta RJ, Shaefer MS, Markin RS, et al. Clinical patterns of cytomegalovirus disease after liver transplantation. *Arch Surg* 1989;124:1443–1450.

39. George MJ, Snydman DR, Werner BG, et al. Use of ganciclovir plus cytomegalovirus immune globulin to treat CMV pneumonia in orthotopic liver transplant recipients. *Transplant Proc* 1993;25[Suppl 4]:22–24.

40. Starzl TE, Porter KA, Iwatsuki S, et al. Reversibility of lymphomas and lymphoproliferative lesions developing under cyclosporin-steroid therapy. *Lancet* 1984;1: 583–587.

41. Touraine JL, Bosi E, El Yafi MS, et al. The infectious lymphoproliferative syndrome in transplant recipients under immunosuppressive treatment. *Transplant Proc* 1985;17:96–98.

42. Riddler SA, Breinig MC, McKnight JLC. Increased levels of circulating Epstein-Barr virus-infected lymphocytes and decreased EBV nuclear antigen antibody responses are associated with the development of posttransplant lymphoproliferative disease in solid-organ transplant recipients. *Blood* 1994;84:972–984.

43. Kenagy DN, Schlessinger Y, Weck K, et al. Epstein-Barr virus DNA in peripheral blood leukocytes of patients with post-transplant lymphoproliferative disease. *Transplantation* 1995;60:547–554.

44. Rowe DT, Qu L, Reyes J, et al. Use of quantitative competitive PCR to measure Epstein-Barr virus genome load in peripheral blood of pediatric transplant recipients with lymphoproliferative disorders. *J Clin Microbiol* 1997;35:1612–1615.

45. Hanto D, Frizzer G, Gajl-Peczalska K, et al. Epstein-Barr virus, immunodeficiency, and B cell lymphoproliferation. *Transplantation* 1985;39:461–470.

46. Cacciarelli TV, Green M, Jaffe R, et al. Management of posttransplant lymphoproliferative disease in pediatric liver transplant recipients receiving primary tacrolimus (FK506) therapy. *Transplantation* 1998;66:1047–1052.

47. McGregor RS, Zitelli BJ, Urbach AH, et al. Varicella in pediatric orthotopic liver transplant recipients. *Pediatrics* 1989;83:256–261.

48. Michaels M, Green M, Wald ER, et al. Adenovirus infection in pediatric orthotopic liver transplant recipients. *J Infect Dis* 1992;165:170–174.

49. Green M, Tzakis A, Reyes J, et al. Infectious complications of pediatric liver transplantation under FK506. *Transplant Proc* 1991;23:3038–3039.

50. Kapelushnik J, Or R, Delukina A, et al. Intravenous ribavirin therapy for adenovirus gastroenteritis after bone marrow transplantation. *J Pediatr Gastroenterol Nutr* 1995;21:110–112.

51. Murphy GF, Wood DP, McRoberts JW, et al. Adenovirus-associated hemorrhagic cystitis treated with intravenous ribavirin. *J Urol* 1993;149:565–566.

52. Liles WC, Cushing H, Holt S, et al. Severe adenovirus nephritis following bone marrow transplantation: successful treatment with intravenous ribavirin. *Bone Marrow Transplant* 1993;14:663–664.

53. Wreghitt TG, Gray JJ, Ward KN, et al. Disseminated adenovirus infection after liver transplantation and its possible treatment with ganciclovir. *J Infect* 1989;19: 88–89.

54. Green M, Michaels M. Adenovirus, parvovirus B19 and papillomavirus. In: Bowden RA, Ljungman P, Paya C, eds. *Transplant infections.* Philadelphia: Lippincott-Raven, 1998:287–294.

55. Dagan R, Schwartz RH, Insel RA, et al. Severe diffuse adenovirus 7a pneumonia in a child with combined immunodeficiency: possible therapeutic effect of human immune serum containing specific neutralizing antibodies. *Pediatr Infect Dis J* 1984;3:246–251.

56. Pohl C, Green M, Wald ER. RSV infection after pediatric liver transplantation. *J Infect Dis* 1992;166–169.

57. Apalsch AM, Green M. Influenza and parainfluenza virus infections in pediatric organ transplant recipients. *Clin Infect Dis* 1995;20:394–399.

58. Hughes WT, Rivera GK, Schell MJ, et al. Successful intermittent chemoprophylaxis for *Pneumocystis carinii* pneumonitis. *N Engl J Med* 1987;316:1627–1632.

59. Leoung GS, Feigal DW, Montgomery B, et al. Aerosolized pentamidine for prophylaxis against *Pneumocystis carinii* pneumonia. *N Engl J Med* 1990;323: 769–775.

60. Hughes WT, Kennedy W, Dugdale M, et al. Prevention of *Pneumocystis carinii* pneumonitis in AIDS patients with weekly dapsone. *Lancet* 1990;2:1066.

61. Strernecik M, Ferrell S, Asher N, et al. Mycobacterial infection after liver transplantation: a report of three cases and review of the literature. *Clin Transplant* 1992; 6:55–61.

62. Higgins R, Kusne S, Reyes J, et al. *Mycobacterium tuberculosis* after liver transplantation: management and guide lines for prevention. *Clin Transplant* 1992;6: 81–90.

63. Lichenstein IH, MacGregor RR. Mycobacterial infections in renal transplant recipients: report of five cases and review of the literature. *Rev Infect Dis* 1983;5: 216–226.

64. Malhorta KK, Dash SC, Dhawan IK, et al. Tuberculosis and renal transplantation: observations from an endemic area. *Postgrad Med J* 1986;62:359–362.

65. Quinibi W, Al-Sibai MB, Taher S, et al. Mycobacterial infection after renal transplantation: report of 14 cases and review of the literature. *Q J Med* 1990;282:1039–1060.

66. Hall KA, Copeland JG, Zukoski CF, et al. Markers of coccidioidomycosis prior to cardiac or renal transplan-

tation and risk of recurrent infection. *Transplantation* 1993;55:1422–1425.

67. Balfour HH, Chace BA, Stapleton JT, et al. A randomized, placebo controlled trial of oral acyclovir for the prevention of cytomegalovirus disease in recipients of renal allografts. *N Engl J Med* 1989;320:1381–1387.

68. Winston DJ, Wirin D, Shaked A, et al. Randomized comparison of ganciclovir and high-dose acyclovir for long-term cytomegalovirus prophylaxis in liver transplant recipients. *Lancet* 1995;246:69–74.

69. Gane E, Saliba F, Valdecasas GJ, et al. Randomized trial of efficacy and safety of oral ganciclovir in prevention of cytomegalovirus disease in liver-transplant recipients. *Lancet* 1997;350:1729–1733.

70. Saliba F, Arulnaden JL, Gugenheim J, et al. CMV hyperimmune globulin prophylaxis after liver transplantation: a prospective randomized controlled study. *Transplant Proc* 1989;21:2260–2262.

71. Fehir KM, Decker T, Samo T, et al. Immune globulin (GAMMAGARD) prophylaxis of CMV infections in patients undergoing organ transplantation and allogeneic bone marrow transplantation. *Transplant Proc* 1989;21:3107–3109.

72. McDiarmid SV, Jordan S, Lee GS, et al. Prevention and pre-emptive therapy of post-transplant lymphoproliferative disease in pediatric liver recipients. *Transplantation* 1998;66:1604–1611.

73. Green M, Reye J, Rowe D. New strategies in the prevention and management of Epstein-Barr virus infection and posttransplant lymphoproliferative disease following solid organ transplantation. *Curr Opin Organ Transplant* 1998; 3:143–147.

74. Abedi MR, Linde A, Christensson B, et al. Preventive effect of IgG from EBV-seropositive donors on the development of posttransplant lymphoproliferative disease in SCID mice. *Int J Cancer* 1997;71:624–629.

8

Heart Transplant Recipients

Sheldon L. Kaplan

Department of Pediatrics, Baylor College of Medicine, Houston, Texas 77030

Since the introduction of cyclosporine, heart transplantation has become increasingly available for children with end-stage cardiac disease. Infection remains an important cause of morbidity and some mortality after heart transplantation. The Pediatric Heart Transplant Study Group prospectively collected data from 22 pediatric centers in the United States from January 1993 to December 1994 (1). Over this 2-year period, 332 children younger than 18 years old (mean age, 5.5 years) underwent heart transplantation. One or more infections (276 total) occurred in 41% of the patients (mean follow-up time, 11.8 months); 22% had one infection, 8% had two infections, and 11% had three or more infections during the study period (Table 8.1). In a similar multicenter study for adults after heart transplantation between January 1990 and June 1991, 31% of 814 patients developed infection; 22% had one infection, and 9% had more than two infections (2). In both pediatric and adult patients, bacterial infections were the most common type after transplantation.

Immunosuppressive therapy after pediatric heart transplantation usually consists of some combination of cyclosporine, azathioprine, and corticosteroids. Cyclosporine predominantly blocks the effect of interleukin-2 on T lymphocytes, resulting in a diminished T-cell response to mitogen stimulation (3). The infections seen in heart transplantation patients outside the postoperative period generally are a result of this block in T-cell function. Because the types of infection seen in these patients vary with the time elapsed since transplantation, this chapter is organized in such a manner.

TABLE 8.1. *Types of infections encountered in 332 children after heart transplantation in a multiinstitutional study*[a]

Type	Number
Bacterial	164
Cytomegalovirus	51
Other viruses (non-Cytomegalovirus)	35
Fungal	19
Protozoal	7

[a]276 infections in 136 patients.
From Schowengerdt KO, Naftel DC, Seib PM, et al. Infection after pediatric heart transplantation: Results of a multiinstitutional study. *J Heart Lung Transplant* 1997;16:1207–1216, with permission.

PRETRANSPLANTATION EVALUATION

Several infectious agents can "reactivate" during transplantation or be transmitted to the patient via the transplanted organ. It is helpful to know the antibody status of the recipient against these agents, so as to anticipate or help diagnose infections occurring after the surgery. Table 8.2 outlines a reasonable pretransplantation evaluation for children. Immunization status is documented, and com-

TABLE 8.2. *Evaluation of children before heart transplantation*

Serology
  Cytomegalovirus
  Varicella
  Epstein-Barr virus
  Toxoplasma gondii
  Human immunodeficiency virus
  Hepatitis A, B, and C
Cultures
  Stool or tracheal aspirates[a]
Skin tests
  Purified protein derivative
  Appropriate control
Freeze extra aliquot of serum
Review immunization status

[a]See text for explanation.

pletion of vaccine administration is performed whenever possible (e.g., hepatitis B vaccine). The conjugate pneumococcal vaccine followed by the 23-valent pneumococcal vaccine is administered to children as outlined by the American Academy of Pediatrics (4). Evidence of an active infection is a contraindication for transplantation. Chemoprophylaxis should be strongly considered for the child with a positive purified protein derivative (PPD) skin test. Dental status is also assessed.

In addition to the routine pretransplantation evaluation outlined in Table 8.2, each patient must be carefully screened for infections particular to the individual circumstances. For example, children from Latin American countries may harbor *Salmonella* or intestinal parasites asymptomatically, and these organisms can cause serious infections after transplantation. Preoperative stool cultures and appropriate examination of the stool for parasites may alert the clinician to the presence of these potential pathogens. If the patient is receiving ventilator support before transplantation, review of tracheal aspirate cultures may be helpful in deciding on initial empiric therapy for suspected sepsis or pneumonia postoperatively.

PROPHYLACTIC ANTIBIOTICS

Administration of prophylactic antibiotics is common in heart transplantation surgery,

and a variety of antibiotics have been employed by various teams. Selection of the antibiotic used for prophylaxis should be individualized for each institution based in part on the organisms associated with postoperative wound infections at that center. A cephalosporin such as cefazolin is usually a reasonable selection for prophylaxis. There is no definite recommendation for the duration of prophylactic antibiotics in these patients, but some centers continue these agents for 2 to 5 days (or longer) postoperatively, or until all lines and chest tubes have been removed.

IMMEDIATE POSTOPERATIVE INFECTIONS

Common Infections

During the month following heart transplantation, the types of infections encountered are the same as those complicating any major thoracic surgery. Pneumonia and bacteremia are the most common postoperative infections. In the multiinstitutional study, 60 episodes of bacteremia occurred among the 136 patients encountering infections (1). Lung abscesses and mediastinitis are seen less frequently. Familiarity with the organisms and antimicrobial susceptibility of isolates recovered from other children in the recovery area or intensive care unit helps direct the initial empiric antibiotic selection.

The bacteremias that develop postoperatively are related predominantly to the indwelling lines required for monitoring and infusion of medications. *Staphylococcus aureus,* coagulase-negative staphylococci, and gram-negative enterics are most commonly isolated from these line-related infections. Other foci of infection (e.g., pneumonia, mediastinitis) also may result in bacteremia (5). Empiric antibiotic therapy for suspected bacteremia in patients who are without focal evidence of infection but have central access lines in place usually consists of a combination such as vancomycin plus an aminoglycoside. Vancomycin should be discontinued as soon as possible if an organism requiring its administration is not isolated (6). Fungemia, usually with *Candida albicans* or other *Candida* species, also may cause line-related infections. Lines must be removed as soon as practical so that catheter-associated infections can be prevented.

As with pediatric oncology patients, bacterial line infection may be eradicated successfully without removing the line, but candidemia is optimally managed by removing the line immediately (7,8). A similar frequency of bacteremia and distribution of organisms is seen in children as in adults after heart transplantation (1,2).

Pneumonia is particularly common in heart transplantation patients because of the operative site, the requirements for intubation and mechanical ventilation, and other factors routinely encountered in critically ill children. In an early study from Pittsburgh, 3 (14%) of 22 children developed definite bacterial pneumonia, all during the first postoperative week (9). In the multiinstitutional study referred to earlier, 56 bacterial lung infections were identified (1). Nosocomial pneumonia caused by gram-negative bacilli such as *Pseudomonas* and *Enterobacter* are especially common in this setting. Chest roentgenograms performed on a daily basis until the patient is out of intensive care may identify a pneumonitis earlier than clinically suspected. As with other intubated patients, Gram stain and culture of a tracheal aspirate helps to guide therapy for a lobar pneumonia. A broad-spectrum combination of antibiotics, such as an extended-spectrum penicillin plus an aminoglycoside, is usually initiated until the pathogen or pathogens are identified. Vancomycin should also be administered if methicillin-resistant *S. aureus* is part of the resident flora in the intensive care unit. If an interstitial pneumonitis is detected, a more aggressive approach to determining a cause is warranted. Bronchoscopy with bronchoalveolar lavage should be strongly considered in these instances. As flexible bronchoscopy (in children with cancer and pulmonary infiltrates) is a safe procedure and, as expected, is more useful for establishing a fungal or viral (rather than a bacterial) cause of pneumonia, because most

of the patients have received broad-spectrum antibiotics before the procedure (10). Lavage fluid is pooled and processed for bacteria, viruses, fungi, and protozoans. Noninfectious causes of pulmonary infiltrates in these children include pulmonary edema, atelectasis, hemorrhage, and adult respiratory distress syndrome. Computed tomography (CT) of the chest is useful for detecting basilar and retrocardiac pneumonia that may not be readily visualized by conventional chest roentgenograms.

Urinary tract infections (UTIs) are also common in children during the month after heart transplantation. Urinary catheterization and use of immunosuppressive agents contribute to the risks of developing UTIs. Typically, gram-negative enteric organisms or enterococci are isolated. Removal of the catheter as soon as possible postoperatively minimizes the potential for development of a UTI. About 10% of adult heart transplantation patients have developed UTIs. Three children (14%) in the Pittsburgh study developed UTIs (*Klebsiella pneumoniae,* 2; enterococcus, 1) during the 2 to 3 weeks after transplantation (9). *Candida* infections of the urinary tract are promoted by the broad-spectrum antibiotics used to treat the other infectious complications of transplantation. Local irrigation of the bladder with amphotericin B (50 mg per liter) in sterile water, a short course of intravenous amphotericin B administration (10 days or less), and fluconazole with careful dosing are three options for treating candidal cystitis (11–13).

Risk factors for the early infections in the pediatric multiinstitutional study were younger recipient age (particularly younger than 6 months), the need for mechanical ventilation at the time of transplantation, cytomegalovirus (CMV)-seropositive donor with CMV-seronegative recipient, and longer donor ischemic time (1).

Sternal Wounds and Mediastinitis

Sternal wound infections and mediastinitis occur in fewer than 5% of adult patients receiving modern immunosuppressive therapy for heart transplantation (2,14,15). Most of these infections manifest during the first postoperative month, usually within the first 2 weeks. Surgical wound infections developed in eight cases in the pediatric multiinstitutional study; it was not noted whether these were at the median sternotomy site (1). Postoperative bleeding requiring reexploration is a risk factor for development of mediastinitis. Fever, incisional pain, and an unstable sternum suggest mediastinitis; however, patients may have no specific evidence of infection including fever. The white blood cell count may be elevated. A pericardial effusion is frequently detected with the development of a mediastinitis, but it is not specific for this infection. Pericardiocentesis may yield purulent material. A fluid collection or abscess within the mediastinum may be demonstrated by CT scan of the chest. Most cases of mediastinitis are caused by *S. aureus,* coagulase-negative staphylococci, or gram-negative bacteria. Median sternotomy wound infections after repair of congenital heart lesions occur in fewer than 1% of children in large centers. Mediastinitis in association with pneumonia and bacteremia developed in 3 of the 22 children in the Pittsburgh series (9). These cases occurred within the first 2 weeks postoperatively, and all three were caused by gram-negative bacilli. Two of the three patients died.

A superficial median sternotomy wound infection not associated with an unstable sternum can be treated with local drainage of the infected subcutaneous tissue and appropriate antibiotics (16). A more aggressive approach is required for more serious infections associated with an unstable sternum, mediastinitis, or osteomyelitis of the sternum (15–17). Adequate drainage and debridement of the area are crucial. Mediastinal drains are usually left in place for several days. Some authorities recommend irrigating the drains with povidone-iodine, but the duration of irrigation is uncertain. Reoperation after the initial drainage procedure may be necessary. Pending culture results, antibiotic therapy is directed against *S. aureus* and gram-negative bacilli, usually with a combination of

antibiotics such as nafcillin or vancomycin plus an aminoglycoside. A 4- to 6-week course of antibiotics typically is recommended. Careful attention to surgical technique to minimize postoperative bleeding and early withdrawal of chest and mediastinal tubes placed intraoperatively decrease the incidence of these potentially fatal infections.

Other Infections Encountered during the First Postoperative Month

Herpes Simplex

Herpes simplex virus (HSV) infections of the oral mucosa and other superficial surfaces are relatively common after heart transplantation. Oral herpes simplex was observed in 21% (11/53) of children undergoing transplantation at Stanford (18). Visceral involvement is unusual, although it may develop (19). HSV infections typically occur at about 13 days (range 0 to 4 months) after transplantation and represent a reactivation process, not newly acquired infections. Pollard et al. (20) observed HSV infection in 95% of HSV-seropositive cardiac transplantation patients but in none of their seronegative patients. *In vitro* assays indicated that a decrease in lymphocyte transformation in response to viral antigen was associated with an increased rate of infection that corresponded to the first 12 weeks after transplantation.

Antiviral therapy for HSV infection is warranted in these immunocompromised patients. The most common antiviral agent for HSV is acyclovir, which can be administered orally or intravenously.

Some authorities recommend providing acyclovir prophylactically for heart transplantation patients who are seropositive for HSV (21). Acyclovir is given intravenously during the perioperative period and then orally for 30 days. Others believe that, because labial or oral herpes simplex is so easily treated, a prophylactic approach is not warranted.

Legionella pneumophila *Infection*

Legionella pneumophila should be considered in the differential diagnosis for fever, respiratory symptoms, and pulmonary infiltrates after heart transplantation (22). *Legionella* pneumonia can develop during the first postoperative month and has been reported more frequently from some transplantation centers than others. Although legionnaire's disease is not common in children, nosocomial infections have been documented at a children's hospital and immunosuppression is a risk factor (23,24). The appropriate cultures and direct fluorescent antibody stains for *Legionella* should be performed on sputum or other respiratory secretions (obtained by invasive techniques) to detect this pathogen in a timely fashion. A *Legionella* urinary antigen test is available and is quite sensitive (25). Macrolides should be considered in empiric therapy if *Legionella* is a serous consideration for nosocomial pneumonia. Macrolides do interact with many of the immunosuppressive agents administered to these patients. Quinolones are also quite active against *Legionella* spp. and avoid many of these interactions; in adult transplantation patients they have become the agent of choice (25). In similar pediatric patients the use of quinolones in this situation should be given consideration. Routine surveillance cultures of the hospital water supply are recommended in hospitals caring for transplantation patients.

Respiratory Syncytial Virus

Ten episodes of respiratory syncytial virus (RSV) infection were noted in the pediatric multiinstitutional study (1). RSV can be acquired in the hospital early after transplantation or as a community-acquired infection after discharge. Too few patients with RSV infections after heart transplantation have been described to comment on the clinical features. Two children with RSV infection were described in the early Pittsburgh study. One child with a heart-lung transplantation developed rapidly progressive, patchy infiltrates on chest radiograph (9). The other had only mild upper respiratory tract symptoms. Both infections manifested on postoperative day 10. RSV infection in 18 pediatric liver transplant recipients was reported from Pittsburgh also (26). Tachypnea, cough, fever, wheezing, and use of accessory muscles were common, as in normal children. In 12 patients, radiographic changes included interstitial and lobar infiltrates, atelectasis, and pleural effusion. Two patients required intubation after the onset of symptoms related to RSV infection. Three others were intubated before acquiring RSV infection and subsequently had complicated courses. In otherwise immunocompetent children with congenital heart disease, especially when associated with pulmonary hypertension, there is an increased risk of morbidity and mortality with RSV infections (27). As with standard nosocomial pathogens, RSV can be acquired in the hospital (28). Therefore, RSV infection should be considered in the young transplantation patient with respiratory symptoms and fever. Respiratory secretions should be cultured for RSV, and rapid detection of RSV infection by enzyme-linked immunosorbent assay (ELISA) or fluorescent antibody testing may be performed.

The decision to administer ribavirin to these patients is based primarily on the severity of the illness. In a small group of children with underlying bronchopulmonary dysplasia or congenital heart disease, aerosolized ribavirin appeared to be associated with more rapid improvement, compared with placebo (29). It is reasonable to administer aerosolized ribavirin to a heart transplantation patient with proven or suspected moderate to severe RSV infection. However, the efficacy of ribavirin in this situation, as in children who require mechanical ventilation because of severe RSV lower respiratory tract infection, is unknown and is unlikely to be documented by rigorous clinical studies (30). The Committee on Infectious Disease of the American Academy of Pediatrics recommends that ribavirin therapy be considered for administration to infants and children undergoing organ transplantation who are at high risk for serious RSV disease (31).

A monoclonal antibody that is effective in preventing serious RSV illness in premature children and those with chronic lung disease has not yet been evaluated in immunocompromised children, including organ transplant recipients (32). Therefore, no specific recommendations can be made regarding its use after heart transplantation (33). The combination of ribavirin and RSV immune globulin (RSV-IG) was administered to pediatric bone marrow transplant recipients who experienced RSV lower respiratory tract infection (34). The outcome in these patients was improved compared with historical controls, but no randomized trials have been conducted. RSV-IG was not efficacious in treating RSV lower respiratory tract infection in children who were younger than 2 years of age with congenital heart disease (35). The value of the humanized monoclonal antibody to RSV for treatment is unknown, but it has been shown to reduce the concentration of RSV in the tracheal aspirates of children with respiratory failure due to RSV (36).

INFECTIONS BETWEEN THE FIRST AND SIXTH POSTOPERATIVE MONTHS

Cytomegalovirus

CMV is the most frequent and perhaps most serious virus that infects immunosuppressed cardiac transplantation patients. In adult series, 12% to 90% of patients with adequate follow-up had evidence of CMV infection postoperatively (2,37,38). Asymptomatic or symptomatic infections are noted most commonly between the first and sixth months after transplantation and rarely after the seventh month. In the Pittsburgh series, seven children (32%) had CMV infections, with onset between 23 and 43 days after transplantation (mean, 33 days). In the multiinstitutional pediatric study, 51 episodes of CMV infection occurred among 332 patients and accounted for 60% of the viral infections, with a peak occurrence in the second month after transplantation (1). Infants younger than 120 days old had CMV infection and disease less commonly than older babies after heart transplan-

tation in one study (39). Maternal antibody to CMV may have been protective in the younger infants.

CMV infection in the transplantation patient arises from three or four possible sources. Primary infection of a seronegative patient occurs through either the transplanted heart or blood transfusions from seropositive donors. Acquisition of CMV in the community is also possible. Seropositive patients can have reactivation of latent CMV infection or be reinfected with a new strain of CMV from the donor heart or from blood products derived from seropositive donors. Evidence that reinfection of a seropositive patient occurs consists of restriction endonuclease analyses of DNA showing identical patterns of CMV isolates from the donor and the patient (40). The exact site within the donor heart where CMV may reside in a latent form is not known, but it may be either cardiac cells or leukocytes that remain within the donor heart. When primary CMV infection is acquired from the donor organ, CMV disease tends to be more severe than when CMV infection is acquired from blood or blood products (41).

A variety of risk factors for development of CMV infection after organ transplantation have been proposed, of which donor and recipient serologic status and the immunosuppressive regimen used are the most significant. Gorensek et al. (38), using multivariate analysis, found that positive recipient CMV serology before transplantation and a larger than average dose of corticosteroids were significant risk factors for CMV infection. Among the group of patients with CMV infection, positive recipient serology was associated with asymptomatic infection, and excessive steroid dose was a risk factor for symptomatic CMV infection.

The clinical manifestations of CMV infection are highly variable. Patients may simply seroconvert or reactivate a latent infection, as determined by positive cultures, but have no symptoms attributable to the CMV infection. Fever, leukopenia, and thrombocytopenia are common postoperative manifestations of systemic CMV infection in the cardiac transplantation patient. Patients may complain of arthralgias, myalgias, and nonspecific abdominal pain. Atypical lymphocytes may be also noted, but they probably are observed more commonly in adult than in pediatric patients. Hepatitis, pneumonitis, gastrointestinal disease including colitis, retinitis, and myocarditis can be caused by CMV infection (37,38,42–45). The retinitis may be asymptomatic, or it may be associated with complaints such as floaters or scotomata. As a result, ophthalmologic screening tests for CMV retinitis are recommended for all patients 3 to 4 months after cardiac transplantation (45).

Of the various tissue invasions by CMV, pneumonitis leads to the greatest mortality rate, 13% in one study (46). CMV pneumonitis is characterized by fever, hypoxemia, and diffuse interstitial infiltrates, although lobar consolidation has been reported (47). Coexisting pulmonary infections with other viruses or bacteria or *Pneumocystis carinii*, as well as other pathologic processes (e.g., infarction), must be kept in mind. Gastrointestinal manifestations that can be documented by endoscopy include gastritis, gastric ulceration, duodenitis, esophagitis, pyloric perforation, and colonic hemorrhage. A 19-year-old transplant recipient developed deteriorating cardiac function, a pericardial effusion, an atrioventricular block, and rising creatine phosphokinase values, all of which were thought to be caused by CMV myocarditis (48). Endomyocardial biopsy results were not consistent with rejection.

The diagnosis of CMV infection can be based on serologic changes in antibody titer to CMV in paired sera run in parallel using established tests, or on the isolation of CMV from a variety of body sites such as urine, blood, bronchial washings, or tissues. Periodic monitoring of CMV serology and cultures in the seronegative recipient helps to anticipate the possibility of active CMV infection. Whether the CMV infection is causing a symptomatic or an invasive illness is more difficult to establish. Histopathologic evidence of CMV infection, such as typical viral inclusions or antigen detection in tissue

by special stains, is required to confirm organ involvement by CMV. Buffy coat cultures are more frequently positive in patients with symptomatic rather than asymptomatic CMV infection, and CMV cultures tend to be positive earlier in the postoperative period for patients with primary CMV infection who develop lung involvement, compared with those who do not (38). In five patients with active CMV infection, monoclonal antibodies to early antigen of CMV detected CMV antigen-positive leukocytes 10 to 28 days before increases in CMV antibody were demonstrated (49). Polymerase chain reaction (PCR) can detect DNA from CMV in blood and other tissues readily and with great sensitivity (50). The antigen and PCR techniques have been applied to early detection of CMV infection for preemptive antiviral therapy strategies (51).

In addition to the CMV infection syndromes, CMV infection itself appears to adversely affect the transplant recipient in other ways. Patients who develop CMV infection, whether symptomatic or asymptomatic, have a higher rate of graft rejection or graft loss, greater risk of fungal infection, more frequent and earlier graft atherosclerosis, and a significantly lower survival rate than patients who do not experience CMV infection (50,52). In the multiinstitutional study, the combination of a CMV-seropositive donor and a CMV-seronegative recipient was a risk factor for earlier infection with any organism (1). Overall, mortality attributed to CMV infection was 6%.

CMV infection of the wide variety of cells it invades leads to the activation of protein synthesis and the production of multiple immunologically active molecules, including cytokines. This adds to the immune deficits induced by the immunosuppressive agents routinely administered to these patients (50). CMV can infect the transplanted organ itself, and this may be associated with allograft injury or rejection (50).

Potentially successful treatment or suppression of visceral CMV infection by ganciclovir, a nucleoside analog active *in vitro* against CMV, requires a timely diagnosis. Ganciclovir alters CMV infection favorably in heart transplantation patients; it is given along with reduction in immunosuppressive therapy if possible. Ganciclovir was administered to 22 heart and heart-lung transplant recipients in a multicenter open-label trial (53). The distribution of the CMV infections was as follows: pneumonitis, 12 patients (54%); gastrointestinal tract, 5 (23%); retinitis, 3 (14%); and multiorgan infection, 2 (9%). The dose of ganciclovir for 18 of these patients was 5 mg per kilogram, given every 12 hours. Retinitis and gastrointestinal CMV infections were treated for a mean of 21.7 ± 7.7 and 28.2 ± 10.0 days, respectively, whereas pneumonitis was treated for a mean of 14.8 ± 2.8 days. Nineteen (86%) of 22 patients experienced a favorable outcome, defined as improvement or stabilization of the CMV infection at necropsy. Six of the 18 patients experienced relapses of CMV infection, and 5 of those 6 showed favorable responses to retreatment with ganciclovir. The most common adverse reactions to ganciclovir are neutropenia (which developed in 4 of the 22 patients in the study cited), thrombocytopenia, impaired renal function, seizures, and other central nervous system (CNS) abnormalities. Because these patients are receiving so many other medications, it is difficult to ascertain which adverse reactions are caused by ganciclovir alone.

The optimal duration of intravenous ganciclovir therapy and the need for maintenance doses are not clear. Treatment of clinical CMV disease usually requires 2 to 4 weeks of ganciclovir. Viremia should be cleared before therapy is discontinued (50). The dose is 5 mg per kilogram, given every 12 hours, with careful monitoring of hematologic parameters and renal function if renal function is initially normal. Modification of the dose is necessary if renal function is impaired. The role of CMV-hyperimmune globulin (CMV-IG) in the treatment of CMV infection in these patients requires further study. The combination of ganciclovir plus CMV-IG may be superior to ganciclovir alone for treatment of CMV pneumonia after bone marrow transplantation (54,55).

In one study, five children developed symptomatic CMV disease after heart transplantation. Blood culture and PCR assays were positive for each (56). Four patients were treated with ganciclovir for 14 days; one received ganciclovir for 30 days. Each also received CMV-IG (150 mg per kilogram) weekly for 3 weeks. In each case symptomatic CMV disease was successfully treated.

If possible, it is optimal to avoid or prevent infections due to CMV in heart transplantation recipients. When the recipient and donor are both CMV-seronegative, only seronegative blood should be used for transfusions. Careful control of immunosuppressive therapy, especially with corticosteroids, may help to avoid some infections. Prophylactic administration of CMV-IG to a seronegative recipient of a heart from a seropositive donor may be useful in some patients but does not appear to be as beneficial as its similar use in renal transplantation (57). In one study ganciclovir was compared with CMV-IG (Cytotec Pharma, Frankurt, Germany) for the prevention of CMV disease in 31 CMV-seropositive heart transplant recipients. OKT3 monoclonal antibody was used for early immunoprophylaxis (58). CMV disease and visceral involvement were higher in the CMV-IG group than in the ganciclovir group (40% versus 6%, respectively; $p = 0.03$). However, CMV-IG would be expected to be more beneficial in recipients who are CMV-seronegative.

In one large, randomized, double-blind, placebo-controlled trial, ganciclovir significantly reduced CMV illness among CMV-seropositive patients during the first 120 days after heart transplantation (9% versus 46% in controls, $p < 0.001$) (59). There was no difference between the study groups for CMV-seronegative recipients. Combination therapy with ganciclovir and CMV-IG for prophylaxis in seronegative recipients of hearts from seropositive donors has been reported. Avery (60) found that the combination was not particularly effective; 50% of patients developed symptomatic CMV syndrome.

Gajarski et al. (56) provided CMV-IG (150 mg per kilogram intravenously at weeks 0, 2, 4, 6, and 8; then 100 mg per kilogram intravenously at weeks 12 and 16) plus ganciclovir

(5 mg per kilogram intravenously every 12 hours for weeks 1 and 2; then 6 mg per kilogram per day intravenously in weeks 3 and 4) to 19 children who were recipients of heart transplants from CMV-seropositive donors. Among the 10 children who were CMV-seronegative, CMV disease occurred in 3; among the 9 who were seropositive, CMV disease occurred in 1. Adverse effects of these agents were not reported. Although dual therapy was not superior to what has been demonstrated in single-agent studies, the authors concluded that larger studies in pediatric transplantation patients should be performed.

CMV resistant to ganciclovir may emerge as a result of ganciclovir prophylaxis or treatment (61). Foscarnet is an alternative agent in this situation.

Epstein-Barr Virus

Epstein-Barr virus (EBV) can cause a spectrum of disease in pediatric heart transplant recipients that includes a mononucleosis-like syndrome, polyclonal lymphoproliferation, and monoclonal lymphoproliferation, usually of B cells. These together are considered post-transplantation lymphoproliferative disorders (PTLD). Boyle et al. (62) from Pittsburgh described the largest reported series in children after heart transplantation. Between January 1982 and December 1995, 7.7% (6/78) of pediatric heart transplant recipients developed PTLD. Being seronegative for EBV before transplantation was a major risk factor for subsequent PTLD. One third (10/30) of the seronegative recipients of thoracic organs who acquired primary EBV infection developed PTLD. None of those children who were seropositive before transplantation developed PTLD. Almost all of these cases occurred within 1 year after transplantation. The transplanted organ was thought to be the most frequent source of EBV.

Symptoms of PTLD may include fever, malaise, sore throat, and lymphadenopathy. Some children have splenomegaly, CNS symptoms such as lethargy or seizures, or gastrointestinal complaints (62,63). Concur-rent opportunistic infections are common. Nodules in the lung may be observed on the chest radiograph.

Diagnosis of PTLD requires biopsy of involved tissues showing lymphoid proliferation with an immunoblastic component. Molecular techniques typically detect EBV nucleic acids in the tissue. EBV serology is also helpful.

Management generally involves decreasing the immunosuppressive regimen or discontinuing it temporarily. Antiviral therapy with acyclovir or ganciclovir is also administered.

Toxoplasma gondii Infection

An increased risk of toxoplasmosis is apparent with heart transplantation, compared with other types of organ transplantation (64). Because *Toxoplasma gondii* has a predilection for muscle, the parasite can be transmitted to the recipient from the heart of a seropositive donor, and active *T. gondii* infections have been observed in donor hearts (65). Reactivation of old infection in the recipient occurs less commonly. The greatest risk occurs in the seronegative recipient of a heart from a seropositive donor. The onset of clinical symptoms is usually after the first postoperative month (66–69). Fever alone with seroconversion may be the only clinical manifestation. However, dissemination of the parasite to the CNS can lead to lethargy, seizures, coma, hemiparesis, and other signs and symptoms of a meningoencephalitis. Chorioretinitis can lead to diminished visual acuity. Unusual manifestations include a sepsis-like picture, pneumonia, and cutaneous lesions (70). Mass lesions may be detected by CT or by magnetic resonance imaging (MRI). A definitive diagnosis of CNS toxoplasmosis requires a demonstration of the organism in tissue by biopsy or at necropsy. Serologic tests help to monitor seronegative patients for seroconversion and perhaps encourage a more aggressive approach for early diagnosis of toxoplasmosis (71). In some instances *T. gondii* can be seen on the endomyocardial biopsies performed routinely to monitor for rejection (72).

Therapy for an established infection with pyrimethamine and sulfadiazine may lead to recovery, and these drugs should be administered if the patient seroconverts (73). Prophylactic administration of pyrimethamine to seronegative recipients of hearts from seropositive donors appears to be beneficial and is recommended (74). Spiramycin is not a useful prophylactic agent (71).

Aspergillus fumigatus Infection

The most common non-*Candida* fungal infection reported outside the immediate postoperative period in most series is *Aspergillus fumigatus*. Frequently this infection is first noted at necropsy. In an early Stanford series, 8 (11%) of 72 cyclosporine-treated patients developed *Aspergillus* infections (pulmonary, 4; disseminated, 4) between 12 to 45 days postoperatively (75). One child in Pittsburgh had disseminated aspergillosis, which is a feature common to all solid organ transplant recipients infected with *Aspergillus* (9,76). In the multiinstitutional study, seven non-*Candida* fungal infections occurred: *Aspergillus* spp., 2; cryptococcus, rhizopus, and rhizomucor, 1 each; unspecified, 2. All patients with disseminated infections died. CNS invasion occurs in many of the patients with pulmonary aspergillosis (67,68). On CT of the head, abnormalities may be seen. Some type of drainage procedure is indicated if CNS aspergillosis is documented or suspected. Response to therapy with amphotericin B is not generally expected. Although in a patient with pneumonitis isolation of *Aspergillus* species from respiratory secretions does not establish a diagnosis, an aspergillosis infection is so often fatal and difficult to establish firmly that amphotericin B administration should be seriously considered based on the culture result alone. The combination of amphotericin B plus flucytosine is recommended for invasive aspergillosis. Liposomal amphotericin B may provide an alternative therapy when treatment fails and for those patients who are intolerant of conventional amphotericin B (77,78). The role of itraconazole for aspergillosis in heart transplant recipients is not clear. In one small study, amphotericin B was superior to itraconazole at a dose of 200 mg twice daily (79). Surgical drainage with debridement plays an important role in the management of most infections (80).

INFECTIONS AFTER THE SIXTH POSTOPERATIVE MONTH

Nocardia asteroides Infection

The complaint of a dry cough and fever and the presence of a solitary pulmonary nodule or abscess on chest roentgenogram are characteristics of infection with *Nocardia asteroides* (81,82). Some patients are asymptomatic despite an abnormal chest roentgenogram. This infection is much less common with cyclosporine than with previous immunosuppressive regimens; it was observed in only 3% of the cyclosporine-treated patients in the early Stanford series (75). The median time to onset of infection was 225 days. A similar incidence of lung nodules or masses caused by *Nocardia* spp. was noted in a more recent series from New York (83). Among pediatric heart transplant recipients, *Nocardia* infections are very unusual. The organism is best isolated from direct lung tissue specimens, but it also may be cultured from bone, skin, or other sites of involvement. Recognition of a cutaneous skin lesion of *Nocardia* should prompt an evaluation for other sites infected (84). Hematogenous dissemination to the CNS can result in abscess formation, which may be sampled by stereotactic techniques (68). Seizures may develop after invasion of brain parenchyma.

Sulfonamides have been the drugs of choice for treating *N. asteroides* infections. Prolonged administration (average duration, 10 months) usually leads to clearing of the pulmonary lesions. An alternative therapy is minocycline, which may be necessary if the patient has adverse reactions to the sulfonamide. Peterson et al. (85) successfully treated five cardiac transplantation patients with *N. asteroides* pulmonary infections using minocycline, but the optimal dose and duration of the drug have not been established.

Pneumocystis carinii Infection

During the postcyclosporine era, *P. carinii* pneumonia (PCP) has been reported in about 3% to 4% of heart transplantation patients (75,86,87). Fever, a nonproductive cough, and tachypnea are typical symptoms, and hypoxemia is characteristic. The chest roentgenogram classically shows a diffuse interstitial infiltrate that can progress rapidly. Methenamine silver or specific antibody stain of fluid or tissue obtained by bronchoalveolar lavage or lung biopsy is usually the most expeditious way to document PCP in children. Coinfection with CMV or other pathogens is common.

Treatment of PCP in the child with a heart transplant is identical to that in other immunocompromised patients. Trimethoprim-sulfamethoxazole prophylaxis for at least 4 months after transplantation has markedly decreased the incidence of this infection in recipients of heart transplants (88). In the multiinstitutional pediatric study, seven episodes of *P. carinii* infection occurred (1).

Other Viruses

Influenza and parainfluenza viruses can cause serious infections at any time after transplantation, but especially in the immediate postoperative period (89,90). Young age and augmentation of immunosuppression are additional risk factors for severe disease leading to death. Symptoms such as fever, cough, rhinorrhea, and pharyngitis are typical for upper respiratory infections. More serious manifestations include adult respiratory distress syndrome, the need for intubation and mechanical ventilation, a sepsis-like picture, and CNS symptoms such as headache, photophobia, and lethargy. Allograft rejection may be enhanced by the viral infections.

For influenza A infections, amantadine or rimantadine should be considered for children with underlying conditions, such as a heart transplant, that predispose the child to a se-

vere or complicated influenza infection (91). A neuraminidase inhibitor can be considered for patients 12 years of age and older for influenza A or B infection. However, experience with either one of these agents in patients with solid organ transplants is limited (92). Experience with aerosolized and intravenous ribavirin for influenza and parainfluenza infections is anecdotal.

Parvovirus B19 infection in heart transplant recipients is recognized to cause severe anemia associated with low or no reticulocytes, similar to the red blood cell suppression in other immunosuppressed patients (93). In one child, severe pneumonia developed in association with fever and a blanching maculopapular rash involving the face, trunk, and extremities (94). Parvovirus B19 genome has also been detected in myocardial biopsies of children with cardiac allograft rejection. Of six children described in one report, one had a diffuse rash and two had persistent rejection despite aggressive therapy (95). Intravenous immunoglobulin is beneficial for treatment of anemia related to parvovirus B19, but its efficacy for treating pneumonia or possible allograft rejection is unknown.

CYCLOSPORINE AND ANTIBIOTICS

Cyclosporine and tacrolimus have made major impacts on the success of organ transplantation. Although morbidity and morality rates remain high among heart transplantation patients, the incidence of infections in general appears to be less since the introduction of cyclosporine, compared with earlier immunosuppressive regimens (96). Cyclosporine serum levels are monitored carefully to ensure that concentrations associated with optimal immunosuppression and minimal adverse effects are maintained. Some antibiotics interfere with the pharmacokinetics of cyclosporine, which may lead to an increase or decrease in the cyclosporine levels (97–105). Table 8.3 outlines these interactions. Because cyclosporine is nephrotoxic, the effects of antimicrobial agents (amphotericin B, aminoglycosides, acyclovir, ceftazidime) adminis-

TABLE 8.3. *Effect of various antibiotics on cyclosporine levels*

Increase cyclosporine level	Decrease cyclosporine level
Clarithromycin	Sulfadiazine
Azithromycin	Rifampin
Erythromycin	Trimethoprim-sulfamethoxazole
Ketoconazole	? Nafcillin
Fluconazole	? Isoniazid
Itraconazole	
? Quinupristin/ dalfopristin	

tered to heart transplantation patients may be additive; therefore renal function must be monitored carefully.

IMMUNIZATIONS

There are no specific guidelines for the immunization of children after heart transplantation. However, it is prudent to follow the recommendations put forth by the Committee on Infectious Diseases of the American Academy of Pediatrics on immunizing immunosuppressed children (104). Ideally, the patient will have received the recommended routine vaccines before transplantation. The pneumococcal conjugate vaccine followed by, when age appropriate, pneumococcal polyvalent vaccine also should be administered before transplantation when feasible (4). Children who undergo heart transplantation after the age of 4 years develop antibody responses to the pneumococcal polyvalent vaccine, whereas those transplanted at a younger age are less likely to respond (105). Most children develop antibodies to the influenza vaccine, but prior exposure predicts a better response (106). In one study, low-level histologic rejection occurred after influenza vaccine administration (107). Depending on the time of year and the approximate date of transplantation, influenza vaccination is appropriate for the patient as well as all household contacts.

After transplantation and the initiation of immunosuppressive therapy, live viral vaccines are contraindicated for the patient. The enhanced inactivated polio vaccine should be given to the child and also to normal siblings. The measles-mumps-rubella and varicella vaccines may be given to siblings. Diphtheria, tetanus, and acellular pertussis inactivated vaccines should be given according to the routine booster schedule, although antibody responses may not be equivalent to those observed in normal children. Use of the live varicella vaccine in these immunocompromised children has not been studied. However, varicella vaccine should be administered before transplantation if varicella antibody is nonexistent on the pretransplantation evaluation. It is unclear whether antibody response data generated in children with leukemia during maintenance chemo therapy can be applied to heart transplant recipients who must continue daily immunosuppressive therapy. Passive immunization with varicella-zoster immune globulin is indicated as recommended for other immunocompromised children.

REFERENCES

1. Schowengerdt KO, Naftel DC, Seib PM, et al. Infection after pediatric heart transplantation; results of a multiinstitutional study. *J Heart Lung Transplant* 1997;16:1207–1216.
2. Miller LW, Naftel DC, Bourge RC, et al. Infection after heart transplantation. A multi-institutional study. *J Heart Lung Transplant* 1994;13:981–993.
3. Goldman MH, Barnhart G, Mohanakumar T et al. Cyclosporine in cardiac transplantation. *Surg Clin North Am* 1985;65:637–659.
4. Committee on Infectious Diseases, American Academy of Pediatrics. Policy statement: recommendations for the prevention of pneumococcal infections, including the use of pneumococcal conjugate vaccine (Prevnar), pneumococcal polysaccharide vaccine, and antibiotic prophylaxis. *Pediatrics* 2000;106:362–366.
5. Wagener MW, Yu VL. Bacteremia in transplant recipients: a prospective study of demographics, etiologic agents, risk factors and outcomes. *Am J Infect Control* 1992;20:239–247.
6. Hospital Infection Control Practices Advisory Committee. Recommendation for preventing the spread of vancomycin resistance. *Infect Control Hosp Epidemiol* 1995;16:105–113.
7. Salzman MB, Rubin LG. Intravenous catheter-related infections. *Adv Pediatr Infect Dis* 1995;10:337–368.
8. Epps SC, Troutman JL, Gutman LT. Outcome of treatment of candidemia in children whose central catheters were removed or retained. *Pediatr Infect Dis J* 1989;8:99–104.
9. Green M, Wald ER, Fricker FJ, et al. Infections in pe-

diatric orthotopic heart transplant recipients. *Pediatr Infect Dis J* 1989;8:87–93.

10. Stokes DC, Shenep JL, Parham D, et al. Role of flexible bronchoscopy in the diagnosis of pulmonary infiltrates in pediatric patients with cancer. *J Pediatr* 1989;115:561–567.

11. Fisher JF, Chew WH, Shadomy S, et al. Urinary tract infections due to Candida albicans. *Rev Infect Dis* 1982;4:1107–1118.

12. Kohn DB, Uehling DT, Peters ME, et al. Short-course amphotericin B therapy for isolated candiduria in children. *J Pediatr* 1987;10:310–313.

13. Como JA, Dismukes WE. Oral azole drugs as systemic antifungal therapy. *N Engl J Med* 1994;330:263–272.

14. Miller R, Ruder J, Karwande SV, et al. Treatment of mediastinitis after heart transplantation. *J Heart Transplant* 1986;5:477–479.

15. Karwande SV, Renlund DG, Olsen SL, et al. Mediastinitis in heart transplantation. *Ann Thorac Surg* 1992;54:1039–1045.

16. Edwards MS, Baker CJ. Median sternotomy wound infections in children. *Pediatr Infect Dis* 1983;2: 105–109.

17. Carrier M, Hudon G, Paquet E, et al. Mediastinal and pericardial complications after heart transplantation: not-so-unusual postoperative problems? *Cardiovasc Surg* 1994;2:395–397.

18. Baum D, Bernstein D, Starnes VA, et al. Pediatric heart transplantation at Stanford: results of a 15-year experience. *Pediatrics* 1991;88:203–214.

19. Kusne S, Schwartz M, Breinig MK, et al. Herpes simplex virus hepatitis after solid organ transplantation in adults. *J Infect Dis* 1991;163:1001–1007.

20. Pollard RB, Arvin AM, Gambert P, et al. Specific cell-mediated immunity and infections with herpes viruses in cardiac transplant recipients. *Am J Med* 1982;73:6 79–687.

21. Gold D, Corey L. Acyclovir prophylaxis for herpes simplex virus infection. *Antimicrob Agents Chemother* 1987;31:361–367.

22. Chow JW, Yu VL. Legionella: a major opportunistic pathogen in transplant recipients. *Semin Respir Infect* 1998;13:132–139.

23. Brady MT. Nosocomial legionnaire's disease in a children's hospital. *J Pediatr* 1989;115:46–50.

24. Carlson NC, Kuskie MR, Dobyns EL, et al. Legionellosis in children: an expanding spectrum. *Pediatr Infect Dis J* 1990;9:133–137.

25. Stout JE, Yu VL. Legionellosis. *N Engl J Med* 1997; 337:682–687.

26. Pohl C, Green M, Wald ER, et al. Respiratory syncytial virus infections in pediatric liver transplant recipients. *Clin Infect Dis* 1992;165:166–169.

27. MacDonald NE, Hall CB, Suffin SC, et al. Respiratory syncytial viral infection in infants with congenital heart disease. *N Engl J Med* 1982;307:397–400.

28. Hall CB, Douglas RG Jr, Geiman JM, et al. Nosocomial respiratory syncytial virus infections. *N Engl J Med* 1975;293:1343–1346.

29. Hall CB, McBride JT, Gala CL, et al. Ribavirin treatment of respiratory syncytial viral infection in infants with underlying cardiopulmonary disease. *JAMA* 1985;254:3047–3051.

30. Smith DW, Frankel LR, Mathers LH, et al. A controlled trial of aerosolized ribavirin in infants receiving

mechanical ventilation for severe respiratory syncytial virus infection. *N Engl J Med* 1991;325:24–29.

31. Committee on Infectious Diseases, American Academy of Pediatrics. Reassessment of the indications for ribavirin therapy in respiratory syncytial virus infections. *Pediatrics* 1996;97:137–140.

32. The Impact-RSV Study Group. Palivizumab, a humanized respiratory syncytial virus monoclonal antibody, reduces hospitalization from respiratory syncytial virus infection in high-risk infants. *Pediatrics* 1998;102:531–537.

33. Committee on Infectious Diseases and Committee on Fetus and Newborn. Prevention of respiratory syncytial virus infections: indications for the use of palivizumab and update on the use of RSV-IGIV. *Pediatrics* 1998;102:1211–1216.

34. DeVincenzo JP, Fuentes RJ, Hirsch RL. Respiratory syncytial virus immune globulin treatment of RSV pneumonia in bone marrow transplant recipients: a compassionate use experience [Abstract 96]. Presented at the 36th Annual Meeting of the Infectious Diseases Society of America, Denver, CO, November 14, 1998.

35. Rodriguez WJ, Gruber WC, Welliver RC, et al. Respiratory syncytial virus (RSV) immune globulin intravenous therapy for RSV lower respiratory tract infection in infants and young children at high risk for severe RSV infections. *Pediatrics* 1997;99:454–461.

36. Malley R, DeVincenzo J, Ramilo O, et al. Reduction of respiratory syncytial virus (RSV) in tracheal aspirates in intubated infants by use of humanized monoclonal antibody to RSV F protein. *J Infect Dis* 1998; 178:1555–1561.

37. Dummer JS, White LT, Ho M, et al. Morbidity of cytomegalovirus infection in recipients of heart or heart-lung transplants who received cyclosporine. *J Infect Dis* 1985;152:1182–1191.

38. Gorensek MJ, Stewart RW, Keys TF, et al. A multivariate analysis of the risk of cytomegalovirus infection in heart transplant recipients. *J Infect Dis* 1988;157: 515–522.

39. Fukushima N, Gundry SR, Razzouk AJ, et al. Cytomegalovirus infection in pediatric heart transplantation. *Transplant Proc* 1993;25:1423–1425.

40. Chou S. Cytomegalovirus infection and reinfection transmitted by heart transplantation. *J Infect Dis* 1987; 155:1054–1056.

41. Wreghitt T. Cytomegalovirus infections in heart and heart-lung transplant recipients. *J Antimicrob Chemother* 1989;23[Suppl E]:49–60.

42. Shuster LD, Cox G, Bhatia P, et al. Gastric mucosal nodules due to cytomegalovirus infection. *Dig Dis Sci* 1989;34:103–107.

43. Kaplan CS, Peterson EA, Icenogle TB, et al. Gastrointestinal cytomegalovirus infection in heart and heart-lung transplant recipients. *Arch Intern Med* 1989;149: 2095–2100.

44. Etheridge SP, Bolman RH, Braunlin EA. Cytomegalovirus colitis in a pediatric heart transplant patient. *Clin Transplant* 1994;8:409–412.

45. Fishburne BC, Mitrani AA, Davis JL. Cytomegalovirus retinitis after cardiac transplantation. *Am J Ophthalmol* 1998;125:104–106.

46. Kirklin JK, Naftel DC, Levine TB, et al. Cytomegalovirus after heart transplantation: risk factors

for infection and death. A multiinstitutional study. *J Heart Lung Transplant* 1994;13:394–404.

47. Shulman LL. Cytomegalovirus pneumonitis and lobar consolidation. *Chest* 1978;91:558–601.

48. Gonwa TA, Capehart JE, Pilcher JW, et al. Cytomegalovirus myocarditis as a cause of cardiac dysfunction in a heart transplant recipient. *Transplantation* 1989;47:197.

49. Van der Bij W, Van Dijk RB, Van Son WJ, et al. Antigen test for early diagnosis of active cytomegalovirus infection in heart transplant recipients. *J Heart Transplant* 1988;7:106–109.

50. Fishman JA, Rubin RH. Infection in organ-transplant recipients. *N Engl J Med* 1998;338:1741–1751.

51. Egan JJ, Lomax J, Barber L, et al. Preemptive treatment for the prevention of cytomegalovirus disease in lung and heart transplant recipients. *Transplantation* 1998;65:747–752.

52. Rubin RH. The indirect effects of cytomegalovirus infection on the outcome of organ transplantation. *JAMA* 1989;261:3607–3609.

53. Keay S, Petersen E, Icenogle T, et al. Ganciclovir treatment of serious cytomegalovirus infection in heart and heart-lung transplant recipients. *Rev Infect Dis* 1988;10[Suppl 3]:S563–572.

54. Emanuel D, Cunningham I, Jules-Elysee K, et al. Cytomegalovirus pneumonia after bone marrow transplantation successfully treated with the combination of ganciclovir and high-dose intravenous immune globulin. *Ann Intern Med* 1988;109:777–782.

55. Reed EC, Bowden RA, Dandliker PS, et al. Treatment of cytomegalovirus pneumonia with ganciclovir and intravenous cytomegalovirus immunoglobulin in patients with bone marrow transplants. *Ann Intern Med* 1988;109:783–788.

56. Garjarski RJ, Rosenblatt HM, Denfield SW, et al. Outcomes among pediatric heart transplant recipients after dual-therapy cytomegalovirus prophylaxis. *Tex Heart Inst J* 1997;24:97–104.

57. Valentine HA. Prevention and treatment of cytomegalovirus disease in thoracic organ transplant: evidence for a beneficial effect of hyperimmune globulin. *Transplant Proc* 1995;27[Suppl 1]:49–57.

58. Aguado JM, Gomez-Sanchez MA, Lumbreras C, et al. Prospective randomized trial of efficacy of ganciclovir versus that of anti-cytomegalovirus (CMV) immunoglobulin to prevent CMV disease in CMV-seropositive heart transplant recipients treated with OKT3. *Antimicrob Agents Chemother* 1995;39:1643–1645.

59. Merigan TC, Renlund DG, Keay S, et al. A controlled trial of ganciclovir to prevent cytomegalovirus disease after heart transplantation. *N Engl J Med* 1992;326:1182–1186.

60. Avery RK. Prevention and treatment of cytomegalovirus infection and disease in heart transplant recipients. *Curr Opin Cardiol* 1998;13:122–129.

61. Baldanti F, Simoncini L, Sarasini A, et al. Ganciclovir resistance as a result of oral ganciclovir in a heart transplant recipient with multiple human cytomegalovirus strains in blood. *Transplantation* 1998;66:324–329.

62. Boyle GJ, Michaels MG, Webber SA, et al. Transplantation lymphproliferative disorders in pediatric thoracic organ recipients. *J Pediatr* 1997;131:309–313.

63. Bernstein D, Baum D, Berry G, et al. Neoplastic disorders after pediatric heart transplantation. *Circulation* 1993;88:230–237.

64. Spiers GE, Hakim M, Calne RY, et al. Relative risk of donor-transmitted Toxoplasma gondii infection in heart, liver and kidney transplant recipients. *Clin Transplant* 1988;2:257–260.

65. Ryning FW, McLeod R, Maddox JC, et al. Probable transmission of Toxoplasma gondii by organ transplantation. *Ann Intern Med* 1979;90:47–49.

66. Luft BJ, Naot Y, Araujo FG, et al. Primary and reactivated Toxoplasma infection in patients with cardiac transplants, clinical spectrum and problems in diagnosis in a defined population. *Ann Intern Med* 1983;99:27–31.

67. Montero CG, Martinez AJ. Neuropathy of heart transplantation: 23 cases. *Neurology* 1986;36:1149–1154.

68. Hall WA, Martinez AJ, Dummer JS, et al. Central nervous system infections in heart and heart-lung transplantation recipients. *Arch Neurol* 1989;46:173–177.

69. Michaels MG, Wald ER, Fricker FJ, et al. Toxoplasmosis in pediatric recipients of heart transplants. *Clin Infect Dis* 1992;14:847–851.

70. Arnold SJ, Kinney MC, McCormick S, et al. Disseminated toxoplasmosis: unusual presentation in the immunocompromised host. *Arch Pathol Lab Med* 1997;121:869–873.

71. Sluiters JF, Balk AHMM, Essed CE, et al. Indirect enzyme-linked immunoassay for immunoglobulin G and four immunoassays for immunoglobulin M to Toxoplasma gondii in a series of heart transplantation recipients. *J Clin Microbiol* 1989;27:529–535.

72. Luft BJ, Billingham M, Remington JS. Endomyocardial biopsy in the diagnosis of toxoplasmic myocarditis. *Transplant Proc* 1986;83:1871–1873.

73. Gallino A, Maggiorini M, Kiowoski W, et al. Toxoplasmosis in heart transplant recipients. *Eur J Clin Microbiol Infect Dis* 1996;15:389–393.

74. Wreghitt TG, Gray JJ, Pavel P, et al. Efficacy of pyrimethamine for the prevention of donor-acquired Toxoplasmosis gondii infection in heart and heart-lung transplant patients. *Transplant Int* 1992;5:197–200.

75. Hofflin JM, Potasman I, Baldwin JC, et al. Infectious complications in heart transplant recipients receiving cyclosporine and corticosteroids. *Ann Intern Med* 1987;106:209–216.

76. Paya CV. Fungal infections in solid-organ transplantation. *Clin Infect Dis* 1993;16:677–688.

77. Walsh TJ, Hiemenz JW, Seibel NL, et al. Amphotericin B lipid complex for invasive fungal infections: analysis of safety and efficacy in 556 cases. *Clin Infect Dis* 1998;26:1383–1396.

78. Ellis M, Spence D, de Pauw B, et al. An EORTC international multicenter randomized trial (EORTC Number 19923) comparing two dosages of liposomal amphotericin B for treatment of invasive aspergillosis. *Clin Infect Dis* 1998;27:1406–1412.

79. Nanas JN, Saroglou G, Anastasion-Nana MI, et al. Itraconazole for the treatment of pulmonary aspergillosis in heart transplant recipients. *Clin Transplant* 1998;12:30–34.

80. Denning DW, Stevens DA. Antifungal and surgical treatment of invasive aspergillosis: review of 2,121 published cases. *Rev Infect Dis* 1990;12:1147–1201.

81. Krick JA, Stinson EB, Remington JS. Nocardia infec-

tion in heart transplant patients. *Ann Intern Med* 1975; 82:18–26.

82. Simpson GL, Stinson EB, Egger MJ, et al. Nocardial infections in the immunocompromised host: a detailed study in a defined population. *Rev Infect Dis* 1981;3: 492–508.

83. Haramati LB, Schulman LL, Austin JH. Lung nodules and masses after cardiac transplantation. *Radiology* 1993;188:491–497.

84. Gentry LO, Zeluff B, Kielhofner MA. Dermatologic manifestations of infectious diseases in cardiac transplant patients. *Infect Dis Clin North Am* 1994;8: 637–654.

85. Peterson EA, Nash ML, Mammana RB, et al. Minocycline treatment of pulmonary nocardiosis. *JAMA* 1983; 250:930–932.

86. Gryzan S, Paradis IL, Zeevi A, et al. Unexpectedly high incidence of Pneumocystis carinii infection after lung heart transplantation: implications for lung defense and allograft survival. *Am Rev Respir Dis* 1988; 137:1268–1274.

87. Fishman JA. Pneumocystis carinii and parasitic infections in transplantation. *Infect Dis Clin North Am* 1995;9:1005–1074.

88. Olsen SL, Renlund DG, O'Connell JB, et al. Prevention of Pneumocystis carinii pneumonia in cardiac transplant recipients by trimethoprim-sulfamethoxazole. *Transplantation* 1993;56:359–362.

89. Mauch TJ, Bratton S, Myers T, et al. Influenza B virus infection in pediatric solid organ transplant recipients. *Pediatrics* 1994;94:225–229.

90. Apalsch AM, Green M, Ledesma-Medina J, et al. Parainfluenza and influenza virus infections in pediatric organ transplant recipients. *Clin Infect Dis* 1995;20:394–399.

91. American Academy of Pediatrics. Influenza. In: Pickering LK, ed. 2000 Red Book: Report of the Committee on Infectious Diseases, 25th ed. Elk Grove Village, IL: American Academy of Pediatrics, 2000:353–354.

92. Sable CA, Hayden FG. Orthomyxoviral and paramyxoviral infections in transplant patients. *Infect Dis Clin North Am* 1994;9:987–1003.

93. Nour B, Green M, Michaels M, et al. Parvovirus B 19 infection in pediatric transplant patients. *Transplantation* 1993;56:835–838.

94. Janner D, Bork J, Baum M, et al. Severe pneumonia after heart transplantation as a result of human Parvovirus B19. *J Heart Lung Transplant* 1994;13:336–338.

95. Schowengerdt KO, Ni J, Denfield SW, et al. Association of parvovirus B19 genome in children with myocarditis and cardiac allograft rejection: diagnosis using the polymerase chain reaction. *Circulation* 1997; 96:3549–3554.

96. Kim JH, Perfect JR. Infection and cyclosporine. *Rev Infect Dis* 1989;11:677–690.

97. Sands M, Brown RB. Interactions of cyclosporine with antimicrobial agents. *Rev Infect Dis* 1989;11: 691–697.

98. Kramer MR, Marshall SE, Denning DW, et al. Cyclosporine and itraconazole interaction in heart and lung transplant recipients. *Ann Intern Med* 1990;113: 327–329.

99. Theisen K. Sulfadiazine therapy for toxoplasmosis in heart transplant recipients decreases cyclosporine concentration. *Clin Investig* 1992;70:752–754.

100. Campana C, Regazzi MB, Buggia I, et al. Clinically significant drug interactions with cyclosporine: an update. *Clin Pharmacokinet* 1996;30:141–179.

101. Osowski CL, Dix SP, Lin SL, et al. Evaluation of the drug interaction between intravenous high-dose fluconazole and cyclosporine or tacrolimus in bone marrow transplant patients. *Transplantation* 1996;61: 1268–1272.

102. Stamatakis MK, Richards JG. Interaction between quinupristin/dalfopristin and cyclosporine. *Ann Pharmacother* 1997;31:576–578.

103. Sadaba B, Lopez de Ocariz A JR, Quiroga J, et al. Concurrent clarithromycin and cyclosporine A treatment. *J Antimicrob Chemother* 1998;42:393–395.

104. American Academy of Pediatrics. Immunocompromised children. In: Pickering LK, ed. 2000 Red Book: Report of the Committee on Infectious Diseases, 25th ed. Elk Grove Village, IL: American Academy of Pediatrics, 2000:56–67.

105. Gennery AR, Cant AJ, Spickett GP, et al. Effect of immunosuppression after cardiac transplantation in early childhood on antibody response to polysaccharide antigen. *Lancet* 1998;351:1778–1781.

106. Mauch TJ, Crouch NA, Freese DK, et al. Antibody response of pediatric solid organ transplant recipients to immunization against influenza virus. *J Pediatr* 1995; 127:957–960.

107. Blumberg EA, Fitzpatrick J, Stutman PC, et al. Safety of influenza vaccine in heart transplant recipients. *J Heart Lung Transplant* 1998;17:1075–1080.

Infections in Patients Undergoing Hematopoietic Stem Cell Transplantation

Jorge Luján-Zilbermann and *Christian C. Patrick

*Departments of Infectious Diseases and *Pathology, St. Jude Children's Research Hospital, Memphis, Tennessee 38105; and the Department of Pediatrics, University of Tennessee College of Medicine, Memphis, Tennessee 38163*

Hematopoietic stem cell transplantation (HSCT) is an increasingly used modality that has become the treatment of choice for patients with certain malignant states and for those with nonmalignant conditions such as congenital immunodeficiencies, hematologic disorders, bone marrow failures, and genetic diseases (1–12 and Statistical Center of the International Bone Marrow Transplant Registry and Autologous Blood and Marrow Transplant Registry, unpublished data, 1999). According to the International Bone Marrow Transplant Registry (IBMTR) and the Autologous Blood and Marrow Transplant Registry (ABMTR), there were more than 15,000 HSCTs performed in North America in 1997.

HSCT can be performed by infusing autologous bone marrow stem cells (autologous BMT), by giving marrow stem cells from a donor who is related (matched allogeneic BMT) or genetically dissimilar (mismatched allogeneic BMT), or, most recently, by infusing peripheral blood stem cells (2,3). Additionally, umbilical cord blood and fetal livers have been used as sources of stem cells.

Infection is a major obstacle affecting the success of HSCT (13–18). Although myeloid recovery can be achieved in 3 to 6 weeks, immune reconstitution may take 2 years or longer, exposing the patient to an increased risk of infection. This recovery of immune function is partially dependent on the source of hematopoietic stem cells (19–21). Syngeneic or autologous stem cell transplant recipients are at a lower risk of infection than their allogeneic counterparts (22). Patients who undergo HSCT in first remission for leukemia have fewer infections than those in relapse. Infections are contingent on the relationship of the donor to the recipient and the changing immunologic recovery after HSCT. Management of infections is based on the anticipation of likely infections based on the immune deficit and the clinical presentation.

This chapter reviews issues leading to the increased risk of infection and the type of organisms and their therapy in BMT patients. Progress in the prevention of viral infections and, most recently, fungal infections is highlighted. Additionally, the use of rapid diagnostic techniques is reviewed.

PATHOPHYSIOLOGY

Infections occurring after HSCT depend on a variety of factors, including the underlying illness and the conditioning regimen (Table 9.1). The underlying illness can itself be an immunodeficiency, leading to deficits in cellular or humoral immunity. The type of trans-

TABLE 9.1. *Factors associated with an increased risk of infection in hematopoietic stem cell transplant recipients*

Underlying disease and its status
  (e.g., remission, relapse)
Type of transplant (e.g. autologous, allogeneic)
Conditioning therapy including radiotherapy
Infectious disease history of recipient and donor
  (if applicable)
Presence of an indwelling medical device
Occurrence and severity of graft versus host disease
  and the immunosuppressive regimens used to
  prevent it
Infections associated with the administration of
  blood products
Epidemiology of hospital and transplantation unit

plant, as stated earlier, affects the rate of infections based on time to engraftment and the development of acute or chronic graft-versus-host disease (GVHD) or therapy to prevent GVHD. Engraftment usually occurs 2 to 3 weeks after allogeneic transplantation, but it can occur as soon as 15 days after transplantation of unmanipulated autologous hematopoietic stem cells or more than 30 days after a cord blood transplant. Natural killer cells re-

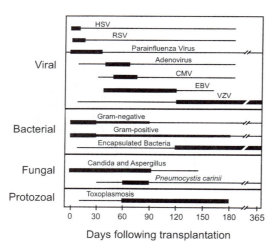

FIG. 9.1. Time frames of infections after hematopoietic stem cell transplantation. Day 0 is the time of the stem cell infusion. The boldness of the line for each infectious agent denotes the frequency of infection with that agent.

turn during the first month after transplantation. CD3+ lymphocytes recover in autologous transplant recipients in 6 to 8 weeks, whereas recovery of this cell type takes an average of 12 weeks in allogeneic transplant recipients. Also, CD8+ cytotoxic T lymphocytes recover earlier than CD4+ helper T lymphocytes, resulting in an inverse CD4+/CD8+ ratio. The infectious disease history of both the donor and the recipient are particularly important because of reactivation of latent infections, predominantly herpesvirus infections. A history of *Aspergillus* infection was reported to result in a 33% relapse rate in one study, with a concomitant high mortality rate (88%) (23). Additionally, the epidemiology of the patient and of the hospital or transplantation unit are important to consider in the recovery of an HSCT patient. The risk of infection is directly proportional to the degree of genetic disparity between the donor and the recipient. For this reason, autologous transplantation carries a much lower risk of infection than does mismatched unrelated donor transplantation. In the latter case, there is a high risk for GVHD. Peripheral blood stem cell transplantation is becoming more routine as stem cell selection techniques improve.

The granulocytopenic period—after the conditioning regimen, with or without irradiation, and before engraftment with concomitant cellular return—is associated with bacterial and fungal infections (Fig. 9.1). The conditioning regimen employs a combination of chemotherapy and total body irradiation (up to approximately 1,320 cGy, usually given in fractions over 4 days with shielding of the lungs). This regimen also causes damage to mucosal integrity, aggravating the risk of infection. The use of colony-stimulating factors can shorten this phase after transplantation (24). The duration of neutropenia can be lengthened by certain manipulations (e.g., antibody or chemotherapy purging of the transplant to remove residual malignant cells) or by the use of marrow-derived cells instead of those harvested by leukapheresis. Administration of cytokines (e.g., granulocyte colony-stimulating factor) enhances cellular return after HSCT (25). The use of selection methods for recovery of CD34+ cells does not affect the granulocyte return, but it does enhance recovery of humoral and cellular immunity.

The middle or early engraftment phase, which lasts until approximately 100 days after HSCT, involves a profound T-cell defect, with herpesviruses being the predominant infecting agents. This immune deficit is enhanced by GVHD and the therapy used to prevent it: cyclosporine, methotrexate, steroids, and the purging of T cells from the graft (3,26). The late engraftment period is associated with selected defects in cellular and humoral immunity along with reticuloendothelial cell dysfunction.

ETIOLOGIC AGENTS

The organisms that cause infection are not dissimilar from those that cause infections in patients with similar immune dysfunctions. HSCT patients have deficits in phagocytic, cellular, and humoral aspects of the immune system. The type of organism infecting these patients depends on the immune dysfunctions that occur in three predictable time periods after transplantation (Fig. 9.1).

In the pretransplantation period, patients can be prone to infections secondary to their underlying diseases (16). Although these infections are rarely fatal, bacterial infections with aerobic gram-negative bacteria do occur, with most localized to the oral cavity, urinary tract, or soft tissue.

A period of neutropenia occurs after the conditioning regimen, usually lasts 3 to 4 weeks, but can last longer in autologous transplant recipients receiving a purged marrow. Bacteria and fungi can cause infection throughout the post-HSCT course, but these infections occur more frequently in the granulocytopenic period (27–29). The most common bacteria are similar to those that occur in bloodstream infections in patients with fever and neutropenia. These bacteria arise from the patient's endogenous microflora. Common infecting organisms include *Staphylococcus epidermidis, Staphylococcus*

aureus, viridans streptococci, and the Enterobacteriaceae (*Escherichia coli, Klebsiella* spp., *Enterobacter* spp.) and *Pseudomonas aeruginosa* (30–39). Other organisms considered in the differential diagnosis include *Serratia* spp., *Xanthomonas* spp., and *Acinetobacter* spp. Also, all patients undergoing HSCT have a central venous line placed, providing a nidus for infection. *S. epidermidis* is isolated most frequently, but organisms such as *Corynebacterium jeikeium, Candida* spp., and *Bacillus cereus* can be problematic and require catheter removal (31). Coagulase-negative staphylococcal infections are associated with the use of central venous catheters and can occur throughout the posttransplantation period, regardless of the neutropenia.

Infections with gram-positive organisms such as viridans streptocococci and *Stomatococcus mucilaginosus* have been increasing in incidence during recent years (33–39). Both of these organisms have been associated with chemotherapy-induced mucositis. Viridans streptococcal infections occurs in up to 28% of HSCT recipients, with a mortality rate of 12%.

Gram-negative bacillary infections occur secondary to mucosal damage with bacterial translocation from the mucosal surface into the bloodstream. Predominant organisms include *E. coli, Klebsiella* spp., *Enterobacter* spp., and *P. aeruginosa. Enterobacter* has a high incidence of inducible β-lactamase activity that alters the approach to therapy.

The most common fungal infections are *Candida* spp. and *Aspergillus* spp. (23, 40–45). These infections are more common in the allogeneic HSCT recipient. Other agents, including those of mucormycosis (e.g., *Mucor, Absidia, Rhizopus*), have been implicated in infections, and other fungal infections, including *Trichosporon, Fusarium, Curvularia,* and *Alternaria*, have been increasingly recognized (46–50). Infections with these organisms usually occur after an extended period of neutropenia accompanied by prolonged administration of broad-spectrum antibiotics. Colonization with *Candida tropicalis* has been shown to be predictive for invasive disease (42,43).

Herpes simplex virus (HSV) and respiratory viruses such as parainfluenza virus can also cause infections during this first time period (51). HSV reactivates in 80% of patients who are HSV-seropositive within the first 5 weeks after transplantation. This reactivation occurs a median of 17 days after transplantation (51).

The second phase of infections occurs after neutrophil recovery and lasts until approximately 100 days after BMT. During this time there is a profound impairment of both humoral and cellular immunity. Although bacterial and fungal infections can still take place, cytomegalovirus (CMV) becomes the major infecting agent. Adenovirus has also become a prominent player. Viral infections can occur because of reactivation of latent infections, by acquisition from infected blood products, or by contact with an infected individual. *Pneumocystis carinii* infection was formerly problematic during this phase, but is not as frequent since the introduction of prophylactic therapy (52). The use of T cell–depleted BMT has increased the risk of Epstein-Barr virus (EBV) infection with associated lymphoproliferative disease (53) (see later discussion).

The third period begins 100 days after the transplantation with deficits in humoral immunity, cellular immune response, and reticuloendothelial function. The encapsulated bacteria, predominantly *Streptococcus pneumoniae*, are major pathogens during this period, as is varicella-zoster virus (VZV) (54).

EPIDEMIOLOGY

The infecting microbial agents in HSCT patients are derived predominantly from the microbial flora or by reactivation of a latent infection. As mentioned previously, the presence of GVHD enhances the infection rate by delaying return of normal immune function and by causing ulceration of the gastrointestinal tract. Additionally, to abrogate GVHD, cyclosporine, methotrexate, glucocorticoids, and/or tacrolimus (FK-506) are administered as prophylactic agents. These agents enhance the infection rate by depressing the cell-mediated immune response and, in the case of methotrexate, by disrupting mucosal barriers. Corticosteroids may also mask fever during an infection.

The conditioning regimen with or without concomitant radiation can also compromise the immune system and disrupt mucosal barriers. The workup of a patient undergoing HSCT includes serologic status analyses of both the donor and the recipient, because infections in transplanted patients can result from reactivation of viruses or fungi (Table 9.2). This is most notable with the herpesvirus group, with CMV being the major cause of pneumonitis during the second phase after allogeneic transplantation. Additionally, other herpesviruses such as HSV, VZV, and EBV, as well as other infecting organisms such as *Toxoplasma* and adenovirus, are prone to reactivate during the posttransplantation period (55).

Knowledge of the epidemiology of the hospital, the transplantation unit, and the patient

TABLE 9.2. *Pretransplantation evaluation of stem cell transplantation patients at St. Jude Children's Research Hospital*

Serology
　Donor—CMV, EBV profile, HAV, HBV Profile, HCV, RPR, HIV
　Recipient—CMV, EBV profile, VZV, HSV, HBV Profile, HCV, RPR, toxoplasmosis, histoplasmosis, *Legionella*, HIV
Laboratory profile
　Donor and recipient—aspartate aminotransferase, alanine aminotransferase, total and direct bilirubin, blood urea nitrogen, creatinine, complete blood count with differential, stool for ova and parasites × 2, and acid-fast bacillus stain
Skin tests
　Donor and Recipient—purified protein derivative (PPD)
Surveillance cultures
　Recipient—Obtain cultures for bacteria and fungi from the anterior nares and rectum
　Send urine for routine bacterial and fungal cultures
Roentgenography
　Recipient—Obtain chest roentgenogram (posteroanterior and lateral) and sinus series if clinically indicated

CMV, cytomegalovirus; EBV, Epstein-Barr virus; HAV, hepatitis A virus; HBV, hepatitis B virus; HCV, hepatitis C virus; HIV, human immunodeficiency virus; RPR, rapid plasma reagin test.

is vital to assess the risk for organisms such as *Aspergillus* and *Legionella*. Additionally, knowledge of the patient's colonizing organism can point out resisting organisms and organisms with high propensity to invade (e.g., *Aspergillus flavus, Aspergillus fumigatus, C. tropicalis, P. aeruginosa*) (56–58). The use of filtered air, such as laminar flow or high-efficiency particulate air (HEPA)–filtered rooms, can be used to reduce the aerosolization of fungal organisms.

A protective environment is controversial. A 1978 study demonstrated no difference in the infection rate when skin cleansing with topical antimicrobial agents, gut decontamination with oral nonabsorbable antibiotics, a sterile food diet, and reverse isolation under laminar flow conditions were used for the first 50 days after BMT; however, the incidence of severe local infections and bacteremias was decreased (59). Protective environments have been observed to decrease the incidence of GVHD in patients with aplastic anemia undergoing BMT (60). At St. Jude Children's Research Hospital, HEPA-filtered air is used without laminar flow. Fresh vegetables are not permitted, to reduce the exposure to gram-negative bacteria, but a sterile diet is not given to patients undergoing HSCT. All patients undergoing HSCT have a central venous catheter placed. Proper maintenance is essential, including careful instructions to the patient and/or their parents.

CLINICAL MANIFESTATIONS

The approach to an HSCT patient should be based on the understanding of infections that occur during each of the at-risk periods. This provides a framework for matching possible etiologic agents with clinical diseases.

Preengraftment (Early) Phase

Bacteremia is the most frequent cause of bacterial infection after HSCT. The portal of entry is usually via disrupted mucosa in the oral or gastrointestinal tract, breakdown of tissue at the perianal site, or the central venous catheter. Because of the uniform use of indwelling central venous catheters for administration of medications, parenteral alimentation, and blood products; and blood sampling, catheter-related infections are common. Infections can manifest as fever with the neutropenia (e.g., *S. epidermidis* infection) or as septic shock (e.g., viridans streptococci, gram-negative infections).

Fungal agents have different portals of entry; for instance, *Aspergillus* spp., agents of mucormycosis, and *Fusarium* spp. enter via the respiratory tract, whereas *Candida* infections originate from the gastrointestinal tract. The prognosis of allogeneic BMT patients with *Aspergillus* is poor, with a 1-year survival rate of 22% (48). GVHD and steroid use are negative risk factors. Diagnosis can be difficult in fungal infections; culture and histopathologic study of material obtained from bronchoscopy, lung aspiration, or open lung biopsy are paramount.

HSV infections can manifest as oral pain or difficulty in swallowing. HSV infection can predispose to bacterial infection (e.g., viridans streptococci). HSV can cause an esophagitis that is difficult to distinguish from CMV or *Candida* infection without a biopsy or cultures. The symptoms of HSV esophagitis include odynophagia, dysphagia, chest pain, hematemesis, nausea, and vomiting (61).

Human herpes virus 6 (HHV-6) has been recovered from 38% to 60% of BMT recipients during the first month after transplantation. Its significance is not clear. It has been linked to bone marrow suppression, interstitial pneumonitis, and encephalitis (62) (see later discussion of pneumonitis).

Hemorrhagic Cystitis

Hemorrhagic cystitis has become more prevalent among transplant patients and can have a variety of infectious and noninfectious causes (63–66) (Table 9.3). Symptoms include suprapubic pain, dysuria, hematuria, and urinary frequency. Chemotherapy-induced cystitis occurs soon after the conditioning regimen, but a multitude of infectious

TABLE 9.3. *Differential diagnosis of hemorrhagic cystitis in hematopoietic stem cell transplant recipients*

Infectious causes
  Bacteria
    Urinary tract infections
  Viruses
    Adenovirus
    Papovavirus (e.g., BK virus)
    Cytomegalovirus
    Herpes simplex virus
  Fungi
    Fungus ball
    Urinary tract infection
Noninfectious causes
  Chemotherapy (e.g., cyclophosphamide)
  Graft-versus-host disease
  Mechanical trauma due to Foley catheter

agents, including adenovirus and papovavirus (BK virus), are common causes. Ultrasound may be a useful modality to monitor the extent of disease (63–66). Ribavirin has been used as therapy, but its efficacy is questionable (67).

Enteric Infections

Enteric infections occur throughout the posttransplantation period. Although diarrhea is common after HSCT, an infectious cause is determined in fewer than 15% of cases (68). Antibiotic-associated diarrhea, including diarrhea secondary to *Clostridium difficile* infection, usually occurs during the granulocytopenic period, when antibiotics are frequently administered (68,69). Other infecting agents include viruses such as adenovirus, rotavirus, and coxsackievirus. CMV infection can manifest as enteritis with pain, diarrhea, nausea, and vomiting. Bacterial and fungal overgrowth can occur as a result of antibiotic-induced selective decontamination (69).

Early Engraftment (Middle Posttransplantation) Phase

This period usually occurs between engraftment and 100 days after transplantation. CMV infection predominated during this phase during the early studies of BMT patients, but its

incidence has diminished with the use of ganciclovir as a prophylactic agent. Bacterial infections become less prominent during this period owing to neutrophil engraftment, but they are seen secondary to use of indwelling catheters. Fungal infections are still possible.

Pneumonitis

Bacterial causes of pneumonia and sinusitis predominate during the neutropenic period; pulmonary infiltrates that occur during the middle period are caused by a variety of infectious or noninfectious agents (70,71) (Table 9.4). Viral infections are more common during this period of time, although the specific organism is not often identified. Idiopathic pneumonia occurs in approximately 30% of patients as a result of the conditioning regimen (72–74).

Sinusitis can occur throughout the posttransplantation periods and may be occult (75,76). Fungal infection with *Aspergillus* or *Mucor* must be considered and treated aggressively.

TABLE 9.4. *Differential diagnosis of pneumonitis in patients undergoing hematopoietic stem cell transplantation*

Infectious causes
  Bacteria
    Staphylococcus aureus
    Legionella pneumophila
    Enterobacteriaceae
  Fungi
    Candida sp.
    Aspergillus sp.
    Pneumocystis carinii
    Mucormycosis
  Viruses
    Adenovirus
    Enteroviruses
    Human parainfluenza virus 1 through 4
    Influenza virus A and B
    Respiratory syncitial virus
Noninfectious causes
  Alveolar hemorrhage
  Bronchiolitis obliterans organizing pneumonia
  Chemotherapy (e.g., bleomycin, busulfan)
  Idiopathic interstitial pneumonitis
  Pulmonary edema
  Pulmonary vascular disease
  Radiation
  Underlying malignancy

CMV infection occurs at a median of 40 to 50 days after transplantation (22,77). This infection is more commonly caused by reactivation of an endogenous virus in seropositive individuals, but it can occur in seronegative patients who received CMV-seropositive stem cells. Risk factors for CMV pneumonia include the seropositivity of the donor, the type of transplant (allogeneic greater than autologous), human leukocyte antigen (HLA)–mismatched transplant, age of the patient (older than 10 years) and development of acute GVHD (78,79). Pneumonitis secondary to CMV occurs because of two critical elements: persistence of viral replication and immune activation linked with GVHD (80). CMV infection occurs in 30% to 50% of patients undergoing allogeneic HSCT, with pneumonia occurring in 10% to 15% of these patients and mortality rate greater than 85% (80). CMV infection and disease do occur among autologous HSCT recipients, but at a much lower incidence (22,77).

The administration of prophylactic ganciclovir to patients who are CMV-seropositive and to those who are CMV-seronegative but are receiving a transplant from a CMV-seropositive donor has substantially reduced the incidence of CMV pneumonia, to less than 5% (81–83). Additionally, the use of CMV-seronegative blood products lowers the risk of CMV disease in CMV-seronegative patients receiving CMV-seropositive blood products (84,85). Prophylaxis usually begins at engraftment and continues to day 100 or 120 after transplantation. Ganciclovir can cause neutropenia, putting the patient at risk for bacterial infections (86). CMV reactivation occurs in 10% to 20% of patients removed from ganciclovir prophylaxis (78,79).

Methods to detect CMV in body fluids to predict disease are changing. Previous methods found that CMV viremia by standard culture had a 60% positive predictive value for disease (87). However, in this same study, 32% of the patients with CMV disease did not have detectable viremia. CMV culture in bronchoalveolar lavage (BAL) fluid is also predictive of CMV pneumonitis, but again

21% of the patients with negative BAL CMV cultures had pneumonitis. The CMV antigenemia test for detecting the presence of the pp65 protein correlates closely with the status of CMV infection (88,89). Viral load, as measured by quantitative polymerase chain reaction from blood, appears promising as an indicator (90,91). No large studies have been done, but this methodology may allow prediction of patients at increased risk.

The clinical manifestations of CMV disease vary considerably. Patients can have from asymptomatic infection or a combination of fever, hepatitis, and leukopenia to life-threatening diseases such as interstitial pneumonitis, esophagitis, or encephalitis.

A variety of other viral infections can cause disease in these patients. Adenovirus that result in a self-limited disease in immunocompetent children can cause life-threatening illness in immunocompromised hosts such as those undergoing HSCT (92–95). A study of 206 patients undergoing BMT at our institution identified 6% with adenoviral infection (94). The most common manifestation was hemorrhagic cystitis, followed by gastroenteritis, pneumonitis, and hepatitis (liver failure) (94,95). Total body irradiation and type of BMT were significant risk factors (94). Of the currently identified 47 types of adenovirus, types of 1, 2, 5, 11, 31, 34, and 35 have been reported as infecting agents in HSCT patients. This virus can become latent in lymphoid tissue and in the kidneys, and as a result can reactivate. Infections most commonly occur with concomitant herpesvirus infection or GVHD. Effective specific therapy is not available.

Respiratory syncytial virus (RSV) is a common cause of lower respiratory tract infection in infants and young children. This virus can cause serious respiratory diseases in adult and pediatric HSCT patients. There are reports of outbreaks that occurred during late fall, winter, and early spring, commensurate with the epidemiology of this virus; however, RSV disease in the immunocompromised patient can occur at any time of the year. RSV infection occurs most commonly during the preengraftment phase, but it can occur throughout the posttransplantation period, depending on the immunologic status of the host (96,97). An outbreak at the Fred Hutchinson Cancer Research Center resulted in diagnosis of RSV infection in 16% of 199 HSCT patients during a 13-week period in 1989 and 1990 (96). Approximately 75% of these infections were nosocomial, and 14 (78% of the 18% that resulted in pneumonia) were fatal. The same type of severe illness has been reported from the University of Minnesota and from M.D. Anderson Cancer Center.

The symptoms of RSV disease show an upper respiratory tract infection syndrome consisting of rhinorrhea, sinus congestion, sore throat, and otitis media that can proceed to pneumonia. Of note, sinusitis has been seen more frequently in patients with parainfluenza and RSV disease than in those with other respiratory viruses. The progression from an upper respiratory tract disease to a pneumonia is highest within the first month after transplantation. The mortality rate is greater than 80% in all transplantation patients, both before and after engraftment.

HSV is the etiologic agent implicated in fewer than 5% of cases of pneumonia after transplantation (61). Oral manifestations of HSV are usually not apparent, making diagnosis difficult without culture results.

The role of HHV-6 in transplantation patients is unclear, but it has been attributed to interstitial pneumonitis (98–109). Viral DNA from HHV-6 has been recovered from 38% to 60% of HSCT recipients, usually within the first month after transplantation.

Parainfluenza is a common cause of croup or laryngotracheobronchitis in young children. Parainfluenza virus types 1 and 3 are the most frequent types seen in immunocompromised patients. Wendt et al. performed a sentinel study highlighting a 16-year retrospective review at the University of Minnesota (110). Approximately 2% of the adults and children were infected with parainfluenza virus; 32% of these patients died. This is sim-

ilar to reports from other transplantation centers. The clinical course and outcome show that sinusitis is a common manifestation of these viruses and that it progresses to pneumonia in the HSCT patient.

Enteroviruses can cause infections in a variety of organ systems, including the lungs, in the post-HSCT period (111). These ubiquitous viruses can manifest with a range of symptoms.

P. carinii was once a devastating cause of pneumonitis in the immunocompromised patient, but its incidence has diminished since the advent of effective prophylaxis. However, it should still be considered in the differential diagnosis of an HSCT recipient with pneumonia (52).

Lymphoproliferative Disease

EBV can cause a posttransplantation lymphoproliferative disease (PTLD) in stem cell recipients. Latent EBV residing in epithelial cells of the oropharynx and in B lymphocytes can reactivate and lead to uncontrolled proliferation. This occurs predominantly in patients receiving T cell—deleted transplants or after intensive immunosuppression (112–114). The incidence of EBV-related PTLD in these high-risk patients is 5% to 25%. It appears as early as 6 to 8 weeks and as late as 6 to 8 months after HSCT. Presentation varies from malaise and low-grade fevers to progressive lymphadenopathy and visceral disease. The disease is invariably fatal if no therapy is given. Antiviral agents are not therapeutic. The use of adoptive immunotherapy with EBV-specific cytotoxic T lymphocytes has been effective (115,116).

Late Posttransplantation Phase

This period occurs from 100 days up to 1 year after transplantation. Bacteremia is less common than in the other two phases, but it continues to be prevalent (117–122). The presence of chronic GVHD with immunosuppression augments the possibility of a bacteremia. Encapsulated bacteria including *S. pneumoniae* are the most common agents, but bacterial infections related to catheter use can still occur (123,124).

VZV occurs in 25% to 40% of HSCT patients (125). Among these patients, reactivation occurs most commonly in those with chronic GVHD, but it can also occur in patients receiving autologous transplants. A prodrome of burning or pain over the involved dermatome can occur. Back pain has also been shown to occur in the immunocompromised patient and may be an indication of VZV reactivation. Groups of vesicles appear in the distribution of one to three sensory dermatomes, as with immunocompromised patients, but atypical zoster with dissemination can occur. If appropriate therapy with acyclovir is not instituted, dissemination can occur in 36% of patients, with a mortality rate of 10%.

Gastrointestinal Disorders and Hepatitis

Diarrhea is common after HSCT. Early in the posttransplantation period, infections with viral agents (e.g., adenovirus, rotavirus, astro-

TABLE 9.5. *Infectious causes of gastroenteritis*

Bacterial
Aeromonas sp.
Campylobacter sp. (rare)
Clostridium difficile
Salmonella sp. (rare)
Shigella sp. (rare)
Bacterial overgrowth (e.g., *Pseudomonas* sp.,
Acinetobacter sp.)
Viral
Astrovirus
Adenovirus
Calicivirus
Cytomegalovirus
Enteroviruses (e.g., coxsackievirus)
Norwalk virus
Rotavirus
Fungal
Cokeromyces recurvatus
Fungal overgrowth (e.g., *Candida* sp.)
Parasitic
Cryptosporidium sp.
Giardia lamblia
Entamoeba histolytica

TABLE 9.6. *Differential diagnosis of hepatitis in patients after hematopoietic stem cell transplantation*

Infectious causes
No reported cases
Viruses
Adenovirus
Cytomegalovirus
Enteroviruses, especially echovirus
Epstein-Barr virus
Hepatitis viruses A through D
Herpes simplex virus
Varicella-zoster virus
Noninfectious causes
Chemotherapy
Drug-induced
Graft-versus-host disease
Total parenteral nutrition
Tumor infiltration
Venocclusive disease

virus, CMV) and *C. difficile* are common (Table 9.5). The conditioning regimen (e.g., busulfan) may also be implicated. After engraftment occurs, acute GVHD can cause bloody diarrhea.

Hepatitis from a variety of infectious and noninfectious causes (Table 9.6) can occur after HSCT. Recently, the ability to detect hepatitis C virus has shown it to be prevalent in the HSCT population, with activation occurring as immunosuppressive therapy is discontinued (126–129). In addition, viral hepatitis is a risk factor for venoocclusive disease.

Central Nervous System Infections

Central nervous system disorders are most commonly a result of noninfectious causes such as drug therapies or metabolic complications. Bacterial meningitis is rare, presumably because of the frequent use broad-spectrum antibiotics. Viral meningitis/encephalitis is also infrequently observed because of the use of antiviral agents with activity against herpesviruses. Brain abscess is caused most commonly by *Aspergillus* spp., followed by *Candida* spp. (130–132). Bacterial causes, including anaerobic bacteria, account for fewer than 10% of the cases.

Toxoplasmosis must be considered in patients who are seropositive.

LABORATORY FINDINGS AND DIAGNOSIS

Laboratory tests, except those for microbiologic evaluations, are of limited value. The absolute neutrophil count defines patients at high risk for bacterial and fungal infections. Microbiologic tests include blood cultures for bacteria, fungi, and viruses. Additionally, Gram stain, acid-fast stains, and other special stains play a predominant role in identifying microorganisms early in the infectious process.

Blood cultures include those for bacteria, fungi, and viruses. The Wampole isolator blood culture system (Wample Laboratories, Cranbury, NJ) can be used to quantitate bacteria when diagnosing central venous catheter–associated infections and to enhance the recovery of fungal organisms. Other sites for cultures are contingent on clinical symptoms (e.g., urine cultures in patients with hemorrhagic cystitis).

Pathologic diagnosis is important because of the modest yield of cultures for fungal causes. Histologic diagnosis of fungal infections can lead to a change in therapy.

Nasopharyngeal swabs or washes play a prominent role in the diagnosis of viral infections, either by direct fluorescent antibody staining or by their growth on specific cell lines. The shell-vial assay has expedited viral diagnosis by putting the sample containing the virus in close proximity to the appropriate cell line, to enhance viral attachment. This has been useful with CMV and the respiratory viruses, including adenovirus.

Nucleic acid detection, including polymerase chain reaction or the amplification of the hybridized product, can provide rapid diagnosis and may be used for quantitation. The latter aspect has shown utility in determining the prognosis of certain infections and in monitoring therapy.

Serologic assays are somewhat limited because patients are immunosuppressed and immunoglobulin therapy is administered to most patients. It can be useful in the diagnosis of *Rochalimaea henselae* and some fungal organisms. Serologic titers for certain pathogens are obtained before transplantation to expedite diagnosis.

MANAGEMENT

Therapy

Therapy for patients undergoing HSCT during the granulocytopenic period mirrors that for patients with chemotherapy-induced fever and neutropenia. A standardized system is essential to ensure adequate coverage of the spectrum of organisms known to colonize the transplantation unit, the hospital, and the community. Knowledge of their associated antibiotic susceptibilities is useful in guiding empiric therapy. This system allows the infection control and infectious disease staff to compare outcomes and provides a rational basis for therapy. There are a variety of different regimens to consider, but an approach tailored to fit the individual hospital is essential (133). At St. Jude Children's Research Hospital, ceftazidime with or without vancomycin is used empirically to provide broad coverage against gram-negative and gram-positive bacteria. The vancomycin is used to provide coverage against viridans streptococci and *S. epidermidis*. If *P. aeruginosa* is suspected, an aminoglycoside should be added. If the patient continues to be neutropenic and febrile after 5 days, a reevaluation may prompt modification of the antibiotic regimen.

If the patient with fever and neutropenia has a persistence of symptoms for 5 to 7 days without the identification of any definite cause, empiric antifungal therapy must be considered. Amphotericin B remains the drug of choice for antifungal therapy, especially true for mold infections. Lipid formulations and azoles also have been introduced that provide options for the practitioner. Lipid formulations reduce the nephrotoxicity of amphotericin B; however, their efficacy varies depending on the infecting fungal agent. Fluconazole has activity against the majority of *Candida* spp. and has good central nervous system penetration. Itraconazole has shown utility in the treatment of invasive *Aspergillus*. Combination therapy is being used but has not been extensively tested. Surgery plays a prominent role in the treatment of mold infection, and in the neutropenic patient it may be the most important aspect of therapy.

Therapy for viral infections, if available, depends on an accurate diagnosis. HSV and VZV are treated with acyclovir. Famciclovir and valacyclovir have activity against HSV and VZV but must be used with caution, because no controlled studies that show their efficacy against VZV in the immunocompromised host are available. The treatment of CMV disease requires the use of ganciclovir; CMV pneumonitis requires ganciclovir plus intravenous immunoglobulin, because the pathogenesis involves viral replication as well as immune-mediated damage. For HSV, VZV, or CMV resistant to acyclovir or ganciclovir, foscarnet is the drug of choice.

Patients with RSV disease may benefit from ribavirin, or anti-RSV antibody (RespiGam), or monoclonal antibody to RSV (palivizumab). Ribavirin has shown some efficacy in infections caused by parainfluenza viruses and anecdotally in hemorrhagic cystitis caused by adenovirus. The neuraminidase inhibitors have joined amantadine and rimantadine as agents used to treat influenza. Amantadine and rimantadine are oral drugs that have efficacy against influenza A, but their usefulness in the immunocompromised host has not been established. The neuraminidase inhibitors, zanamivir and oseltamivir, have activity against influenza A and B, but again data are lacking to support their utility in the immunocompromised host. Adoptive immunotherapy using virus-specific cytotoxic T cells has been used to treat and prevent infections in patients receiving allogeneic stem cell transplants against EBV and CMV infections.

Prophylaxis

Prophylaxis plays a key role in HSCT, but it must be weighed against the toxicity and drug interactions of the prophylactic drug. Regular hand washing is the time-tested method for reducing infections.

No standard method is employed to reduce bacterial infections. Studies involving the use of the quinolone class of antibiotics show decreased infections with gram-negative bacteria, but breakthrough gram-positive bacterial infections have been observed (134–136). The quinolones provide the ability to decrease the aerobic flora in the gastrointestinal tract while preserving the anaerobes (selective decontamination); this results in less bacteria available to cause disease (136).

Fungal prevention is desirable because infections are difficult to treat, require toxic drugs, and usually have high morbidity and/or mortality rates. Oral fluconazole and low-dose amphotericin B have been shown to be effective in preventing superficial fungal infections and systemic infections with *Candida albicans* (137,138). Fluconazole use is problematic because of the emergence of resistant organisms, such as *Candida krusei* and other non-*albicans Candida* strains, and the fact that it has no activity against certain molds such as *Aspergillus* (138). The use of aerosolized amphotericin B has not shown any benefit for prophylaxis in small studies.

Antiviral prophylaxis has been important in HSCT to prevent primary or reactivation herpesvirus infection. Acyclovir has been used during the granulocytopenic period to prevent HSV infection. This prevention is practiced by most adult HSCT centers but must be tempered in the pediatric patient by evaluating the risks of acyclovir compared with the minimal risk of HSV mortality. Ganciclovir has produced a remarkable reduction in the incidence of CMV disease during the middle period af-

TABLE 9.7. *St. Jude Children's Hospital's schema for administering immunizations after HSCT*

Recommended time after HSCT (mo)	Type of immunization
12	Td[a], IPV, Hib, and pneumoccal
14[b]	Td, IPV, Hib, pneumococcal and hepatitis B
16	Td, IPV, Hib, pneumococcal and hepatitis B
24	MMR[c]

HBV, hepatitis B virus; Hib, *Haemophilus influenzae* type b vaccine; HSCT, hematopoietic stem cell transplant; IPV, inactivated poliomyelitis vaccine; MMR, measles-mumps-rubella vaccine; Td, tetanus and diphtheria toxoid.
[a]Diphtheria and tetanus toxoids and acellular perlussis (DTaP) vaccine if patient is <6 y of age.
[b]If there is an antibody response to any vaccine at 12 mo after autologous HSCT, no further immunization is necessary.
[c]Live virus vaccines are contraindicated in patients with graft-versus-host disease and patients receiving steroids.

ter allogeneic HSCT. Ganciclovir prophylaxis is usually administered from engraftment until day 100 or 120 after transplantation. Prophylaxis in periods of community or nosocomial outbreaks of influenza for HSCT patients less than 6 months beyond transplantation consists of amantadine or rimantadine. Vaccination and prophylaxis are needed for patients who have been exposed to influenza but were never vaccinated.

Intravenous immunoglobulin (IVIG) is administered during the first few months after allogeneic HSCT to prevent infections and acute GVHD (139–142). The utility of IVIG is not clear in all transplant recipients. The dosage is not standardized. Prolonged administration may delay immune reconstitution.

Vaccination

Patients undergoing autologous or allogeneic HSCT lose immunity to common childhood diseases and should be regarded as unvaccinated (143–154). Reimmunization begins at 1 year after HSCT, although this is an arbitrary time point to consider vaccination based on published data (Table 9.7). The inactivated polio vaccine should be used in the post-HSCT patient (143). Measles-mumps-rubella vaccination should be considered at 2 years after HSCT; however the use of steroids and chronic GVHD delays these immunizations (146). New guidelines for vaccinated patients after HSCT are being developed by the Centers for Disease Control and Prevention and the American Society for Bone Marrow Transplantation.

ACKNOWLEDGMENT

This work was supported by the National Cancer Institute Cancer Center Support Grant P30 CA 21765 and by the American Lebanese Syrian Associated Charities.

REFERENCES

1. Thomas ED, Storb R, Clift RA, et al. Bone marrow transplantation. *N Engl J Med* 1975;292:832–843, 895–902.
2. Hong R. Bone marrow transplantation. *Adv Pediatr* 1993;40:101–124.
3. Armitage JO. Bone marrow transplantation. *N Engl J Med* 1994;330:827–838.
4. Walters MC, Patience M, Leisenring W, et al. Bone marrow transplantation for sickle cell disease. *N Engl J Med* 1996;335:369–376.
5. Krivit W, Lockman LA, Watkins PA, et al. The future for treatment by bone marrow transplantation for adrenoleukodystrophy, metachromatic leukodystrophy, globid cell leukodystrophy and Hurler syndrome. *J Inherit Metab Dis* 1995;18:398–412.
6. Shpall EJ, Stemmer SM, Bearman SI, et al. Role of autotransplantation in treatment of other solid tumors. *Hematol Oncol Clin North Am* 1993;7:663–686.
7. Tyndall A, Gratwohl A. Haemotopoietic stem and progenitor cells in the treatment of severe autoimmune diseases. *Ann Rheum Dis* 1996;55:149–151.
8. Brenner MK. Gene transfer to hematopoietic cells. *N Engl J Med* 1996;335:337–339.
9. Casper J, Camitta B, Truitt R, et al. Unrelated bone marrow donor transplants for children with leukemia or myelodysplasia. *Blood* 1995;85:2354–2363.
10. Kurtzburg J, Laughlin M, Graham ML, et al. Placental blood as a source of hematopoietic stem cells for transplantation into unrelated recipients. *N Engl J Med* 1996;335:157–166.
11. Gluckman E. The therapeutic potential of fetal and

neonatal hematopoietic stem cells. *N Engl J Med* 1996;335:1839–1840.

12. Wagner JE, Kernan NA, Steinbuch M, et al. Allogeneic sibling umbilical-cord blood transplantation in children with malignant and nonmalignant disease. *Lancet* 1995;346:214–219.

13. Winston DJ, Gale RP, Meyer DV, et al. Infectious complications of human bone marrow transplantation. *Medicine (Baltimore)* 1979;58:1–31.

14. Wingard JR. Advances in the management of infectious complications after bone marrow transplantation. *Bone Marrow Transplant* 1990;6:371–383.

15. Van de Meer JWM, Goguiot H, et al. Infections in bone marrow transplant recipients. *Semin Hematol* 1984;21:123–128.

16. Sable CA, Donowitz GR. Infections in bone marrow transplant recipients. *Clin Infect Dis* 1994;19:273–284.

17. Ellison RT. Infections associated with bone marrow transplantation. In: Gorbach S, Bartlett JG, Blacklow N, eds. *Infectious diseases,* 2nd ed. Philadelphia: Saunders, 1998:1237–1242.

18. Patrick CC. Infections in bone marrow transplant recipients. In: Long SS, Pickering LK, Prober CG, eds. *Principles and practice of pediatric infectious diseases.* New York: Churchill Livingstone, 1997:634–639.

19. Korbling M, Huh YO, Durett A, et al. Allogeneic blood stem cell transplantation: peripheralization and yield of donor-derived primitive hematopoietic cells (CD34+ and Thy−1dim) and lymphoid subsets, and possible predictors of engraftment and graft-versus-host disease. *Blood* 1995;86:2842–2848.

20. Roberts MM, To LB, Gillis D, et al. Immune reconstitution following peripheral blood stem cell transplantation, autologous bone marrow transplantation and allogeneic bone marrow transplantation. *Bone Marrow Transplant* 1993;12:469–475.

21. Charbonnier A, Sainty D, Faucher C, et al. Immune reconstitution after blood cell transplantation. *Hematol Cell Ther* 1997;39:261–264.

22. Wingard JR, Chen DY, Burns WH, et al. Cytomegalovirus infection after autologous bone marrow transplantation with comparison to infection after allogeneic bone marrow transplantation. *Blood* 1988;71:1432–1437.

23. Offner F, Cordonnier C, Ljungman P, et al. Impact of previous *Aspergillus* on the outcome of bone marrow transplantation. *Clin Infect Dis* 1998;26:1098–1103.

24. Nemunaitis J, Rabinowe SN, Singer JW, et al. Recombinant granulocyte-macrophage colony-stimulating factor after autologous bone marrow transplantation for lymphoid cancer. *N Engl J Med* 1991;324:1773–1778.

25. Bensinger WI, Clift RA, Ansasetti C, et al. Transplantation of allogeneic peripheral blood stem cells mobilized by recombinant human granulocyte colony stimulating factor. *Stem Cells* 1996;14:90–105.

26. Ferrarra JLM, Deeg HJ. Graft versus host disease. *N Engl J Med* 1991;324:667–674.

27. Bodey, GP, Buckley M, Sathe YS, et al. Quantitative relationship between circulating leukocytes and infection in patients with acute leukemia. *Ann Intern Med* 1966;64:328–340.

28. Gurney H. The problem of neutropenia resulting from cancer therapy. *Clinician* 1989;7:2–10.

29. Sickles EA, Green WH, Wiernick PH. Clinical presentation of infection in granulocytopenic patients. *Arch Intern Med* 1975;135:715–719.

30. Engelhard D. Bacterial and fungal infections in children undergoing bone marrow transplantation. *Bone Marrow Transplant* 1998;21[Suppl 2]:S78–S80.

31. Engelhard D, Elishoov H, Strauss N, et al. Nosocomial coagulase-negative staphylococcal infections in bone marrow transplantation recipients with central vein catheter: a 5-year prospective study. *Transplantation* 1996;61:430–434.

32. Dell'Orto MG, Rovelli A, Barzaghi A, et al. Febrile complications in the first 100 days after bone marrow transplantation in children: a single center's experience. *Pediatr Hematol Oncol* 1997;14:335–347.

33. Classen DC, Burke JP, Ford CD, et al. *Streptococcus mitis* sepsis in bone marrow transplant patients receiving oral antimicrobial prophylaxis. *Am J Med* 1990;89:441–446.

34. Villablanca JG, Stiner M, Kersey J, et al. The clinical spectrum of infections with viridans streptococci in bone marrow transplant patients. *Bone Marrow Transplant* 1990;6:387–393.

35. Valteau D, Hartmann O, Brugieres L, et al. Streptococcal septicaemia following autologous bone marrow transplantation in children treated with high-dose chemotherapy. *Bone Marrow Transplant* 1991;7:415–419.

36. Steiner M, Villablanca JG, Kersey J, et al. Viridans streptococcal shock in bone marrow transplantation patients. *Am J Hematol* 1993;42:3540–3558.

37. Bochud PY, Eggiman Ph, Calandra T, et al. Bacteremia due to viridans streptococcus in neutropenic patients with cancer: clinical spectrum and risk factors. *Clin Infect Dis* 1994;18:25–31.

38. Bochud P, Calandra T, Francioli P. Bacteremia due to viridans streptococci in neutropenic patients: a review. *Am J Med* 1994;97:256–264.

39. Henwick S, Koehler M, Patrick CC. Complications of bacteremia due to *Stomatococcus mucilaginosus* in neutropenic children. *Clin Infect Dis* 1993;17:667–671.

40. Meyers JD. Fungal infections in bone marrow transplant patients. *Semin Oncol* 1990;17:10–13.

41. Wingard JR. Fungal infections after bone marrow transplant. *Biol Blood Marrow Transplant* 1999;5:55–68.

42. Verfaille C, Weisdorf D, Haake R, et al. *Candida* infections in bone marrow transplant recipients. *Bone Marrow Transplant* 1991;8:177–184.

43. Goodrich JM, Reed EC, Mori M, et al. Clinical features and analysis of risk factors for invasive candidal infection after marrow transplantation. *J Infect Dis* 1991;164:731–740.

44. Wald A, Leisenring W, van Burik JA, et al. Epidemiology of *Aspergillus* infections in a large cohort of patients undergoing bone marrow transplantation. *J Infect Dis* 1997;175:1459–1466.

45. Morrison VA, Haake RJ, Weisdorf DJ. The spectrum of non-*Candida* fungal infections following bone marrow transplant. *Medicine (Baltimore)* 1993;72:78–89.

46. Morrison VA, McGlave PB. Mucormycosis in the BMT population. *Bone Marrow Transplant* 1993;11:383–388.

47. Gamis AS, Gudnason T, Giebink GS, et al. Dissemi-

nated infection with *Fusarium* in recipients of bone marrow transplants. *Rev Infect Dis* 1991;13, 1077–1088.

48. Ribaud P, Chastang C, Latge J-P, et al. Survival and prognostic factors of invasive aspergillosis after allogeneic bone marrow transplantation. *Clin Infect Dis* 1999;28:322–330.

49. Cartivarian SE, Anaissie EJ, Bodey GP. Emerging fungal pathogens in immunocompromised patients: classification, diagnosis and management. *Clin Infect Dis* 1993;17[Suppl 2]:S487–S491.

50. Wingard JR. Oral complications of cancer therapies: Infectious and noninfectious systemic consequences. *NCI Monogr* 1990;9:21–26.

51. Wasserman R, August CS, Plotkin SA. Viral infections in pediatric bone marrow transplant patients. *Pediatr Infect Dis J* 1988;7:109–115.

52. Tuan I, Dennison D, Weisdorf DJ. *Pneumocystis carinii* pneumonitis following bone marrow transplantation. *Bone Marrow Transplant* 1992;10:267–272.

53. Lucas KG, Pollok KE, Emanuel DJ. Post-transplant EBV induced lymphoproliferative disorders. *Leuk Lymphoma* 1996;25:1–8.

54. Atkinson K, Storb R, Prentice RL, et al. Analysis of late infections in 89 long-term survivors of bone marrow transplantation. *Blood* 1979;53:720–731.

55. Slavin MA, Meyers JD, Remington JS, et al. *Toxoplasma gondii* infection in marrow transplant patients: a 20-year experience. *Bone Marrow Transplant* 1994; 13:549–557.

56. Wingard JR, Dick JD, Charache P, et al. Antibiotic-resistant bacteria in surveillance stool cultures of patients with prolonged neutropenia. *Antimicrob Agents Chemother* 1986;30:435–439.

57. Riley DK, Pavia AT, Beatty PG, et al. Surveillance cultures in bone marrow transplant recipients: worthwhile or wasteful? *Bone Marrow Transplant* 1995;15: 469–473.

58. Schimpff SC. Oral complications of cancer therapies: surveillance cultures. *NCI Monogr* 1990;9:37–42.

59. Buckner CD, Clift RA, Sanders JA, et al. Protective environment for marrow transplant recipients: a prospective study. *Ann Intern Med* 1978;89:893–901.

60. Storb RA, Prentice RL, Buchner CD. Graft-versus-host disease and survival in patients with aplastic anemia treated by marrow grafts from HLA-identical siblings: beneficial effect of protective environment. *N Engl J Med* 1983;308:302–307.

61. Bustamante CI, Wade JC. Herpes simplex virus infection in the immunocompromised cancer patient. *J Clin Oncol* 1991;9:1903–1915.

62. Singh N, Carrigan DR. Human herpesvirus-6 in transplantation: an emerging pathogen. *Ann Intern Med* 1996;124:1065–1071.

63. Ambinder RF, Burns W, Forman M, et al. Hemorrhagic cystitis associated with adenovirus infection in bone marrow transplantation. *Arch Intern Med* 1986;146; 1400–1401.

64. Arthur RR, Shak KV, Baust SJ, et al. Association of BK viruria with hemorrhagic cystitis in recipient of bone marrow transplants. *N Engl J Med* 1986;315:230–234.

65. Russell SJ, Vowels MR, Vale T. Hemorrhagic cystitis in pediatric bone marrow transplant patients: an association with infective agents, GVHD and prior cy-

66. Childs R, Sanchez C, Engler H, et al. High incidence of adeno- and polyomavirus-induced hemorrhagic cystitis in bone marrow allotransplantation for hematological malignancy following T cell depletion and cyclosporine. *Bone Marrow Transplant* 1998;33: 889–893.

67. Cassano WF. Intravenous ribavirin therapy for adenovirus cystitis after allogeneic bone marrow transplantation. *Bone Marrow Transplant* 1991;7:247–248.

68. Cox GJ, Matsui SM, Lo RS, et al. Etiology and outcome of diarrhea after marrow transplant: a prospective study. *Gastroenterology* 1983;107:1398–1407.

69. Yolken RH, Bishop CA, Townsend TR, et al. Infectious gastroenteritis in bone marrow transplant recipients. *N Engl J Med* 1982;306:1010–1012.

70. Meyers JD, Flournoy N, Thomas ED. Nonbacterial pneumonia after allogeneic marrow transplantation: a review of ten year's experience. *Rev Infect Dis* 1982;4: 1119–1132.

71. Pannuti C, Gingrich R, Pfaller MA, et al. Nosocomial pneumonia in patients having bone marrow transplant: attributable mortality and risk factors. *Cancer* 1992; 69:2643–2662.

72. Wingard JR, Mellits ED, Sostrin MB, et al. Interstitial pneumonia after allogeneic marrow transplantation: nine-year experience at a single institution. *Medicine (Baltimore)* 1988;67:175–186.

73. Ljungman P, Cleaves CA, Meyers JD. Respiratory virus infections in immunocompromised patients. *Bone Marrow Transplant* 1984;4:35–40.

74. Wingard JR. Viral infections in leukemia and bone marrow transplant patients. *Leuk Lymphoma* 1993;11 [Suppl 2]:115–125.

75. Gussack GSA, Burson JG, Hudgins P, et al. Sinusitis in the bone marrow transplant patient: diagnosis and management. *Am J Rhinol* 1995;9:1–5.

76. Deutsch JH, Hudgins PA, Siegel JL, et al. The paranasal sinuses in patients with acute graft-versus-host disease. *Am J Neuroradiol* 1995;16:1287–1291.

77. Enright H, Haake R, Weisdorf D, et al. Cytomegalovirus pneumonia after bone marrow transplantation. *Transplantation* 1993;55:1339–1346.

78. Meyers JD, Flournoy N, Thomas ED. Risk factors for cytomegalovirus infection after human marrow transplantation. *J Infect Dis* 1990;162:478–488.

79. Enright H, Haake R, Weisdorf D, et al. Cytomegalovirus pneumonia after bone marrow transplantation: risk factors and response to therapy. *Transplantation* 1993;55:1339–1346.

80. Zaia JA. Epidemiology and pathogenesis of cytomegalovirus disease. *Semin Hematol* 1990;27[Suppl 1]:5–10.

81. Schmidt GM, Horak DA, Niland JC, et al. A randomized, controlled trial of prophylactic ganciclovir for cytomegalovirus pulmonary infection in recipients of allogeneic bone marrow transplants. *N Engl J Med* 1991;324:1005–1011.

82. Goodrich JM, Bowden RA, Fisher L, et al. Ganciclovir prophylaxis to prevent cytomegalovirus disease after allogeneic marrow transplant. *Ann Intern Med* 1993; 118:173–178.

83. Goodrich JM, Mori M, Gleaves CA, et al. Early treat-

ment with ganciclovir to prevent cytomegalovirus disease after allogeneic bone marrow transplantation. *N Engl J Med* 1991;325:1601–1607.

84. Miller WJ, McCollough J, Balfour HH, et al. Prevention of cytomegalovirus infection after bone marrow transplantation: a randomized trial of blood product screening. *Bone Marrow Transplant* 1991;7:227–234.

85. Bowden RA, Slichter SJ, Sayers M, et al. A comparison of filtered leukocyte-reduced and cytomegalovirus (CMV) seronegative blood products for the prevention of transfusion-associated CMV infection after marrow transplant. *Blood* 1995;86:3598–3603.

86. Salzberger B, Bowden RA, Hackman RC, et al. Neutropenia in allogeneic marrow transplant recipients receiving ganciclovir for prevention of cytomegalovirus disease: risk factors and outcome. *Blood* 1997;90: 2502–2508.

87. Meyers JD, Ljungman P, Fisher LD. Cytomegalovirus excretion as a predictor of cytomegalovirus disease after marrow transplantation: importance of cytomegalovirus viremia. *J Infect Dis* 1990;162:373–380.

88. Boeckh M, Gooley TA, Myerson D, et al. Cytomegalovirus pp65 antigenemia-guided early treatment with ganciclovir versus ganciclovir at engraftment after allogeneic marrow transplantation: a randomized double-blind study. *Blood* 1996;10: 4063–4071.

89. Boeckh M, Bowden RA, Gooley T, et al. Successful modification of a pp65 antigenemia-based early strategy for prevention of cytomegalovirus disease in allogeneic marrow transplant recipients. *Blood* 1999;93: 1781–1782.

90. Zaia JA, Gallez-Hawkins GM, Tegtmeier BR, et al. Late cytomegalovirus diseases in marrow transplantation is predicted by virus load in plasma. *J Infect Dis* 1997;176:782–785.

91. Boeckh M, Gallez-Hawkins GM, Myerson D, et al. Plasma polymerase chain reaction for cytomegalovirus DNA after allogeneic marrow transplantation: comparison with polymerase chain reaction using peripheral blood leukocytes, pp65 antigenemia, and viral culture. *Transplantation* 1997; 64:108–113.

92. Shields AF, Hackman RC, Fife KH, et al. Adenovirus infections in patients undergoing bone marrow transplantation. *N Engl J Med* 1985;312:529–533.

93. Hierholzer JC. Adenovirus in the immunocompromised host. *Clin Microbiol Rev* 1992;5:262–274.

94. Hale GA, Heslop HE, Krance RA, et al. Adenovirus infection after pediatric bone marrow transplantation. *Bone Marrow Transplant* 1999;23:277–282.

95. Howard DS, Phillips GL III, Reece DE, et al. Adenovirus infections in hematopoietic stem cell transplant recipients. *Clin Infect Dis* 1999;29:1494–1501.

96. Harrington RD, Hooton TM, Hackman RC, et al. An outbreak of respiratory syncytial virus in a bone marrow transplant center. *J Infect Dis* 1992;165: 987–993.

97. Hertz MI, Englund JA, Snover D, et al. Respiratory syncytial virus-induced acute lung injury in adult patients with bone marrow transplants: a clinical approach and review of the literature. *Medicine (Baltimore)* 1989;68:269–281.

98. Drobyski WR, Knox KK, Mayenski D, et al. Brief report: fatal encephalitis due to a variant B human herpesvirus-6 infection in a bone marrow transplant recipient. *N Engl J Med* 1994;330:1356–1360.

99. Knox KK, Carrigan DR. Chronic myelosuppression associated with persistent bone marrow infection due to human herpes virus 6 in a bone marrow transplant recipient. *Clin Infect Dis* 1996;22:174–175.

100. Cone RW, Huang ML, Hackman RC, et al. Coinfection with human herpes virus 6 variants A and B in lung tissue. *J Clin Microbiol* 1996;34:877–881.

101. Kadakia MP, Rybka WB, Stewart JA, et al. Human herpes virus 6: infection and disease following autologous and allogeneic bone marrow transplantation. *Blood* 1996;87:5341–5354.

102. Chan PKS, Peiris JSM, Yuen KY, et al. Human herpesvirus-6 and human herpesvirus-7 infections in bone marrow transplant recipients. *J Med Virol* 1997; 53:295–305.

103. Rieux C, Gaustheret-Dejean A, Challine-Lehmann D, et al. Human herpesvirus-6 meningoencephalitis in a recipient of an unrelated allogeneic bone marrow transplantation. *Transplantation* 1998;65:1408–1411.

104. Bosi A, Zazzi M, Amantini A, et al. Fatal herpes virus 6 encephalitis after unrelated bone marrow transplant. *Bone Marrow Transplant* 1998;22:285–288.

105. Kadakia MP. Human herpes virus 6 infection and associated pathogenesis following bone marrow transplantation. *Leuk Lymphoma* 1998;31:251–266.

106. Cone RW, Huang MC, Corey L, et al. Human herpes virus 6 infections after bone marrow transplantation: clinical and virologic manifestations. *J Infect Dis* 1999;179:311–318.

107. Wang FZ, Linde A, Hagglund H, et al. Human herpes virus 6 DNA in cerebrospinal fluid specimens from allogeneic bone marrow transplant patients: does it have clinical significance? *Clin Infect Dis* 1999;28: 562–568.

108. Maeda Y, Teshima T, Yamada M, et al. Monitoring of human herpes viruses after allogeneic peripheral blood stem cell transplantation. *Br J Haematol* 1999;1: 295–302.

109. Cone RW, Hackman RC, Huang M-LW, et al. Human herpes virus 6 in lung tissue from patients with pneumonitis after bone marrow transplantation. *N Engl J Med* 1993;329:156–161.

110. Wendt CH, Weisdorf DJ, Jordan MC, et al. Parainfluenza virus respiratory infection after bone marrow transplantation. *N Engl J Med* 1992;326:921–926.

111. Biggs, DD, Toorkey BC, Carrigan DR, et al. Disseminated echovirus infection complicating bone marrow transplantation. *Am J Med* 1990;88:421–425.

112. Lucas KG, Pollok KE, Emanuel DJ. Post-transplant EBV induced lymphoproliferative disorders. *Leuk Lymphoma* 1996;25:1–8.

113. Shapiro RS, McClain K, Frizzera G, et al. Epstein-Barr virus associated B-cell lymphoproliferative disorders following bone marrow transplantation. *Blood* 1988;71:1234–1243.

114. Zutterr MM, Martin PJ, Sale GE, et al. Epstein-Barr virus lymphoproliferation after bone marrow transplantation. *Blood* 1988;72:520–529.

115. Papadopoulos EB, Ladayani M, Emmanuel D, et al. Infusions of donor leukocytes as treatment of Epstein-Barr virus associated lymphoproliferative disorders

complicating allogeneic marrow transplantation. *N Engl J Med* 1994;330:1185–1191.

116. Rooney CM, Smith C, Ng CY, et al. Use of gene modified virus specific T lymphocytes to control Epstein-Barr-virus-related lymphoproliferation. *Lancet* 1995; 345:9–13.

117. Sullivan KM, Mori M, Sanders J, et al. Late complications of allogeneic and autologous marrow transplantation. *Bone Marrow Transplant* 1992;10:127–134.

118. Hoyle C, Goldman JM. Life-threatening infections occurring more than 3 months after BMT. *Bone Marrow Transplant* 1994;14:247–252.

119. Sullivan KM, Agura E, Anasetti C, et al. Chronic graft-versus-host disease and other late complications of bone marrow transplantation. *Semin Hemat* 1991;28: 250.

120. Atkinson K, Farewell V, Storb R, et al. Analysis of late infections after human bone marrow transplantation: role of genotypic nonidentity between marrow donor and recipient and of nonspecific suppressor, cells in patients with chronic graft-versus-host disease. *Blood* 1982;60:714–720.

121. Ochs L, Shu XO, Miller J, et al. Late infections after allogeneic bone marrow transplantation: comparison of incidence in related and unrelated donor transplant recipients. *Blood* 1995;86:3979–3986.

122. Sullivan KM, Nims J, Leisenring W, et al. Determinants of late infection following marrow transplantation for aplastic anemia and myelodysplastic syndrome. *Blood* 1995;86[Suppl 1]:213a(abst).

123. Aucouturier P, Barra A, Intrator L, et al. Long lasting IgG subclass and antibacterial polysaccharide antibody deficiency after allogeneic bone marrow transplantation. *Blood* 1987;70:779–785.

124. Winston DJ, Shiffman G, Wang D, et al. Pneumococcal infections after human bone marrow transplantation. *Ann Intern Med* 1979;91:835–841.

125. Han CS, Miller W, Haake R, et al. Varicella zoster infection after bone marrow transplantation: incidence, risk factors and complications. *Bone Marrow Transplant* 1994;13:277–283.

126. Fan FS, Tzeng CH, Hsiao KI, et al. Withdrawal of immunosuppresive therapy in allogeneic bone marrow transplantation reactivates chronic viral hepatitis C. *Bone Marrow Transplant* 1991;8:417–420.

127. Kolho E, Ruutu P, Ruutu T. Hepatitis C in BMT patients. *Bone Marrow Transplant* 1993;11:119–123.

128. Strasser SI, Myerson D, Spurgeon CL, et al. Hepatitis C virus infection and bone marrow transplantation: a cohort study with a 10-year follow-up. *Hepatology* 1999;29:1893–1899.

129. Frickhofen N, Wiesneth M, Jainta C, et al. Hepatitis C virus infection is a risk factor for liver failure from veno-occlusive disease after bone marrow transplantation. *Blood* 1994;83:1998–2004.

130. Lipton SA, Hickey WF, Morris JH, et al. Candidal infection in the central nervous system. *Am J Med* 1984;76:101–108.

131. Walsh TJ, Hier DB, Caplan LR. Fungal infections of the central nervous system: comparative analysis of risk factors and clinical signs in 57 patients. *Neurology* 1985;35:1654–1657.

132. Abbassi S, Shenep JL, Hughes WT, et al. *Aspergillus* in children with cancer: a 34-year experience. *Clin Infect Dis* 1999;29:1210–1219.

133. Hughes WT, Armstrong D, Bodey GP, et al. 1997 Guidelines for the use of antimicrobial agents in neutropenic patients with unexplained fever. *Clin Infect Dis* 1997;25:551–573.

134. Storring RA, Jameson B, Mcelwain TJ, et al. Oral nonabsorbable antiobiotics prevent infection in acute lymphoblastic leukemia. *Lancet* 1977;2:837–840.

135. Lew MA, Keohoe K, Ritz J, et al. Prophylaxis of bacterial infections with ciprofloxacin in patients undergoing bone marrow transplantations. *Transplantation* 1991;51;630–636.

136. Patrick CC. Use of fluoroquinolones as prophylactic agents in patients with neutropenia. *Pediatr Infect Dis J* 1997;16:135–139.

137. Goodman JL, Winston DJ, Greenfield RA, et al. A controlled trial of fluconazole to prevent fungal infections in patients undergoing bone marrow transplantation. *N Engl J Med* 1992;3:845–851.

138. Wingard JR, Mertz WG, Rinaldi MG, et al. Increase in *Candida krusei* infection among patients with bone marrow transplantation and neutropenia treated prophylactically with fluconazole. *N Engl J Med* 1991; 325:1274–1277.

139. Sullivan KM, Kopecky KJ, Jocom J, et al. Immunomodulatory and antimicrobial efficacy of intravenous immunoglobulin in bone marrow transplantation. *N Engl J Med* 1990;323:705–712.

140. Casper JT, Sedmak G, Harrie RE. Intravenous immunoglobulin: use in pediatric bone marrow transplantation. *Semin Hematol* 1992;29:[Suppl 2]: 100–105.

141. Winston DJ, Ho WG, Lin C-H, et al. Intravenous immunoglobulin for prevention of interstitial pneumonia after bone marrow transplantation. *Ann Intern Med* 1987;106:12–18.

142. Woff SN, Fay JW, Herzig RH, et al. High-dose weekly intravenous immunoglobulin to prevent infections in patients undergoing autologous bone marrow transplantation or severe myelosuppressive therapy: a study of the American Bone Marrow Transplant Group. *Ann Intern Med* 1993;118:937–942.

143. Ljungman P, Duraj V, Magnius L. Response to immunization against polio after allogeneic marrow transplant. *Bone Marrow Transplant* 1991;7:89–93.

144. Engelhard D, Nagelar, Hardan I, et al. Antibody response to a two-dose regimen of influenza vaccine in allogeneic T cell-depleted and autologous BMT recipients. *Bone Marrow Transplant* 1993;11:1–5.

145. Ljungman P, Fridell E, Lonnqvst B, et al. Efficacy and safety of vaccination of marrow transplant recipients with a live attenuated measles, mumps, and rubella vaccine. *J Infect Dis* 1989;159:610–615.

146. Molrine D, Guinan E, Antin J, et al. Donor immunizations with *Haemophilus influenzae* type B (HIB)-conjugate vaccine in allogeneic bone marrow transplantation. *Blood* 1996;87:3012–3018.

147. Avanzini M, Carra A, Maccario R, et al. Antibody response to pneumococcal vaccine in children receiving bone marrow transplantations. *J Clin Immunol* 1995; 15:137–144.

148. Guinan E, Molrine D, Antin J, et al. Polysaccharide conjugate vaccine response in bone marrow transplant recipients. *Transplantation* 1994;57:677–684.

149. Hammarstrom V, Pauksen K, Azinge J, et al. The influence of graft versus host reaction on the response to

pneumococcal vaccination in bone marrow transplant patients. *Support Care Cancer* 1993;1:195–199.

150. Barra A, Cordonnier C, Preziosi M, et al. Immunogenicity of *Haemophilus influenzae* type B conjugate vaccine in allogeneic bone marrow recipients. *J Infect Dis* 1992;166:1021–1028.

151. Lortan JE, Vellodi A, Jurges ES, et al. Class- and subclass-specific pneumococcal antibody levels and response to immunization after bone marrow transplantation. *Clin Exp Immunol* 1992;88:512–519.

152. Ljungman P, Wiklund HM, Duraj V, et al. Response to tetanus toxoid immunization after allogeneic bone marrow transplantation. *J Infect Dis* 1990;162:496–500.

153. Parkkali T, Olander R, Ruutu T, et al. A randomized comparison between early and late vaccine with tetanus toxoid vaccine after allogeneic BMT. *Bone Marrow Transplant* 1997;19:933–938.

154. Giebink GS, Warkentin PI, Ramsay NKC, et al. Titers of antibody to pneumococci in allogeneic bone marrow transplant recipients before and after vaccination with pneumococcal vaccine. *J Infect Dis* 1992;166:1021–1028.

10

Vascular Access Device Infections

Patricia M. Flynn

Department of Infectious Diseases, St. Jude Children's Research Hospital, Memphis, Tennessee 38105;
Department of Pediatrics, Division of Infectious Diseases, University of Tennessee,
Memphis, Tennessee 38103

Since the introduction of the Broviac catheter in 1973 (1), the use of this and similar long-term catheters has increased greatly. Initially designed for the administration of parenteral nutrition, these catheters are now widely used in oncology patients, in neonates, and in patients infected with human immunodeficiency virus (HIV), cystic fibrosis, hemophilia, and other chronic medical conditions that require frequent venous access. In general, these catheters are well tolerated, convenient, and accepted by patients, parents, and medical staff. The two major complications are thrombosis and infection. This chapter focuses on infections in Broviac and Hickman catheters and in totally implanted vascular access devices (VADs).

HISTORICAL PERSPECTIVE

In 1973, Broviac et al. (1) reported the use of a silicone rubber central venous catheter that was tunneled subcutaneously before exiting the skin. In addition to the subcutaneous tunnel, a polyester cuff was located proximal to the skin exit site. Fibrotic tissue developed around this cuff and potentially provided both stability and a barrier to infection (Fig. 10.1A). This prototype catheter was used successfully to administer parenteral nutrition, but because it had a small lumen, withdrawing blood samples was difficult. Hickman et al. (2) modified the

Broviac catheter in 1979 for use in bone marrow transplant recipients. The internal diameter of this catheter was significantly larger, thereby aiding the administration of blood products and withdrawing blood samples. Hickman catheters are now available with two lumens.

During the past decade, the totally implantable VAD has become popular (3). This device is similar to the Broviac/Hickman (B/H) catheter except that the distal end of the catheter, a portal, lies in a surgically created subcutaneous pocket (Fig. 10.1B). The catheter is accessed by using a noncoring needle to puncture the diaphragm of the subcutaneous portal through the skin (Fig. 10.2). These devices are desirable, particularly in adolescent patients, because they preserve body image. Additionally, they require flushing less often than B/H catheters and thus may be less susceptible to infection.

Catheter-related infections can be divided into superficial infections (those involving the exit site or tunnel tract) and septic infections. The latter can occur with or without evidence of superficial infection. The generally agreed on definition of exit-site infection is the presence of erythema, tenderness, induration, and purulence within 2 cm of the skin exit of the catheter (4) or within 2 cm from any edge of a subcutaneous port (5). The latter also is called a "pocket" infection (6). Tunnel tract infection is the development of erythema, ten-

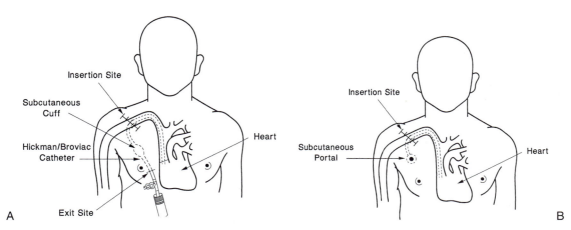

FIG. 10.1. A: Broviac/Hickman catheter. The catheter is tracked subcutaneously to exit the skin at a distant site. A polyester cuff lies within the tract. **B:** Totally implantable vascular access device. A portal lies in a surgically created subcutaneous pocket.

derness, and induration along the subcutaneous tract of the B/H catheter at a distance greater than 2 cm from the skin exit site with or without signs of inflammation or purulence at the exit site (4). Similarly, this definition can include the subcutaneous port (5).

The definition of catheter-related sepsis has changed over time. These definitions have included (a) all septic episodes in patients with central venous catheters (7), (b) episodes of clinical sepsis that resolve after removal of the catheter (8), (c) episodes of sepsis when the same organism has been cultured from both the catheter tip and the blood (9), and (d) the presence of significantly higher concentrations of organisms in blood obtained via the catheter than from a peripheral vein (10,11).

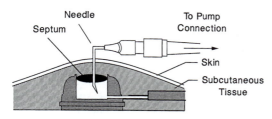

FIG. 10.2. A noncoring needle is inserted at a 90-degree angle through the skin and septum of the portal.

Although standardization of a definition of catheter-related sepsis has not been achieved, most current studies employ comparison of blood cultures obtained via the catheter with that obtained from a peripheral vein.

ETIOLOGY OF INFECTIONS

The organisms involved in catheter-related infections can be divided into those that cause septic infections and those that cause superficial infections. Gram-positive cocci predominate in both categories. In a comprehensive review, Decker and Edwards (12) summarized 13 studies of etiologic agents of catheter-related sepsis in pediatric patients. It should be noted that various definitions of catheter-related sepsis were used in these studies. Gram-positive cocci accounted for 64% of all isolates, of which more than half were coagulase-negative staphylococci. Gram-negative bacilli accounted for 28% of all isolates with *Klebsiella* sp. and *Escherichia coli* predominating. Fungal organisms, namely *Candida* spp. and *Malassezia furfur,* represented 6% of all isolates. Multiple organisms were involved in 12% of presumed catheter-related septicemic episodes. There is no apparent association of infecting organisms with underlying diseases; however, Piedra et al.

(13) noted that gram-negative bacilli were more commonly isolated from children with short bowel syndrome compared with those from children with malignancies. Recent reports suggested that the relative frequency of gram-negative bacillary infections may be increasing (14,15). Additional surveillance is necessary to confirm changing epidemiology rather than isolated differences.

Decker and Edwards also summarized six studies of isolates from superficial infections in pediatric patients (12). Again, gram-positive cocci were most frequently isolated and accounted for 51% of all isolates. *Staphylococcus aureus* (16% of all isolates) and coagulase-negative staphylococci (14%) were the most common. Gram-negative bacilli accounted for 41% of the isolates. *Pseudomonas aeruginosa* was the most frequently isolated gram-negative organism (16% of all isolates). Fungal organisms were noted only rarely (2%) in the studies reviewed (12). In a review of VAD-infections in a pediatric oncology hospital, however, *Candida* spp. were isolated from 35% of exit-site and tunnel-tract infections (5). The frequency of *Candida* spp. infections in this patient population may have been associated with the use of topical antibiotic ointment on the exit sites of B/H catheters in that institution. Whereas the relationship between use of antibiotic ointment and fungal colonization of the skin exit site has not been evaluated for B/H catheters, studies of other intravenous catheters demonstrated an association between *Candida* spp. colonization and antibiotic ointment use (16,17).

Fewer reports of infections associated with totally implanted VADs have appeared (5, 18–23). As with B/H catheters, gram-positive organisms were the most frequently isolated. Coagulase-negative staphylococci were the predominant organism in both septic and superficial infections, accounting for more than half of all isolates in both categories. *S. aureus* was isolated in 20% and 15% of septic and superficial infections, respectively.

Several unusual pathogens deserve special attention because of their role in VAD infections. *Malassezia furfur* and *M. pachyderma-* *tis* are lipophilic yeasts that can be present on human skin. *M. furfur* is the causative agent of tinea versicolor. These organisms have gained notoriety as pathogens in neonates with central venous catheters who are receiving lipid emulsion infusions (24). The rapidly growing atypical mycobacteria *Mycobacterium fortuitum* and *M. chelonae* also have been reported recently to cause both exit-site infections and bacteremia in patients fitted with B/H catheters (25–27). No common source has been identified, and they are thought to be sporadic and arise from environmental sources.

PATHOPHYSIOLOGY

As with all foreign material and prostheses, the presence of a VAD induces changes in host factors that could predispose to the development of infection. These factors were reviewed by Dickinson and Bisno (28). All catheters induce chronic inflammation, the so-called foreign-body reaction. After placement, a thrombin sheath, which is rich in fibrin and fibronectin, coats the catheter. Additionally, some catheter materials, such as Teflon, may decrease the phagocytic and bactericidal properties of neutrophils (29).

Microorganisms can gain access to the catheter in several ways (30). They can (a) be introduced at the time of catheter placement, (b) colonize the skin surface and migrate along the catheter tract (31,32), (c) be introduced by contaminated infusates (30), (d) contaminate the catheter hub as a result of manipulation (30,33), or (e) seed the catheter from distant sites of infection (4,31). Although all these methods can result in catheter-related infection, most VAD infections most likely are caused by intraluminal colonization by microorganisms resulting from manipulation by medical staff or the patients themselves or the migration of microorganisms along the external surface of the catheter from colonized skin surfaces (34). The timing of infection may also be related to the source of the infecting microorganism; early infections more likely are caused by skin microorganisms and late infections via the catheter hub or lumen contamination (34).

Once the microorganism reaches the catheter, several complex and poorly understood factors are involved with adherence. Current knowledge of these factors was reviewed by Dickinson and Bisno (28). *S. aureus* and *Candida albicans* can adhere tightly to the fibrin-rich and coagulase-negative staphylococci to the fibronectin-rich layer of the catheter's biofilm (35). Coagulase-negative staphylococci and their role in adherence to catheter materials has been investigated most thoroughly (36). The results of these studies suggest that the bacterial organisms actually can embed themselves in the catheter and reproduce without external nutrients. In addition, these organisms can produce a slime-like substance that might further enhance adherence to the catheter surface and potentially act as a barrier from antibiotics and host defenses (36).

EPIDEMIOLOGY

The epidemiology of VAD-related infections varies greatly according to the patient population being studied as well as the design, maintenance, and usage patterns of the catheter (Table 10.1). For purposes of this review, disease-related risk in pediatric populations, if available, will be used.

Oncology Patients

Single-Lumen Broviac/Hickman Catheters

Extensive experience with B/H catheters in pediatric oncology patients has been reported. Despite similar surgical placement and care plans, the rate of infection varies greatly among studies (23,37–52). When all infections were tallied, the overall rate was 2.86 infections per 1,000 days of catheter use and the rate of septic infections was 1.82 infections per 1,000 days of catheter use. In some of these studies, a relatively indiscriminate definition of catheter-related sepsis was used (any positive blood culture from a patient with a catheter in place) and may have falsely inflated the catheter-related sepsis rate.

Most authors report infection rates as episodes per days of catheter use or provide data to do so; however, others prefer to report time to infection by using Kaplan–Meier estimates (5,48). This method is useful for representing the rate of catheter-related infection as it changes with the duration of catheterization (Fig. 10.3). Wurzel et al. (48) found the risk of catheter-related infection during the first month after placement to be three times greater than in the second month and more than 100 times greater than after 2 months. Similar increases in risk during the first month of catheter placement also were noted by King et al. (39) and Mirro et al. (5).

TABLE 10.1. *Reported infection rates[a] for vascular access devices in pediatric patients*

	Total no. of catheters	Total no. of catheter days	Sepsis rate	Overall infection rate[b]
Oncology patients with Broviac Hickman catheters[c]	1,131	223,659	1.82	2.86
Oncology patients with totally implanted VADs[d]	174	37,177	0.56	0.83
Patients receiving TPN[e]	116	8,974	4.90	5.01
Neonates with Broviac catheters[f]	532	24,797	4.64	4.64

TPN, total parenteral nutrition; VAD, vascular access device.
[a]Rates reported as episodes per 1,000 catheter days.
[b]Includes superficial and septic infections.
[c]See refs. 23, 37–52.
[d]See refs. 19–23, 48.
[e]See refs. 37, 54, 55.
[f]See refs. 39, 58–62.

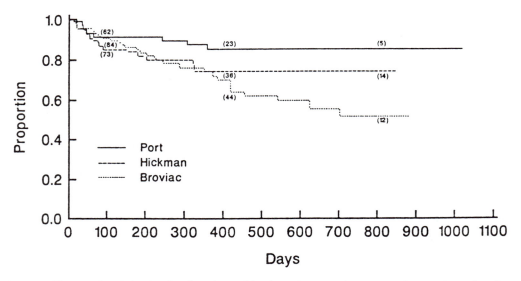

FIG. 10.3. Time to first infection in all patients. Numbers in parentheses are the number of patients analyzed at 100, 400, and 700 days of use for each catheter type. (From Mirro J Jr, Rao BN, Stokes DC, et al. A prospective study of Hickman/Broviac catheters and implantable ports in oncology patients. *J Clin Oncol* 1989;7:214, with permission.)

Significantly high infection rates also have been demonstrated in younger age groups. Johnson et al. (43) and Wurzel et al. (48) noted that toddlers and children younger than 2 years of age were at higher risk than older oncology patients. This increased risk has been attributed to the proximity of the externalized catheter tip to the diaper area and the ability of toddlers to disrupt the catheter dressing.

The role of neutropenia in catheter-related infection is controversial. To date, conflicting reports have been published (45,46). It does appear, however, that catheters placed during neutropenia are more likely to become infected (45).

Double-Lumen Hickman Catheters

Hickman-style catheters with two lumens have become an important device for critically ill cancer patients, especially bone mar-

row transplant recipients. Although these catheters are commonly used in cancer patients, no randomized, controlled study comparing single- and double-lumen catheters has been done. In a nonrandomized study of pediatric cancer patients, Shulman et al. (53) found single- and double-lumen catheters to have similar infection rates.

Totally Implanted Vascular Access Device

Although experience with implanted devices in pediatric oncology patients is limited, sufficient reports have been published to discuss these devices (19–23,48). When all infections are combined, the overall rate of infection in totally implanted VADs is 0.83 infections per 1,000 days of catheter use. Although this is substantially less than that for B/H catheters (2.86 infections per 1,000 patient days), no study has randomized patients with comparable risk factors to receive either catheter type. In studies conducted at three different centers, the infection rates were lower for implantable devices than for B/H catheters, but the difference was not statistically significant (5,23,48). Even when independent factors that can affect infection rates, such as age, were controlled, implanted ports fared better. As with B/H catheters, the infection rates with ports were greatest in the initial period after catheter placement. Mirro et al. (5) noted a statistically significant increase in infection rates in patients with Broviac catheters compared with implanted ports but only after 400 days of catheter use.

Patients Receiving Total Parenteral Nutrition

Little available data are available to calculate an infection rate for pediatric patients receiving only total parenteral nutrition (TPN). Combining data from several studies (39,54,55) results in an overall rate of 5.01 infections per 1,000 days of catheter use. Apparently, this rate is truly higher than that for pediatric oncology patients with similar catheters receiving comparable clinical care. Indeed, the infection rate in pediatric patients receiving TPN was more than twice that of cancer patients in a study by King et al. (39). Additionally, children with cancer receiving TPN have a 2.4-fold greater risk of developing a catheter-related infection compared with those not receiving TPN (56). Lipid infusions also may increase the risk of catheter-related infection in neonates (57).

Neonates

Infection rates are uniformly higher in neonates with Broviac catheters than in pediatric cancer patients. When six studies are combined (39,58–62), the incidence of sepsis in neonates is 4.64 per 1,000 catheter days. Most patients were critically ill and had many risk factors for infection. Very low-birth-weight infants had an especially high incidence of infection (62).

Patients Infected with Human Immunodeficiency Virus

Scanty evidence exists to indicate that catheter-related infections occur more frequently in HIV-positive adults than HIV-negative adults (63). Pizzo et al. (64) reported that HIV-positive children receiving continuous infusion zidovudine had a slightly higher incidence of catheter-related infection than children with cancer at the same institution.

CLINICAL MANIFESTATIONS

The hallmark of superficial infection of VADs is erythema, tenderness, induration, or purulence at the catheter exit site, overlying the subcutaneous portal, or extending along the subcutaneous path of the catheter. Fever is the most common manifestation of septic VAD-related infections and was noted in 91% of infections reported by King et al. (39). Of important note is the occurrence of chills that might occur after manipulation of the catheter, suggesting that flushing the catheter causes the release of microorganisms into the bloodstream.

Tachycardia, lethargy, apnea, and bradycardia have been noted to occur much less often than fever and usually affect fewer than 20% of all patients (39). Unfortunately, no data are available regarding whether neonates respond to catheter-related infection differently than older children.

LABORATORY DIAGNOSIS

The diagnosis of superficial catheter-related infection usually is usually made by physical examination. Gram's stain, acid-fast stain, and culturing the site or drainage can be helpful in establishing the etiologic agent(s).

The difficulty of diagnosing a catheter-related septic infection is in distinguishing it from septic episodes unrelated to the catheter. Because most patients with VADs are immunocompromised, they are inherently at increased risk of developing sepsis. Procedures to discriminate septic episodes can be divided into those that require catheter removal and those that can be performed with the catheter in place.

Initial efforts to diagnose catheter-related infections included a semiquantitative culture of the catheter tip. Maki et al. (65) noted a high correlation of catheter-related sepsis with the presence of more than 15 colony-forming units isolated after the catheter tip was rolled across a 5% sheep-blood agar plate. Several other authors have sought to make rapid diagnoses of catheter-related infections by using Gram stain (66) or acridine orange stain (67) of the catheter tip. All these methods were performed on a variety of intravascular catheters and their usefulness in the diagnosis of long-term VAD infections is limited because they require removal of the catheter.

To circumvent removing the catheter, several investigators suggested using comparative quantitative cultures of blood obtained via both the catheter and a peripheral vein (10,11,68–72). An infection is considered to be catheter-related when colony counts are greater than fourfold higher in blood obtained via the catheter than from a peripheral vein. Using this technique, comparative quantitative cultures have been shown to have a sensitivity of 94%, a specificity of 100%, and a positive predictive value of 100% (72). Quantitative cultures can be performed by using pour plates (68), direct plating of small aliquots of blood (10), serial quantitative dilutions of blood (11), or the DuPont Isolator (69–71). Although comparative quantitative cultures are relatively complex, this is the most specific method of diagnosing catheter-related sepsis.

THERAPY

Initially, it was thought that all VADs should be removed if sepsis or signs of local infection were present (73,74). With the widespread use of surgically placed B/H catheters, however, this notion was challenged because the catheters are intended for long-term use and additional surgical procedures are re-

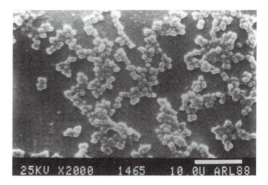

FIG. 10.4. Scanning electron microscopy reveals adherence of coagulase-negative staphylococci to a subcutaneous port septum following an unsuccessful course of in situ antibiotic therapy (2,000×). (Courtesy of Drs. W. Ghesquiere, A. Hayashi, and I.W. Killam, Hospital for Children, Halifax, Nova Scotia, Canada.)

quired to replace them. There has been considerable experience with in situ therapy for infections in pediatric patients. When information from available studies was pooled (5, 11,23,38,39,41,43,44,46,55,62,75), approximately 76% of all B/H catheter-related infections were successfully treated with antibiotics, without catheter removal.

The data regarding infections related to totally implanted devices in pediatric patients are limited. Whereas some investigators report successful treatment of these infections in situ (5,21), others noted that they are more difficult to resolve (19,23,76). Pegelow et al. (19) suggested that the dead space of the portal provides a sanctuary for microorganisms that is not readily accessible by antibiotics. Indeed, Ghesquiere et al. (76) presented scanning electron micrographs illustrating the presence of many bacteria adhering to the septum of the portal after an unsuccessful course of in situ antibiotic therapy (Fig. 10.4).

Therapy for Presumed Septic Infections

Because fever is the most common clinical symptom of catheter-related sepsis, all febrile episodes in children with catheters must be investigated. Particular attention should be given to those patients who develop chills or fever or both associated with catheter flushing. When possible, blood samples for quantitative culture should be obtained via both the catheter and a peripheral vein. For neutropenic patients, empiric antibiotic therapy should be started. Therapy should include broad-spectrum antibiotics as is usual in this population; vancomycin for coagulase-negative staphylococci coverage also should be considered.

The necessity for empiric antibiotic therapy is not clear in nonneutropenic patients because there are several other causes of fever in this population. Prince et al. (55) noted that catheter-related sepsis caused only about one third of febrile episodes in children with Broviac catheters who were receiving TPN. The decision to administer antibiotics to nonneutropenic patients must be made on an individual basis (12,45). When antibiotic therapy is given, it should include vancomycin plus an aminoglycoside (12,55,75,77) or vancomycin plus a third-generation cephalosporin (77,78).

If catheter-related sepsis is diagnosed, appropriate changes in antibiotic therapy can be made. Antibiotics should be administered through the catheter for 10 to 14 days (11,12). If the catheter is no longer necessary, the patient's clinical condition deteriorates, or blood cultures continue to be positive after the patient has received 48 to 72 hours of appropriate therapy, the catheter should be removed (55,77,78). Antibiotic administration to these patients should be determined by the patient's clinical status and pathogenicity of the isolate.

Although about three fourths of catheter-related infections can be managed without catheter removal, several organisms are particularly difficult to eradicate. In general, successful treatment of *Candida* spp. and *Malassezia* spp. infections require catheter removal (24,39,46,62,77,80). Eppes et al. (79) reviewed candidemia in patients with several types of central catheters and noted that persistent fungemia, morbidity, and mortality were associated with attempts to maintain the catheters in patients with candidemia. They recommend prompt removal of the central catheter and initiation of antifungal therapy for children with catheter-related candidemia.

Other organisms that may prove difficult to eradicate include *Bacillus* sp. (11,12,81), methicillin-resistant *S. aureus* (62) and atypical mycobacteria (25–27). The presence of multiple organisms also may decrease the likelihood of successful in situ therapy (41).

The use of urokinase as adjuvant therapy to antibiotics has been proposed. Urokinase may dissolve the fibrin sheath around the catheter that harbors microorganisms, making them susceptible to circulating antibiotics and host defenses. To date, adequate controlled trials have not been completed. A recent pediatric trial was halted because of possible adverse events. Among 41 patients is a placebo-controlled trial, no difference in bacterial clearance was detected (82). A larger study of 63 patients failed to demonstrate improved infection clearance with urokinase (83).

Several centers recommended the use of antibiotic "dwell" or "lock" therapy in lieu of, or in addition to, conventional infused antibiotic therapy. In this approach, concentrated solutions of select antibiotics are instilled into the catheter for up to 24 hours. Although no controlled trials have been performed, many investigators have reported success (84–87). Caution should be exercised when using this technique, especially in immunocompromised patients, who may have seeding of distant sites during catheter-related bacteremia.

Therapy for Superficial Infections

Usually, infection limited to the exit site can be managed with local care with or without the addition of antibiotic (44). If appropriate oral agents are not available or the patient is neutropenic, antibiotics should be administered parenterally (12). Exit-site infection caused by *Pseudomonas aeruginosa* may be more difficult to eradicate than infections caused by other organisms (5,43,45). Whereas fungemia most likely requires catheter removal, *Candida* spp. exit-site infections without extension into the tunnel tract may be successfully treated with topical therapy (5).

Tunnel-tract (5,11,44,46) and portal infections (23) have proven to be much more difficult to treat with in situ therapy. Available data suggest that only one third of tunnel tract infections (4) and one half of portal infections (5,23) will be cured without catheter removal. Decisions to attempt in situ therapy of these infections must be made on an individual basis.

COMPLICATIONS

Although most VAD infections can be treated successfully in situ, complications resulting from these infections can occur. The most severe are septic thrombophlebitis and endocarditis. Septic thrombophlebitis has been reported to account for 3.5% of catheter-related infections in adults with Hickman catheters (4). The frequency of this complication in pediatric patients is unknown. Treatment consists of catheter removal, antibiotic therapy, and possible surgical resection of the involved venous segments (4).

Endocarditis is a rare complication of catheter-related infection. It is difficult to determine an incidence rate because most cases appear in case reports rather than epidemiologic studies (88–90). Treatment requires removal of the catheter, long-term antibiotic therapy, and possible surgery if a large infected thrombus is present (89). All patients with catheter-related sepsis who develop septic emboli or have persistent or recurrent bacteremia should have echocardiographic examinations (90).

PREVENTION

Education and consistency in catheter care are undoubtedly the mainstays of preventing infection. Trained personnel to educate patients, parents, and other health care professionals about catheter care have proven beneficial (91). Different regimens for exit-site care of B/H catheters have been adapted from studies of short-term central venous catheters and peripheral cannulae. Most centers prefer a dry gauze dressing over the exit site. This dressing is associated with significantly lower rates of site colonization, site infection, and catheter-related sepsis compared with transparent occlusive dressings in central venous catheters (92). Infection risk may be less with new semipermeable dressings compared with occlusive dressings, but comparative studies need to be performed (93). Occlusive dressing can be reserved for bathing and swimming in chlorinated pools. Topical povidone–iodine is commonly applied to the exit site of B/H catheters in some centers. Antibiotic ointment is used less commonly. Whereas antibiotic ointment may decrease the number of sites colonized by pathogenic bacteria (94), higher rates of *Candida* spp. colonization may occur (17). Both ointments decreased the number of local infections of peripheral cannulae, but only antibiotic ointment did so significantly (17).

Routine flushing of the catheter with a mixture of heparin and vancomycin has significantly reduced the incidence of catheter-related bacteremia with vancomycin-susceptible organisms when the combination was compared with heparin alone (95,96). Larger trials of this combination regimen are needed before general use can be recommended.

Long-term VADs have been in general use for more than a decade and have proven advantageous despite the risk of infection. Further studies of pathogenesis, adjuvant therapy, and prevention of infections are needed to enhance our knowledge of how these useful devices can be used more safely and efficiently.

REFERENCES

1. Broviac JW, Cole JJ, Scribner BH. A silicone rubber atrial catheter for prolonged parenteral alimentation. *Surg Gynecol Obstet* 1973;136:602–606.
2. Hickman RO, Buckner CD, Clift RA, et al. A modified right atrial catheter for access to the venous system in marrow transplant recipients. *Surg Gynecol Obstet* 1979;148:871–875.
3. Gyves J, Ensminger W, Niederhuber J, et al. Totally implanted system for intravenous chemotherapy in patients with cancer. *Am J Med* 1982;73:841–845.
4. Mirro J Jr, Rao BN, Stokes DC, et al. A prospective study of Hickman/Broviac catheters and implantable ports in oncology patients. *J Clin Oncol* 1989;7:214–222.
5. Press OW, Ramsey PG, Larson EB, et al. Hickman catheter infections in patients with malignancies. *Medicine* 1984;63:189–200.

6. Centers for Disease Control and Prevention. Intravascular device-related infection. *Federal Register* 1995;60: 49978–50006.

7. Dillon JD Jr, Schaffner W, Van Way CW III, et al. Septicemia and total parenteral nutrition. Distinguishing catheter-related from other septic episodes. *JAMA* 1973; 223:1341–1344.

8. Ryan JA Jr, Abel RM, Abbott WM, et al. Catheter complications in total parenteral nutrition: a prospective study of 200 consecutive patients. *N Engl J Med* 1974; 290:757–761.

9. Abrahm JL, Mullen JL. A prospective study of prolonged central venous access in leukemia. *JAMA* 1982; 248:2868–2873.

10. Raucher HS, Hyatt AC, Barzilai A, et al. Quantitative blood cultures in the evaluation of septicemia in children with Broviac catheters. *J Pediatr* 1984;104:29–33.

11. Flynn PM, Shenep JL, Stokes DC, et al. In situ management of confirmed central venous catheter-related bacteremia. *Pediatr Infect Dis J* 1987;6:729–734.

12. Decker MD, Edwards KM. Central venous catheter infections. *Pediatr Clin North Am* 1988;35:579–612.

13. Piedra PA, Dryja DM, LaScolea LJ Jr. Incidence of catheter-associated gram-negative bacteremia in children with short bowel syndrome. *J Clin Microbiol* 1989; 27:1317–1319.

14. Castagnola E, Garaventa A, Viscoli C, et al. Changing pattern of pathogens causing broviac catheter-related bacteremias in children with cancer. *J Hosp Infect* 1995; 29:129–133.

15. Groeger JS, Lucas AB, Thaler HT, et al. Infectious morbidity associated with long-term use of venous access devices in patients with cancer. *Ann Intern Med* 1993; 119:1168–1174.

16. Norden CW. Application of antibiotic ointment to the site of venous catheterization—a controlled trial. *J Infect Dis* 1969;129:611–615.

17. Maki DG, Band JD. A comparative study of polyantibiotic and iodophor ointments in prevention of vascular catheter-related infection. *Am J Med* 1981;70:739–744.

18. Lokich JJ, Bothe A Jr, Benotti P, et al. Complications and management of implanted venous access catheters. *J Clin Oncol* 1985;3:710–717.

19. Pegelow CH, Narvaez M, Toledano SR, et al. Experience with a totally implantable venous device in children. *Am J Dis Child* 1986;140:69–71.

20. Shulman RJ, Rahman S, Mahoney D, et al. A totally implanted venous access system used in pediatric patients with cancer. *J Clin Oncol* 1987;5:137–140.

21. McDowell HP, Hart CA, Martin J. Implantable subcutaneous venous catheters. *Arch Dis Child* 1986;61: 1037–1038.

22. Soucy P. Experiences with the use of the Port-a-Cath in children. *J Pediatr Surg* 1987;22:767–769.

23. Ross MN, Haase GM, Poole MA, Burrington JD, et al. Comparison of totally implanted reservoirs with external catheters as venous access devices in pediatric oncologic patients. *Surg Gynecol Obstet* 1988;167:141–144.

24. Powell DA, Aungst J, Snedden S, et al. Broviac catheter-related *Malassezia furfur* sepsis in five infants receiving intravenous fat emulsions. *J Pediatr* 1984;105:987–990.

25. Flynn PM, Van Hooser B, Gigliotti F. Atypical mycobacterial infections of Hickman catheter exit sites. *Pediatr Infect Dis J* 1988;7:510–513.

26. Svirbely JR, Buesching WJ, Ayers LW, et al. *Mycobacterium fortuitum* infection of a Hickman catheter site. *Am J Clin Pathol* 1983;80:733–735.

27. Hoy JF, Rolston KVI, Hopfer RL, et al. *Mycobacterium fortuitum* bacteremia in patients with cancer and long-term venous catheters. *Am J Med* 1987;83:213–217.

28. Dickinson GM, Bisno AL. Infections associated with indwelling devices: concepts of pathogenesis; infections associated with intravascular devices. *Antimicrob Agents Chemother* 1989;33:597–601.

29. Zimmerli W, Lew PD, Waldvogel FA. Pathogenesis of foreign body infection. Evidence for a local granulocyte defect. *J Clin Invest* 1984;73:1191–1200.

30. Liñares J, Sitges-Serra A, Garau J, et al. Pathogenesis of catheter sepsis: a prospective study with quantitative and semiquantitative cultures of catheter hub and segments. *J Clin Microbiol* 1985;21:357–360.

31. Bjornson HS, Colley RN, Bower RH, et al. Association between microorganism growth at the catheter insertion site and colonization of the catheter in patients receiving total parenteral nutrition. *Surgery* 1982;92:720–727.

32. Snydman DR, Gorbea HF, Pober BR, et al. Predictive value of surveillance skin cultures in total-parenteral-nutrition-related infection. *Lancet* 1982;2:1385–1388.

33. Weightman NC, Simpson EM, Speller DCE. Source of infection in Hickman catheters. *J Clin Pathol* 1986;39: 1046.

34. Sherertz RJ. Pathogenesis of vascular catheter-related infections. In: Seifert H, Jansen B, Farr BM, eds. *Catheter-related infections.* New York: Marcel Dekker, Inc, 1997:1–29.

35. Raad II, Safar H. Long-term central venous catheters: Infectious complications and cost. In: Seifert H, Jansen B, Farr BM, eds. *Catheter-related infections.* New York: Marcel Dekker, Inc, 1997:307–324.

36. Peters G, Locci R, Pulverer G. Adherence and growth of coagulase-negative staphylococci on surfaces of intravenous catheters. *J Infect Dis* 1982;146:479–482.

37. Merritt RJ, Ennis CE, Andrassy RJ, et al. Use of Hickman right atrial catheter in pediatric oncology patients. *J Parenter Enteral Nutr* 1981;5:83–85.

38. Shapiro ED, Wald ER, Nelson KA, et al. Broviac catheter-related bacteremia in oncology patients. *Am J Dis Child* 1982;136:679–681.

39. King DR, Komer M, Hoffman J, et al. Broviac catheter sepsis: the natural history of an iatrogenic infection. *J Pediatr Surg* 1985;20:728–733.

40. Colombani PM, Dudgeon DL, Buck JR, et al. Multipurpose central venous access in the immunocompromised pediatric patient. *J Parenter Enteral Nutr* 1985;9:38–41.

41. Darbyshire PJ, Weightman NC, Speller DCE. Problems associated with indwelling central venous catheters. *Arch Dis Child* 1985;60:129–134.

42. Cairo MS, Spooner S, Sowden L, et al. Long-term use of indwelling multipurpose silastic catheters in pediatric cancer patients treated with aggressive chemotherapy. *J Clin Oncol* 1986;4:784–788.

43. Johnson PR, Decker MD, Edwards KM, et al. Frequency of broviac catheter infections in pediatric oncology patients. *J Infect Dis* 1986;154:570–578.

44. Cameron GS. Central venous catheters for children with malignant disease: surgical issues. *J Pediatr Surg* 1987; 22:702–704.

45. Hartman GE, Shochat SJ. Management of septic complications associated with Silastic catheters in childhood malignancy. *Pediatr Infect Dis* 1987;6:1042–1047.

46. Viscoli C, Garaventa A, Boni L, et al. Role of Broviac catheters in infections in children with cancer. *Pediatr Infect Dis J* 1988;7:556–560.

47. Yokoyama S, Fujimoto T, Tajima T, et al. Use of Broviac/Hickman catheter for long-term venous access in pediatric cancer patients. *Jpn J Clin Oncol* 1988;18:143–148.

48. Wurzel CL, Halom K, Feldman JG, Rubin LG. Infection rates of Broviac-Hickman catheters and implantable venous devices. *Am J Dis Child* 1988;142:536–540.

49. Das I, Philpott C, George RH. Central venous catheter-related septicaemia in paediatric cancer patients. *J Hosp Infect* 1997;36:67–76.

50. Uderzo C, D'Angelo PD, Rizzari C, et al. Central venous catheter-related complications after bone marrow transplantation in children with hematologic malignancies. *Bone Marrow Transplant* 1992;9:113–117.

51. Van Hoff J, Berg AT, Seashore JH. The effect of right atrial catheters on infectious complications of chemotherapy in children. *J Clin Oncol* 1990;8:1255–1262.

52. Rizzari C, Palamone G, Corbetta A, et al. Central venous catheter-related infections in pediatric hematology-oncology patients: role of home and hospital management. *Pediatr Hematol Oncol* 1992;9:115–123.

53. Shulman RJ, Smith EO, Rahman S, et al. Single- vs. double-lumen central venous catheters in pediatric oncology patients. *Am J Dis Child* 1988;142:893–895.

54. Byrne WJ, Halpin TC, Asch MJ, et al. Home total parenteral nutrition: an alternative approach to the management of children with severe chronic small bowel disease. *J Pediatr Surg* 1977;12:359–366.

55. Prince A, Heller B, Levy J, et al. Management of fever in patients with central vein catheters. *Pediatr Infect Dis* 1986;5:20–24.

56. Christensen ML, Hancock ML, Gattuso J, et al. Parenteral nutrition associated with increased infection rate in children with cancer. *Cancer* 1993;72:2732–2738.

57. Freeman J, Goldmann DA, Smith NE, et al. Association of intravenous lipid emulsion and coagulase-negative staphylococcal bacteremia in neonatal intensive care units. *N Engl J Med* 1990;323:301–308.

58. Loeff DS, Matlak ME, Black RE, et al. Insertion of a small central venous catheter in neonates and young infants. *J Pediatr Surg* 1982;17:944–949.

59. Grisoni ER, Mehta SK, Connors AF. Thrombosis and infection complicating central venous catheterization in neonates. *J Pediatr Surg* 1986;21:772–776.

60. Warner BW, Gorgone P, Schilling S, et al. Multiple purpose central venous access in infants less than 1,000 grams. *J Pediatr Surg* 1987;22:820–822.

61. Lally KP, Hardin WD Jr, Boettcher M, et al. Broviac catheter insertion: operating room or neonatal intensive care unit. *J Pediatr Surg* 1987;22:823–824.

62. Sadiq HF, Devaskar S, Keenan WJ, et al. Broviac catheterization in low birth weight infants: incidence and treatment of associated complications. *Crit Care Med* 1987;15:47–50.

63. Raviglione MC, Battan R, Pablos-Mendez A, et al. Infections associated with Hickman catheters in patients with acquired immunodeficiency syndrome. *Am J Med* 1989;86:780–786.

64. Pizzo PA, Eddy J, Falloon J, et al. Effect of continuous intravenous infusion of zidovudine (AZT) in children with symptomatic HIV infection. *N Engl J Med* 1988;319:889–896.

65. Maki DG, Weise CE, Sarafin HW. A semiquantitative culture method for identifying intravenous-catheter-related infection. *N Engl J Med* 1977;296:1305–1309.

66. Cooper GL, Hopkins CC. Rapid diagnosis of intravascular catheter-associated infection by direct Gram staining of catheter segments. *N Engl J Med* 1985;312:1142–1147.

67. Zufferey J, Rime B, Francioli P, et al. Simple method of rapid diagnosis of catheter-associated infection by direct acridine orange staining of catheter tips. *J Clin Microbiol* 1988;26:175–177.

68. Wing EJ, Norden CW, Shadduck RK, et al. Use of quantitative bacteriologic techniques to diagnose catheter-related sepsis. *Arch Intern Med* 1979;139:482–483.

69. Flynn PM, Shenep JL, Barrett FF. Differential quantitation with a commercial blood culture tube for diagnosis of catheter-related infection. *J Clin Microbiol* 1988;26:1045–1046.

70. Ruderman JW, Morgan MA, Klein AH. Quantitative blood cultures in the diagnosis of sepsis in infants with umbilical and Broviac catheters. *J Pediatr* 1988;112:748–751.

71. Benezra D, Kiehn TE, Gold JWM, et al. Prospective study of infections in indwelling central venous catheters using quantitative blood cultures. *Am J Med* 1988;85:495–498.

72. Capdevila JA, Planes AM, Palomar M, et al. Value of differential quantitative blood cultures in the diagnosis of catheter-related sepsis. *Eur J Clin Microbiol Infect Dis* 1992;11:403–407.

73. Thomas JH, MacArthur RI, Pierce GE, et al. Hickman-Broviac catheters. Indications and results. *Am J Surg* 1980;140:791–796.

74. Pollack PF, Kadden M, Byrne WJ, et al. 100 patient years' experience with the Broviac Silastic catheter for central venous nutrition. *J Parenter Enteral Nutr* 1981;5:32–36.

75. Wang EEL, Prober CG, Ford-Jones L, et al. The management of central intravenous catheter infections. *Pediatr Infect Dis* 1984;3:110–113.

76. Ghesquiere W, Hanakowski M, Swift M, et al. Central line infections involving totally implantable venous devices in a pediatric population. *Twenty-ninth Interscience Conference on Antimicrobial Agents and Chemotherapy,* Houston, Texas, 1989:285.

77. Shenep JL, Flynn P. Infections associated with long-term intravascular and cerebrospinal fluid shunt catheters. In: Aronoff SC, ed. *Advances in pediatric infectious diseases.* Chicago: Year Book Medical Publishers, Vol 145, 1986:145–162.

78. Hiemenz J, Skelton J, Pizzo PA. Perspective on the management of catheter-related infections in cancer patients. *Pediatr Infect Dis* 1986;5:6–11.

79. Eppes SC, Troutman JL, Gutman LT. Outcome of treatment of candidemia in children whose central catheters were removed or retained. *Pediatr Infect Dis J* 1989;8:99–104.

80. Powell DA, Marcon MJ. Failure to eradicate Malassezia furfur broviac catheter infection with antifungal therapy. *Pediatr Infect Dis J* 1987;6:579–580.

81. Saleh RA, Schorin MA. *Bacillus* sp. sepsis associated with Hickman catheters in patients with neoplastic disease. *Pediatr Infect Dis J* 1987;6:851–856.

82. LaQuaglia MP, Caldwell C, Lucas A, et al. A prospective randomized double-blind trial of bolus urokinase in

the treatment of established Hickman catheter sepsis in children. *J Pediatr Surg* 1994;29:742–745.

83. Atkinson JB, Chamberlin K, Boody BA. A prospective randomized trial of urokinase as an adjuvant in the treatment of proven Hickman catheter sepsis. *J Pediatr Surg* 1998;33:714–716.

84. Messing B, Peitra-Cohen S, Debure A, et al. Antibiotic-lock technique: a new approach to optimal therapy for catheter-related sepsis in home-parenteral nutrition patients. *J Parenter Enteral Nutr* 1988;12:185–189.

85. Johnson DC, Johnson FL, Goldman S. Preliminary results treating persistent central venous catheter infections with the antibiotic lock technique in pediatric patients. *Pediatr Infect Dis J* 1994;10:930–931.

86. McCarthy A, Byrne M, Breathnach F, et al. "In-situ" teicoplanin for central venous catheter infection. *Ir J Med Sci* 1995;164:125–127.

87. Rao JS, O'Meara A, Harvey T, Breatnach F. A new approach to the management of Broviac catheter infection. *J Hosp Infect* 1992;22:109–116.

88. Liepman MK, Jones PG, Kauffman CA. Endocarditis as a complication of indwelling right atrial catheters in leukemic patients. *Cancer* 1984;54:804–807.

89. Haddad W, Idowu J, Georgeson K, et al. Septic atrial thrombosis. A potentially lethal complication of Broviac catheters in infants. *Am J Dis Child* 1986;140:778–780.

90. Tsao MMP, Katz D. Central venous catheter-induced endocarditis: human correlate of the animal experimental model of endocarditis. *Rev Infect Dis* 1984;6: 783–790.

91. Keohane PP, Jones BJM, Attrill H, et al. Effect of catheter tunneling and a nutrition nurse on catheter sepsis during parenteral nutrition: a controlled trial. *Lancet* 1983;2:1388–1390.

92. Conly JM, Greives K, Peters B. A prospective, randomized study comparing transparent and dry gauze dressings for central venous catheters. *J Infect Dis* 1989;159: 310–319.

93. Treston-Aurand J, Olmsted RN, Allen-Bridson K, et al. Impact of dressing materials on central venous catheter infection rates. *J Intraven Nurs* 1997;20:201–206.

94. Zinner SH, Denny-Brown BC, Braun P, et al. Risk of infection with intravenous indwelling catheters: effect of application of antibiotic ointment. *J Infect Dis* 1969; 120:616–619.

95. Schwartz CL, Henrickson KJ, Powell KR. Prevention of intraluminal catheter infections by vancomycin. *Pediatr Res* 1989;25:156A.

96. Randolph AG, Cook DJ, Gonzales CA, et al. Benefit of heparin in central venous and pulmonary artery catheters: a meta-analysis of randomized controlled trials. *Chest* 1998;113:165–171.

11

Sickle Cell Disease and Other Hemoglobinopathies

Winfred C. Wang

Department of Pediatrics, Division of Infectious Diseases, University of Tennessee, Memphis, Tennessee 38103

Hemoglobinopathies result from genetic mutations that cause either a change in the amino-acid sequence of one of the globin chains of the hemoglobin molecule (e.g., sickle cell anemia) or decreased globin synthesis (e.g., β-thalassemia). The prevalent abnormal hemoglobin (Hb) in the population of the United States is Hb S, in which valine is substituted for glutamic acid in the sixth position of the globin chain. Sickle cell trait (Hb AS) is present in about 8% of the African-American population. Sickle cell disease refers to any clinically significant hemoglobinopathy involving Hb S. The most common types are sickle cell anemia (Hb SS), Hb SC disease, and Hb S-β thalassemia (1). One in 350 black newborns in the United States is affected with sickle cell disease; it is therefore one of the most commonly encountered genetic conditions.

Thalassemia results from diminished α or β globin chain synthesis. β-thalassemia major occurs when genes for diminished or absent β-globin synthesis are inherited from both parents. In the United States, most cases occur in families of Italian, Greek, or Southeast Asian ethnic background.

This chapter focuses on infections associated with sickle cell disease because they are a leading cause of mortality and morbidity in children with this condition. Sepsis caused by *Streptococcus pneumoniae* previously was responsible for most fatalities in the first few years of life, but this mortality rate has decreased with the use of penicillin prophylaxis. Children with sickle cell disease are also susceptible to osteomyelitis, meningitis, pneumonia, and urinary tract infections. The susceptibility to infection appears to result primarily from compromised splenic function, but other aspects of the immune system may be involved as well. In addition, B-19 parvovirus infection may have life-threatening consequences from suppression of bone marrow erythropoiesis.

HISTORICAL INFORMATION

Although sickle cell anemia was first described by James Herrick in 1910, it was not until the mid-1960s that susceptibility to severe bacterial infection from *S. pneumoniae* was recognized in children with this condition (2). An increased incidence of infection with *Haemophilus influenzae* was noted in the mid-1970s (3). Although excessive bone infection was noted earlier, an association of *Salmonella* osteomyelitis with sickle cell disease was reported in the 1950s (4). Several mechanisms for the increased susceptibility to infection among sickle cell patients have been proposed. Defective opsonization, possibly as a result of an abnormality in the complement system, was suggested in 1968 (5). Perhaps the most important factor, functional asplenia, was described 1 year later (6).

Prevention of serious infections in children with sickle cell disease has been a major objective during the past two decades. Initial experience with pneumococcal vaccine was reported in 1977 (7). More recently, conjugated *H. influenzae* vaccine has virtually eliminated this infection in young infants with sickle cell disease (8). The most significant advance in recent years has been the utilization of penicillin in preventing pneumococcal sepsis (9).

PATHOPHYSIOLOGY AND IMMUNOLOGY

B-Cell Function

B-cell function appears to be closely linked to the status of the spleen in sickle cell disease. Levels of circulating immunoglobulin (Ig) have been measured in children and adults (10,11). In children, IgG and IgA levels are normal or increased, possibly secondary to hemolysis and chronic stimulation of the reticuloendothelial system. By contrast, serum IgM is often decreased. In one study, a normal serum IgM level was associated with visualization of the spleen on spleen scan and decreased IgM with a lack of visualization (12). Patients who undergo splenectomy for hereditary spherocytosis or β thalassemia also have decreased levels of IgM, suggesting that the spleen is a major source of this Ig (13). Serum IgM was increased in some patients with Hb S-β thalassemia and Hb SC disease, in whom functional asplenia is less likely to occur. Levels of Ig were unchanged during pain crises (10).

The number of circulating B-lymphocytes in sickle cell patients is normal or increased (11,14). Studies of Ig synthesis *in vitro* by peripheral blood mononuclear cells, however, demonstrated diminished IgM (but not IgG) production (14). The same pattern has been found in patients who have undergone splenectomy (15). *In vitro* mixing experiments using fractionated B and T cells indicated that diminished IgM synthesis is related to decreased B-cell function rather than to excessive T-suppressor or inadequate T-helper function (15). Why do functional or anatomic splenectomy result in decreased IgM synthesis? It is possible that the loss of the spleen's intimate anatomic arrangement of macrophages, germinal center B cells, and marginal zone T cells eliminates important local intercellular or humoral interactions, which may result in reduced IgM production *in vivo* and a diminished capacity of circulating B cells to synthesize IgM *in vitro*.

T-Cell Function

Most analyses of circulating lymphocyte subpopulations in patients with sickle cell disease have shown a diminished proportion of T cells (14,16–18). Because of an increased absolute lymphocyte count, however, the absolute number of T cells has been normal or increased (14,16,17). The proportion of T-helper (CD4) cells has been normal or decreased, whereas the absolute number may be increased (16). T-suppressor (CD8) cells have been reported to be increased, decreased, or normal (14,17,18). In most reports, the ratio of CD4:CD8 cells is normal or increased (14,17,18). Cell-mediated immunity measured by lymphocyte blast cell transformation with the mitogens phytohemagglutinin, concanavalin A, and pokeweed mitogen *in vitro* and skin test reactivity *in vivo* initially were thought to be decreased (16). More recently, it has been shown that mitogen stimulation of peripheral blood mononuclear cells and lymphocyte-mediated antibody-dependent cell cytotoxicity are normal (17,18).

Patients who have undergone splenectomy have increased numbers of lymphocytes, B cells, and CD3, CD4, and CD8 cells (15,17, 18). The loss of a functioning splenic microenvironment has been blamed for a lack of differentiation of B cells to Ig-secreting cells, a decreased primary immune response to intravenous antigens, a delayed secondary response to pneumococcal antigen, and decreased *in vitro* IgM antipneumococcal antibody production (18). The similarities of the lymphocyte abnormalities in sickle cell patients to those in splenectomized patients are striking, but quantitative differences are still present (15,18).

The role of zinc deficiency in the immune function of sickle cell patients is controversial; the diagnosis may depend on the tissue measured (e.g., plasma vs. red blood cell count). In children with sickle cell disease, zinc deficiency has been associated with an increased risk of infection and an increased proportion of hypofunctional neutrophils (19) but a normal lymphocyte response to most mitogens (20). Zinc supplementation improved delayed hypersensitivity and DNA synthesis in subgroups of patients (21).

Immunologic function in sickle cell disease has been evaluated by response to vaccination. More than 90% of children with Hb SS who were immunized with a bivalent influenza vaccine developed protective antibody titers (22) and 96% responded to hepatitis B vaccine (23).

Complement

Abnormalities in the complement system in children with sickle cell disease first were reported by Winkelstein and Drachman in 1968 (5). Heat-labile serum opsonizing activity for pneumococcus was decreased, although hemolytic complement activity was normal. It was suggested that splenic dysfunction resulted in impairment of splenic clearance and heat-labile opsonin synthesis. Five years later, Johnston et al. found that when the classic pathway of complement activity is blocked, the alternative pathway cannot fully restore activity (24). Several other investigators sought to identify specific abnormalities in the alternative pathway, but the results have been conflicting. Both diminished (25,26) and normal (27,28) activity of the alternative pathway have been described. Specific components of the alternative pathway, including factors B, D, and P, may be de-

creased or normal (25,26). More recently, increased activation of the alternative pathway was suggested by decreased C3 levels and increased C3d and C3b,P complexes (27,28). Chronic activation of the alternative pathway of complement may lead to its deficient function in the opsonization process.

A series of studies by Bjornson and Lobel led to different conclusions (29,30). They suggested that the diminished opsonization of *S. pneumoniae* was not due to abnormalities in the classic or alternative pathways of complement but to decreased IgG (and possibly IgM) anticapsular polysaccharide antibody.

Spleen

During early life, children with Hb SS have splenomegaly with congestion of the splenic pulp by masses of sickled red cells. By late childhood, vascular occlusion and infarction have occurred, and the spleen becomes atrophic and fibrotic. Functional asplenia in sickle cell anemia was suggested by the presence of Howell–Jolly bodies in red blood cells. Spleen scans using technetium-99 (^{99}Tc) sulfur colloid demonstrated absent or decreased splenic uptake in infants as young as 5 months of age (6). It has been postulated that sickled cells in the splenic sinusoids produce relative obstruction of blood flow leading to diversion of flow through intrasplenic shunts and bypass of the phagocytic, reticuloendothelial elements of the organ. Reticuloendothelial blockade by saturation of phagocytic cells from chronic hemolysis may be a contributing factor to splenic hypofunction. In successive stages, the spleen initially is enlarged and hyperactive, then enlarged and hypoactive, and finally atrophic. This process occurs earlier in children with Hb SS than in other types of sickle cell disease. Splenic enlargement before 1 year of age was believed to be an indicator of greater susceptibility to severe bacterial infection in one study (31), but confirmation has not yet occurred.

A semiquantitative method of evaluation of splenic function is the measurement by interference phase-contrast microscopy of "pocks" or "pits" in circulating red blood cells (32). In the red blood cells of persons who have undergone splenectomy, 20% to 30% contain at least one of these surface indentations, whereas fewer than 1% of the circulating red cells of normal persons are pitted. Investigators in the Cooperative Study of Sickle Cell Disease (CSSCD) examined developmental patterns of splenic dysfunction in a large cohort of infants with sickle cell disease (33). Nonvisualization of the spleen correlated strongly with a pitted red cell count >3.5%. In Hb SS, this occurred at a mean age of 1 to 2 years, and the count reached a plateau of 12% at 3 to 5 years of age. An elevated pit count occurred later and less frequently in Hb S-β+ thalassemia, and an intermediate pattern was seen in Hb SC disease. Increased pitted red cell levels also were associated with decreased Hb F levels (33). Relatively low pit counts have been found in young children with splenomegaly and splenic sequestration (34), but increased pitted cells are almost always present in children who have had pneumococcal sepsis or osteomyelitis (34). In summary, pitted red blood cell counts are a relatively sensitive and specific indicator of the presence of splenic dysfunction.

Neutrophils

The total white blood cell count (WBC) and absolute neutrophil count are moderately increased in sickle cell disease. Neutrophil function, as measured by nitroblue tetrozolium reduction, hexose monophosphate shunt activation, peroxide generation, chemiluminescence, and killing of *Staphylococcus aureus* and *Candida,* is normal (35). Thus, neutrophil dysfunction does not appear to contribute to infection in sickle cell disease.

Summary

Normal healthy infants have a relatively immature immune system and little type-specific antibody; however, they are protected against severe pneumococcal disease by two additional defense mechanisms: (a) the alter-

native pathway of complement and (b) the filtering action and antibody-producing ability of the spleen. In the absence of specific antibody, the alternate complement pathway activates complement and fixes C3b to the surface of the organism, thereby increasing opsonic activity in the blood. Removal of pneumococci that are coated with activated complement components then takes place primarily in the spleen. The spleen is also the site of production of antibody, which allows the classic complement pathway to assist in the clearing of these bacteria.

Children with sickle cell disease, particularly those with Hb SS, have defective splenic filtering function from an early age. They have diminished opsonization capacity for encapsulated organisms as a result of abnormalities in B-cell function and probably in the alternative pathway of complement. If they are young, they do not have antibody to capsular polysaccharide because of a lack of exposure to the appropriate antigens and immature IgG antibody responses. The net result of impaired opsonic activity and hypofunction of the reticuloendothelial cells of the spleen is a severe problem in clearance of pneumococci and other encapsulated bacteria from the blood.

CLINICAL MANIFESTATIONS AND LABORATORY DIAGNOSIS

Sepsis

A comprehensive evaluation of bacteremia in sickle cell disease was reported by the CSSCD before the widespread use of penicillin prophylaxis (36). Of 3,451 patients with follow-up, 178 cases of bacteremia occurred in 134 patients. Bacteremia in Hb SS patients was frequent during the first 3 years of life (seven or eight cases per 100 patient-years); the risk in Hb SC disease during the first 2 years of life was five or six cases per 100 patient-years. In older children, the incidence of bacteremia was much lower. *S. pneumoniae* accounted for 60% of the cases of bacteremia in children younger than 6 years but only 19% of cases in children older than 6 years.

Infections caused by *S. pneumoniae* often are characterized by an extremely rapid and fulminant course, which can be fatal in less than 12 hours. Patients may present with severe hypotension and disseminated intravascular coagulation. Convulsions, ataxia, and a disordered sensorium are common. Occasionally, the clinical presentation is deceptively mild, but then the infection progresses rapidly. The presence of diarrhea is an ominous symptom. In one series, four deaths occurred among six septic children who had diarrhea around the time of presentation (37). The mortality rate among 24 children who had pneumococcal bacteremia without diarrhea was 12.5%.

Most septic sickle cell patients are seen initially in an emergency department for fever. Six episodes of septicemia occurred among 182 episodes of fever in 22 children with sickle cell disease who were studied prospectively (38). In all six cases, the child's temperature was above 39.5°C, and in five cases it was above 40.5°C. Other physical findings and laboratory studies were not useful as indicators of sepsis. Although the total WBC and the absolute neutrophil count usually are increased above baseline levels, they are not valuable for differentiating infection from vasoocclusive crisis or for differentiating bacterial from nonbacterial infection (39). In a review of 27 bacteremic children with sickle cell disease, the mean age was 4.7 years, 36% had a temperature of 40°C or higher at presentation (but 21% had a temperature of 38°C or higher), the mean WBC was $24 \times 10^3/\text{mm}^3$, 79% of cultures were positive for *S. pneumoniae,* and five patients had meningitis (40).

Although most cases of fatal pneumococcal septicemia have been associated with Hb SS, particularly during the first 3 years of life, older children with Hb SC disease may be at relative high risk, perhaps related to loss of splenic function at an older age. Among seven anecdotal cases of fatal pneumococcal septicemia in children with Hb SC disease, six occurred in children who were 3 1/2 to 15 years of age (41).

A previous episode of pneumococcal sepsis in a child with sickle cell disease may indicate a higher risk for subsequent infection (42). In a recent report, 8 of 30 patients had recurrent sepsis, suggesting that patients who have had an initial episode should continue penicillin prophylaxis indefinitely and should not be candidates for outpatient management of febrile illness (see later discussion herein).

A major threat to successful therapy of invasive infection that is due to *S. pneumoniae* is the emergence of antibiotic-resistant (nonsusceptible) organisms (43,44). In the sickle cell population, regional epidemiologic patterns appear to determine antibiotic resistance. A recent report cited 16 cases of bacteremia/sepsis attributable to *S. pneumoniae* with intermediate or high resistance to penicillin in U.S. children with sickle cell anemia (45). The median age of the patients was 2 years, and the children had a spectrum of presentations ranging from appearing well (except for fever) to being highly toxic. A temperature higher than 40.0°C (seen in 12 of 16) and a WBC count greater than $30 \times 10^3/\text{mm}^3$ (in 5 of 16 patients) often were associated with invasive infection. Two patients developed clinical evidence of meningitis despite 4 to 5 days of treatment with intravenous cephalosporin (plus 2 1/2 days of vancomycin treatment in one). Many of the organisms were also nonsusceptible to extended-spectrum cephalosporins and other antibiotics, including erythromycin, trimethoprim–sulfamethoxazole, and chloramphenicol. None was resistant to vancomycin. Of the four patients who had highly resistant organisms, two died; however, the mortality rate (12.5%) was not unusually high.

Perhaps the second most frequent cause of bacteremia/sepsis at this time, *Salmonella* sp, is commonly associated with osteomyelitis (see later discussion herein). *Salmonella* bacteremia was not observed in children younger than 3 years of age in the CSSCD but accounted for 30% of cases of bacteremia in children 6 to 9 years of age (36). In a recent article reporting 55 Jamaican patients with *Salmonella* infection, 28 initially had osteomyelitis and 27 had bacteremia/septicemia (46). Although the large majority of patients with bacteremia did not develop osteomyelitis, 23% died, suggesting that suspected sepsis in sickle cell disease should be managed with anti-salmonellae agents pending culture results.

Meningitis

Approximately 80% of cases of meningitis in young children with sickle cell disease are caused by *S. pneumoniae*. Meningitis may occur in infants as young as 5 months of age, and repeated episodes are common (2). The clinical presentation of meningitis in these children is usually unremarkable, but the disease can progress rapidly (47). On initial lumbar puncture, there may be few cells as well as normal glucose and protein concentrations in the cerebrospinal fluid.

Osteomyelitis

The overall incidence of osteomyelitis in sickle cell disease is approximately 2% to 5% (48). Although a predominance of *S. aureus* among the organisms responsible for osteomyelitis has been described in small series, a recent review of international and national reports over the last two decades indicated that the predominant organism remains salmonellae, which accounted for more than twice as many cases as *S. aureus* (49). An increased rate of intestinal salmonellae carriage in patients with sickle cell disease has not been found, but salmonellae may enter the bloodstream through microinfarctions in the intestinal mucosa (4). Organisms in the circulation can lodge and proliferate in areas of infarcted bone, as occurred in a case of osteomyelitis at the site of a healed fracture in a sickle cell patient (50). Blockade of the reticuloendothelial system by red cell fragments may be another contributory factor. The immune response to *Salmonella* vaccine in sickle cell anemia appears to be normal, but defective opsonization of salmonellae has been reported (51). Other investigators have described normal opsonization of *Salmonella* lipopolysaccharide in an assay mediated by the alternative pathway of complement (52). The possible interrelationship of these factors in the pathophysiology of *Salmonella* osteomyelitis is shown in Fig. 11.1.

Osteomyelitis usually starts in the medullary cavity of the humerus, radius, tibia, femur, or ulna (in descending order of frequency) (53). Multiple sites of bone involvement are common, and lesions may be bilateral and symmetric. In infants, the metacarpals and metatarsals are frequently involved, and osteomyelitis may present as a case of "hand–foot syndrome" that fails to resolve (54). The presentation of osteomyelitis with fever, bone pain, and local swelling is usually acute; in some cases, however, the only indication may be a persistent fever without findings referable to bone (55). Septic arthritis may complicate osteomyelitis, or it can occur by itself (55). Blood cultures are positive in 20% to 50% of cases in which the etiologic agent is *Salmonella* (56). A definitive diagnosis can be made when the organism is isolated from bone by aspiration or open biopsy at the site of infection; however, a positive blood culture for *Salmonella* organisms in a patient with localized bone findings or persistent fever is strongly suggestive of osteomyelitis.

Without a positive culture, it may be extremely difficult to differentiate between bone infarction and osteomyelitis. A marked increase in WBC, a leftward shift of the white cell differential, and an elevated sedimentation rate favor the latter but are nonspecific. Persistent fever or fever exceeding 39°C also favors osteomyelitis. Radiographs are of limited value because bone infarction is often indistinguishable from osteomyelitis. Radionuclide scans with technetium diphosphonate (bone scan), technetium sulphur colloid (bone marrow scan), and gallium, either individually or in combination, have been used to differentiate the two conditions (57,58). The timing of these scans is important because infarction may resemble osteomyelitis after the process has continued for several days.

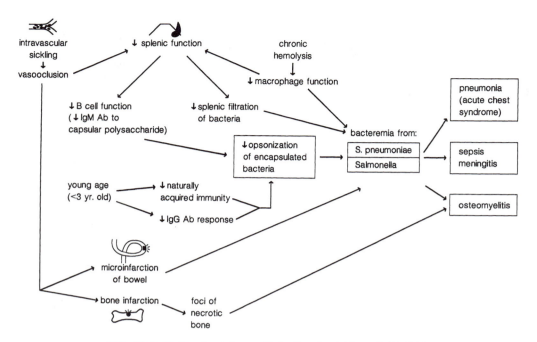

FIG. 11.1. Pathophysiology of infection in sickle cell disease.

Scans may be falsely positive or falsely negative. In general, bone scans show increased uptake with osteomyelitis and decreased uptake with infarction early in the course of these conditions. Bone marrow scans usually show decreased uptake with infarction (58). When bone marrow and gallium scans were performed in tandem, greater uptake with the gallium scan favored osteomyelitis, but congruent uptake of the two scans favored infarction (57,58). In general, magnetic resonance imaging has been of limited value in the diagnosis of osteomyelitis (59).

Pneumonia (Acute Chest Syndrome)

The combination of fever or respiratory symptoms and a new pulmonary infiltrate has been referred to as the acute chest syndrome (ACS). It is usually impossible to distinguish pulmonary infarction from pneumonia, and the two processes are likely to coexist. In children under age 5 years, pneumonia is common, whereas, in older children and adults,

pulmonary infarction is more frequent (60). Temperature, WBC count, and arterial oxygenation level are not helpful in differentiating infarction and infection. In a recent review of 1,100 episodes of ACS from the CSSCD, bacteremia occurred in 14% of infants but in only 1.8% of patients older than 10 years of age (60). Younger children presented with fever and cough, had a greater tendency to have upper lobe disease, required shorter hospitalization and less frequent transfusion, and were less likely to have a preceding painful event. The mortality rate was four times higher in adults than in children.

The National Acute Chest Syndrome Study Group evaluated nearly 700 adults and children using bronchoscopy and comprehensive microbiologic methods; the most common identifiable etiologies were pulmonary fat emboli, mycoplasma, and chlamydia (E.P. Vichinsky and the National Acute Chest Syndrome, *personal communication*, 1999). Secretory phospholipase A$_2$ (sPLA$_2$), an enzyme that cleaves phospholipids and liberates potentially toxic free fatty acids, has been found to be markedly increased in patients with ACS, and its concentration has been directly correlated with the severity of the disease (61). Severe *Mycoplasma pneumoniae* infection is characterized by a prolonged high fever, multiple pulmonary infiltrates, leukocytosis, negative blood cultures, a positive cold agglutinin screening test, and an elevated complement-fixing antibody titer (62). In a series of 30 children with sickle cell disease and ACS, *Chlamydia pneumoniae* was isolated from the nasopharynx in four children (13%), and two others had serologic evidence of infection (63). Acute infection with B19 parvovirus has been recognized as a cause of severe ACS. In a recent series, three patients with Hb SC disease, acute parvovirus infection, and ACS died of respiratory failure (64).

Aplastic Crisis/Parvovirus

An aplastic (hypoplastic) crisis in a patient with a hereditary hemolytic anemia is defined as a transient episode of pure red cell aplasia with virtual absence of erythroid precursors in the bone marrow and reticulocytes in the circulation (65). Because of the shortened red cell life span in sickle cell disease, hereditary spherocytosis, β-thalassemia major, pyruvate kinase deficiency, and other conditions in which aplastic crises have been reported, a temporary interruption of erythropoiesis leads to a precipitous fall in hemoglobin level. The occurrence of aplastic crises in sickle cell disease has been well recognized since the 1940s; however, identification of an infectious etiologic agent did not occur until 1981. Six cases in London (66) and 24 cases in Jamaica (67) were linked to a parvovirus-like agent, subsequently identified as human parvovirus (HPV) B19. In Jamaica, outbreaks of aplastic crises had been occurring every 4 to 5 years since 1956. More recent prospective studies confirmed that HPV is the etiologic agent of aplastic crises in sickle cell disease in 80% to 100% of cases (65,68). Because evidence of previous HPV infection in children (27%) (68) and in adults (50%) (66) is con-

siderably higher than the incidence of aplastic crisis in sickle cell disease, it is clear that not all infected patients develop this condition.

The most well-studied outbreak of HPV in patients with hereditary hemolytic anemia involved 26 patients, primarily children with sickle cell disease, in northeastern Ohio from March to August 1984 (65,69). The risk of aplastic crisis was 7.2% for Hb SS children and 4.5% for Hb SC children. All patients had prodromal symptoms of fever, chills, lethargy, or malaise for 1 to 17 days (median, 4 days) before manifestations of red cell aplasia were seen. Severe anemia and reticulocytopenia were the predominant hematologic features. The reticulocyte count decreased to below 1% in 85% of the cases, compared with baseline reticulocyte counts of 8% to 24% in Hb SS and 3% to 6% in Hb SC disease. The nadir of the hematocrit was 7% to 18% in Hb SS and 17% to 32% in Hb SC disease. Reticulocytopenia lasted up to 14 days from the time of presentation. Twenty-two of 26 patients received red cell transfusions; three of the four patients who did not require transfusion had Hb SC disease.

Recently, other sequelae of HPV were noted in children with sickle cell disease. In a series from Jamaica, seven patients developed glomerulonephritis with proteinuria and symptoms of nephrotic syndrome within 7 days following an aplastic crisis resulting from HPV (70). Chronic, potentially fatal renal failure appears to be a common consequence of this complication. In addition, HPV may result in severe pulmonary complications (see preceding discussion) (64).

Other Infections

Urinary tract infections are common in persons with sickle cell trait as well as in those with sickle cell disease; the incidence appears to be highest among young pregnant women. Abnormalities such as glomerular scarring, hyposthenuria, and functional obstruction may predispose to infections. *Escherichia coli* is the most common cause of urinary tract infection and often is associated with bacteremia as well (36). Recurrent abdominal pain in a child with sickle cell anemia may be caused by gastritis due to *Helicobacter pylori* (71).

Transfusion-transmitted infections are a significant problem in children with Hb SS because most of these children require red cell transfusions at some point in their lives and about 15% require chronically administered regular transfusions for several months to many years. Newly acquired transfusion-transmitted HIV infection has not been reported since the 1980s. A recent analysis of the status of HIV-positive patients with sickle cell disease noted that 44% had a stable infection with a relatively high CD4 lymphocyte level and low viral load (compared with 14% of controls) and suggested that the absence of splenic function prior to infection with HIV might have had an ameliorating effect (72).

Hepatitis C infection was analyzed in 99 patients with sickle cell disease in New York City (73). Although the overall prevalence of antibody to hepatitis C virus (HCV) was 10%, the frequency was 23% in those who received more than 10 U of packed red blood cells, 8% in those who received 1 to 10 U, and 0% in those who did not receive any transfusions. Two of seven liver biopsies showed significant liver damage (cirrhosis in one and chronic active hepatitis in the other). The prevalence of HCV antibody appeared to be directly related to the number of blood transfusions received.

Because peripheral vein access is often a problem in patients with sickle cell disease, central venous access devices, including implantable ports and partially implanted catheters, have been used increasingly more often, which has created another potential site of infection; however, whether catheters in children with sickle cell disease are more likely to become infected than those in other patients is controversial (74–76). One report (74) cited an incidence of fewer than one episode of catheter-associated bacteremia per 1,000 catheter-patient days, whereas the others noted an incidence of four to five episodes per 1,000 catheter-patient days. Infecting or-

ganisms included coagulase-negative staphylococcus, *S. aureus,* and *E. coli.*

TREATMENT

Sickle cell patients are susceptible to *S. pneumoniae, Haemophilus influenzae, E. coli, S. aureus,* and *Salmonella* species (36). The blood, lungs, bone, meninges, and urinary tract are the most frequently involved sites. Antibiotic coverage must be aimed particularly at *S. pneumoniae* when sepsis, pneumonia, or meningitis are possibilities. The most common situation requiring consideration of antibiotics is the child with sickle cell disease who comes to the emergency department with fever. It is essential to: (a) educate families to bring the child with fever to medical attention, (b) aggressively evaluate the patient to determine the etiology of fever, and (c) provide prompt antibiotic coverage when indicated (77). Because of the rapidity with which pneumococcal sepsis progresses, intravenous antibiotic therapy should begin soon after initial evaluation of patient, ideally, within 3 hours of documenting fever. In most recent cases, we initiated antibiotic therapy with intravenous ceftriaxone, 50 mg/kg.

The success of prophylactic penicillin in reducing the incidence of pneumococcal sepsis led to the concept that not all febrile children with sickle cell disease require hospitalization for intravenous antibiotic coverage until cultures are confirmed to be negative (78–81). In a randomized trial, children with sickle cell hemoglobinopathies aged 6 months to 12 years, were assigned to treatment as either inpatients or outpatients on presentation with a temperature exceeding 38.5°C (79). Excluded from randomization were those who were thought to be at higher risk for invasive infection because they had a toxic appearance, a temperature above 40.0°C, a WBC count greater than $30 \times 10^3/mm^3$ or lower than $5 \times 10^3/mm^3$, or a history of pneumococcal sepsis or splenectomy; those with certain complications, including severe pain, ACS, or a hemoglobin level lower than 5.0 g/dL; and those with social contraindications (Table 11.1). Children who were

TABLE 11.1. *Exclusion criteria for outpatient management of febrile children with sickle cell disease*

Toxic appearance, hypotension, dehydration
Significant pain
Temperature ≥40.0°C
WBC >30.0 or <5.0 × 10³/cu.³
Hemoglobin level <5.0 g/dL or reticulocyte count <1%
New infiltrate on chest radiography
  (acute chest syndrome)
History of sepsis
History of splenectomy
History of poor compliance with medical treatment
Lack of available transportation
Lack of telephone or effective means of
communication.

WBC, white blood cell count.

randomized to outpatient management received an initial dose of ceftriaxone, 50 mg/kg administered intravenously, and returned 24 hours later for a second dose. None of the 86 patients in the randomized groups had a bloodstream infection. Outpatient treatment saved a mean of approximately $1,200 per febrile episode (in 1993). It was concluded that at least half the children with sickle cell disease who present with fever can be treated safely on an outpatient basis. A follow-up study of 107 febrile episodes in 80 patients at low risk for sepsis were treated with an initial dose of intravenous ceftriaxone followed by a 5-day course of an oral antibiotic (80). No patient had sepsis, but 11 required hospitalization over the 14-day period following initial evaluation, including one patient who developed a splenic sequestration crisis and several who had persistent or recurrent fever. Our present policy is to manage febrile children with sickle cell disease as outpatients following a dose of intravenous ceftriaxone and 4 to 8 hours of observation in the emergency department unless they meet the exclusion criteria indicated in Table 11.1. We have not found it necessary to modify our indications for hospitalization, despite the increasing prevalence of antibiotic-resistant organisms.

Empiric antibiotic therapy nonetheless must be tailored to the incidence of penicillin and cephalosporin resistance among the prevalent strains of *S. pneumoniae* in the community. We add vancomycin to the initial cephalosporin regimen if the patient meets one or more of these criteria: (a) toxic appearance; (b) presence of another potentially serious focus of infection, such as ACS or meningitis; (c) temperature of 40°C or higher; and (d) WBC count below 5.0 × 10³/mm³ or greater than 30.0 × 10³/mm³. When *S. pneumoniae* is cultured and its antibiotic sensitivities have been identified, the algorithm shown in Fig. 11.2 is recommended (45). An extended-spectrum cephalosporin such as ceftriaxone is used alone only if the organism is fully sensitive. If the organism is nonsusceptible to cephalosporin, vancomycin is added or substituted. Few drugs are available to treat penicillin and cephalosporin-resistant pneumococcal meningitis. Treatment failures have been described for chloramphenicol, and, rarely, vancomycin. If meningitis has been diagnosed, a repeat lumbar puncture after 24 to 36 hours of therapy is performed as an *in vivo* measure of the effectiveness of the antimicrobial regimen; follow-up blood cultures also may be indicated. If all cultures are negative after 72 hours and fever resolves, the patient is discharged without additional antibiotics; it is emphasized to the parent that the child must resume taking prophylactic penicillin (if the child had been taking penicillin previously).

Sickle cell patients with ACS are presumed to have pneumonia as part of their pulmonary process. Antibiotic coverage for *S. pneumoniae* may be provided with parenteral ceftriaxone and vancomycin. Because *M. pneumoniae* and *Chlamydia* sp. are common pathogens among identifiable causes of ACS, it may be appropriate to add erythromycin or azithromycin treatment, particularly if these organisms are prevalent in the community or the patient does not respond to initial antibiotic therapy. Supportive care with oxygen and red cell transfusion may be necessary if the patient is hypoxemic, unusually anemic, or in significant respiratory distress. Parenteral antibiotics should be administered for 4 to 5 days or longer if the patient continues to be symptomatic. The patient then may receive an oral antibiotic (e.g., amoxicillin, cefaclor) to

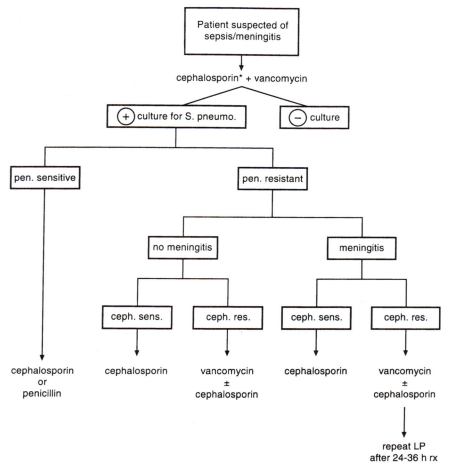

*intravenous cephalosporin
(e.g., ceftriaxone, cefotaxime, cefuroxime)

FIG. 11.2. Algorithm for treatment of invasive infection with *S. pneumoniae.* (From Wang WC, Wong W-Y, Rogers ZR, Wilimas JA, Buchanan GR, Powars DR. Antibiotic-resistant pneumococcal infection in children with sickle cell disease in the United States. *J Pediatr Hematol Oncol* 1996;18:140, with permission.)

complete a 10-day course. After several weeks, a follow-up chest radiogram should be performed to determine whether the pulmonary process has resolved and to provide a baseline for evaluation of future febrile episodes. Recently, a randomized double-blind, placebo-controlled trial demonstrated that intravenous dexamethasone (0.3 mg/kg every 12 hours for 4 doses) in children with mild to moderate ACS resulted in a shorter hospital stay, less blood transfusion, and a

shorter duration of fever (82). There was an increased frequency of readmissions after discharge, and further study of this modality is needed.

Successful therapy of osteomyelitis is greatly enhanced through identification of the etiologic organism from a positive blood culture or direct culture of the infected bone. Initial treatment should include coverage of *Salmonella, S. aureus* and *H. influenzae.* A combination of a penicillinase-resistant penicillin and a drug that provides coverage for salmonellae (e.g., cefotaxime, ampicillin, chloramphenicol) may be indicated before sensitivities become available. Because of the tendency of salmonellae to establish chronic infection in necrotic bone, a prolonged intravenous course of antibiotics is necessary. A recent article described the emergence of ciprofloxacin resistance during the course of treatment of three patients with *Salmonella* osteomyelitis, a worrisome finding in this era of increasing antibiotic resistance (83).

PREVENTION

Pneumococcal Vaccine

Attempts to develop a vaccine against *S. pneumoniae* date back to the early part of the century. In 1977, an octavalent vaccine containing purified polysaccharide antigens of serotypes of pneumococcus that frequently are associated with disease (types 1, 3, 6, 7, 14, 18, 19, and 23 by the American system) was reported to be efficacious in sickle cell disease. This was replaced by a 14-valent vaccine containing the additional serotypes 2, 4, 9, 12, and 25 (and eliminating type 18). In 1983, a 23-valent vaccine became available; this is currently in use and "covers" 87% of the pneumococcal isolates from clinical specimens submitted to the Centers for Disease Control and Prevention for serotyping.

Unfortunately, the current vaccine has several problems. Not all clinically significant pneumococcal serotypes are represented. The efficacy of the different antigens in generating a protective antibody response is variable, and antibody responses are poor in young children, especially those younger than 2 years of age (84). Sepsis or meningitis may occur with serotypes of pneumococcus that are contained in the vaccine. The most frequent vaccine breakthroughs occurred with types 6, 19, and 23 (84,85). Pneumococcal antibody levels in these patients almost invariably have been less than a theoretic protective level of 300 ng/mL (86). Reimmunization of children with sickle cell anemia who received pneumococcal poly-

saccharide vaccine at age 5 years induced limited production of serotype-specific IgG antibodies, regardless of previous pneumococcal vaccine history (87). Current practice is to administer the 23-valent vaccine at age 2 years and a second dose at age 5 years.

Particularly promising is the development of a heptavalent pneumococcal saccharide vaccine containing serotypes 4, 6B, 9V, 14, 18C, 19F, and 23F individually conjugated to CRM_{197} and administered at 2, 4, 6, and 12 to 15 months of age (88). In a small preliminary trial in children with sickle cell disease who were 2 years of age or older, subjects who received two doses of pneumococcal-conjugate vaccine followed by the 23-valent vaccine achieved higher antibody concentrations for all serotypes contained in the conjugate vaccine than those who received the 23-valent vaccine alone (89). It is anticipated that within the next 2 years, the use of a conjugated pneumococcal vaccine will become part of standard immunization practice in children with sickle cell disease in the first few months of life in a manner analogous to the use of the *H. influenzae* B polysaccharide (HIB) vaccine (90).

Penicillin Prophylaxis

With the introduction of pneumococcal vaccine in the late 1970s, the prompt use of antibiotics for febrile illnesses, and closer supervision of infants with sickle cell disease, it was hoped that a significant reduction in the incidence of pneumococcal septicemia would occur. Unfortunately, data generated by the CSSCD in the United States and by the Jamaican Sickle Cell Program indicated no change in the infection rate in children with sickle cell disease in the early 1980s (9,91). Although penicillin prophylaxis was proposed in the 1970s, it did not gain widespread acceptance because of concerns about parental compliance, development of penicillin-resistant pneumococci, inhibition of naturally acquired immunity, and the necessary duration of coverage.

The most convincing evidence for benefit from penicillin prophylaxis came from a multicenter, randomized, double-blind, placebo-controlled trial to test whether the regular daily administration of oral penicillin would reduce the incidence of pneumococcal septicemia in children with sickle cell anemia who were under the age of 3 years at the time of entry (9). Two hundred fifteen children were randomized at a median age of 15 months and received either oral Penicillin VK, 125 mg, or a placebo twice daily. Thirteen of 110 patients given placebo developed pneumococcal septicemia compared with two of 105 treated with penicillin prophylaxis ($p = 0.0025$). This 84% reduction in the incidence of pneumococcal sepsis, along with similar results from a randomized trial in Jamaica using prophylaxis with long-acting penicillin administered by monthly injection (91), led to the consensus recommendation to initiate penicillin prophylaxis by 3 months of age in children with Hb SS or Hb Sβ^0-thalassemia. More recently, a second multicenter trial addressed the question of whether penicillin prophylaxis should be continued beyond the fifth birthday (92). Children with Hb SS or Sβ^0-thalassemia who had been receiving penicillin prophylaxis and who had not had prior invasive pneumococcal infection or splenectomy were randomized at age 5 years to continue penicillin or placebo. Over an average follow-up of 3.2 years, no significant difference between those receiving penicillin (two cases of invasive infection among 200 patients) and those receiving placebo (four cases among 200 patients) was found. The study's conclusion was that it is safe to stop prophylactic penicillin therapy at 5 years of age in patients who meet the criteria described above, but parents must continue to be aggressively counseled to seek medical attention for their children's febrile events.

The routine use of penicillin prophylaxis in young children with sickle cell disease led to decreased mortality. The incidence of pneumococcal bacteremia in children with Hb SS in the first 3 years of life is now approximately 2.5 cases per 100 patient years of follow-up (43,44). The mortality rate has been approximately 12%. Although the incidence

of invasive infection due to *S. pneumoniae* has decreased approximately threefold since the widespread use of penicillin prophylaxis began in the late 1980s, it is still significant, as is the mortality rate for those infected.

Poor compliance with twice daily administration of penicillin may be the most significant risk factor for the occurrence of pneumococcal sepsis (93). Reported compliance by structured interview was 67%, but measured compliance by urine assay was only 43% in one series (94). In another study, 60% of mothers reported that they were strictly compliant with obtaining prescribed refills, but pharmacy records indicated only a 12% adherence rate; the perceived burdens of having to obtain refills and remembering to give the medication were the most important reasons cited for lack of compliance (95). A structured education program remains the most effective means of optimizing compliance (96), but this approach is not always successful (97).

Several questions regarding penicillin prophylaxis remain. Does prophylaxis lead to the development of penicillin-resistant strains? Penicillin use reduces the nasopharyngeal colonization rate of *S. pneumoniae* to about 10% (98), but in three recent reports, it had no statistically significant effect on the frequency of antibiotic resistance, which was present in 33% to 55% of isolates (99–101). By contrast, in another recent study, nasopharyngeal colonization with penicillin nonsusceptible *S. pneumoniae* was associated with penicillin prophylaxis (102) and penicillin nonsusceptible pneumococci have been approximately twice as frequent in patients with invasive infection who were receiving penicillin prophylaxis compared with those who were not on penicillin or were poorly compliant (T. Adamkiewicz and the Pneumococcal Infection Registry, *personal communication*, 1999). Will penicillin prophylaxis from an early age prevent acquisition of natural immunity? Serotypes not included in the pneumococcal vaccine may be of particular concern, but no change in invasive serotypes has been documented. Should children with sickle cell disease other than Hb SS or Hb

Sβ⁰-thalassemia also receive penicillin prophylaxis? In young children with Hb SC disease and Hb Sβ+-thalassemia, the need for penicillin prophylaxis is less certain because of their substantially lower risk of life-threatening septicemia (103). Nevertheless, many centers maintain children with these types of sickle cell disease on penicillin until age 5 years. In fact, it might be appropriate to continue penicillin prophylaxis in children with Hb SC disease beyond age 5 years because the relatively rare fatal infections that do occur in these patients typically take place after 5 years of age (41).

H. influenzae B Vaccine

The HIB vaccine is not consistently immunogenic in children with sickle cell disease who are younger than 6 years old; however, conjugated HIB vaccines introduced in the late 1980s yielded excellent antibody responses in infants with sickle cell disease 2 to 6 months of age (8). After two doses, 90% of infants had protective HIB antibody levels (>1.0 g/mL); after three doses, 100% had protective levels. HIB vaccination is now part of routine pediatric immunization practice.

In summary, current recommendations for prevention of infection in young children with sickle cell anemia are:

1. Penicillin prophylaxis: Penicillin VK, 125 mg orally twice daily, age 3 months to 3 years; 250 mg adminstered twice daily, age 3 to 5 years. Continue after 5 years if history of pneumococcal sepsis or splenectomy.
2. Pneumococcal vaccine (23-valent): Primary vaccination at age 24 months; booster vaccination at age 5 years. (Replacement by conjugated pneumococcal vaccine, when available.)
3. Conjugated HIB vaccine: ages 2, 4, 6, and 15 months.

PROGNOSIS

A significant mortality was associated with bacteremia in the CSSCD report (36). Eigh-teen deaths occurred in 148 cases of bacteremia in patients with Hb SS; 16 of the 18 were older than 10 years of age, and 15 had pneumococcal sepsis. In bacteremic subjects, mortality was not associated with age, sex, degree or duration of fever, previous administration of vaccine, use of prophylactic penicillin, or the presence of splenomegaly. Mortality was associated with manifestations of disseminated intravascular coagulation and an initial WBC lower than $15 \times 10^3/mm^3$. When death occurred, the course was extremely rapid; 75% died within 24 hours of their arrival at the hospital.

The mortality rate from pneumococcal meningitis has been 18% to 38%, although a decline in this rate, ascribed to earlier diagnosis and more prompt treatment, has been reported (104). Sequelae of meningitis have included mental retardation, hemiparesis, nerve palsies, deafness, and blindness, but they do not appear to be more common in Hb SS disease than in patients without hemoglobinopathies (105).

Overall mortality from sickle cell disease has dropped markedly since the mid-1960s, when it was estimated that 50% of patients with Hb SS would not live to the age of 20 years. In the CSSCD, between 1979 and 1987, 73 deaths occurred among 14,670 person-years of follow-up, a probability of survival to age 20 of 89%, and an overall mortality rate of 2.6% (106). Thirty-eight percent of the deaths were due to bacterial infection, and *S. pneumoniae* was the cause in 23 of 28 cases. The other leading identifiable causes of death were stroke (12%) and ACS (8%). A significant beneficial effect from newborn screening for sickle cell disease has been seen (107). Coupled with extensive parental education, this led to markedly improved treatment of life-threatening events such as sepsis and acute splenic sequestration. In children with sickle cell disease identified by newborn screening, the mortality rate was 1.8%, compared with an 8% rate in children who were diagnosed at a median age of 21 months. The beneficial role of prophylactic penicillin has been described above.

INFECTIONS IN THALASSEMIA

Patients with β-thalassemia major and other severe forms of thalassemia such as Hb E-β thalassemia have an increased risk of infection, especially if they are receiving inadequate transfusion support (108). Pneumonia was a frequent complication of thalassemia until blood transfusion regimens were improved in the late 1960s. Transfusion-transmitted infections (e.g., HIV, HCV) are described in Chapters 3 and 19. Among more than 1,000 Italian patients with β-thalassemia major, the prevalence of HIV was 2.9% in 1990 at the beginning of a prospective study (109). Subsequently, the incidence of HIV infection was 1.7 per 10,000 person-years of follow-up, and the risk of HIV infection was 1 in 190,000 U, reflecting the greatly diminished risk of acquiring HIV in the 1990s. Patients with β-thalassemia major frequently require splenectomy in late childhood for hypersplenism associated with an increased transfusion requirement. After splenectomy, these patients are particularly susceptible to *S. pneumoniae* sepsis and therefore require penicillin prophylaxis. The increased susceptibility may be related in part to compromise of the reticuloendothelial system from the products of chronic hemolysis.

Yersinia enterolitica infection has been seen in iron-overloaded subjects, particularly chronically transfused patients with thalassemia (110). Deferoxamine, the iron-chelating agent required by these patients, may be used by *Yersinia* to incorporate iron needed for its growth. Clinical manifestations of systemic yersiniosis include fever, diarrhea, mesenteric lymphadenitis, and abdominal abscesses. The diagnosis is made by isolation of the organism from blood, stool, or abscess culture or by an increased serologic titer. Broad-spectrum antibiotics, including coverage that is effective against *Yersinia,* is indicated for thalassemic children with a serious acute infection.

ACKNOWLEDGMENT

This work was supported in part by the American Lebanese Syrian Associated Charities (ALSAC).

REFERENCES

1. Serjeant GR. *Sickle cell disease.* Oxford: Oxford University Press, 1992.
2. Robinson MG, Watson RJ. Pneumococcal meningitis in sickle-cell anemia. *N Engl J Med* 1966;274:1006–1008.
3. Ward J, Smith AL. *Haemophilus influenzae* bacteremia in children with sickle cell disease. *J Pediatr* 1976; 88:261–263.
4. Hook EW, Campbell CG, Weens HS, et al. *Salmonella* osteomyelitis in patients with sickle cell anemia. *N Engl J Med* 1957;257:403.
5. Winkelstein JA, Drachman RH. Deficiency of pneumococcal serum opsonizing activity in sickle-cell disease. *N Engl J Med* 1968;279:459–466.
6. Pearson HA, Spencer RP, Cornelius EA. Functional asplenia in sickle-cell anemia. *N Engl J Med* 1969; 281:923–926.
7. Ammann AJ, Addiego J, Wara DW, et al. Polyvalent pneumococcal-polysaccharide immunization of patients with sickle-cell anemia and patients with splenectomy. *N Engl J Med* 1977;297:897–900.
8. Gigliotti F, Feldman S, Wang WC, et al. Immunization of young infants with sickle cell disease with a *Haemophilus influenzae* type b saccharide-diphtheria CRM197 protein conjugate vaccine. *J Pediatr* 1989; 114:1006–1010.
9. Gaston MH, Verter JI, Woods G, et al. Prophylaxis with oral penicillin in children with sickle cell anemia. *N Engl J Med* 1986;314:1593–1599.
10. Bjornson AB, Lobel JS, Lampkin BC. Humoral components of host defense in sickle cell disease during painful crisis and asymptomatic periods. *J Pediatr* 1980;96:259–262.
11. Venkataraman M, Westerman MP. B-cell changes occur in patients with sickle cell anemia, *Am J Clin Pathol* 1985;84:153–158.
12. Gavrilis P, Rothenberg SP, Guy R. Correlation of low serum IgM levels with absence of functional splenic tissue in sickle cell disease syndromes. *Am J Med* 1974;57:542–545.
13. Constantoulakis M, Trichopoulos D, Avgoustaki O, et al. Serum immunoglobulin concentrations before and after splenectomy in patients with homozygous β-thalassemia. *J Clin Pathol* 1978;31:546–550.
14. Wang W, Herrod H, Presbury G, et al. Lymphocyte phenotype and function in chronically transfused children with sickle cell disease. *Am J Hematol* 1985;20:31–40.
15. Wang WC, Herrod HG, Valenski WR, et al. Lymphocyte and complement abnormalities in splenectomized patients with hematologic disorders. *Am J Hematol* 1988;28:239–245.
16. Hernández P, Cruz C, Santos MN, et al. Immunologic dysfunction in sickle cell anaemia. *Acta Haematol* 1980;63:156–161.
17. Escalona E, Malave I, Rodriguez E, et al. Mitogen induced lymphoproliferative responses and lymphocyte sub-populations in patients with sickle cell disease. *J Clin Lab Immunol* 1987;22:191–196.
18. Donadi EA, Falcao RP. Are the changes of lymphocyte subsets in sickle cell anemia due to the loss of splenic function? *Acta Haematol* 1988;80:91–94.
19. Carpentieri U, Smith L, Daeschner CW III, et al. Neutrophils and zinc in infection-prone children with sickle cell disease. *Pediatrics* 1983;72:88–92.

20. Daeschner CW III, Carpentieri U, Goldman AS, et al. Zinc deficiency and blood lymphocyte function with sickle cell disease. *Scand J Haematol* 1985;35:186–190.

21. Ballester OF, Prasad AS. Anergy, zinc deficiency, and decreased nucleoside phosphorylase activity in patients with sickle cell anemia. *Ann Intern Med* 1983; 98:180–182.

22. Steinberg E, Overturf GD, Portnoy B, et al. Serologic and clinical response of children with sickle cell disease to bivalent influenza A split virus vaccine. *J Pediatr* 1978;92:823–825.

23. Sarnaik SA, Merline JR, Bond S. Immunogenicity of hepatitis B vaccine in children with sickle cell anemia. *J Pediatr* 1988;112:429–430.

24. Johnston RB, Newman SL, Struth AG. An abnormality of the alternate pathway of complement activation in sickle-cell disease. *N Engl J Med* 1973;288:803–808.

25. Wilson WA, Thomas EJ, Sissons JGP. Complement activation in asymptomatic patients with sickle cell anaemia. *Clin Exp Immunol* 1979;36:130–139.

26. Larcher VF, Wyke RJ, Davis LR, et al. Defective yeast opsonization and functional deficiency of complement in sickle cell disease. *Arch Dis Child* 1982;57:343–346.

27. Bjornson AB, Gaston MH, Zellner CI. Decreased opsonization for *Streptococcus pneumoniae* in sickle cell disease: studies of selected complement components and immunoglobulins. *J Pediatr* 1977;91:371–378.

28. De Ceulaer K, Forbes M, Maude GH, et al. Complement and immunoglobulin levels in early childhood in homozygous sickle cell disease. *J Clin Lab Immunol* 1986;21:37–41.

29. Bjornson AB, Lobel JS. Lack of a requirement for the Fc region of IgG in restoring pneumococcal opsonization via the alternative complement pathway in sickle cell disease. *J Infect Dis* 1986;154:760–769.

30. Bjornson AB, Lobel JS. Direct evidence that decreased serum opsonization of *Streptococcus pneumoniae* via the alternative complement pathway in sickle cell disease is related to antibody deficiency. *J Clin Invest* 1987;79:388–398.

31. Rogers DW, Vaidya S, Serjeant GR. Early splenomegaly in homozygous sickle-cell disease: an indicator of susceptibility to infection. *Lancet* 1978;2:963–965.

32. Casper JT, Koethe S, Rodey GE, et al. A new method for studying splenic reticuloendothelial dysfunction in sickle cell disease patients and its clinical application: a brief report. *Blood* 1976;47:183–188.

33. Pearson HA, Gallagher D, Chilcote R, et al., and the Cooperative Study of Sickle Cell Disease. Developmental pattern of splenic dysfunction in sickle cell disorders. *Pediatrics* 1985;76:392–397.

34. Grover R, Wethers DL. Spleen dysfunction in hemoglobinopathies determined by pitted red cells. *Am J Pediatr Hematol Oncol* 1988;10:340–343.

35. Strauss RG, Johnston RB Jr, Asbrock R, et al. Neutrophil oxidative metabolism in sickle cell disease. *J Pediatr* 1976;89:391–394.

36. Zarkowsky HS, Gallagher D, Gill FM, et al., and the Cooperative Study of Sickle Cell Disease. Bacteremia in sickle hemoglobinopathies. *J Pediatr* 1986;109:579–585.

37. Seeler RA, Jacobs NM. Diarrhea in *Streptococcus pneumoniae* bacteremia. *Am J Hematol* 1980;8:309.

38. McIntosh S, Rooks Y, Ritchey AK, et al. Fever in young children with sickle cell disease. *J Pediatr* 1980;96:199–204.

39. Buchanan GR, Glader BE. Leukocyte counts in children with sickle cell disease. *Am J Dis Child* 1978; 132:396–398.

40. Holzmann G, Berman B. Bacteremia in children with sickle cell disease: a twelve year single institutional experience. *Int J Pediatr Hematol Oncol* 1988;5:411.

41. Lane PA, Rogers ZR, Woods GM, et al. Fatal pneumococcal septicemia in hemoglobin SC disease. *J Pediatr* 1994;124:859–862.

42. Hongeng S, Wilimas JA, Harris S, et al. Recurrent *Streptococcus pneumoniae* sepsis in children with sickle cell disease. *J Pediatr* 1997;130:814–816.

43. Adamkiewicz TV, Buchanan GR, Facklam RR, et al. 1997–98 survey of invasive *Streptococcus pneumoniae* (PN) infection in children with sickle cell disease (SCD). *Blood* 1998;92:526a (abst 2161).

44. Hord J, Smith-Whitley K, Byrd R, et al. *Streptococcus pneumoniae* sepsis and meningitis in children with sickle cell disease in the penicillin prophylaxis era. *Blood* 1998;92:526a (abst 2160).

45. Wang WC, Wong W-Y, Rogers ZR, et al. Antibiotic-resistant pneumococcal infection in children with sickle cell disease in the United States. *J Pediatr Hematol Oncol* 1996;18:140–144.

46. Wright J, Thomas P, Serjeant GR. Septicemia caused by salmonella infection: an overlooked complication of sickle cell disease. *J Pediatr* 1997;130:394–399.

47. Landesman SH, Rao SP, Ahonkhai VI. Infections in children with sickle cell anemia: special reference to pneumococcal and salmonella infections. *Am J Pediatr Hematol Oncol* 1982;4:407–418.

48. Syrogiannopoulos GA, McCracken GH Jr, Nelson JD. Osteoarticular infections in children with sickle cell disease. *Pediatrics* 1986;78:1090–1096.

49. Burnett MK, Bass JW, Cook BA. Etiology of osteomyelitis complicating sickle cell disease. *Pediatrics* 1998;101:296–297.

50. Ebong WW. Acute osteomyelitis three years after a closed fracture in an adult with sickle-cell anemia: a case report. *J Bone Joint Surg Am* 1980;62A:1196–1198.

51. Hand WL, King NL. Serum opsonization of Salmonella in sickle cell anemia. *Am J Med* 1978;64:388–395.

52. Field RJ, Overturf GD, Strunk R. Opsonization of Salmonella enteriditis lipopolysaccharide in sickle cell disease. *Pediatr Res* 1981;15:107–111.

53. Adeyokunnu AA, Hendrickse RG. *Salmonella* osteomyelitis in childhood: a report of 63 cases seen in Nigerian children of whom 57 had sickle cell anaemia. *Arch Dis Child* 1980;55:175–184.

54. Noonan WJ. *Salmonella* osteomyelitis presenting as 'hand-foot syndrome' in sickle cell disease. *BMJ* 1982;248:1464–1465.

55. Ortiz-Neu C, Marr JS, Cherubin CE, et al. Bone and joint infections due to *Salmonella*. *J Infect Dis* 1978; 138:820–828.

56. Specht EE. Hemoglobinopathic Salmonella osteomyelitis: orthopedic aspects. *Clin Orthop* 1971;79:110–118.

57. Amundsen TR, Siegel MJ, Siegel BA. Osteomyelitis and infarction in sickle cell hemoglobinopathies: differentiation by combined technetium and gallium scintigraphy. *Radiology* 1984;153:807–812.

58. Kim HC, Alavi A, Russell MO, et al. Differentiation of bone and bone marrow infarcts from osteomyelitis in sickle cell disorders. *Clin Nucl Med* 1989;14:249–254.

59. Mankad VN, Yang Y-M, Williams JP, et al. Magnetic

resonance imaging of bone marrow in sickle cell patients. *Am J Pediatr Hematol Oncol* 1988;10:344–347.

60. Vichinsky EP, Styles LA, Colangelo LH, et al., and the Cooperative Study of Sickle Cell Disease. Acute chest syndrome in sickle cell disease: clinical presentation and course. *Blood* 1997;89:1787–1792.

61. Styles LA, Schalkwijk CG, Aarsman AJ, et al. Phospholipase A$_2$ levels in acute chest syndrome of sickle cell disease. *Blood* 1996;87:2573–2578.

62. Shulman ST, Bartlett J, Clyde WA, et al. The unusual severity of mycoplasmal pneumonia in children with sickle-cell disease. *N Engl J Med* 1972;287:164–167.

63. Miller ST, Hammerschlag MR, Chirgwin K, et al. Role of *Chlamydia pneumoniae* in acute chest syndrome of sickle cell disease. *J Pediatr* 1991;118:30–33.

64. Lowenthal EA, Wells A, Emanuel PD, et al. Sickle cell acute chest syndrome associated with parvovirus B19 infection: case series and review. *Am J Hematol* 1996; 51:207–213.

65. Saarinen UM, Chorba TL, Tattersall P, et al. Human parvovirus B19-induced epidemic acute red cell aplasia in patients with hereditary hemolytic anemia. *Blood* 1986;67:1411–1417.

66. Pattison JR, Jones SE, Hodgson J, et al. Parvovirus infections and hypoplastic crises in sickle-cell anaemia. *Lancet* 1981;1:664–665.

67. Serjeant GR, Topley JM, Mason K, et al. Outbreak of aplastic crises in sickle cell anaemia associated with parvovirus-like agent. *Lancet* 1981;2:595–597.

68. Gowda N, Rao SP, Cohen B, et al. Human parvovirus infection in patients with sickle cell disease with and without hypoplastic crisis. *J Pediatr* 1987;110:81–84.

69. Chorba T, Coccia P, Holman RC, et al. The role of parvovirus B19 in aplastic crisis and erythema infectiosum (fifth disease). *J Infect Dis* 1986;154:383–393.

70. Wierenga KJJ, Pattison JR, Brink N, et al. Glomerulonephritis after human parvovirus infection in homozygous sickle-cell disease. *Lancet* 1995;346:475–476.

71. Kennedy L, Mahoney DH, Redel CA. *Helicobacter pylori* gastritis in a child with sickle cell anemia and recurrent abdominal pain. *J Pediatr Hematol Oncol* 1997;19:163–164.

72. Bagasra O, Steiner RM, Ballas SK, et al. Viral burden and disease progression in HIV-1-infected patients with sickle cell anemia. *Am J Hematol* 1998;59:199–207.

73. Hasan MF, Marsh F, Posner G, et al. Chronic hepatitis C in patients with sickle cell disease. *Am J Gastroenterol* 1996;91:1204–1206.

74. Abdul-Rauf A, Gauderer M, Chiarucci K, et al. Long-term central venous access in patients with sickle cell disease. Incidence of thrombotic and infectious complications. *J Pediatr Hematol Oncol* 1995;17:342–345.

75. McCready CE, Doughty HA, Pearson TC. Experience with the Port-A-Cath in sickle cell disease. *Clin Lab Haematol* 1996;18:79–82.

76. Jeng M, Vichinsky E, Feusner J. Complications of central venous catheters in pediatric sickle cell disease. *Blood* 1998;92:526a (abst 2159).

77. Reid CD, Charache S, Lubin B, eds. Management and therapy of sickle cell disease. NIH Publication 95-2117, 1995.

78. Rogers ZR, Morrison RA, Vedro DA, et al. Outpatient management of febrile illness in infants and young children with sickle cell anemia. *J Pediatr* 1990;117:736–739.

79. Wilimas JA, Flynn PM, Harris S, et al. A randomized study of outpatient treatment with ceftriaxone for selected febrile children with sickle cell disease. *N Engl J Med* 1993;329:472–476.

80. Williams LL, Wilimas JA, Harris SC, et al. Outpatient therapy with ceftriaxone and oral cefixime for selected febrile children with sickle cell disease. *J Pediatr Hematol Oncol* 1996;18:257–261.

81. Platt OS. The febrile child with sickle cell disease: A pediatrician's quandary. *J Pediatr* 1997;130:693–694.

82. Bernini JC, Rogers ZR, Sandler ES, et al. Beneficial effect of intravenous dexamethasone in children with mild to moderately severe acute chest syndrome complicating sickle cell disease. *Blood* 1998;92:3082–3089.

83. Workman MR, Philpott-Howard J, Bragman S, et al. Emergence of ciprofloxacin resistance during treatment of salmonella osteomyelitis in three patients with sickle cell disease. *J Infect* 1996;32:27–32.

84. Overturf GD, Rigau-Perez JG, Honig G, et al. Pneumococcal polysaccharide immunization of children with sickle cell disease. II. Serologic response and pneumococcal disease following immunization. *Am J Pediatr Hematol Oncol* 1982;4:25–35.

85. Broome CV, Facklam RR, Fraser DW. Pneumococcal disease after pneumococcal vaccination: an alternative method to estimate the efficacy of pneumococcal vaccine, *N Engl J Med* 1980;303:549–552.

86. Kaplan J, Frost H, Sarnaik S, et al. Type-specific antibodies in children with sickle cell anemia given polyvalent pneumococcal vaccine. *J Pediatr* 1982;100:404–406.

87. Bjornson AB, Falletta JM, Verter JI, et al. Serotype-specific immunoglobulin G antibody responses to pneumococcal polysaccharide vaccine in children with sickle cell anemia: effects of continued penicillin prophylaxis. *J Pediatr* 1996;129:828–835.

88. Rennels MB, Edwards KM, Keyserling HL, et al. Safety and immunogenicity of heptavalent pneumococcal vaccine conjugated to CRM197 in United States infants. *Pediatrics* 1998;101:604–611.

89. Vernacchio L, Neufeld EJ, MacDonald K, et al. Combined schedule of 7-valent pneumococcal conjugate vaccine followed by 23-valent pneumococcal vaccine in children and young adults with sickle cell disease. *J Pediatr* 1998;133:275–278.

90. Rubin LG, Voulalas D, Carmody L. Immunization of children with sickle cell disease with *Haemophilus influenzae* type b polysaccharide vaccine. *Pediatrics* 1989;84:509–513.

91. John AB, Ramlal A, Jackson H, et al. Prevention of pneumococcal infection in children with homozygous sickle cell disease. *BMJ* 1984;288:1567–1570.

92. Falletta J, Woods GM, Verter JI, et al., for the Prophylactic Penicillin Study II. Discontinuing penicillin prophylaxis in children with sickle cell anemia. *J Pediatr* 1995;127:685–690.

93. Buchanan GR, Smith SJ. Pneumococcal septicemia despite pneumococcal vaccine and prescription of penicillin prophylaxis in children with sickle cell anemia. *Am J Dis Child* 1986;140:428–432.

94. Teach SJ, Lillis KA, Grossi M. Compliance with penicillin prophylaxis in patients with sickle cell disease. *Arch Pediatr Adolesc Med* 1998;152:274–278.

95. Elliott VE, Day SW, Wang W, et al. The health belief

model as a predictor of compliance with prophylactic penicillin treatment for young children with sickle cell disease. National Sickle Cell Disease Program, 23rd Annual Meeting, San Francisco, CA 1999 (abst).

96. Day SW, Brunson GE, Wang WC. A successful newborn sickle cell trait counseling program utilizing health department nurses. *Pediatr Nurs* 1997;23:557–561.

97. Berkovitch M, Papadouris D, Shaw D, et al. Trying to improve compliance with prophylactic penicillin therapy in children with sickle cell disease. *Br J Clin Pharmacol* 1998;45:605–607.

98. Anglin DL, Siegel JD, Pacini DL, et al. Effect of penicillin prophylaxis on nasopharyngeal colonization with *Streptococcus pneumoniae* in children with sickle cell anemia. *J Pediatr* 1984;104:18–22.

99. Daw NC, Wilimas JA, Wang WC, et al. Nasopharyngeal carriage of penicillin-resistant *Streptococcus pneumoniae* in children with sickle cell disease. *Pediatrics* 1997;99:http://www.pediatrics.org/cgi/content/full/99/4/e7.

100. Woods GM, Jorgensen JH, Waclawiw M, et al., for the Ancillary Nasopharyngeal Culture Study of Prophylactic Penicillin Study II. Influence of penicillin prophylaxis on antimicrobial resistance in nasopharyngeal *S. pneumoniae* among children with sickle cell anemia. *J Pediatr Hematol Oncol* 1997;19:327–333.

101. Norris CF, Mahannah SR, Smith-Whitley K, et al. Pneumococcal colonization in children with sickle cell disease. *J Pediatr* 1996;129:821–827.

102. Steele RS, Warrier R, Unkel PJ, et al. Colonization with antibiotic-resistant *Streptococcus pneumoniae* in children with sickle cell disease. *J Pediatr* 1996;128:531–535.

103. Rogers ZR, Buchanan GR. Bacteremia in children with sickle hemoglobin C disease and sickle beta+-thalassemia: is prophylactic penicillin necessary? *J Pediatr* 1995;127:348–354.

104. Powars D, Overturf G, Weiss J, et al. Pneumococcal septicemia in children with sickle cell anemia: changing trend of survival. *JAMA* 1981;245:1839–1842.

105. Griesemer DA, Winkelstein JA, Luddy R. Pneumococcal meningitis in patients with a major sickle hemoglobinopathy. *J Pediatr* 1978;92:82–84.

106. Leikin SL, Gallagher D, Kinney TR, et al., and the Cooperative Study of Sickle Cell Disease. Mortality in children and adolescents with sickle cell disease. *Pediatrics* 1989;84:500–508.

107. Vichinsky E, Hurst D, Earles A, et al. Newborn screening for sickle cell disease: effect on mortality. *Pediatrics* 1988;81:749–755.

108. Modell B, Berdoukas V. *The clinical approach to thalassaemia.* London: Grune & Stratton, 1984:140.

109. Prati D, Capelli C, Rebulla P, et al., for the Cooleycare Cooperative Group. The current risk of retroviral infections transmitted by transfusion in patients who have undergone multiple transfusions. *Arch Intern Med* 1998;158:1566–1569.

110. De Montalembert M, Girot R. Infections in thalassemic patients. In: Buckner CD, ed. *Advances and controversies in thalassemia therapy: bone marrow transplantation and other approaches.* New York: Alan R. Liss, 1989:231–238.

12

Infections in Children with Renal Disease

Bettina H. Ault, Deborah P. Jones, and Robert J. Wyatt

Department of Pediatrics, Division of Nephrology, University of Tennessee,
Memphis, Tennessee 38103

Children with renal disease may have increased susceptibility to infection for various reasons. Uremia by itself produces alterations in immune function. Hemodialysis, particularly when an indwelling vascular access is present, carries an increased risk for sepsis. Central line infections are discussed in Chapter 7. Children on peritoneal dialysis are at risk for peritonitis as a result of the presence of a catheter connecting the peritoneal cavity with the outside environment, loss of serum proteins from the peritoneal surface, and metabolic abnormalities of the intraperitoneal milieu related to the instillation of dialysate. The immunosuppressive regimen used for renal transplant recipients is associated with an increased risk for a variety of infections (discussed in Chapter 11). Children with the nephrotic syndrome have a markedly increased susceptibility to bacterial infections, particularly spontaneous peritonitis. Because of the increased susceptibility of children with renal disease to infection, specific guidelines for immunization related to the particular condition have been developed.

END-STAGE RENAL DISEASE

Prior to the widespread use of dialysis and transplantation, the incidence of infection for patients hospitalized with chronic renal failure (CRF) was 60%, with infection the cause of death in 38% (1). End-stage renal disease (ESRD) is defined as a glomerular filtration rate (GFR) below 10% of normal on a chronic basis and denotes the need for dialysis or renal transplantation. Chronic renal insufficiency (CRI) is associated with a GFR that is 10% to 75% of normal. The most recent data continue to show that infectious disease is a major cause of death among both adult and pediatric patients with ESRD, whether they are treated with chronic dialysis or with renal transplantation (2).

The incidence for new cases of ESRD for the years 1994 through 1996 in the U.S. pediatric population is only 15 cases per one million population (children aged 0–19 years) per year (3). Prevalence of ESRD, which includes both children on chronic dialysis and those with a functioning renal transplant, is 65 cases per one million children aged 0 through 19 years (3). The death rate for pediatric patients with ESRD is 17 per 1,000 patient-years (3). Infection is listed as the leading cause of death, accounting for at least 22% of those deaths (3). Both incidence of new cases of ESRD and overall death rates are considerably lower for pediatric patients than for adult patients (2,4).

Immunologic Abnormalities in Uremia

Patients with ESRD appear to have a variety of defects of the immune system related to uremia (5,6). Numerous clinical observations support the concept that immune function is not normal in uremic individuals. These include increased susceptibility to infection, increased risk for cancer, development of skin anergy, decreased activity of autoimmune processes, and decreased response to vaccination (7). Although infection is the most common cause of serious morbidity and mortality in the dialysis patient population, most serious infections are related to the presence of a foreign body for dialysis access. When infections related to dialysis access are excluded, the rate of mortality resulting from infection in patients with ESRD is less than 3% (8). Most studies of immune function in renal failure have been conducted in uremic adults. Different investigators have found conflicting results in some cases, and the contribution of the different abnormalities to the increased susceptibility to infection seen in these patients is unclear.

T Cell Abnormalities

T cells from uremic patients exhibit a decreased response to mitogens and allogeneic cells, despite the fact that they show signs of activation. The most striking abnormality of uremic T cells is their increased expression of membrane-associated and soluble interleukin-2 (IL-2) receptors in the face of decreased production of IL-2 (9). The uremic milieu appears to be responsible for this abnormality because cultured peripheral blood mononuclear cells from normal individuals also exhibit increased synthesis of IL-2 receptors, decreased IL-2 synthesis, and decreased response to mitogens in the presence of uremic serum. Addition of IL-2 to the supernatant restores mitogenic responsiveness to these cells (10). Initiation of dialysis in uremic individuals partially restores ability of their T cells to produce IL-2 (10). In addition to the observed abnormalities in IL-2 and IL-2 receptor expression, patients with uremia have abnormalities in interaction between T cells and monocytes. Activation of T cells requires both antigen presentation and secondary modulating signals. Uremia might alter any or all of these pathways. In a series of experiments using peripheral blood mononuclear cultures from uremic patients on hemodialysis the normal T-cell proliferative response was partially restored by incubation with cells bearing the B7 molecule, which is the ligand for CD28 on T cells (11).

B Cell Abnormalities

Antibody response to viral (hepatitis B, influenza) and bacterial antigens (pneumococci) is quantitatively lower than normal in adults on hemodialysis, although the absolute number of circulating B cells is not different from controls. Levels of circulating immunoglobulins (Ig) are also comparable (12). The poor responses to vaccines and the increase in infections primarily controlled by antibodies in patients on maintenance hemodialysis indicate defective humoral immunity, most probably because of impaired T- and B-cell interaction. Adults with renal failure have markedly decreased rates of seroconversion to the recombinant hepatitis B vaccine (13); there is evidence that an abnormal IL-2 response plays a role. Those with the poorest responses to the vaccine tend to have the highest expression of IL-2 receptors on their T cells (14). The administration of recombinant IL-2 with hepatitis B vaccine increased the seroconversion rate in one study (15); subsequent studies, however, have not borne this out (16, 17).

Natural Killer Cells

Natural killer (NK) cell function in uremia has received considerable attention because of the increased incidence of malignancy in uremic adults. Some studies have shown no difference in NK cell activity between normal and uremic persons, whereas others have shown a decrease in NK number and function in patients on dialysis (6). Zaoui and Hakim showed a marked decrease in NK function after hemodialysis with cuprophane membranes (18). Although abnormalities in NK function are speculated to be a factor in the increased incidence of malignancy among uremic patients, no clear association has been established.

Neutrophils

Neutrophil dysfunction is probably one of the most important immunologic factors in the increased susceptibility to infection of patients with kidney failure. Abnormalities in neutrophil chemotaxis, phagocytosis, bactericidal activity, and metabolic functions have been reported in uremic patients (19). Hemodialysis causes neutrophil activation, mainly through generation of complement fragments following contact of the cells with dialysis membranes. This activation is especially marked with the use of cuprophane membranes. Phagocytic response was assessed in renal failure patients at initiation of hemodialysis using one of two membranes: cuprophane or a synthetic polysulfone membrane. All patients experienced a transient decrease in their neutrophil metabolic response to phagocytic stimuli, which reached its lowest level 2 to 3 weeks after initiation of dialysis. The group using the cuprophane membrane had a more profound decrease with a 29% to 37% decrease from baseline compared with 4% to 12% in the polysulfone group. In addition, three of eight patients dialyzed with the cuprophane membrane developed bacterial sepsis within the first 20 weeks, whereas none of the seven using the polysulfone membrane had infections (20). Numerous granulocyte inhibitory proteins have been isolated from uremic serum. Some of these proteins have homology to immunoglobulin light chains, β_2-microglobulin, and complement factor D. These proteins inhibit various neutrophil functions including chemotaxis, degranulation, and metabolic processes (5). In addition, iron overload and increased cytosolic calcium, which is a consequence of hyperparathyroidism, may contribute to decreased phagocytic function (5). Neutrophils from uremic patients show acceleration of apoptosis *in vitro* and plasma from uremic patients accelerates apoptosis of nor-

mal neutrophils (21). Apoptosis may play a role in the neutrophil dysfunction found in uremic patients.

Cytokines

Patients with uremia have abnormal levels of a variety of cytokines, including interleukin-1 (IL-1), tumor necrosis factor-α (TNF-α), and interleukin-6 (IL-6). Numerous factors are probably responsible for the increased levels of these mediators. The kidney is at least partly responsible for the clearance of a variety of cytokines, and plasma levels may rise because of decreased GFR (22,23). The hemodialysis procedure may increase levels of cytokines through two mechanisms. Complement activation by dialysis membranes, especially cuprophane membranes, can be significant and may stimulate mononuclear cells to produce these cytokines. Exposure to endotoxin and other bacterial products diffusing across the dialysis membrane may trigger an intense acute phase response with elevated levels of these cytokines. Elevated cytokine levels in patients with renal failure are responsible for a variety of constitutional symptoms and may contribute to immune dysfunction by their effects on neutrophils and on T- and B-cell functions (6).

Studies of Immune Function in Uremic Children

An early study used mixed lymphocyte culture to evaluate cellular immune function in children with chronic renal failure, some of whom were on dialysis. The mean mitogen proliferative response was lower in children with CRI and markedly abnormal in children on dialysis, particularly hemodialysis, compared with healthy age-matched controls (24). In another study, however, no significant differences in the percentages of B and T cells, T-cell subsets, or mitogenic responses to lectins were found in 26 children with CRF and ESRD on both hemodialysis and peritoneal dialysis (25). Few other studies are available in the pediatric age group.

PERITONEAL DIALYSIS

In peritoneal dialysis, the peritoneal membrane is used for transport of solute from the microcirculation into dialysate within the peritoneal cavity. Fluid removal is accomplished by increasing the tonicity, or the glucose concentration of the dialysate. The modality of peritoneal dialysis uses a Tenckhoff catheter, which is surgically inserted into the peritoneal cavity and tunneled through the subcutaneous tissue. Currently, Tenckhoff catheters have one or two Dacron cuffs to provide material for fibroblast adhesion and mechanical barrier formation.

The dialysate solution is composed of glucose and electrolytes with the addition of lactate as the standard buffer to maintain a pH of 5.2 to 5.5. Sterile technique is used to connect or disconnect the patient at the time of dialysis. An exchange or cycle is accomplished by a manual technique in continuous ambulatory peritoneal dialysis (CAPD), whereby 2 to 3 L of dialysate are infused, allowed to dwell, and then drained four or five times within a 24-hour period. In small children and infants, continuous cycling peritoneal dialysis (CCPD) is more commonly prescribed because the smaller dwell volumes and frequent connect and disconnects are impractical. CCPD usually is performed over 8 to 10 hours at night, during sleep, by an automated machine that infuses and then drains the dwell volume, allowing a dwell of 30 to 60 minutes with a long daytime dwell at the end of cycling.

Peritoneal Environment

The peritoneum is composed of mesothelial cells that function as a barrier as well as a lipid-producing lubricant (26). The mesothelial cells are arranged in a confluent monolayer along a basement membrane. Macrophages are present within the peritoneal cavity as well as beneath the mesothelial layer within the stroma of connective tissue. Within the stroma are vessels that are surrounded by dendritic cells and lymphocytes. Dialysis, or removal of uremia-related substances, occurs between the vessels, the stroma, and the peritoneal cavity itself.

Macrophages/monocytes are the principal cells found in peritoneal fluid; relatively fewer lymphocytes are found. Under normal conditions, polymorphonuclear neutrophils (PMNs) constitute less than 5% of the total population under normal conditions. Once the peritoneum is used for dialysis, the resident cell population tends to change, with fewer mature macrophages and a greater percentage of lymphocytes. The proportion of PMNs may increase toward 30%, and eosinophils also may increase.

Bacteria within the peritoneal cavity may be phagocytized by opsonin-dependent or -independent mechanisms. Intracellular defenses then kill the organism, with eventual removal by the lymphatics. The normal volume of peritoneal fluid is about 50 mL, with opsonin concentrations (IgG, C3 and fibronectin) equal to those in plasma (26). When the peritoneal cavity is filled with glucose-containing dialysate, the concentration of opsonins decreases to only 1% to 3% of the plasma concentration. In addition, mature macrophages are constantly being removed by cycles of dialysis and replaced with less mature cells, which may be less efficient at phagocytosis.

Phagocytosis and Bactericidal Activity of Peritoneal Leukocytes

Dialysate fluid inhibits the ability of resident macrophages and infiltrating PMNs to phagocytose and kill invading bacteria. The ability of peritoneal macrophages to mount a respiratory burst and release reactive oxygen species and hypochlorite is impaired (26). This process is opsonin dependent. Thus, reduced levels of opsonins in peritoneal fluid may be responsible, in part, for reduced killing by macrophages in dialysis patients. The dialysate itself and the length of its dwell time also may play a role in the patient's response to bacterial invasion. The longer the dwell time, the less inhibition of phagocytosis occurs, such that dialysate from an overnight dwell may not appear to inhibit phagocytosis. Numerous studies have shown that acidic pH, the use of lactate as buffer, and high dialysate concentration of glucose adversely affect macrophage, PMN, and mesothelial cell function (27).

Chemotaxis by peripheral blood and peritoneal PMNs was significantly lower in children on peritoneal dialysis compared with healthy controls (28). Both mean chemotactic response and mean chemiluminescence of peritoneal PMNs increased during an episode of peritonitis. Infusion of IgG into the peritoneal cavity causes an increase in chemotactic response and mean chemiluminescence, probably as a result of enhanced opsonization (28).

PERITONITIS

Peritonitis remains a major complication for children undergoing either CCPD or CAPD. In addition to complications related to acute infection, long-term sequelae include the loss of peritoneal transport capacity as a result of mesothelial fibrosis, which sometimes forces a change in the dialysis modality to hemodialysis. Compared with the older child or adult, in infants and children younger than 6 years of age, the rate of peritonitis episodes is higher; in this young group of patients, peritoneal dialysis is the only practical method for dialysis in some centers.

Incidence

The incidence of peritonitis is higher in children than adults mainly because of the high rate among children less than 6 years of age. Comparison of peritonitis rates among adults and children on CCPD and CAPD from a single center revealed that, whereas the incidence of peritonitis was significantly lower in adults than in children on CAPD, there was no significant age-related difference in those using CCPD (29). Peritonitis-free survival according to age was 50% at 18 months after start of peritoneal dialysis in children older than 6 years of age compared with only 20%

in children younger than 6 years of age (30). Data from the European multicenter study reported one episode every 16.9 patient-months (30), and the North American Pediatric Renal Transplant Cooperative Study (NAPRTCS) multicenter study reported one episode every 13.3 months (31). Analysis of the 1998 NAPRTCS data by age showed an annual peritonitis rate of 1.09 (one episode each 11 patient-months) for children aged 1 year or younger, 0.96 (one episode every 12.5 patient-months) for those aged 2 to 5 years, 0.89 (one episode every 13.5 patient-months) for those aged 6 to 12 years, and 0.85 (one episode every 14 patient-months) for those aged 12 years or older. About 50% of all children on peritoneal dialysis will develop peritonitis, and 10% to 20% will have three or more episodes.

Diagnosis

Peritonitis comes to the attention of the caretaker/patient when signs of peritoneal irritation, fever, or cloudy fluid are observed. A cell count of greater than 100 PMNs per mm^3 is highly suggestive of peritonitis. In a series of 166 children with peritonitis, 78% had abdominal pain, 62% had fever, and in 17% cloudy dialysate was the only sign. The mean initial peritoneal cell count was 1,750 cells/mm^3, with a range of 800 to 5,000 (29). Patients and parents are taught to recognize subtle signs of peritonitis and to contact their physician or dialysis center for further diagnostic studies. In the face of clinical symptoms, empiric therapy is begun based on the previous history of the patient and the results from Gram stain of the peritoneal fluid cell pellet.

Predisposing Factors

Peritonitis usually is acquired by one of two routes: touch contamination at the time of connection (intraluminal route) or exit-site infection or colonization with entry of organisms along the tunnel tract (periluminal route) (32). Urinary diversion (vesicostomy, ureterostomy) also may increase the risk for gram-negative peritonitis because of the frequency of colonization of these diversions and proximity to the catheter. Pelvic infection with *Neisseria gonorrheae* may spread to the peritoneum. Occasionally, peritonitis may be related to an intraabdominal event, such as transmural migration of bacteria after enema, or as a result of visceral injury. In addition to these extrinsic factors, individual host factors, which have been discussed already, also may predispose to peritonitis. Recently, children on peritoneal dialysis underwent evaluation of lymphocyte subpopulations. Fourteen children had no history of peritonitis, and seven had one or more peritonitis episodes. The children with peritonitis had a significantly lower percentage of NK cells and a higher CD3, CD4, and CD4:CD8 ratio (33).

Exit-Site Infection

Exit-site or tunnel infections are the single most important predisposing factor to the development of peritonitis by the periluminal route. Exit-site colonization without overt infection also may increase the risk for contamination along the tunnel tract. Exit-site infection manifests as erythema, exudate, or increased granulation tissue around the site. Trauma, irritation at the exit site, water immersion, the presence of urinary diversion, and the presence of a gastrostomy tube may increase the likelihood of bacterial contamination and exit-site infection. *Staphylococcus aureus* is the most common causative agent for exit site infections. In a series of children with peritonitis reported by the Mid-European Pediatric Peritoneal Dialysis Study Group, 53% of children with *S. aureus* peritonitis had colonization with the same organism at their exit site compared with only 5.3% of those with non-*S. aureus* peritonitis (30). In addition, *S. aureus* nasal carriage is associated with exit-site infections. In a series of 21 children on chronic peritoneal dialysis who were screened at intervals for *S. aureus* nasal carriage, 13 (62%) developed nasal *S. aureus* carriage, and seven of these, or 54%, devel-

oped exit-site infections; one developed peritonitis (34). Those without demonstration of *S. aureus* nasal carriage did not develop *S. aureus* exit-site infections or peritonitis. The other organism cultured from the exit site with significant frequency is *Pseudomonas*, which has been successfully treated in most patients with oral ciprofloxacin (35).

Intraperitoneal Response to Bacterial Invasion

After the introduction of significant quantities of bacteria into the peritoneal cavity, peritoneal macrophages generate inflammatory cytokines IL-1, IL-6, IL-8 and TNF-α and chemotactic agents. The production of prostaglandins (TXB_2, PGE_2) is decreased, and production of leukotrienes increased in response to bacterial challenge. Macrophages from chronically dialyzed patients appear to be already primed with greater than normal constitutive cytokine synthesis (36). In response to cytokines and to bacterial invasion, mesothelial cells increase: (a) production of vasodilatory prostaglandins, which increase the permeability of the membrane to proteins; and (b) transcription and release of cytokines, such as IL-8, which augments the recruitment of PMNs from the peripheral circulation into the peritoneal cavity. Exposure of PMNs to dialysate inhibits the production of leukotrienes. Cell function, however, is partially restored by either increasing the acidic pH to neutral or by reduction of osmolality. Dialysate also reduces cytokine mRNA transcription by mesothelial cells (37).

Spectrum of Infecting Organisms

In most series of children with peritonitis, gram-positive organisms account for the majority of infections. *S. aureus* and *S. epidermidis* account for about half the initial episodes and more than three fourths of the relapses (30). *S. epidermidis* may invade after colonization of the external catheter, with entry into the peritoneum at the time of connection through touch contamination (32). *S. aureus* peritonitis has been linked most commonly to colonization of the exit site and tunnel with organisms matching those in the nares of the caretaker or patient (see preceding discussion of exit-site infections). *S. aureus* usually is associated with much more severe and prolonged clinical symptoms and may be more common among patients on CAPD compared with those on CCPD, presumably because of the increased number of connections made during a 24-hour period. Other gram positive organisms include enterococcus, nonenterococcal streptococci, and diphtheroids (30,32,38,39). Occasionally, gram-positive rods such as *Bacillus* species and *Oerskovia* are cultured.

Gram-negative infections account for approximately one fourth of the organisms recovered during peritonitis (31,32,38,39). Various pathogens are reported among the pediatric center case series; *Escherichia coli, Acinetobacter, Pseudomonas* sp, and *Klebsiella* sp are the most common. Gram-negative organisms encountered rarely include *Citrobacter, Serratia, Haemophilus, Neisseria,* or *Morganella* sp.

Fungal peritonitis accounts for 1% to 5% of acute peritonitis (31,32,37–39). Fungal peritonitis is the most serious and potentially life-threatening type of peritonitis. *Candida* spp. were the cause of fungal peritonitis in 78% of children in the NAPRTCs database (40) and 76% of adult patients reported from a single center (41). *Candida* spp. recovered from peritoneal fluid cultures included *C. albicans, C. parapsilopsis*, *C. tropicalis*, *C. rugosa*, *C. krussei,* and *C. guillermondi*. Less common fungi include *Cryptococcus, Torulopsis, Histoplasma, Paccilomyces, Coccidiodes,* and *Ustilago* spp. (39–43). Risk factors for fungal peritonitis include recent bacterial peritonitis, recent antibiotic administration, immunosuppressive drugs, and gastrostomy tube (44), although no one single factor is consistently recognized in the various case series.

Occasionally, acid-fast bacteria, such as atypical mycobacteria, cause peritonitis (45). In some series, clinical peritonitis with negative culture may account for up to 25% of cases. The likelihood for yield is increased if 5 to 10 mL of peritoneal fluid is immediately placed into bottles containing broth for anaerobic and aerobic culture in a manner similar to that of blood culture technique (39).

Treatment

Treatment of peritonitis should be started as quickly as possible and may begin with three rapid exchanges with dialysate containing heparin but without antibiotic in an attempt to remove physically cells, bacteria, and fibrin. Initial treatment is empiric unless the Gram stain can guide the choice of antimicrobial agent. Because the most common cause of peritonitis is staphylococci, coverage for gram-positive organisms is prudent. Usually, coverage for gram-negative organisms is included as well. A survey of 49 pediatric nephrologists found that vancomycin is the initial therapy chosen by 29 (59%), an aminoglycoside is initial therapy chosen by 28 (57%), and a cephalosporin is chosen as initial therapy by 20 (41%), with even distribution among first, second, and third generation (46). To avoid the overzealous use of vancomycin, the ad hoc guidelines for initial therapy were revised and now recommend a first-generation cephalosporin plus aminoglycoside (47); however, this combination would be inadequate for approximately one third of the cases of gram-positive peritonitis. If the patient recently had an infection with resistant staphylococci, or if the patient is particularly symptomatic, vancomycin might be warranted as the choice for initial therapy. Otherwise, the initial use of vancomycin has been discouraged for fear that resistance might increase because vancomycin resistance is transferable to staphylococci. Once the culture results are available, antimicrobial therapy is selected according to the sensitivity profile. Most bacterial peritonitis can be adequately treated with a single agent; however, in the case of *Serratia, Acinetobacter,* or *Pseudomonas* organisms, two agents usually are recommended. The length of therapy varies between 10 and 14 days.

In addition to the choice of initial antimicrobial, one may choose to provide continuous or intermittent antibiotics (30). This issue is primarily in children on CAPD rather than CCPD, in which the bags of dialysate for treatment are prepared at the time of treatment rather than throughout the day. Loading doses of antibiotics are favored by many investigators in the treatment of CAPD and CCPD patients with peritonitis. Others, however, add antibiotic to dialysate in a concentration similar to that desired for plasma. Because most patients on CCPD are left with a "dwell" of dialysate containing antibiotics at the end of therapy, treatment is continuous. One concern about continuous therapy is ototoxicity resulting from vancomycin or aminoglycoside. In one study, however, children who received treatment with intraperitoneal but not intravenous aminoglycoside had no significant alteration in audiograms (48).

Relapses of peritonitis may occur as a result of the sequestration of bacteria along the catheter within a slime layer or fibrin accumulation. Regimens to decontaminate the Tenckhoff catheter may be useful in such cases. There were no relapses of peritonitis in a group of children treated with infusion of urokinase followed by instillation of intraluminal antibiotics at high concentrations once daily for three consecutive days and change of the transfer set. This compared favorably with a 76% recurrence rate and a 37% rate of catheter removal among historical controls (49).

Fungal Peritonitis

Of 55 adults with fungal peritonitis, 47 underwent catheter removal, and eight had their catheters left in place; mortality was 15% and 50%, respectively (41). Removal of the Tenckhoff catheter within 1 week of diagnosis is usually recommended, although some advocate continuation of peritoneal dialysis during the initiation of systemic antifungal therapy in hope that the presence of fluid within the cavity will reduce the likelihood for formation of adhesions. Some reports of successful same-day removal and reinsertion of the catheter in the case of fungal peritonitis have appeared, but most centers remove the

catheter for a period of 2 to 4 weeks in addition to systemic antifungal therapy. Following removal of the peritoneal dialysis catheter, a temporary, and sometimes a permanent, change in dialysis modality to hemodialysis is required. Approximately 50% of patients successfully return to peritoneal dialysis after adequate treatment.

The use of single versus double antifungal treatment is controversial. Intravenous amphotericin B is the most commonly used single agent. Intravenous amphotericin B alone was used in 30 of 51 (59%) episodes of fungal peritonitis in children and in 37 of 55 (67%) adults with fungal peritonitis. Intraperitoneal amphotericin B is painful; nonetheless, it was used during 11 of 51 (22%) episodes in children but in only 5 of 55 (9%) of adults (40,41). Oral, intravenous, and intraperitoneal fluconazole has been used alone or in combination with other antifungals. Flucytosine occasionally has been given orally alone or in combination with fluconazole. The duration of treatment for fungal peritonitis is typically 2 weeks.

Prevention

Treatment with prophylactic antibiotics at the time of catheter placement has been reported to reduce the early development of peritonitis (50). Treatment of nasal carriage of *S. aureus* with intranasal mupirocin as well as daily exit-site care with mupirocin will reduce the frequency of peritonitis (31). A novel approach to prevent the inital colonization of the tunnel via external contamination implants the Tenckhoff catheter completely subcutaneous for the first several months after surgery. This type of approach is practical only for patients who are currently on hemodialysis or whose ESRD is anticipated well in advance. Using the swan-neck presternal catheter in infants at risk for contamination from diaper soiling is another potential method for prevention of exit-site infection and peritonitis (51). Of children enrolled in the NAPRTCS database, 17.5% have swan neck catheters (31). In addition, the use of a catheter with two cuffs appears to delay the time to first episode of peritonitis, as does lateral or downward direction of the exit sites from insertion site.

Prevention of Exit-Site Infections

Prevention of exit site infections starts with meticulous postimplantation care to prevent colonization and trauma during the early healing period. The catheter site should receive a sterile dressing at the completion of implantation while still in the operating room. The dressing should remain in place for 1 to 2 weeks unless the gauze becomes wet. The catheter should be immobilized to prevent trauma. The site may be cleansed with a mild antiseptic, taking care not to allow the antiseptic to enter the sinus space between the catheter and subcutaneous tissue. Once the site has healed, it can be cleansed with antibacterial soap and carefully dried with application of mupirocin.

Prophylaxis for *S. aureus* nasal carriage using mupirocin or rifampin also may prevent peritonitis and exit-site infections (52). Treatment of six children on peritoneal dialysis who had nasal carriage using rifampin/cloxacillin was successful in eradicating nasal carriage but recolonization occurred in two thirds of cases. The use of intranasal mupirocin for 3 days each month plus exit site care with mupirocin is a reasonable alternative to systemic therapy.

CHILDHOOD NEPHROTIC SYNDROME

Definitions and Classifications

Children with nephrotic syndrome have a greatly increased risk of serious bacterial infections. The nephrotic syndrome is characterized by large urinary protein loss (40 mg/m² per hour; normal is less than 4), hypoalbuminemia (< 2.5 g/dl) and hyperlipidemia (53). The child with nephrotic syndrome usually has generalized edema, often with marked ascites. An affected child is at high risk for the development of bacterial sepsis or peritonitis as a result of encapsulated organisms, particularly *Streptococcus pneumoniae,* due to decreased serum levels of IgG and complement factor B.

For children between the ages of 1 and 16 years who have the nephrotic syndrome, more than 85% will have primary idiopathic nephrosis, whereas others will have nephrotic syndrome as a result of glomerulonephritis, such as membranoproliferative or membranous glomerulonephritis (53). Of children aged 1 to 16 years with idiopathic nephrotic syndrome, 93% will achieve remission, defined by complete loss of proteinuria, in response to treatment with prednisone given in a dose of 60 mg/24 hours/m² (maximum dosage 80 mg every 24 hours) (54). Such patients are classified as having steroid-responsive idiopathic nephrotic syndrome (SRINS). Most of these children have normal light microscopic findings on renal biopsy: this is termed *minimal change lesion nephrosis* (MCLN) (54). The incidence of SRINS for white children aged 1 through 9 years is nearly two cases per 100,000 children per year (55). The long-term prognosis for children with SRINS is excellent, and the time in relapse for these patients is short (56). Children with idiopathic nephrosis who do not achieve remission in response to prednisone are at high risk for having focal segmental glomerulosclerosis (FSGS) or chronic glomerulonephritis. These children often have long periods of marked hypoalbuminemia and most eventually progress to ESRD (53). Because longer duration of proteinuria tends to increase the risk of bacterial peritonitis, such children are more likely to develop bacterial peritonitis than children with SRINS.

Immunologic Alterations in Nephrotic Syndrome

The first immunologic defect found to be present in the nephrotic syndrome was the marked depression of serum gamma globulin concentration (57). Subsequently, the pattern for serum immunoglobulin concentrations in the nephrotic syndrome consisted of markedly depressed IgG, normal or depressed IgA, and normal or elevated IgM (58–60). Depression of the serum IgG concentration occurs in nephrotic syndrome from all causes. Serum IgG concentrations in patients with SRINS will rise after remission is achieved with corticosteroid therapy but will not always rise into the normal range even after many years of remission (59,60). Because IgG has been recovered from the urine of patients with nephrotic syndrome (61), urinary losses are felt to contribute in part to the depression of the serum levels (59,61). Children with the nephrotic syndrome have a reduction of IgG_2 subclass levels disproportionate to the reduction of the other IgG subclass levels (62).

In addition to depression of serum IgG levels, children with active nephrotic syndrome have low serum levels of the complement proteins factors B and I (63). Opsonization of encapsulated bacteria is a prerequisite for efficient phagocytosis. Perhaps the most important serum opsonins are IgG (64,65) and C3b (66). Although serum C3 levels are normal or increased in children with active nephrosis (63,67–69), low factor B levels are suspected to limit the generation of C3b through the C3b amplification loop, resulting in impaired opsonization of encapsulated bacteria (63,69,70). McLean et al. found that serum from children with nephrotic syndrome had a decreased capacity for opsonization of *E. coli,* which was restored by the addition of factor B (69). Children with nephrotic syndrome who develop peritonitis have significantly lower serum levels of factor I (71), factor B (70), and IgG (72) during relapse than those who do not develop peritonitis. Factor B is also important for macrophage spreading; low serum levels may enhance susceptibility to bacterial infection by impairing macrophage function (73).

Spectrum of Bacterial Infection

Considerable evidence exists that the pathogenesis of idiopathic childhood nephrosis involves a basic defect in cellular immunity (74–76). None of the described defects, however, has been linked to the increased susceptibility to infection associated with the nephrotic syndrome. Opportunistic infections attributable to viruses and fungi rarely, if ever, occur in association with childhood nephrosis. The infections clearly related to the nephrotic sydrome alone are bacterial, and defective opsonization appears to be the main risk factor.

Numerous clinical series have been published on peritonitis in childhood nephrosis, from the period during the mid-1950s, when corticosteroids first were used to induce prompt remission for most children with nephrosis, until the mid-1980s, when pneumococcal vaccine was routinely administered to such patients. These studies showed that *S. pneumoniae* was the predominant causative organism, isolated in more than 50% of the cases (77–82). For 20% of the cases, symptoms and signs (>50 PMNs per mm^3 of peritoneal fluid or a positive blood culture) of peritonitis were present, and the response to antibiotic therapy was good, and yet the peritoneal culture was negative (77). Other organisms that frequently cause peritonitis in children with nephrotic syndrome include streptococci other than *S. pneumoniae, E. coli, Enterobacteriaceae,* and *H. influenzae* (72,77–82).

For the period 1967 through 1986, 37 of 214 (17.3%) of children with follow-up for nephrotic syndrome in Dallas developed peritonitis (80). In that study, 16% of the children with MCLN had at least one episode of peritonitis. A much lower rate for peritonitis of 5.4% of 351 children with nephrotic syndrome occurred in Boston at about the same time (1970–1980) (72). In that series, black children were significantly more likely to develop peritonitis than were white children (72), which may be in part because of a high prevalence of steroid-resistant FSGS among African-American children. Recurrent episodes of peritonitis occur in 20% of children with nephrotic syndrome who had an initial episode (77), which suggests an underlying predisposition in these children.

In addition to spontaneous bacterial peritonitis, children with active nephrotic syndrome are at increased risk for invasive tissue infections (83,84). *S. pneumoniae* has been reported to cause a rapidly spreading erysipelas in patients with nephrotic syndrome (85).

The frequency of bacterial infection and the spectrum of causative organisms may differ in children from underdeveloped countries compared with children from North America and Europe (84). In countries where tuberculosis is endemic, the treatment of nephrotic syndrome with corticosteroids can unmask latent disease. Tuberculosis occurred in 9% of Indian children with nephrotic syndrome compared with a 1% prevalence in the general population (86). Tuberculosis generally developed while the child was being treated with corticosteroids and other immunosuppressive medications and often resulted in the inability to treat the renal disease adequately, sometimes resulting in death or progression to renal failure (86).

Treatment

Based on the spectrum of causative organisms, the traditional initial therapy for septicemia or peritonitis in children with the nephrotic syndrome has been penicillin plus an aminoglycoside (77). With the recent increase in frequency of penicillin- and cephalosporin-resistant pneumococcal infections, however, such treatment may not be adequate.

Penicillin-resistant *S. pneumoniae* caused peritonitis in two infants with congenital nephrotic syndrome (87) and in two chidren with nephrosis, one with steroid-resistant FSGS and the other at the onset of SRINS (88). In areas where the incidence of penicillin- and cephalosporin-resistant *S. pneumoniae* infections is high, vancomycin may be advisable for initial therapy for peritonitis in children with the nephrotic syndrome.

Congenital Nephrotic Syndrome

Congenital nephrotic syndrome becomes apparent in the first 3 months of life (89) and has numerous causes, including congenital infections such as cytomegalovirus and syphilis (90,91), maternal systemic lupus erythematosus (92), and hereditary conditions. The two most common causes of congenital nephrotic syndrome are diffuse mesangial sclerosis, which is associated with abnormalities in the Wilms' tumor 1 (*WT-1*) gene (93) and Finnish-type congenital nephrotic syndrome, which has special infectious considerations (94–100).

Finnish-type congenital nephrotic syndrome is so named because it has an extremely high incidence (i.e., 1 per 8,000 live births) in Finland (94), although cases have been reported in all other ethnic groups (95). This autosomal recessive disorder results from mutations in the gene for nephrin, a transmembrane protein of the immunoglobulin family of cell adhesion molecules, which is crucial in maintaining the integrity of the glomerular filtration barrier (96). Infants with Finnish-type congenital nephrotic syndrome have massive proteinuria beginning in utero (97). Because of the unique molecular defect in the glomerular basement membrane, children with this syndrome have much greater losses of IgG in the urine than in typical childhood nephrotic syndrome. Serum levels of IgG may be as low as seen in children with agammaglobulinemia (98). Serum IgM levels are usually normal or elevated, probably because the larger size of these immunoglobulins results in their retention. IgA levels are usually normal (99,100). Loss of opsonic activity undoubtedly contributes to the extremely high rate of bacterial sepsis in these infants. Mahan et al. reported 67 episodes of serious bacterial infection in 41 infants with this syndrome (96). In a review by Ljungberg, 21 infants with congenital nephrotic syndrome had 64 confirmed and 61 suspected episodes of sepsis over a 1.1-year follow-up (99). Most common pathogens included *S. epidermidis* (40%), *S. aureus* (16%), *E. coli* (12%), and *S. pneumoniae* (9%) (98). Episodes of sepsis in these infants are often notable for a lack of acute phase signs and symptoms (99,100). Attempts to replace IgG in these patients with intravenous infusions have been unsuccessful because the immunoglobulin is lost in the urine in a matter of hours (98,99). Infusions of intravenous immunoglobulin do not appear to prevent the occurrence of bacterial sepsis (98). Prophylactic antibiotics appear to have no efficacy (99). Care for infants with congenital nephrotic syndrome involves careful observation for signs and symptoms of sepsis and prompt institution of antibiotic therapy (99). In addition, some centers, including ours, administer intravenous IgG when sepsis is diagnosed, although this therapy is unproven (98). At present, infants with congenital nephrotic syndrome are cared for with albumin infusions and aggressive nutrition in the first year of life, and nephrectomy and dialysis in the second year (100). Nephrectomy results in normalization of serum protein levels (100).

IMMUNIZATION IN CHILDHOOD RENAL DISEASE

Children with renal disease merit special considerations with regard to immunization. Those with certain types of renal disease may respond suboptimally to vaccines, and the use of immunosuppressive drugs for treatment may also affect response to vaccines. In addition, some fear that the immune stimulation associated with certain immunizations might trigger a relapse of nephrotic syndrome in some children.

Chronic Renal Insufficiency and End-Stage Renal Disease

Although only a few studies of response to vaccination in children with CRI have been conducted, available data suggest that the response to diphtheria, tetanus, rubella, hepatitis B, and pneumococcal and influenza vaccines is normal (101–104). In addition to standard vaccines recommended by the American College of Immunization Practices (ACIP) for healthy children (105), influenza and pneumococcal vaccines are recommended by most pediatric nephrologists for children with CRI (106,107). Children with CRI are likely to undergo future renal transplantation. Thus, it is important to

demonstrate that such children have protective antibody titers to varicella and mumps, measles, and rubella vaccines, particularly because live virus vaccines may not be safe to administer after transplantation (106–108).

Vaccine recommendations for pediatric patients undergoing chronic dialysis are similar to those for children with CRI (106,107). Good response to diphtheria and tetanus toxoids, rubella, and *Haemophilus influenzae* type B vaccine (HIB) have been demonstrated for infants immunized while on CCPD (109–111); however, children on dialysis may not respond as well as normal controls to the measles and mumps component of the measles, mumps, and rubella (MMR) vaccine (111). Adults on dialysis have a decreased rate of seroconversion with the hepatitis B vaccine (13), whereas children appear to have a better response (102). One solution to this problem is doubling the recommended dose of hepatitis B vaccine. This approach produced a 97% seroconversion rate after three doses among pediatric patients on peritoneal dialysis (112). Hepatitis B surface antibody levels should be followed, and the patient should be reimmunized if levels fall below 10 mIU/mL (107). Greenbaum and Salusky showed a poor response to the varicella vaccine by children on dialysis, with only two of nine dialysis patients mounting a protective response after one dose of vaccine (113). Others, however, showed a good response to two doses of the vaccine (107). For patients on dialysis, it is advisable to measure varicella and mumps, measles, and rubella titers before renal transplantation and reimmunize if levels are not protective (107). A prospective study on efficacy of pneumococcal vaccine in children on dialysis has shown a good initial antibody response to the limited number of strains tested, with persistence over at least 2 years (107). Earlier studies showed a significant decline in antibody titers with time in pediatric patients on dialysis (114,115). Booster immunizations may be indicated in patients at high risk for pneumococcal disease (107). There are currently no studies on the effects of the conjugate pneumococcal vaccine (Prevnar) in children with renal insufficiency.

Nephrotic Syndrome

Although there are special considerations for the immunization of children with the nephrotic syndrome, most pediatric nephrologists agree that such children should be adequately protected against common childhood diseases (116). There is no contraindication to administration of inactive vaccines to children with nephrotic syndrome, although there are no data on response rates to these vaccines in children with nephrotic syndrome compared with normal controls. In general, pediatric nephrologists follow the ACIP guidelines for administration of vaccines to the immunosuppressed host (108). No data are presently available on response rates to the MMR vaccine in patients with nephrotic syndrome. In one study, children with the nephrotic syndrome showed poor response to the varicella vaccine, even though all patients were in remission and off corticosteroid therapy at the time of vaccination (117). A multicenter investigation of antibody response to varicella following two-dose administration of the vaccine is currently in progress. Boys with SRINS had a poor response to the hepatitis B vaccine (118). Septicemia resulting from *H. influenzae* type b occurred in a child with active nephrotic syndrome despite prior administration of the HIB vaccine (119). The absence of additional reports of failure of the HIB vaccine to protect against invasive *H. influenzae* type B infection suggests that children with nephrotic syndrome maintain immunity to the HIB vaccine.

Pneumococcal infection can be a life-threatening problem in children with idiopathic nephrotic syndrome. Two studies showed adequate response to a 14-valent pneumococcal vaccine in children with steroid-responsive nephrotic syndrome in remission (120,121). Wilkes et al. (121) found no difference in the ability to mount a protective response to most capsular types included in the vaccine between patients receiving daily prednisone and those on alternate-day steroid therapy. Spika et al. (120) found no difference between patients on steroid therapy and those not receiving steroids; however, in that study, two patients who were either currently or recently treated with an alkylating agent (chlorambucil or cyclophosphamide) had significantly lower levels of capsular antibody than normal controls or patients with nephrotic syndrome in remission (120), and patients with steroid-resistant nephrotic syndrome and heavy proteinuria had significantly lower levels of capsular antibody than their steroid-responsive counterparts (120).

Several studies reported failures of the pneumococcal vaccine to protect against disease caused by a certain serotype in the 14-valent vaccine (122–124). Moore et al. documented a case of pneumococcal peritonitis caused by strain 19, found in the vaccine, in a girl who had previously received the vaccine (122). Serologic studies documented a poor antibody response to strain 19 following immunization. Children with nephrotic syndrome in remission showed a significantly poorer response to strain 19F than to other strains in the vaccine (120). Pneumococcal disease in previously immunized children with nephrotic syndrome also has been associated with strains 4 and 14 (123,124). There are at present no data on response to the conjugate vaccine for children with nephrotic syndrome.

We currently recommend that patients with SRINS receive the polyvalent pneumococcal vaccine during their first remission, whether or not they are still receiving prednisone. Although the likelihood of a protective antibody response is much less in patients with steroid-resistant nephrotic syndrome, vaccination of these patients also is recommended because the persistent hypoalbuminemia and proteinuria increase their risk for peritonitis. The study of Spika et al. (120) suggests that pneumococcal vaccine should not be administered during or for several months after treatment with alkylating agents.

Because immune stimuli (e.g., bee sting, respiratory infections) may act as triggers for relapse of SRINS, some controversy exists as to whether to provide routine immunization of children with frequently relapsing nephrotic syndrome at all. Because the mean age of presentation with the nephrotic syndrome is 3 years, most children who develop nephrotic syndrome will have partially completed their childhood immunization schedule. In a survey of North American pediatric nephrologists, nearly half recommended delaying or deferring at least some immunizations because of the risk of relapse, despite the fact that there are no published data to support this practice (116). More studies on this issue are clearly needed. Most pediatric nephrologists believe the risk of relapse of the nephrotic syndrome must be weighed against the risk of not protecting the child adequately against childhood diseases. Our current practice is to keep patients with infrequent relapses on a standard immunization schedule. In children who have frequent relapses but who have received all recommended immunizations through 18 months, we recommend deferring booster immunizations until the child has been in remission and off corticosteroids for 2 years.

REFERENCES

1. Montgomerie JZ, Kalmanson GM, Guze LB. Renal failure and infection. *Medicine* 1968;47:1–32.
2. United States Renal Data System. 1998 Annual Data Report: VI. Causes of death. *Am J Kidney Dis* 1998; 32:S81–83.
3. United States Renal Data System. 1998 Annual Data Report: VIII. Pediatric end-stage renal disease. *Am J Kidney Dis* 1998;32:S98–103.
4. United States Renal Data System. 1998 Annual Data Report: II. Incidence and prevalence of ESRD. *Am J Kidney Dis* 1998;32:S38–49.
5. Cohen G, Haag-Weber M, Horl WH. Immune dysfunction in uremia. *Kidney Int* 1997;52:S79–82.
6. Descamps-Latscha B, Herbelin A. Long-term dialysis and cellular immunity: a critical survey. *Kidney Int* 1993;43:S135–142.
7. Chatenoud L, Herbelin A, Beaurain G, et al. Immune deficiency of the uremic patient. *Adv Nephrol Necker Hosp* 1990;19:259–274.
8. Khan IH, Catto GR. Long-term complications of dialysis: infection. *Kidney Int* 1993;41:S143–148.
9. Donati D, Degiannis D, Homer L, et al. Immune deficiency in uremia: Interleukin-2 production and responsiveness and interleukin-2 receptor expression and release. *Nephron* 1991;58:268–275.
10. Donati D, Degiannis D, Raskova J, et al. Uremic serum effects on peripheral blood mononuclear cell and purified T lymphocyte responses. *Kidney Int* 1992;42:681–689.
11. Girndt M, Kohler H, Schiedhelm-Weick E, et al. T cell activation defect in hemodialysis patients: evidence for a role of the B7/CD28 pathway. *Kidney Int* 1993; 44:359–365.
12. Descamps-Latscha B, Chatenoud L. T cells and B cells

in chronic renal failure. *Semin Nephrol* 1986; 16:183–191.
13. Stevens CE, Alter HJ, Taylor PE, et al. Hepatitis B vaccine in patients receiving hemodialysis. Immunogenicity and efficacy. *N Engl J Med* 1984;11:496–501.
14. Dumann H, Meuer S, Meyer zum Buschenfelde KH, et al. Hepatitis B vaccination anad interleukin 2 receptor expression in chronic renal failure. *Kidney Int* 1990; 38:1164–1168.
15. Meuer SC, Dumann H, Meyer zum Buschenfelde KH, et al. Low dose interleukin-2 induces systemic immune responses against HbsAg in immunodeficient non-responders to hepatitis B vaccination. *Lancet* 1989;I:15–18.
16. Jungers P, Devillier P, Salomon H, et al. Randomised placebo-controlled trial of recombinant interleukin-2 in chronic uraemic patients who are non-responders to hepatitis B vaccine. *Lancet* 1994;344:856–857.
17. Mauri JM, Valles M. Effects of recombinant interleukin-2 and revaccination for hepatitis B in previously vaccinated, non-responder chronic uraemic patients. Collaborative Group of Girona. *Nephrol Dial Transplant* 1997;12:729–732.
18. Zaoui P, Hakim RM. Natural killer-cell function in hemodialysis patients: Effect of the dialysis membrane. *Kidney Int* 1993;43:1298–1305.
19. Lewis SL, van Epps DE. Neutrophil and monocyte alterations in chronic dialysis patients. *Am J Kidney Dis* 1987;9:381–395.
20. Vanholder R, Ringoir S, Dhondt A, et al. Phagocytosis in uremic and hemodialysis patients: A prospective and cross sectional study. *Kidney Int* 1991;39:320–327.
21. Cendoroglo M, Jaber BL, Balakrishnan VS, et al. Neutrophil apoptosis and dysfunction in uremia. *J Am Soc Nephrol* 1999;10:93–100.
22. Pereira BJ, Shapiro L, King AJ, et al. Plasma levels of IL-1 beta, TNF alpha and their specific inhibitors in undialyzed chronic renal failure, CAPD and hemodialysis patients. *Kidney Int* 1994;45:890–896.
23. Cavaillon JM, Poignet JL, Fitting C, et al. Serum interleukin-6 in long-term hemodialyzed patients. *Nephron* 1992;60:307–313.
24. Manca F, Perfumo F, Kunkl A, et al. *In vitro* evidence for impaired cellular immune responsiveness in children with chronic renal failure. *Acta Paediatr Scand* 1989;78:597–600.
25. Drachman R, Schlesinger M, Shapira H, et al. The immune status of uraemic children/adolescents with chronic renal failure and renal replacement therapy. *Pediatr Nephrol* 1989;3:305.
26. Cameron JS. Host defenses in continuous ambulatory peritoneal dialysis and the genesis of peritonitis. *Pediatr Nephrol* 1995;9:647.
27. Jörres A, Gahl G, Frei U. Peritoneal dialysis fluid biocompatibility: Does it really matter? *Kidney Int* 1994; 48:S79–86.
28. Akman S, Guven AG, Ince S, et al. Effect of intraperitoneal immunoglobulin infusion on neutrophil function in CAPD children with and without peritonitis. *Adv Peritoneal Dial* 1998;14:239–242.
29. Howard RL, Millspaugh J, Teitelbaum I. Adult and pediatric peritonitis rates in a home dialysis program: comparison of continuous ambulatory and continuous cycling peritoneal dialysis. *Am J Kidney Dis* 1990; 16:469–472.

30. Schaefer F, Klaus G, Müller-Wiefel DE, et al., and the Mid-European Pediatric Peritoneal Dialysis Study Group (MEPPS). Intermittent versus continuous intraperitoneal glycopeptide/ceftazidime treatment in children with peritoneal dialysis-associated peritonitis. *J Am Soc Nephrol* 1999;10:136.

31. Warady BA, Sullivan EK, Alexander SR. Lessons from the peritoneal dialysis patient database: a report of the North American Pediatric Renal Transplant Cooperative Study. *Kidney Int* 1996;49:S68–71.

32. Piraino B. Peritonitis as a complication of peritoneal dialysis. *J Am Soc Nephrol* 1998;9:1956–1964.

33. Aksu N, Keskinoglu A, Erdogan H, et al. Does immunologic status predict peritonitis in children treated with CAPD? *Adv Perit Dial* 1998;14:243–246.

34. Kingwatanakul P, Warady BA. *Staphylococcus aureus* nasal carriage in children receiving long-term peritoneal dialysis. *Adv Perit Dial* 1997;13:281–284.

35. Kazmi HR, Raffone FD, Kliger AS, et al. Pseudomonas exit site infections in continuous ambulatory peritoneal dialysis patients. *J Am Soc Nephrol* 1992; 2:1498.

36. Topley N, Williams JD. Role of the peritoneal membrane in the control of inflammation in the peritoneal cavity. *Kidney Int* 1994;46:S71–78.

37. Saklayen MG. CAPD peritonitis: incidence, pathogens, diagnosis and management. *Med Clin North Am* 1990;74:997.

38. Kuison B, Melocoton TL, Holloway M, et al. Infectious and catheter-related complications in pediatric patients treated with peritoneal dialysis at a single institution. *Pediatr Nephrol* 1995;9:S12–17.

39. Powell D, San Luis I, Calvin S, et al. Peritonitis in children undergoing continuous ambulatory peritoneal dialysis. *Am J Dis Child* 1985;139:29–32.

40. Warady BA, Bashir M, Donaldson LA. Fungal peritonitis in children receiving long term peritoneal dialysis: a report of the NAPRTCS. *Kidney Int* 2000;58: 384–389.

41. Goldie SJ, Kiernan-Troidle L, Torres C, et al. Fungal peritonitis in a large chronic peritoneal dialysis population: a report of 55 episodes. *Am J Kidney Dis* 1996; 28:86.

42. Enriquez JL, Kalia A, Travis LB. Fungal peritonitis in children on peritoneal dialysis. *J Pediatr* 1990;117: 830.

43. Ampel NM, White JD, Varanasi UR, et al. Coccidioidal peritonitis associated with continuous ambulatory peritoneal dialysis. *Am J Kid Dis* 1988;11:512–514.

44. Murugasu B, Conley SB, Lemire JM, et al. Fungal peritonitis in children treated with peritoneal dialysis and gastrostomy feeding. *Pediatr Nephrol* 1991;5:620.

45. Paul E, Devarajan P. *Mycobacterium phlei* peritonitis: a rare complication of chronic peritoneal dialysis. *Pediatr Nephrol* 1998;12:67.

46. Tranaeus A. Update on peritonitis incidence and treatment. 15th Annual Conference on Peritoneal Dialysis, Baltimore, MD 1995.

47. Keane WF, Alexander SR, Bailie GR. Peritoneal dialysis-related peritonitis treatment recommendations: 1996 update. *Perit Dial Int* 1996;16:557.

48. Warady BA, Reed L, Murphy G, et al. Aminoglycoside ototoxicity in pediatric patients receiving long term peritoneal dialysis. *Pediatr Nephrol* 1993;7:178.

49. Klaus G, Schäfer F, Querfeld U, et al. Treatment of relapsing peritonitis in pediatric patients on peritoneal dialysis. *Adv Perit Dial* 1992; 8: 302–305.

50. Sardegna KM, Beck AM, Strife FC. Evaluation of perioperative antibiotics at the time of catheter placement. *Pediatr Nephrol* 1998;12:149–152.

51. Sieniawska M, Roszkowska-Blaim M, Warchol S. Swan neck presternal catheter for continuous ambulatory peritoneal dialysis in children. *Pediatr Nephrol* 1993;7:557.

52. Hanevold CD, Fisher MC. Waltz R, et al. Effect of rifampin on *Staphylococcus aureus* colonization in children on chronic peritoneal dialysis. *Pediatr Nephrol* 1995;9:609–611.

53. International Study of Kidney Disease in Children. Nephrotic syndrome in children: prediction of histopathology from clinical and laboratory characteristics at time of diagnosis. *Kidney Int* 1978;13:159–165.

54. International Study of Kidney Disease in Children. The primary nephrotic syndrome in children: identification of patients with minimal change nephrotic syndrome from initial response to prednisone. *J Pediatr* 1981;98:561–564.

55. Wyatt RJ, Marx MB, Kazee M, et al. Current estimates of the incidence of steroid responsive idiopathic nephrosis in Kentucky children 1–9 years of age. *Int J Pediatr Nephrol* 1982;3:63–65.

56. Trompeter RS, Lloyd BW, Hicks J, et al. Long-term outcome for children with minimal-change nephrotic syndrome. *Lancet* 1985;1:368–370.

57. Longsworth LG, MacInnes DA. An electrophoretic study of nephrotic sera and urine. *J Exp Med* 1940;71: 77–82.

58. Momma K. Immunochemical semiquantitative estimation of gamma-M- and gamma-A-immunoglobulins in healthy and diseased children. *Acta Paediatr Jpn* 1965; 7:13–22.

59. Giangiacomo J, Cleary TG, Cole BR, et al. Serum immunoglobulins in the nephrotic syndrome. A possible cause of minimal-change nephrotic syndrome. *N Engl J Med* 1975;293:8–12.

60. Sobel AT, Intrator L, Lagrue G. Serum immunoglobulins in idiopathic minimal-change nephrotic syndrome. *N Engl J Med* 1976;294:50–51.

61. Peterson PA, Berggard I. Urinary immunoglobulin components in normal, tubular, and glomerular proteinuria: quantities and characteristics of free light chains, IgG, IgA and FC γ fragment. *Eur J Clin Invest* 1971;1:255–264.

62. Shakib F, Hardwicke J, Stanworth DR, et al. Asymmetric depression in the serum level of IgG subclasses in patients with nephrotic syndrome. *Clin Exp Immunol* 1977;28:506–511.

63. Forristal J, Iitaka K, Vallota EH, et al. Correlations between serum factor B and C3b inactivator levels in normal subjects and in patients with infections, nephrosis and hypocomplementemic glomerulonephritis. *Clin Exp Immunol* 1977;28:61–71.

64. Rowley D, Turner KJ. Number of molecules of antibody required to promote phagocytosis of one bacterium. *Nature* 1966;210:496–498.

65. Quie PG, Messner RP, Williams RC Jr. Phagocytosis in subacute bacterial endocarditis. Localization of the primary opsonic site to the Fc fragment. *J Exp Med* 1968;128:553–570.

66. Fearon DT. Cellular receptors for fragments of the third

component of complement. *Immunol Today* 1984; 5:105.

67. Wyatt RJ, Forristal J, Davis CA, et al. Control of serum C3 levels by beta 1H and C3b inactivator. *J Lab Clin Med* 1980;95:905–917.

68. Strife CF, Jackson EC, Forristal J, et al. Effect of the nephrotic syndrome on the concentration of serum complement components. *Am J Kidney Dis* 1986;8:37–42.

69. McLean RH, Forsgren A, Bjorksten B, et al. Decreased serum factor B concentration associated with decreased opsonization of *Escherichia coli* in the idiopathic nephrotic syndrome. *Pediatr Res* 1977;11:910–916.

70. Anderson DC, York TL, Rose G, et al. Assessment of serum factor B, serum opsonins, granulocyte chemotaxis, and infection in nephrotic syndrome of children. *J Infect Dis* 1979;140:1–11.

71. Matsell DG, Wyatt RJ. The role of I and B in peritonitis associated with the nephrotic syndrome of childhood. *Pediatr Res* 1993;34:84–88.

72. Krensky AM, Ingelfinger JR, Grupe WE. Peritonitis in childhood nephrotic syndrome: 1970–1980. *Am J Dis Child* 1982;136:732–736.

73. Götze O, Bianco C, Cohn ZA. The induction of macrophage spreading by factor B of the properdin. *J Exp Med* 1979;32:372–386.

74. Shalhoub RJ. Pathogenesis of lipoid nephrosis: a disorder of T-cell function. *Lancet* 1974;2:556–560.

75. Fodor P, Saitua MT, Rodriguez E, et al. T-cell dysfunction in minimal change nephrotic syndrome of childhood. *Am J Dis Child* 1982;136:713–717.

76. Matsumoto K. Impaired local graft-versus-host reaction in lipoid nephrosis. *Nephron* 1982;31:281–282.

77. Feinstein EI, Chesney RW, Zelikovic I. Peritonitis in childhood renal disease. *Am J Nephrol* 1988;8:147–165.

78. Wilfert CM, *Katz SL. Etiology of bacterial sepsis in nephrotic children 1963–1967.* Pediatrics 1968;42: 840–843.

79. Speck WT, Dresdale SS, McMillan RW. Primary peritonitis and the nephrotic syndrome. *Am J Surg* 1974; 127:267–269.

80. Gorensek MJ, Lebel MH, Nelson JD. Peritonitis in children with nephrotic syndrome. *Pediatrics* 1988;81: 849–856.

81. O'Regan S, Mongeau J, Robitaile P. Primary peritonitis in the nephrotic syndrome. *Int J Pediatr Nephrol* 1980;1:216.

82. Rubin HM, Blau EB, Michaels RH. Hemophilus and pneumococcal peritonitis in children with the nephrotic syndrome. *Pediatrics* 1975;56:598–601.

83. Asmar BI, Bashour BN, Fleischmann LE. *Escherichia coli* cellulitis in children with idiopathic nephrotic syndrome. *Clin Pediatr* 1987;26:592–594.

84. Gulati S, Kher V, Gupta A, et al. Spectrum of infections in Indian children with nephrotic syndrome. *Pediatr Nephrol* 1995;9:431–434.

85. Varghese R, Melo JC, Chun CH, et al. Erysipelas-like syndrome caused by *Streptococcus pneumoniae*. *South Med J* 1976;72:757.

86. Gulati S, Kher V, Gulati K, et al. Tuberculosis in childhood nephrotic syndrome in India. *Pediatr Nephrol* 1997;11:695–698.

87. Milner LS, Berkowitz FE, Ngwenya E, et al. Penicillin resistant pneumococcal peritonitis in nephrotic syndrome. *Arch Dis Child* 1987;62:964–965.

88. Ilyas M, Roy S III, Abbasi S, et al. Serious infection due to penicillin-resistant *Streptococcus pneumoniae* in two children with nephrotic syndrome. *Pediatr Nephrol* 1996;10:639–641.

89. Hoyer JR, Anderson CE. Congenital nephrotic syndrome. *Clin Perinatol* 1981;8:333–346.

90. Papaioannou AC, Asrow GG, Schuckmell NH. Nephrotic syndrome in early infancy as a manifestation of congenital syphilis. *Pediatrics* 1961;27:636–641.

91. Shahin B, Papadopoulou ZL, Jenis EH. Congenital nephrotic syndrome associated with congenital toxoplasmosis. *J Pediatr* 1974;85:366–370.

92. Ty A, Fine B. Membranous nephritis in infantile systemic lupus erythematosus associated with chromosomal abnormalities *Clin Nephrol* 1979;2:137–141.

93. Jeanpierre C, Denamur E, Henry I, et al. Identification of constitutional WT1 mutations, in patients with isolated diffuse mesangial sclerosis, and analysis of genotype/phenotype correlations by use of a computerized mutation database. *Am J Hum Genet* 1998;62:824–833.

94. Huttunen NP. Congenital nephrotic syndrome of the Finnish type. Study of 75 patients. *Arch Dis Child* 1976;51:344–348.

95. Kestila M, Lenkkeri U, Mannikko M, et al. Positionally cloned gene for a novel glomerular protein—nephrin—is mutated in congenital nephrotic syndrome. *Mol Cell* 1998;1:575–582.

96. Mahan JD, Mauer SM, Sibley RK, et al. Congenital nephrotic syndrome: evolution of medical management and results of renal transplantation. *J Pediatr* 1984;105: 549–557.

97. Kjessler B, Johansson SG, Sherman M, et al. Alphafetoprotein in antenatal diagnosis of congenital nephrosis. *Lancet* 1975;1:432–433.

98. Harris HW Jr, Umetsu D, Geha R, et al. Altered immunoglobulin status in congenital nephrotic syndrome. *Clin Nephrol* 1986;25:308–313.

99. Ljungberg P, Holmberg C, Jalanko H. Infections in infants with congenital nephrosis of the Finnish type. *Pediatr Nephrol* 1997;11:148–152.

100. Holmberg C, Antikainen M, Ronnholm K, et al. Management of congenital nephrotic syndrome of the Finnish type. *Pediatr Nephrol* 1995;9:87–93.

101. Fivush B, Case B, May M, et al. Hypogammaglobulinemia in children undergoing continuous ambulatory peritoneal dialysis. *Pediatr Nephrol* 1989;3:186–188.

102. Vazquez G, Mendoza-Guevara L, Alvarez T, et al. Comparison of the response to the recombinant vaccine against hepatitis B virus in dialyzed and nondialyzed children with CRF using different doses and routes of administration. *Adv Perit Dial* 1997;13: 291–296.

103. Furth SL, Neu AM, Case B, et al. Pneumococcal polysaccharide vaccine in children with chronic renal disease: a prospective study of antibody response and duration. *J Pediatr* 1996;128:99–101.

104. Furth SL, Neu AM, McColley SA, et al. Immune response to influenza vaccination in children with renal disease. *Pediatr Nephrol* 1995;9:566–568.

105. Recommended childhood immunization schedule—United States, 1998. *MMWR Morb Mortal Wkly Rep* 1998;7:8–12.

106. Furth SL, Neu AM, Sullivan EK, et al. Immunization practices in children with renal disease: a report of the North American Pediatric Renal Transplant Cooperative Study. *Pediatr Nephrol* 1997;11:443–446.

107. Fivush BA, Neu AM. Immunization guidelines for pediatric renal disease. *Semin Nephrol* 1998;18:256–263.

108. Advisory Committee on Immunization Practices. Use of vaccines and immune globulins in persons with altered immunocompetence. *MMWR Morb Mortal Wkly Rep* 1993;42(Suppl 4):1–18.

109. Neu AM, Warady BA, Furth SL. Antibody levels to diphtheria, tetanus and rubella in infants vaccinated while on peritoneal dialysis: a study of The Pediatric Peritoneal Dialysis Study Consortium. *Adv Perit Dial* 1997;13:297–299.

110. Neu AM, Lederman HM, Warady BA. *Hemophilus influenza* type b immunization in infants maintained on peritoneal dialysis. *Pediatr Nephrol* 1996;10:84–85.

111. Schulman SL, Deforest A, Kaiser BA, et al. Response to measles-mumps-rubella vaccine in children on dialysis. *Pediatr Nephrol* 1992;6:187–189.

112. Watkins SL, Hogg RJ, Alexander SR. Response to recombinant hepatitis B virus vaccine in children with chronic renal failure, with and without dialysis. *J Am Soc Nephrol* 1994;5:344.

113. Greenbaum LA, Salusky IB. Poor humoral response to the varicella vaccine in a pediatric dialysis population. *J Am Soc Nephrol* 1996;7:1447.

114. Nikoskelainen J, Koskela M, Forsstrom J. Persistence of antibodies to pneumococcal vaccine in patients with chronic renal failure. *Kidney Int* 1985;28:672–677.

115. Fuchshuber A, Kuhnemund O, Keuth B. Pneumococcal vaccine in children and young adults with chronic renal disease. *Nephrol Dial Transplant* 1986;11:468–473.

116. Schnaper HW. Immunization practices in childhood nephrotic syndrome: a survey of North American pediatric nephrologists. *Pediatr Nephrol* 1994;18:4–6.

117. Quien RM, Kaiser BA, DeForest A, et al. Response to the varicella vaccine in children with nephrotic syndrome. *J Pediatr* 1997;131:688–690.

118. La Manna A, Polito C, Foglia AC, et al. Reduced response to hepatitis B virus vaccination in boys with steroid-sensitive nephrotic syndrome. *Pediatr Nephrol* 1992;6:251–253.

119. Allen U, Wang E. *Haemophilus influenzae* type B infection after nephrotic syndrome in a previously vaccinated child. *CMAJ* 1989;141:310–311.

120. Spika JS, Halsey NA, Fish AJ, et al. Serum antibody response to pneumococcal vaccine in children with nephrotic syndrome. *Pediatrics* 1982;69:219–223.

121. Wilkes JC, Nelson JD, Worthen HG, et al. Response to pneumococcal vaccination in children with nephrotic syndrome. *Am J Kidney Dis* 1982; 2:43–46.

122. Moore DH, Shackelford PS, Robson AH, et al. Recurrent pneumococcal sepsis and defective opsonization after pneumococcal capsular polysaccharide vaccine in a child with nephrotic syndrome. *J Pediatr* 1980; 96:882–885.

123. Primack WA, Rosel M, Thirumoorthi MC, et al. Failure of pneumococcal vaccine to prevent *Streptococcus pneumoniae* sepsis in nephrotic children. *Lancet* 1979; 2:1192.

124. Broome CV, Facklam RR, Fraser DW. Pneumococcal disease after pneumococcal vaccination: an alternative method to estimate the efficacy of pneumococcal vaccine. *N Engl J Med* 1980;303:549–552.

13

Infections in Children with Cystic Fibrosis

Marc D. Foca, Sujatha Rajan, and Lisa Saiman

*Department of Pediatrics, Division of Pediatric Infectious Diseases,
Columbia University, New York, New York 10032*

Cystic fibrosis (CF) is the most common life-shortening autosomal recessive disease among the white population, and it affects approximately 25,000 persons in the United States with an estimated seven million asymptomatic carriers (1). Traditionally, CF has not been thought of as an immunologic disorder. Yet, for decades, it has been known that chronic, progressive lung infections with a predictable cascade of pathogens are the major cause of morbidity and mortality for CF patients. With the exception of sinusitis, CF patients rarely develop bacteremia or infections outside the airway. Thus, CF patients may be considered to have a regional immunodeficiency of the respiratory tract.

Identification of the gene responsible for CF, the cystic fibrosis transmembrane conductance regulator (*CFTR*), has improved our understanding of the links between the pathogenesis of lung disease and abnormal *CFTR*. Although much remains to be learned, there is an increasing appreciation of the deranged inflammation within the lung. An enhanced understanding of the function of CFTR led to the development of possible therapeutic interventions by targeting specific aspects of abnormal pathophysiology. The management of CF can be considered a model for other genetic diseases as well as acquired respiratory tract diseases.

THE CYSTIC FIBROSIS GENE: CYSTIC FIBROSIS TRANSMEMBRANE CONDUCTANCE REGULATOR

Using positional cloning and chromosome jumping, the *CFTR* gene was discovered in 1989 on chromosome 7 q21-31 (2–4). It codes for a 1,480 amino acid protein with a molecular weight that varies from 140 to 170 kD. The protein consists of two transmembrane (anchoring) domains that form a pore, two intracellular nucleotide-binding domains that regulate opening and closing of the channel, and a central regulatory domain termed the *R domain,* which is rich in phosphorylation sites (Fig. 13.1). *CFTR* is a Cl⁻ channel, and transition from the closed to the open state is mediated by a cyclic adenosine monophosphate (cAMP)-dependent protein kinase that phosphorylates the R domain; adenosine triphosphate (ATP) interacts with one of the nucleotide-binding domains. The characteristics of *CFTR* place it among the adenine nucleotide binding cassette (ABC) transport protein superfamily.

The cystic fibrosis conductance regulator has many functions (5,6). It regulates other ion channels, including (a) another Cl⁻ channel (termed the *outwardly rectifying chloride*

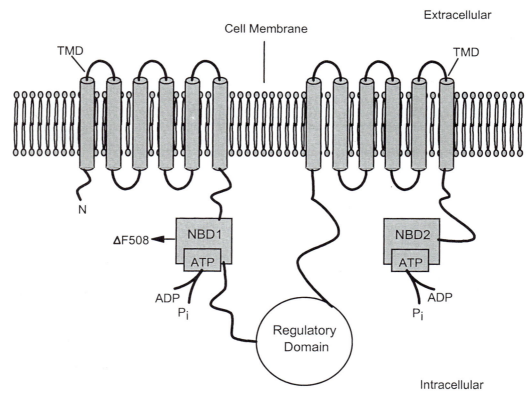

FIG. 13.1. Schematic representation of the cystic fibrosis transmembrane conductance regulator (CFTR), which contains two transmembrane domains (TMD), each with six membrane-spanning segments; two nucleotide-binding domains (NBD), which bind adenosine triphosphate (ATP); and a regulatory (R) domain. ΔF_{508}, shows the approximate location of this deletion mutation.

channel), (b) the amiloride-sensitive Na⁺ channel, and (c) perhaps a Ca^{2+} channel. CFTR also may transport ATP. Located in the apical membrane, CFTR is actively recycled to the membranes of the intracellular organelles. It is speculated that CFTR located in the intracellular organelles serves to maintain the optimal pH for enzymatic function of sialyltransferases that glycosylate lipids and proteins found on the epithelial cell surface. This would lead to abnormal glycosylation, which may provide bacterial receptors on respiratory epithelial cells as will be described later; however, there is controversy regarding this role for CFTR.

Classification of *CFTR* Mutations

Mutations of *CFTR* are numerous and complex and may lead to decreased production of the CFTR protein, impaired delivery of CFTR to the appropriate site in the cell, or impaired function of *CFTR*. It is now appreciated that mutations in *CFTR* can be divided into five classes (Table 13.1). Approximately 60% of U.S. patients have been genotyped, and about 50% are homozygous for the ΔF_{508} mutation, which deletes a phenylalanine from the normal protein. Whereas 70% of CF alleles encode ΔF_{508}, 15 to 20 other mutations are also relatively common and responsible for most

TABLE 13.1. *Classes of mutations in the cystic fibrosis transmembrane conductance regulator*

Class	Description
I	No protein production secondary to premature mRNA termination either by introducing a premature signal for termination of translation or by altering mRNA
II	Defective intracellular processing and/or trafficking. ΔF_{508} is a class II mutation and is temperature sensitive; at body temperature CFTR encoding the ΔF_{508} does not properly dissociate from molecular chaperones in the endoplasmic reticulum, presumably because of improper folding. The CFTR protein is pathologically retained in the endoplasmic reticulum, not properly glycosylated, and is subsequently degraded
III	Properly trafficked to the apical membrane but cannot be activated because of defective ATP- or phosphorylation-dependent regulation of CFTR
IV	Defective Cl⁻ channel conductance despite normal placement and regulation of CFTR
V	Splice site mutations in the RNA that reduce the efficiency of protein translation

ATP, adenosine triphosphate; CFTR, cystic fibrosis transmembrane conductance regulator.

of the non-ΔF_{508} mutations (5,6). More than 600 mutations in *CFTR* have been described, not all of which are associated with the CF phenotype.

Sites of CFTR Expression in the Lung

Although the bronchial lumens are the major site of pathology in CF, respiratory epithelial cells contain little *CFTR* mRNA, with the exception of the terminal airways (6). In contrast, high levels of CFTR protein are detectable in airway submucosal glands, particularly in serous cells. Serous cells are thought to secrete a watery fluid that transports mucins produced by proximal mucous cells through the ducts and into the airway lumen. Thus, mutations in *CFTR* may impact the function of the submucosal glands more directly than respiratory epithelial cells.

PATHOPHYSIOLOGY

Cystic fibrosis is characterized by a neutrophil-dominated inflammatory response of the airways rather than the interstitium or the alveoli (7–9). Recent work in young infants suggested that inflammation may occur in the absence of detectable infection, perhaps as a direct consequence of abnormal *CFTR*. Thus, there is a growing understanding of the viscious cycle of inflammation and infection; this understanding led to the development of

several therapeutic strategies that will be described subsequently. Several factors contribute to this cycle, including (a) excessive inflammatory response, (b) failure to clear bacterial infection, and (c) the consequences of the local host response. This multifactorial pathogenesis is shown in Fig. 13.2.

Excessive Inflammatory Response in Cystic Fibrosis

Excessive or persistent inflammation plays an important role in CF lung disease. Numerous studies demonstrate high levels of interleukin-8 (IL-8, a potent chemoattractant) in the airways of CF patients at virtually all stages of the disease (7–10). More recently, bronchoalveolar lavage (BAL) studies performed in young infants and children with minimal or no obvious clinical lung disease demonstrated markers of inflammation even in the absence of colonization or infection with traditional CF pathogens (11). These CF infants had elevated numbers of neutrophils and increased concentrations of neutrophil elastase and the proinflammatory cytokines IL-1, IL-8, and tumor necrosis factor-α (TNF-α). Khan and colleagues compared 16 CF infants (mean age, 6 months) with 11 control infants (mean age, 12 months) and documented similar markers of inflammation as early as 4 weeks of age (12). To date, the mechanisms for this early inflammation are not well understood, but possible expla-

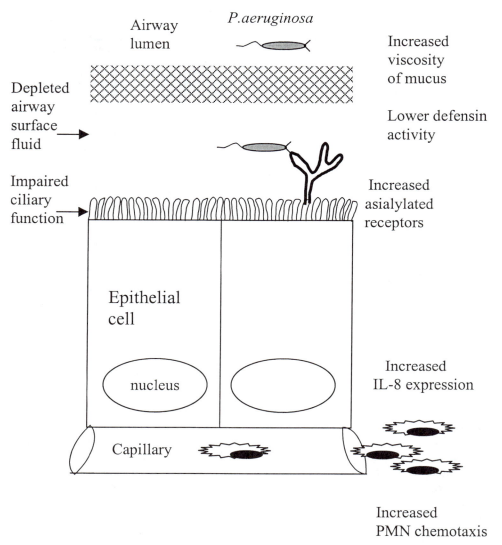

FIG. 13.2. Schematic representation of hypotheses proposed to explain the pathogenesis of cystic fibrosis airway disease.

nations include (a) innate upregulation of cytokine production as a result of increased transcription of factors regulating cytokines in CF epithelial cells (13), (b) persistence of inflammatory cells during the recovery phase of subclinical infection, and (c) bronchoscopic sampling may not detect possible viral and bacterial pathogens. Thus, inflammation may not be a consequence of infection, but it may be present before infection.

Excessive inflammation of the airways of chronically infected patients also may be due to persistent cytokine production as a result of antigenic stimulation from bacteria. *In vitro* studies have shown that epithelial cells express IL-8 in response to adherent organisms (14). Alternatively, the underproduction of antiinflammatory factors, that is, IL-10, could be responsible for excessive inflammation. IL-10 suppresses macrophage production of the proinflammatory cytokines TNF-α and IL-1 (15). Berger et al. showed that CF epithelial cells have decreased IL-10 production compared with non-CF cells (16). Thus, the downregulation of IL-10 may contribute to the continued production of proinflammatory cytokines in the CF airway.

Failure to Clear Organisms as a Result of Impaired Mucociliary Clearance

Normal mucociliary clearance cleanses inhaled particles from the bronchopulmonary epithelium by upward flow of the mucus layer positioned on the tips of the cilia that freely move within a watery layer. In CF, it is thought that a net deficiency of water hinders the flow of the mucus "blanket" as a result of electrolyte transport abnormalities from *CFTR* dysfunction (17). CF respiratory epithelial cells have increased basal and increased β-agonist-stimulated absorption of Na⁺, but lack β-agonist-stimulated Cl⁻ secretion. The decreased secretion and increased absorption of electrolytes by the CF epithelium are thought to lead to the dehydration of secretions because normally water flows passively with electrolytes to maintain isotonicity (18–20). Most recently, elegant *in vitro* studies confirmed this by demonstrating that CF airway epithelial cells have abnormally high rates of airway surface liquid absorption, which depletes the periciliary liquid layer and is thought to abolish mucus transport by impairing ciliary function (21). *In vivo* studies, in part, have supported this *in vitro* observation: infected CF patients with moderate lung disease had decreased clearance of tagged particles from the lung compared with normal volunteers (22). Such studies should be repeated in young infants to examine the impact of disordered electrolyte transport on mucociliary clearance in uninfected patients. Finally, *Pseudomonas aeruginosa* lipopolysaccharide can upregulate mucin transcription by airway epithelial *cells,* which further contributes to the increased viscosity of airway secretions (23).

P. aeruginosa Binding within the Lung

Several *in vitro* models suggest that there is increased bacterial binding to CF respiratory epithelial cells. CF cells have increased asialylated glycolipid receptors on their surface compared with normal cells, and asialoganglioside GM_1 is a receptor for both the pilus and flagella of *P. aeruginosa* (24,25). Studies have shown also that binding to epithelial cells increases when such cells are derived from patients homozygous for ΔF_{508} compared with cells derived from patients with other *CFTR* mutations or heterozygote carriers (26). It should be noted that in pathologic specimens from CF patients, bacteria are found within the airway lumen, but they are not adherent to epithelial cells. Thus, adherence may represent an initial phase of infection that is followed by biofilm formation within the airways.

Pier and colleagues suggested an alternative explanation for the unique predisposition of *P. aeruginosa* for the CF lung. They postulated that *CFTR* functions as a receptor for *P. aeruginosa* on normal respiratory epithelial cells. Following bacterial adherence, the cells internalize the bacteria, slough, and are removed by mucociliary clearance (27). This proposed mechanism of host defense is therefore impaired in CF cells, which lack apical *CFTR*. This theory remains controversial because of concern that this result may reflect experimental artifact rather than a true *in vivo* phenomenon.

Mucin is the major glycoprotein found in the airway fluid. Studies suggested that glycosylation or sulfation of glycoproteins is altered in CF and that these glycosylated mucins may act as bacterial receptors (28); however, an increase in specific binding to CF mucins compared with normal mucins has not been shown (29,30), although a structural component of flagellum has been shown to bind to mucin (31). Thus, the role of mucin in bacterial adherence remains unclear.

Impaired Opsonophagocytosis

Opsonophagocytosis appears to be impaired in the CF respiratory tract. Glucose is required for nonopsonic phagocytosis of *P. aeruginosa* by macrophages (32). Unfortunately, glucose is present at extremely low concentrations in bronchial fluid, which may impair efficient phagocytosis and promote initial colonization by *P. aeruginosa*. In addition, surface components of *P. aeruginosa*, such as pili and flagella, mediate nonopsonic phagocytosis by macrophages and neutrophils (33). These virulence factors are lost in chronic infection, which may account for the persistence of *P. aeruginosa*.

Role of Defensins

There has been much interest in the innate immune system, particularly in the defensins, which are small antimicrobial peptides found in many sites in many species (34). Human β-defensin-1 (hβD-1) is expressed in the respiratory tract from the trachea to alveoli and has broad antimicrobial activity, including activity against *P. aeruginosa* (35). Studies suggested that the airway surface liquid from cultured CF airway cells lacked bactericidal activity compared with that of normal cells and that this activity could be restored when the liquid was made hypotonic (36). These researchers suggested that the CF airway is relatively hypertonic, which adversely impacts on the bactericidal activity of the salt-sensitive peptides. The relative importance of these *in vitro* findings is unclear, however. Sampling airway surface liquid is difficult *in vivo*, and the precise osmolarity remains controversial, particularly because recent studies indicated that the airway surface liquid of normal cells is isotonic, not hypotonic (21).

Consequences of Local Host Response and the Role of Neutrophils in Tissue Damage

Neutrophils are the predominant inflammatory cell in the CF airway, and they cause extensive damage. The major mechanisms causing such damage are (a) the highly reactive toxic metabolites of molecular oxygen produced by the "respiratory burst" that accompanies cell activation or phagocytosis and (b) the potent digestive enzymes and proteases present in neutrophil granules. Following stimulation, oxidase enzyme systems (e.g., myeloperoxidase) are activated and combine with oxygen to produce highly reactive toxic species, including singlet oxygen, hydroxyl radicals, superoxide, and hydrogen peroxide (37). Studies have shown that the severity of lung disease correlates with sputum peroxidase activity (38).

Cystic fibrosis sputum and BAL fluid have free protease activity (39–42) that is due to neutrophil elastase and cathepsin G. Both these enzymes can hydrolyze connective tissue proteins; elastase degrades elastin, and both elastase and cathepsin G hydrolyze proteoglycans and solubilize collagen, making the latter susceptible to further degradation by neutrophil collagenase. Proteolysis of lung connective tissue occurs relentlessly, and fragmented elastin fibers in bronchial-based inflammatory lesions, ulcers, and abscesses are seen at postmortem examination (43). Protease concentrations have been shown to correlate with clinical status and pulmonary exacerbations.

In addition, these enzymes may have other effects. *In vitro*, neutrophil elastase and cathepsin G stimulate the release of mucin from serous gland cells, although the mechanism is unknown (44,45). Neutrophil elastase also inhibits the beating of cilia *in vitro* (46).

The lung normally is protected against proteolytic damage by the α-1-protease inhibitor, α-1-antitrypsin, secretory leukocyte protease inhibitor, and, to a lesser extent, by α-2-macroglobulin. These protease inhibitors are fragmented and inactivated by (a) excess neutrophil elastase, (b) reactive oxygen species released during neutrophil activation, and (c) bacterial elastase (37). Thus, lung damage in CF is thought to occur as a result of the imbalance between the excess proteases overwhelming naturally occurring antiproteases.

Effects of Neutrophil Proteases on Phagocytic Host Defenses

Ironically, neutrophil proteases may adversely effect in phagocytosis. Activation of neutrophils leads to a rapid increase in surface expression of complement receptors that promote adherence to the endothelium, migration of the neutrophils into tissues, and efficient phagocytosis of complement-coated particles. Tosi et al. showed that neutrophil proteases, and not bacterial proteases, cleave the complement receptor CR1 (the receptor for C3b) on neutrophils (47). This decrease in CR1 expression can interfere with efficient complement-mediated phagocytosis. In addition, neutrophil elastase cleaves opsonins, such as fibronectin, IgG, and C3bi, another major complement receptor ligand, and further decreases bactericidal activity by creating an "opsonin-receptor mismatch." Serum and bronchial washings from chronically infected CF patients do not promote phagocytosis of *P. aeruginosa* by alveolar macrophages.

Cleavage of IgG significantly inhibits uptake of immune complexes by phagocytes. Specific anti-*Pseudomonas* antibodies bind bacteria, but they do not promote binding of the bacteria to alveolar macrophages. These IgG antibodies are smaller than normal as a result of cleavage by neutrophil elastase (39,48).

Antibody Response in Cystic Fibrosis

Responses to most standard antigens are normal in CF (49). In general, older CF patients have high levels of immunoglobulins as a result of chronic antigen exposure in the respiratory tract and increased IL-6 production in the lung. Cowen et al. showed that CF patients colonized with *P. aeruginosa* have elevated IgG subclass titers to this pathogen compared with normal subjects and noncolonized CF patients (50). Most patients develop IgG, IgA, and IgM antibodies against a wide array of bacterial antigens, including exoenzymes, pili, lipopolysaccharide (LPS), alginate, and outer-membrane proteins. The titers

of these antibodies increase after pulmonary exacerbation (51). The formation of immune complexes containing pseudomonal antigens may enhance the inflammatory response in the lung, further exacerbating inflammation-associated lung damage (52).

Pier et al. suggested that a subset of older patients who were not infected chronically with *P. aeruginosa* made anti-mucoexopolysaccharide (MEP) antibodies that facilitated opsonophagocytic killing by neutrophils. Chronically infected patients with CF and controls also made antibodies to MEP, but these anti-MEP antibodies did not promote killing in this assay (53); however, other studies showed that both chronically infected and apparently uninfected patients with CF made opsonic as well as nonopsonic antibodies but that neither were protective (54). In view of the high proportion of CF patients harboring *P. aeruginosa*, it seems likely that antibody response does not prevent infection in CF patients.

Role of T Cells

Functional consequences of *CFTR* mutations in lymphoid cells have not been described. Harper et al. studied T-lymphocyte function, immediate hypersensitivity skin responsiveness, and serum IgE levels in children with CF (55). Their studies demonstrated evidence of increased IgE sensitization thought to be due to the disrupted mucosal barrier, but they did not demonstrate quantitative or functional T-lymphocyte abnormalities. The lack of increased susceptibility to protozoans or other opportunistic infections suggest that cell-mediated immunity is intact (55); however, neutrophil elastase can cleave surface antigens on T cells, including CD4, CD8, and the α-β-heterodimer of the T-cell antigen receptor complex, thereby inhibiting lymphocyte activation and consequently decreasing production of γ-interferon (56,57). The clinical impact of these observations is not evident, especially in view of the major impact of neutrophil-mediated inflammation.

PATHOGENS IN CYSTIC FIBROSIS

There is a predictable cascade of lung pathogens in CF (Table 13.2). Young children with CF are initially colonized with *Staphylococcus aureus* and nontypeable *Haemophilus influenza,* and *S. aureus* is the predominant pathogen during the first decade of life (58); however, *P. aeruginosa* may be the first pathogen isolated even from children younger than 1 year of age, and by 18 years of age about 80% of American patients are infected with *P. aeruginosa.* Notably, multiple antibiotic-resistant *P. aeruginosa* and methicillin-resistant *S. aureus* are being identified with increasing frequency (59,60).

The epidemiology of CF pathogens appears to be changing during the past decade. *Burkholderia cepacia* has been described as a pathogen in CF for nearly two decades, but other intrinsically antibiotic resistant bacteria, such as *Stenotrophomonas maltophilia* and *Alcaligenes xylosoxidans,* are recovered from the respiratory tract of CF patients with increasing frequency, as are *Aspergillus* spp. and nontuberculous mycobacteria (NTM). The etiologies behind these emerging pathogens are multifactorial and include (a) the increased longevity of CF patients, (b) more frequent and prolonged antimicrobial therapy, (c) nosocomial acquisition, and (d) improved laboratory techniques that utilize selective media.

Pseudomonas aeruginosa Infection

The most important pathogen in CF is *P. aeruginosa.* Infection with this organism clearly is associated with a decline in respiratory function. Recent studies of infants with CF showed that children infected with *P. aeruginosa* are more likely to have cough and lower chest-radiograph scores than uninfected children. Hudson et al. showed that infants younger than 2 years of age infected with both *S. aureus* and *P. aeruginosa* have lower pulmonary function, lower chest radiograph scores, and lower 10-year survival rates than uninfected children (61). Some investigators showed that the mucoid phenotype of *P. aeruginosa* is responsible for the marked decline in pulmonary function (62).

Initial colonization of the airways usually is due to nonmucoid strains of *P. aeruginosa* that express pili, flagella, and exoproducts. In chronic infection, as a result of incompletely defined environmental pressures, these organisms convert to the mucoid phenotype because of overproduction of alginate (63). Mucoid strains grow as microcolonies in the lung and create biofilms. Bacteria in biofilms not only avoid ciliary clearance but also evade phagocytosis and antibiotics. In chronic infection, the organisms also lose lipopolysaccharide O-side chains, thereby becoming insensitive to serum.

The exotoxins produced by *P. aeruginosa* may contribute to virulence. These exotoxins

TABLE 13.2. *Microbiology of the respiratory tract of CF patients, 1997 CF National Patient Registry (n = 17,996 patients)[a]*

Organism	Percentage	No. of patients
"Normal" flora	10.9	1,969
Haemophilus influenza	15.4	2,777
Staphylococcus aureus	40.7	7,326
Methicillin-resistant *Staphylococcus aureus*	2.6	473
Pseudomonas aeruginosa[b]	60.9	10,951
Burkholderia cepacia	3.5	636
Stenotrophomonas maltophilia	5.1	926
Alcaligenes xylosoxidans	2.7	480
Nontuberculous mycobacteria sp.	0.9	165
Aspergillus sp.	8.6	1,547

CF, cystic fibrosis.
[a]These data represent 92% of all CF patients cared for at accredited CF centers. One patient may harbor more than one organism; 68.9% of specimens were sputum, 29.4% throat cultures, and 1.7% bronchoalveolar lavage.
[b]67% of strains are mucoid.

have been studied in variety of animal models, including sepsis, acute lung infections, and bacteremia (64,65). These products include exotoxin A and exoenzyme S, leukocidin, phospholipase C, elastase, and alkaline protease (66). These exoproducts contribute to pathophysiology by increasing the viscosity of secretions and impairing ciliary clearance as well as by causing small airway obstruction, which ultimately leads to lung destruction.

Burkholderia cepacia Infection

During the 1980s, *B. cepacia* emerged as an important pathogen in CF. Infection with this multiply antibiotic-resistant gram-negative rod can be associated with a particularly virulent clinical course known as the *cepacia syndrome*, which is characterized by high fever, bacteremia, rapid deterioration in pulmonary function, and death (67). It is now appreciated that only one third of patients harboring *B. cepacia* experience a rapid decline in lung function, one third decline in a pattern expected with *P. aeruginosa,* and the remainder appear to be merely "colonized."

Five distinct genomovars or subspecies, collectively termed the *B. cepacia complex*, have been described by taxonomists, which may help to account for the differences in clinical course associated with this pathogen (68). Most CF isolates are genomovar II or III, which appear to be associated with a more rapidly progressive course, whereas patients harboring *B. multivorans* appear to be clinically stable. Spread from one CF patient to another of *B. cepacia* has occurred and may become apparent years after contact with an infected patient (69). Most recently, plans by biotechnology companies to apply *B. cepacia* to commercial crops as a herbicide have been halted because of concern by the CF medical community (70).

Other Potential Pathogens

The significance of *A. xylosoxidans* and *S. maltophilia* in CF remains unclear (60). Progression of lung disease almost always occurs in patients concomitantly colonized with *P. aeruginosa,* and patient-to-patient transmission has not yet been documented among CF patients. There is much concern, however, that, as has been noted in intensive care unit settings, these organisms are emerging in CF under the selective pressure of antimicrobial agents used to treat more traditional pathogens.

Approximately 10% of CF patients develop allergic bronchopulmonary aspergillosis (ABPA) (71). This immunologically mediated syndrome is marked by a brisk IgE response, specific antibody to *A. fumigatus,* eosinophilia, and symptoms of reactive airway disease. Short-lived pulmonary infiltrates may be noted on chest radiograph. Whereas *Aspergillus* spp. normally do not invade the parenchyma, the airways can become impacted with mucus-containing fibrin, eosinophils, and mononuclear cells, which can result in permanent damage, including airway obstruction and proximal bronchiectasis.

Nontuberculous mycobacteria have been reported to be associated with clinical exacerbations in CF patients, but it is difficult to differentiate between colonization and actual disease (72). Isolation of these organisms may be due to increased survival of CF patients (73) as well as ascertainment bias because special culture techniques are required to isolate these organisms (74). Signs and symptoms of mycobacterial disease are nonspecific and may mimic pulmonary exacerbations, as described subsequently herein, although night sweats and recurrent fever may provide clues to this diagnosis. Radiographic signs are generally nonspecific, but small nodules in the lung periphery demonstrable on high resolution computed tomography scan have proven helpful in making the diagnosis (75).

Viral Pathogens

The ability of viral pathogens to induce inflammation in the CF lung and adversely impact on the clinical course of lung disease has been the subject of increasing interest (76). It has been thought that the early inflammation noted in young infants prior to detectable bacterial pathogens may be induced by viral pathogens. Abman et al. found that infants infected with respiratory syncytial virus (RSV) in the first year of life had severe morbidity including the need for prolonged oxygen supplementation, mechanical ventilation, and signs of chronic lung disease (77).

EPIDEMIOLOGY

In the United States, there are about 25,000 CF patients. The U.S. CF Foundation maintains the National CF Patient Registry, which compiles data from approximately 21,000 patients cared for at CF Foundation accredited care centers (S. FitzSimmons, CF Foundation National Patient Registry, 1997) (78). The incidence of disease is approximately 1/2,500 live births in the white population, 1/17,000 live births in the African-American population, and 1/12,000 live births in the Hispanic population. In the U.S. National Registry, 96% of patients are white, whereas only 3.5% are African-Americans. Approximately 53% are male, and 70% are diagnosed in the first year of life; the mean age at diagnosis is 3 years (S. FitzSimmons, CF Foundation National Patient Registry, 1997). With a growing appreciation of mild, atypical CF and the ability to perform genotypic analysis, about 7% of patients are 18 years or older at the time of diagnosis. The average life expectancy has been increasing and is currently 31 years of age; as a result, 36% of CF patients are over 18 years of age.

CLINICAL MANIFESTATIONS

Historical Perspective

Cystic fibrosis was recognized as a distinct disorder by Anderson in 1938 (79). In her series of 49 patients, 5 infants died in the first week of life "from some form of intestinal obstruction," 19 children died between 1 week and 6 months of age from bronchopneumonia with evidence of failure to thrive and bulky stools, and 25 children died at 6 months to 14 years of age from chronic pulmonary infection and evidence of celiac disease. The pathologic findings included cystic changes in the pancreas with evidence of fibrosis, bronchiectasis, vitamin A deficiency, osteoporosis, and intestinal atresia. In 1945, Farber described inspissation of the secretions of many organs (80), and in 1953, Di Sant'Agnese et al. developed the diagnostic sweat test after noting increased secretion of Na^+ and Cl^- while investigating the acute collapse of CF patients during a heat wave (81).

Pulmonary Disease

Most patients present during the first 4 years of life either with acute or persistent respiratory symptoms (82). Pulmonary disease usually is heralded by the onset of a nonproductive cough that evolves into a loose, productive cough with purulent secretions. There is much variability in the clinical course of CF patients; some remain clinically asymptomatic for long periods, and others develop a chronic cough; still others suffer from repeated pulmonary exacerbations and clinical deterioration. Clinical symptoms associated with pulmonary exacerbations include exercise intolerance, shortness of breath, and failure to gain weight secondary to increased metabolic demand. Initially, pulmonary exacerbations may be mild, and some patients may be managed as outpatients. With time, however, these exacerbations become more debilitating and may be associated with as much as a 10 - 15% decline in forced expiratory volume in 1 second (FEV_1).

Physical signs of CF include barrel chest, digital clubbing, scattered rales, and eventually cyanosis (82). Pulmonary function tests initially show an obstructive pattern, with the earliest changes in the forced expiratory flow $(FEF)_{25\%-75\%}$ indicative of small airway disease. As the disease progresses, there is a shift to a restrictive pattern as fibrosis accumulates. Whereas the rate of disease progression is variable, overall it is estimated that the annual decline in FEV_1 in children can be as much as 3% to 4% predicted. Radiographically, there may initially be evidence of hyperinflation, flattening of the diaphragms, and a narrowing of the cardiac silhouette. Patients with advanced disease develop bronchiectasis, atelectasis, hilar adenopathy, and pulmonary artery dilatation. End-stage respiratory disease consists of cor pulmonale and respiratory failure and is the cause of death in more than 95% of patients.

Gastrointestinal Disease

Numerous gastrointestinal manifestations can cause substantial morbidity in CF patients. About 16% of newly diagnosed CF patients present with either meconium ileus or intestinal obstruction at birth. Failure to thrive as a result of pancreatic exocrine dysfunction and malnutrition, particularly from fat-soluble vitamins, are found at presentation in 43% of patients. The mean height and weight of American CF patients are in the 20th percentile, but 24% of all patients are below 5% for weight (83). Most CF patients have pancreatic insufficiency (93%), and symptoms include failure to thrive, bulky stools occasionally with visible fat droplets, decreased muscle mass, and a protuberant abdomen. About 20% of patients have some liver involvement that is frequently asymptomatic; only about 2% advance to cirrhosis (84). Ultimately, 4% of patients develop diabetes, and older patients can have severe gastroesophogeal reflux or rectal prolapse. Pancreatitis can occur after fatty meals, alcohol intake, or antibiotic therapy.

Correlation of *CFTR* Genotype with CF Phenotype

Correlation of specific mutations in *CFTR* with the manifestations of CF and disease progression has been the focus of many investigators (5). The classic triad of elevated sweat Cl^-, pancreatic insufficiency, and chronic pulmonary disease occurs in most patients homozygous for the ΔF_{508} mutation; however, it appears that class IV mutations are associated

with a milder form of CF in which pancreatic function remains unimpaired, the diagnosis of CF is made later in life, and sweat Cl^- levels are lower.

Corey et al. showed that patients homozygous for the ΔF_{508} mutation have a more rapid pulmonary decline than patients who are either heterozygous for ΔF_{508} or who have non-ΔF_{508} mutations (85). This evidence led researchers to postulate that the organ system manifestations of CF depend on the level of *CFTR* function (6). Carriers of the disease have a 50% reduction in the level of *CFTR* and are clinically unaffected. Genital tract disease alone manifested as obstructive aspermia secondary to congenital absence of the vas deferens occurs if the level of *CFTR* is 10% of normal. Lung and sweat gland dysfunction occur at approximately 5% of normal levels, and severe pulmonary manifestations and pancreatic disease occur if the level of *CFTR* expression is below 1%.

DIFFERENTIAL DIAGNOSIS

The differential diagnosis of CF includes disorders of ciliary function, immunodeficiency, allergy, and infection.

Laboratory Diagnosis

With the discovery of abnormal *CFTR* in 1987, the laboratory diagnosis of CF has continued to improve, although the traditional sweat test continues to be the "gold standard." A consensus panel convened in 1997 recommended that the diagnosis of CF be made by pairing a laboratory diagnosis with classic clinical manifestations (Table 13.3) (86). Alternatively, a sibling of a child with CF or an infant with a positive newborn screen also should have one of the following laboratory tests that provide evidence of *CFTR* dysfunction: (a) a positive sweat test using pilocarpine ionoelectrophoresis documenting elevated Cl^- levels, (b) mutations in the *CFTR* gene known to be associated with clinical manifestations of CF, or (c) electrolyte transport abnormalities across the nasal epithelium

TABLE 13.3. *Criteria for the diagnosis of CF*

One or more of the following four clinical features:
  Chronic pulmonary or sinus disease with
    Persistent infection with typical CF pathogens
    Chronic cough and sputum production
    Persistent chest radiograph abnormalities (e.g., bronchiectasis, atelectasis)
    Airway obstruction
    Nasal polyp or sinus abnormalities
    Clubbing
  Gastrointestinal and nutritional abnormalities
    Intestines (e.g., meconium ileus, obstruction syndrome, rectal prolapse)
    Pancreas (e.g., insufficiency or recurrent pancreatitis)
    Liver (e.g., chronic focal biliary or multilobular cirrhosis)
    Nutritional (e.g., failure to thrive, fat soluble vitamin deficiency)
  Salt-loss syndromes (e.g., acute salt depletion, metabolic alkalosis)
  Obstructive azospermia due to congenital absence of the vas deferens
Plus:
  One or more of the following laboratory evidence of abnormal CFTR
    Elevated sweat Cl
    Mutations in both alleles of CFTR
    Characteristic abnormalities in nasal potential difference

CF, cystic fibrosis; CFTR, cystic fibrosis transmembrane regulator; Cl, chloride.
Adapted from Rosenstein BJ, Zeitlin PL. Cystic fibrosis. *Lancet* 1998;351:277–288, with permission.

measured by nasal potential difference. In general, a sweat Cl^- concentration greater than 60 mmol/L is considered consistent with the diagnosis of CF, but in children younger than 3 months of age, a concentration greater than 40 mmol/L is suspicious. Nasal potential difference measures the known abnormalities in electrolyte transport exhibited by CF epithelial cells and generally is reserved for assessment of patients with borderline sweat tests, only one known *CFTR*-associated mutation, or atypical clinical manifestations because this testing modality is not widely available.

Screening for CF during Pregnancy and Newborn Screening

With the discovery of *CFTR,* the usefulness of prenatal and postnatal screening for CF has been explored. Because of the large number of mutations described in *CFTR* (not all of which are associated with clinical disease), it has not been possible to recommend prenatal screening for the general population. At present, only eight to ten of the most common mutations are included in commercially available screening assays, and different *CFTR*

mutations are found in different ethnic groups. Thus prenatal DNA testing, although a powerful tool, is not yet considered sensitive enough for universal population-based screening and should be reserved for families with an affected child and planning to have another child.

Statewide newborn screening studies have been performed in pilot studies in Wisconsin and Denver (87). Thus far, these studies have shown that earlier diagnosis led to improved nutritional status; the weight gain of infants diagnosed by newborn screening was greater compared with infants diagnosed conventionally when symptoms developed. The impact of newborn screening on lung function is under investigation and requires a longer follow-up period. The Centers for Disease Control and Prevention recommend that more states develop newborn-screening pilot programs to determine the accuracy of such testing and the implications of early intervention (49,88). Such screening studies use heel-stick immunoreactive trypsinogen test (IRT) to screen for CF and to perform analysis for *CFTR* mutations in infants with elevated IRT. The *CFTR* mutational analysis for a given state must include the most common genetic mutations found in that state's population. A negative newborn screening test cannot be considered to rule out CF definitively, especially if clinical symptoms are present.

MANAGEMENT AND TREATMENT OF LUNG DISEASE

The clinical management of patients with CF has evolved into a multidisciplinary team approach because of the multiorgan nature of the disease. CF patients throughout the world are cared for in CF centers that promote standards of care and new research and maintain national registries of patient data. Many available treatments and investigational strategies are being explored to impact on different aspects of the pathophysiology of CF lung disease (Table 13.4).

ANTIMICROBIAL TREATMENT

The increasing longevity of CF patients has paralleled the development of effective anti-*Pseudomonas* antibiotics. Antibiotics are used in several stages of the natural history of lung disease, including (a) to prevent the acquisition of pathogens, (b) to delay chronic infection, (c) to treat pulmonary exacerbations, and (d) as suppressive therapy in chronically infected patients (89). Antimicrobial agents may be given orally, intravenously, or by aerosolization and are selected for use based on their activity against the pathogens isolated from the respiratory tract. The goals of antibiotic therapy in CF have been to decrease the antigenic burden by reducing the number of organisms in the lung and thereby reduce inflammation rather than completely eradicate bacterial pathogens.

Prophylaxis to Prevent Acquisition of Pathogens

There has been much interest in prophylactic administration of antimicrobial agents in an effort to slow the cascade of infection and inflammation in CF. From 1985 through 1992, British investigators randomized 42 newly diagnosed infants to receive flucloxacillin for 12 months (250 mg per day) versus antibiotics when clinically indicated

TABLE 13.4. *Currently available treatments and investigational strategies for the management of the lung disease of CF*

Abnormality	Solution	Approach	
		Available treatment	Investigational strategy
Abnormal CFTR gene	Provide normal gene		Gene therapy
Abnormal CFTR protein	Provide normal protein		Chemical chaperons (e.g., glycerol, phenylbutyrate)
	Activate mutant form		Milrinone, geninstein, CPX
	Prevent premature termination of mRNA		Gentamicin
Abnormal electrolyte transport	Block Na⁺ uptake		Amiloride
	Increase Cl⁻ efflux		UTP
Impaired clearance of respiratory secretions	Augment clearance	Airway clearance techniques	
Abnormal mucus	Decrease viscosity	rhDNase	Gelsolin
Infection	Decrease bacterial density	Antibiotics	Anti-*Pseudomonas* vaccine
	Prevent viral infections	Vaccinations	RSV monoclonal antibody and vaccine
Abnormal inflammatory response	Decrease host inflammatory reaction	Steroids Ibuprofen	α-1-antitrypinase Pentoxifylline
Bronchiectasis	Replace irreversibly damaged lung	Lung transplant	Living related donor transplant

CF, cystic fibrosis; CFTR, cystic fibrosis transmembrane conductance regulator; CPX, 8-Cyclophenyl-1,3-dipropylxanthine; RSV, respiratory syncytial virus; UTP, uridine triphosphate.

(90). The infants who received flucloxacillin had lower rates of *S. aureus* infection and fewer hospitalizations, but both groups had similar pulmonary function (91). In a placebo-controlled trial of 119 newly diagnosed American CF patients (mean age at enrollment, 16 months), cephalexin was used for 5 to 7 years to prevent *S. aureus* infection. No differences in pulmonary function, pulmonary exacerbations, nutritional status, or chest radiograph scores were detected in the two groups. Altough CF patients treated with cephalexin did have decreased *S. aureus* colonization, they also had increased *P. aeruginosa* infection (personal communication, HC Stutman). Thus anti-staphylococcal prophylaxis, which is practiced in the United Kingdom, has not been widely endorsed in the United States because of concerns about the emergence of resistance, the possible increased risk of *P. aeruginosa* acquisition, and the lack of impact on pulmonary function.

Another prophylactic strategy that has been used, particularly in Europe, is the utilization of antibiotics to prevent acquisition of *P. aeruginosa*. Some centers advocate routine, quarterly treatment with agents such as colistin and ciprofloxacin (92). These studies are flawed in that the outcomes of historic controls were compared with the treatment group rather than the outcomes of placebo-treated controls. The emergence of resistance is an important concern, and this approach merits further study.

Prevention of Chronic Infection

Until quite recently, many in the CF community considered that asymptomatic patients harboring *P. aeruginosa* were merely "colonized" and that successful eradication of this organism is not possible; however, some European CF physicians advocate routine administration of antibiotics every 3 months after the first isolation of *P. aeruginosa* to prevent chronic infection, to slow lung deterioration, and to decrease mortality (93,94). Again, in these studies, the outcomes of treated patients were compared with historic

controls. Thus, whereas treated patients had improved pulmonary function and improved survival, controlled trials supporting this practice are lacking, and there is concern about the emergence of strains of *P. aeruginosa* that is resistant to multiple antibiotics.

Treatment of Pulmonary Exacerbations

Currently, treatment of pulmonary exacerbations is the most accepted indication for use of antimicrobial agents. In a landmark study, Regelmann and colleagues demonstrated that patients with pulmonary exacerbations randomized to receive antibiotics and adjuvant therapies such as intensified bronchodilators and chest physiotherapy improved more than patients randomized to adjuvant therapies alone (95).

Treatment of pulmonary exacerbations is a blend of science and art. Antibiotic agents are chosen based on the susceptibility of bacteria identified in the sputum. In children who are too young to expectorate sputum, oropharyngeal cultures may be useful but do not always accurately predict lower airway pathogens (96). A large number of treatment trials for antibiotic management of pulmonary exacerbations have been published. Most enrolled small numbers of patients and concluded that the comparative treatment regimens were equivalent in efficacy. However, most of these trials were inadequately powered to detect differences in treatment groups (97). Appropriate treatment of a pulmonary exacerbation consists of using two parenteral agents from different antibiotic classes in efforts to provide "synergy" and to delay the emergence of resistance (59). Most commonly, a β-lactam agent with activity against *P. aeruginosa,* such as ticarcillin, piperacillin, or ceftazidime, and an aminoglycoside agent are selected. No doubt, this is a logical strategy, but controlled data supporting this practice are absent. *In vitro* synergy studies also have been performed to guide clinical care for multiple antibiotic-resistant strains, but studies of clinical efficacy have not been performed (59).

Antibiotic dosages must be higher in CF patients because their volume of distribution and clearance are increased (98). Serum levels of aminoglycosides must be monitored closely to prevent toxicities such as loss of hearing and renal function, especially given the repeated antibiotic courses that CF patients receive. Agents are administered for 2 to 3 weeks, and response to therapy is multifaceted and consists of an improved sense of well-being, improved pulmonary function, and a reduction in the density of bacteria in the sputum.

The CF community has not yet arrived at a consensus regarding the equivalency of inpatient versus outpatient management of pulmonary exacerbations. Outpatient management no doubt has advantages: lower costs, less disruptive to patients and their families, and less risk of acquiring nosocomial pathogens; however, recent work suggested that patients actually have greater improvement with hospitalization, which may be due to better compliance with bed rest, chest physiotherapy, and bronchodilator treatments (99).

Chronic Suppressive Therapy or Maintenance Therapy

Antibiotics are frequently used to treat patients known to be colonized with *P. aeruginosa* in efforts to prolong the time between pulmonary exacerbations and to slow the progression of lung deterioration. This strategy is termed *chronic suppressive therapy* or *maintenance therapy*. A wide variety of oral agents that may not kill *P. aeruginosa* are used empirically with anecdotal support from patients and physicians (89).

For two decades, aerosolized agents have been used for the management of chronic infections; these agents include tobramycin, colistin, gentamicin, amikacin, and various β-lactams, including carbenicillin and cephaloridine (100). Most recently, a phase 3 double-blind, placebo-controlled, randomized treatment trial of aerosolized tobramycin (TOBI,

Pathogenesis, Seattle, WA, U.S.A.) was performed (101). Patients received 300 mg of tobramycin delivered by a jet nebulizer twice daily every other month for 6 months. Treated patients had a 10% improvement in FEV_1 compared with a 2% decline in pulmonary function among patients receiving placebo. Treated patients also had a reduction in bacterial density, particularly during the first two cycles; however, patients receiving tobramycin had increased tinnitus and hoarseness during treatment cycles.

Although this study confirmed the efficacy of aerosolized tobramycin, several concerns remain: (a) Clinicians are concerned about the emergence of resistance to tobramcyin with long-term aerosol use. This did not occur to a significant extent in the 6-month trial, but there was a trend toward higher minimum inhibitory concentrations (MICs) in the treated group. (b) There is concern that if resistance does occur, intravenous tobramycin will not be effective for treatment of pulmonary exacerbations. (c) The CF community is concerned that intrinsically tobramcyin-resistant pathogens such as *B. cepacia, S. maltophilia, A. xylosoxidans* as well as *Aspergillus* spp. or NTM will emerge on treatment. Notably, increased emergence of intrinsically resistant organisms was not seen during the 6-month trial or during the 12-month open-label study that followed (102). (d) Currently, the clinical significance of increased MICs is unclear because higher MICs were not associated with lack of response in the 6-month trial, although few patients were studied. (e) Conventionally, an organism is considered resistant to tobramcyin if the MIC is greater than 8 µg/mL because of concern about toxicity when this agent is given systemically. Concentrations 10- to 100-fold higher can be delivered by the aerosol route, however; so the conventional breakpoint for tobramycin resistance may be irrelevant for drug delivered by nebulization. (f) Finally, how will resistance be detected using commercially available susceptibility tests that do not measure MICs above 16 µg/mL? It is critical that ongoing studies address these concerns.

Treatment of Allergic Bronchopulmonary Aspergillosis

Treatment of allergic bronchopulmonary aspergillosis can be difficult. Although steroids are thought to be the treatment of choice (because this disorder is immunologically mediated), response to steroids is variable. Some investigators attempted to use antifungal therapy, such as itraconazole or aerosolized amphotericin, and reported response, but no controlled trials have been performed (89).

Treatment of Nontuberculous Mycobacteria

To date, it is uncertain whether NTM is a pathogen in CF, but a case–control study is ongoing to address the potential role of this organism. At this time, some general principles for treatment have been advocated but not rigorously studied. If serial sputum cultures and stains for acid-fast bacilli are positive, if a decline in pulmonary function coincides with the isolation of NTM, and if the patient does not respond to conventional management for traditional CF pathogens, then a trial of antimycobacterial agents can be initiated based on the mycobacteria species that is isolated. Drug levels can be obtained because there are no pharmacokinetic studies of these agents in CF patients (103). Duration of treatment is uncertain, but if the patient responds, the treatment should be continued for 1 year. *In vitro* susceptibility testing can be performed for patients who do not respond.

CLEARANCE OF ABNORMAL SECRETIONS

Mechanical Mobilization of Secretions

For decades, it has been known that CF patients cannot readily clear their secretions. To mobilize the secretions, chest physiotherapy has been used. Conventional chest physiotherapy uses manual percussion, or "clapping," over various regions of the lungs accompanied by postural drainage; however,

this process can be time consuming and labor intensive, and it requires a person other than the patient to perform the chest physiotherapy. As more CF patients are living into adulthood, independence from a caregiver is desirable. In addition, the quality of this method and compliance are uncertain (104). More recently, a pipe-like Flutter Valve (Scandi-Pharm, Birmingham, AL, U.S.A.) and automated percussive vests (ThAIRapy Bronchial Drainage System, American Biosystems, Inc., St. Paul, MN, U.S.A.) were introduced. The percussive vests use high-frequency chest compression to generate pulsating waves at varying frequencies that are transmitted externally to the patient's chest. During treatment for pulmonary exacerbations, conventional chest physiotherapy and the vest were shown to have similar effects on clinical status (104), but a more prolonged comparative trial of different chest physiotherapy modalities is ongoing.

Pharmocologic Mobilization of Secretions

The viscoelastic properties of CF secretions is due largely to the DNA of degenerating neutrophils, and mucolytic agents have been used to mobilize the thick, tenacious secretions (105). Inhaled human recombinant DNase (Pulmozyme, Genentech, San Francisco, CA, U.S.A.) reduces the viscosity of CF sputum *in vitro* by cleaving the neutrophil DNA into shorter segments, which promotes expectoration. Two placebo- controlled, randomized phase 3 trials studied 2.5 mg of rhDNase given once or twice daily for 24 weeks (106). Both treatment groups had improvement in FEV_1 of 5.8% and 5.6% compared with 0% in the placebo group. Treated patients had a reduction of parenteral antibiotic use (28%–37%), fewer hospital days (1.2 days), decreased shortness of breath, and an improved sense of well-being. Dose-related upper-airway irritation has been described as voice changes and laryngitis (107). By 1997, 44.3% of U.S. CF patients were being treated with rhDNase (S. FitzSimmons, CF Foundation National Patient Registry, 1997).

Gelsolin is an investigational human protein that reduces the viscosity of CF sputum *in vitro* by severing actin filaments (108). Actin filaments constitute 10% of leukocyte protein and form viscoelastic filaments. Experimental studies have shown that gelsolin, DNase, and Gc globulin are additive in lowering the vicosity of CF sputum.

MODIFYING THE INFLAMMATORY RESPONSE

Steroids

For longer than a decade, it has been appreciated that an overexuberant host inflammatory response could be responsible for much of the damage in CF lungs. Efforts to control the inflammatory response have focused largely on children in an attempt to preserve lung function.

The efficacy of steroids was studied in a multicenter randomized, placebo-controlled trial that included 285 CF children aged 6 to 14 years. Subjects were treated with alternate-day prednisone 2 mg/kg/day, 1 mg/kg/day versus placebo for 24 months (109). Pulmonary function declined more slowly in the steroid treatment groups, but adverse events, including glucose intolerance, height retardation, and cataracts, were unacceptably frequent, and the 2 mg/kg/day treatment arm was prematurely terminated. Treated children also had increased acquisition of *P. aeruginosa*. Although these investigators concluded that their findings suggested a possible role for the lower treatment dose, this therapeutic strategy generally has not been used because of concerns about toxicity.

Ibuprofen

More recently, ibuprofen (Upjohn, Kalamazoo, MI, U.S.A.) was studied in CF patients to "blunt" the inflammatory response and preserve lung function (110). High concentrations of ibuprofen can inhibit neutrophil migration, adherence, aggregation, and release of lysosomal enzymes. Conversely, lower concentrations may potentiate the inflammatory response. Konstan and colleagues performed a double-blind, placebo-controlled trial wherein 85 CF patients aged 5 to 39 years with mild to moderate lung disease (FEV_1 >60) were randomized to receive ibuprofen versus placebo twice daily for 4 years. The investigators sought peak serum levels of 50 to 100 μg/mL, which required high doses of ibuprofen that ranged from 16.2 to 31.6 mg/kg. Ibuprofen slowed deterioration of lung function ($p = 0.02$) and prevented weight loss ($p = 0.02$). These benefits occurred only among children who were less than 13 years of age when initially enrolled in the trial. Adverse effects such as abdominal pain or use of antacids or H_2 receptor antagonists occurred with equal frequency in both groups; however, conjunctivitis and epistaxis were clearly related to ibuprofen and required discontinuing the drug.

Despite the promise of ibuprofen therapy and its low cost (estimated $200 annually), ibuprofen is not being widely used by CF clinicians at this time. In 1997, only 6.6% of American patients were being treated with ibuprofen (S. FitzSimmons, CF Foundation National Registry, 1997). There are several probable explanations for this lack of enthusiasm: (a) Serum levels for ibuprofen are not widely available. (b) Dosage adjustment is unfamiliar to many physicians. (c) There has been concern about adverse effects, including ulcers and gastrointestinal tract bleeding. (d) Benefit has been shown in only a small subset of children, and many clinicians are concerned that this study should be repeated by others to confirm the findings.

Investigational Agents α-1-Antitrypsin and Pentoxifylline

The investigational use of α-1-antitrypsin, the major inhibitor of neutrophil elastase, has been studied in CF patients. In a preliminary study, α-1-antitrypsin (1.5 mg/kg) was administered by aerosol to 17 CF patients and 12 healthy controls (111). After 7 days of treatment, *in vivo* concentrations of elastase decreased, α-1-antitrypsin levels increased, and the BAL fluids increased *P. aeruginosa* killing activity *in vitro*.

The proposed mechanism of action of the investigational agent pentoxifylline is to inhibit the macrophage-derived cytokines TNF-α and IL1-β. In preliminary studies, Aronoff and colleagues administered pentoxifylline (Hoecht-Roussel Pharmaceuticals, Inc., Somerville, NJ, U.S.A.) to 16 CF patients over 11 years of age for 6 months and showed unchanged concentrations of neutrophil elastase in treated patients compared with increased concentrations in patients who received placebo ($p = 0.05$) (112). No statistically significant changes in pulmonary function were demonstrated.

MODIFYING THE ELECTROLYTE IMBALANCE

With the understanding that *CFTR* is a Cl⁻ channel, investigators attempted to improve the function of other channels and thereby normalize electrolyte physiology. In so doing, the rheologic properties of CF sputum would be improved, leading to clearance of the respiratory tract secretions. These strategies potentially included the use of (a) aerosolized amiloride, a Na^+ channel blocker, to decrease Na^+ absorption by CF airway epithelial cells; and (b) nucleotides, such as uridine triphosphate, which utilize the Ca^{2+} calmodulin-dependent pathway to bypass abnormal *CFTR* (113,114).

To date, only a small double-blind crossover pilot study of 14 patients treated with aerosolized amiloride has been published (114). Fourteen patients aged 18 to 37 years were treated with amiloride delivered to the airway surface four times daily for 25 weeks. Loss of forced vital capacity was slowed during amiloride treatment, but FEV_1 was unaffected. *In vitro* measures of sputum viscosity and elasticity improved with treatment, as did calculated indexes of mucociliary and cough clearance. No adverse effects on sputum microbiology or toxicity were observed. A longer-acting compound is being developed to facilitate treatment.

LUNG TRANSPLANTATION

Lung transplantation is currently considered a last resort for the end-stage pulmonary disease of CF. Bilateral lung and, less commonly, heart lung and single lung transplantation, have been performed in CF patients. By 1997, 847 American CF patients and approximately 300 CF patients from Canada, the United Kingdom, and France had undergone lung transplantation (115). Available lungs are in short supply. Thus, from 1990 to 1997, approximately 50 CF patients had living related donor lobes transplanted. This strategy is controversial because of the risk to the donor and the implications for the multi-CF patient family. Overall, the 5-year survival for CF patients who underwent transplantation since 1992 is 48%.

Cystic fibrosis patients present unique challenges for lung transplantation. On the one hand, they are relatively young and have many years of productive life ahead, the life-threatening manifestations of their underlying disease is limited to their lungs, and CF patients have been capable of compliance with complex medical regimens. On the other hand, transplantation in CF patients can be complex. The optimal time to list a patient for a lung transplant is difficult to determine because the natural history of CF cannot be precisely predicted (116), and there can be an 18- to 24-month wait for available lungs (117). Whereas the transplanted lungs do not develop CF, they can become infected with the pretransplant pathogens (118) or newly acquired pathogens (119). Complications following transplant include rejection, opportunistic infections, and high rates of bronchiolitis obliterans (115,120).

GENE THERAPY

Gene therapy holds much promise, but it has not progressed beyond phase 1 safety trials because of the enormous technical hurdles. These hurdles include (a) developing suitable vectors to deliver the gene and avoid the host immune response, (b) defining the appropriate target cells, and (c) safety, if adenovirus vectors are used (121). Phase 1 trials to evaluate safety have been performed and demonstrated successful introduction of wild-type *CFTR* into nasal and respiratory tract epithelial cells. These trials included adenovirus vectors, adeno-associated vectors, and liposomes to deliver normal *CFTR*. The duration of *CFTR* expression has been short lived, however, and antibodies against the adenovirus vectors have developed.

PROGNOSIS

The outlook for CF patients and their families has never been brighter. The mean life expectancy during the 1960s was 10 years and is now 31 years of age. More than one third of patients are 18 years of age or older, and many patients are living into their fourth and fifth decade of life.

PREVENTION

Vaccine Strategies

There is no effective vaccine against *P. aeruginosa,* although several investigational vaccines are currently under study. Appropriate use of currently available vaccines is advocated. Annual influenza vaccination is recommended, but CF patients are not at increased risk of *Streptococcus pneumoniae* infections, and the pneumococcal vaccine is not recommended. There is an ongoing trial of RSV monoclonal antibody to prevent RSV disease in young infants (Palivizumab, Medimmune Inc., Gaithersburg, MD, U.S.A.) and a trial of an RSV subunit vaccine to prevent recurrent RSV disease in older CF patients (122).

Infection Control

Preventing the acquisition of respiratory tract pathogens has not been generally feasible because of the ubiquitous nature of these organisms. As a result of the widespread recognition of patient-to-patient spread of *B.*

cepacia, however, it is recommended that patients harboring this pathogen be segregated from other CF patients and not cohorted together (123). More recently, concern about possible patient-to-patient spread of *P. aeruginosa* (124), particularly multiple antibiotic-resistant strains, led some CF centers to favor further cohorting and segregation of patients.

SUMMARY

With the growing understanding of the pathogenesis of CF, several recent phase 3 trials led to important contributions to our therapeutic armamentarium, and numerous investigational strategies are being developed. A discussion of treatment of the lung disease of CF patients would be incomplete without emphasizing the time, effort, and financial resources expended by CF patients, their family and friends, and the multidisciplinary medical care team. Thus, therapeutic additions must be carefully studied in well-designed clinical trials to allow a rational evaluation of the risks and benefits for each patient.

REFERENCES

1. Ramsey BW. Management of pulmonary disease in patients with cystic fibrosis. *N Engl J Med* 1996;333:179–188.
2. Rommens JM, Iannuzzi MC, Kerem B, et al. Identification of the cystic fibrosis gene: chromosome walking and jumping. *Science* 1989;245:1059–1065.
3. Riordan JR, Rommens JM, Kerem B, et al. Identification of the cystic fibrosis gene: cloning and characterization of complementary DNA. *Science* 1989;245:1066–1073.
4. Kerem B, Rommens JM, Buchanan JA, et al. Identification of the cystic fibrosis gene: genetic analysis. *Science* 1989;245:1073–1080.
5. Rosenstein BJ, Zeitlin PL. Cystic fibrosis. *Lancet* 1998;351:277–282.
6. Ma J, Davis PB. What we know and what we do not know about cystic fibrosis transmembrane conductance regulator. *Clin Chest Med* 1998;19:459–471.
7. Standiford TJ, Kunkel SL, Basha MA, et al. Interleukin expression by a pulmonary epithelial cell line. *J Clin Invest* 1990;86:1945–1953.
8. Bonfield TL, Panuska JR, Konstan MW, et al. Inflammatory cytokines in cystic fibrosis lungs. *Am J Respir Crit Care Med* 1995;152:2111–2118.
9. Konstan MW, Hilliard KA, Norvell TM, et al. Bronchoalveolar lavage findings in cystic fibrosis patients with stable, clinically mild lung disease suggest ongoing infection and inflammation. *Am J Respir Crit Care Med* 1994;150:448–454.

10. Noah TL, Black HR, Cheng P-W, et al. Nasal and bronchoalveolar lavage fluid cytokines in early cystic fibrosis. *J Infect Dis* 1997;175:638–647.

11. Armstrong DS, Grimwood K, Carlin JB, et al. Lower airway inflammation in infants and young children with cystic fibrosis. *Am J Respir Crit Care Med* 1997; 156:1197–1204.

12. Khan TZ, Wagener JS, Bost T, et al. Early pulmonary inflammation in infants with cystic fibrosis. *Am J Respir Crit Care Med* 1995;151:1075–1082.

13. Dimango E, Ratner AJ, Bryan R, et al. Activation of NF-kB by adherent *Pseudomonas aeruginosa* in normal and cystic fibrosis respiratory epithelial cells. *J Clin Invest* 1998;101:2598–2606.

14. DiMango E, Zar HJ, Bryan R, Prince A. Diverse *Pseudomonas aeruginosa* gene products stimulate respiratory epithelial cells to produce interleukin-9. *J Clin Invest* 1995;96:2204–2210.

15. Moore KW, O'Garra A, Malefyt R, et al. Interleuken-10. *Ann Rev Immunol* 1993;11:165–190.

16. Bonfield TL, Konstan MW, Burfeind P, et al. Normal bronchial epithelial cells constitutively produce the anti-inflammatory cytokine interleukin-10, which is down-regulated in cystic fibrosis. *Am J Respir Cell Mol Biol* 1995;13:257–261.

17. Koch C, Hoiby N. Pathogenesis of cystic fibrosis. *Lancet* 1993;341:1065–1069

18. Boucher RC, Stutts MJ, Knowles MR, et al. Na+ transport in cystic fibrosis respiratory epithelia: abnormal basal rate and response to adenylate cyclase activation. *J Clin Invest* 1986;78:1245–1252.

19. Wilumsen NJ, Boucher RC. Transcellular sodium transport in cultured cystic fibrosis human nasal epithelium. *Am J Physiol* 1991;261:C332–C341.

20. Clarke LL, Grubb BR, Gabriel S, et al. Defective epithelial chloride transport in a gene-targeted mouse model of cystic fibrosis. *Science* 1992;257: 1125–1128.

21. Matsui H, Grubb BR, Tarran R, et al. Evidence for periciliary liquid layer depletion, not abnormal ion composition in the pathogenesis of cystic fibrosis airways disease. *Cell* 1998;95:1005–1007.

22. Bennett WD, Olivier KN, Zeman KL, et al. Effect of uridine 5'-triphosphate plus amiloride on mucociliary clearance in adult cystic fibrosis. *Am J Respir Crit Care Med* 1996;153:1796–1801.

23. Li JD, Dohrman AF, Gallup M, et al. Transcriptional activation of mucin by *Pseudomonas aeruginosa* lipopolysaccharide in the pathogenesis of cystic fibrosis lung disease. *Proc Natl Acad Sci USA* 1997;94: 962–967.

24. Saiman L, Prince A. *Pseudomonas aeruginosa* pili bind to asialoGM1 which is increased on the surface of cystic fibrosis epithelial cells. *J Clin Invest* 1993;92: 1875–1880.

25. Immundo L, Barasch J, Prince A, et al. Cystic fibrosis cells have a receptor for pathogenic bacteria on their apical surface. *Proc Natl Acad Sci USA* 1995;92: 3019–3023.

26. Zar H, Saiman L, Quittell L, et al. Binding of *Pseudomonas aeruginosa* to respiratory epithelial cells from patients with various mutations in the cystic fibrosis transmembrane regulator. *J Pediatr* 1995;126: 230–233.

27. Pier GB, Grout M, Zaidi TS. Cystic fibrosis trans-

membrane conductance regulator is an epithelial cell receptor for clearance of *Pseudomonas aeruginosa* from the lung. *Proc Natl Acad Sci USA* 1997;94: 12088–12093.

28. Ramphal R, Pyle M. Evidence for mucins and sialic acid as receptors in the lower respiratory tract. *Infect Immun* 1983;41:339–344.

29. Reddy MS. Human tracheobronchial mucin: purification and binding to Pseudomonas aeruginosa. *Infect Immun* 1992;60:1530–1535.

30. Sajjan U, Reisman J, Doig RT, et al. Binding of non-mucoid *Pseudomonas aeruginosa* to normal human intestinal mucin and respiratory mucin from patients with cystic fibrosis. *J Clin Invest* 1992;89;657–665.

31. Arora SK, Ritchings BW, Almira EC, et al. The *Pseudomonas aeruginosa* flagellar cap protein, FliD, is responsible for mucin adhesion. *Infect Immun* 1998; 66:1000–1007.

32. Speert DP, Gordon S. Phagocyosis of unopsonized *Pseudomonas aeruginosa* by murine macrophages is a two-step process requiring glucose. *J Clin Invest* 1992;90:1085–1092.

33. Mahenthiralingam E, Speert DP. Nonopsonic phagocytosis of *Pseudomonas aeruginosa* by macrophages and polymorphonuclear leukocytes requires the presence of the bacterial flagellum. *Infect Immun* 1995;63: 4519–4523.

34. Ganz T, Lehrer RI. Defensins. *Pharmacol Ther* 1995;66:191–205.

35. Goldman MJ, Anderson GM, Stolzenberg ED, et al. Human β-defensin-1 is a salt-sensitive antibiotic that is inactivated in CF. *Cell* 1997;88:553–560.

36. Smith JJ, Travis SM, Greenberg EP, et al. Cystic fibrosis airway epithelia fail to kill bacteria because of abnormal airway surface fluid. *Cell* 1996;85:229–236.

37. Berger M. Inflammation in the lung in cystic fibrosis. *Clin Rev Allergy Immunol* 1991;9:119–142.

38. Regelmann WE, Siefferman CM. Sputum peroxidase activity correlates with the severity of lung disease in cystic fibrosis. *Pediatr Pulmonol* 1995;19:1–9.

39. Fick RB Jr, Naegel GP, Squier SU, et al. Proteins of the cystic fibrosis respiratory tract: fragmented immunoglobulin G opsonic antibody causing defective opsonophagocytosis. *J Clin Invest* 1984;74:236–248.

40. Bruce MC, Poncz L, Klinger JD, et al. Biochemical and pathologic evidence for proteolytic destruction of lung connective tissue in cystic fibrosis. *Am Rev Respir Dis* 1985;132:529–535.

41. Suter S, Schaad UB, Tegner H, et al. Levels of free granulocyte elastase in bronchial secretions from patients with cystic fibrosis: effect of antimicrobial treatment against *Pseudomonas aeruginosa. J Infect Dis* 1986;153:902–909.

42. Berger M, Sorensen RU, Tosi MF, et al. Complement receptor expression on neutrophils at an inflammatory site, the *Pseudomonas*-infected lung in cystic fibrosis. *J Clin Invest* 1989;84:1302–1313.

43. Tomashefski JF, Vawter GF, Reid L. Pulmonary pathology. In: Hodson ME, Norman A, Batten JC, eds. *Cystic fibrosis.* London: Bailliere Tindall, 1983:31–51.

44. Sommerhoff CP, Nadel JA, Basbaum CB, et al. Neutrophil elastase and cathepsin G stimulate secretion from cultured bovine airway gland serous cells. *J Clin Invest* 1990;85:682–699.

45. Klinger JD, Tandler B, Liedtke CM, et al. Proteinases

of *Pseudomonas aeruginosa* evoke mucin release by tracheal epithelium. *J Clin Invest* 1984;74:1669–1678.

46. Smallman LA, Hill SL, Stockley RA. Reduction of ciliary beat frequency *in vitro* by sputum from patients with bronchiectasis: a serine proteinase effect. *Thorax* 1984;39:663–667.

47. Tosi MF, Zakem H, Berher M. Neutrophil elastase cleaves C3bi on opsonized pseudomonas as well as CR1 on neutrophils to create a functionally important opsonin receptor mismatch. *J Clin Invest* 1990;86: 300–308.

48. Fick RB Jr, Baltimore RS, Squier SU, et al. IgG proteolytic activity of *Pseudomonas aeruginosa* in cystic fibrosis. *J Infect Dis* 1985;151:589–598.

49. Abman SH, Ogle JW, Harbeck RJ, et al. Early bacteriologic, immunologic, and clinical courses of young infants with cystic fibrosis identified by neonatal screening. *J Pediatr* 1991;119:211–217.

50. Cowen RG, Winnie GB. *Anti-Pseudomonas* IgG subclass titers in patients with cystic fibrosis: correlations with pulmonary function, neutrophil chemotaxis, and phagocytosis. *J Clin Immunol* 1993;13:359–370.

51. Hollsing AE, Granstrom M, Vasil ML, et al. Prospective study of serum antibodies to *Pseudomonas aeruginosa* exoproteins in cystic fibrosis. *J Clin Microbiol* 1987;25:1868–1974.

52. Hoiby N, Schiotz PO. Immune complex mediated tissue damage in the lungs of cystic fibrosis patients with chronic *Pseudomonas aeruginosa* infection. *Acta Pediatr Scand* 1982;301:S63–S73.

53. Pier GB, Saunders JM, Ames P, et al. Opsonophagocytic killing antibody to *Pseudomonas aeruginosa* mucoid exopolysaccharide in older noncolonized patients with cystic fibrosis. *N Engl J Med* 1987;317: 793–798.

54. Tosi MF, Zaken-Cloud H, Demko CA, et al. Cross-sectional and longitudinal studies of naturally-occuring antibodies to *Pseudomonas aeruginosa* in cystic fibrosis indicated absence of antibody mediated protection and decline in opsonic quality after infection. *J Infect Dis* 1995;172:453–461.

55. Harper TB, Gaumer HR, Waring W, et al. Cell mediated immunity and suppressor T cell function in children with cystic fibrosis. *Lung* 1980;157:219–228.

56. Horvat RT, Clabaugh M, Duval-Jobe C, et al. Inactivation of human gamma interferon by *Pseudomonas aeruginosa* proteases: elastase augments the effects of alkaline protease despite the presence of α-macroglobulin. *Infect Immun* 1989;57:1668–1674.

57. Pedersen BK, Kharazmi A. Inhibition of human natural killer cell activity by *Pseudomonas aeruginosa* alkaline protease and elastase. *Infect Immun* 1987; 55:986–989.

58. Gilligan PH. Microbiology of airway disease in patients with cystic fibrosis. *Clin Microbiol Rev* 1991; 4:35–51.

59. Saiman L, Mehar F, Niu WW, et al. Antibiotic susceptibility of multiply resistant *Pseudomonas aeruginosa* isolated from patients with cystic fibrosis, including candidates for transplantation. *Clin Infect Dis* 1996; 23:532–537.

60. Burns JL, Emerson J, Stapp JR, et al. Microbiology of sputum from patients at cystic fibrosis centers in the United States. *Clin Infect Dis* 1998;27:158–163.

61. Hudson VL, Wielinski CL, Regelmann WE. Prognos-

tic implications of initial oropharyngeal bacterial flora in patients with cystic fibrosis diagnosed before the age of two years. *J Pediatr* 1993;122:854–860.

62. Henry RL, Mellis CM, Petrovic L. Mucoid *Pseudomonas aeruginosa* is a marker of poor survival in cystic fibrosis. *Pediatr Pulmonol* 1992;12:158–161.

63. Deretic V, Schurr MJ, Hongwei Y. *Pseudomonas aeruginosa,* mucoidy and the chronic infection phenotype in cystic fibrosis. *Trends Microbiol* 1995;3: 351–356.

64. Cash HA, Woods DE, McCullough B, et al. A rat model of chronic respiratory infection with Pseudomonas aeruginosa. *Am Rev Respir Dis* 1979;119: 453–459.

65. Tang H, Kays M, Prince A. Role of *Pseudomonas aeruginosa* pili in acute pulmonary infection. *Infect Immun* 1995;63:1278–1285.

66. Sorensen RU, Waller RL, Klinger JD. Infection and immunity to Pseudomonas. *Clin Rev Allergy Immunol* 1991;9:47–74.

67. Burns J, Saiman L. *Burkholderia cepacia* infections in cystic fibrosis. *Pediatr Infect Dis J* 1999:18:155–156.

68. LiPuma JJ. *Burkholderia cepacia* epidemiology and pathogenesis: implications for infection control. *Curr Opin Pulm Med* 1998;4:337–341.

69. Lipuma JJ, Marks-Austin KA, Holsclaw DS, et al. Inapparent transmission of *Pseudomonas* (*Burkholderia*) *cepacia* among patients with cystic fibrosis. *Pediatr Infect Dis J* 1994;13:716–719.

70. Govan JR, Vandamme P. Agricultural and medical microbiology: a time for bridging gaps. *Microbiology* 1998;144:2373–2375.

71. Elliot MW, Newman Taylor AJ. Allergic bronchopulmonary Aspergillosis. *Clin Exp Allergy* 1997;27: 55–59.

72. Wood RE, Boat TF, Doershuk CF. Cystic fibrosis. *Am Rev Respir Dis* 1976;113:833–878.

73. Kilby JM, Gilligan PH, Yankaskas JR, et al. Nontuberculous mycobacteria in adult patients with cystic fibrosis. *Chest* 1992;102:70–75.

74. Whittier S, Olivier K, Gilligan P, et al. Proficiency testing for clinical microbiology laboratories using a modified decontamination procedure for detection of non-tuberculous mycobacteria in sputum samples from cystic fibrosis patients. *J Clin Microbiol* 1997; 35:2706–2708.

75. Olivier KN, Yankaskas JR, Knowles MR. Nontuberculous mycobacterial pulmonary disease in cystic fibrosis. *Semin Respir Infect* 1996;11:272–284.

76. Prober CG. The impact of respiratory viral infections in patients with cystic fibrosis. *Clin Rev Allerg Immunol* 1991;9:87–102.

77. Abman SH, Ogle JW, Butler-Simon N, et al. Role of respiratory syncytial virus in early hospitalizations for respiratory distress in young infants with cystic fibrosis. *J Pediatr* 1988;113:826–830.

78. FitzSimmons SC. The changing epidemiology of cystic fibrosis. *J Pediatr* 1993;122:1–9.

79. Anderson DH. Cystic fibrosis of the pancreas and its relation to celiac disease: clinical and pathological study. *Am J Dis Child* 1938;56:344–399.

80. Farber S. Some organic digestive disturbances in early life. *J Mich Med Soc* 1945;44:587–594.

81. Di Sant-Agnese PA, Darling RC, Perera GA, et al. Abnormal electrolyte composition of sweat in cystic fi-

brosis of the pancreas: clinical significance and relationship to disease. *Pediatrics* 1953;12:549–563.

82. Boat TF. Cystic fibrosis. In: Behrman RE, Kleigman RM, Arvin AM, eds. Nelson WE, senior ed. *Nelson textbook of pediatrics,* 15th ed. Philadelphia: WB Saunders, 1996:1239–1250.

83. Lai H-C, Kosorok MR, Sondel SA, et al. Growth status in children with cystic fibrosis based on the National Cystic Fibrosis Patient Registry Data: evaluation of various criteria used to identify malnutrition. *J Pediatr* 1998;132:478–485.

84. Colombo C, Battezzati PM, Podda M. Hepatobiliary disease in cystic fibrosis. *Semin Liver Dis* 1994;14: 259–269.

85. Corey M, Edwards L, Levison H, et al. Longitudinal analysis of pulmonary function decline in patients with cystic fibrosis. *J Pediatr* 1997;131:809–814.

86. Rosenstein BJ, Cutting GR. The diagnosis of cystic fibrosis: a consensus statement. Cystic Fibrosis Foundation Consensus Panel. *J Pediatr* 1998;132:563–565.

87. Farrell PM, Kosorok MR, Laxova A, et al. Nutritional benefits of neonatal screening for cystic fibrosis: Wisconsin Cystic Fibrosis Neonatal Screening Study Group. *N Engl J Med* 1997;337:997–999.

88. Proceedings of a 1997 Workshop. Newborn screening for cystic fibrosis: a paradigm for public health genetics policy development. *MMWR Morb Mortal Wkly Rep* 1997;48(RR-16):1–24.

89. Moss RB. Cystic fibrosis: pathogenesis, pulmonary infection, and treatment. *Clin Infect Dis* 1995;21: 839–851.

90. Beardsmore CS, Thompson JR, Williams A, et al. Pulmonary function in infants with cystic fibrosis: the effect of antibiotic treatment. *Arch Dis Child* 1994;71: 133–137.

91. Weaver LT, Green MR, Nicholson K, et al. Prognosis in cystic fibrosis treated with continuous flucloxacillin from the neonatal period. *Arch Dis Child* 1994;70: 84–89.

92. Frederiksen B, Koch C, Hoiby N. Antibiotic treatment of initial colonization with *Pseudomonas aeruginosa* postpones chronic infection and prevents deterioration of pulmonary function in cystic fibrosis. *Pediatr Pulmonol* 1998;23:330–335.

93. Valerius NH, Koch C, Hoiby N. Prevention of chronic *Pseudomonas aeruginosa* colonisation in cystic fibrosis by early treatment. *Lancet* 1991;338:725–726.

94. Vazquez C, Municio M, Corera M, et al. Early treatment of Pseudomonas aeruginosa colonisation in cystic fibrosis. *Acta Paediatr* 1993;82:308–309.

95. Regelmann WE, Elliott GR, Waarwick WJ, et al. Reduction of sputum *Pseudomonas aeruginosa* density by antibiotics improves lung function in cystic fibrosis more than do bronchodilators and chest physiotherapy alone. *Am Rev Respir Dis* 1990;141:914–921.

96. Ramsey BW, Wentz KR, Smith AL. Predictive value of oropharyngeal cultures for identifying lower airway bacteria in cystic fibrosis patients. *Am Rev Respir Dis* 1991;144:331–337.

97. Ramsey B, Boat T. Outcome measures for clinical trials in cystic fibrosis: summary of a cystic fibrosis foundation consensus conference. *J Pediatr* 1994;124:177–82.

98. de Groot R, Smith AL. Antibiotic pharmacokinetics in cystic fibrosis: differences and clinical significance. *Clin Pharmacol* 1987;13:228–253.

99. Bosworth DG, Nielson DW. Effectiveness of home versus hospital care in the routine treatment of cystic fibrosis. *Pediatr Pulmonol* 1997;24:42–47.

100. Saiman L. Use of aerosolized antibiotics in patients with cystic fibrosis. *Pediatr Infect Dis J* 1998;17: 217–224.

101. Ramsey BW, Pepe MS, Quan JM, et al. Intermittent administration of inhaled tobramycin in patients with cystic fibrosis. *N Engl J Med* 1999;340:23–30.

102. Burns JL, Van Dalfsen JM, Shawar RM, et al. Effect of chronic intermittent administration of inhaled tobramycin on respiratory microbial flora in patients with cystic fibrosis. *J Infect Dis* 1999;179:1190–1196.

103. Peloquin C. *Mycobacterium avium* complex infection. *Clin Pharmacokinet* 1997;32:132–144.

104. Arens R, Gozal D, Omlin KJ, et al. Comparison of high frequency chest compression and conventional chest physiotherapy in hospitalized patients with cystic fibrosis. *Am J Respir Crit Care Med* 1994;150:1154–1157.

105. Ramsey BW, Astley SJ, Aitken ML, et al. Efficacy and safety of short-term administration of aerosolized recombinant human deoxyribonuclease in patients with cystic fibrosis. *Am Rev Respir Dis* 1993;148:145–151.

106. Fuchs HJ, Borowitz DS, Christiansen DH, et al. Effect of aerosolized recombinant human DNase on exacerbations of respiratory symptoms and on pulmonary function in patients with cystic fibrosis. *N Eng J Med* 1994;331:637–642.

107. Ramsey BW, Dorkin HL, and the Consensus Committee. Consensus conference: practical applications of pulmozyme. *Pediatr Pulmonol* 1994;17:404–408.

108. Vasconcellos CA, Allen PG, Wohl ME, et al. Reduction in viscosity of cystic fibrosis sputum *in vitro* by gelsolin. *Science* 1994;263:969–971.

109. Eigen H, Rosenstein BJ, FitzSimmons S, et al. A multicenter study of alternate day prednisone therapy in patients with cystic fibrosis: Cystic Fibrosis Foundation Prednisone Trial Group. *J Pediatr* 1995;126:515–523.

110. Konstan MW, Byard PJ, Hoppel CL, Davis PB. Effect of high-dose ibuprofen in patients with cystic fibrosis. *N Engl J Med* 1995;332:848–854.

111. McElvaney NG, Hubbard RC, Birrer P, et al. Aerosol alpha-1-antitrypsin treatment for cystic fibrosis. *Lancet* 1991;337:392–394.

112. Aronoff SC, Quinn FJ, Carpenter LS, et al. Effects of pentoxifylline on sputum neutrophil elastase and pulmonary function in patients with cystic fibrosis: preliminary observations. *J Pediatr* 1994;125:992–994.

113. Knowles MR, Church NL, Waltner WE, et al. A pilot study of aerosolized amiloride for the treatment of lung disease in cystic fibrosis. *N Engl J Med* 1990; 322:1189–1194.

114. Knowles MR, Clarke LL, Boucher RC. Activation by extracellular nucleotides of chloride secretion in the airway epithelia of patients with cystic fibrosis. *N Engl J Med* 1991;325:533–538.

115. Yankaskas JR, Mallory GB, and the Consensus Committee. Lung transplantation in cystic fibrosis: consensus conference statement. *Chest* 1998;113:217–226.

116. Milla CE, Warwick WJ. Risk of death in cystic fibrosis patients with severely compromised lung function. *Chest* 1998;113:1230–1234.

117. Zuckerman JB, Kotloff RM. Lung transplantation for cystic fibrosis. *Clin Chest Med* 1998;19:535–554.

118. Kanj SS, Tapson V, Davis D, et al. Infections in pa-

tients with cystic fibrosis following lung transplantation. *Chest* 1997;112:924–930.

119. Snell GI, de Hoyos A, Krajden M, et al. *Pseudomonas cepacia* in lung transplant recipients with cystic fibrosis. *Chest* 1993;103:466–471.

120. Steinbach S, Sun L, Jiang RZ, et al. Transmissibility of *Pseudomonas cepacia* infection in clinic patients and lung-transplant recipients with cystic fibrosis. *N Engl J Med* 1994;331:981–987.

121. Wilson JM. Vectors—shuttles vehicles for gene therapy. *Clin Exp Immunol* 1997;107:31–32.

122. Piedra PA, Grace S, Jewell A, et al. Sequential annual administration of purified fusion protein vaccine against respiratory syncytial virus in children with cystic fibrosis. *Pediatr Infect Dis J* 1998;17:217–224.

123. LiPuma JJ. *Burkholderia cepacia* epidemiology and pathogenesis: implications for infection control. *Curr Opin Pulm Med* 1998;4:337–341.

124. Farrell PM, Shen GH, Splaingard M, et al. Acquisition of *Pseudomonas aeruginosa* in children with cystic fibrosis. *Pediatrics* 1997;100:E21–29.

14

Malnutrition, Immunocompetence, and the Risk of Infection

José Ignacio Santos

National Child Health Program, Ministry of Health, Mexico City, Mexico, D.F. 01600

Clinical, metabolic, and biochemical evidence derived from numerous clinical field studies and laboratory animal experiments substantially support the concept that malnutrition affects host susceptibility to infection and that the latter, once established, can further deteriorate the nutritional status of the host. In general, these studies point to the immune system's acute sensitivity to alterations in the host's nutritional status; however, not every organ or cell type is equally affected by a given nutrient's deficiency or excess. These observations increased interest in the interactions between nutrition and infection and in the role of nutritional support to bolster the immunity or host defenses of seriously ill patients. Physicians are increasingly aware of the association between malnutrition (deficiencies or excesses) and various conditions, including sepsis, multiple trauma, cancer, acquired immunodeficiency syndrome (AIDS), renal disease, hepatic failure, cystic fibrosis, prematurity, and aging. An acute or chronic disease can be exacerbated by associated nutritional deficiencies, placing affected persons at increased risk of severe, often fatal, infections (1).

EPIDEMIOLOGY, DIAGNOSIS, AND CLASSIFICATION OF MALNUTRITION

Among the most widespread nutritional deficiency states are protein-calorie malnutri-

tion, vitamin A deficiency, and the nutritional anemias.

Protein-Calorie Malnutrition

The worldwide prevalence of malnutrition, although difficult to ascertain, is accentuated in developing countries with fragile economies, in new emerging democracies plagued by civil strife causing the displacement of people into refugee camps in both developing and developed countries (e.g., Somalia, Rwanda, Yugoslavia) and among the marginated people of affluent countries. In the Western hemisphere, infectious diseases are the leading cause of morbidity and mortality in children under the age of 5 years, and malnutrition contributes directly or indirectly to this process (2–11).

Depending on the precise composition of the diet, protein-calorie deficiency results in the three main clinical syndromes: marasmus, kwashiorkor, and marasmic kwashiorkor. Marasmus denotes starvation and results from a deficiency in total calories. It is clinically characterized by an absence of subcutaneous fat and wasted muscle. In contrast, kwashiorkor is considered to result from consumption of a diet deficient in protein relative to calories and is characterized by muscle wasting and edema. It should be noted that the most important precipitating factor in the pathogenesis of kwashiorkor is an acute infection in the already semistarved or marasmic child. Other clinical manifestations of this clinical entity include growth failure, hepatomegaly, hair changes, and dermatoses. Hypoalbuminemia and a decrease in the total serum proteins are always found. Kwashiorkor has its main incidence during the second year of life or after weaning from the breast. Diets inadequate in total calories, with a disproportionate lack of protein, will result in either marasmus or kwashiorkor or in a mixed type, *marasmic–kwashiorkor.* In nutritional growth failure, or *dwarfing,* there are no clinical signs other than low weight that correspond to age (2,6,12–14). Table 14.1 shows the classification of malnutrition used by the Food and Agriculture Organization and the World Health Organization.

Although severe forms of protein-calorie malnutrition can be diagnosed clinically, nutritional assessment provides an objective characterization that is useful for the diagnosis and management of morbid and premorbid states. Anthropometric measurements include weight and height as a percent of standard, deficit in height for weight, head circumference, triceps skinfold thickness, arm-muscle circumference, body mass index, and age. These measurements, compared with a recognized standard, have been useful in identifying moderate and severe malnutrition (12). The clinical diagnosis of malnutrition can be further substantiated with the aid of a biochemical profile, including the measurement of serum albumin, transferrin, and the creatinine height index; these laboratory tests provide additional objective information (15). Persistent low serum total protein and albu-

min levels suggest an inadequate protein intake, a protein-losing state such as renal disease, or inadequate synthesis resulting from hepatic insufficiency. In nutritional surveys, in addition to measurement of serum albumin levels and albumin–globulin ratios, serum electrophoretic patterns may serve as an additional diagnostic adjunct in the evaluation of protein nutriture.

Part of any nutritional assessment should include an evaluation of dietary intake and the comparison of results to a recognized standard. The use and careful interpretation of several biochemical and immunologic measurements, coupled to anthropometric assessment, can provide a reasonable evaluation of the nutritional state.

Vitamin A Deficiency

Epidemiologically, vitamin A deficiency does not occur in an isolated form and generally is found in association with protein-calorie malnutrition. Globally, more than 250 million children under the age of 5 years are at risk of vitamin A deficiency. Africa has the highest prevalence of clinical vitamin A deficiency; however, Southeast Asia has the highest numbers of clinically and subclinically affected. More than 90% of children with vitamin A deficiency have only subclinical signs, and more than three million have clinical signs of xeropthalmia in those who are subclinically affected (16).

Sufficient evidence exists to indicate that, in addition to affecting mucosal integrity, vitamin A deficiency affects several cellular immune mechanisms, resulting in an increased incidence of gastrointestinal and respiratory infec-

TABLE 14.1. *Simplified classification of protein-calorie malnutrition*

Condition	Body weight as % of standard	Edema	Deficit in weight for height
Underweight child	80–60	0	Minimal
Nutritional dwarfing	<60	0	Minimal
Kwashiorkor	80–60	+	++
Marasmus	<60	0	++
Marasmic kwashiorkor	<60	+	++

+, present; ++, moderate.

tions in affected persons. It is estimated that improving the vitamin A status of all deficient children worldwide would prevent one to three million childhood deaths annually (1,16).

Although night blindness is a reliable clinical indicator of vitamin A deficiency, it is difficult to test for in young children. In this age group. The presence of Bitot spots provide more objective evidence. The definitive diagnosis is the determination of serum retinol; levels below 10 μg/dL are considered deficient.

Nutritional Anemias

Anemia is best defined in functional or physiologic terms rather than quantitatively and generally is expressed as a hemoglobin mass suboptimal for the oxygen transport needs of an individual. *Nutritional anemia is* is defined as the deficiency of one or more essential nutrients (minerals or vitamins) required for the synthesis of hemoglobin and the production of erythrocytes.

Nutritional anemias represent the second most common group of deficiency disorders after protein-calorie malnutrition. Nutritional anemias occur when there is a deficiency of one or more essential nutrients required for hemoglobin synthesis and erythropoiesis (17). They constitute the second largest group of nutritional disorders after protein-calorie malnutrition. The time of greatest vulnerability is during infancy, pregnancy, and lactation, when the requirements are increased because of the demands for growth (16–20). In addition to protein, several nutrients are required for erythropoiesis, including iron, folic acid, vitamin B_{12}, pyridoxine, ascorbic acid, copper, and vitamin E. Among these, iron, B_{12}, and folic acid are the most important.

Iron deficiency is the most common nutritional anemia throughout the world. In most instances, it results from a primary dietary deficiency that produces a combination effect: intake inadequate to meet the demands of growth and chronic blood loss resulting from chronic infections or intestinal parasitism (17–19,21).

Iron deficiency has both hematologic and nonhematologic manifestations. The hematologic manifestations are the most frequently used by the clinician for diagnosis because of the relative ease by which a complete blood count is performed, or simply the hemoglobin and hematocrit are determined. There are, however, pitfalls in using the hematocrit or hemoglobin to separate anemic from nonanemic subjects. In addition to performing a blood smear and determining the mean cell volume, serum ferritin is considered the best marker. The nonhematologic manifestations are often more subtle and include spooning of nails, glossitis, and angular stomatitis (22).

Folic acid deficiency is probably the second most common cause and is generally seen in women during pregnancy. Anemia resulting from the other micronutrients is less common and generally is characterized by specific clinical conditions, especially malabsorption. The deficiency state of each of these nutrients also impinges to a greater or lesser degree on host defense mechanisms.

CAUSES OF MALNUTRITION AND DEFICIENCY STATES

In developing as well as in industrialized countries, the causes of malnutrition are similar, sometimes only changing the order of their frequency. Causes include the following:

- An insufficient amount of nutrients, whether the result of inadequate intake, poor feeding habits, anorexia nervosa, bulemia, food fadism, or cultural and religious restrictions
- Increased loss or inadequate use of nutrients as a result of diarrhea, malabsorption, or gastrointestinal inflammatory diseases, among others
- Increases in the demand for certain nutrients, as in the case of neoplasms, hyperthyroidism, acute infections, and stressful conditions such as trauma and surgery
- Chronic diseases, such as cystic fibrosis, degenerative collagen vascular diseases, congenital cardiopathies, chronic renal fail-

ure, primary or acquired immunodeficiencies, including AIDS resulting from human immunodeficiency virus (HIV), where malnutrition or cachexia is a closely associated factor.

- Intrauterine growth retardation due to poor maternal diet, maternal infection during pregnancy, or congenital infections (22–29).

ACUTE-PHASE RESPONSE TO INFECTION AND ITS IMPACT ON NUTRITIONAL STATUS

The *acute-phase response* is the initial nonspecific host response to infection and consists of a series of metabolic, endocrine, neurologic, and immunologic changes that serve to reestablish homeostasis (30,31,32). The acute-phase response, depending on the host's nutritional status, may be normal, weak, or absent, which is why its clinical and laboratory expression (fever, anorexia, hypoalbuminemia, hypoferremia) may be inapparent. In a similar fashion, the clinical manifestations of infected malnourished children are unspecific, weak, or absent. In a study carried out in Mexico, a clinical–pathologic discordance was found when comparing the respective diagnoses of the autopsy findings of 119 children with third-degree malnutrition who died with a clinical diagnosis of being infected. In this study, the investigators found that 41.6% of cases with peritonitis and 55.5% with amebiasis were not diagnosed based on clinical and laboratory data. These researchers concluded that, in the malnourished person, specific clinical and laboratory studies used to diagnose infections may not always offer the best results (33).

Systemic infections, except for differences due to the causative organism, are accompanied by a series of highly predictable biochemical, hormonal, and metabolic responses. Some of these responses occur during the incubation period, and most are triggered by interleukin 1 (IL-1) from monocytes (31), as depicted in Fig. 14.1.

The response to infection is associated with increased energy requirement. For example,

for every degree of fever, there is a 7% increase in the basal metabolic rate; sweating also causes the loss of nutrients. Another response to infection is anorexia, which decreases the intake of nutrients. The net effect of increased nutrient requirements, increased losses, and decreased intake is altered nutritional status (30–32,34–43). The endocrine response is characterized by an increase in the production of glucocorticoids, mineral corticoids, growth hormone, glucagon, and insulin, among others. Accompanying changes in the catabolism of skeletal muscle, via the alanine pathway, provide amino acids used for gluconeogenesis, tissue repair, and the synthesis of new proteins needed for enzymes, acute phase proteins, immunoglobulins, and other host defense mechanisms. All these additional requirements result in a negative nitrogen balance at the expense of skeletal muscle (34,35).

In the presence of an acute infection, carbohydrate metabolism undergoes important changes necessary to provide quickly the energy requirements for the host immune and none immune response mechanisms. The carbohydrate caloric reserve, based on glycogen stores, is only 1,000 kcal, which in the adult is consumed in 12 to 24 hours, depending on the metabolic demand; in a child, on the other hand, this amount of reserve is rapidly consumed in 8 to 12 hours. Carbohydrate metabolism is confounded by the paradoxic impairment of glucose tolerance resulting from a relative insulin resistance state that results in *pseudodiabetes*. Thus, the energy source provided by glycogen will be the first to be consumed, placing a demand on alternate energy sources (34,44).

The major energy reserve in humans is found in lipids. When faced with an infectious process, the changes in lipid metabolism differs, depending on the etiologic agent. In infections caused by gram-negative bacteria, bacterial lipopolysaccharide triggers the release of tumor necrosis factor (TNF), which in turn inhibits serum lipoprotein lipase activity with the consequent decrease in the clearance of triglycerides; the net result is less use

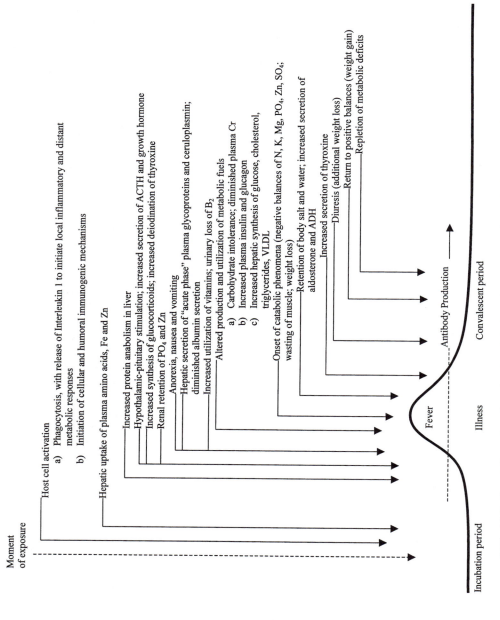

FIG. 14.1. Onset time of various host metabolic responses in relation to the sequential phases of a "model" acute, self-limited, generalized infectious illness. (From Beisel WR. Magnitude of the host nutritional responses to infection. *Am J Clin Nutr* 1977;30:1236, with permission.)

of fats and greater catabolism of structural proteins. In sepsis caused by gram-positive organisms, the activity of the serum lipoprotein lipase may be normal and hypertriglyceridemia less pronounced. During an acute infection, mineral metabolism also undergoes varied changes; iron, magnesium, potassium, phosphates, zinc, and sulfur are either sequestered or lost, whereas vitamins are rapidly used or excreted (30,31,40–50).

For example, acute infection is associated with a significant decline in serum iron levels, usually before other signs of infection, such as fever, develop. The iron is not lost from the body but accumulates in cellular storage forms and is sequestered in the liver, reticuloendothelial system, and bone marrow. Although this does not represent an absolute loss, this sequestration does represent functional wastage because the nutrient is essentially nonavailable for its normal metabolic or physiologic purposes. It has been suggested by many investigators that the decrease in serum iron might reduce the growth of pathogenic microorganisms. In fact, many studies have shown that certain species of bacteria grow poorly in media containing low concentration of iron and that iron supplements increase the growth of bacteria *in vitro* and *in vivo*.

Similarly, during the acute-phase response to infection, the liver, bone marrow, and lymphocytes show an increased uptake of zinc. This redistribution is more accentuated when the infection is severe (17,49,50). The decline in serum zinc to microbiostatic levels is also due to the production of a zinc-binding protein, calprotectin, by polymorphonuclear leukocytes.

Vitamin A metabolism is affected dramatically in response to infection by yet a different mechanism. In addition to increased utilization, during acute infections, there is impaired absorption and, paradoxically, a higher percent of absorbed vitamin A is excreted by the kidney, resulting in decreased serum retinol and its storage form in the liver (16–18).

These examples reflect the metabolic changes in nutrient utilization absorption and redistribution, which are common responses to most acute infections. Their relative impact on nutritional status obviously will be greater in the nutritionally compromised host.

EFFECT OF RECURRENT OR CHRONIC INFECTIONS ON NUTRITIONAL STATUS

The nutritional cost of an acute or recurrent infection in a well-nourished child may well not be associated with clinically overt manifestations or loss of specific function. In the marginally nourished child, the child with chronic illness, or in settings where the prevailing diet is barely sufficient to sustain normal growth, recurrent bouts of infection will precipitate or aggravate protein-calorie malnutrition and can result in impaired growth, particularly in its linear expression. The relationship between the frequency of infection and growth and development has been the subject of several longitudinal field studies, including one by Mata, which is illustrated in Fig. 14.2 (7).

As depicted in the figure, during the first 6 months, while still being breast fed, the infant who is born with evidence of intrauterine growth retardation, weighing less than his or her expected potential because of maternal undernutrition, does quite well and actually is able to surpass the standard median weight for age. Coincident with being weaned from the breast and being introduced to a grain-based or milk-formula diet prepared in water, often from a nonpotable source, the child experiences recurrent and prolonged bouts of diarrhea and other infectious illnesses. The nutritional wastage and metabolic cost associated with these recurrent infections result in a net energy deficiency that culminates in growth failure; so by 3 years of age, the child's body weight is less than 60% of the reference standard (50–54).

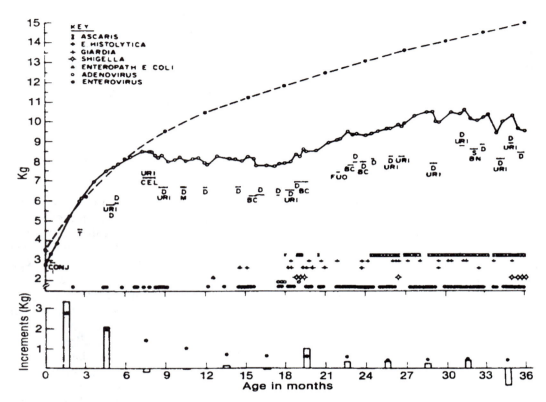

FIG. 14.2. The effect of repeated infections on the nutritional status and growth of a male infant in the first 3 years of life. The *solid line* is the weight of the child, and the *broken line* represents the median of the reference standard. The length of each horizontal line indicates duration of infection. Each mark represents 1 week positive for specific infectious agent. The bottom portion shows observed weight gain (*vertical bars*) versus median increments of the standard (*solid circles*). BC, bronchitis; BN, bronchopneumonia; CEL, cellulitis; CONJ, conjunctivitis; D, diarrhea; FUO, fever of unknown origin; I, impetigo; M, measles; S, stomatitis; T, oral thrush; URI, upper respiratory tract infection. (From Mata LJ. Influence of recurrent infection on growth of children in Guatemala. *Am J Clin Nutr* 1972;25:1267, with permission.)

Risk and Severity of Infection

Susceptibility to infectious diseases is multifactorial and depends on native and acquired immunity, which are in turn influenced by the host's genetic constitution, sex, and age. The nutritional status of an individual has a profound effect on both host susceptibility to specific infectious diseases and on their outcome. Diarrheal disease, respiratory infection, or measles may be a self-limited process in a well-nourished person but may cause significant morbidity or even death of a malnourished host.

Defining the effects of an infection such as whooping cough or measles on the nutritional status of a child has proved to be relatively easy. When nutrition or specific nutrient deficiencies are isolated from other environmental factors, however, it is more difficult to determine their influence on susceptibility to infection. Furthermore, the nutritional status of the host, specifically malnutrition, may have a profound effect on the outcome of specific infectious diseases.

For example, the walling-off process initiated by the inflammatory response to an infecting agent requires the synthesis of fibrin polysaccharides and collagen. This process will be retarded if there is a lack of essential precursors such as protein. In this situation, the inflammatory response is compromised, the walling off process is retarded or not fully developed, greatly increasing the risk that the infection will spread, increasing both the severity of the disease and the utilization of additional nutrients.

This synergistic relationship between nutrition and infection accounts for most of the morbidity in the world. The mortality from pneumonia and gastroenteritis is 10 and 30 times higher, respectively, in malnourished children. In Mexico, the leading cause of morbidity and mortality in children under the age of 5 years is infectious diseases; malnutrition is eight times more frequent as a multiple cause of death (55,56). In Latin America, 60.9% of deaths from infectious diseases are associated with malnutrition (57).

Malnutrition also significantly increases the risk of infection in hospitalized patients (29,58–63). Studies of patients admitted to a children's hospital demonstrated an increased risk for nosocomial infections in malnourished children. In three separate studies, we found that the greatest risk of hospitalized children who acquired nosocomial infections corresponded to patients with varying degrees of malnutrition. The risk of developing varicella or cryptosporidiosis was 5.9 and 4.3 times greater, respectively, in the presence of malnutrition. Moreover, during the 1989 through 1990 measles pandemic, the greatest numbers of attributed complications and deaths were found in severely malnourished children (64–66).

Similarly, in a retrospective, hospital-based, case–control study, Sarabia et al. (67) found that Peruvian children hospitalized for diarrhea were more likely to be infected with *Cryptosporidium* organisms if they were malnourished than were noninfected controls. They also found that nosocomial infection with *C. parvurn* occurred in three severely malnourished children, two of whom died.

MALNUTRITION: AN ACQUIRED IMMUNODEFICIENCY

The malnourished host is more susceptible to infection. Studies of malnourished subjects, however, usually have dealt with generalized malnutrition involving multiple deficiency states. Therefore, it is difficult to attribute changes in the immune status to any specific nutrient deficiency. The most one can do is document the changes in the different arms of the immune system and determine whether these changes are reversible with improved nutrient intake. It is only recently that we have begun to understand the pivotal role that the immune system plays in the interactions between nutritional status and susceptibility to infectious disease. We now appreciate that any compromise in what might be considered an optimal nutritional state may have varying effects on immunity. Such compromise may be expected to reduce the host's ability to cope with exposure to an infectious agent and may increase his or her risk to disease.

Clinical, laboratory, and field epidemiologic studies have demonstrated that malnutrition affects the most of the host's defense mechanisms, which leads us to consider the malnourished patient as an immunocompromised host. The major alterations of the immune mechanisms in the malnourished host include the following: (a) cell-mediated immunity, including a decrease in the number and *in vitro* response of T cells and cutaneous anergy; (b) humoral immunity, including levels of antibodies being either normal or increased, specific antigenic response that is variable, and deficient secretion of serum immunoglobulin A (sIgA); (c) T-helper cell (Th) subpopulations in which specific nutrient-deficiency states appear to favor or supress the development of either the Th1 or Th2 responses; (d) changes in complement, including a decrease in CH50 and variable levels of specific components; (e) alterations in phagocytic cells (polymorphonuclear, mononuclear, macrophages [MO]) and a decrease in chemotaxis, phagocytosis, and microbicidal capacity; (f) functional and structural changes in the respiratory and gastrointestinal epithelium, causing tissue damage and decreasing local resistance to infection because the first barrier microorganisms encountered in the host is the physical integrity of the skin and mucosal membranes (1,17,20,68–82).

Anatomic Barriers and the Mucosal Immune System

The structural integrity of the skin and mucous membranes coupled to the mucosal immune system constitute the primary line of defense by preventing invasion of host tissues by pathogenic microoganisms. In malnutrition, protein and micronutrient deficiency states cause atrophic changes in the skin and impinge on the physiochemical barriers and endogenous secretions, including mucus and lysozyme, increasing host susceptibility to colonization, penetration, and invasion by pathogenic as well as opportunistic microorganisms. Chronic deficiency states of vitamin A, ascorbic acid, riboflavin, and pyridoxine result in abnormal keratinization, poor wound healing, cheilosis, and angular stomatitis. Deficiencies in zinc and methionine also are associated with poor wound healing. Although circulating levels of IgA may be normal in malnourished persons, both local production and mucosal levels of secretory IgA are diminished, which results in an increased susceptibility to gastrointestinal and respiratory pathogens (67,83–89).

Cell-Mediated Immunity

Malnutrition has its most profound effect on cell-mediated immunity. According to histopathologic postmortem studies in children and adults, malnutrition causes thymic involution with atrophy of the thymic–lymphatic system. From functional, clinical, and laboratory points of view, anergy or negativization of delayed hypersensitivity skin tests has been demonstrated; the lymphocytes from malnourished children exhibit a decrease in the blast transformation and incor-

poration of thymidine into DNA in the presence of specific mitogens. It also has been shown that there is an abnormal subpopulation of circulating T lymphocytes in malnourished children. Persons with clinical malnutrition are more susceptible to intracellular opportunistic infections, sepsis caused by gram-negative microorganisms, and disseminated herpetic infections. There have been reports of defects in cell-mediated immunity in specific micronutrient deficiencies, including pyridoxine, pantothenic acid, vitamin B_{12}, folate, vitamin A, vitamin E, iron, and zinc (24,42,65,84,90–102).

Humoral Immunity

With regard to humoral immunity, although the levels of secretory IgA are usually decreased, the serum immunoglobulin concentrations are usually normal or elevated in malnourished persons. Increased serum IgD and IgE levels have been reported; however, because most of the data are from developing countries, it is presumed that the increased levels of IgE are due to concurrent parasitic infestation or altered T-cell function. Even though serum immunoglobulin levels are normal to elevated, their functional capacity has always been subject to question. Finally, data regarding the production of immunoglobulins in response to specific antigen challenge in malnourished individuals are conflicting, showing quantitatively normal responses to several antigens, including bacterial polysaccharides, poliovirus, and measles and deficient responses to typhoid vaccine and viral vaccines against yellow fever and influenza A (103–110).

T-Helper Cell Subpopulations

Although the effects of overt protein-calorie malnutrion on T-helper cell function has not been elucidated, numerous micronutrient deficiencies appear to create a prime environment conducive to the development of T-cell subpopulations. Of these, the most studied have been the T-helper cell subpopu-

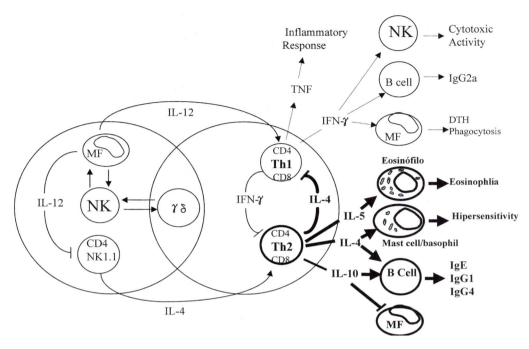

FIG. 14.3. Effects of vitamin A deficiency on the Th1–Th2 response.

lations: Th1 and the Th2 lymphocytes and their respective cytokines. Deficiencies of vitamin A, D_3, and possibly B_{12} lead to an excess T-cell secretion of interferon gamma (IFN-γ), which is important in phagocytic and cell-mediated immunity, and in a decreased secretion of IL-4 and IL-5. These micronutrient deficiencies favor the development of the Th1 response and limit Th2 cell growth and differentiation (111) (Fig. 14.3).

In contrast, deficiencies in vitamin E, C , B_6, and possibly folate and zinc lead to decreased production of IFN-γ and increased production of IL-4 and IL- 5, which are important in the development of a Th2 humorally mediated immune response and limitation of the Th1 cell-mediated response (111–115).

Complement

The levels of complement, as determined by immunodiffusion technique or by hemolytic activity, are decreased in malnutrition, especially in the presence of active infection. Although the opsonizing and bactericidal activity of whole serum has been reported to be impaired in malnourished children, details concerning the chemotactic and opsonic serum activity of the C3 complement fraction are less convincing. The complent levels return to normal levels with nutritional recovery (103,105,107–109).

Phagocytic Cell Function

The phagocytic cells play a pivotal role in the host defense against bacterial and some fungal infections. In recent years, the functional activities of phagocytic cells in several clinical immunodeficiency states, including malnutrition, have been studied. PMN leukocyte functional studies carried out in our laboratory and by other investigators demonstrated changes in adherence, chemotactic activity, phagocytosis, and the microbicidal capacity of these cells in malnourished children in the presence or absence of an acute infection (Table 14.2). In infected patients, some of these

TABLE 14.2. *Neutrophil function in severely malnourished children*

Function	Nourished	Malnourished	p Value
Adherence (%)	69.6 ± 14.1	86.2 ± 5.6	≤0.001
Chemotaxis (μm)	101 ± 5.19	87.0 ± 6.19	≤0.05
NBT dye reduction (OD)	0.463 ± 0.02	0.367 ± 0.03	≤0.01
Bactericidal capacity (CFU)	2.16 ± 0.18	1.71 ± 0.13	≤0.05

CFU, colony forming units; NBT, nitroblue tetrazolium; OD, once daily.

defects persist for several days despite specific therapy and nutritional support (74,116–120).

Specific deficiencies in vitamin B_{12} and iron also decrease PMN function. Because of the technical difficulties involved in obtaining a sufficient number of cells needed for the specific assays, the information available on the function of phagocytic cells of the phagocytic-MN system in malnourished children is limited and controversial. There is evidence to suggest a decrease in the metabolic activity associated with macrophage phagocytic capacity and bacterial clearance in experimental models of protein-calorie malnutrition (1,121). In recent years, studies on mediators of the acute responses to infection have become more important, and, as previously mentioned, it has been shown that there is a decrease in the synthesis and the release of IL-1 by macrophages from malnourished children, which may suggest possible damage in the entire chain reaction needed for the defense against various microorganisms (74,122). Experimental data from animal studies carried out by our group showed that nutritional deprivation of rats for 72 hours produces acute malnutrition, with a 30% weight deficit and increased mortality from experimental sepsis by *Salmonella typhimurium*, despite receiving a normal diet during the experimental infection. Bacteremia was greater, and there was a diminished leukocyte response in malnourished animals. The *in vitro* evaluation of the chemotactic and phagocytic response as well as the metabolism associated with phagocytosis and the microbicidal capacity of peritoneal macrophages in malnourished animals showed all these cell functions to be decreased (123).

Other studies showed that both cellular immunity and phagocytic cell function are al-tered as a result of the acute effects of malnutrition. Thus, based on the preceding, we may conclude that the individual's nutritional status appears to be a key determinant in modulating the immune response.

Proinflammatory Cytokines

During the last two decades, a group of hormone-like substances, generically named *cytokines,* have become the research focus of scientists worldwide. Three cytokines implicated in playing a key role in the production and regulation of the inflammatory process are TNF-α (or *cachectin*), IL-1, and IL-6 (32,44,124–126). There does not seem to be a consensus in the medical literature about the capacity of the malnourished child to produce proinflammatory cytokines. To date, there are no reports concerning the role of TNF-α and IL-6 in malnutrition. What is known can be summarized as follows:

- With an adequate stimulus, malnourished animals and human adults are incapable of synthesizing IL-1. This ability is regained when they are refed (44,123,126).
- Critically ill adults with chronic malnutrition do not synthesize IL-1, and this is associated with a greater mortality. Patients who could synthesize IL-1 in response to nutritional support showed improved survival (44,123,126).
- The monocytes from severely malnourished children do not produce IL-1 *in vitro,* and this is another factor that contributes to the immunodeficiency characteristic of these children (127).
- In animal models, the response to the exogenous administration of IL-1 requires the

availability of metabolic substrates to obtain its effect (126).

• Finally, the response of macrophages and PMNs from malnourished children to some cytokines is altered or deficient. Some of these functions may be corrected *in vitro* by the addition of cytokines (127).

Weight Loss, Cachexia, and AIDS

Infection by HIV has become a prototype of the profound effect of infection on host nutritional status. Weight loss is the hallmark and most sensitive indicator of a patient's accelerated downhill course from HIV infection to AIDS. The weight loss in patients with HIV infection follows the same pattern of wasting and cachexia seen in patients with cancer and is characterized by a disproportionate loss of lean body mass and less of an effect on lipid stores. Depending on the stage of HIV infection, the causes or mechanisms of weight loss are similar to those triggered by an acute intercurrent opportunistic infection (23–27).

Severe weight loss, known in Africa as *Slim's disease*, is part of the World Health Organization's case definition of AIDS (23). As early as 1987, the Centers for Disease Control and Prevention modified the case definition for AIDS to include more than 10% weight loss in an HIV-positive person. Conversely, observations from our pediatric AIDS clinic reveal that once specific antiretroviral therapy is instituted, the best predictor for a decrease in intercurrent infections and repeat hospitalizations is not the CD4 counts but the increase in the patient's height and weight, attesting to improved nutritional status.

Although the specific causes of cachexia in persons with AIDS are not known, it is fair to assume that many factors contribute to the HIV wasting syndrome, including poor dietary intake due to decreased appetite, nausea, increased metabolic requirements, malabsorption and the presence of concomitant opportunistic infections.

Many similarities are found when comparing the immune response of severely malnourished persons with that of subjects who have HIV/AIDS, even in the absence of clinical infection. These findings have been described in both the absence of clinical evidence of malnutrition or opportunistic infections in the case of patients with HIV/AIDS. These observations should increase the awareness of the clinician to think

TABLE 14.3. *Postmortem diagnosis of infection in 39 children with malnutrition and 22 children with AIDS*

Postmortem-culture (+) group	Malnutrition	AIDS	Histopathologic dx group	Malnutrition	AIDS
Subjects with (+) cultures	28 (71.7%)	12 (54.5%)	*Chlamydia* sp.	1	—
1 Isolate/patient	10 (35.7%)	7 (58.3%)	Acid-fast organisms	4	1
2 Isolates/patient	11 (39.2%)	3 (25%)	*Bacteroids* sp.	—	1
>2 Isolates/patient	7 (24.1%)	2 (16.6%)	Cytomegalovirus	2	5
Negative cultures	5 (12.8%)	5 (22.7%)	Epstein-Barr virus	2	—
			Herpes virus	1	—
Bacterial infections			Measles	2	2
Enterobacteriaceae	30	13	Varicella	1	—
P. aeruginosa	6	2	RSV	1	—
S. maltophilia	1	—	Adenovirus	—	1
S. aureus	4	—	*Histoplasma* sp.	1	2
Staphylococcus coag (–)	4	1	*Cryptococcus* sp.	—	3
Haemophilus influenzae	1	—	Mucormycosis	1	—
Non group A, B hemolytic *Streptococcus*	1	—	*Aspergillus* sp.	—	3
Enterococcus sp.	1	—	*Candida* sp.	5	6
Campylobacter sp.	1	—	*Pneumocystis carinii*	—	6
Candida sp.	7	2	*Cryptosporidium*	1	6
			Entamoeba hystolitica	1	

AIDS, acquired immunodeficiency syndrome; DX, diagnosis; RSV, respiratory syncytial virus.

TABLE 14.4. *Comparison of the focus of infection at time of autopsy in 39 malnourished children and 22 children with AIDS*

Focus of infection	Malnutrition	AIDS
Pneumonia	23	17
GI tract	19	14
Sepsis	15	13
Tracheitis	7	4
Heart	4	3
Oral cavity	4	1
Liver	2	2
Central nervous system	2	3
Kidney	2	1
Skin	2	—

AIDS, acquired immunodeficiency syndrome; GI, gastrointestinal.

of both immune deficiencies in countries where malnutrition and AIDS are prevalent (23–27,128–137).

The similarities in the alterations of the immune system also were illustrated in the postmortem findings of 39 children who died with the diagnosis of severe malnutrition and 22 who died with AIDS. In this as yet unpublished study, Beltran and co-workers compared the microbiologic diagnoses determined either by postmortem microbiologic cultures or histopathologic findings (138). Although bacterial infections were a more commonly associated cause of death in malnourished children (Table 14.3), there was a remarkable similarity in the frequency, etiology, types of infections, and organ systems affected in malnourished children and children with AIDS (Table 14.4).

MANAGEMENT OF MALNUTRITION AND SPECIFIC DEFICIENCY STATES

The treatment of protein-calorie malnutrition depends on the severity of disease and on whether a life-threatening infectious disease is present. All patients with severe kwashiorkor should be hospitalized. Severe dehydration should be treated with oral rehydration therapy by trained personnel. If an infection is present, appropriate diagnostic studies ideally should be performed before administering empiric therapy against the likely offending organisms. Adequate intake of calories and protein generally can be accomplished orally or through an intragastric tube. The intake should include protein-rich foods such as skim milk or a mixture of skim milk, vegetable oil, and casein. As associated symptoms of diarrhea and anorexia subside and the child is able to eat, the diet can be modified. With the assistance of the mother or other family member, the diet can be changed to get the child discharged from the hospital as soon as appropriate. There has been a strong interest in stressing aggressive nutritional support to curve or reverse weight loss in AIDS patients in efforts to improve survival (23,25,26).

Considerable progress has been made in improving vitamin A status in children under 5 years of age. In many countries throughout the world where subclinical vitamin deficiency is suspected, vitamin A supplementation has been linked to periodic immunization activities. In 1994, the World Health Organization adopted a policy of integrating the administration of vitamin A as part of the expanded program of immunization. In Mexico, for example, vitamin A is administered to children over 6 months of age and under 5 years of age living in rural or marginated areas in conjunction with immunization and other health activities programmed as National Health Weeks at 6-month intervals.

With regard to nutritional anemias, management generally is targeted at meeting iron requirements. Iron can be supplemented in many forms, of which the ferrous salts are preferable. Dosage should be calculated in terms of elemental iron. The recommended allowances range from 10 mg daily for infants to 18 mg daily for adults. Pregnancy and lactation demand 18 mg daily. When those conditions exist, a supplemental iron source is generally required. Finally, the other micronutrient deficiencies are best addressed through national policies that guarantee the fortification of foods and flours.

Improving Host Defenses in the Malnourished Host with Specific Nutrients: Benefits and Risks

Recently, there has been greater interest in the role of nutritional support and the direct effect of single nutrients and other compounds on the immune function. The extensive research on the role of micronutrients in child survival in developing countries has clearly established that supplementation with specific nutrients can reduce morbidity and mortality of specific infectious diseases (17,18,22)

Impact of Vitamins on the Regulation of the Immune Response

Nutritional therapy directed toward correcting a specific nutritional deficiency has been related to the use of minerals and vitamins. In other situations, the capacity of the nutrients in correcting the *in vitro* defects of the phago-cytic cells has been evaluated. Shigeoka and co-workers (127) found that vitamin E and 2,3-dihydrobenzoic acid can correct the respiratory burst of PMNs from stressed neonates (1,18). In an experimental murine model, vitamin E supplementation also has been shown to enhance lymphocyte proliferation in response to mitogen stimulation, enhance T-helper cell activity, and increased natural killer cell cytotoxicity (111).

Experimental evidence shows that vitamin A deficiency is associated with functional damage of PMNs and cells belonging to the mononuclear system and that vitamin A supplementation increases the functional activity of macrophages (125,126). Shenai et al. (29)

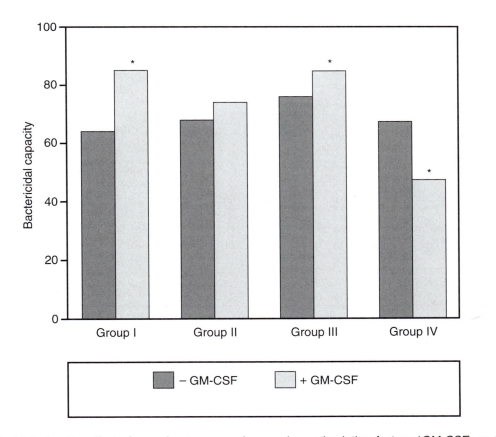

FIG. 14.4. *In vitro* effect of granulocyte macrophage colony stimulating factors (*GM-CSF*) on the bactericidal capacity of polymorphonuclear leukocytes against *Staphylococcus aureus*. Group I, well nourished. Group II, malnourished. Group III, well nourished with infection. Group IV, malnourished with infection. (From Garcia Lloret MI, Santos JI, *unpublished data*, with permission.)

reported that vitamin A supplementation in children with low birth weight decreases the mortality associated with bronchopulmonary dysplasia. It would be of great interest to determine the exact functional activity of macrophages and circulating monocytes as well as the PMNs of children treated the same way. Community-based prophylaxis trials have shown that vitamin A supplementation in deficient populations can reduce mortality in children under the age of 5 years by an average of 35% (16). Furthermore, hospital-based treatment trials with vitamin A in children with measles revealed a reduction of at least 50% of measles-associated mortality in African children. Studies that evaluated its impact on the regulation of the immune response are fairly consistent and strongly suggest that, as demonstrated schematically in Fig. 14.4, vitamin A inhibits a Th1 response and promotes a Th2 response (111).

The structural and functional similarity between vitamin D and a number of steroid hormones is well established. There is also laboratory evidence to support the immunoregulatory role of vitamin D_3 once it is converted to 1,25-dihydroxi vitamin D_3. This metabolite inhibits T-cell proliferation and the *in vitro* production of immunoglobulins by primed B cells. Moreover, both vitamin D_3 and its metabolite inhibit natural killer cell activity in a dose-dependent manner.

Finally, the metabolite has varying effects on Th1 and Th2 responses as evidenced by its capacity to decrease the production of IFN-γ and the synthesis of IL-2 and IL-12 and increase the synthesis of IL-4, IL-5, and IL-10 as well as secretory IgA and serum IgG1 levels. In sum, vitamin D_3 and its metabolite appear to inhibit Th1 response and promote Th2 response (111).

Studies in experimental animal models and in humans have linked vitamin C deficiency to various alterations in immune cellular functions, including depressed cell mediated immunity, PMN phagocytosis, and microbicidal activity. Whereas increased levels of this vitamin have been associated with elevated levels of immunoglobulins and increased neutrophil function in cattle, some studies in humans demonstrated increased mitogenic response in T cells and increased antibody production. There is also a limited body of evidence to support increased IFN-γ production, suggesting in part that vitamin C may be important in promoting a Th1 response while suppressing the Th2 response (111).

Vitamin B₆

Laboratory and clinical studies suggest that vitamin B_6 deficiency suppresses Th1 activity while promoting Th2 response and that supplementation reverses these responses. Table 14.5 summarizes the impact of vitamin B_6 as well as of other vitamins on the Th1–Th2 response.

TABLE 14.5. *Summary of the impact of vitamin deficiencies and supplementation on the Th1-Th2 response*

Vitamins	Th1 response		Th2 response	
	Deficient	Supplemented	Deficient	Supplemented
A	++		– – –	++
D		– – – –		+
B₁₂		–		
E		+++	– –	
C	–	++		
B₆	– –	++		+
Folate	–			

Th1, T-helper cell type 1; Th2, T-helper cell type 2.
+, increase; –, reduction; each symbol represents two studies.
From Long K, Santos JI. Vitamins and the regulation of the immune response. *Pediatr Infect Dis J* 1999;18:223, with permission.

Fatty Acids and the Inflammatory Response

The etiology behind the infectious process is varied but is due predominantly to bacterial infections and partly favored by functional phagocytic defects (PMN and monocyte–macrophage cells) considered of the utmost importance in the defense against these types of microorganisms. The PMN cells of malnourished patients show a decrease in their movement, opsonic recognition, and, even more importantly, their bactericidal capacity (1,74,116,120). Given these deficiencies, the development of new therapeutic modalities that include the exogenous modulation of the phagocytic function as a coadjuvant treatment for infections in the malnourished host is of great importance.

The mechanism through which fatty acids can influence the cellular immune response include their direct incorporation into the cell membrane or the utilization of eicosanoids as precursors for the biologically active lipid mediators, derived from arachidonic acid. The eicosanoids, thromboxane, and especially prostacycline and leukotrienes are highly active compounds, mediators of the inflammatory response and of hypersensitivity reactions. Leukotriene B4 is a potent mediator that triggers chemotaxis, adherence, aggregation, and the degranulation of neutrophils. In addition, there is evidence that leukotriene B4 is a direct mediator of oxidative metabolism within the granulocyte and that human monocytes produce the release of arachidonic acid, thus promoting the formation of eicosanoids (128).

Lee et al. (129) evaluated the effect dietary enrichment with fish-derived fatty acids (eicosapentaenoic and docosahexaenoic acids) on monocyte and nutrophil function and demonstrated changes in the biosynthesis of thromboxane and prostaglandins by PMNs and monocytes and the decrease in the adherence and migration of PMNs. These observations suggested a possible dietary manipulation to decrease the inflammatory response in cases where it produces greater damage than benefit (129).

We evaluated the effect of a dietary supplement of linoleic acid, as soy phosphatidylcholine (PC) or as triglyceride, on PMN leukocyte function, arachidonate (AA) concentrations and release, and leukotriene B4 (LTB4) generation in normal adults. Eight subjects were fed PC (27 g) or placebo for 3 days in a blinded crossover experiment with PMN assays at baseline and at 4, 7, and 14 days (128).

The results of this study demonstrated that a dietary lipid soy PC can modify the composition and concentration of a major fatty acid of the PMNs. Added to a normal unrestricted diet, PC enhanced neutrophil phagocytosis and killing of *Candida albicans* in an *ex vivo* system. The mechanism of action may be related to alterations in the membrane lipid composition of the PMN, leading to the release of vasoactive eicosanoids, which are bioregulators of immune responses. The oral ingestion of PC, which contains no AA, resulted in increased concentrations of AA in the PMNs. In addition, LTB4, a potent chemotactic agent for PMNs, which also stimulates aggregation, degranulation, and hexose transport in PMNs, was generated in response to the formylmethionyl peptide and to the calcium ionophore A23187 by PMNs from subjects fed PC (129).

In contrast, neutral fats that provided equivalent amounts of the precursor fatty acid linoleic acid had no effect on PMN function or PMN fatty acid composition in this study. The possibility that an equivalent amount of choline, glycerol, or phosphate added to a neutral fat preparation would have resulted in the same effects as produced by PC feeding seems unlikely. PC was added to the routine diet, which was assumed to contain more than adequate amounts of choline, phosphorus, and glycerol, albeit in different forms (128).

Coupled with data from animal experiments, these results suggested a potential immunomodulatory role for phosphatidylcholine in humans who have increased risks of bacterial or fungal infections. It should be stressed from the present study that the quality rather than the quantity of fat may be im-

TABLE 14.6. *Effect of iron deficiency and supplementation on outcome of experimental Salmonella typhimurium[a] infection*

	Controls (n = 20)	↓ Fe (n = 20)	↓ Fe + Fe IM[b] (n = 19)
Mean HCT	48%	28%	34%
Bacteremia	2/20 (10%)	6/20 (30%)	7/19 (37%)
Mortality	0	0	0
Mean spleen wt	0.7 g	0.9 g	0.9 g
Spleen culture	11/20 (55%)	12/20 (60%)	14/19 (74%)

HCT, hematocrit.
[a]Infecting dose, 5×10^6 colony-forming units.
[b]2.5 μg Fe/g body weight.

portant in how dietary lipids affect host defenses and immune functions.

The administration of specific nutrients does not always have a beneficial effect. The administration of iron in patients with severe protein malnutrition should be deferred if the patient is suspected of having an underlying inapparent chronic infection, such as tuberculosis or malaria, because these diseases may be suppressed by malnutrition and iron supplementation may lead to reactivation. In the case of malaria, iron may precipitate cerebral complications. In these high-risk patients, iron supplementation also may predispose to gramnegative sepsis (25,139–155).

The risk of iron supplementation during an acute infectious process is exemplified in Table 14.6, which summarizes the results of *S. typhimurium* infection in two groups of rats subjected to experimental iron-deficiency diet after weaning, resulting in a 40% reduction in mean hematocrit compared with controls. The three groups were infected intravenously with 5×10^6 colony-forming units of *S. typhimurium* and one of the iron deficient groups was given, concomitantly, 2.5 μg Fe/g of body weight (142).

Although no difference in mortality was observed among the three groups, two observations are worth pointing out. First, iron deficiency definitely was associated with greater morbidity in the iron-deficient groups, as evidenced by the greater incidence of bacteremia. Second, altered clearance demonstrated by the persistence of positive spleen cultures was greater in the iron-supplemented group (142).

The addition of fats rich in essential fatty acids is an integral part of the parenteral feeding of premature children or those with gastrointestinal and surgical ailments that impede the oral administration of food. There are reports of *in vitro* and *in vivo* studies with respect to the adverse effect of the administration of lipids on the natural function of PMNs and macrophages; therefore, controversies surrounding the route and index of administration of these lipids is a key point for the presentation of these events because the enteral administration of fatty acids does not alter the phagocytic function (156–161).

From a nutritional point of view, the process of nutrient loss and redistribution has the potential of being exploited to the benefit of the host. Two treatment techniques may be used to improve the host response to infection. Nutrients that are essential to optimal immune function and that are being rapidly metabolized may be selectively replaced. Nutrients that the parasite or invading organism needs may be withdrawn. Treatment can include either of these techniques or a combination of the two (16,17,20,39,78,125,138, 141,161).

IS THERE A ROLE FOR IMMUNOMODULATORS IN THE MALNOURISHED HOST?

Recently, interest has developed as to the role of immunomodulators in improving host defense mechanisms in patients with cancer, AIDS, or other immunocompromised states, including the malnourished host. A varied array of substances have been used, from cytokines and complex sugars to antibiotics.

Cytokines

The granulocyte and macrophage colony-stimulating factor (GM-CSF) is a cytokine whose main action is to stimulate the proliferation and function of PMNs and monocytes–macrophages (162). Results from several preliminary studies carried out in our laboratory suggested that the PMNs from malnourished patients exhibit a response to stimulation with this cytokine (1). Coincubation with GM-CSF stimulates the production of intermediate oxygen metabolites and the bactericidal capacity against *S. aureus* in cells from healthy adults and well-nourished children with acute infections. In contrast, GM-CSF does not seem to have any effect and in others may have an inhibitory action on the function of PMNs in malnourished children with infections (Fig. 14.4). Similar results were obtained when the effects of another cytokine (M-CSF) on the activity of monocytes were analyzed. These observations suggested that changes in the synthesis or response to certain cytokines can be determining factors of the poor inflammatory response frequently observed in malnourished infected patients.

Complex Sugars

The β-glucans, complex sugars originally derived from *Saccharomyces cerevisiae* yeast, are potent stimulators of nonspecific defense mechanisms. Their administration increased resistance to infection in diverse experimental models (119). Recently, similar synthetic soluble compounds with biologic properties related to those of the glucans were developed. These seem to have fewer side effects than the original compound. It has been shown that poly(1,6)-B-D-glucopyronosyl-(1-3)-B-D-glucopyranose (PGG) (a ramified polymer composed entirely of glucose monomers) links to glucan receptors present in membranes of the mononuclear phagocytes and stimulates its mi-

crobial function, probably through the induction of the synthesis of several cytokines (119).

We studied the effect of PGG on the *in vivo* cell migration determined by the number of cells that migrate toward sterile sponges implanted in the subcutaneous tissue and the *ex vivo* opsonophagocytic capacity of the PMNs in an experimental model using malnourished rats. Administration of a single dose of PGG (15 mg/kg) increased the migration as well as the bactericidal capacity of peripheral neutrophils and those present in tissues. The recruitment and activation of PMNs to the bloodstream resulted in a more effective elimination of circulating bacteria as observed in an experimental sepsis in a malnourished rat model using *S. aureus* (Fig. 14.4). Based on these findings and with the purpose of evaluating the possibility of using the PGG as a therapeutic immunomodulator in immunocompromised patients, we studied the *in vitro* effect of this compound on the function of PMNs from malnourished children. Through these experiments, we were able to document that the *in vitro* incubation of PMNs from malnourished children with PGG significantly increases their bactericidal capacity. The mechanism for this increase does not seem to be through an increase in the respiratory burst or through the secretion of lysozyme.

Antibiotics

Besides their antiinfective activity against specific microorganisms, antibiotics interact in several ways with host cells. In some cases, this interaction results in the development of toxic and undesirable effects of these drugs; in others, it may have the ability to modulate some aspects of the inflammatory responses that can have a beneficial result in the treatment of the infection (79,115,163,164).

In general, the elimination of an invading microorganism depends on the recognition, ingestion, and digestion of the microorganism by the phagocytic cells. These specific cell functions may be modified by some antimicrobial drugs, which, as a result of their action on the bacterial wall and even in subtherapeutic concentrations, favor the ingestion of microorganisms. Other antibiotics, particularly those that diffuse and concentrate intracellularly, can exert a specific action on phagocytes, modulating their function at different levels (1). Certain antibiotics, such as the aminoglycosides, rifampin, amphotericin, and tetracyclines, are characteristically inhibitors of phagocytic cell activity, whereas others, like the lincosinamides, macrolides, and vancomycin, stimulate the function of these cells (118).

Clindamycin is a wide-spectrum antibiotic that belongs to the lincosinamide group. This liposoluble drug penetrates the PMN cells through active transport, concentrating intracellularly (especially within the lysosomes) between 10 and 100 times the serum concentration (117,153). Given these circumstances, we carried out a series of experiments to determine the effect of several antibiotics, including clindamycin, on the *in vitro* and *in vivo* microbicidal function on PMNs from well-nourished and malnourished persons. Preliminary studies showed that the *in vitro* coincubation of clindamycin with human PMNs from healthy adults had a stimulating effect on chemotaxis, respiratory burst, and the microbicidal capacity of these cells (78,118,164). Stimulation of the phagocytic function was observed when low concentrations (2 pg/mL) of the antibiotic were used, whereas when higher concentrations (10 pg/mL) of the antibiotic were used, there was an inverse effect. Similar results were obtained in studies using an animal model with sepsis caused by *Klebsiella pneumoniae*.

We subsequently studied the effect of a subtherapeutic dose (5 mg/kg) or a low therapeutic dose (10 mg/kg) of clindamycin for 48 hours on the *ex vivo* phagocytic function of malnourished patients diagnosed with an infection and admitted to the hospital. Patients were randomly divided into three groups: group 1 (20 children) received 10 mg/kg daily of clindamycin; group 2 (20 children) received 5 mg/kg daily, and group 3 (10 children) served as the control group and was not given clindamycin. All patients were given specific treatment using diverse antimicro-

bials for their illness based on their physician's orders. Three fundamental aspects concerning PMN activity were assessed: chemotaxis, chemiluminescence (as an indicator of the magnitude of the respiratory burst), and *in vitro* bactericidal capacity against a strain of *Staphylococcus aureus* resistant to clindamycin with a minimal inhibitory concentration (MIC) greater than 128 μg/mL. Analysis of the PMN functions studied showed a significant increase in the three parameters compared with the pretreatment values of patients who received 5 mg/kg. This improvement was not seen in the control group. This increase in phagocytic activity was documented through an increase in chemotaxis in the generation of intermediate oxygen metabolites and, more importantly, by significant increases in the bactericidal capacity of PMNs after 48 hours of treatment with clindamycin. All together, these observations suggested that clindamycin potentially can be used as an immunomodulator at low dosages in infected malnourished children (118,154).

NUTRITIONAL AND PHARMACOLOGIC TREATMENT OF THE HIV WASTING SYNDROME

Despite aggressive nutritional support measures for children and adults with AIDS, the presence of esophagitis, chronic diarrhea, vomiting, and malabsorption of nutrients will contribute to muscle wasting, exacerbating the malnourished state (22–28). In a prospective study of the patterns of weight change in advanced stages of AIDS, Macallan and co-workers showed that decreased food intake is one of the primary causes of weight losing episodes (165). Abrams et al. carried out a prospective study of dietary intake in AIDS patients and found that a high nutrient intake at baseline was associated with higher CD4 count and slower progression from HIV seropositivity to AIDS over a 6-year follow-up (166). Thus, it is reasonable to assume that, by improving the nutritional status of persons who have AIDS, it could be possible to improve the immune system and delay the progression of disease.

Several clinical trials are currently under investigation in adult patients with AIDS in efforts to improve their nutritional status and prevent onset of the wasting syndrome. These trials include the use of different nutritional regimens to improve lean body mass, such as whole protein and long-chain triglycerides plus multivitamins or partially hydrolyzed protein and medium-chain triglyceride mixtures plus multivitamins or multivitamins alone.

The use of pharmacologic agents to improve nutritional status or prevent the HIV-related wasting syndrome included oral anabolic agents such as testosterone, nandrolone decanoate, an appetite stimulant (megace), and human growth hormone, all of which have been shown to improve lean body mass and overall nutritional status (167,168). Thalidomide, initially marketed as a sedative and withdrawn because of its teratogenic effects, is known to have antiinflammatory and immunosupressive effects and has been shown to reverse wasting in patients with advanced AIDS (169).

Finally, there are several National Institute of Allergy and Infectious Diseases (NIAID)-supported trials that look carefully at nutrition and AIDS, including AIDS Clinical Trial Group (ACTG) 892, which attempts to correlate viral load with body composition and total body weight; ACTG 313, which compares a regimen of an appetite stimulant, megace, and testosterone enenthane with megace alone on the increase of lean body mass; and ACTG 329, which is enrolling women with HIV wasting syndrome and using nandrolone, a male hormone with minimal masculinizing effects, to assess weight gain and increases of lean body mass.

The presentation and evolution of HIV disease are heterogeneous, and therapeutic approaches that are successful in adults may not be appropriate for children. Thus, it will be necessary to evaluate different nutritional and pharmacologic interventions for the prevention and treatment of the HIV-associated wasting syndrome, including specific approaches in children (22–24).

CONCLUSIONS

A person's nutritional status is a determining factor in his or her susceptibility to infection. Infection by itself is the cause of energy and nutrient losses that can induce malnutrition, and in the case of a previously malnourished host, there may be a worsening of this already precarious nutritional status. Therefore, the interrelation of the concepts of nutrition and infection immunity can become part of a vicious cycle that directly and totally affects the morbidity and mortality rates of the malnourished host (154). The possible pathways by which an infectious agent may trigger the vicious cycle and alter nutritional status, which in turn alters immunocompetence and increases susceptibility to infection, are depicted in Fig. 14.5.

The limitation of an infectious process depends fundamentally on a vigorous inflammatory response. To carry out such a response, the host must have an integral immune system and an adequately available amount of energetic substrates. A malnourished subject has a variable deficit of both requirements and not only is more easily infected but follows a more severe and prolonged course. Infection itself has a negative effect on the nutritional state of the patient because of the needs generated by energetics and the catabolism of circulating proteins.

The proposal to use immunomodulators as a treatment for severely ill patients, particularly in cases of malnutrition, acquires relevance when we take into consideration that this reiterative cycle of malnutrition and infection is the main cause of morbidity and mortality in children from underdeveloped countries (93,153). The study of clinically applicable immunomodulators should include not only those nutrients or compounds that stimulate the inflammatory response but also those capable of limiting it because in many cases it is the uncontrollable inflammatory response that results in permanent damage. Our observations, as well as those of many other researchers, support the idea of using not only classic immunomodulators but other modali-

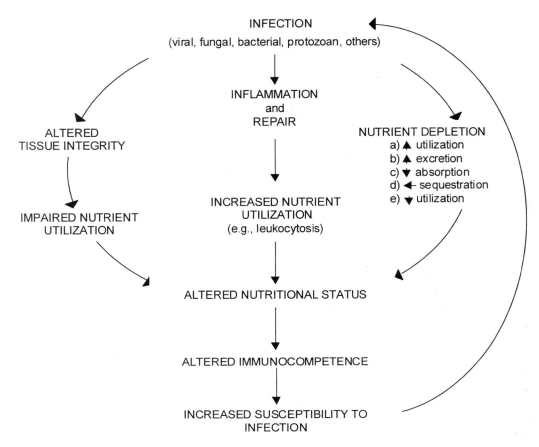

FIG. 14.5. Possible pathway by which an infectious agent may trigger the vicious cycle altering nutritional status, which in turn alters immunocompetence.

ties such as single nutrients for exogenously modulating the host's response to infection. In addition, there is some evidence for the possibility of selective modulation (increased or decreased) of the immune response, depending on the host's needs, through the intervention with specific nutrients, drugs, and biologic response modifiers.

In summary, the concepts mentioned herein explain the need to increase energy consumption when the malnourished host is faced with an acute infectious process to mount an adequate immune response against the invading agent and also help explain the repercussion of the acute infectious process on the nutritional status of the individual. Available data suggest that specific, mixed, chronic, and acute nutritional deficiencies produce damage to the host's immune response, which in turn increases susceptibility to infection. The immunologic characteristics of the malnourished patient are similar to those observed in AIDS patients, especially when malnutrition is associated with disseminated opportunistic infections.

REFERENCES

1. Santos JI. Nutrition, infection and immunocompetence. In: *Infectious disease clinics of North America* 1994;8:243–267.
2. Gomez F. Chronic severe infantile malnutrition. *Ann NY Acad Sci* 1956;69:969.
3. Gomez F, Ramos RG, Frenk S, et al. Mortality in second and third degree malnutrition. *J Trop Pediatr* 1956;2:77.

4. Ramos RG, Cravioto J, Navanete A. Letalidad en nino desnutrido: analisis de 1100 casos internados en el servicio de Nutricion del Hospital Infantil de Mexico durante los anos 1953 a 1957, inclusive. *Bol Med Hosp Infant Mex* 1957;16:875.

5. Cravioto J, Ramos RG, Renteria RR. Correlacion clinico-patologica de algunos hallazgos en 119 autopsias de ninos con desnutricion cronica de tercer grado, internados en el Hospital Infantil de Mexico. *Bol Med Hosp Infant Mex* 1958;15:1009.

6. Ramos RG, Miranda JC. Deaths among children with third degree malnutrition. *Am J Clin Nutr* 1965;16:351.

7. Mata LJ. Infuence of recurrent infections on nutrition and growth of children in Guatemala. *Am J Clin Nutr* 1972;25:1267.

8. Toole MS, Waldman RI. An analysis of mortality trends among refugee populations in Somalia and Sudan. *Bull World Health Organ* 1988;66:237.

9. Martinez C. Nutrition and development of children from poor rural areas. VII. Effects of nutritional status on the frequency and severity of infections. *Nutr Rep Int* 1979;19:307.

10. Sepuveda JA, Lezana M, Tapia TC. Estado nutricional de preescolares y mujeres en Mexico: resultados de una encuesta probabilistica nacional. *Gac Med Mex* 1990;126:201.

11. Health in the Americas: Child Health. PAHO Scientific Publication No.565 65, 1998.

12. Lewinter LS, Suskind D, Murthy KK, et al. The malnourished child. In: Suskind RM, Lewinter LS, eds. *Textbook of pediatric nutrition,* 2nd ed. New York: Raven Press, 1993:127.

13. Sorensen RU, Leiva LE, Kuvidila S. Malnutrition and the immune response. In: Suskind RM, Lewinter LS, eds. *Textbook of pediatric nutrition,* 2nd ed. New York: Raven Press, 1993:141.

14. Whitehead RC. Protein and energy requirements of young children living in the developing countries to allow for catch-up growth after infections. *Am J Clin Nutr* 30:1545, 1977.

15. Mac Lean WC Jr, Graham G. *Pediatric nutrition in clinical practice.* Menlo Park, CA: Addison-Wesley Publishing, 1982:198–217.

16. Sommer A. Vitamin A, infectious disease, and childhood mortality: a solution. *J Infect Dis* 1993;167:1003.

17. Clark S. Kamen R. The human hematopoietic colony stimulating factors. *Science* 1987;236:1229.

18. Beisel WR. Single nutrients and immunity. *Am J Clin Nutr* 35:417, 1982.

19. Beisel WR, Edelman R, Nauss K, et al. Single nutrient effects on immunological functions. *JAMA* 245:53, 1981.

20. Wilkinson JD, Pollack MM, Glass NL, et al. Mortality associated with multiple organ system failure in sepsis in pediatric intensive care unit. *J Pediatr* 11:324, 1987.

21. Suskind R. *The immune response in the malnourished child: nutrition, disease resistance and immune function.* New York: Marcel Dekker, 1984:233–254.

22. Bentler M, Stanish M. Nutrition support of the pediatric patient with AIDS. *J Am Diet Assoc* 1987;87:488–491.

23. Dworkin M, Wormser P, Axelrod F, et al. Dietary intake in patients with acquired immunodeficiency syndrome (AIDS), patients with AIDS-related complex, and serologically positive human immunodeficiency virus patients: correlation with nutritional status. *JPEN J Parenter Enter Nutr* 1990;14:605.

24. Wheeler D, Gilbert C, Launer C, Muurahainen N, et al. Weight loss as a predictor of survival and disease progression in HIV infection. *J Acqir Immun Defic Syndr Hum Retrovirol* 1998;18:80.

25. Gruenfeld C, Feingold KR. Metabolic disturbances and wasting in the acquired immunodeficiency syndrome. *N Engl J Med* 1992;327:329.

26. Kotler DP, Wang J, Pienon RN Jr. Body composition studies in patients with the acquired immunodeficiency syndrome: 1–3. *Am J Clin Nutr* 1985;42:1255.

27. Arditi M, Kabat W, Yogev R. Serum tumor necrosis factor, alpha interleukin 1-beta, p24 antigen concentration and CD4+cells at various stages of human immunodeficiency syndrome. *Pediatr Infect Dis J* 1991;10:450.

28. Gorbach SL, Tamsin A. Weight loss and human immunodeficiency virus infection: cachexia versus malnutrition. *Infect Dis Clin Pract* 1992;1:224.

29. Mariscalco MM. Infection and the host response. In: Fuhrman BP, Zimmerman JJ, eds. *Pediatric critical care.* St. Louis, MO: Mosby Yearbook, 1992:917–927.

30. Shenai JP, Kennedy KA, Chytil F, et al. Clinical trial of vitamin A supplementation in infants susceptible to bronchopulmonary dysplasia. *J Pediatr* 1987;11:269.

31. Beisel WR. Effects of infection on nutritional status and immunity. *Fed Proc* 1980;39:3105.

32. Beisel WR. Magnitude of the host nutritional responses to infection. *Am J Clin Nutr* 1977;30:1236.

33. Dinarello CA, Wolf SM. The role of interleukin-1 in disease. *N Engl J Med* 1993;328:106.

34. Beisel WR, Wannemacher RW Jr. Gluconeogenesis, ureagenesis, and ketogenesis during sepsis. *JPEN J Parenter Enteral Nutr* 1980;4:277.

35. Cerra FB, Siegel JH, Coleman B. Septic autocannibalism. *Ann Surg* 1980;192:570.

36. Dinacello CA. Interleukin-1. *Rev Infect Dis* 1984;6:51.

37. Dinarello CA. The proinflammatory cytolkines interleukin-1 and tumor necrosis factor and the treatment of septic shock. *J Infect Dis* 1991;163:1177.

38. Dinarello CA, Cannon JG, Wolff SM. New concepts in fever pathogenesis. *Rev Infect Dis* 1988;10:168.

39. Drabik MD, Schnure FC, Mok KT, et al. Effect of protein depletion and short term parenteral refeeding on the host response to interleukin 1 administration. *J Lab Clin Med* 1987;109:509.

40. Hoffman LG, Kluger MJ. Protein deficiency: its effects on body temperature in health and disease states. *Am J Clin Nutr* 1979;32:1423.

41. Hoffman LG, McFarlane DD, Bistrian BR, et al. Febrile and plasma iron responses of rabbits injected with endogenous pyrogen from malnourished patients. *Am J Clin Nutr* 1981;34:1109.

42. Keenan RA, Moldawer LL, Yang RD, et al. An altered response by peripheral leukocytes to synthesize or release leukocytic endogenous mediator in critically ill, protein- malnourished patients. *J Lab Clin Med* 1982;100:844.

43. Beutler B. Tumor necrosis, cachexia, shock and inflammation: a common mediator. *Ann Rev Biochem* 1988;57:505.

44. Wannemacher RW, Beall FA, Canonico PG, et al. Glu-

cose and alanine metabolism during bacterial infections in rats and rhesus monkeys. *Metabolism* 1980; 39:201.

45. Conejero R, Lorenzo A, Amal F, et al. Significance of the changes in plasma amino-acid levels in meningococcal infection. *Crit Care Med* 1987;139:337–345.

46. Klugger MJ. Fever revisited. *Pediatrics* 1992;90:846.

47. Saenz XL, Laputta F. The acute phase host reaction during bacterial infection and its clinical impact in children. *Pediatr Infect Dis J* 1993;12:S3.

48. Sherry B, Cerami A. Cachectin/tumor necrosis factor exerts endocrine, paracrine, autocrine control of inflammatory responses. *J Cell Biol* 1988;101:1269.

49. Henkin RI, Smith FR. Zinc and copper metabolism in acute viral hepatitis. *Am J Med Sci* 1972;264:401.

50. Keusch GT. Micronutrients and susceptibility to infection. *Ann NY Acad Sci* 1990;587:181.

51. Cole TJ. Infection and its effect on the growth of young children: A comparison of the Gambia and Uganda. *Trans R Soc Trop Med Hyg* 1977;71:197.

52. Mata LJ. *The children of Santa Maria Clinic.* Boston: MIT Press, 1978.

53. Mata LJ. The malnutrition-infection complex and its environmental factors. *Proc Nutr Soc* 1979;38:29.

54. Cooper WC. Effects of protein insufficiency on immune responsiveness. *Am J Clin Nutr* 1974;21:647.

55. Bustamante PM, Villa AR, Lezana MF, et al. Analysis de la desnutricion como causa multiple de muerte. *Salud Publica Mex* 1991;33:475.

56. Chavez A, Martinez C. Nutricion en edades tempranas y morbilidad infantil. In: Naranjo BA, Chavez A, Madrigal H, eds. *Doce años de programas y proyectos:* contribuciones a las actividades Nacionales de Nutricion. Mexico City, Mexico: INNNSZ, 1987:92.

57. Puffer RR, Serrano J. *Patterns of mortality in childhood.* Washington DC: Pan American Health Organization, 1973: PAHO Science Publication 262.

58. Bristrian BR. Protein status of general surgical patients. *JAMA* 1974;230:BSB.

59. Bristrian BR. Prevaience of malnutrition in general medical patients. *JAMA* 1976;135:1567.

60. Christou NV. Host defense mechanism in surgical patients: A correlative study of the delayed hypersensitivity skin test response granulocyte function and sepsis in 2202 patients. *Can J Surg* 1983;28:39.

61. Johnson WC. Role of delayed hypersensitivity in predictive postoperative morbidity and mortality. *Am J Surg* 1979;137:536.

62. Meakins JL. Clinical importance of host defense resistance to infection in surgical patients. *Adv Surg* 1981; 15:225.

63. Shizgal HM, Martin MF. Caloric requirements of the critically ill septic patient. *Crit Care Med* 1988;16:312.

64. Navarrete NS, Avila FC, Ruiz GE, et al. Sarampion nosocomial: Propuesta para su control en hospitales. *Bol Med Hosp Infant Mex* 1990;47:49S.

65. Navarrete NS, Schirmann Gl, Avila FC, et al. Disminucion del riesgo de adquirir varicella nosocomial despues de un programa de control. *Bol Med Hosp Infant Mex* 1992;49:151.

66. Navarrete NS, Stetler HC, Avila FC, et al. An outbreak of *Cryptosporidium* diarrhea in a pediatric hospital. *Pediatr Infect Dis* 1991;10:248.

67. Sarabia AS, Salazar LE, Giiman RH, et al. Case–control study of *Cryptosporidium parvum* infection in Peruvian children hospitalized for diarrhea: possible association with malnutrition and nosocomial infection. *Pediatr Infect Dis J* 1990;9:627.

68. Baskbaram P, Sivakhumar B. Interleukin-1 in malnutrition. *Arch Dis Child* 1986;61:182.

69. Billiar TR, Curran RD. Kupffer cell and hepatocyte interactions: a brief overview. *JPEN J Parenteral Enteral Nutr* 1990;14(Suppl):175S.

70. Bradley SF, Kauffman CA. Effect of malnutrition on salmonellosis and fever. *Infect Immun* 1988;56:1000.

71. Chandra RK. Serum complement and inununoconglutinin in malnutrition. *Arch Dis Child* 1975;50:225.

72. Chandra RK. Immunocompetence in nutritional assessment. *Am J Clin Nutr* 1980;33:2694.

73. Keusch CT. Nutrition as a determinant of host response to infection and the metabolic sequelae of infection. *Am Infect Dis* 1979;2:265.

74. Douglas SD, Schopfer K. Phagocyte function in protein-calorie malnutrition. *Clin Exp Immunol* 1974;17: 121.

75. Garcia MI, Santos Jl. Las citocinas y su papel como mediadores de salud y enfermedad. *Bol Hosp Infant Mex* 1990;47:12.

76. Gelfand J. Profound depression of the alternative complement pathway in protein-energy malnutrition: a reversible defect of host defenses. In: *Programs and abstracts from the Proceedings of the 22nd ICCAC*; Washington, DC: American Society for Microbiology, 1982:157.

77. Golden MH. Effect of zinc on thymus of recently malnourished children. *Lancet* 1077;2:1057.

78. Wood GH, Watson RR. Interrelationships among nutritional status, cellular immunity and cancer. In: Watson RR: *Nutrition resistance and immune function.* New York: Marcel Dekker, 1984.

79. Santos JI, Arbo A. The *in vitro* effects of sublactam on polymorphonuclear phagocyte function. *Diagn Microbiol Infect Dis* 1989;12:147S.

80. Santos Jl, Arredondo JL, Gnehm H, et al. The effects of iron deficiency on experimental *Haemophilus influenzae* type b pneumonia. In: *Programs and abstracts from the 22nd Interscience Conference on Antimicrobial Agents and Chemotherapy,* Miami Beach, FL: October 4–6, 1982.

81. Sorensen RU, Leiva LE, Kuvidla S. Malnutrition and the immune response. In: Suskind RM, Lewinter LS, eds. *Textbook of pediatric nutrition,* 2nd ed. New York: Raven Press, 1993:141–160.

82. Wood GH, Watson RR. Interrelationships among nutritional status, cellular immunity, and cancer. In: Watson RR, ed. *Nutrition resistance and immune function.* New York: Marcel Dekker, 1984:53–59.

83. Hunter AM. The nutritional status of patients with chronic obstructive pulmonary disease. *Am Rev Respir Dis* 1989;124:256.

84. Morley D. Severe measles in the tropics. *BMJ* 1969; 1:197.

85. Phillips I. Acute bacterial infection in kwashiorkor and marasmus. *BMJ* 1958;1:407.

86. Morley D. Severe measles: some unanswered questions. *Rev Infect Dis* 1983;5:460.

87. Roster FT, Curlin GE, Aziz KMA, et al. Synergistic impact of measles and diarrhea on nutrition and mortality in Bangladesh. *Bull World Health Org* 1981;59: 901.

88. Seth V, Chandra RK. Opsonic activity, phagocytosis, and bactericidal capacity of polymorphs in undernutrition. *Arch Dis Child* 1972;47:282.

89. Smythe PM. Changes in intestinal bacterial flora and the role of infection in kwashiorkor. *Lancet* 1968;2:724.

90. Bell RG. Influence of dietary protein restriction on immune competence: effect on lymphoid tissue. *Clin Exp Immunol* 1976;26:314.

91. Chandra RK. Nutrition as a critical determinant in susceptibility to infection. *World Rev Nutr Diet* 1997;25:166.

92. Chandra RK. Serum thymic hormone activity in protein-energy malnutrition. *Clin Exp Immunol* 1979;38:228.

93. Chandra RK. T and B lymphocyte subpopulations and leukocyte terminal deoxynucleotidyl transferase in protein-energy undernutrition. *Acta Paediatr Scand* 1979;8:841.

94. Edelman R. Mechanisms of defective delayed cutaneous hypersensitivity in children with protein-calorie malnutrition. *Lancet* 1973;1:506.

95. Forse RA. Reliability of skin testing as a measure of nutritional state. *Arch Surg* 1981;116:1284.

96. Keusch GT, Cruz J, Torun B, et al. Immature circulating lymphocytes in malnourished Guatemalan children. *J Pediatr Gastroenterol Nutr* 1987;6:387.

97. Koster F. Recovery of cellular immune competence during treatment of protein-calorie malnutrition. *Am J Clin Nutr* 1981;34:887.

98. Olusi, SO. Effect of thymosin on T-lymphocyte rosette formation in children with kwashiorkor. *Clin Immunol Immunopathol* 1980;15:687.

99. Powel GM. Response to live attenuated measles vaccine in children with severe kwashiorkor. *Am J Trop Pediatr* 1982;2:143.

100. Wabon RR. The effects of malnutrition on secretory and cellular immune processes. *Crit Rev Food Sci Nutr* 1979;12:113.

101. Whittle HC. Cell-mediated immunity during natural measles infection. *J Clin Invest* 1978;62:678.

102. Whittle HC. Immunity to measles in malnourished children. *Clin Exp Immunol* 1980;42:144.

103. Chandra RK. Serum complement and immunoconglutinin in malnutrition. *Arch Dis Child* 1975;50:225.

104. Dillon BC. Opsonic fibronectin deficiency in the etiology of starvation-induced reticuloendothelial phagocytic dysfunction. *Exp Mol Pathol* 1982;36:177.

105. Haller L. Plasma levels of complement components and complement haemolytic activity in protein-energy malnutrition. *Clin Exp Immunol* 1978;34:248.

106. Howard LJ. Plasma fibronectin (opsonic glycoprotein) as an index of nutritional deficiency and repletion of human subjects. *JPEN J Parenter Enteral Nutr* 1981;5:558.

107. Keusch GT. Serum opsonic activity in acute protein-energy malnutrition. *Bull World Health Organ* 1981;59:923.

108. Sirisinha S. Complement and C3 proactivator levels in children with protein-caloric malnutrition and effect of dietary treatment. *Lancet* 1973;1:1016.

109. Stiehm ER. Humoral immunity in malnutrition. *Fed Proc* 1980;39:3093.

110. Suskind RM. Immunoglobulins and antibody response in children with protein calorie malnutrition. *Am J Clin Nutr* 1976;29:836.

111. Long K, Santos JI. Vitamins and the regulation of the immune response. *Pediatr Infect Dis J* 1999;18:223.

112. Xu-Amano J, Beagley KW, Mega J, et al. Induction of T helper cells and cytokines from mucosal IgA. *Adv Exp Med Biol* 1992;3:480.

113. Fitch FW, McKisic MD, Lancki DW, et al. Differential regulation of murine T lymphocyte subsets. *Ann Rev Immunol* 1993;11:29.

114. Sazawal S, Jalla S, Mazumder S, et al. Effect of zinc supplementation on cell mediated immunity and lymphocyte subsets in preschool children. *Indian Pediatr* 1997;34:589.

115. Clerici M, Shearer GM. A Th1-Th2 switch is a critical step in the etiology of HIV infection. *Immunol Today* 11993;4:107.

116. Arbo A, Monroy V, Soria C. Altered polymorphonuclear adherence in malnourished children is corrected *in vitro* with pentoxifylline. In: *Program and Abstracts from the 28th Interscience Conference on Antimicrobial Agents and Chemotherapy,* 1988 (abst 1276).

117. Arbo A, Santos JI. The *in vitro* effects of clindamycin on polymorphonudear leukocyte function. *Drug Invest* 1990;2:235.

118. Santos JI, Arbo A, Pavia N. *In vitro* and *in vivo* effects of clindamycin on polymorphonuclear leukocyte function. *Clin Ther* 1992;14:578.

119. Santos JI, Garcia MIL, Arbo A. Farmacomodulacion de la Respuesta Inflamatoria en la Desnutricion. *Enferm Infecc Microbiol Clin* 1992;7(ed esp):14.

120. Santos JI, Gifaldi A, Alpuche Cl. Neutrophil function in malnourished children recovering from infection. *Enferm Infect Microbiol Clin* 1992;17:21–26.

121. Keusch GT. Macrophage antibacterial functions in experimental protein-calorie malnutrition. II. Cellular and humoral factors for chemotaxis, phagocytosis, and intracellular bactericidal activity. *J Infect Dis* 1978;125:134.

122. Alpuche CM, Pavia NM, Arbo AH, et al. The effect of acute starvation on macrophage function and host susceptibility to *Salmonella typhimurium* infection. IV Congress, Asoc. Panamericana de Infectologia; February 21–24, 1989; Caracas, Venezuela.

123. Hoffman G. Lymphokines and monokines in protein-energy malnutrition. In: *Nutrition and immunology.* New York: Alan R. Liss, 1988:9–16.

124. Hall GM, Desborough JP. Interleukin-6 and the metabolic response to surgery. *Br J Anaesth* 1992;69:337.

125. Hatchigian EA, Santos JI. Vitale: enhanced phagocytosis with vitamin A during experimental *Salmonella* infection. *Soc Exp Biol Med* 1989;191:47.

126. Ongaskul M, Sirisinha S, Lamb A. Impaired blood clearance of bacteria and phagocytic activity in vitamin A deficient rats (41999). *Proc Soc Exp Biol Med* 1985;178:204.

127. Shigeoka AO, Charette RP, Wyman ML. et al. Defective oxidative metabolic responses of neutrophils from stressed neonates. *J Pediatr* 1981;98:392.

128. Jannace PW, Lerman RM, Santos JI, et al. Effects of oral soy phosphatidylcholine on phagocytosis, arachidonate concentrations, and killing by human polymorphonuclear leukocytes. *Am J Clin Nutr* 1992;56:599.

129. Lee TH, Hoover RI, Austen KF. Effect of dietary enrichment with eicoaapentaenoic acid and monocyte leukotriene generation and neutrophil function. *N Engl J Med* 1985;312:1217.

130. Movat HZ. Tumor necrosis factor and interleukin-1: role in acute inflammation and microvascular injury. *J Lab Clin Med* 1987;110:668.

131. Sullivan JS, Kilpatrick I, Caetarino AL, et al. Correlation of plasma cytokine elevations with mortality rate in children with sepsis. *J Pediatr* 1992;120:910.

132. Aylestock J, Gould E, Yogev R. Failure to thrive in HIV-infected children: incidence, prevalence and clinical correlates. *Pediatric AIDS and HIV Infection* 1996;7:83–90.

133. Simpser E. Nutritional support in children with HIV: some answers, many questions. *J Pediatr Gastroenterol Nutr* 1994;18:426.

134. Melchior J, Salmon D, Rigaud D, et al. Resting energy expenditure is increased in stable malnourished HIV-infected patients. *Am J Clin Nutr* 1990;53:437.

135. Alfaro M, Siegel R, Baker R, et al. Resting energy expenditure and body composition in pediatric HIV infection. *Pediatric AIDS and HIV Infection* 1995;6:276.

136. Sharkey SJ, Sharkey KA, Sutherland LR, et al. Nutritional status and food intake in human immunodeficiency virus infection. *J Acquir Immune Defic Syndr Hum Retroviol* 1992;5:1091.

137. Schwenck A, Burger B, Wessel D, et al. Clinical risk factors for malnutrition in HIV-1 infected patients. *AIDS* 1993;7:1213.

138. Beltran S, Peña R, Mayoral PV, et al. Hallazgos histopatológicos en estudios post mortem de ninos desnutridos y ninos con SIDA. Programa Congreso Panamericano de Infectologia, Resumen 123. Cartagena, Colombia, 1995.

139. Murray J. Suppression of infection by famine and its activation by refeeding a paradox? *Perspect Biol Med* 1977;20:47.

140. Murray MJ, Murray C. The adverse effect of iron repletion on the course of certain infections. *BMJ* 1978;2:1113.

141. McGregor IA. Malaria: nutritional implications. *Rev Infect Dis* 1982;4:798.

142. Santos JI, Hatchigian E, Vitale JJ. The effect of iron deficiency and supplementation on experimental *Salmonella typhimurium* infection. *FASEB J* 1984.

143. Schopfer K, Douglas SD. Neutrophil function in children with kwashiorkor. *J Lab Clin Med* 1976;88:450.

144. Sever JL, Fuccillo DA, Ellanberg J, et al. Infection and low birth weight in industrialized society. *Am J Dis Child* 1975;129:557.

145. Calandra T, Gerain J, Heumann D. High circulating levels of interleukin-6 in patients with septic shock: evolution duxing sepsis, prognostic value, and interplay with other cytokines. *Am J Med* 1991;91:23.

146. Damas P, Ledoux D, Nys M, et al. Cytokine serum level during severe sepsis in human IL-6 as a marker of severity. *Ann Surg* 1992;215:356.

147. Dofferhoff AS, Bom VJ, Vriers-Hospers HG. Patterns of cytokines, plasma endotoxin plasminogen activator inhibitor, acute phase proteins during the treatment of severe sepsis in humans. *Crit Care Med* 1992;20:185.

148. Gasson J. Molecular physiology of granulocyte-macrophage colony stimulating factor. *Blood* 1991;77:1131.

149. Hirano T, Kishimoto T. Interleukin-6. In: Zembella M, Asherson GLo, eds. *Human monocytes.* London: Academic Press, 1989:211.

150. Nathan CF. Secretory products of macrophages. *J Clin Invest* 1987;79:319.

151. Nawroth PP, Stern DM. Modulation of endothelial cell hemostatic properties by tumor necrosis factor. *J Exp Med* 1986;163:740.

152. Old UJ. Polypeptide mediator network. *Nature* 1987;326:330.

153. Ruef C, Coleman DL. Granulocyte-macrophage colony stimulating factor: pleiotropic cytokine with potential clinical application. *Rev Infect Dis* 1990;12:41.

154. Stanley ER. Macrophage colony stimulating factor (CSF-I). *J Cell Physiol* 1985;98:123.

155. Tracey Kf, Lowry SF, Cerami A. Cachectin: a hormone that triggers acute shock and chronic cachexia *Infect Dis* 1988;157:413.

156. Stahl GE, Spear ML, Hannosh M. Intravenous administration of emulsions to premature infants. *Clin Perinatol* 1986;13:133.

157. Stronk RC, Munow BW, Thilo E. Macrophage function in infants receiving intralipid by low-dose intermittent infusion. *J Pediatr* 1985;106:640.

158. Wheeler JG, Boyle RJ, Abraawm JS. Intralipid infusion in neonates. Effects on polymorphonuclear function. *J Pediatr Gastroenterol Nutr* 1985;4:453.

159. Wiernlk A, Jastrand C, Julander I. The effect of intralipid on mononuclear and polymorphonuclear phagocytes. *Am J Clin Nutr* 1983;37:256.

160. Wing EJ. Acute starvation protects mice against Listeria monocytogenes. *Infect Immun* 1980;28:771.

161. Santos JI, Arredondo JL, Vitale JJ. Nutrition, infection and immunity. *Pediatr Ann* 1983;12:182.

162. Weiebart RH. Human granulocyte macrophage colony-stimulating factor is a neutrophil activator. *Nature* 1985;314:361.

163. Salimonou R. Effects of IFN on the activation of NK cells in malnourished children. *Clin Exp Immunol* 1984;56:775.

164. Arbo A, Mancilla J, Alpuche C, Santos Jl. *In vitro* and *in vivo* effects of subinhibitory concentrations of clindamycin on experimental *Klebsiella pneumonia* sepsis. *Chemotherapy* 1990;36:337.

165. Macallan DC, Noble C, Baldwin C. Prospective analysis of patterns of weight change in stage IV HIV infection. *Am J Clin Nutr* 1993;58:417–424.

166. Abrams B, Duncan D, Hertz-Picciotto I. A prospective study of dietary intake and acquired immune deficiency syndrome in HIV seropositive homosexual men. *J Acquir Immune Defic Syndri Hum Retrovirol* 1993;6:949–958.

167. Berger JR, Pall L, Hall CD. Oxandrolone in AIDS wasting myopathy. *AIDS* 1996;10:1657–1662.

168. Gold J, High HA, Li Y. Safety and efficacy of nandrolone decanoate for treatment of wasting in patients with HIV infection. *AIDS* 1996;10:745–752.

169. Reyes-Teran G, Sierra-Madero JG, Martinez del Cerro V, Ruiz-Palacios G. Effects of thalidomide on HIV wasting syndrome: a randomized, double-blind, placebo-controlled clinical trial. *AIDS* 1996;10:1501–1507.

15

Asplenia

P. Joan Chesney

Department of Pediatrics, Division of Infectious Diseases,
University of Tennessee, Memphis, Tennessee 38103

As the largest lymphatic organ in the body, representing one quarter of the body's lymphoid tissue, the spleen is also the only lymphatic structure designed to filter blood rather than lymph. The spleen is not necessary for life because almost all of its functions can be subsumed by other organs. Three important functions of the spleen are (a) the filtering and phagocytosis of particulate matter, such as bacteria from the blood of nonimmune hosts; (b) removal of foreign material, such as parasites and inclusions from erythrocytes; and (c) the production of antigen-specific immonoglobuin M (IgM) immune responses. Functional asplenia or hyposplenia is associated with (a) graft versus host disease following bone marrow transplants; (b) with a variety of autoimmune diseases, chronic hemolytic disorders, and malignancies; and (c) following surgical splenectomy or the congenital absence of the spleen.

In the absence of splenic function and in nonimmune hosts, the risk of fulminant infection caused by bacteria with polysaccharide capsules is significantly increased, and half of these infected patients die. Fulminant sepsis can occur many decades after the loss of splenic function. The risk of sepsis can be decreased through the use of chemoprophylaxis in selected patients, immunoprophylaxis (immunization), rapid evaluation and treatment of febrile illnesses, and, most importantly, ed-

ucation and frequent reinforcement for persons with functional asplenia about the risk of fulminant infection.

Recent developments include the introduction of polysaccharide-protein-conjugate vaccines for *Haemophilus influenzae* type b and for seven of the 90 serotypes of *Streptococcus pneumoniae* (pneumococcus), conservative management of splenic trauma, and surgical techniques to preserve splenic function. Unresolved issues include whether to continue chemoprophylaxis in an era of increasingly antibiotic-resistant pneumococci, what antibiotics to use empirically in patients suspected of being infected in this era of antibiotic resistance, how to protect partially immunized infants who are at increased risk, how to protect against the pneumococcal serotypes not present in the new vaccines, and how often to reimmunize functionally asplenic patients with the pneumococcal and meningococcal polysaccharide vaccines.

CAUSES OF ASPLENIA

Anatomic

Congenital Asplenia Syndromes

Congenital agenesis of the spleen may occur as an isolated finding, and familial cases of probable autosomal recessive inheritance have been well described (1–4). In the mouse, an orphan homeobox gene *HOX11* appears to control splenogenesis. In humans, mutations of this gene may be responsible for isolated congenital asplenia (5).

Ivemark syndrome (*asplenia syndrome*) is characterized by developmental abnormalities in laterality or heterotaxy (3). These include splenic abnormalities (absence, hypoplasia, lobulation, polysplenia, dextroposition) in association with cardiovascular anomalies (monoventricular or monoatrial heart, persistent truncus arteriosus, pulmonary stenosis or atresia with or without transposition of the great arteries, anomalous pulmonary venous return), trilobulated or bilobulated lungs, and isomerism of the liver with median position of the gallbladder and malrotation of the gastrointestinal tract. Although most cases are sporadic, familial occurrence is well described (6). This syndrome of visceroatrial heterotaxy is clinically and genetically heterogeneous, suggesting that normal laterality develops by complex mechanisms. Mutations in the connexin 43 gap-junction gene, which lead to abnormally regulated cell-to-cell communication in heart tissue, and buffy-coat preparations from affected children are associated with visceroatrial heterotaxia (5). Up to the age of 12 years, these children may have other immune defects, including decreased numbers of total T and T- helper lymphocytes and decreased antigen-specific lymphoproliferative responses (7).

In one series of 59 children with congenital asplenia (7 with isolated asplenia and 52 with the asplenia syndrome), 16 cases of sepsis (27%) were documented in children under 6 months of age (4). The organism was most often gram-negative, and the course of the infection was similar to that of unaffected infants. In children aged 6 months to 13 years, however, the organism most often was encapsulated, the fulminant nature of the illness was dramatic, and death occurred within 24 hours of onset in five of the 11 children who died. From 1950 through 1975, the greatest number of patients with the asplenia syndrome died of heart disease. If they survived the first year of life, they were at greater risk of dying of infection than of heart disease.

Splenectomy

For children, the major indications for splenectomy are trauma, malignancy, massive size, and hypersplenism. Congenital abnormalities, portal hypertension, Wiskott–Aldrich syndrome, and acute splenic sequestration syndrome in sickle cell disease are rare indications. For all ages, hypersplenic states account for 5% to 50% of splenectomies, trauma for 10% to 30%, incidental to other surgery 20% to 36%, and malignancy 19% to 34% (8). Although the same has not been described in children, adults infected with human immunodeficiency virus (HIV) have demonstrated improved survival and time to acquired immunodeficiency syndrome (AIDS) (9,10) and remission of progressive multifocal encephalopathy following splenectomy (11).

TABLE 15.1. *Causes of functional hyposplenism*

Developmental
  Normal newborn
Hematologic
  Hemoglobinopathies
  Idiopathic thrombocytopenic purpura
  Malignant histiocytosis
Gastrointestinal
  Celiac sprue
  Inflammatory bowel disease
  Portal hypertension
  Acute alcoholism
  Dermatitis herpetiformis
Immunologic
  Systemic lupus erythematosus
  Rheumatoid arthritis
  Grave's disease
  Polyarteritis nodosa
Infiltrative
  Storage diseases (Gaucher's, Niemann–Pick)
  Amyloidosis
  Sarcoidosis
Miscellaneous
  Graft vs. host disease post bone marrow transplant
  Splenic irradiation
  HIV infection
  Total parenteral nutrition

HIV, human immunodeficiency virus.
Adapted from Bridgen M, Patullo A. Prevention and management of overwhelming postsplenectomy infection: an update. *Crit Care Med* 1999;27:836–842, with permission.

Functional

Functional hyposplenism, a poorly functioning but intact spleen associated with several underlying diseases, also places persons at increased risk for fulminant sepsis (Table 15.1) (12). Decreased function may be the result of infarction of tissue (sickle cell disease), infiltrative disease (Hodgkin's or Gaucher's), or hypocomplementemia (systemic lupus erythematosus) (13,14). For other diseases, the reasons for the hyposplenia are more difficult to discern (15–20).

PATHOPHYSIOLOGY

Normal Anatomy and Physiology

The adult spleen normally contains 25 mL of blood and weighs approximately 135 g at puberty. Although this represents only 0.1% of body weight, 300 mL of blood/minute pass through the spleen, which represents 5% to 6% of cardiac output (21,22).

The spleen is surrounded by peritoneum and a fibrous capsule that contains numerous elastic fibers and some smooth muscle. The dense connective tissue of the fibrous capsule enters the splenic parenchyma to form numerous branching and incompletely anastomosing channels (Fig. 15.1). The splenic pulp lies between the fibers and is designated red or white based on the presence or absence of erythrocytes and on the color of fresh tissue (23,24).

At the hilum, the trabecular artery and vein and nonmyelinated axons of the sympathetic system enter the connective tissue trabeculae (Fig. 15.2). The trabecular artery branches into many central arteries, which acquire a periarterial sheath of reticular tissue and predominantly T lymphocytes. At various points, the amount of this lymphatic tissue increases to form densely packed lymphoid nodules composed of macrophages and B lymphocytes. In the nodules, branches of the central artery come off at right angles to "skim" plasma from the blood to supply nutrition and soluble antigens to the densely packed cells. The branching arterioles end at the periphery of the nodule in the marginal zone. This zone

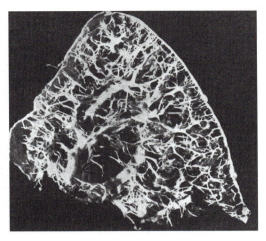

FIG. 15.1. Trabecular framework and capsule of human spleen after removal of pulp. (From Weiss L. *Histology: cell and tissue biology*, 5th ed. New York: Elsevier Science Publishing Co., 1983:545, with permission.)

is composed of many activated macrophages loosely attached to reticular cells and a few scattered T lymphocytes. Germinal centers may be present in the center of the lymphoid nodules.

The central artery ends by emptying 90% of its hemoconcentrated blood into the red pulp. The remainder enters directly into a venous sinusoid or into the trabecular vein (Fig. 15.2). This vein, which has no valves or muscular wall, is an endothelium-lined channel hollowed out in the trabecular connective tissue, which enters directly into the portal vein. Arterial blood may pass quickly through the spleen with direct flow into the trabecular vein, thus providing only nutrients, or it may pass slowly through the filtration system of the red pulp in the splenic cords, where circulation is slow and congested.

The red pulp is composed of the extravascular splenic cords and the venous sinusoids. The cords are composed of loosely arranged reticular fibers, reticular cells, macrophages, and all elements of circulating blood. The venous sinusoids (Fig. 15.2) make up an anastomosing plexus within the red pulp. All the sinusoids ultimately unite to form the trabecular vein (Fig. 15.2).

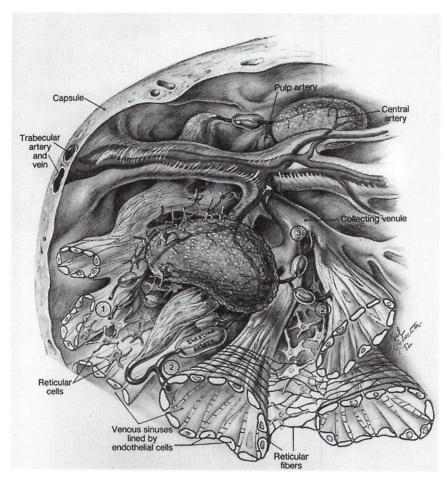

FIG. 15.2. Structure of the spleen and the central arteries may terminate in the substance of the splenic cord or red pulp (1), in a venous sinusoid (2), or directly into a collecting trabecular vein (3). (From Kelly DE, Wood RL, Enders AC. *Bailey's textbook of microscopic anatomy,* 18th ed. Baltimore: Williams & Wilkins, 1984:460, with permission.)

The venous sinusoids are uniquely arranged, with parallel and elongated endothelial cells surrounded by circumferential reticular fibers (Fig. 15.2). Macrophages may be present between the endothelial cells. The basement membrane is incomplete, providing for many intercellular clefts of 1 to 3 μm, which allow erythrocytes and white blood cells to pass from the red pulp into the sinusoids (Fig. 15.3). It is at this interface that white blood cells and normal erythrocytes enter the circulation and imperfect erythrocytes are prevented from entering the circulation.

When a radiolabeled particulate antigen is introduced into the circulation, it is taken up first by the macrophages of the red pulp splenic cords. After 1 hour, the label moves to the marginal zone of the lymphoid nodules, which contains activated macrophages and T lymphocytes. At 2 hours, the label moves into the small lymphocytes surrounding the germinal centers of the nodules, the B lymphocytes. By 4 hours, the germinal center itself has been penetrated. Within 48 hours, antigen persists only in the germinal center. The cellular response to antigen is twofold. After 24

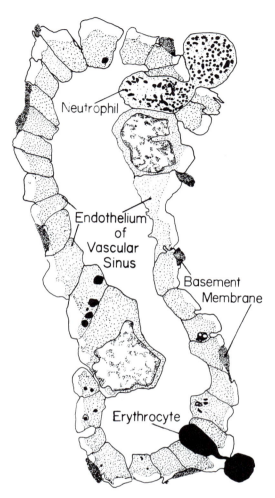

FIG. 15.3. Venous sinusoid from red pulp showing entrance of an erythrocyte (**bottom**) and neutrophil (**top**). (From Weiss L. *Histology: cell and tissue biology*, 5th ed. New York: Elsevier Science Publishing Co., 1983:559, with permission.)

hours, large plasmablasts appear in the periarterial sheath. Within 2 days, they have moved to the perimeter of the sheath and out into the red pulp, and by 4 days, there are many plasma cells in the red pulp (24). Simultaneously, the germinal centers enlarge and contain many mitotic cells. The centers slowly diminish in size over 10 days and return to normal within 4 weeks. Thus, activated B cells travel to the center of the nodule to give rise to memory B cells and plasma cells, which then travel to the red pulp to release antibody into the blood (25).

Normal Development

In utero, the spleen is first recognizable at 5 weeks of life. The pluripotent stem cells, which originate in the yolk sac at 2.5 to 3 weeks of life, reach the fetal liver by 5 weeks. By way of the thymus, stem cells reach the spleen, lymph nodes, and appendix by 8 weeks. In utero, hematopoiesis is the major function of the spleen until the fetus reaches the age of 6 to 8 months. At birth, the spleen weighs 11 g and will resume its hematopoietic function only under pathologic conditions. The spleen does not reach its full weight until adulthood, unlike all other lymphoid structures, which are histologically mature by 1 year of age (21–24).

Normal Function

The spleen is a multifunctional organ (Table 15.2). In addition to its potential hematopoietic function, it is the organ that controls circulating erythrocyte numbers and quality. Cells that are not easily deformed cannot move from the splenic cords through the slits in the venous sinuses to reenter the circulation. Thus, *senescent cells,* or cells deformed by abnormal hemoglobin, are broken down by activated macrophages. The globin protein is broken into amino acids, iron is removed from heme and returned to the circulation, and the iron-free heme molecule is broken down to bilirubin. Erythrocytes containing particulate material, that is, Howell–Jolly bodies (nuclear remnants), Heinz bodies, vesicles, or parasites, can slide partway through the slits in the sinusoids. Macrophages

TABLE 15.2. *Potential functions of the spleen*

Hematopoiesis of all blood elements
Regulation of erythrocyte number and shape
Storage and volume changes
Cellular differentiation
Antigen processing of intravascular antigens
Production of antibody and cytokines
Phagocytosis

then remove the particulate material, a phenomenon known as *pitting* (1). The cell membrane reseals, and the erythrocytes enter the circulation.

The spleen also functions as a storage organ. The elasticity of the splenic capsule, which also contains smooth muscle, the nonrigidity of the cords, and the reticular composition of the spleen allow it to distend to hold as much as 45% of the body's red cell mass under pathologic conditions such as splenic sequestration in sickle cell disease. Normally, 30% of the body's platelets and factor VIII are stored here.

The immune functions of the spleen include serving as a large reservoir of fixed tissue macrophages derived from circulating monocytes. Although the spleen is capable of initiating primary and secondary immune responses to soluble antigens, its most important immune function is that of responding to blood-borne particulate antigens in the nonimmune host. In animal models, blood-borne bacteria opsonized with specific antibody or complement are cleared efficiently by the liver phagocytes, as are small particles of 0.01 to 0.001 µm. For bacteria with amorphous polysaccharide capsules and no attached opsonins and for larger particulate matter, however, the spleen provides the most effective organ for initiating a primary IgM immune response (26) and for phagocytosing the particulate matter. This appears to be the result of a combination of factors. The slow, congested, and viscous nature of flow through the splenic cords, which are rich in macrophages, reticular, dendritic, and plasma cells, provides for maximal exposure of the antigen to lymphocytes and macrophages, which then synthesize antibodies, cytokines, and other mediators. The spleen also provides a critical number of phagocytes to surround and phagocytose organisms that have no attached opsonins. The spleen is also uniquely capable of making IgM antibody, alternate complement components, and other opsonins, such as tuftsin, rapidly and efficiently.

Pathophysiology

In early studies in rabbits (27), when virulent pneumococci were injected intravenously into immune animals, the bacteria were rapidly and efficiently removed by the phagocytic cells of the liver. In nonimmune animals, the organisms continued to circulate. If the nonimmune animals were given 5×10^3/mL killed pneumococci intravenously 8 hours before the live organisms were injected, protection was demonstrated, and the virulent bacteria were rapidly cleared. This same protective effect was not present in splenectomized rabbits. Thus, the spleen was critical for the early production of protective opsonins, now known to be IgM antibody, properdin, tuftsin, and other alternate complement components (25).

ETIOLOGIC AGENTS

The organisms responsible for fulminant sepsis in persons with nonfunctioning or ab-

TABLE 15.3. *Frequency distribution of the most commonly cultured organisms in 178 episodes of bacteremia among 3,451 patients with sickle hemoglobinopathies expressed as a percent of total episodes[a]*

Age (yr)	<3	3–5	6–9	10–19	≥20
Streptococcus pneumoniae	75[a]	43	25	30	10
HITB	10	18	8	12	8
Escherichia coli	5	8	25	28	40
Salmonella	0	18	25	13	4
Staphylococcus aureus	2	4	0	12	8
Other	8	7	17	5	30

HITB, *Haemophilus influenzae* type B.
[a]Fatality rate was 24% for the 46 cases in children younger than 3 years of age.
From Zarkowsky HS, Gallagher D, Gill FM, et al. Bacteremia in sickle hemoglobinopathy. *J Pediatr* 1986;109: 579–585, with permission.

TABLE 15.4. *Capnocytophaga canimorsus*

Fastidious gram-negative rod
Follows close contact with dog or cat saliva
Splenectomy significant risk factor
Can cause fulminant sepsis in all hosts
Rare in children
Mortality rate of 33%
Susceptible to penicillins
Sepsis may occur even on antibiotic prophylaxis

From Pers C, Gahrn-Hansen B, Frederiksen W. *Capnocytophaga canimorsus* septicemia in Denmark, 1982–1995: review of 39 cases. *Clin Infect Dis* 1996; 23:71–75; Scully RE. Case records of the Massachusetts General Hospital. *N Eng J Med* 1999;340: 1819–1826; and Chaudhuri AK, Hartley RD, Maddocks AC. Waterhouse–Friderichsen's syndrome caused by DF-Z bacterium in a splenectomized patient. *J Clin Pathol* 1981;34:172–173, with permission.

sent spleens are most commonly those with a thick polysaccharide capsule, that is, *S. pneumoniae, Klebsiella* sp., *H. influenzae* type b and *Escherichia coli* (Table 15.3). Overall, pneumococci cause 50% to 90% of all these infections (8). Most series of splenectomized patients with fulminant sepsis include patients with infections caused by *Neisseria meningitidis, Salmonella* sp., *Staphylococcus aureus* and other streptococcal species (25–35). It is not clear, however, that the incidence of these infections is increased in these patients, although the severity may be greater. Splenectomized patients are also at increased risk for infections caused by *Capnocytophaga canimorsus* (Table 15.4), a fastidious gram-negative rod (36–38) and the intraerythrocytic protozoan *Babesia* sp. (Table 15.5) (39) and may have more severe infections with these organisms. It is not clear whether splenectomy increases the incidence or severity of malaria.

EPIDEMIOLOGY

Although an increased risk of septicemia following splenectomy is well defined in all age groups, the specific incidence, type of organism, and mortality rate are clearly related to age (Tables 15.3 and 15.6) and underlying disease state (Tables 15.6 and 15.7). For example, in children under the age of 6 years who have sickle hemoglobinopathies, the incidence of bacteremia depends on the type of hemoglobinopathy (Table 15.6), and the type of organism depends on age (Table 15.3). In children with congenital asplenia, the type of organism and course of infection are age dependent (4). For children over 6 months of age in whom protective maternal antibody levels have declined, infection is fulminant and most often caused by encapsulated organisms. The high mortality rates in children younger than 2 years of age presumably relate to their age-related inability to form antibodies to polysaccharide encapsulated organisms in addition to the absence of a functioning spleen.

Splenectomized children under 15 years of age have a greater overall risk of overwhelming infection (0.13%–8.1%) compared with adults (0.28%–1.9%) (30). This appears to be in part a function of the previous exposure of adults to encapsulated bacteria with development of specific opsonizing antibodies.

The lowest incidence of overwhelming sepsis follows splenectomy for trauma, estimated

TABLE 15.5. Babesia *species*

Intraerythrocytic protozoan carried by deer tick *Ixodes dammini*
Borrelia burgdorferi also carried by *Ixodes dammini* in endemic areas
Asplenia significant risk factor for severe disease
Diagnosis: Giemsa-stained thin blood films: PCR for Babesia sp. DNA: IFA for IgM and IgG is specific/sensitive
Erythrocyte lysis results in clinical manifestations of
    Fever: jaundice: renal insufficiency: hemolytic anemia: hemoglobinemia: hemoglobinuria and complications
      of ischemia caused by obstruction of blood vessels
    Splenomegaly: hepatomegaly: hepatic dysfunction: cerebral abnormalities
Treatment: Clindamycin and quinine orally or azithromycin and atovaquone

IFA, interferon A; IgG, immunoglobulin G; IgM, immunoglobulin M; PCR, polymerase chain reaction.
From Rosner F, Zarrahi MH, Benach JL, et al. Babesiosis in splenectomized adults. *Am J Med* 1984:765: 696–700, with permission.

TABLE 15.6. *Age-specific incidence rates of septicemia/meningitis in patients with sickle cell disease expressed as events/100 patient years and compared with nonsplenectomized populations[a]*

	Age (yr)							
	≤2	<3	2–4	3–5	5–19	6–19	10–19	≥20
HBSS								
Attack rate	9.68	7.98	4.10	2.54	1.40	1.05	0.63	0.40
Reference	35	21	35	21	35	21	35	21
HBSC								
Attack rate	—	3.54	—	0	—	0.27	0.48	0.19
Reference		21		21		21	21	21
Normal children								
Attack rate	0.0035	—	—	—	—	—	—	—
White Mountain Apache children								
Attack rate	2.40	—	—	—	—	—	—	—
Alaskan Native American children								
Attack rate	0.62	—	—	—	—	—	—	—

HBSC, sickle cell hemoglobin C; HBSS, sickle cell hemoglobin S.
From Overturf GD. Infections and immunizations of children with sickle cell disease. *Adv Pediatr Infect Dis* 1999;14:191–213, with permission.

to be 15.7% for infants and 10.4% for children under 5 years of age (32). For children overall, it has been estimated to be between 0.9% (31) and 1.45% (30). For adults, the incidence of sepsis following splenectomy for trauma may be no greater than sepsis for the general population, but infection is 58 times more likely to be fatal (30). Overall, the highest incidence of sepsis (10%–24%) and highest mortality rates (50%) occur in patients who have undergone a splenectomy for underlying hemoglobinopathies (thalassemia) (30) or for malignancy (40,41).

Sickle Cell Disease

Before pneumococcal vaccine was introduced in 1978, and before the use of penicillin prophylaxis and neonatal screening for hemoglobinopathies, the rates of invasive pneumo-

TABLE 15.7. *Incidence of postsplenectomy sepsis and sepsis-related mortality*

Cause of mortality (no. of patients)	Sepsis	Sepsis-related mortality	Increase[a]
Trauma (688)	2%	40%	58×
Incidental to other surgery (233)	2%	40%	86×
ITP (489)	2%	70%	70–140×
Congenital spherocytosis (850)	4%	63%	200×
Hemolytic anemia (67)	8%	40%	300×
Portal hypertension (221)	8%	72%	600×
Primary anemia (70)[b]	9%	83%	700×
Reticuloendothelioses (69)[c]	12%	88%	300×
Thalassemia (109)	25%	44%	1,100×

ITP, idiopathic thrombocytopenic purpura.
[a]Increase in sepsis-related mortality compared to sepsis-related mortality in normal individuals.
[b]Included some patients with Fanconi's anemia, some with sickle cell disease, and some with undertemined etiology.
[c]Included patients with Letterer-Siwe disease, myeloproliferative syndromes, Gaucher's disease and Niemann-Pick disease.
From Singer DB. Postsplenectomy sepsis. *Perspectives in Pediatric Pathology* 1973;1:285–311, with permission.

coccal infections in children with sickle cell disease exceeded those of normal children by 30- to 300-fold (28,42,43). The greatest risk was in children under 5 years of age (Table 6). The total case fatality rate was 26.8% (28,42), and 10% to 20% of children died of pneumococcal sepsis before their second birthday (43). Continuing high rates of invasive pneumococcal disease (3.0–3.5/100 child years) were documented recently despite the availability of pneumococcal polysaccharide vaccines and chemoprophylaxis (44). The incidence of infection in children under 2 years of age did not change after the introduction of the polysaccharide pneumococcal vaccine. Children with sickle cell hemoglobinopathy and some forms of thalassemia have less risk than children with sickle cell disease, but overwhelming infections do occur in these patients (45) (Table 15.7).

The risk of invasive pneumococcal disease in other children with congenital or surgical splenectomy never has been precisely defined. It has been assumed that children under 2 years of age have risks similar to patients with SSD who are autosplenectomized uniformly by 18 months of age.

CLINICAL MANIFESTATIONS

Overwhelming and fulminant infection in persons with absent or decreased splenic function has been called *overwhelming postsplenectomy infection* by some researchers (8,29). A brief prodrome of fever and chills and nonspecific symptoms of myalgias, malaise, sore throat, headache, nausea, vomiting, diarrhea, and abdominal pain progress rapidly to hypotension, respiratory distress, disseminated intravascular coagulation, diffuse purpura, severe hypoglycemia, and coma. Many patients have no focal site of infection. For others, pneumonia and meningitis are common sites of infection. Convulsions, cardiovascular collapse, peripheral gangrene of fingers, toes, ears, nose and lips are common. Bilateral adrenal hemorrhage with necrosis similar to the Waterhouse–Friderichsen syndrome frequently is found at autopsy. Death in up to 75% of patients occurs within 48 hours of presentation despite aggressive treatment and support (29–35).

DIFFERENTIAL DIAGNOSIS

The differential diagnosis of fever and other nonspecific symptoms may have many etiologies in the asplenic host. Fulminant sepsis always should be suspected and the first dose of antibiotics given rapidly. Time then can be taken to explore other possible diagnoses.

LABORATORY DIAGNOSIS

The unique laboratory findings in fulminant sepsis in patients with compromised splenic function are a high degree of bacteremia and the presence of circulating erythrocytes, reflecting the absence of splenic function. Organisms may be seen in the peripheral smear within neutrophils or in extracellular fluid in a buffy-coat preparation (8,29). The degree of bacteremia is usually greater than 10^6 organisms per milliliter of blood compared with 10^2 per milliliter in nonfulminant cases. The blood smear will also show Howell-Jolly bodies (Fig. 15.4A), and there will be greater than 12% of "pocked" erythrocytes as examined by interference phase-contrast microscopy (Fig. 15.4B) (1,46). These surface indentations or membrane vesicles are removed only in the spleen. Normally, there are fewer than 2% pocked erythrocytes. Other laboratory tests should be performed to detect, evaluate, and manage multisystem organ involvement (Table 15.8).

An ultrasound or computed tomography (CT) examination of the abdomen can be performed rapidly to determine whether a spleen is present. Splenic function can be evaluated by scanning with technetium-99 metastable sulfur colloid (^{99m}Tc).

MANAGEMENT AND THERAPY

The cornerstone of management is to recognize the patient at risk and to regard any fever as a medical emergency. Although

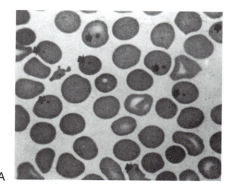

A

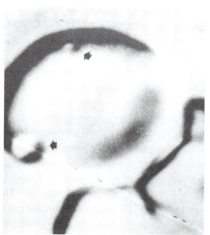

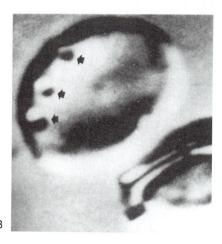

B

FIG. 15.4. A: Howell–Jolly Bodies (*arrows*) within red blood cells. **B:** Red blood cells with surface indentations or "pocks" by interference phase-contrast microscopy. (From Feder HM, Pearson HA. Assessment of splenic function in familial asplenia. *N Engl J Med* 1999:341:211, with permission.)

there is no proof that early treatment will delay or prevent low-grade bacteremia from progressing to high-grade bacteremia and septic shock, empiric broad-spectrum antimicrobial therapy should be administered as soon as possible. Blood, urine, cerebrospinal fluid (CSF), if indicated, and other cultures from potential foci of infection should be obtained rapidly, and therapy should not be delayed.

Initial therapy should be directed at the organisms responsible for most reported cases of fulminant sepsis: *S. pneumoniae, H. influenzae* type b, *N. meningitidis, E. coli, Salmonella* sp., and groups B and D streptococci. Other antibiotics for less common gram-negative organisms such as *Enterobacter* sp., *P. aeruginosa,* and anaerobic organisms can be added, but they are rarely associated with fulminant sepsis in this situation. Initial therapy also should be directed to possible foci of infection, most importantly the meninges. Therapy should take into account possible antimicrobial resistance of the organism and the pharmacokinetics of the antimicrobials. Thus, an antimicrobial combination that rapidly achieves high bactericidal levels in both blood and meninges with activity against potentially antibiotic resistant organisms would be the combination of choice. Pneumococci causes 50% to 90% of episodes in both children and adults, and because 40% to 50% of pneumococci cases in the United States are now nonsusceptible to penicillin (47), the combination of vancomycin and cefotaxime (or ceftriaxone) at doses appropriate for meningitis should be used initially when sepsis associated with a nonfunctioning spleen is suspected (40) (Table 15.9). This combination also should be effective initially for *S. aureus* sepsis and most episodes of gram-negative sepsis as well as that caused by groups B and D streptococci if pneumococci are isolated. Management based on the susceptibilities of the organism is provided in Table 15.9.

The management of children with sickle cell disease and fever, particularly the highest risk population under 5 years of age, is diffi-

TABLE 15.8. *Diagnosis of asplenia or functional hyposplenism*

Definite
  Pitted RBC numbers increased by interference contrast microscopy[a]
  No spleen by ultrasound or computed tomography examination
  Poorly functioning spleen by radionuclide scanning using technetium-99 metastable sulfur colloid
Possible (rule out asplenia)
  Congenital asplenia in other family members
  Congenital heart disease with heterotaxy syndrome and abnormal heart position
  Fulminant sepsis caused by encapsulated organism
  Repeated invasive pneumococcal infections
  Abdominal scar suggesting splenectomy
  Abnormal blood smear with increased number RBCs with inclusions

RBC, red blood cells.

[a]Strong correlation between presence of ≥3.5% "pocked or vesiculated" RBC's on peripheral smear and inability to visualize the spleen on ^{99m}Tc scans.

From Feder HM, Pearson HA. Assessment of splenic function in familial asplenia. *N Engl J Med* 1999;341: 210–211, with permission.

TABLE 15.9. *Intravenous antimicrobial therapy for pneumococcal sepsis with or without meningitis in the asplenic or hyposplenic child*

	Antimicrobial	Dose	Interval
Initial empiric therapy[a]			
Meningitis	Cefotaximer[b] or	250–300 mg/kg/D	q6–8 h
	ceftriaxone[b]	100 mg/kg/D	q12–24 h
	Plus vancomycin	60 mg/kg/D	q6 h
Bacteremia or other non-CNS invasive infections	Cefotaxime or ceftriaxone	As above	
Follow-up therapy once antimicrobial susceptibilities available			
Meningitis			
Penicillin-susceptible (S) (MIC <0.1 µg/mL)	Penicillin	250–400,000 µ/kg/D	q4 h
Penicillin nonsusceptible (NS) (MIC ≥0.1 µg/mL) Cefotaxime S (MIC ≤0.1 µg/mL)	Cefotaxime or ceftriaxone	As above	
Penicillin NS (MIC ≥0.1 µg/mL) Cefotaxime NS (MIC >0.1 µg/ml + <2 µg/mL)	Cefotaxime or ceftriaxone + Vancomycin	As above 60 mg/kg/D	q6 h
Penicillin NS (MIC >0.1 µg/ml) Cefotaxime highly resistant (HR) (MIC >2 µg/mL)	Cefotaxime or ceftriaxone + Vancomycin + Rifampin (consult infectious disease specialist)	As above 60 mg/kg/D 20 mg/kg/D (p.o.)	q6 h q12 h
Bacteremia and/or other non-CNS invasive infection			
Penicillin S	Penicillin	As above	
Penicillin NS + cefotaxime S	Cefotaxime or ceftriaxone	As above	
Penicillin NS + cefotaxime HR	Cefotaxime or ceftriaxone + Vancomycin (consult infectious disease specialist)	As above 40 mg/kg/D	q6h q6 h

CNS, central nervous system; MIC, minimum inhibitory concentration; p.o., by mouth (orally).

[a]For severe allergy to β-lactam antibiotics, vancomycin plus rifampin can be used initially for suspect pneumococcal infections.

[b]Antimicrobial susceptibilities of cefotaxime and ceftriaxone are generally the same, and either drug can be selected.

From the Committee on Infectious Diseases of the American Academy of Pediatrics. Therapy for children with invasive pneumococcal infections. *Pediatrics* 1997;99:289–299, with permission.

cult (48). Pneumococcal bacteremia may present with nonspecific symptoms and progress rapidly to death within a few hours. On the other hand, children with sickle cell disease may have simple colds. Aggressive repeated episodes of treatment, hospitalization, and the accompanying trauma to the child can have significant emotional, financial, and social costs. Criteria that can help to define which children should be managed aggressively in the hospital are listed in Table 15.10 (48,49).

Children at lower risk for bacterial sepsis may include those who are older than 5 years, who have a form of sickle hemoglobin but not sickle cell disease, who are known to be compliant with penicillin prophylaxis, and who are not toxic. If the rest of the family has the same symptoms, the child has been mildly ill without change for several days, and the caregivers are reliable, they also may be at lower risk.

In all cases, the caregivers should be well educated with respect to symptoms, signs, and complications of fulminant sepsis. The evaluation of children with the risk factors listed in Table 15.10 should be rapid, and intravenous antibiotics at appropriate high doses (Table 15.9) should be started without delay.

PROGNOSIS AND SEQUELAE

Most published cases of fulminant sepsis occur within the first few years after splenectomy averaging 50% to 70% of episodes within 2 years, particularly in young children (32). Earlier infections appear to have a high mortality: Approximately 80% of fatal infections occur within 2 years of splenectomy (8). Overall, half of all patients with fulminant sepsis die. The risk of sepsis is lifelong, however, and cases as late as 59 years after splenectomy have been reported (8,50). Whereas strict compliance with chemoprophylaxis and immunization with current vaccines will decrease the incidence of disease and mortality, fulminant disease still can occur (51–57).

Patients who survive fulminant sepsis frequently have necrotic digits, nose, and ear lobes. Sequelae of severe organ-system failure would be expected, but no systematic follow-up study of survivors has been reported. Gangrene, amputations, deafness following meningitis, mastoid osteomyelitis, and aortic insufficiency following endocarditis have been reported (29).

PREVENTION

Preservation of Splenic Tissue

Splenic injury in children results most often from motor-vehicle accidents, and the spleen is the most commonly injured abdominal organ. Other forms of blunt abdominal trauma, such as sports injuries or bicycle accidents, also may result in splenic lacerations or rupture. Because 5% to 6% of cardiac out-

TABLE 15.10. *Criteria defining children with sickle cell disease, asplenia, and fever who are at increased risk for bacterial sepsis and require hospitalization*

Age <6 mo	Hemoglobin value <5 gm/dL
Prior history of sepsis	Leucocyte count >30,000 or <5,000/mm^3
Seriously ill or toxic appearance	Platelet count <100,000/mm^3
Dehydration by history or examination	New pulmonary infiltrate
Concurrent severe pain	No prior training in early warning
Temperature ≥40°C (particularly if	signs and complications
sudden onset and rapid rise)	Poor history of compliance
Hypotension	No telephone or immediate access to the hospital
Poor perfusion	Allergy to penicillin or cephalosporin

From Wilimas JA, Flynn PM, Harris S, et al. A randomized study of outpatient treatment with ceftriaxone for selected febrile children with sickle cell disease. *N Engl J Med* 1993;329:472–476; and Wang WC, Wong WY, Rogers ZR, et al. Antibiotic-resistant pneumococcal infection in children with sickle cell disease in the United States. *J Pediatr Hematol Oncol* 1996;18:140–144, with permission.

put passes through the spleen each minute, blood loss into the peritoneal cavity may be significant and rapidly result in hemodynamic instability.

Recognition of the risk of postsplenectomy sepsis has resulted in a more conservative approach to the management of splenic injury in children. A trend to repair rather than to remove the spleen following trauma resulted in a decrease in the number of splenectomies performed for trauma from 20% in 1970 through 1980 to 4% in 1981 through 1990 according to one report (30). Currently, up to 80% of such injuries in children are managed nonoperatively with bed rest, fluid support (which may include transfusion), and careful observation, often in the intensive care unit for the first 24 to 48 hours.

When the child is hemodynamically unstable and surgery is necessary, every attempt is made to repair the spleen (splenorrhaphy), to perform a partial splenectomy, or to perform a splenectomy with autotransplantation of splenic tissue (58–61). In the latter procedure, intact cubes of splenic tissue no larger than than 5 mm to preserve some of the reticular structure are fixed in the highly vascularized greater omentum with a pursestring suture.

Patients studied after a splenectomy frequently have ectopic splenic tissue present, either as (a) accessory spleens (found in 15% of this population) randomly localized in the abdomen, which may undergo compensatory hypertrophy (62), or splenosis, which involves autotransplanted splenic cells seeded after splenic rupture (63–66).

The reticular structure of these accidentally implanted cells or autotransplanted fragments is inadequate to restore the normal clearance function of the spleen (59,60,64-66); however, immunoglobulin responses of both the IgM and IgG classes to five serotypes in the 23-valent pneumococcal polysaccharide vaccine were demonstrated in adult patients 6 months after splenic autotransplantation. Splenectomized patients with ectopic splenic tissue had lower antibody responses to fewer serotypes, and patients with no splenic tissue had no responses to the five vaccine serotypes

tested (59). Thus, although autotransplants do not restore the clearance function of the spleen, they can partially restore the humoral immune response to pneumococcal polysaccharide antigens.

Antibiotic Prophylaxis (Chemoprophylaxis)

Penicillin prophylaxis is recommended for all children with sickle cell disease and should begin before the child is 3 months of age. This recommendation is based on a prospective placebo-controlled, multicenter trial in children younger than 3 years of age with sickle cell disease. Using 125 mg twice daily, the children had follow-up for 15 months. In the placebo group of 110 children, 15 episodes of invasive pneumococcal infection occurred, resulting in three deaths. There were two episodes in the 105 children who received prophylaxis, representing an 84% reduction of pneumococcal infection in the treatment group ($p = 0.0025$) (69). The explanation for the success of prophylaxis is unclear. Decreased nasopharyngeal carriage rates of *S. pneumoniae* have been documented in patients on prophylaxis but were lower than for normal children even before prophylaxis was initiated (43). The efficacy of penicillin prophylaxis in other asplenic or hyposplenic populations at any age has not been studied.

Prophylaxis is problematic with respect to compliance, the effect on development of antibiotic resistance by pneumococci, and duration. Compliance has been the major problem. One study documented compliance rates of only 66% (68). Monthly benzathine injections to infants resulted in no infections in sickle cell disease patients who received injections compared with 18 infections in a comparably sized group in which children failed to appear for injections or were not receiving prophylaxis (69). Two additional studies documented noncompliance with oral prophylaxis and ratios of pneumococcal sepsis of 3.2 per 100 patient-years, or half the rate defined for children before the use of vaccine or prophylaxis (43) (Table 15.6).

Markedly increased and increasing rates of penicillin and cephalosporin resistance in invasive pneumococcal isolates from children within the United States over the last 10 years (47) have raised concern regarding the continued efficacy and potential risks of penicillin prophylaxis. Several studies documented high rates of nasopharyngeal colonization with penicillin-resistant pneumococci in patients with sicklecell disease (70–72). Patients with sickle cell disease and pneumococcal sepsis caused by penicillin-resistant isolates also have been reported (49,73). As yet, however, no centers have reported rates of infection with penicillin-resistant pneumococci greater than expected or greater than the rates in normal children.

It is not clear whether and when penicillin prophylaxis can be discontinued in children with sickle cell disease without increasing the risk for overwhelming sepsis. A recent study found no difference in attack rates when children over 5 years of age were randomized to continue penicillin prophylaxis (250 mg twice daily) or to discontinue it. Children who had undergone splenectomy or had previous episode of pneumococcal sepsis were excluded (74). The number of children enrolled and the overall incidence of pneumococcal disease were both low; therefore, a general consensus as to the duration of prophylaxis has not yet been developed (43). The risk of pneumococcal sepsis after chemoprophylaxis is discontinued increases over the next 2 years to the rates of sepsis over the 2 years following a splenectomy when no prophylaxis is given (69,75). Finally, cases of pneumococcal sepsis have been reported in patients receiving prophylaxis (51–57). Thus, a penicillin prophylaxis regimen alone may decrease but does not eliminate the risk of pneumococcal sepsis. Most experts recommend penicillin prophylaxis for congenital asplenia, for patients who have had autosplenectomies (as in sickle cell disease) or splenectomies for hemolytic anemias, malignancies, liver transplants, or for any reason in patients under 5 years of age and for at least the first year following splenectomy at any age.

Antibody Responses to Immunization

Pneumococcal capsular polysaccharides, like capsular polysaccharides of all bacteria, are thymus independent (TI) antigens. Proteins and protein–polysaccharide conjugate vaccines are thymus-dependent (TD) antigens. Antibody responses to TI antigens compared with those to TD antigens are characterized by being oligoclonal, dependent on age, exhibiting poor antibody subclass switching, and generating no memory cells. Polysaccharide antigens induce primarily IgM and IgA responses (26,76). TI antigens, however, are able to activate preexisting memory cells, as shown by the ability of polysaccharide vaccines to induce booster responses after priming with TD protein–polysaccharide conjugate vaccines (77,78).

Pneumococcal polysaccharide vaccines elicit relatively long-lasting antibody and protection in healthy adults, but revaccination does not result in an anamnestic response because no memory B cells were generated. In children, antibody levels decline rapidly to probable nonprotective levels within 2 to 5 years (79–82).

In addition, the vaccine is poorly immunogenic in the population groups at highest risk for pneumococcal disease (i.e., in patients with asplenia, patients infected with HIV, elderly and very young patients. Children produce smaller amounts of antipolysaccharide antibody than adults and substantive responses to the most common pediatric serotypes (serotypes 6A, 14, 19, and 23F) are observed only after the age of 4 to 5 years. The molecular mechanisms behind the activation and differentiation of B cells by TI antigens are poorly understood but appear to involve at least two signals on the surface of the B cell. The immunoglobulin receptor and the complement receptor CR2 recognize the polysaccharide and complement component C3d deposited on the polysaccharide. They respond by increasing the number of B cells secreting antipolysaccharide IgM. Marginal-zone B cells in the spleen are involved in the initiation of TI responses, which do not occur frequently in children under 2 years of age. B cells of the marginal zone in the spleen of infants have a low expression of CR2 receptors. The delay in the ontogeny of the immune response to TI antigens may thus be a result of the inability of neonatal B cells to be triggered via CR2, a signal necessary for full activation (83,84).

The efficacy of the pneumococcal polysaccharide vaccine has been documented for adults with asplenia to be 77% (85–87). A controlled, prospective trial of efficacy has never been performed in children with sickle cell disease. Limited prospective, open, or retrospective trials have been performed (43). The limited studies have confirmed that pneumococcal antibody and opsonic activity are dependent on age, serotype, and splenic function. Many investigators have reported failures of pneumococcal polysaccharide vaccine to protect children with sickle cell disease (43). Calculated efficacy rates for the vaccine in young children with SSD based on reported serotypes causing invasive infection are zero (43,85).

The timing of booster doses of pneumococcal polysaccharide vaccines is unclear because antibody levels clearly decline over time (85). The current Advisory Committee on Immunization Practices (ACIP) recommendation is for reimmunization once in asplenic patients (88). Although antibody levels continue to decline, repeated reimmunizations have not been recommended because there are no data available that describe the risks of frequent reimmunization. Although a high incidence of reactions to booster doses has been documented in children (43), some experts suggest routine reimmunization every 5 years for asplenic patients to minimize the risk for serious disease (89,90). It is recommended that a booster dose in children aged 2 to 10 years be given 2 to 5 years after the first dose because antibody to selected serotypes falls rapidly after initial immunization, and there is a reasonable response to reimmunization (79–82).

Although the TD pneumococcal protein–polysaccharide conjugate vaccines may be available in the United States after the year 2000, it is unlikely they will be available for children in underdeveloped countries for several years.

Immunization (Immunoprophylaxis)

The absent antibody responses to the TI polysaccharide capsules of encapsulated bacteria in children under 2 years of age resulted in a lack of efficacy of the available polysaccharide vaccines for pneumococci, meningococci, and *H. influenzae* type b (HITB). The success of the HITB protein conjugate vaccines has been dramatic (91). All children should now be immunized at 2, 4, and 6 months of age with a booster at 12 to 15 months of age. Systemic disease caused by HITB is now rare and is seen almost exclusively in infants too young to be fully immunized.

Unlike systemic disease caused by *H. influenzae*, for which serotype b caused more than 95% of cases, invasive pneumococcal disease in children under 6 years of age can be caused by any of the 90 different serotypes. Seven serotypes, however, account for 80% of isolates from blood and from CSF in children under 6 years of age (85). These seven serotypes constitute the heptavalent pneumococcal protein–polysaccharide conjugate vaccine newly approved by the U.S. Food and Drug Administration (FDA) (Table 15.11) (92–94). In subjects over 6 years of age, these seven serotypes account for only 50% of isolates (85).

A dramatic response resulted when the heptavalent conjugate vaccine given at 2, 4, and 6 months with a booster at 12 to 15 months was 100% effective in preventing invasive disease (positive culture in blood or CSF) when randomized to 38,000 children who received full immunization (92). The duration of immunity is not yet known, but immunologic memory was present 20 months after the initial immunization in children 2 to 3 years of age (77). Persons over the age of 6 years are infected 50% of the time with serotypes not present in the conjugate but present in the polysaccharide vaccine, and children over 6 years can respond better to TI antigens; therefore, booster doses using the polysaccharide vaccine may be recommended, particularly for populations at increased risk for overwhelming pneumococcal sepsis (93).

In infants with sickle cell disease, the conjugate vaccine was immunogenic when given at 2, 4, and 6 months of age (93). In children over 2 years of age, antibody levels were compared for children receiving only one dose of the 23-valent polysaccharide vaccine with those receiving two doses of the conjugate vaccine given 8 weeks apart followed by the 23-valent polysaccharide vaccine 8 weeks later (78). The geometric mean antibody titers were higher for all seven serotypes in the group who received both the conjugate and polysaccharide vaccines. For two serotypes not contained in the conjugate vaccine, antibody titers were the same for both groups, indicating that the conjugate vaccine did not interfere with responses to the polysaccharide vaccine.

The recommendations of the Committee on Infectious Diseases of the American Academy of Pediatrics and the ACIP for universal use of the heptavalent conjugate vaccine likely will be similar to those listed in Table 15.12 (94). For asplenic and hyposplenic individuals, booster doses of the 23-valent pneumococcal vaccine to cover the 16 serotypes not included in the heptavalent vaccine that are responsible for 50% of cases of pneumococcal sepsis in persons over 5 years of age may be recommended. Previous ACIP recommendations suggested that revaccination with the 23-valent vaccine be considered after 2 to 5 years for children under 10 years of age (88, 95). Some experts recommend revaccination every 5 years as long as the risk persists (89,90). No official recommendation exists, however, because the incidence of severity of adverse reactions to repeated revaccination is not known.

Quadrivalent meningococcal vaccine (Menomune-A,C,Y,W-135, Connaught Laboratories) contains 50 μg each of four purified polysaccharides in a dose of 0.5 mL. In older children and adults, serogroups A and C have efficacies of 85% to 100% in controlling epidemics (96). Bactericidal antibodies result from immunization of older children and adults with types Y and W-135, although clinical protection has not been documented. Measurable antibody levels to types A and C decline markedly over 3 years for older children and adults. This decrease in antibody is even more marked for children under 4 years of age. For infants under 2 years of age, type A is immunogenic, whereas type C is poorly immunogenic. Revaccination can be considered within 3 to 5 years for those at high risk (96). The incidence and severity of adverse reactions to revaccination have not been determined.

TABLE 15.11. *Serotype composition of pneumococcal vaccines*

Purified polysaccharide[a] (23 valent)			Protein-polysaccharide conjugate[b] (7 valent)	
1	9N	*18C*	4	*18C*
2	*9V*	19A	6B	19F
3	10A	*19F*	*9V*	23F
4	11A	20	14	
5	12F	22F		
6B	*14*	*23F*		
7F	15B	33F		
8	17F			

[a]One dose (0.5 mL) contains 25 μg of each capsular polysaccharide antigen (575 μg total) in normal saline with either phenol (0.25% MSD) or thimerosal (0.01% Lederle) available as Pneumovax 23 (Merck, Sharpe, Dohme, Inc.) and Pnuimmune 23 (Lederle Laboratories).

[b]One dose (0.5 mL) contains 2 μg of each polysaccharide (except for 6B, which has 4 μg) conjugated to 20 μg of cross-reactive material 197 (CRM197), a mutant, nontoxic diphtheria toxin available as Prevenar (Wyeth-Ayerst Laboratories) (available in fall 2000).

TABLE 15.12. *Suggested regimens for immunization of children with heptavalent pneumococcal polysaccharide–protein conjugate vaccine (Prevnar)*

Age at first dose (mo)	Primary series	Booster
2–6	3 doses, 2 mo apart[a]	1 dose at 12-<16 mo
7–11	2 doses, 2 mo apart[a]	1 dose at 12-<16 mo
12–23	2 doses, 2 mo apart[a]	—
24–35	1 dose[b]	[b]

[a]No less than 6 wk apart.
[b]One dose followed by a booster dose 2 months later, followed by 23-valent polysaccharide vaccine 2 mo later. From Black S, Shinefield H, Ray P, et al. Efficacy of heptavalent conjugate pneumococcal vaccine in 37,000 infants and children: results of the Northern California Kaiser Permanente efficacy trial. In: Abstracts of the 39th Annual Meeting of the Interscience Conference on Antimicrobial Agents and Chemotherapy. San Francisco, CA, 1999:379. Abst 1398; and Rennels MB, Edwards KM, Keyserling HL, et al. Safety and immunogenicity of heptavalent pneumococcal vaccine conjugated to CRM$_{197}$ in United States infants. *Pediatrics* 1998;104:604–611, with permission.

Immune responses to antigens are better when given before than after removal of the spleen or bone marrow transplants (97). Patients with scheduled transplants and splenectomies should have all immunizations completed two weeks before the procedure whenever possible.

Rapid Antibiotic Administration

For splenectomized patients of all ages and in those who anytime following splenectomy develop fever and other nonspecific signs of infection, medical care should be sought immediately. This is true even for patients who have been appropriately immunized and who are receiving antibiotic prophylaxis. If medical care cannot be accessed within 1 hour, the patient should have a high dose of an appropriate oral antibiotic such as Augmentin at home, which can be taken while medical care is being accessed. MediAlert bracelets should be worn by asplenic or hyposplenic patients (8,12,98,99).

SUMMARY

Universal immunization of infants with the polysaccharide–protein conjugate vaccine for *S. pneumoniae* is expected to reduce the incidence of invasive pneumococcal infections as dramatically as has been seen for *H. influenzae* b infections. Similar conjugate vaccines are under development for *N. meningitidis*.

The impact of these vaccines for splenectomized adults and children is anticipated to be equally dramatic. Until these vaccines and recommendations for their administration are available, patients should be warned repeatedly about the risk of fulminant infection, and appropriate measures must be instituted to prevent and treat such infections as early as possible.

REFERENCES

1. Feder HM, Pearson HA. Assessment of splenic function in familial asplenia. *N Engl J Med* 1999;341:210–211.
2. Gillis J, Harvey J, Isaacs D, et al. Familial asplenia. *Arch Dis Child* 1992;67:665–666.
3. Rose V, Izukawa T, Moes CAF. Syndromes of asplenia and polysplenia: a review of cardiac and noncardiac malformations. *Br Heart J* 1975;37:840–852.
4. Waldman JD, Rosenthal A, Smith AL, et al. Sepsis and congenital asplenia. *J Pediatr* 1977;90:555–559.
5. Britz-Cunningham SH, Shah MM, Zupan CW, et al. Mutations of the connexin 43 gap-junction gene in patients with heart malformations and defects of laterality. *N Engl J Med* 1995;332:1323–1329.
6. Cesko I, Hajdud J, Toth T, et al. Ivemark syndrome with asplenia in siblings. *J Pediatr* 1997;130:822–824.
7. Wang K, Hsieh KH. Immunologic study of the asplenia syndrome. *Pediatr Infect Dis J* 1991;10:819–822.
8. Lynch A, Kapila R. Overwhelming post-splenectomy infections. *Infect Dis Clin North Am* 1996;10:693–707.
9. Bernard NF, Chernott DN, Tsoukas CM. Effect of splenectomy on T-cell subsets and plasma HIV viral titers in HIV-infected patients. *J Hum Virol* 1998;1:338–345.
10. Tsoukas CM, Bernard NF, Abrahamowicz M, et al. Effect of splenectomy on slowing Human immunodeficiency virus disease progression. *Arch Surg* 1998;133:25–31.
11. Power C, Nath A, Aoki FY, et al. Remission of progressive multifocal leukoencephalopathy following splenectomy and antiretroviral therapy in a patient with HIV infection. *N Engl J Med* 1997;336:661–662.

12. Brigden M, Patullo A. Prevention and management of overwhelming postsplenectomy infection, an update. *Crit Care Med* 1999;27:836–842.

13. Scerpello EG. Functional asplenia and pneumococcal sepsis in patients with systemic lupus erythematosus. *Clin Infect Dis* 1995;20:194–195.

14. Muller AF, Toghill PJ. Hyposplenic patients need prophylactic penicillin. *Br Med J* 1994;308:132–133.

15. Kalhs P, Panzer S, Kletter K, et al. Functional asplenia after bone marrow transplantation. *Ann Intern Med* 1988;109:461–464.

16. Guertler AT, Carter CT. Fatal pneumococcal septicemia in a patient with a connective tissue disease. *J Emerg Med* 1996;14:33–38.

17. VanderHoeven JG, Koning JD, Masclee AM, et al. Fatal pneumococcal septic shock in a patient with ulcerative colitis. *Clin Infect Dis* 1996;22:860–861.

18. Rege K, Mehta J, Treleaven J, et al. Fatal pneumococcal infections following allogeneic bone marrow transplant. *Bone Marrow Transplant* 1994;14:903–906.

19. Janoff EN, Rubins JB. Invasive pneumococcal disease in the immunocompromised host. *Microb Drug Resist* 1997;3:215–232.

20. Cuthbert RJG, Agbal A, Cates A, et al. Functional hyposplenism following allogeneic bone marrow transplantation. *J Clin Pathol* 1995;48:257–262.

21. French J, Camitta BM. Anatomy and function of the spleen: In: Behrman RE, Kliegman RM, Jenson HB, eds. *Nelson: textbook of pediatrics*, 16th ed. Philadelphia: WB Saunders, 1999;1525–1529.

22. Sills RH. The spleen and lymph nodes. In: Oski FA, DeAngelis CD, Feigin RD, et al., eds. *Principles and practice of pediatrics*. Philadelphia: JB Lippincott, 1990;1540–1545.

23. Kelly DE, Wood RL, Enders AC. Lymphatics. In: *Bailey's textbook of microscopic anatomy*. Baltimore: Williams & Wilkins, 1984;457–471.

24. Weiss L. *Histology: cell and tissue biology*, 5th ed. New York: Elsevier Science Publishing, 1983.

25. Amlot PL, Grennan D, Humphrey JH. Splenic dependence of the antibody response to thymus-independent (TI-2) antigens. *Eur J Immunol* 1985;15:508–512.

26. Sullivan JL, Ochs HD, Schiffman G, et al. Immune response after splenectomy. *Lancet* 1978;1:178–181.

27. Ellis EF, Smith RT. The role of the spleen in immunity. *Pediatrics* 1966;37:111–117.

28. Zarkowsky HS, Gallagher D, Gill FM, et al. Bacteremia in sickle hemoglobinopathy. *J Pediatr* 1986;109:579–585.

29. Styrt B. Infection associated with asplenia: risks, mechanisms and prevention. *Am J Med* 1990;18:5-33N–5-42N.

30. Singer DB. Postsplenectomy sepsis. *Perspect Pediatr Pathol* 1973;1:285–311.

31. Eraklis AJ, Filler RM. Splenectomy in childhood—a review of 1,413 cases. *J Pediatr Surg* 1972;7:382–388.

32. Holdsworth RJ, Irving AD, Cuschieri A. Postsplenectomy sepsis and its mortality rate: Actual versus perceived risks. *Br J Surg* 1991;78:1031–1034.

33. Posey DL, Marks CM. Overwhelming postsplenectomy sepsis in childhood. *Am J Surg* 1983;145:318–321.

34. Zarrabi MH, Rosner F. Serious infections in adults following splenectomy for trauma. *Arch Intern Med* 1984;144:1421–1424.

35. Pedersen FK. Postsplenectomy infections in Danish children splenectomized 1969–1978. *Acta Paediatr Scand* 1983;72:589–595.

36. Pers C, Gahrn-Hansen B, Frederiksen W. *Capnocytophaga canimorsus* septicemia in Denmark, 1982–1995: review of 39 cases. *Clin Infect Dis* 1996;23:71–75.

37. Scully RE. Case records of the Massachusetts General Hospital. *N Engl J Med* 1999;340:1819–1826.

38. Chaudhuri AK, Hartley RD, Maddocks AC. Waterhouse-Friderichsen's syndrome caused by DF-2 bacterium in a splenectomized patient. *J Clin Pathol* 1981;34:172–173.

39. Rosner F, Zarrabi MH, Benach JL, et al. Babesiosis in splenectomized adults. *Am J Med* 1984;765:696–700.

40. Chilcote RR, Baehner RL, Hammond D, and The Investigators and Special Studies Committee of the Children's Cancer Study Group. Septicemia and meningitis in children splenectomized for Hodgkin's disease. *N Engl J Med* 1976;295:798–800.

41. Donaldson SS, Kaplan HS. Complications of treatment of Hodgkin's disease in children. *Cancer Treat Rep* 1982;66:977–989.

42. Wong WY, Powars DR, Chan L, et al. Polysaccharide encapsulated bacterial infection in sickle cell anemia: a thirty year epidemiologic experience. *Am J Hematol* 1991;39:176–182.

43. Overturf GD. Infections and immunizations of children with sickle cell disease. *Adv Pediatr Infect Dis* 1999;14:191–213.

44. Buchanan GR, Smith SJ. Pneumococcal septicemia despite pneumococcal vaccine and prescription of penicillin prophylaxis in children with sickle cell anemia. *Am J Dis Child* 1986;140:428–432.

45. Lane PA, Rogers ZR, Woods GM, et al. Fatal pneumococcal septicemia in hemoglobin SC disease. *J Pediatr* 1994;124:859–862.

46. Traub A, Giebink GS, Smith C, et al. Splenic reticuloendothelial function after splenectomy, spleen repair, and spleen autotransplantation. *N Engl J Med* 1987;317:1559–1564.

47. Committee on Infectious Diseases of the American Academy of Pediatrics. Therapy for children with invasive pneumococcal infections. *Pediatrics* 1997;99:289–299.

48. Wilimas JA, Flynn PM, Harris S, et al. A randomized study of outpatient treatment with ceftriaxone for selected febrile children with sickle cell disease. *N Engl J Med* 1993;329:472–476.

49. Wang WC, Wong WY, Rogers ZR, et al. Antibiotic-resistant pneumococcal infection in children with sickle cell disease in the United States. *J Pediatr Hematol Oncol* 1996;18:140–144.

50. Waghorn DJ, Mayon-White RT. A study of 42 episodes of overwhelming post-splenectomy infection: Is current guidance for asplenic individuals being followed? *J Infect* 1997;35:289–294.

51. Klinge J, Hammersen G, Scharf J, et al. Overwhelming postsplenectomy infection with vaccine-type *Streptococcus pneumoniae* in a 12 year old despite vaccination and antibiotic prophylaxis. *Infection* 1997;25:368–371.

52. Abildgaard N, Nielsen JL. Pneumococcal septicemia and meningitis in vaccinated splenectomized adult patients. *Scand J Infect Dis* 1994;26:615–617.

53. Evans DIK. Fatal post-splenectomy sepsis despite pro-

phylaxis with penicillin and pneumococcal vaccine. *Lancet* 1984;1:1124.

54. Hostetter MK, Schwartz AL, Siber GR. Pneumococcal vaccine failure. *Am J Dis Child* 1981;135:1149–1150.

55. Zarrabi, Rosner F. Rarity of failure of penicillin prophylaxis to prevent postsplenectomy sepsis. *Arch Intern Med* 1986;146:1207–1208.

56. Konradsen HB, Henrichsen J. Pneumococcal infections in splenectomized children are preventable. *Acta Paediatr Scand* 1991;80:423–427.

57. Brivet F, Herer B, Frewmaux A, et al. Fatal postsplenectomy pneumococcal sepsis despite pneumococcal vaccine and penicillin prophylaxis. *Lancet* 1984;ii: 356–357.

58. Holdsworth RJ. Regeneration of the spleen and splenic autotransplantation. *Br J Surg* 1991;78:270–278.

59. Leemans R, Manson W, Snijder JAM, et al. Immune response capacity after human splenic autotransplantation: restoration of response to individual pneumococcal vaccine subtypes. *Ann Surg* 1999;229:279–285.

60. Pabst R, Westermann J, Rothkötter HJ. Immunoarchitecture of regenerated splenic and lymph node transplants. *Int Rev Cytol* 1991;128:215–220.

61. Pisters PWT, Pachter HL. Autologous splenic transplantation for splenic trauma. *Ann Surg* 1994;219:225–235.

62. Rudowski WJ. Accessory spleens: clinical significance with particular reference to the recurrence of idiopathic thrombocytopenic purpura. *World J Surg* 1985;9: 422–430.

63. Stovall TG, Ling FW. Splenosis: report of a case and review of the literature. *Obstet Gynecol Surg* 1988;43: 69–72.

64. Rice HM, James PD. Ectopic splenic tissue failed to prevent fatal pneumococcal septicemia after splenectomy for trauma. *Lancet* 1980;1:565–566.

65. Carr NJ, Twik EP. The histological features of splenosis. *Histopathology* 1992;21:549–553.

66. Hathaway JM, Harley RA, Self S, et al. Immunological function in post-traumatic splenosis. *Clin Immunol Immunopathol* 1995;74:143–150.

67. Gaston MH, Verter JI, Woods G, et al. Prophylaxis with oral penicillin in children with sickle cell anemia. A randomized trial. *N Engl J Med* 1986;314:1593–1599.

68. Buchanan GR. Chemoprophylaxis in asplenic adolescents and young adults. *Pediatr Inf Dis J* 1993;12: 892–893.

69. John AB, Ramal A, Jackson H, et al. Prevention of pneumococcal infection in children with homozygous sickle cell disease: A randomized trial. *BMJ* 1984;288: 1567–1570.

70. Norris CF, Mahannah SR, Smith-Whitley K, et al. Pneumococcal colonization in children with sickle cell disease. *J Pediatr* 1996;129:821–827.

71. Steele RW, Warrier R, Unkel PJ, et al. Colonization with antibiotic-resistant *Streptococcus pneumoniae* in children with sickle cell disease. *J Pediatr* 1996;128: 531–535.

72. Daw NC, Wilimas JA, Wang WC, et al. Nasopharyngeal carriage of penicillin-resistant *Streptococcus pneumoniae* in children with sickle cell disease. *Pediatrics* 1997;99(electronic pages).

73. Chesney PJ, Wilimas JA, Presbury G, et al. Penicillin and cephalosporin-resistant strains of *Streptococcus pneumoniae* causing sepsis and meningitis in children with sickle cell disease. *J Pediatr* 1995;127:526–532.

74. Falletta JM, Woods GM, Verter JI, et al. Discontinuing penicillin prophylaxis in children with sickle cell anemia. *J Pediatr* 1995;127:685–690.

75. Bestak M. Splenectomy for red cell membrane disorders should be accompanied by prophylactic measures to prevent sepsis. *Pediatr Rev* 1994;15:274–275.

76. Wara DW. Host defense against Streptococcus pneumoniae: The role of the spleen. *Rev Infect Dis* 1981;3: 299–309.

77. Obaro SK, Huo Z, Banya WAS, et al. A glycoprotein pneumococcal conjugate vaccine primes for antibody responses to a pneumococcal polysaccharide vaccine in Gambian children. *Pediatr Infect Dis J* 1997;16: 1135–1140.

78. Vernacchio L, Neufeld EJ, MacDonald K, et al. Combined schedule of 7-valent pneumococcal conjugate vaccine followed by 23-valent pneumococcal vaccine in children and young adults with sickle cell disease. *J Pediatr* 1998;133:275–278.

79. Konradsen HB, Pedersen FK, Henrichsen J. Pneumococcal revaccination of splenectomized children. *Pediatr Infect Dis J* 1990;9:258–263.

80. Giebink GS, Le CT, Schiffman G. Decline of serum antibody in splenectomized children after vaccination with pneumococcal capsular polysaccharides. *J Pediatr* 1984;105:576–584.

81. Weintrub PS, Schiffman G, Addiego JE Jr, et al. Long-term followup and booster immunization with polyvalent pneumococcal polysaccharide in patients with sickle cell anemia. *J Pediatr* 1984;105:261–263.

82. Bjornson AB, Falletta JM, Verter JI, et al. Serotype-specific immunoglobulin G antibody responses to pneumococcal polysaccharide vaccine in children with sickle cell anemia: effects of continued penicillin prophylaxis. *J Pediatr* 1996;129:828–835.

83. Timens W, Boes A, Rozeboom-Uiterwijk T, et al. Immaturity of the human splenic marginal zone in infancy: possible contribution to the deficient infant immune response. *J Immunol* 1989;143:3200–3206.

84. Alonso de Velasco E, Verheul AFM, Verhoef J, et al. *Streptococcus pneumoniae:* virulence factors, pathogenesis and vaccines. *Microbiol Mol Biol Rev* 1995;59: 591–603.

85. Butler JC, Breiman RF, Campbell JF, et al. Pneumococcal polysaccharide vaccine efficacy: an evaluation of current recommendations. *JAMA* 1993;270:1826–1831.

86. Shapiro ED, Berg AT, Austrias R, et al. The protective efficacy of polyvalent pneumococcal polysaccharide vaccine. *N Engl J Med* 1991;325:1453–1460.

87. Broome CV, Facklam RR, Fraser DW. Pneumococcal disease after pneumococcal vaccination. *N Engl J Med* 1980;303:549–552.

88. Centers for Disease Control and Prevention. Prevention of pneumococcal disease. *MMWR Morb Mortal Wkly Rep* 1997;46(RR-8):1–24.

89. Molrine D, Siber G, Samra Y, et al. Normal IgG and impaired IgM responses to polysaccharide vaccines in asplenic patients. *J Infect Dis* 1998;179:513–517.

90. Chan CY, Molrine DC, George S, et al. Pneumococcal conjugate vaccine primes for antibody responses to polysaccharide pneumococcal vaccine after treatment of Hodgkin's disease. *J Infect Dis* 1996;173:256–258.

91. Centers for Disease Control and Prevention. Progress toward elimination of *Haemophilus influenzae* type b disease among infants and children—United States,

1987–1995. *MMWR Morb Mortal Wkly Rep* 1996;45:901–906.

92. Black S, Shinefield H, Ray P, et al. Efficacy of heptavalent conjugate pneumococcal vaccine in 37,000 infants and children: results of the Northern California Kaiser Permanente efficacy trial. Presented at: 39th Annual Meeting of the Interscience Conference on Antimicrobial Agents and Chemotherapy; San Francisco, CA; 1999:379(abst 1398).

93. O'Brien KL, Steinhoff MC, Edwards K, et al. Immunologic priming of young children by pneumococcal glycoprotein conjugate, but not polysaccharide, vaccines. *Pediatr Infect Dis J* 1996;15:425–430.

94. Committee on Infectious Diseases. Policy Statement: recommendations for the prevention of pneumococcal infections, including the use of pneumococcal conjugate vaccine (Prevnar), pneumococcal polysaccharide vaccine, and antibiotic prophylaxes (RE9960). *Pediatrics* 2000;106:362–366.

95. Centers for Disease Control and Prevention. Use of vaccines and immune globulins for persons with altered immunocompetence. *MMWR Morb Mortal Wkly Rep* 1993:42(RR-4):1–18.

96. Centers for Disease Control and Prevention. Control and prevention of meningococcal disease. *MMWR Morb Mortal Wkly Rep* 1997;46(RR-5):1–21.

97. Parkkali T, Kayhty H, Ruutu T, et al. A comparison of early and late vaccination with *Haemophilus influenzae* type b conjugate and pneumococcal polysaccharide vaccines after allogeneic BMT. *Bone Marrow Transplant* 1996;18:961–967.

98. Kind EA, Craft C, Fowles JB, et al. Pneumococcal vaccine administration associated with splenectomy: missed opportunities. *Am J Infect Control* 1998;26: 418–422.

99. Staat ME, Roberts N, England L, et al. Documentation of pneumococcal *H. influenzae* type b and meningococcal vaccine use in asplenic patients. Presented at: 36th Annual Meeting Infectious Diseases Society of America, Denver, CO; 1998.

16

Infections in Burn Patients

Lisa M. Hunsicker, John P. Heggers, and *Janak A. Patel

*Department of Surgery, Division of Plastic Surgery; *Department of Pediatrics, Division of Pediatric Infectious Diseases, University of Texas Medical Branch, Galveston, Texas 77555*

Improvement in the mortality rate from burns is a direct result of the maturation of the science of burn care comprising developments in fluid resuscitation, wound care, surgical care, nutritional support, and antimicrobial therapy. In 1998, the mortality rate in children with burns at the Shriners Burns Hospital, Galveston, Texas, was 5 of 377 admissions (1.3%). Specifically, the mortality rate attributable to infection was 0.5%. Even infants, who previously were reported to have poorer chances of survival than older children, now fare better (1).

THE BURN WOUND

Mechanism of Burn Injury

The effects of extreme heat on the skin lead to cellular and subcellular impairment. The determining factors of how severe a burn will be are the temperature, length of exposure, and actual burning agent. Moritz and Henrique showed that the skin can withstand temperatures up to 40°C (104°F) for relatively long periods before an injury becomes apparent (2). As the temperature increases, tissue destruction progresses. As temperatures exceed 45°C, protein denaturation supersedes the cell's reparative capabilities. Plasma membrane necrosis has been observed in cells exposed to 45°C for 1 hour (3). If the heat source is removed and the tissue is cooled rapidly, progressive damage may be avoided,

thereby determining the cell's survivability. Delay in cooling results in dermal ischemia and progression of injury. Other cytologic findings in thermal injury are redistributions of solid and fluid components of the cell nuclei. Fluid imbibition results in nuclear swelling, membrane rupture, and pyknosis. As denaturation proceeds, vital cellular metabolic processes are injured and the metabolic response can vary. If enzyme activity is decreased to below 50% of its normal level, cell death occurs. In lesser degrees of enzyme impairment, cell recovery may be possible.

Local Tissue Changes

Jackson's classic description of local burn injury included three concentric zones (4). As temperatures increase, protein denaturation results in severe protein alterations, leading to coagulation. The protein architecture is destroyed, and new aberrant macromolecules are formed. The central area of a burn wound is that which is in direct contact with the heat source. Cell necrosis is complete and is called the *zone of coagulation*. Cellular recovery is impossible, and injury severity decreases from the surface to the deeper levels. This zone is the burn eschar. At the peripheral margins of the zone of coagulation, a less injured zone is present. These cells in the *zone of stasis* show direct injury from the heat, but the damage is not lethal; however, blood flow to this area becomes progressively impaired. Ischemia to the already compromised cells may lead to necrosis and conversion to dead eschar. Circulatory impairment occurs via vessel wall neutrophil adherence, fibrin deposition, platelet microthrombus formation, vasoconstriction, and endothelial swelling. Heat-compromised erythrocytes lose their ability to deform, and their passage through microvessels is impeded. The circulatory embarrassment may be delayed for up to 24 hours, and the ischemia may progress for up to 48 hours postburn. If stasis conditions are minimal, injury may be halted and cell recovery may occur within 1 week; however, this tissue is fragile, and further insults such as infection, hypovolemia, pressure, and overresuscitation can lead to further necrosis. Finally, the *zone of hyperemia* lies peripheral to the zone of stasis. This zone sustains minimal injury and often recovers within 7 to 10 days. There is notable vasodilation resulting from potent vasoactive mediators secondary to the inflammatory response. Complete recovery is expected in this zone barring further trauma or infection.

Burn Wound Depth

In addition to injury zones, burn wounds are categorized by their depth (3). *First-degree* burns consist of epidermal damage only. These wounds are painful and erythematous as a result of local vasodilation. These wounds heal spontaneously, usually scarless, within 7 days. *Second-degree* burns are partial-thickness injuries, further categorized as *superficial* or *deep*. The epidermis and superficial portion of the dermis is injured in superficial second-degree burns. These wounds are painful and often blister. Healing occurs via epithelial migration from the wound edges, hair follicles, and sebaceous glands. There is relatively little scarring, and reepithelization occurs within 2 weeks. Deep second-degree burns are much more serious. Most of the dermis is destroyed, sparing the bases of the epidermal appendages. The nerve endings also are destroyed, making the wound insensate. Blisters usually are not present because of the thicker eschar formation. These wounds are treated as full-thickness injuries. Reepithelialization is tenuous and slow. The protracted inflammatory phase often results in excessive collagen deposition and extensive scarring. Third-degree burns are full-thickness injury to the skin. Healing occurs by contraction and reepithelialization from the wound edges. As with deep second-degree burns, these wounds are insensate and without blistering. Treatment for third-degree burns is with excision and skin grafting. *Fourth-degree* burns extend into the deep tissue, including muscle, bone, and viscera. Treatment is debridement and possible amputation. Closure of these wounds may vary from primary closure postamputation to skin grafting and possible flap reconstruction.

Burn Inflammation

Many of these processes are either partly or entirely results of the inflammatory process. Cellular infiltration, initiated by local inflammatory mediators such as prostanoids and leukotrienes, and proinflammatory cytokines from the burn wound begins with the arrival of neutrophils at 4 to 5 days postburn, followed by macrophages (5). The neutrophils further mediate damage by the release of oxygen free radicals (6). Reestablishment of blood flow in the zone of stasis is yet another setting wherein oxygen free radicals are produced, leading to further injury. This phenomenon of ischemia–reperfusion injury occurs as oxygen is restored to the tissues (7). Inflammation becomes prominent at 7 to 10 days. Consequently, blood flow is maximal at this stage, creating a troublesome and hazardous setting for surgical excision of the eschar.

Inhalation Injury

Burn victims, especially those trapped in enclosed areas, injure the respiratory tract on inhalation of toxic gases from surrounding burning materials. It is rare to have an actual thermal airway injury. The upper airway is rather effective in cooling and warming inspired air. Also, air has a low heat capacity. To cause direct injury to the airway, the flames must come into direct contact with them. Injury to the oropharynx after inhalation resembles thermal injury elsewhere in the body (8). Protein denaturation, inflammatory mediator release, and increased cellular and microvascular permeability all occur, leading to airway edema and consequent airway obstruction. Intubation may be nearly impossible, even to the most experienced anesthesiologist.

The chemical injury from toxic gases is almost instantaneous. First, separation of ciliated epithelial cells from the basement membrane occurs (9). Next, the systemic circulation to the lung as well as the bronchial circulation is increased as a result of vasodilation. Shortly thereafter, edema is evident. The inflammatory phase then is followed by an exudative phase (10). Furthermore, the protein component of this fluid is composed of lung lymph and induces bronchoconstriction. As postburn time increases, fibrin casts are formed from the exudates, which may lead to airway obstruction. As the epithelium sloughs and fibrin cast formation increases, susceptibility to infection increases. Pneumonia leading to sepsis and death is well documented. Finally, pseudomembrane formation proceeds and squamous metaplasia follows (11). Healing make take weeks to initiate, and permanent airway damage, that is, stenosis and tracheal granuloma formation, may occur.

IMMUNE RESPONSES IN BURNS

A combination of impaired local and systemic host defenses and loss of the skin barrier are major factors responsible for the increased susceptibility to infections in burn patients. The major elements initially contributing to the inflammatory response following burns include the plasma proteins, mast cells, tissue macrophages, and systemically recruited neutrophils and monocytes.

Alterations in the host defenses include induction of local and systemic cytokine synthesis, decreased immunoglobulin levels, changes in the concentration and activity of both the classic and alternative complement pathways, reduced levels of circulating plasma fibronectin, depressed serum opsonic activity, and impairment of the macrophages, lymphocytes, neutrophils, and the reticuloendothelial system. The immunologic status of the burned patient has a measurable impact on outcome in terms of survival, death, and major morbidity. It is important to note that much of the work on immunologic aspect of burns has been conducted in adult humans or in experimental animals, whereas little work has been performed in children.

Cytokine Cascade

Following burn injury, numerous cytokines are induced rapidly. Many cytokines relate to the severity of burn injury and prognosis, whereas others correlate with infection. Studies to date can be summarized as follows:

- Tumor necrosis factor-α (TNF-α) is detectable early during the period of shock, at which time the serum levels cannot be correlated with prognosis. By contrast, the maximum TNF level over the entire clinical course is of prognostic significance (12). Patients with high TNF levels (>540 pg/mL) have a poor prognosis, although the absolute level of TNF does not correlate with burn size (13).
- Peripheral blood lymphocytes of patients with large burns produce significantly lesser quantities of interleukin-2 (IL-2), which correlates with length of time from injury (14). Studies of plasma cytokines show that the concentrations of IL-1 and IL-1 receptor antagonist (IL-1ra) are increased in all patients and are highest at the time of admission (15). Concentrations of IL-1ra correlated with the total burn surface area and the area of third-degree burn as well as plasma C-reactive protein. Concentrations of IL-1 and IL-1ra are higher in patients who develop infective complications. Patients who survive have significantly

higher IL-1β concentrations than those who die. These results suggest that IL-1ra may be influenced by the size of the burn and the acute phase response, IL-1β and IL-1ra may play a role in host's response to infection, and IL-1β may influence the outcome.

- Peripheral blood monocytes are superstimulated to produce large amounts of IL-1, leading to exhaustion of monocyte function (16). Reduced IL-1 production by monocytes is found in patients with complicated organ injury, multiorgan failure, and systemic infection.
- Endothelin-1, which activates monocytes to produce cytokines, is elevated in the early phase of burn injury (17).
- Initially, there is little or no interferon-gamma (IFN-γ), but increases are evident from day 5 to day 10 in all patients (15).
- Serum levels of IL-6 increase rapidly after burns and correlate with the induction of acute phase reactants (18). In animal models of burn, levels of IL-6 in unburned skin adjacent to a burn are elevated within 30 minutes and seem to be regulated by local IL-1α (19).
- IL-8 is released from the unburned skin adjacent to a burn (20). Serum IL-8 levels are elevated in some burn patients but do not correlate with the severity of burns. On the other hand, IL-8 levels are elevated in burn patients with sepsis (21).
- The production of granulocyte colony stimulating factor (G-CSF) and of granulocyte macrophage colony stimulating factor (GM-CSF) is impaired (22).
- Blood monocytes of burn patients produce significantly more IL-10 at 7 to 10 days after burn injury, which correlates with subsequent septic events (23). Animal experiments showed that burn injury induces the loss of antigen-specific T-helper 1 (Th1) lymphocytes function and that IL-10 acts as a trigger to downregulate Th1 activity after injury(24).

Neutrophils

Thermal injury induces neutropenia and myeloid maturation arrest despite elevated G-

CSF levels (25). The degree of neutropenia correlates with the reduction in bone marrow G-CSF receptor expression. The neutrophils of burn patients are also functionally altered (25): The Fc receptor expression is decreased, intracellular killing capacity is depressed (this is a differential suppression, more for some organisms than others), and this suppression is accompanied by a brief increase in neutrophil respiratory burst response. There is also failure of initial alkalization of the phagolysosome and alteration of subsequent kinetics of acidification (27). This depression of oxygen-independent bactericidal mechanism may impair the capacity of the neutrophil for intracellular killing following thermal injury. Expression of CD16 [FcR, Fc, immunoglobulin G (IgG) receptor] and CD11 (adhesion molecule) on neutrophils is impaired following major injury; and this reduction appears to be directly related to the appearance of bacteremia or pneumonia (28). These changes in adhesion molecule expression, which is closely related to chemotaxis, may play a part in the failure of delivery of neutrophils in adequate numbers to the local site of a burn. Furthermore, there is a defect in actin polymerization in burn patients' neutrophils, a basic mechanism of chemotaxis, which also may contribute to a failure of motility (29).

There is an impairment in leukotriene generation from the neutrophils of severely burned patients. This impairment appears to be based on the availability, or lack of availability, of the metabolizable substrate-free arachidonic acid (30). Because leukotriene B is also a potent neutrophil chemotactic agent, this may further contribute to the failure of neutrophil function.

Complement

The burn blister fluid shows much lower opsonic activity for bacteria such as *Pseudomona aeruginosa* than patient's own serum (31). There is a mild impairment of C3 production and release by macrophages of burn patients *in vitro*. Systemically, both the classic and the aternative pathways are depleted, but the alternative pathway is more profoundly perturbed. Following bacteremia, there is additional complement activation and depletion (32).

Macrophages

Suppression of the ability of the reticuloendothelial system to take up particulate material was among the original observations of burn immunology made in the 1960s. In the more recent reports, however, a differentially increased uptake of colloid in alveolar macrophages compared with other organs has been demonstrated, perhaps indicating alveolar macrophage activation. Macrophages and monocytes appear to be activated in a fashion similar to lymphocytes following thermal injury. Macrophage activation, as measured by the serum neopterin level, is increased following thermal injury (33). This activation is confirmed by increased expression of the monocyte cell surface antigen C3b and iC3b (34). At the same time, there is a reduction in human leukocyte antigen (HLA) HLA-DR, HLA-DQ, and HLA-DP expression by monocytes, and these class II antigens are obligatory for many cell-mediated immunologic processes, thereby implying a possible loss of monocyte function following thermal injury (35). C3 production by burned patients' macrophages is suppressed, but the synthetic ability for key cytokines such as IL-6 is increased (36).

T Lymphocytes and Cell-Mediated Immunity

Early T-cell studies in burn patients showed a variety of changes: impairment in mitogenic and antigenic responsiveness of lymphocytes, burn size–related suppression of graft versus host reactivity, suppression of delayed cutaneous sensitivity tests, and diminution in both peripheral lymphocyte numbers and thoracic duct lymphocyte concentration. Currently, controversy exists as to whether the failure of T-cell functions is due to an intracellular defect related to thermal injury, the result of "overuse," or indirectly the result of downregulation by the cytokine cascade or other products of the inflammatory reaction.

Analysis of peripheral blood T cells supports the theory that, rather than an absolute reduction in CD4 and an increase in CD8 cells, there may be a redistribution of lymphocyte traffic (37). Suppression in the numbers of the total lymphocyte population is the only consistent overall change. Furthermore, not only is there lymphocyte traffic between central lymphocyte stores and the peripheral blood following thermal injury, but the responsiveness of these lymphocyte populations also varies according to site; for example, splenic lymphocytes of experimentally burned animals remain most profoundly depressed in response to antigenic stimulation compared with the peripheral blood and other organs (38). In addition, in peripheral blood, the appearance of "activation" antigens on CD4 and CD8 cells (HLA-DR, IL-2R, and transferrin receptor) is significantly depressed as early as 1 day postburn (39). This finding has not been universally confirmed by others.

The addition of recombinant IL-2 does not appear to reverse the suppression of the appearance of surface markers such as IL-2R in burned patients, although it does not improve the response of natural killer cells to stimulation (40). In experimental preparations, at least some of the observed T-cell suppression can be alleviated by early removal of the burn wound, thereby creating another argument for the prompt closure of the burn wound (41).

B Lymphocytes and Humoral Immunity

The function of B cells following thermal injury is less well documented than that of macrophages or T cells. The expression of this major histocompatability complex is impaired; therefore, some diminution of B-cell function can be expected as a result of diminished recognition of antigenic presentation (42). Under the influence of stress-induced corticosteroids, there is a relative increase of circulating B cells compared with T cells in peripheral blood (43). Spontaneous cytokine (IL-4 and IL-2)-induced expression of the activation antigen CD23 is reduced significantly during the second to fifth week postburn (44).

If the products of B-cell activation, namely, the immunoglobulins, are measured *in vivo,* the results are somewhat difficult to interpret because of the increased catabolism of protein and the leakage through the burn wound. Briefly, there is marked diminution of serum IgG concentration, total and all subclasses, and these levels return to normal between 10 and 14 days postburn. Extremely low levels of IgG on admission (300–400 mg%) are predictors of a poor prognosis. IgM and IgA levels appear to be relatively unaffected. Overall, it seems that the defective immunoglobulin production following thermal injury is probably a factor of macrophage/lymphocyte interaction rather than a failure of intrinsic activity by B cells (45).

BURN-WOUND MICROBIOLOGY

A working knowledge of the common flora of burn wounds is essential to tailor therapy appropriately. Pathogens peculiar to thermal injuries are basically no different from the normal flora of the environment.

Gram-Positive Bacteria

The gram-positive bacteria predominance is consistent with the normal inhabitants of the skin prior to the thermal injury. *Staphylococcus, Micrococcus, Peptococcus, Streptococcus, Enterococcus*, and *Peptostreptococcus* organisms are common gram-positive cocci in burn wounds. These organisms can be life threatening as invasive infections or simply local colonization alone. Table 16.1 shows the distribution of gram-positive bacteria at the Shriners Burns Hospital for Children at Galveston, which receives patients from all over the world. For the year 1998, the gram-positive cocci accounted for 60% of the isolates; however, staphylococci were more prevalent (73.5%) than enterococci, which accounted for 17.1%. Among the staphylococci,

TABLE 16.1. *Gram-positive bacteria isolated from 377 pediatric burn patients admitted to the Shriners Burns Hospital, Galveston, for acute burn care (January 1998–December 1998)*

Organism	No.	%
Staphylococcus aureus MS	81	11.4
Staphylococcus aureus MR	40	5.6
Staphylococcus epidermidis MS	186	26.1
Staphylococcus epidermidis MR	216	30.3
Enterococcus faecalis	85	12.1
Enterococcus faecium	36	5.1
Other gram-positives[a]	67	9.4
Total	712	100.0
Total gram-positives among all isolates	1,187	60.0

MS, methicillin sensitive; MR, methicilin resistant.
[a]Includes other streptococci, diphtheroids, and *Bacillus* sp.

there appeared to be an equal distribution of methicillin sensitive (51%) and methicillin resistant (49%) isolates.

Cook stressed the importance of microbial surveillance and epidemiologic studies, which are thought to reduce methicillin-resistant *Staphylococcus aureus* (MRSA) prevalence but concedes that this may be inadequate for eradicating or preventing outbreaks (46). Minimizing transmission and infection is emphasized; however, Reardon et al. suggested that this process is time consuming and requires extensive resources for little gain (47). Methicillin-susceptible *S. aureus* (MSSA)/MRSA colonization in 86 patients was studied and found to have no significant changes on length of stay, number of operations, or mortality between these two organisms. It is acknowledged, however, that the presence of *Staphylococcus* (MSSA or MRSA) did significantly increase both the number of operations and the length of stay. Many burn units report frequent colonization of burn patients with toxic shock toxin (TSS-1) producing strains of staphylococci; however, their presence does not correlate well with increased morbidity or mortality rates (48).

Group A β-hemolytic *Streptococcus,* although common in the past as a cause of epidemics in burn units, now is encountered infrequently as a result of the frequent empiric use of antibiotics for burn wound manipulations. Other β-hemolytic streptococci belonging groups B, C, E, F, and G can be encountered as well (49). Significant vigilance of infection control still is needed because occasional clusters of outbreak of group A streptococcal infection continue to be reported (50,51). Fortunately, group A streptococcus still remains uniformly sensitive to penicillins; hence prophylaxis and treatment are easily accomplished.

Enterococcal infections account for fewer than 20% of burn-wound infections from gram-positive bacteria (Table 16.1); however, a significant cause for concern is the emergence of vancomycin-resistant enterococcus (VRE) in burn units (52–53). Whereas additional morbidity to VRE itself is not clear, when it occurs as a polymicrobial bacteremia, mortality rates as high as 20% have been noted (52).

Other Gram-positive bacilli include the aerobic *Corynbacterium* and *Listeria* sp. as well as the spore-forming *Bacillus* (aerobe) and *Clostridium* (anaerobe) sp. *Bacillus* and *Clostridium* sp. are associated with burn wounds that have come in contact with contaminated soil. In avascular muscle injuries, for example, electrical injuries or crush injuries combined with burns, there is a high risk for developing tetanus (*C. tetani*) (54), which has led to the practice of use of tetanus immunoprophylaxis and booster vaccines (55).

Gram-Negative Bacteria

The presence of the gram-negative bacteria in burn wounds is due in part to translocation of bacteria from the gastrointestinal tract of patients (56). In a study of children with burns, we found that patients with large wounds (>50% total body surface area) were significantly more likely to be colonized with their fecal gram-negatives than those with smaller wounds (57). Whereas the gram-negatives accounted for only 40% of the total bacterial isolates of the wound, they represented a formidable adversary (Table 16.2). Most of this group of organisms were extended β-lactam-resistant bacteria. Although

TABLE 16.2. *Total gram-negative bacteria isolated from 377 pediatric burn patients admitted to the Shriners Burns Hospital, Galveston, Texas, for acute burn care (January 1998–December 1998)*

Organism	No.	%
Enterics		
Enterobacter cloacae	53	11.2
Escherichia coli	49	10.3
Klebsiella pneumoniae	45	9.5
Other enterics[a]	179	37.7
Noncarbohydrate fermentors		
Pseudomonas aeruginosa	91	19.2
Acinetobacter sp.	28	5.9
Stenotrophomonas maltophia	9	1.8
Other nonfermentors[b]	21	4.4
Total	475	100.0
Total gram-negatives among all isolates	1,187	40.0

[a]Includes *Serratia, Enterobacter, Klebsiella, Proteus* and *Citrobacter* sp.
[b]Includes *Aeromonas, Achromobacter, Vibrio,* and *Alkaligines* sp.

the carbohydrate fermenting enterics seem to account for 68.7% of the Gram-negative isolates as a whole, *P. aeruginosa,* a nonfermenter, is the most common gram-negative pathogen in burn patients. Other important gram-negative bacteria include the Enterobacteriaceae such as *Escherichia coli, Enterobacter cloacae, Klebsiella pneumoniae,* and *Serratia marcescens.* The Enterobacteriaceae also are encountered as a cause of nosocomial pneumonia in patients who have inhalation injury and are on ventilators, and as a cause of urinary tract infection in patients with indwelling urinary catheters.

Even without invasive infections, gram-negative bacteria have been implicated in systemic inflammatory diseases, including shock and disseminated intravascular coagulation, secondary to the circulation of bacterial endotoxin from the gut and the burn wound (58,59). Often, gut decontamination is instituted to reduce the incidence of endotoxin-mediated disease.

Fungi

Until the advent of topical antimicrobials and systemic antibiotics, fungal infections were not common in burn patients. The burn wound is the most commonly infected site, although fungemia and dissemination to the respiratory tract in patients on ventilators and to the urinary tract in patients with indwelling catheter are frequently encountered. *Candida* spp. are the most common fungal colonizers of the wound (Table 16.3); however, fewer than 20% of patients develop widespread candidiasis. Overall, there is a 3% to 5% rate of candidemia in the burn population and a comparable rate of burn-wound invasion. A study of burned children at our center showed that those developing candidemia did so during the first week postburn and 7 days after excision of burn eschar (60). It is hypothesized that patients with massive burns are further suppressed by repeated surgical intervention, anesthesia, and perioperative use of broad-spectrum antibiotics, thereby predisposing these patients to early development of *Candida* septicemia. With early recognition of burn-wound invasion through routine biopsies, wound swabs, and early amphotericin therapy, the mortality has been reduced to fewer than 10% compared with 60% to 90% reported in earlier series (61).

Unlike *Candida,* true fungal infections with *Aspergillus, Penicillium, Rhizopus, Mucor, Rhizomucor, Fusarium,* and *Curvularia* organisms occur early in the hospital course, specifically in those exposed to the spores on the ground or in water at the time of injury. Once colonized, broad nonbranching hyphae extend into subcutaneous tissue and stimulate an inflammatory response. Vascular invasion is common and often is accompanied by thrombosis and avascular necrosis, clinically observed as rapidly advancing dark discolorations of the wound margin. Systemic dissemination occurs with the invasion of the vaculature.

Viruses

Linnemann and MacMillan performed a retrospective survey of serum for viral antibodies in pediatric burn patients (62), of whom 22% had fourfold increases in antibodies to cytomegalovirus (CMV), 8% had increases to herpes simplex virus (HSV) and to Epstein-Barr virus (EBV), and 5% to varicella-zoster virus (VZV). None of the patients had evidence of adenovirus or hepatitis B virus infection. On the basis of these observations, a prospective study of viral infections, using both serologic and viral culture techniques, was performed. This study showed that CMV infection developed in 33% of children, herpes simplex infection in 25%, and adenovirus infection in 17%. In all of the most severely burned children, CMV infections developed, and both primary and reactivation infections were observed. Most primary CMV infections are likely to occur from the transfusion of blood products. CMV infection typically occurs about 1 month after burn and clinically presents as fever of unknown origin with lymphocytosis; however, it rarely alters the patient's clinical course (63). Kealey et al. showed that 56% of burned patients initially seropositive for CMV had a fourfold or greater increase in CMV antibodies as evidence of CMV reactivation (64). These patients tended to be younger, to have a larger burn area, and to have a longer hospital stay. No patient who experienced CMV infection, whether primary or reactivated, had serious complications attributable to CMV.

Another transfusion-related infection is hepatitis C virus (HCV). Coursaget et al. studied anti-HCV antibodies in 45 burn patients at the time of burn injury and more than 6 months after burn injury (65). HCV infection was detected in 18% as a consequence of

TABLE 16.3. *Medically important fungi isolated from 377 pediatric burn patients admitted to the Shriners Burn Hospital, Galveston, Texas, for acute burn care (January 1998–December 1998)*

Organism	No.	%
Candida spp.	32	63.0
Fusarium spp.	8	15.6
Aspergillus spp.	5	9.8
Penicillium spp.	3	5.8
Rhizomucor spp.	2	3.8
Zygometes spp.	1	2.0
Total	51	100.0

the numerous transfusions of blood or blood derivatives used during the postburn treatment. Five patients displayed evidence of anti-C100, anti-C33c, and anti-Core antibodies together; two patients had only anti-C100 and anti-C33c antibodies, and the last one showed only anti-Core antibodies. Chronic hepatitis was observed in 83% of HCV infections. Kinetics of appearance of anti-HCV antibodies varied between patients. Anti-Core is generally the first to be detected at high levels; however, in at least one case, it was detected only 2.5 months after C100 and C33c antibodies. The incidence of HCV using the newer polymerase chain reaction technique to detect the viral genome has not been evaluated in burn patients. Nonetheless, the current blood-banking procedures decreased the transmission of HCV by blood products.

Another transfusion-related agent is human immunodeficiency virus (HIV), which has become extremely rare as a result of the screening of donors that began in 1987 in the United States. Significant risk existed prior to that period, however. A retrospective review of burned children at our center who had received blood or blood products between 1978 and 1985 identified 52 patients at risk for HIV infection (66). More than 50% of the identified population had received 3 U or more of blood or blood products during their acute hospital stay. A total of 214 patients (36.8%) were tested for HIV seroconversions: five tested HIV positive by enzyme-linked immunosorbent assay (ELISA), and four were confirmed by Western blot, yielding a 1.9% incidence. The four confirmed patients received 2 to 9 total body blood volume turnovers during their postburn period in hospital.

In burn units, HSV is of significant concern because it is a dermatopathologic virus. A review of the literature suggested that patients under 10 years of age are at greater risk of an HSV infection when the total body surface area is greater than 15% (83%) (67); however, the role of HSV in wound healing is unclear. Bourdarias et al. (68) showed that in 11 patients with burns, local areas of active epidermal regeneration were most commonly affected. Acyclovir ther-

apy was not used, and the duration of hospitalization was normal compared with other children. Nonetheless, HSV in the lungs may worsen morbidity. Byers et al. showed that the relative risk for HSV infection was higher for cases with adult respiratory distress syndrome but not with pneumonia. Disseminated HSV infection also can be fatal (69).

Another dermatopathologic virus is VZV. Miniepidemics of VZV have occurred within pediatric burn units (70,71). The characteristic fluid-filled lesions appear in healed or healing partial-thickness burns as well as uninjured epithelium and mucous membranes. The vesicles are much more destructive in injured than in uninjured skin and may present as hemorrhagic, oozing pockmarks that are prone to secondary infection and subsequent scarring. Neovascularized skin grafts may be lost; therefore, further grafting procedures should be delayed until the lesions are quiescent.

Morbidity attributable to respiratory virus infections, particularly in those with inhalation injury, has not been well studied. More than 100 pediatric burn patients at our center were tested for respiratory syncytial virus (RSV) during the winter seasons of 1995 and 1996. Only six patients were positive for RSV, and one death occurred in this group (1% mortality rate).

Parasites

Parasitic infestation also is seen, especially in children from the developing world. We recently evaluated 32 admissions of children with burns at our center, of whom 64% were from Mexico (Table 16.4). Of these children's

TABLE 16.4. *Parasitic infestations in 377 pediatric burn patients admitted to Shriners Burn Hospital, Galveston, Texas, for acute burn care (January 1998–December 1998)*

Organism	No.	%
Entamoeba coli	2	25.0
Blastocystis hominis	2	25.0
Ascaris lumbricoides	2	25.0
Ancylostoma duodenale	1	12.5
Endolimax nana	1	12.5
Total	8	100.0

stools, 9.8% were positive for parasites. We also have described three cases of *Ascaris* pneumonitis that exacerbated the smoke-induced lung injury (72).

CLINICAL MANIFESTATIONS

Local Signs

An open burn wound is a favorable target for bacterial colonization. The progression from simple eschar colonization to the invasive process is favored by a series of factors related to the patient, such as extension and depth of the burn, age, presence of previous disease, and local conditions of the wound; or to the microorganism, such as density, motility, toxins, and antimicrobial resistance; or to iatrogenic causes, such as prosthetic devices and nosocomial spread of bacteria. It is essential to recognize the early signs of local burn-wound infection by examining the wound at least once a day.

The local signs of burn wound infection can be summarized as follows (73–74):

- Black or dark brown focal areas of discoloration
- Partial-thickness injury converted to full-thickness necrosis
- Subcutaneous tissue with hemorrhagic discoloration
- Enhanced sloughing of burned tissue or eschar
- Purplish discoloration or edema of skin around the margins of the wound
- Pyocyanotic appearance of subeschar tissue
- The presence of ecthyma gangrenosa in *Pseudomonas* infection (Fig. 16.1)
- Variable-sized abscess formation and focal subeschar inconsistency
- Green pigment (pyocyanin) visible in subcutaneous fat in *Pseudomonas* infection
- Centrifugal advance of subcutaneous edema with central ischemic necrosis in fungal infection
- Hemorrhagic saponification of subcutaneous fat in fungal infection
- Vesicular lesions in healing or healed partial-thickness burns in viral infection

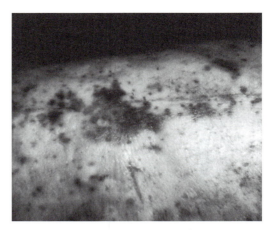

FIG. 16.1. Photograph of dark purplish discoloration of burned skin characteristic of ecthyma gangrenosa due to *Pseudomonas aeruginosa.*

- Crusted serrated margins of partial-thickness burns in viral infection

Systemic Signs

Progression from local to systemic invasion can occur rapidly, which correlates with the size of the burn wound, the extent of environmental contamination, and surgical procedures. Early recognition of systemic invasion is critical to avoid the high rates of mortality. Many of the signs of sepsis resemble complications of burn itself; for example, fevers, tachycardia, shock, and elevated or depressed neutrophil count can occur in burned patients with or without infection. Certain patterns of clinical signs and symptoms, however, may help to recognize the systemic bacterial invasion (Table 16.5) (75). An increase in C-reactive protein serum levels has been found useful in predicting systemic infection, although increases in the first 2 days after the burn or the day after surgery may occur without infection (76). When sepsis did occur, it always was preceded by increased C-reactive protein about 2 days before the patient was deemed septic clinically. Elevated levels of certain cytokines (reviewed above) may be useful markers, but they remain largely research tools.

TABLE 16.5. *Signs and symptoms of progression from local invasion to systemic illness*

Gram-negative sepsis	Gram-positive sepsis
Burn wound biopsy >10^5 organisms/g tissue or histologic tissue invasion	Same
Rapid onset, well to ill in 8–12 h	Gradual
Temp. 37–39°C can be normal, followed by hypothermia (34°–35°C), plus decrease in WBC	Temperature >40°C
WBC may be elevated	WBC 20–50 K, HCT decrease
Ileus	Same
Decreased BP and urinary output	Same
Wounds develop focal gangrene, satellite lesions away from burn wound	Macerated wounds, ropy, tenacious exudate
Mental obtundation	Anorexic and irrational

BP, blood pressure; HCT, hematocrit; WBC, white blood cell count.
From Heggers JP, Linares H, Edgar P, et al. Treatment of infections in burns. In: Herndon DN, ed. *Total burn care*. London: W.B. Saunders, 1996:98–135, with permission.

Other than the infection of the burn skin, several types of infectious complications in burned patients have been recognized:

1. Bacteremia is a frequent complication. Surgical burn-wound manipulations are responsible for bacteremias in about 50% of cases, but routine instrumentation and intravascular catheter devices also can cause bacteremia (77,78). Sasaki et al. showed that patients with a positive blood culture had an average total body surface area injury of 46.6%, whereas those with a 25.5% injury had negative blood cultures (79).

2. Subacute bacterial endocarditis is a risk associated with persistent bacteremia from any cause, including repeated instrumentation, surgical intervention, and placement of central venous catheters (80,81). *S. aureus* and gram-negative bacilli are the most frequent causes. In most cases, antemortem diagnosis is rarely suspected in burned children (80,82). In addition to local valvular damage, infected vegetations may dislodge septic emboli.

3. Suppurative thrombophlebitis occurs at the site of catheter insertion. It may occur in up to 5% of patients with burns over 20% of their total body surface area (83).

4. Suppurative chondritis occurs in patients with full-thickness burn of the ear. Because of the auricle's relatively low level of blood supply, chondritis frequently follows the progression of tissue ischemia, usually 3 to 5 weeks after burn injury (84). *P. aeruginosa* and *S. aureus* are the most common pathogens; however, with the use of mafenide acetate as topical agent, the incidence of suppurative chondritis has decreased significantly.

5. Suppurative sinusitis is seen in patients with long-term nasotracheal intubation. In one study, 8% of patients with burns who had nasotracheal intubation for more than 7 days developed sinusitis (85).

6. Pneumonia may occur with or without inhalation injury, although those with inhalation injury have a substantially higher risk (86). Bronchopneumonia is the most common type of pulmonary infection, usually occurring in the second week of burn injury. Predisposing factors are the size of burn wound (hematogenous spread), aspiration, the presence of tracheostomy or nasotracheal tube (nosocomial spread from burn wound), the existence of inhalation injury, and disturbances of fluid and electrolyte balance. Most deaths from infection in burned patients today are caused by pneumonia rather than wound infection (86).

7. Urinary tract infection occurs in association with prolonged and often unnecessary catheterization (87).

8. Osteomyelitis can occur when bones are exposed by the burn, by open fracture accompanying the burn, by extension of infection from a septic joint, introduction of organisms

along traction pins, internal fracture fixation devices, or bacteremia. Clinically significant osteomyelitis in burn patients is rare, however (88).

9. Septic arthritis occurs when a joint is exposed by a burn or by removal of burn eschar (88). The joints most frequently exposed are the knee, the elbow, the proximal interphalangeal joints of the hand, and the metacarpophalangeal joints on the dorsal surfaces of the hand. The incidence of septic arthritis is obscured by its frequent association with signs and symptoms of severe burns that are rarely separable. Rarely, in burns a joint may become infected from adjacent metaphysial osteomyelitis. In children, most joints can be salvaged. Adult joints are less resilient.

10. Central nervous system infections in burned patients include meningitis, microabscesses, and septic infarcts. In one review, *Candida* spp., *S. aureus,* and *P. aeruginosa* caused almost 80% of infections, occurring most frequently in patients with extensive burn with wound infection or endocarditis (89).

11. Toxic shock syndrome resulting from TSS toxin producing strains of *S. aureus* has been identified in acutely burned children. Childs found that 13% of children developed a toxic shocklike illness; however, its effect on overall burn mortality was not clear (48).

12. Multiorgan failure in burn patients is most commonly initiated by wound infection and systemic sepsis. One single overwhelming infection is not required; rather, small repetitive infections may initiate the cascade, perhaps by priming immune cells.

CLINICAL INVESTIGATIONS

There are three major approaches to determine burn wound infection: (a) quantitative burn-wound cultures (BWCs), (b) histologic assessment of bacterial invasion, and (c) bronchioalveolar lavage (BAL) fluid.

Quantitative BWC by Biopsy

Teplitz demonstrated that quantitative bacterial counts of BWCs correlated with histologic

specimens showing invasion or colonization (90). Burn-wound infection (often referred to as *burn wound sepsis* in surgical literature) is suspected when proliferating microorganisms exceed 10^5/g tissue and when there is invasion of subjacent unburned tissue (Fig. 16.2). The presence of microorganisms within the necrotic eschar cannot be considered evidence of burn-wound infection. Furthermore, although a bacterial count of 10^5/g of tissue is likely to indicate bacterial invasion, this is not invariably true. Only the histologic sections can indicate the level of infection. Therefore, BWCs always should be accompanied by histologic sections from the same area (91,92).

At the time of surgery, the potentially infected tissues should be excised with a punch biopsy (Fig. 16.3) and divided into equal aliquots (93). One aliquot should be placed into saline and delivered to the microbiology section for quantitative assessment. These biopsies are weighed aseptically and homogenized in a sterile tube in 3 mL of sterile saline. Known dilutions of the homogenate then are plated using precalibrated loops (10 µL) on blood agar, colistin-neomycin agar, MacConkey agar, and Sabourauds agar for identification in the initial dilutions of 0.1 mL with a 1 mL sterile pipette. After 24 hours, the

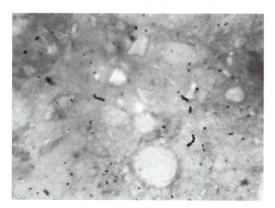

FIG. 16.2. Photomicrograph of a homogenized biopsy stained with Gram stain. Gram-positive cocci are seen (cultures grew group A *Streptococcus* at greater than 10^5 colony-forming units per gram of tissue).

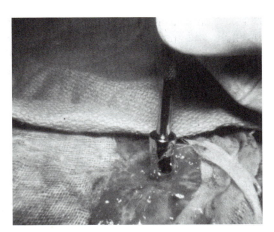

FIG. 16.3. Photograph showing the use of a 6-mm punch for collecting a skin biopsy for tissue histology and quantitative culture.

TABLE 16.6. *Staging of microbial status of the burn wound by biopsy histology*

Stage I: colonization
  A. Superficial: microorganisms present only on burn wound surface
  B. Penetrating: variable depth of microbial penetration of eschar
  C. Proliferating: variable level of microbial proliferation at nonviable-viable tissue interphase (subeschar space)
Stage II: invasion
  A. Microinvasion: microorganisms present in viable tissue immediately subjacent to subeschar space
  B. Deep invasion: penetration of microorganisms to variable depth and expanse within viable subcutaneous tissue
  C. Microvascular involvement: microorganisms within small blood vessels and lymphatics (thrombosis of vessels common)

From Pruitt BA Jr, McManus AT, Kim SH, et al. Burn infections: current status. *World J Surg* 1998; 22:135–145, with permission.

colony numbers are counted, and the quantitative BWC is calculated according to the following formula.

CFU/g of tissue = number of colonies × volume × dilution/weight of biopsy (g),

where CFU = colony-forming units.

Histologic Procedures

Standard histologic procedures as well as cryostat examination are necessary (91). The tissues should be examined for morphologic

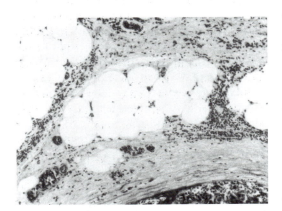

FIG. 16.4. Photomicrograph of a cross-section of tissue stained with hematoxylin and eosin showing invasion of *Pseudomonas aeruginosa.*

changes as well as for the presence of pathogens (Fig. 16.4). Many bacterial and fungal pathogens can be identified by staining with Gram stain and Gomori-methamine-silver stains. More specialized stains may be necessary to identify other fastidious bacteria and fungi. Tzanck stain can be used to identify inclusion bodies suggestive of HSV or VZV invasion. Viral specific antibodies also can be used to detect these viruses by immunohistochemistry. The microbial status of the burn wound as assessed by histologic examination of a biopsy specimen can be graded on the basis of the density and depth of penetration of microorganisms (Table 16.6) (74,91).

BRONCHOALVEOLAR LAVAGE

It is essential that BAL be collected by personnel experienced in the evaluation of patients with inhalation injury who are at risk for airway edema and obstruction. BAL should be processed as previously described (Fig. 16.1). BAL fluids also can be processed for respiratory viruses such RSV and influenza by rapid antigenic detection by immunoassays, which are within the capability of most laboratories, or by culture, which requires an onsite virology laboratory to process highly labile virus such as RSV.

TREATMENT MODALITIES OF INFECTION

Wound care is the mainstay of burn care. The goal is to minimize infection and facilitate burn-wound healing. Wound care addresses both partial- and full-thickness burn injuries until all wounds are closed.

Wound Dressing

The superficial epidermal layer provides a barrier to microorganisms, and the deeper lipid epidermal layer provides protection against water-vapor loss. In full-thickness burns, the eschar may extend beyond the skin into the subcutaneous fat and muscle. Wound closure cannot occur until this is removed. Bacterial proteases lead to eschar pseudoseparation and are slowed with antiseptic therapies. The eschar is allowed to fragment and slough, with resultant decrease in wound size. This is called *wound contraction*, and it also can be excised and skin grafted. Full-thickness skin grafts have the least contraction. Deep dermal wounds that are allowed to heal spontaneously lead to hypertrophic scarring. Compression garments are used for the prevention and treatment of scarring.

When approaching burn-wound care, first a plan must be decided. Outer burn dressings provide comfort, metabolic enhancement, and protection. First, superficial burns are exquisitely sensitive to air currents, as are deeper burns after some healing. Also, dressings provide splinting as well as drainage containment. Next, occlusive dressings help eliminate shivering, cold stress, and evaporative heat loss. In open, granulating wounds, water vapor loss is maximal. Finally, the protective component deals with the control of topical organisms. Supplies consist of large 9×9 burn gauze, Kerlex wraps, Ace wraps, and topical antimicrobials. Gentle wound cleansing with daily debridement is also important.

Buttock burn wounds should be examined carefully and frequently for the presence of deep stool staining, an ominous predictor of burn wound sepsis and death (94). Such wounds should be emergently excised.

Topical Antimicrobials

Topical antimicrobial agents are used extensively in burn patients. Most patients with stage I and stage II A and B wounds (Table 16.6) can be treated with topical or subeschar antimicrobials alone.

Silver Sulfadiazine

Silver sulfadiazine (Silvadene, SSD, Thermazine, Flamazine, Burnazine) is a 1% water-soluble cream combining sulfadiazine with silver (Ag+). The Ag^+ ion binds with the DNA of an organism and, consequently, releases sulfonamide, which interferes with the intermediary metabolic pathway of the microbe. It is most effective against *P. aeruginsosa* and the enterics and equally as effective as any antifungal drug against *Candida albicans. S. aureus,* and some strains of *Klebsiella* sp. have been less effectively controlled (75). Antimicrobial effectiveness has been observed to last for up to 24 hours. More frequent changes are required if a creamy exudate forms on the wound. The benefits of this topical agent are its ease of use and its ability to reduce pain. It has some tissue-penetrating ability but is limited to the surface epidermis. It is not associated with acid-base disturbances or pulmonary fluid overload, as is Sulfamylon.

Silvadene can be used separately or in combination with other antibacterials or enzymatic escharotomy compounds. It can be combined with nystatin, which enhances the antifungal capability of this agent. By itself, it has been shown to retard wound healing; however, in conjunction with nystatin or aloe vera, the wound-retardant effect is reversed. The breaking strength is not affected. Granulocyte reduction has been reported; however, this appears to be reversible.

Cerium Nitrate–Silver Sulfadiazine

Lanthanide salt cerium nitrate has been added to silver sulfadiazine (Silvadene) since the 1970s and has been shown to have increased efficacy for wound bacteriostasis in large burn wounds. The antimicrobial spectrum is similar to that of silver nitrate or silvadene. Its efficacy is thought to be due to, in part, its preservation of the cell-mediated immune response. Methemoglobinemia has been seen only rarely, and there are no associated electrolyte disturbances. There is only minimal cerium absorption noted in patients with large burns treated for weeks. Its use is somewhat limited because it is not commercially available in the United States. It is, however, available in several west European countries as Flammacerium. Koller and Orsag studied the effects of cerium sulfadiazine in 20 burn patients and found it to be safe and effective in the treatment of deep, extensive burn wounds (95). This was found to be easy to use, with painless application and removal. It was also noted that the eschar turned yellow and developed a leathery consistency with good resistance to infection. This enabled serial excisions to be performed when early total burn excisions were not possible. Recently, there have been reports of *P. aeruginosa* resistance to sulfadiazine (96).

Silver Nitrate (AgNO₃)

Formerly used as a 10% solution and found to be toxic at this concentration, it has now been reinstated as a 0.5% solution that is nontoxic. In this dilute form, it does not injure regenerating epithelium in the wound and is bacteriostatic against *S. aureus, E. coli,* and *P. aeruginosa* (75). $AgNO_3$ is most effective when the wound is carefully cleansed of all emollients and other debris and debrided of all dead tissue. Multilayered coarse mesh dressings should be placed over the wound and saturated with the $AgNO_3$ solution. Like Silvadene, $AgNO_3$ has limited penetration because the Ag^+ ion is rapidly bound to the body's natural chemical substances, such as Cl^-. Because it is hypotonic in nature, it can cause osmolar dilution, resulting in hyponatremia and hypochloremia. Serum electrolytes should be monitored carefully.

Notable detriments to the use of $AgNO_3$ are that it is expensive, light sensitive, and turns black on contact with tissues and other Cl^--containing compounds. Further, it also requires special handling; if allowed to dry or if it is covered with an impervious dressing, hyperpyrexia could occur. *Klebsiella* and *Providencia* species and other *Enterobacteriaceae* are not as susceptible to it as are other bacteria. *E. cloacae* can cause methemoglobinemia by converting nitrite to nitrate as well as other nitrate-positive organisms.

Mafenide Acetate

Mafenide acetate (Sulfamylon) is available both in a 10% water-soluble cream and a 5% solution and has more substantial bacteriologic data to support its efficacy than do any of the other topical antimicrobials (97,98). It has been shown to be effective against a broad range of microorganisms, especially against all strains of *P. aeruginosa* and *Clostridium* organisms (75). After a wound has been cleansed of debris, Sulfamylon is applied to the wound like "butter." The treated burn surface is left exposed for maximal antimicrobial potency. The cream is applied a minimum of twice a day and is reapplied between applications if it is rubbed off the wound.

Advantages of the cream include its ability to control *P. aeruginosa* wound infections, its ease of application, and the absence of the need for dressings. Additionally, it has an ability to permeate burn eschar and thereby to circumvent the colonization of a burn. The 5% solution is applied every 8 hours. It has been proclaimed to have effective tissue-penetrating ability and appears to be especially effective after dead tissue is removed from the granulating bed.

Unfortunately, several detrimental aspects are associated with the use of mafenide acetate. Protracted use, with a low environmental pH, favors the growth of *C. albicans.* Mafenide acetate is converted to *p*-sulfamylvanzoic acid by monamine oxidase, which is a carbonic anhydrase inhibitor; this subsequently causes metabolic acidosis in patient. In the unburned patient, respiratory alkalosis is present; therefore, an imbalance is not present. On the other hand, if an inhalation injury exists with its concomitant respiratory acidosis and is associated with metabolic acidosis initiated by this drug, the end result can be fatal. This also can be seen when treatment occurs during septic episodes with metabolic acidosis or if it is applied over a large area of the body surface. Another detrimental problem is that it is painful when applied to superficial partial-thickness burns with intact free nerve endings. Also, its requirement to remain uncovered for antimicrobial activity may be considered a disadvantage. The 5% aqueous solution of mafenide acetate can be used in a wet dressing covered by a splint.

Other investigators have shown that fatality in major burns can be reduced by 33% by the use of Sulfamylon. Like Silvadene, it can be used individually or in conjunction with other antimicrobials (nystatin); however, Sulfamylon retards wound healing and reduces the breaking strength of healed wounds.

Gentamicin Sulfate

Gentamicin sulfate is available as a 0.1% water-soluble cream and is chemically similar to the other aminoglycosides, such as kanamycin and neomycin. It has a broad spectrum of antimicrobial activity. It is used based on its capabilities against *P. aeruginosa.* Unfortunately, its topical use has rapidly stimulated gentamicin resistance (99).

Bacitracin and Polymyxin

Topical antibiotics, such as bacitracin and polymyxin, have been unproductive in controlling infection, specifically in grafting procedures. These two antibiotics have little or no effect on localized burn-wound infections (75).

Nitrofurantoin

Although initially its therapeutic value was questioned, nitrofurantoin has been shown to be effective in the treatment of MRSA. It is also effective 75% of the time for most gram-negative organisms other than *P. aeruginosa* (75).

Mupirocin (Bactroban)

Studies at our center have shown mupirocin to be superior to Silvadene in treating MSSA/MRSA (100). Although mupirocin is weaker against gram-negative bacteria, it is also comparable to Silvadene and Sulfamylon against *P. aeruginosa, E. coli,* and *K. pneumonia* (75). Mupirocin inhibits wound healing compared with controls by a half-life of 2 days, and its breaking strength is significantly enhanced over controls.

Nystatin (Mycostatin, Nilstat)

Combining nystatin and Silvadene or nitrofurantoin results in effective prevention of local and systemic *Candida* infections as well as burn-wound sepsis (101); however, in combination therapy of Sulfamylon and nystatin, Sulfamylon actually loses its antimicrobial activity. Therefore, use with Sulfamylon is discouraged. Our investigators also studied concentrated nystatin powder on the effect of angioinvasive fungi (*Fusarium, Aspergillus*) refractory to systemic amphotericin B and serial excisions including amputations (102). A concentrated form of nystatin (6,000,000 U/g) was used every 6 hours and wet to dry dressings laid overtop. The nystatin was applied as a dried aerosol. Within 14 days, all four of the children studied recovered with the eradication of their invasive fungal infections. Also, all areas previously autografted underneath the nystatin powder healed nicely, and all other open areas showed excellent granulation and subsequent autografting.

Sodium Hypochlorite (0.025% Heggers Solution)

Currently, the most effective topical antibacterial agent for cleansing a wound is sodium hypochlorite (NaOCl). It transcends the topical antimicrobial effects and tissue toxicity of products such as povidone–iodine (Betadine), acetic acid, and hydrogen peroxide. Acetic acid is toxic to fibroblasts and not bactericidal. Betadine is fibroblast toxic as well. Hydrogen peroxide (3%) is bactericidal but also toxic to fibroblasts.

The efficacy of NaOCl has been determined to be at a concentration of 0.025%, which is bactericidal, nontoxic to fibroblasts, and does not inhibit wound healing, provided buffers are used (103). It is a broad-spectrum antiseptic and is bactericidal for *P. aeruginosa*, *S. aureus* (MRSA and MSSA), enterococci, as well as other gram-negative and gram-positive organisms (75).

Povidine–Iodine

The active antimicrobial component in this compound is the iodine. It has a broad spectrum of antibacterial and antifungal activities; however, there are disadvantages, and its use is generally discouraged. It is painful when applied. It is often inactivated by wound exudates. Renal dysfunction and acidosis have been noted in association with systemic absorption when applied to open wounds (104). Therefore, povidine–iodine is a highly effective disinfectant when used on intact skin.

Chlorhexidine

Chlorhexidine, when combined with 0.5% silver nitrate, has similar efficacy as Silvadene (105). Some variants of this product have broader antimicrobial activities, but pain on application has limited its use. Unlike the sulfonamides, plasma-mediated resistance has not occurred.

Subeschar Antibiotics

Moncrief described the technique of subeschar antibiotic infusion (106). Its use in the face of microbial invasion into unburned tissue when topical therapies are not effective or in cases where treatment has been delayed. The most common drugs used are tobramycin, gentamicin, and kanamycin. These are administered via multiple needle infusions by subcutaneous lysis. The results of this technique are more rapid eschar separation. The fluid infusion limit is 2,000 mL (adult dose) and should be accounted for in patient's fluid requirements. The infusion fluid should consist of 0.25 to 0.45 N saline to avoid salt overload. Lactated Ringer's solution should be avoided because some of the drugs are incompatible with calcium. Erythromycin has been studied, but it is too painful to use. Colistin, novobiocin, and cephaloridine have been used but were ineffective.

New and Unusual Antimicrobial Alternatives

Tredget et al. investigated a new product called Acticoat (107). This silver-coated dressing was easier to use and had less pain on removal than 0.5% silver nitrate; however, 2 hours after the application, the pain was comparable. Also, burn-wound sepsis was less in the Acticoat group, as was secondary bacteremia. This study was limited, and its authors recommended further investigation. Finally, Mepitel is a new gridlike silicone-coated nylon dressing used in partial-thickness burn wounds. Both Bugmann et al. (108) and Gotschall et al. (109) found this product to decrease pain on dressing change, wound-healing time, and overall hospital stay compared with Silvadene. Bugmann et al. observed no effect on infection in the 70 children studied. Similarly, Gotschall et al. (109) found no significant difference in wound infection between Mepitel and Silvadene.

Other, rather unusual substances have been evaluated for burn-wound care, especially when resources for the use of expensive antimicrobials are limited. Nagoba et al. reported on the use of citric acid (3%) in multidrug-resistant *Pseudomonas* in a case of severe electric burns (110). This organism was completely eradicated, and infection was controlled in 14 days. Subramanyam found that 100% of wounds treated with honey healed within 15 days compared with only 50% in wounds treated with boiled potato-peel dressings (111).

Systemic Antimicrobials

Whereas stage I and stage II A and B wounds (Table 16.6) can be treated with topical or subeschar antimicrobials alone, stage II C wounds require the immediate institution of systemic antibiotic therapy. Systemic antimicrobials also are indicated for the various systemic infectious complications, as discussed earlier. Information on the selection of appropriate systemic antimicrobials for the specific infectious agents is available from standard references on infectious diseases; hence, this issue is not to be discussed herein. Several newer antimicrobial agents are available whose controlled use in burn patients has not been properly studied. Nonetheless, the following general principles may help guide the use of antimicrobial therapy:

- Each antimicrobial agent must be selected for its specificity for the microbe present.
- Such decisions should be made on appropriately collected culture and susceptibility data.
- Colonizing flora should be distinguished from those responsible for inflammation and invasion.
- The time, dosage, route of administration, and duration of treatment should be in accordance with what is required to make the organism nonpathogenic.
- The need for broad-spectrum antibiotics should be balanced with the risk of promoting fungal infections.

Antibiotic Prophylaxis

Prophylactic use of antibiotics remains a highly controversial topic in burn literature. Penicillin prophylaxis is used commonly in many burn centers during outbreaks of group A streptococcal infections (50,51). Prophylactic antibiotics are also used prior to surgical manipulation or instrumentation because the risk of bacteremia is as high as 50%. The choice of perioperative antibiotics is dependent on the knowledge of existing microorganisms that are present not only on injured skin but also in the wound, which is ready for surgery. Nonetheless, carefully controlled studies are needed to identify the value of prophylactic antibiotics. In a placebo-controlled study of cefazolin use in burn children, for children with less than 35% burn, cefazolin was not necessary and, for those with greater than 35% burn, it was not effective (112). Studies with larger numbers of patients are needed to evaluate properly the need for prophylactic antibiotics under various settings.

Gut Support and Decontamination

The gut microflora have been implicated in the development of multiorgan failure when the gut barrier fails. Hence, it has been theorized that early enteral feeding of the gut, which promotes gut barrier function, is important for the prevention of multiorgan failure. A decontaminated gut with nonabsorbable broad-spectrum antibiotics might diminish the impact of gastrointestinal barrier failure. Although there is suggestion that the rate of pneumonia may be decreased by such maneuvers, there is no apparent impact on mortality (113). Overall, convincing human data on the beneficial effect of enteral feeding and gut decontamination on sepsis and multiorgan failure are lacking.

Immunomodulators

In view of the intricate relationship between altered immune defenses in burn patients and increased susceptibility to infections, various types of immunotherapies have been tried in burned patients:

- In an Italian study, treatment with intravenous pooled immunoglobulins (IVIG) had a beneficial effect on septic phenomena and recovery (114); however, in two U.S. studies, no change in infection rates or mortality was shown. Overall, the beneficial role of IVIG as prophylaxis or treatment remains unproven (115,116).

- In a German study, prophylaxis with intravenous *anti-Pseudomonas* immunoglobulin did not appear to be beneficial to burn patients in general; however, it was shown to be effective in burn patients with inhalation injury (117).
- In a South African study, prophylaxis with high-titer anti-lipopolysaccharide IgG reduced the incidence of burn wound infection but did not affect mortality (118).
- Benefits of plasmaphoresis have not been proven.
- Fresh-frozen plasma to improve opsonic activity has been not been studied properly.

INFECTION CONTROL

Hospital-acquired infections in burn patients are common. In burned children, wound infections, ventilator-related pulmonary infections, central line bacteremias, and catheter-associated urinary tract infections are the most common nosocomial infections (87,119). The rates of infections may be lower than those seen in adults, but urinary tract infections are more common in children (87).

Surveillance of infection in a burn patient is performed to implement prompt treatment based on surveillance cultures and antimicrobial sensitivities at the earliest sign of invasion. Such surveillance requires cultures of sputum, urine, and wounds about three times weekly; however, the need for such cultures and the frequency of monitoring remain controversial. Additional infection control measures involve surveillance of spread of pathogens among burn patients in a unit. In dealing with the burn wound, strict infectious disease precautions must be maintained to prevent contamination and worsening infection in these already immunocompromised patients.

In the past, poor handwashing and shared hydrotherapy tubs were the source of many infections, some of which were life threatening. Strict enforcement of handwashing and the use of gowns, gloves, and masks led to decreased patient contamination rates. Also, disposable hydrotherapy tub liners are used without the risk of patient to patient transmission of infections (120). Furthermore, isolation of burn patients in a single room compared with an open ward scenario dramatically affected infection rates. McManus et al. studied this in 2,519 patients and found significantly lower incidence and mortality rates associated with gram-negative bacteremia in the isolated patients. Also, the open ward bacterial isolates showed significantly more antimicrobial resistance compared with those of the patients in isolation (121).

Additional infection-control measures include the use of germicidal solutions to clean daily all the hardware in patient rooms, such as intravenous poles and pumps, monitoring equipment, bedside tables, and beds. On discharge of the patient, the whole room, including floors, walls, ceilings and mattresses, need to be cleaned with germicidal solutions. Air filters should be repeatedly monitored for fungal and bacterial growth.

Lai et al. studied the effects of strict isolation of patients with VRE, the use of vancomycin, and the cost to benefit analysis of barrier precautions (53). Their findings showed that pharyngeal swabs were poor for surveillance but that rectal swabs were more useful. Also, vancomycin-use guidelines were adhered by 85% of the staff. The overall cost for these implementations was $11,000, including the barrier supplies and cleaning protocols. Despite all this, VRE was not eradicated. On the other hand, van Rijn showed that isolation in a quarantine unit was highly effective in preventing outbreaks of multiresistant bacteria (122).

REFERENCES

1. Sheridan R, Remesnyder J, Perlack K, et al. Treatment of seriously burned infant. *J Burn Care Rehabil* 1998; 19:115–118.
2. Moritz AR, Henrique FC, Jr. Studies of thermal injury: the relative importance of time and surface tempera-

ture in the causation of cutaneous burns. *Am J Pathol* 1947;23:695–720.

3. Williams WG, Phillips LG. Pathophysiology of the burn wound. In: Herndon DN, ed. *Total burn Care.* Philadelphia: WB Saunders, 1996:63–70.

4. Jackson DM. The diagnosis of the depth of burning. *Br J Surg* 1953;40:588–596.

5. Shilling JA. Burn healing. *Physiol Rev* 1968;48:374–423.

6. Gasser H, Paul E, Redl H, et al. Loss of plasma antioxidants after burn injury. *Circ Shock* 1991;34:13 (abst).

7. Kaufman T, Neuman RA, Weinberg A. Is postburn dermal ischemia enhanced by oxygen free radicals? *Burns* 1989;15:291–294.

8. Abdi S, Herndon DN, McGuire J, et al. Time course of alterations in lung lymph and bronchial blood flows after inhalation injury. *J Burn Care Rehabil* 1990;11:510–515.

9. Barro RE, Wang CZ, Cox RA, et al. Cellular sequence of tracheal repair in sheep post smoke inhalation injury. *Lung* 1992;170:331–338.

10. Herndon DN, Traber LD, Linares H, et al. Etiology of the pulmonary pathophysiology associated with inhalation injury. *Resuscitation* 1986;14:43–59.

11. Toor AH, Tomashefski JF, Kleinerman J. Respiratory tract pathology in patients with severe burns. *Hum Pathol* 1990;21:1212–1220.

12. Endo S, Inada K, Yamada Y, et al. Plasma tumor necrosis factor-α (TNF-α) levels in patients with burns. *Burns* 1993;19:12–17.

13. Marano MA, Fong Y, Moldawer LL, et al. Serum cachectin/tumor necrosis factor in critically ill patients with burns correlates with infection and mortality. *Surg Gynecol Obstet* 1990;170:32–38.

14. Wood JJ, Rodrick ML, O'Mahony JB, et al. Inadequate interleukin 2 production: a fundamental immunological deficiency in patients with major burns. *Ann Surg* 1984;200:311–320.

15. Vindenes HA, Ulvestad E, Bjerkens R. Concentrations of cytokines in plasma of patients with large burns: their relation to time after injury, burn size, inflammatory variables, infection, and outcome. *Eur J Surg* 1998;164:647–656.

16. Liu XS, Yang ZC, Luo ZH, et al. Clinical significance of the change in blood monocyte interleukin-1 production *in vitro* in severely burned patients. *Burns* 1994; 20:302–306.

17. McMillen MA, Huribal M, Cunningham ME, et al. Endothelin-1, interleukin-6, and interleukin-8 levels increase in patients with burns. *J Burn Care Rehabil* 1996;17:384–389.

18. Ninsten MWN, DeGroot ER, TenDuis HJ, et al. Serum levels of IL-6 and acute phase responses. *Lancet* 1987;2:921.

19. Kawakami M, Terai C, Okada Y. Changes in interleukin-6 levels in skin at different sites after thermal injury. *J Trauma* 1998;44:1056–1063.

20. Garner WL, Rodriguez JL, Miller CG, et al. Acute skin injury releases neutrophil chemoattractants. *Surgery* 1994;116:42–48.

21. Yeh, FL, Lin WL, Shen HD, et al. Changes in levels of serum IL-8 in burned patients. *Burns* 1997;23:565–572.

22. Peterson V, Hansbrough J, Buerk C, et al. Regulation

of granulopoiesis following severe thermal injury. *J Trauma* 1983;23:19–24.

23. Kelly JL, Lyons A, Soberg CC, et al. Anti-interleukin-10 antibody restores burn-induced defects in T-cell function. *Surgery* 1997;122:146–152.

24. Lyons A, Kelly JL, Rodrick ML, et al. Major injury induces increased production of interleukin-10 by cells of the immune system with a negative impact on resistance to infection. *Ann Surg* 1997;226:450–458.

25. Shoup M, Weisenberger JM, Wang JL, et al. Mechanisms of neutropenia involving myeloid maturation arrest in burn sepsis. *Ann Surg* 1998;228:112–122.

26. Munster AM. Alterations of the host defense mechanism in burns. *Surg Clin North Am* 1970;50:1217–1225.

27. Bjerknes R, Vindenes H. Neutrophil dysfunction after thermal injury—alteration of phagolysosomal acidification in patients with large burns. *J Trauma* 1989;15:71–81.

28. Babcock GF, Alexander JW, Warden GD. Flow cytometric analysis of neutrophil subsets in thermally injured patients developing infection. *Clin Exp Immunol* 1990;54:117–125.

29. Vindenes HA, Bjerknes R. Impaired actin polymerization and depolymerization in neutrophils from patients with thermal injury. *Burns* 1997;23:131–136.

30. Koller M, Konig W, Brom J. et al. Studies on the mechanisms of granulocyte dysfunctions in severely burned patients—evidence for altered leukotriene generation. *J Trauma* 1989;29:43–45.

31. Ono Y, Kunii O, Suzuki H, et al. Opsonic acitivity of sera and blister fluid from severely burned patients evaluated by a chemiluminescence method. *Microbiol Immunol* 1994;38:373–377.

32. Utoh J, Utsunomiya T, Imamura T, et al. Complement activation and neutrophil dysfunction in burned patients with sepsis—a study of two cases. *Jpn J Surg* 1989;19:462–467.

33. Balogh D, Lammer H, Kornberger E, et al. Neopterin plasma levels in burn patients. *Burns* 1992;18:185–188.

34. Moore FD Jr, Davis CF. Monocyte activation after burns and endotoxemia. *J Surg Res* 1989;46:350–354.

35. Gibbons RA, Martinez OM, Lim RC, et al. Reduction in HLA-DR, HLA-DQ, and HLA-DP expression by Leu-M3+ cells. *Clin Exp Immunol* 1989;5:371–735.

36. Zhou D, Munster AM, Winchurch RA. Inhibitory effects of interleukin 6 on immunity: possible implications in burns. *Arch Surg* 1992;127:65–69.

37. Organ BC, Antonacci AC, Chio J, et al. Changes in lymphocyte number and phenotype in seven lymphoid compartments after thermal injury. *Ann Surg* 1988; 210:78–89.

38. Dietich EA, Xu D, Qi L. Different lymphocyte compartments respond differently to mitogenic stimulation after thermal injury. *Ann Surg* 1990;211:72–77.

39. Maldonado MD, Venturoli A, Franco A, et al. Specific changes in peripheral blood lymphocyte phenotype from burn patients: probable origin of the thermal injury-related lymphocytopenia. *Burns* 1991;17:188–192.

40. Gadd MA, Hansbrough JF, Hoyt DB, et al. Defective T-cell surface antigen expression after mitogen stimulation: an index of lymphocyte dysfunction after controlled murine injury. *Ann Surg* 1989;29:112–118.

41. Hansbrough JF, Zapata-Sirvent R, Hoyt D. Postburn immune suppression: an inflammatory response to the burn wound? *J Trauma* 1990;30:671–675.

42. Noelle RJ, Snow EC. T Helper cell-dependent B cell activation. *FASEB J* 1991;5:2770–2776.

43. Kagan RJ, Bratescu A, Jonason O, et al. The relationship between the percentage of circulating B cells, corticosteroid levels, and other immunologic parameters in thermally injured patients. *J Trauma* 1989;29: 208–213.

44. Schluter B, Konig W, Koller M, et al. Differential regulation of T- and B-lymphocyte activation in severely burned patients. *J Trauma* 1991;31:239–246.

45. Faist E, Ertel W, Baker CC, et al. Terminal B-cell maturation and immunoglobulin (Ig) synthesis *in vitro* in patients with major injury. *J Trauma* 1989;29:2–9.

46. Cook N. Methicillin-resistant *Staphylococcus aureus* versus the burn patient. *Burns* 1998;24:91–98.

47. Reardon CM, Brown TP, Stephenson AJ, et al. Methicillin-resistant *Staphylococcus aureus* in burns patients—why all the fuss? *Burns* 1998;24:393–397.

48. Childs C, Edwards-Jones V, Heathcote DM, et al. Patterns of *Staphylococcus aureus* colonization, toxin production, immunity and illness in burned children. *Burns* 1994;20:514–521.

49. Lesseva M, Girgitzova BP, Bojadjiev C. Beta-hemolytic streptococcal infections in burned patients. *Burns* 1994;20:422–425.

50. Gruteke P, van Belkum A, Schouls LM, et al. Outbreak of group A streptococci in a burn center: use of pheno- and genotypic procedures for strain tracking. *J Clin Microbiol* 1996;34:114–118.

51. Ridgway EJ, Allen KD. Clustering of group A streptococcal infections on a burn unit: important lessons in outbreak management. *J Hosp Infect* 1993;25: 173–182.

52. Law EJ, Blecher K, Still JM. Enterococcal infection as cause of morbidity and mortality in patients with burns. *J Burn Care Rehabil* 1994;15:236–239.

53. Lai KK, Kelley AL, Melvin ZS, et al. Failure to eradicate vancomycin-resistant enterococci in a university hospital and the cost of barrier precautions. *Infect Control Hosp Epidemiol* 1998;19:647–652.

54. Larkin JM, Moylan JA. Tetanus following a minor burn. *J Trauma* 1975;15:546–548.

55. Sherman RT. The prevention and treatment of tetanus in the burn patient. *Surg Clin North Am* 1970;50: 1277–1281.

56. Baron P, Traber LD, Traber DL, et al. Gut failure and translocation following burn and sepsis. *J Surg Res* 1994;57:197–204.

57. Fleming RY, Zeigler ST, Walton MA, et al. Influence of burn size on the incidence of contamination of burn wounds by fecal organisms. *J Burn Care Rehabil* 1991;12:510–515.

58. Konigova R, Konickova Z, Bouska I. Clinical forms of endotoxin in burns. *Scand J Plast Reconstr Surg* 1979; 13:61–62.

59. Ljunghusen O, Lundahl J, Nettelblad H, et al. Endotoxemia and complement activation after severe burn injuries—effect on leukocytes, soluble selectins, and inflammatory cytokines. *Inflammation* 1996;20:229–241.

60. Desai MH, Herndon DN, Abston S. *Candida* infection in massively burned patients. *J Trauma* 1987;27: 1186–1188.

61. Sheridan RL, Weber JM, Budkevich LG, et al. Candidemia in pediatric patients with burns. *J Burn Care Rehabil* 1995;16:440–443.

62. Linnemann CC Jr, MacMillan BG. Viral infections in pediatric burn patients. *Am J Dis Child* 1981;135: 750–753.

63. Deepe GS Jr, MacMillan BC, Linnemann CC Jr. Unexplained fever in burned patients due to cytomegalovirus infection. *JAMA* 1982;248:2299–301.

64. Kealey GP, Bale JF, Strauss RG, et al. Cytomegalovirus infection in burn patients. *J Burn Care Rehabil* 1987;8:543–545.

65. Coursaget P, Lesage G, Simpson B, et al. Incidence of hepatitis C virus infection in burn patients: detection of anti-C100, anti-C33c and anti-Core antibodies. *Biomed Pharmacother* 1991;45:445–449.

66. Rutan RL, Bjarnason DL, Desai MH, et al. Incidence of HIV seroconversion in paediatric burn patients. *Burns* 1992;18:216–219.

67. Hayden FG, Himmel HN, Heggers JP. Herpes virus infections in burn patients. *Chest* 1994;106(Suppl): 15S–21S.

68. Bourdarias B, Perro G, Cutillas M, et al. Herpes simplex virus infection in burned patients: epidemiology of 11 cases. *Burns* 1996;22:287–290.

69. Byers RJ, Hasleton PS, Quigley A, et al. Pulmonary herpes simplex in burns patients. *Eur Respir J* 1996; 9:2313–2317.

70. Weintrub WH, Lilly AB, Randolph JG. A chickenpox epidemic in a pediatric burn unit. *Surgery* 1974;76: 490–494.

71. Sheridan RL, Weber JM, Pasternak MM, et al. A 15-year experience with varicella infections in a pediatric burn unit. *Burns* 1999;25:353–356.

72. Heggers JP, Muller MJ, Elwood E, et al. Ascariasis pneumonitis: a potentially fatal complication in smoke inhalation injury. *Burns* 1995;21:149–51.

73. Hegger JP, Robson MC. Infection control in burn patients. *Clin Plast Surg* 1986, 13:39–47.

74. Pruitt BA Jr, McManus AT, Kim SH, et al. Burn infections: current status. *World J Surg* 1998, 22:135–45.

75. Heggers JP, Linares H, Edgar P, et al. Treatment of Infections in Burns. In: Herndon DN, ed. *Total burn care.* Philadelphia: WB Saunders, 1996:98–135.

76. Neely AN, Smith WL, Warden GD. Efficacy of a rise in C-reactive protein serum levels as an early indicator of sepsis in burned children. *J Burn Care Rehabil* 1998;19:102–105.

77. Beard CH, Ribeiro CD, Jones DM. The bacteremia associated with burns surgery. *Br J Surg* 1975;62: 638–641.

78. Hamory BH. Nosocomial sepsis related to intravascular access. *Crit Care Nurs J* 1989;11:58–65.

79. Sasaki TM, Welch OW. Herndon DN, et al. Burn wound manipulation induced bacteremia. *J Trauma* 1979;19:46–48.

80. Baskin TW, Rosenthal A, Pruitt BA. Acute bacterial endocarditis: a silent source of sepsis in the burn patient. *Ann Surg* 1976;184:618.

81. Cartotto RC, Macdonald DB, Wasan SM. Acute bacterial endocarditis following burns: case report and review. *Burns* 1998;24:363–373.

82. Albertson S, Greenhalgh DG, Breeden MP, et al. Cardiac abnormalities in children with burns: an autopsy analysis. *J Burn Care Rehabil* 1994;15:401–404.

83. Stein JM, Pruitt BA Jr. Suppurative thrombophlebitis: a lethal iatrogenic disease. *N Engl J Med* 1970, 282: 1452–1455.

84. Mills DC II, Roberts LW, Mason AD Jr, et al. Suppurative chondritis: its incidence, prevention, and treatment in burn patients. *Plast Reconstr Surg* 1988;82: 267–276.

85. Bowers BL, Purdue GF, Hunt JL. Paranasal sinusitis in burn patients following nasotracheal intubation. *Arch Surg* 1991;126:1411–1412.

86. Shiranin KZ, Pruitt BA Jr, Mason AD Jr. The influence of inhalation injury and pneumonia on burn mortality. *Ann Surg* 1987;205:82–87.

87. Schlager T, Sadler J, Weber D, et al. Hospital-acquired infections in pediatric burn patients. *South Med J* 1994;87:481–484.

88. Evans EB. Musculoskeletal changes secondary to thermal burns. In: Herndon DN, ed. *Total burn care.* Philadelphia: WB Saunders, 1996:265–278.

89. Winkelman MD, Galloway PG. Central nervous system complications of thermal burns. A postmortem study of 139 patients. *Medicine (Baltimore)* 1992;71: 271–283.

90. Teplitz C. The pathology of burns and the fundamentals of burn wound sepsis. In: Artz CP, Moncrief JA, Pruitt BA Jr, eds. *Burns: a team approach.* Philadelphia: WB Saunders, 1979:45.

91. Pruitt BA, Foley FD. The use of biopsies in burn patient care. *Surgery* 1973;73:887–897.

92. Parks DH, Linares HA, Thompson PD. Surgical management of burn wound sepsis. *Surg Gynecol Obstet* 1982;153:374–376.

93. Heggers JP, Robson MC, eds. *Quantitative bacteriology: its role in the armamentarium of the surgeon,* 1st ed. Boca Raton, FL: CRC Press, 1991:1–139.

94. Renz BM, Sherman R. Exposure of buttock burn wounds to stool in scald-abused infants and children: stool-staining of eschar and burn wound sepsis. *Am Surg* 1993;59:379–383.

95. Koller J, Orsag M. Our experience with the use of cerium sulphadiazine in the treatment of extensive burns. *Acta Chir Plast* 1998;40:73–75.

96. Heggers JP, Robson MC. The emergence of silver sulfadiazine resistant *Pseudomonas aeruginosa. Burns* 1978;5:184–187.

97. Mendelson JA. The management of burns under conditions of limited resources using topical aqueous Sulfamylon (mafenide) hydrochloride spray. *J Burn Care Rehabil* 1997;18:238–244.

98. Kucan JO, Smoot EC. Five percent mafenide acetate solution in the treatment of thermal injuries. *J Burn Care Rehabil* 1993;14:158–153.

99. Desai MH, Rutal ML, Heggers JP, et al. The role of gentamicin iontophoresis in the treatment of burned ears. *J Burn Care Rehabil* 1991;12:521–524.

100. Strock LL, Lee M, Rutan RL, et al. Topical Bactroban (Mupirocin): efficacy in treating MRSA wounds infected with methicillin-resistant staphylococci. *J Burn Care Rehabil* 1990;11:454–459.

101. Heggers JP, Robson MC, Herndon DN, et al. The efficacy of nystatin combined with topical microbial agents in the treatment of burn wound sepsis. *J Burn Care Rehabil* 1989;10:508–511.

102. Barrett JP, Ramzy PI, Heggers JP, et al. Topical nystatin powder in severe burns: a new treatment for angioinvasive fungal infections refractory to other topical and systemic agents. *Burns* 1999;25:505–508.

103. Heggers JP, Sazy JA, Stenberg BD, et al. Bactericidal and wound healing properties of sodium hypochlorite: the 1991 Lindberg Award. *J Burn Care Rehabil* 1991;12:420–424.

104. Krizek TJ, Davis JH, DesPrez JD, et al. Topical therapy of burns—experimental evaluation. *Plast Reconstr Surg* 1967;39:248–255.

105. Lawrence JC, Cason JS, Kidson A. Evaluation of phenoxetol-chlorhexidine cream as prophylactic agent in burns. *Lancet* 1982;24:524–525.

106. Moncrief JA. Topical therapy for control of bacteria in the burn wound. *World J Surg* 1978;2:151–165.

107. Tredget EE, Shankowsky HA, Groeneveld A, et al. A matched-pair, randomized study evaluating the efficacy and safety of acticoat silver-coated dressing for the treatment of burn wounds. *J Burn Care Rehabil* 1998;19:531–537.

108. Bugmann P, Taylor S, Gyger D, et al. A silicone-coated nylon dressing reduces healing time in burned pediatric patients in comparison with standard sulfadiazine treatment: a prospective randomized trial. *Burns* 1998; 24:609–612.

109. Gotschall CS, Morrison MI, Eichelberger MR. Prospective, randomized study of the efficacy of Mepitel on children with partial-thickness scalds. *J Burn Care Rehabil* 1998;19:279–283.

110. Nagoba BS, Gandhi RC, Wadher BJ, et al. Citric acid treatment of severe electric burns complicated by multiple antibiotic resistant *Pseudomonas aeruginosa. Burns* 1998;24:481–483.

111. Subrahmanyam M. Honey dressing versus boiled potato peel in the treatment of burns: a prospective randomized study. *Burns* 1996;22:491–493.

112. Rodgers GL, Fisher MC, Lo A, et al. Study of antibiotic prophylaxis during burn wound debridement in children. *J Burn Care Rehabil* 1997;18:342–346.

113. Mackie DP, van Hertum WA, Schumburg T, et al. Prevention of infection in burns: preliminary experience with selective decontamination of the digestive tract in patients with extensive injuries. *J Trauma* 1992;32: 570–575.

114. Mian EU, Gianfaldoni R, Mian M. The use of intravenous immunoglobulins in patients with severe burns. *Clin Ter* 1992;141:75–81.

115. Waymack JP, Jenkins ME, Alexander JW, et al. A prospective trial of prophylactic intravenous immune globulin for the prevention of infections in severely burned patients. *Burns* 1989;15:71–76.

116. Munster AM, Moran KT, Thupari J, et al. Prophylactic intravenous immunoglobulin replacement in high-risk burn patients. *J Burn Care Rehabil* 1987;8: 376–380.

117. Stuttmann R, Hebebrand D, Hartert M, et al. [Prevention with pseudomonas immune globulin in burn injury patients with inhalation trauma: does it have an effect on lung function and outcome]? *Klin Wochenschr* 1991;69(Suppl 26):168–177.

118. Jones EB. Prophylactic anti-lipopolysaccharide freeze-dried plasma in major burns: a double blind controlled trial. *Burns* 1995;21:267–272.

119. Weber JM, Sheridan RL, Pasternack MS, et al. Nosocomial infections in pediatric patients with burns. *Am J Infect Control* 1997;25:195–201.

120. Tredget EE, Shankowsky HA, Joffe AM, et al. Epidemiology of infections with *Pseudomonas aeruginosa* in burn patients: the role of hydrotherapy. *Clin Infect Dis* 1992;15:941–949.
121. McManus AT, Mason AD Jr, McManus WF, et al. A decade of reduced gram-negative infections and mortality associated with improved isolation of burned patients. *Arch Surg* 1994;129:1306–1309.
122. van Rijn RR, Kuijper EC, Kreis RW. Seven-year experience with a 'quarantine and isolation unit' for patients with burns: a retrospective analysis. *Burns* 1997;23:345–348.

PART III

Infectious Complications as Defined by Anatomic Location

17

Assessment and Management of Suspected Infection in Neutropenic Patients

Jonathan A. McCullers and Jerry L. Shenep

Department of Infectious Diseases, St. Jude Children's Research Hospital, Memphis, Tennessee 38105; Department of Pediatrics, Division of Infectious Diseases, University of Tennessee, Memphis, Tennessee 38103

HISTORICAL PERSPECTIVE

The fundamental knowledge underlying our approach to infection in the neutropenic cancer patient can be traced back to the end of the nineteenth century, when physicians first began to recognize that bacteria in the blood were responsible for some illnesses. A German pathologist, Felix Birch-Hirschfeld, demonstrated in 1872 that bacteria injected into the blood could be found within leukocytes (1). In 1874, the Danish pathologist Peter Panum hypothesized that leukocytes destroy invading bacteria (1). A decade later, the Russian pathologist Élie Metchnikoff coined the term *phagocytosis* to describe the process by which leukocytes ingest and digest bacteria (1). Metchnikoff was subsequently given credit as the founder of the phagocytic theory of immunity. Despite the early appreciation of these basic concepts, it was not until the landmark article by Bodey and colleagues in 1966 that the relationship between neutropenia and infection was rigorously documented (2). This study established that the risk of infection increased perceptibly when the absolute neutrophil count (ANC) dropped below 1,000 cells/μL and increased markedly when the ANC was less than 500 cells/μL. Patients with ANCs less than 100 cells/μL were at even greater risk compared with patients with ANCs between 100 and 500 cells/μL.

Bodey's work provided essential quantitative information to support what at the time was a radical departure from the accepted practice of infectious diseases. Rather than await culture evidence of infection, and direct therapy according to the identification of bacterial isolates, Schimpff and colleagues administered therapy empirically to neutropenic cancer patients, even though life-threatening infection was not yet clinically apparent (3). Using this approach resulted in a significant decrease in the mortality of patients with *Pseudomonas aeruginosa* infection. This sentinel study encouraged other investigations of this approach (4–7), and soon the use of empiric therapy became accepted practice in the febrile, neutropenic patient, leading to increased survival of the cancer patient in the 1970s (8).

In the setting of significant ototoxicity and nephrotoxicity associated with aminoglycoside therapy, the issue of the optimal duration of empiric therapy of the neutropenic patient with fever soon came to the forefront. Two studies addressing this issue were performed at the National Cancer Institute in the 1970s and continue to influence practice today.

In the initial study, 33 neutropenic cancer patients who had become afebrile following prolonged fever were randomized to continue or discontinue empiric therapy after 7 days of treatment (9). None of the 16 patients who continued therapy developed problems. In contrast, 7 of the 17 patients who stopped therapy developed febrile illnesses. There were five culture-positive infections in this latter group, including two that were fatal.

The second study involved 50 neutropenic patients with cancer who were persistently febrile after 7 days of therapy, although no infection could be identified. These patients were randomized to one of three treatment arms: antibiotic therapy stopped, antibiotic therapy continued, or antibiotic therapy continued with the addition of amphotericin B (10). Of the 16 patients who stopped antibiotic therapy, 9 developed infections (6 developed septic shock, and 1 developed disseminated fungal infection), an outcome concordant with the results of the first study. With continued antibiotic therapy, 6 of 16 patients developed overt infections, including five that were caused by fungi. In contrast, no bacterial or conventional fungal infections occurred in the 18 patients who continued antibiotics with the addition of amphotericin B; however, one patient in this third group developed disseminated cytomegalovirus infection, and another developed fatal pneumonia as a result of *Pseudallescheria boydii* infection, a rare fungal pathogen resistant to amphotericin B. Despite the occurrence of these two opportunistic diseases, infections in this group were significantly reduced compared with infections in the group where antibiotic therapy was discontinued ($p = 0.013$). These two studies are the basis for our continued reluctance today to discontinue empiric therapy in the persistently neutropenic patient.

Although neutropenia occurs in circumstances other than cancer and chemotherapy, the vast majority of the medical literature addressing issues in febrile neutropenia is based on studies in neutropenic cancer patients. Therefore, this chapter is based largely on studies of neutropenic cancer patients. Virtually all the principles of assessment and management of neutropenic cancer patients appear to be applicable to neutropenic patients with underlying conditions other than cancer. Nonetheless, it is important to recognize that neutropenia may be only one component of a patient's immunologic deficit. For example, management of infectious complications in neutropenic bone marrow transplantation patients extends beyond management that targets neutropenia.

PATHOGENESIS OF INFECTION IN THE NEUTROPENIC PATIENT

Although the degree of neutropenia is the predominant determinant of the risk of infection in the cancer patient, several other factors strongly influence the likelihood of infection. The rate of increased risk of infection becomes greater with time. Thus, with prolonged neutropenia, the risk for infection is not linear with time but is greatest in the latter period of neutropenia (11–14). Dynamically, rapidly developing neutropenia appears to carry a greater risk of infection than neutropenia that develops more slowly, although this relation could be merely a marker for increased mucosal barrier disruption associated with conditions that cause rapid development of neutropenia (2,15).

Mucositis may be an underappreciated risk factor for neutropenic cancer patients. In one analysis of the risk of infection in pediatric cancer patients, the risk of infection correlated with the degree of mucositis better than with the degree of neutropenia (16). Mucositis, including inflammation of the oral, nasopharyngeal, esophageal, and gastrointestinal mucous membranes, permits access of organisms to the bloodstream, and the lack of neutrophils allows microbial proliferation. Cytarabine is especially implicated in damage to the oral mucosa, which helps explain how this agent predisposes in particular to viridans streptococci, the major group of organisms colonizing the oral cavity (17–20). Mucositis associated with cancer chemotherapy may explain in part the significantly higher risk for infection of the cancer patient compared with that of the patient with congenital or acquired chronic neutropenia. The integument is another important barrier to infection that is frequently compromised in cancer patients, most often by intravascular catheters. The observation that most pathogenic isolates in cancer patients originate in the patient's own flora reflects the importance of the skin and mucous membranes in the pathogenesis of infection in these patients (21).

Intravascular catheters are commonly related to infections in the neutropenic patient. Intravascular catheter-related infections can be classified into four categories based on the site of infection and its pathogenesis. An *exit site* infection is a cellulitis that occurs within the tissue immediately surrounding the exit site. A *tunnel-tract* infection is an infection that extends along the tunnel tract, originating either at the exit site or within the tunnel. An *intraluminal* infection is a focus of infection within the lumen of the catheter, which therefore has a direct connection to the circulation. A fourth category of catheter-related infection is the *intravascular pericatheter* infection in which fibrin and clot adhering to the tip or outer surface of the catheter support a nidus of infection that has direct contact with the circulation. An important distinction between this category and the intraluminal infection category is that microorganisms may not be concentrated in blood drawn through the catheter lumen in the case of the pericatheter infection.

The cancer patient frequently suffers from malnutrition as a consequence of both the cancer and its treatment. The relative role of malnutrition regarding the risk of infection is not well defined in this setting, but malnutrition adversely affects immune function (22) and likely contributes to the infection risk to some degree.

The particular type of cancer and the remission status of the cancer affect both the risk of infection and the pattern of infecting organisms. For example, leukemia patients in relapse are at higher risk than leukemia patients in remission independent of the ANC, and patients with leukemia are at higher risk than are patients with lymphoma or solid tumors independent of the ANC (23). Infection is not only more common in the neutropenic patient, but the rapidity at which it progresses and the level of severity that is attained are generally exacerbated in the setting of neutropenia (24–26).

INITIAL ASSESSMENT OF THE FEBRILE NEUTROPENIC PATIENT

In general, about 10% to 20% of neutropenic patients who develop fever but are otherwise well will have bacteremia, and an equal number may be found to have a focus of infection during their febrile episode. Thus, most patients with febrile episodes during neutropenia will not have a documented infection (27–29), but this observation does not necessarily indicate an absence of infection. Untreated, many more febrile neutropenic patients would manifest infection at the cost of increased morbidity and mortality (30). The ability to identify accurately which neutropenic patient is infected has remained an elusive goal (31). Given the lack of the ability to target therapy, the outstanding success of empiric therapy in reducing infectious complications in febrile neutropenic patients with regimens having low toxicity and acceptable cost is all the more remarkable.

Fever is a cardinal and frequently lone sign of infection in the neutropenic patient. In nonneutropenic patients, acute fever in the absence of other signs or symptoms is commonplace and in isolation is not alarming. Therefore, precise definitions and measurement of fever are generally not critical in this setting. In contrast, the febrile, neutropenic patient with no other symptoms or signs usually will be admitted to the hospital and receive broad-spectrum antibiotics. Thus, the determination of fever in the setting of neutropenia has particular significance. A temperature that is above the normal range for a given neutropenic patient is generally cause for instituting empiric therapy. Practically, the clinician will not be able to determine a given patient's normal temperature range, and in the past clinicians have varied considerably in the threshold temperature that is considered to represent fever. Recent guidelines (32) define fever as a single oral temperature greater than 38.3°C (101°F), or 38.0°C (101.4°F) over at least 1 hour. Although the individual patient may vary considerably, an axillary temperature is a median of 0.6°C lower than an oral temperature, whereas a rectal temperature is a median of 0.6°C higher than an oral temperature (use of the rectum for temperature measurement is usually avoided in the neutropenic patient) (33). Core body temperature is similar to rectal temperature. Measurements using tympanic thermometry are highly dependent on the particular instrument used and the mode in which the instrument is operated (33). When there is a question regarding measurement of temperature, use of an oral glass mercury thermometer held under the tongue for 10 minutes in a patient who has had no oral intake for at least 30 minutes yields a highly reproducible result. Fever in the neutropenic patient should not be attributed to reactions to blood products, neoplasms, or drugs, including hematopoietic growth factors, because needed therapy may be delayed with potentially disastrous consequences (30,34). It is also important to note that infection can occur in the neutropenic host without fever; the absence of fever should not delay therapy when infection is suspected.

Neutropenia is usually defined as an absolute neutrophil count below 500/μL of blood or 1,000/μL with a predicted decline to below 500/μL (4,32,35). An ANC below 100/μL, an ANC less than 500/μL for more than 10 days, and a rapidly falling ANC are particularly associated with the occurrence of infection.

Customary signs and symptoms of localized infection may be diminished or even absent in the setting of neutropenia (25,31,36–39). In the neutropenic patient, meningeal signs are not reliably present in meningitis, and inflammation may not be apparent in infections of the skin, subcutaneous tissues, and mucous membranes. Thus, even minor signs must be considered potential indicators of infection. On the other hand, pain does not seem to be diminished in neutropenia to the degree that inflammation is, and therefore pain becomes a more important symptom in neutropenic patients (36). A history of tooth pain may be indicative of an odontogenic infection (40). Dysphagia and retrosternal pain may point toward esophagitis. (41). Pain over the sinuses or chest pain may be an indicator of *Aspergillus* infection (42–44). Perianal pain should be of particular concern because it is frequently indicative of perirectal cellulitis, a serious complication of neutropenia (37,38,45). Myalgias and arthralgias occasionally precede the diagnosis of disseminated fungal infection (46–48). A history of fever, chills, or rigors within 2 hours following accessing and flushing of an indwelling vascular catheter should increase suspicion of an intraluminal catheter-related infection (49).

The physical examination generally can be focused on common sites of infection, including the oral cavity, skin, nails, catheter exit sites, lungs, abdomen, and perirectal area (24). Careful and thorough examination of the oral cavity is an important part of the physical examination of the neutropenic patient because the oral mucosa is thought to be one of the most common portals of entry for microbes in systemic infection (16–20,50). The presence of redness, tenderness, swelling, ulcers, aphthae, white plaques, vesicles, pseudomembranes, and hemorrhage may be indicative of localized disease requiring treatment (e.g., candidiasis or herpetic stomatitis) and may indicate a portal for systemic infection (40). Careful examination of the skin and nails may reveal clues of serious infection. Scattered or isolated small macular papular lesions may represent septic emboli of bacterial or fungal origin. Ecthyma gangrenosum, a necrotic skin lesion most commonly associated with *P. aeruginosa* infections, has a predilection for the axillary and inguinal regions (26,30,51). Ecthyma should not be presumed to be caused by *P. aeruginosa* because similar lesions have been described, not only with *Aeromonas* and non-*aeruginosa* species of *Pseudomonas* (52) but also with mycoses, including *Candida* (53), *Aspergillus* (54), *Mucor* (55,56), and *Fusarium* (46) sp. Because a rather ordinary appearing skin lesion or rash may be indicative of septicemia or disseminated fungal infection, consideration should be given to performance of a skin biopsy for any lesion of questionable etiology (57–59). Skin lesions that occur in association with pulmonary disease may be indicative of certain opportunistic pathogens (e.g., *Cryptococcus, Nocardia, Fusarium)*, and skin biopsy may avoid more invasive procedures such as an open lung biopsy (52,56). As in the immunocompetent host, skin rashes also may be a manifestation of viral infection, which are of special concern in the immunocompromised host. Although many chemotherapeutic agents have cutaneous manifestations, consideration should be given to possible infectious causes before attributing the etiology of a rash to an antineoplastic agent or antibiotic. The nails should be examined carefully for the presence of discoloration or tenderness because they are frequently sites of fungal infection, especially with dermatophytes or molds such as *Aspergillus* and *Fusarium* (60). Onychomycosis often presents as a spreading white hue under the proximal nail bed, with or without accompanying paronychia (61).

Particular attention should be focused on breaks in the integument, both surgical and accidental. Catheter exit sites should be examined for the presence of erythema, tenderness, vesicles, or drainage. Atypical mycobacteria should be considered in culture-negative exit-site infections, especially if the drainage has a greenish tint or the infection has had a subacute course (62, 63). The tunnel tract should be inspected and palpated from the exit site to the insertion site. Erythema, tenderness, and swelling are usually indicative of infection, although tenderness may be the only symptom or sign present in a neutropenic host. Bone-marrow biopsy sites should be inspected for erythema and palpated for tenderness and fluctuance. The perirectal area should be checked for erythema, fissures, swelling, hemorrhoids, tenderness, and fluctuance (37,38,45). During neutropenia, a gentle digital examination should be performed only if the potential impact on management justifies the slight but not negligible risk of mucosal injury, which could lead to cellulitis or bacteremia.

Cultures should be obtained while the initial dose of antibiotic(s) is being prepared. A minimum of two blood cultures from separate locations should be obtained when feasible. If an intravascular catheter is present, blood for culture should be obtained through every catheter lumen as well as from a peripheral site. The time of collection and source of each sample should be identified (e.g., 8:00 a.m., red lumen). When obtained before antibiotic therapy, quantitative cultures frequently permit distinction of catheter-related intraluminal and periluminal infections from those having another focus of infection (64,65). This information may be helpful in cases where infection is focused in a single lumen of a triple-lumen catheter because delivery of antibiotics through the infected lumen may be necessary for treatment to be effective. Any suspected site of infection, including the oral cavity, wounds, and catheter exit sites, should be cultured. If there are signs or symptoms localizing to the oral cavity, cultures for bacteria and fungi (especially *Candida*) and herpes simplex virus are indicated. Surface cultures of areas of cellulitis have limited value (e.g., isolation of *P. aeruginosa* on the surface of an area of perirectal cellulitis does not necessarily indicate that this is the causative agent, but coverage should generally include any pathogenic isolate at the site of infection); when feasible, a skin biopsy is preferable. Suspected catheter exit-site infections should be cultured for atypical mycobacteria (62,63) as well as for routine bacterial and fungal organisms. Infrequently, herpes simplex may cause catheter exit-site infection, and culture for this virus should be obtained when its presence is suspected on the basis of physical examination or concomitant orolabial herpes simplex infection or in cases when initial cultures fail to yield an etiology. If the upper respiratory tract is a potential source, cultures and stains for respiratory viral pathogens are indicated. If the genitourinary tract is suspect, a urine culture is indicated, but catheterization for culture generally should be avoided because of the increased risk of inducing infection during neutropenia.

The value and use of routine surface cultures are among the most controversial issues in the management of neutropenic patients with unexplained fever. Because a large portion of infections are derived from the patient's own microbial flora, knowledge of the composition of the flora is potentially helpful (66,67); however, management of the specific patient cannot be guided solely by the results of surveillance cultures. Empiric therapy is generally initiated before the results of surface cultures are available, and the presence of pathogens on surface cultures does not reliably predict infection with these organisms or exclude nondetected organisms (21,66,67). On the other hand, knowledge of the presence of colonizing multiresistant bacterial pathogens, *P. aeruginosa,* commonly pathogenic *Aspergillus* spp. (*flavus, fumigatus, niger,* and *terreus* are the common pathogenic species), *Candida tropicalis* and *Candida krusei* may reasonably influence the clinician's management of a patient. For example, because *C. tropicalis* is about tenfold more likely than *Candida albicans* to invade systemically during empiric therapy of fever in the neutropenic cancer patient (68–74), one might elect to start empiric amphotericin B sooner rather than later when *C. tropicalis* is present. Likewise, because *C. krusei* organisms are resistant to fluconazole, this drug generally would be avoided if colonization were detected (75). These limited advantages of routine surveillance cultures must be weighed against the substantial cost and time required for their collection and processing (76). For epidemiologic investigations or targeted infection-control processes, the use of surveillance cultures is more widely accepted (77,78).

Until recently, a routine chest radiograph was recommended for all patients with neutropenia and unexplained fever; however, several newer studies cast doubt on the utility of this practice (79–83). A chest radiograph should be obtained in patients with respiratory symptoms at the onset of fever or if respiratory symptoms develop during the neutropenic episode. Computed tomography of the chest and abdomen is especially helpful in identifying disseminated fungal disease (84,85). Ultrasound, magnetic resonance imaging, and radionucleotide scans may be useful in specific situations; however, infection can be present in neutropenic patients despite negative results from all these tests, and the absence of a specific finding from a diagnostic imaging study does not exclude the possibility of infection.

Although continuing to hold promise, development of rapid diagnostic tests for identifying infecting microorganisms has yet to achieve widespread clinical utility. Newer modalities, such as the polymerase chain reaction, an assay on whole blood for the 16S ribosomal subunit common to many invasive fungi, and specific antigenic tests that indicate active infection by opportunistic pathogens are under study and warrant continued research.

COMMON PATHOGENS IN NEUTROPENIC PATIENTS

Because empiric therapy of the neutropenic patient is targeted to the likely pathogens, knowledge of the common pathogens in neutropenic patients is essential. Given that neutropenia is the overriding risk factor for infection in the neutropenic host, the pattern of infecting microorganisms is by and large similar in adults and children alike, regardless of locale. There are some notable exceptions to this generalization. The incidence of viridans streptococcal sepsis varies significantly from center to center, related in part to the fact that this infection is more common in neutropenic children than in neutropenic adults and because of its association with high-dose cytarabine, based on the prevalence of use of this chemotherapeutic modality in a particular institution (17–20). Histoplasmosis and coccid-

TABLE 17.1. *Common microbial causes of fever in the neutropenic host*

Microbial category	Initial pathogens	Secondary pathogens
Gram-positive bacteria	Coagulase-negative staphylococci	Coagulase-negative staphylococci
	Viridans streptococci	Viridans streptococci
	Staphylococcus aureus	*Staphylococcus aureus*
	Stretopcoccus pyogenes	*Enterococcus* sp.
	Enterococcus sp.	*Corynebacterium* sp.
	Corynebacterium sp.	
	Streptococcus pneumoniae	
Gram-negative bacteria	*Escherichia coli*	*Escherichia coli*
	Pseudomonas aeruginosa	*Pseudomonas aeruginosa*
	Klebsiella sp.	*Klebsiella* sp.
	Enterobacter sp.	*Enterobacter* sp.
	Acinetobacter sp.	
	Stenotrophomonas maltophilia	
Anaerobic bacteria	*Bacillus cereus*	*Bacillus cereus*
	Bacillus sp.	*Bacillus* sp.
	Clostridium septicum	*Clostridium septicum*
	Clostridium sp.	*Clostridium* sp.
	Capnocytophaga sp.	*Capnocytophaga* sp.
Fungi	*Pneumocystis carinii*	*Candida* spp.
	Candida spp.	*Aspergillus* sp.
	Cryptococcus neoformans	*Fusarium* sp.
	Histoplasma capsulatum	*Mucor* sp.
	Coccidioides immitis	*Rhizopus* sp.
	Aspergillus sp.	*Pseudallescheria boydii*
Viruses	Cytomegalovirus	Cytomegalovirus
	Herpes simplex virus	Herpes simplex
	Varicella zoster virus	Adenovirus
	Influenza virus	
	Parainfluenza virus	
	Respiratory syncytial virus	
	Adenovirus	
	Enterovirus	
	Coxsackie virus	
Protozoa	*Cryptosporidium parvum*	

ioidomycosis occur most commonly in neutropenic patients who live in the Mississippi and San Joaquin valleys, respectively, which are the endemic areas of the etiologic fungi. Atypical mycobacterial infections associated with use of intravascular catheters are common only in warm climates. Of greater significance, bacterial susceptibilities may vary from institution to institution. Thus, to some extent, the clinician must be familiar with the common infecting pathogens and their susceptibility patterns in the local center. Nonetheless, certain generalities are valid.

The pattern of infection changes markedly depending on the duration of prior antibiotic therapy. Therefore, it is useful to classify common pathogens into two categories (Table 17.1): those occurring prior to administration of broad-spectrum antibiotics (initial pathogens) and those occurring during empiric therapy (secondary pathogens).

Bacteria

Bacteria have consistently been the major initial infectious hazard and, together with fungi, are the most common cause of secondary infections in the neutropenic host (8,86). Updated from the previous edition of this textbook (87), Table 17.2 summarizes the bacterial pathogens isolated from 11,193 episodes of fever and neutropenia. As reported in 37 studies of empiric antibiotic therapy for febrile neutropenic patients over the last two decades (27,28,88–122), 2,213 occurrences of primary bacteremia and 177

TABLE 17.2. *Blood isolates in 11,193 episodes of fever and neutropenia[a]*

Study period	Primary infections		Secondary infections	
	1977–1985	1986–1995	1981–1985	1986–1995
No. patient episodes	2,946	8,247	954	3,037
No. bacteremias (%)	620	1,593	47	130
Gram-negative				
Escherichia coli	168 (27)	291 (18)	2 (4)	7 (5)
Pseudomonas aeruginosa	106 (17)	153 (10)	2 (4)	9 (7)
Klebsiella sp.	81 (13)	83 (5)	1	7
Enterobacter sp.	15	40	1	12
Other	50	114[b]	8	8[c]
Subtotal	420 (68)	681 (43)	14 (30)	43 (33)
Gram-positive				
Coagulase-negative staphylococci	45 (7)	312 (20)	8 (17)	41 (32)
Staphylococcus aureus	85 (14)	200 (13)	5 (11)	4 (3)
Streptococcus sp.	25 (13)	270 (31)[d]	1 (3)	11 (14)
Streptococcus pneumoniae	14	17	0	0
Corynebacterium sp.	10	24	8	8
Group D streptococci	7	22	9	12
Listeria monocytogenes	4	3	0	0
Other	3	34	0	0
Subtotal	193 (31)	882 (55)	31 (66)	76 (58)
Anaerobes				
Bacillus cereus	1	3	0	2
Bacillus sp.	2	3	0	1
Clostridium septicum	0	0	2	1
Clostridium sp.	2	5	0	1
Capnocytophaga sp.	0	3	0	3
Other	2	16	0	3
Subtotal	7 (1)	30 (2)	2 (4)	11 (9)

[a]Pooled data from 37 studies (1977 to 1995). See text for references.
[b]Most common isolates were *Proteus* sp. (n = 18), *Salmonella* sp. (n = 10), *Pseudomonas* sp. (n = 9), and *Serratia* sp. (n = 6).
[c]Most common isolate was *Stenotrophomonas maltophilia* (n = 6).
[d]Most common isolates were viridans streptococci (n = 131) or undefined (n = 139); absolute numbers are not available because of differences in reporting.

occurrences of secondary bacteremia (superinfections and breakthrough bacteremias) transpired during these episodes of febrile neutropenia. During this period, a major change has taken place in the relative frequency of the gram-negative rods compared with the gram-positive bacteria, with the latter becoming gradually more frequent (27,93,99,123–125). Gram-positive organisms now account for more than half of documented bacterial infections in febrile neutropenic patients, as opposed to fewer than one third just two decades ago. Potential reasons to account for this shift include the increased use of indwelling vascular catheters (126–128), the use of prophylactic antibiotic regimens for selective bowel decontamination (124–126,129), and the decreased antistaphylococcal activity of the third-generation cephalosporins commonly used in current empiric regimens compared with the activity of first-generation cephalosporins (126,130).

Roughly 60% of all gram-positive isolates are staphylococci, mainly coagulase-negative staphylococci (*Staphylococcus epidermidis* is the most common species), together with the considerably less common *Staphylococcus aureus* (Table 17.2). Coagulase negative staphylococci have increased in incidence more than gram-positive bacteria as a whole, whereas the incidence of *S. aureus* has remained relatively constant. Thus, coagulase-negative staphylococci, which at one time were considered nonpathogenic, account for a large portion of the increased occurrence of gram-positive bacterial infections (124,125,131). Although infections with coagulase-negative staphylococci are occasionally life threatening or even fatal (49,124), these bacteria typically do not cause fulminant infection. Most coagulase-negative staphylococcal isolates are methicillin resistant, whereas most *S. aureus* remain methicillin susceptible. *S. aureus* is becoming more resistant over time, however, with 30% or more of hospital strains being methicillin resistant, increasing to 50% during outbreaks (132–134). In addition, in some areas, 10% or more of community isolates of *S. aureus* are methicillin resistant.

Perhaps creating the most concern about gram-positive bacterial infections in the neutropenic cancer patient is the emergence over the past two decades of viridans streptococci as major pathogens (7–20,135). Further heightening this concern is the increasing resistance to penicillin observed among these diverse and ubiquitous microorganisms (135). Sepsis with viridans streptococci may be complicated by multiorgan failure or the adult respiratory distress syndrome (ARDS) (136,137). Among pediatric patients, who are at increased risk of manifesting disease from this pathogen compared with adults, the manifestations may include prolonged high fever, severe pulmonary or cardiac failure, shock, encephalopathy, pneumonia, and renal impairment (135,137). Factors associated with viridans streptococcal infections include administration of cytarabine, which causes severe mucositis; use of certain prophylactic antibiotics, such as ciprofloxacin; and the presence of central venous catheters (17–20, 135). Apparently, because of mucosal disruption, herpes simplex has been associated with viridans streptococcal infections, and acyclovir has been advocated to reduce mucosal injury and therefore susceptibility to viridans streptococcal infections in this setting (138,139).

Other gram-positive bacteria that are important pathogens in neutropenic patients are *Streptococcus pneumoniae*, *Streptococcus pyogenes*, *Enterococcus faecalis* and *faecium*, and *Corynebacterium* sp. (Table 17.2). Enterococcal species are isolated more frequently as a cause of superinfection, especially in patients treated with cephalosporins (111,112). The emergence of vancomycin-resistant enterococcal strains has been problematic in many centers and presents difficulty in treatment and infection control (140–143). Concern that vancomycin resistance may spread to other pathogens led to a major effort to curtail the use of vancomycin based on the assumption that restricted use will lessen the chance of emergence of resistant organisms (144). *Corynebacterium jeikeium* has emerged as a pathogen in patients with prolonged neutropenia, prolonged hospitalization, multiple antibiotic treatment, and disruption of the integument (145,146). *Corynebacterium equi* should be considered in the differential diagnosis of cavitary pneumonia in cancer patients (147). *Listeria monocytogenes* and *Stomatococcus mucilaginous* are uncommon gram-positive bacteria that sporadically cause infection in neutropenic patients. Stomatococcus seems to be increasing in incidence and can present with sepsis, ARDS, and meningitis (148,149).

Historically, three gram-negative rods—*Escherichia coli, P. aeruginosa,* and *Klebsiella pneumoniae*—have been responsible for approximately 85% of all gram-negative infections in neutropenic hosts. Although the frequency of these three pathogens has remained stable, selective antibiotic pressure has allowed a number of other gram-negative bacteria to assume more prominent roles in infections associated with neutropenic patients. These include *Enterobacter cloacae, Acinetobacter anitratus, Stenotrophomonas maltophilia, Proteus* sp., and *Citrobacter* sp. Prior to the advent of empiric antibiotic therapy, bacteremia with gram-negative rods resulted in a high mortality, approaching 100% in patients with cancer (24,39). This changed dramatically with the increased use of empiric broad-spectrum antibiotics. *S. maltophilia,* which is resistant to the antibiotics typically used in empiric regimens for neutropenia and fever, may be emerging as a frequent cause of secondary or breakthrough infections (Table 17.2).

Anaerobic infections have been uncommon over the years, accounting for only 1% to 2% of isolated organisms (Table 17.2) (8,30,86, 150). *Clostridium* sp are most common (150, 151), followed by *Bacillus* sp. and *Bacteroides* sp. (151,152). *Clostridium septicum* is the most common species among clostridial anaerobic infections, followed by *Clostridium perfringens*. The portal of entry for *C. septicum* is typically the gastrointestinal tract, frequently in association with typhlitis or leukemic infiltrates of the intestine (153,154). *C. septicum* infection also may present with distal myonecrosis, which carries a high mortality (79%) (154). Other patients may present with intravascular hemolysis, which may be rapidly fatal. *Clostridium tertium* is an emerging anaerobic pathogen that is resistant to β-lactams, clindamycin, and metronidazole (155). *Bacteroides fragilis* accounts for about two thirds of infections from *Bacteroides* sp. (151). The most common portals of entry for anaerobic bacteria are intraabdominal abscesses, soft tissue infections, and occasionally the oropharynx. Other emerging anaerobic pathogens are the *Bacillus* sp. (152). *Bacillus cereus* may cause characteristic skin vesicles on the extremities, seen most commonly during the summer, or may be associated with central venous catheters (156). Capnocytophaga sp and *Leptotrichia buccalis,* microorganisms that constitute normal oropharynx flora, occasionally cause sepsis in the neutropenic patient (157,158).

Clostridium difficile infection, a common complication of both antibiotic and cytotoxic therapy that affects the gut microbial flora, typically manifests as diarrhea caused by production of a microbial toxin (159). Fulminant infection manifesting as pseudomembranous colitis is uncommon in children; a syndrome resembling typhlitis (without diarrhea) also has been described (160–163). Outbreaks of *C. difficile* disease in oncology units have been reported (164,165). Treatment of *C. difficile* has become a contentious topic because the presence of *C. difficile* in the stool is a risk factor for the presence of vancomycin-resistant enterococci, and treatment of *C. difficile* with oral vancomycin can lead to development of resistance among enterococci colonizing patients with leukemia (166). Oral metronidazole is generally the preferred treatment for *C. difficile* toxin-induced diarrhea because efficacy with this therapy is similar to that with vancomycin, but metronidazole is not as likely to induce resistance (144). Restriction of certain antibiotics has been demonstrated to reduce *C. difficile* colonization and *C. difficile* associated diarrhea (167).

Mycobacteria are unusual pathogens in neutropenic patients, with the notable exception of intravascular exit-site and tunnel-tract infections due to rapid-growth mycobacteria (*Mycobacterium chelonae, Mycobacterium fortuitum*) (62,63). These infections are often indolent and resistant to treatment, requiring catheter removal and wide excision of involved skin. Antibiotic treatment with clarithromycin may be an effective adjunct to surgery (62,63).

Fungi

Before antibiotic therapy is administered, fungal infections are so uncommon in the neutropenic patient that empiric antimicrobial regimens usually do not include antifungal drugs at the onset of fever in the absence of specific indications. After a few days of broad-spectrum antibiotic therapy, which favors mucosal overgrowth of fungi, mycoses become a major concern in the neutropenic patient (168–172).

Overall, the most common fungal pathogens are *Candida* and *Aspergillus* spp. (171–173), but before antibiotic therapy, one is as likely to encounter cryptococcus, *Pneumocystis carinii,* or, in endemic areas, *Histoplasma capsulatum* or *Coccidioides immitis* (51,174–176). *P. carinii,* formerly considered to be a protozoan but recently reclassified as a fungus based on genetic evidence (177), would be much more common were it not for the use of trimethoprim-sulfamethoxazole (TMP-SM) prophylaxis (178). *Candida* spp. account for the great majority of mucosal infections and a large portion of invasive fungal infections following antibiotic therapy. Infections with *Candida* usually originate in the gastrointestinal tract (179). *C. albicans* is the most commonly encountered species, followed by *C. tropicalis, Candida parapsilosis, Torulopsis (Candida) glabrata, Candida lusitaniae,* and *C. krusei* (179,180). The frequencies of *C. tropicalis* (68,69) and *C. parapsilosis* (181) as agents of fungemia have been increasing in recent years and may approach that of *C. albicans* at some institutions. Although *C. tropicalis* is an infrequently isolated agent in surveillance cultures, it is responsible for a disproportionate amount of fungal disease in the neutropenic host (68,69), implying that it is a more invasive or pathogenic organism than *C. albicans* (70). This is supported by animal models of *Candida* infection (71,72) and is manifested in the neutropenic host by an increased frequency of fungemia (68,69), meningitis (73), and osteomyelitis (74) relative to *C. albicans.* Although not seen commonly, invasive disease with *C. krusei* is noteworthy because this species is typically resistant to fluconazole and may be responsible for outbreaks in the setting of widespread use of fluconazole (75). Isolation of even a single colony of a *Candida* sp from a blood culture should be regarded as an indication of infection in a neutropenic patient because failure to treat early with an antifungal agent may result in disseminated and focal disease (e.g., arthritis), leading to increased morbidity and mortality (182).

Among hundreds of species of *Aspergillus,* only *A. fumigatus* and *A. flavus* are frequent causes of invasive aspergillosis in the immunocompromised host; *A. terreus* and *A. niger* are relatively rare (173). Risk factors for acquisition are granulocytopenia and high-dose corticosteroid therapy. *Aspergillus* is usually acquired through the respiratory tract. Outbreaks of aspergillosis in susceptible hosts have been reported in association with construction, especially within hospitals; building materials and air ducts are potential sources of *Aspergillus* spores (183). Invasive pulmonary aspergillosis and disseminated aspergillosis have an ominous prognosis in the setting of prolonged neutropenia or bone marrow transplant (78,184).

Fusarium, well known for causing keratitis and onychomycosis (185), has become a more frequent cause of disseminated infection in immunocompromised hosts (46,60,186,187). Unlike *Aspergillus, Fusarium* commonly can be detected in the bloodstream by culture or by newer antigenic and lysis centrifugation techniques (188). Many isolates of *Fusarium* are resistant to currently available antifungals. *Mucor* is a less common but well-described pathogen in the neutropenic patient (189). *Malassezia furfur* is another emerging fungal pathogen, and it has a propensity to cause infection in patients receiving intravenous lipids (190). Although uncommon, infection with *P. boydii* is especially significant because this organism is resistant to amphotericin B treatment, but it may be susceptible to certain imidazoles (191).

Fungi once thought to be nonpathogenic have on numerous occasions been observed to cause infection in neutropenic patients, not just of the skin or mucous membranes, but in many cases having invaded deeply (173). Among the infections reported are phaeohyphomycoses with the dematiaceous fungi (*Curvularia, Bipolaris, Exserohilum, Alternaria, Exophiala, Phialophora*) (185). Other new fungal opportunists include *Acremonium* sp., *Scedosporium apiospermum* (teleomorph *P. boydii*), *Trichosporon beigelii, Blastoschizomyces capitatus,* and *Saccharomyces.*

Viruses

Although bacterial and fungal infections receive the greatest attention in the neutropenic host, viral infections may account for up to one fourth of infectious episodes, depending on the age of the child and the degree of immunosuppression (30). Although most viral infections are no more severe in the neutropenic host than in the nonneutropenic host, these infections may take on greater significance because their associated fever leads to empiric antibiotic therapy and hospitalization.

Moreover, some viral infections are of greater severity in the immunosuppressed host (15). Primary varicella in the neutropenic host can cause visceral dissemination to the lung, liver, and central nervous system, with 7% to 30% mortality (192–194). The use of varicella vaccine may decrease this complication in the near future, but zoster will remain as problematic as it has been for many years to come. Zoster, although more common than varicella, is not life threatening to the degree that varicella is; however, zoster also may disseminate to the liver, central nervous system, or, uncommonly, to the lung, as with varicella (195–197). Measles rarely occurs in the immunocompromised host today, but giant cell pneumonitis and encephalitis may complicate the patient's course when it does occur.

Primary herpes simplex infections are uncommon among neutropenic patients, who tend to have reduced exposure to infectious agents; however, reactivation of latent infection is common (198). Within 3 weeks after bone marrow transplantation or intensive chemotherapy, 50% or more of seropositive patients will have reactivation of their infection (198–200). Dissemination is unusual, but these infections cause breakdown of mucosal barriers that may lead to fatal bacterial or fungal infections with organisms such as *Candida* and viridans streptococci (198,201). Esophagitis or tracheitis in the intubated patient is occasionally observed (194,202). Acyclovir prophylaxis can reduce the incidence of herpetic gingivostomatitis, but resistance to acyclovir may develop, limiting the usefulness of this approach (203, 204).

Cytomegalovirus (CMV) infection is consequential in the neutropenic host not only because of somewhat greater severity on average but also because of the fact that CMV-induced fever and worsened neutropenia can combine leading to a prolonged course of antibiotic therapy and associated complications, such as fungal infections. In one study, CMV was cultured from the urine and saliva of 27% of children with acute leukemia. Less frequently, CMV may be isolated from the blood of children with leukemia, but it only rarely disseminates in the non-bone marrow transplant patient (205). In the absence of prophylaxis, CMV causes interstitial pneumonitis in approximately 17% of patients undergoing allogeneic bone marrow transplantation, resulting in mortality in 85% of patients (206). Use of prophylaxis with ganciclovir has resulted in a sharp decrease in the incidence of interstitial pneumonitis in this population (207), and early treatment with a combination of ganciclovir and intravenous immunoglobulin has reduced mortality significantly when CMV pneumonia does occur (208,209).

Children receiving chemotherapy have increased susceptibility to respiratory syncytial virus (210), an important observation considering that this agent is the most common cause of pneumonia in the United States in children aged 6 months to 3 years. Adenoviruses are responsible for more severe disease in immunosuppressed patients compared with immunocompetent hosts, causing diffuse pneumonia, hepatitis, and hemorrhagic cystis (211–213). Parainfluenza and influenza viruses also may have more severe courses in children with cancer, especially those undergoing allogeneic bone marrow transplant (214,215).

Parasites

As with immunocompetent children in the United States, parasites are the least common class of pathogens in neutropenic children, accounting for about 1% of all infectious episodes (24,61). *P. carinii,* once classified as a protozoan, is now considered a fungus based on genetic studies (177); therefore, it is considered in the antecedent section on fungi. *Cryptosporidium parvum* is the most commonly encountered opportunistic protozoan causing severe disease in neutropenic children, and it should always be considered in the differential diagnosis of diarrhea (216). Rarely, *Cryptosporidium* is associated with pulmonary disease, which, as is the case with enterocolitis causing diarrhea, requires a modified acid-fast stain of secretions for diagnosis (217). *Toxoplasma gondii* rarely present with lymphadenopathy and fever or with brain abscess (218). *Strongyloides stercoralis* hyperinfection also may occur sporadically, manifesting as pulmonary infiltrates and respiratory symptoms (219,220).

ANTIMICROBIAL MANAGEMENT OF THE FEBRILE NEUTROPENIC PATIENT

Principles of Antibiotic Therapy in the Neutropenic Host

The last 20 years brought an expanding number of potent new antibiotics and changes in the predominant organisms responsible for infections in cancer patients (31); however, the principles of empiric therapy remained essentially unaltered in the management of cancer patients with neutropenia (221). Several principles of empiric antimicrobial therapy provide a framework on which approaches to specific patient cohorts or specific patients can be developed; these are detailed below and summarized in Table 17.3.

1. Empiric, broad-spectrum antimicrobial therapy is necessary at the outset of fever in the neutropenic patient. Criteria for the initiation of empiric antimicrobial therapy should reflect the risk for morbidity and mortality relative to the observed clinical signs and symptoms. Empiric parenteral antimicrobial therapy is rarely used in the well-appearing immunocompetent child because the risk of life-threatening infection in this setting is remote. The risk in the neutropenic patient for life-threatening infection is increased sufficiently such that broad-spectrum empiric antibiotic therapy is justified at the onset of fever when no other signs or symptoms are seen.

2. The choice of antibiotics for initial empiric therapy should be based on the likely infecting organisms and the relative morbidity and mortality observed with these organisms. Providing antimicrobial coverage for all the potential infecting organisms in a particular patient is generally not feasible. The probability of morbidity and mortality associated with the likely infecting organisms is used to guide antimicrobial selection. For example, coagulase-negative staphylococci are the most common blood isolate in children with fever and neutropenia, whereas *P. aeruginosa* infections are uncommon; however, the much higher mortality associated with *P. aeruginosa* compared with coagulase-negative staphylococcal infections argues that priority be given to cov-

TABLE 17.3. *Principles of antibiotic therapy in the neutropenic host*

I. Empiric, broad-spectrum antibiotic therapy is necessary at the outset of fever in the neutropenic patient.
II. Initial empiric therapy should be based on likely infecting organisms.
    Cover pathogens with high morbidity and mortality
    Be familiar with local antibiotic susceptibility patterns
III. Analysis of factors associated with the specific patient may guide empiric therapy.
    Take into account host factors, including mucositis, presence of an indwelling catheter, or antecedent viral infection
    Know patient's flora and inquire regarding exposures
    Examine for focus of infection
IV. Antimicrobial regimens should minimize toxicity and emergence of resistance.
    Withdraw antibiotics when they are not needed
    Minimize number and duration of antimicrobials while maintaining broad spectrum coverage
V. Empiric therapy should be modified to reflect the changing pattern of infections during therapy.
    Deterioration should prompt change to optimize both gram-positive and gram-negative coverage
    Isolation of a specific pathogen may allow directed therapy while maintaining broad-spectrum coverage
    Withdraw unnecessary antibiotics when practical
    Add antifungal coverage when needed
VI. Optimal therapy requires balancing need to reduce morbidity and mortality against the goal of minimizing use of antibiotics.
VII. Prevention of infection is preferable to treatment of infection.

erage of *P. aeruginosa* infections. Coverage for coagulase-negative staphylococci can be added based on culture results with little risk of additional mortality. It is necessary to be familiar with the susceptibility patterns of bacterial organisms common in the hospital or community where the patient is receiving treatment. Antibiotic resistance or the prevalence of a particular microorganism serotype, species, or strain may be an important factor in infection of the neutropenic patient. Local antibiotic susceptibility patterns of the targeted organisms, which vary considerably by institution, may alter the choice of initial empiric therapy.

3. Analysis of factors associated with a specific patient's neutropenia can facilitate prediction of the likely infecting organisms, thereby helping to guide initial empiric antimicrobial selection. Epidemiologic information regarding the likely infecting organisms may help to guide the selection of a specific empiric antimicrobial regimen. For example, if severe oral mucositis accompanies neutropenia, coverage for oral flora should be especially considered. Frequently, microorganisms infecting neutropenic hosts are derived from the host's normal flora; however, clinicians should be especially alert to the possibility that a pathogen may be acquired from another patient, hospital personnel, or as a result of airborne transportation potentially related to hospital construction. Clinicians also should inquire about unusual exposures such as contact with an animal or food potentially harboring pathogens or environmental exposures to recognized sources of pathogens, such as soil contaminated with large amounts of avian feces, which foster growth of *H. capsulatum.* Often the portal of entry of a microorganism is predictable even when the nature of the encounter is obscure. Knowledge of the portal may influence the choice of empiric therapy. Among neutropenic children with cancer, as many as half or more of the bacteremias may be catheter related; so this source should always be considered. For multilumen catheters, infection may be present in only one of the lumens. Breaks in the skin or

mucous membranes are other common sources. Other potential foci of infection should be sought, including pneumonia, urinary tract infection, perirectal erythema, pharyngitis, or typhlitis (infection of the cecum or nearby bowel wall). If the nasopharynx or gastrointestinal tract is the suspected portal of infection, infection with *S. pneumoniae* or *Salmonella* sp., respectively, should be considered.

4. Antimicrobial regimens should be selected that minimize toxicity to the patient and minimize the risk of emergence of resistance. Antibiotics should not be initiated when there is no clear need, or they should be discontinued as soon as it is clear that they are not needed. Antimicrobial choices should take into account not only the potential pathogens but also the possible toxicities of the agents used. The risk for emergence of antimicrobial resistance is related to the number and duration of courses of antimicrobials. In the presence of antimicrobials, the colonizing flora will be altered because of proliferation or new colonization of resistant organisms. The occurrence of thrush caused by the proliferation of *Candida* during antimicrobial therapy is a good example. Neutropenia without antimicrobial therapy does not predispose to thrush. Change in the pattern of infections may reflect change in colonization patterns because colonization and proliferation of organisms is the first step in the pathogenesis of many infections. Toxicity and emergence of resistance are important limitations of empiric antimicrobial therapy. A major challenge in management of neutropenic patients is properly balancing the appropriate use of empiric therapy with the potential for adverse effects to the patient or future patients who may encounter resistant organisms. The clinician has the responsibility to withhold antibiotics when they are not warranted; however, when antimicrobials are warranted, they should be given at an appropriate dosage and for an appropriate duration to help ensure eradication of the pathogen.

5. Empiric therapy should be modified to reflect the changing pattern of infections dur-

ing therapy. Particularly with prolonged neutropenia, modification of the initial empiric therapy is the rule rather than the exception in the febrile, neutropenic patient. The course of infection in the febrile neutropenic patient is often dynamic, requiring constant vigilance by the treating physician and appropriate responses to changes in the patient's situation. Deterioration in the patient's condition should prompt broadening of the empiric antimicrobial regimen to include additional coverage for both gram-positive and gram-negative organisms if optimal coverage was not already present in the empiric regimen. The addition of antifungal agents should also be considered. Continued fever in the neutropenic patient without an identified source also may be an indication for the addition of empiric antifungal agents. Isolation of a specific pathogen from blood cultures or other sterile sites should allow modification of the initial empiric regimen to direct therapy more specifically to the organism being isolated; however, the conventional practice of selecting the antibiotic with the narrowest spectrum, all other factors being equal, may not always hold in the neutropenic patient. Limiting the spectrum of coverage to gram-positive bacteria is associated with a significantly increased risk of gram-negative bacterial infections in the neutropenic cancer patient (222) and generally should be avoided. Failure to isolate a specific pathogen as a cause of fever in the neutropenic patient may lead to modifications in the empiric regimen as well. If potentially toxic antimicrobials or antibiotics targeted to a specific organism that was not isolated in cultures were included in the initial empiric regimen, these may be discontinued before resolution of the fever and neutropenia. An example would be inclusion of vancomycin in the initial regimen as a result of concern over gram-positive, catheter-associated bacteremia. Failure to isolate such a pathogen in an otherwise stable patient with continued neutropenia and fever might be an indication to withdraw the vancomycin to avoid nephrotoxicity or selection of vancomycin resistant strains of *Enterococcus*.

6. Optimal empiric antimicrobial therapy of the neutropenic host requires balancing the need to reduce morbidity and mortality against the goal of minimizing the use of antibiotics. Antimicrobial use entails considerable costs, both direct and indirect. These include the toxicities associated with the drug, the induction of antimicrobial resistance, the cost of the antibiotic itself, and the cost of administration. For optimization of antimicrobial therapy, these costs must be carefully balanced against the benefits of antimicrobial use. Currently, minimizing resistance and containing monetary costs are the greatest challenges in this field.

7. *Prevention* of infection is preferable to *treatment* of infection. Prevention of infection in the neutropenic patient can be accomplished by avoiding contact with the organism or by bolstering host defense. Prophylactic antibiotics may be useful in some circumstances, although their use is tempered by the possibility of inducing antibiotic-resistant organisms.

Standardized Approach to Empiric Therapy

When patient cohorts are treated by a standardized plan, an opportunity exists to determine the weaknesses and strengths of the approach. In the absence of a standardized approach, little can be learned because of the inability to distinguish trends from random events in an environment when multiple empiric regimens are used based on individual preferences. Because of sufficiently large cohorts of patients and the willingness of investigators in the field to conduct randomized trials and use standardized treatment schemes, great strides have been made during the past three decades in the management of the neutropenic child with cancer and unexplained fever. This progress has culminated in the development and publication of national guidelines of antimicrobial management for these patients (32). A final advantage of the standardized management plan is that this strategy facilitates research because potential

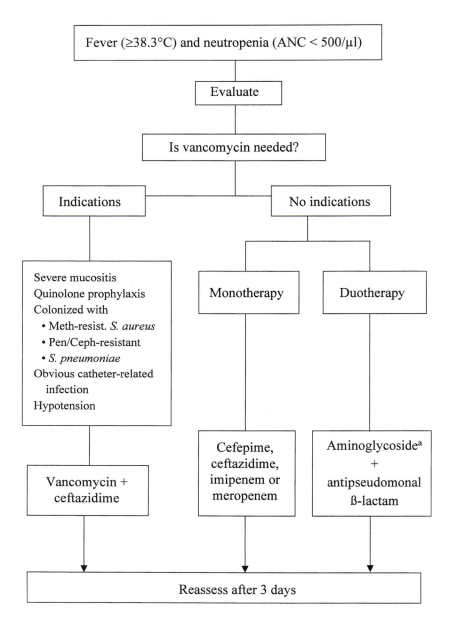

FIG. 17.1. Three general approaches to antimicrobial therapy were recently endorsed by the Infectious Diseases Society of America through its Practice Guidelines Committee: single-drug therapy (monotherapy), two-drug therapy (duotherapy) without vancomycin, and vancomycin plus one or two other drugs. In the absence of indications for vancomycin or duotherapy, monotherapy is generally the most cost-effective regimen when including the cost of preparation and administration of drugs, and monotherapy typically has fewer associated serious adverse effects. [a]Avoid aminoglycosides if the patient is receiving other nephrotoxic, ototoxic, or neuromuscular blocking agents. (Modified from Hughes WT, Armstrong D, Bodey GP, et al. 1997 Guidelines for the use of antimicrobial agents in neutropenic patients with unexplained fever. Infectious Diseases Society of America. *Clin Infect Dis* 1997;25:551–573, with permission of the University of Chicago Press.)

shortcomings of a particular regimen are more readily apparent and randomized trials are easier to conceive, design, and implement.

For some neutropenic patients, the underlying condition or special circumstances are so uncommon that standardized regimens, if feasible at all, are possible only at a national or international level. Lessons learned from larger cohorts of neutropenic patients can be extrapolated to these singular patients, albeit cautiously.

The optimal empiric antibiotic regimen for the cancer patient with neutropenia and fever remains a matter of debate. There is a consensus that the regimen should be broad spectrum, covering most of the predominant gram-positive and gram-negative bacterial pathogens, and should be bactericidal, with few serious adverse effects and lacking a propensity to induce or select resistant microorganisms (31,32,223). Allergies and renal function of the patient as well as the antimicrobial spectrum of resistance at the institution where the patient is being treated should be considered. Three general schemes have been developed for empiric therapy and have been refined by the Infectious Diseases Society of America through its Practice Guidelines Committee (32): single-drug therapy (monotherapy), two-drug therapy (duotherapy) without vancomycin, and vancomycin plus one or two other drugs (Fig. 17.1).

Selection of the Initial Empiric Antibiotic Regimen

Monotherapy

Although not an option in the early history of empiric therapy for neutropenic patients, the new broad-spectrum antibiotics with good antipseudomonal activity and a high serum bactericidal activity make monotherapy a popular choice today for initial empiric therapy of neutropenia and fever (224). Two classes of antibiotics can be considered candidates for monotherapy: the antipseudomonal third-generation cephalosporins (ceftazidime) (27,95,108,109,122,225–233) and the car-

bapenems (imipenem/cilastatin) (28,113,116, 122,228,234–240) and meropenem (241–243). Newer agents under study for monotherapy include cefpirome (244), cefoperazone/sulbactam (245), and cefepime, a drug related to the cephalosporins with enhanced activity against both gram-positive and gram-negative organisms (246–249). Quinolones have been used as monotherapy in neutropenic adults, but they are not recommended for use in children and may predispose to the development of viridans streptococcal sepsis (250), which is more common in neutropenic children than adults (251,252).

Limitations of monotherapy are due mainly to suboptimal activity against gram-positive bacteria, especially *S. aureus,* coagulase-negative staphylococci, *Enterococcus,* some strains of penicillin-resistant *S. pneumoniae, Corynebacterium,* and viridans streptococci. This can result in gram-positive superinfections, an issue that is particularly relevant in view of the shift toward predominance of gram-positive pathogens in neutropenic hosts and their increased resistance to methicillin. Other reservations regarding monotherapy include resistance developing among gram-negative rods and a lack of synergistic effect on gram-negative rods, especially for patients whose granulocyte count remains below 100/mm^3 (253). Despite these concerns, there are no striking differences between monotherapy and multidrug combinations for initial empiric therapy of fever in the neutropenic patient (27,108,115,116,233,237). Regardless of whether monotherapy or multidrug regimens are used, the patient must be monitored closely for nonresponse, emergence of secondary infections, adverse effects, and the development of drug-resistant organisms. Modifications of the initial empiric regimen because of these considerations may become necessary during the course of treatment and are discussed subsequently.

Duotherapy without Vancomycin

Regimens using two drugs without the use of vancomycin may be appropriate in certain settings. Possibilities include use of an amino-glycoside (gentamicin, tobramycin, or amikacin) with an antipseudomonal carboxy penicillin or ureidopenicillin (ticarcillin with or without clavulanate, azlocillin, mezlocillin, or piperacillin), an aminoglycoside with a third-generation antipseudomonal cephalosporin (ceftazidime), or a combination of two β-lactam agents, particularly the combination of aztreonam or ceftazidime with a β-lactam drug possessing good gram-positive activity (nafcillin or oxacillin). Ceftazidime is the preferred cephalosporin because of its antipseudomonal activity, but studies suggested that once-daily dosing of ceftriaxone and an aminoglycoside is as effective as multiple daily doses of these two agents (254) or as effective as monotherapy with ceftazidime (232). In general, different two-drug regimens yield similar results when compared head to head (for a summary of publications on this subject, see ref. 32). The choice of empiric regimens should be based not only on theoretic considerations but also on the knowledge of the prevalence and pattern of resistance in the particular institution.

Duotherapy overcomes many of the potential limitations of monotherapy, but it has some disadvantages as well. Advantages include potential synergistic killing against some gram-negative bacilli and gram-positive bacteria (255), activity against anaerobes with certain combinations, minimal emergence of resistant strains during treatment (256,257), and less need for early modifications of therapy. Most combination regimens, however, excluding vancomycin, lack activity against certain gram-positive bacteria, and there are toxic effects associated with use of aminoglycoside antibiotics and carboxy penicillins, including nephrotoxicity, ototoxicity, and hypokalemia. Aminoglycoside serum levels should be monitored as needed, and dosages should be adjusted until optimal therapeutic concentrations are achieved.

Studies of quinolone drugs in combination with other antibiotics are limited and may be problematic in the pediatric patient because of potential toxicity. The role of macrolide drugs

such as erythromycin, clarithromycin, and azithromycin in the empiric management of fever in the neutropenic host has not been delineated.

Vancomycin Plus One or Two Drugs

Initial management of the febrile neutropenic patient should not include vancomycin except in cases where life-threatening infections from gram-positive organisms susceptible only to vancomycin are suspected or are common (Fig. 17.1). The increased incidence of infections with gram-positive organisms such as coagulase-negative staphylococci, viridans streptococci, penicillin, cephalosporin-resistant *S. pneumoniae,* and methicillin-resistant *S. aureus,* which may require vancomycin for effective treatment, has made the issue of when to include vancomycin in the initial regimen a contentious one. Although the use of vancomycin has not been demonstrated to decrease overall mortality from infections with gram-positive bacteria as a group, the mortality associated with viridans streptococcal infections may be higher among patients who are not initially treated with vancomycin (103,250); however, the excessive use of vancomycin in the hospital setting has been associated with emergence of vancomycin-resistant organisms, especially enterococci, which present treatment dilemmas as a result of multidrug resistance. Therefore, at institutions where fulminant infections with organisms susceptible only to vancomycin are rare, vancomycin should be used only for life-threatening, culture-proven infections or pending definitive culture results in cases where resistant gram-positive organisms are postulated to exist.

Indications for inclusion of vancomycin in the initial empiric regimen for fever in high-risk patients are summarized in Fig. 17.1. Vancomycin therapy should be used initially in patients with clinically obvious, serious, catheter-related infections; intensive chemotherapy that produces substantial mucosal damage (i.e., high-dose cytarabine), known colonization with methicillin-resistant *S. au-*

reus or pneumococci known to be resistant to penicillin and cephalosporins, hypotension, or other evidence of cardiovascular impairment, or a blood culture positive for gram-positive bacteria before final identification and susceptibilities are known. If no infection needing vancomycin is identified, the drug should be discontinued after 48 to 72 hours.

Vancomycin has been studied in combination with a number of drugs in neutropenic patients with fever and can be added to most single agents or two-drug combinations that are used for empiric therapy (103,114,239, 258–266). Because the combination of vancomycin with ceftazidime has been studied most extensively and has been demonstrated to provide broad-spectrum coverage and to have a wide margin of safety, it is recommended as the combination of choice for initial therapy when vancomycin is needed. Teicoplanin has been evaluated in a limited number of trials as an alternative to vancomycin, but additional studies are required to assess its proper use in empiric therapy (259,264,267–271).

Modification of the Initial Empiric Antibiotic Regimen

As more patients remain neutropenic for longer periods, the concept of empiric therapy has extended beyond the initial management to include the modifications or additions to the primary antibiotic therapy that are necessary to maximize the survival of the patient. Strategies are evolving to deal with problems such as prolonged fever despite antibiotic therapy and prolonged neutropenia with or without fever as well as decisions on stopping antibiotic therapy when no pathogen is identified.

In perhaps up to two thirds of febrile neutropenic children with cancer, neutropenia will resolve without either identification of the cause of fever or modification of the initial empiric regimen. When a specific etiology of fever is identified, in many cases, the initial regimen will be altered, but often no change is indicated. The longer the patient re-

mains neutropenic and on broad-spectrum antibiotics, however, the more likely it is that a modification of the initial regimen will be required because of the risk of secondary infectious complications (30). The precipitating agents can be bacteria, viruses, or protozoa, but beyond the first few days of antibiotic therapy, fungi become the major threat.

Although modification to the empiric regimen requires more individualization than the initial regimen, a degree of standardization to empiric therapy modification is possible. Deterioration of the patient's condition should signal a need to add vancomycin if it was not part of the empiric regimen and to consider adding a second drug with activity against gram-negative organisms if monotherapy was used initially. Isolation of an organism from cultures may require alteration of the initial regimen. If coagulase-positive staphylococci, viridans streptococci, or methicillin-resistant *S. aureus* are found to be causative, the addition of vancomycin may be warranted. If *P. aeruginosa* is isolated, even from surface cultures, the addition of a second anti-pseudomonas antibiotic should be considered. In the setting of fever beyond 3 to 6 days of broad-spectrum antibiotics, the addition of empiric antifungal therapy, typically with amphotericin B, is generally recommended. In the presence of gingivostomatitis, cultures for herpes simplex virus should be obtained, and the empiric addition of acyclovir may be considered pending outcome of culture results.

These modifications of the empiric antibiotic therapy are essential to the management of the febrile neutropenic patient. This emphasizes the need for scrupulous monitoring of the patient to detect new signs of infection, necessitating at least daily examination, blood cultures when the patient is febrile, and cultures of any potential site(s) of infection.

Afebrile within Three Days of Initiation of Empiric Therapy

Although the time to defervescence after initiation of empiric antibiotics varies from 2 to 7 days, recent guidelines advocate reassessment on day 4 or 5 to determine whether modifications should be made in the initial therapy. The patient who has defervesced within the first 72 hours and who has no identified infection can be assessed for the need to continue the chosen empiric regimen in its present form (Fig. 17.2). Consideration should be given at this time to discontinuation of vancomycin if it was part of the initial regimen. If an organism is identified, the antibiotic regimen can be changed to achieve optimum therapy, but broad-spectrum coverage should be maintained because secondary or breakthrough infections are common (222). Treatment with a broad-spectrum regimen should continue for a minimum of 7 days and ideally until the absolute neutrophil count is above 500/μL. If neutropenia is prolonged, however, consideration can be given to discontinuation of therapy prior to granulocyte recovery, particularly if recovery is anticipated within the next 5 days. Patients who are considered to be at low risk for infectious complications in whom this can be considered

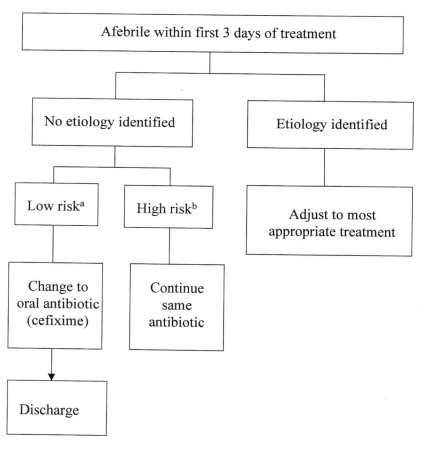

FIG. 17.2. Management of the patient who has no identified infection and has defervesced within the first 72 hours of empiric therapy as suggested by the Infectious Diseases Society of America through its Practice Guidelines Committee. [a]Clinically well, absolute neutrophil count (ANC) greater than 100/μL. [b]Clinically symptomatic or ANC below 100/μL. (Modified from Hughes WT, Armstrong D, Bodey GP, et al. 1997 Guidelines for the use of antimicrobial agents in neutropenic patients with unexplained fever. Infectious Diseases Society of America. *Clin Infect Dis* 1997;25:551–573, with permission of the University of Chicago Press.)

must be able to be carefully observed, must have intact integument and mucous membranes (e.g., no mucositis, ulcerations, or evidence of catheter-site infections), and should not have incipient invasive procedures or ablative chemotherapy planned (32).

If all cultures are negative and there is no discernible source of infection, treatment for compliant patients may be changed after more than 2 days of intravenous therapy to an oral antibiotic such as cefixime, a quinolone such as ciprofloxacin or ofloxacin, or a drug combination of clindamycin and ciprofloxacin or amoxicillin/clavulanic acid plus perfloxacin, and the patient can be observed closely as an outpatient (272). This approach is not advocated for patients who had signs of sepsis (chills, hypotension, and requirement for fluid resuscitation) at admission. Oral therapy also may not be generally advisable in patients who are febrile at 48 hours or who have a neutrophil count below 100/μL. An alternative to outpatient oral antibiotics is to continue intravenous antibiotics at home for patients who qualify.

Fever beyond the First Three Days of Treatment

The patient who remains febrile despite empiric antibiotic treatment may or may not need modifications to the initial regimen. The patient should be reassessed on day 4 or 5 after initiation of therapy in an attempt to identify the possible sources of persistent fever. Common reasons for persistent fever without identification of a causative organism include a nonbacterial infection, a bacterial infection resistant to the antibiotics being used, a secondary infection, drug fever, or an avascular focus of infection such as an abscess or catheter site (32). Infections treated with appropriate antibiotics may take longer than 4 or 5 days to defervesce, and resistant organisms may be partially suppressed but not eliminated by the antibiotic regimen in use.

Reassessment should include a careful physical examination including any catheter site(s), reculture of blood and specific sites of

infection, and diagnostic imaging of any organ suspected of infection. Examination of the sinuses by plain film or computed tomography (CT) scan or of the viscera by ultrasound or CT scan may be valuable in detecting bacterial or fungal disease. Additional studies to identify nonbacterial, atypical, or uncommon infectious agents such as herpes simplex virus, CMV, Epstein-Barr virus, enterovirus, enteric protozoa, *Mycobacterium tuberculosis,* and nontuberculous mycobacteria should be undertaken if the presence of these organisms is suggested by clinical features. If reassessment suggests a possible source of infection not adequately covered by the initial empiric regimen, a change should be made accordingly.

If fever persists beyond 4 or 5 days of empiric antibiotic therapy and no cause is evident, three options may be considered: (a) to continue treatment with the initial regimen, (b) to change or add antibiotic(s), or (c) to add amphotericin B to the regimen, with or without changing antibiotics. If the patient has remained stable during the initial 4 to 5 days of initial antibiotic treatment and reevaluation has not identified a source of the infection, the initial regimen could be continued (Fig. 17.3), especially if the neutropenia is expected to resolve within 5 days (32). If the patient has new findings on reevaluation or is becoming progressively more ill, consideration should be given to adding or changing antibiotic(s).

If the initial regimen included vancomycin and initial cultures have not yielded an organism for which vancomycin is needed, deliberation should be given to discontinuing this agent to minimize bacterial resistance to this drug. If blood or site-specific isolates yield coagulase-negative staphylococci, methicillin-resistant *S. aureus, Corynebacterium* species, enterococcus, or viridans streptococci, or if there is evidence of life-threatening sepsis, vancomycin should be continued. If the initial regimen did not include vancomycin and these criteria are met, it should be either added to the initial antibiotic(s) or included in any new regimen.

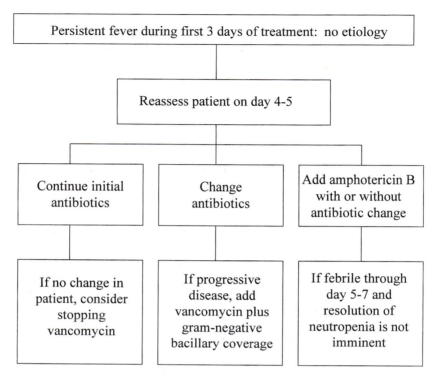

FIG. 17.3. Management of the patient who has no identified infection and has persistent fever beyond the first 72 hours of empiric therapy as suggested by the Infectious Diseases Society of America through its Practice Guidelines Committee. (Modified from Hughes WT, Armstrong D, Bodey GP, et al. 1997 Guidelines for the use of antimicrobial agents in neutropenic patients with unexplained fever. Infectious Diseases Society of America. *Clin Infect Dis* 1997;25:551–573, with permission of the University of Chicago Press.)

The third alternative is the addition of amphotericin B, either with or without other changes in the empiric antibiotic regimen. Evidence of fungal infection should be carefully sought prior to institution of this agent because the decision to discontinue treatment is often more difficult than the decision to begin it empirically. A careful physical examination, including the skin and the nails, biopsy of any suspicious lesions, CT of the chest and abdomen, either radiographs or CT of the sinuses, cultures of blood and suspected sites of infection including sinus cultures at endoscopy if sinus disease is suspected, and serological or antigen tests for fungal agents should all be done before amphotericin B is started.

Most experts are of the opinion that the patient who has been febrile and profoundly neutropenic for 5 to 7 days despite the administration of broad-spectrum antibiotics is a candidate for empiric amphotericin B therapy (10). Some patients may benefit from earlier administration (273,274), and there is currently debate as to exactly when and under what circumstances antifungal agents should be used. Individual cases where the patient has no clinical features suggestive of fungal infection and is expected to recover neutrophil counts rapidly may be monitored carefully and amphotericin B therapy withheld.

Several recently marketed preparations of liposomal amphotericin B appear to be less nephrotoxic than amphotericin B and induce less hypokalemia (275). Currently, there are no definitive studies to assess the relatively efficacies of these agents. The higher cost of liposomal amphotericin preparations and the lack of randomized comparative therapeutic trials with amphotericin B have limited the use and endorsement of liposomal amphotericin B. These agents are most often used in patients requiring antifungal therapy who demonstrate intolerance to and do not respond to conventional amphotericin B. Patterns of use of liposomal preparations of amphotericin B will evolve when comparative trials become available.

Antifungal azoles may be an alternative to amphotericin B in some institutions where mold infections and drug-resistant *Candida* species (i.e., *C. krusei* and *T. glabrata*) are uncommon, especially if the patient does not have evidence of sinus or pulmonary disease (276). Current data are insufficient to recommend empiric therapy with azoles for routine use. Fluconazole use should be avoided if the patient has received fluconazole prophylactically; has clinical features suggestive of keratitis, sinusitis, or systemic mycoses; or is being treated at institutions where fluconazole-resistant species are common. In the absence of these conditions, fluconazole may provide an alternative to amphotericin B in patients in whom renal function is impaired. Itraconazole may also be considered in some circumstances, offering more activity against molds, but less activity against *Candida* species.

Duration of Therapy

When an infection is documented in the neutropenic patient, it usually is satisfactory to treat the patient for 10 to 14 days. Exceptions to this are patients with persistent fever, particularly those who remain neutropenic. If no source of infection can be identified in the patient who is neutropenic, the appropriate duration of antimicrobial therapy is controversial. The risk of stopping antibiotic therapy prematurely should be balanced against the risks associated with continuing broad-spectrum antibiotics unnecessarily, especially that of developing a resistant bacterial or fungal superinfection.

The most important determinant of the duration of therapy is the patient's neutrophil count (Fig. 17.4). If the neutrophil count exceeds 500/µl and the patient is afebrile, antibiotic therapy may be stopped after a minimum of 7 days. In the case of persistent fever and a neutrophil count returning to greater than 500/µL, it is probably safe to stop antibiotics and reassess after the neutrophil count has been greater than 500/µl for 4 to 5 days (32). Assessment for fungal and viral infections should be undertaken to explain the source of persistent fever (277).

It is more difficult to decide on a course of action in patients who remain neutropenic. If no signs of infection except fever are present on physical examination and laboratory and radiographic studies, and the patient can be closely monitored, it is reasonable to stop antibacterial therapy and observe closely after the patient has been afebrile for 5 to 7 days (32). Clinicians should consider continuous antibacterial therapy for patients whose absolute neutrophil count is below 100/µL, have mucous membrane lesions of the mouth or gastrointestinal tract, or whose vital signs are unstable (9). In patients whose neutrophil count remains below 500/µL and who remain persistently febrile and in whom no source of fever can be documented, the patient should be reassessed after 2 weeks. If no source of infection can be found at that time and the patient is clinically well, some authorities suggest that antibiotics can be discontinued at that time (32,278).

It is similarly difficult to recommend a length of therapy for empiric amphotericin B. If a fungal infection has been identified, then length of therapy will depend on the causative agent, the extent of disease, and the response to treatment. If fungal infection is suspected, but not identified, there are little data to support a firm time for discontinuation of therapy. It has been suggested that if no lesions can be found by physical examination, chest radiography, and CT of the abdominal organs, empiric amphotericin B can be stopped after 2 weeks (32,84,85). In cases where suspicious lesions are present or ablative chemotherapy is planned, it may be more prudent to continue

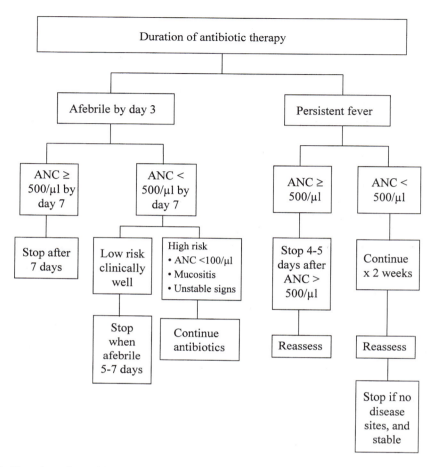

FIG. 17.4. Duration of empiric antibiotic therapy as suggested by the Infectious Diseases Society of America through its Practice Guidelines Committee. (Modified from Hughes WT, Armstrong D, Bodey GP, et al. 1997 Guidelines for the use of antimicrobial agents in neutropenic patients with unexplained fever. Infectious Diseases Society of America. *Clin Infect Dis* 1997;25:551–573, with permission of the University of Chicago Press.)

amphotericin B until resolution or recovery after neutropenia.

ADJUNCTS TO ANTIMICROBIAL THERAPY OF FEBRILE, NEUTROPENIC PATIENTS

Hematopoietic Growth Factors

Hematopoietic growth factors are the most commonly used adjunct to antimicrobial therapy of neutropenic patients. These factors are glycoprotein hormones that stimulate the proliferation and differentiation of blood cells (279,280). Two of these growth factors, granulocyte colony-stimulating factor (G-CSF) and granulocyte macrophage stimulating growth factor (GM-CSF), have been most frequently used in managing the neutropenic cancer patient. In addition to increasing number of neutrophils, G-CSF and GM-CSF also enhance phagocytic function (e.g., phagocytosis, chemotaxis, oxidative burst, and antibody-dependent cytotoxicity) and the function of macrophages in the lung (281). Thus, CSF augments neutropenic patients' host defenses both by shortening the duration of neutropenia after chemotherapy or bone marrow transplantation and by enhancing the response to invading microorganisms (282,283). Relative to G-CSF, GM-CSF acts on a broader range of blood cells, including eosinophils, monocytes, and their lineages in addition to granulocytes. GM-CSF is also more likely to be associated with fever, a particularly vexing adverse effect in the neutropenic patient.

Administration of G-CSF and GM-CSF decreases the incidence and duration of febrile neutropenic episodes after chemotherapy in some, but not all, circumstances (282,283). The routine use of CSFs is not recommended for neutropenic children; however, use of these agents may be considered on a case-by-case basis when the predicted duration of neutropenia is several days and there is life-threatening bacterial or fungal infection such as pneumonia, hypotensive episodes, or organ dysfunction related to sepsis, cellulitis, or sinusitis, and systemic fungal infections, especially if these infections fail to respond to appropriate antibiotic therapy as expected (32). Therapy with CSFs should also be considered for patients who remain severely neutropenic and have infection or colonization with a high risk of infection with antibiotic- or antifungal-resistant organisms.

Granulocyte Transfusions

Despite sporadic reports of successful use of granulocyte infusions to prevent infection or augment antimicrobial therapy in neutropenic patients (284,285), widespread use of this adjuvant therapy has never been advocated. In part, lack of endorsement of granulocyte transfusions is based on the occurrence of substantial complications from this modality and the need for large numbers of willing donors to extend treatment beyond the occasional child in special circumstances. Among the adverse effects that weigh against routine use of granulocyte transfusions are immediate reaction to the infusion, including rash and

hypotension, transmission of viral infections—most notably CMV infection, development of pulmonary infiltrates of unclear pathogenesis, and, rarely, development of graft versus host disease (286,287). Harvesting granulocytes from donors requires the use of anticoagulants and, in some cases, the use of marrow stimulants to enhance recovery of granulocytes, and therefore adverse effects occasionally occur in the donor.

Antimicrobial Prophylaxis

It is critical to distinguish empiric therapy, which is antimicrobial administration for suspected infection, from prophylactic therapy, which is antimicrobial therapy in a high-risk setting for infection, but without evidence such as fever to suggest infection. Antibiotic and antifungal empiric therapy continues to receive universal support in the setting of neutropenic patients with suspected infection. In contrast, recently sentiment has turned decidedly against the prolonged use of prophylactic antibiotics in neutropenic patients (32). Although the short-term benefits of prophylaxis of neutropenic patients has been well documented (32), the emergence of serious problems of antimicrobial resistance with once universally and exquisitely susceptible microorganisms has caused thoughtful reevaluation of prophylaxis. If used at all, prophylaxis should be administered for as short a time as possible, and the targeted population should be as small as possible (32). Among prophylactic regimens that one could consider, TMP-SM is appealing because this drug prevents pneumonia due to *P. carinii,* it is well tolerated by children with cancer, it does not have a strong propensity to cause overgrowth of fungi, and it is not generally used as a front-line treatment drug; so antibacterial resistance to it may not be critical. In an effort to limit adverse effects of TMP-SM, 3 days a week (Monday, Tuesday, Wednesday) administration was evaluated in children with cancer. An unanticipated result of that study was that 3 days per week TMP-SM prevented bacterial infection at least as effectively as daily administration (178). Counter to the use of TMP-SM as prophylaxis is that its administration may select for organisms with other important antibiotic resistances, it may prolong neutropenia, and it can cause serious allergic reactions, although these are distinctly uncommon in the immunosuppressed cancer patient. Quinolones have been shown to be effective prophylaxis in neutropenic adults, but the use of quinolones in children without a specific indication is still avoided because of possible damage to growing cartilage. Although quinolones may be superior to TMP-SM in preventing gram-negative bacterial infections (288), these agents have been associated with increased risk to viridans streptococcal sepsis (250) of particular concern in children, although varying considerably in incidence among institutions. Nonabsorbable regimens designed to modulate selectively the intestinal flora are often poorly tolerated by cancer patients and tend to induce fungal overgrowth and antimicrobial resistance.

In contrast to data that strongly support the use of empiric antifungal therapy in the patient with suspected fungal infection, prophylaxis against fungal infection has not been convincingly shown to be beneficial. Use of prophylactic fluconazole has been associated with increased incidence of colonization and infection with molds and resistant yeasts, such as *C. krusei*. Itraconazole has relatively better activity against molds, but experience with this agent is still quite limited. The toxicity of amphotericin B compromises any advantage that might be gained from its prophylactic use. Thus, currently, antifungal prophylaxis is not generally recommended.

In conclusion, given the present concerns regarding the emergence of antimicrobial resistance, antimicrobial prophylaxis is not routinely recommended other than the coincidental antibacterial prophylaxis in the course of TMP-SM prophylaxis against *P. carinii* pneumonia.

Antiviral Drugs

With the exception of prophylactic ganciclovir or foscarnet administration in patients undergoing bone marrow transplantation, empiric use of antiviral agents in the febrile neutropenic patient is seldom used in the absence of evidence of viral infection. Because bacterial or fungal invasion may be facilitated in the presence of skin or mucous membrane disruption by herpes simplex virus (139) or varicella zoster virus, acyclovir treatment is indicated to hasten healing of the lesions, even in the absence of fever. Valacyclovir and famciclovir are new agents that are better absorbed orally than acyclovir and require less frequent dosing, offering reasonable alternatives to oral acyclovir. Although lack of response or resistance to acyclovir is uncommon with herpes simplex virus, resistance does occur. Foscarnet is generally effective for treating lesions from acyclovir-resistant herpes simplex virus. The role of the new antiviral drug cidofovir has not been adequately studied yet. Certain respiratory tract infections caused by viral agents (e.g., influenza) may benefit from specific antiviral therapy in febrile neutropenic patients.

SUMMARY

Recognition that fever may be the sole indication of a life-threatening infection combined with standardized approaches to empiric therapy and the availability of safe, effective broad-spectrum antibiotics has had a major impact on mortality and morbidity in the cancer patient. The vast majority of neutropenic children can be managed successfully with the principles and regimens outlined in this chapter.

Whereas standardization of approach is desirable, successful management of the neutropenic child also requires individual focus, including at least daily physical examination and assessment of the patient's course once fever has occurred. The patterns of infectious agents and the susceptibilities of the local institution also must be judiciously factored into the management of the individual patient. One must stand ready to modify therapy at any point during the course of the neutropenia, reflecting the increasingly dynamic course of infection as the duration of neutropenia lengthens. Perhaps in no other cohort of patients is constant vigilance so unequivocally linked to outcome.

ACKNOWLEDGMENTS

Supported in part by grant P30 CA 21765 from the National Cancer Institute and by the American Lebanese Syrian Associated Charities (ALSAC).

REFERENCES

1. Bullock W. *The history of bacteriology.* New York: Dover Publications, 1979:259.
2. Bodey GP, Buckley M, Sathe YS, et al. Quantitative relationships between circulating leukocytes and infection in patients with acute leukemia. *Ann Intern Med* 1966;64:328–340.
3. Schimpff S, Satterlee W, Young VM, et al. Empiric therapy with carbenicillin and gentamicin for febrile patients with cancer and granulocytopenia. *N Engl J Med* 1971;284:1061–1065.
4. Bodey GP, Middleman E, Umsawadi T, et al. Infections in cancer patients: results with gentamicin sulfate therapy. *Cancer* 1972;29:1697–1701.
5. Feld R, Bodey GP, Rodriguez V, et al. Causes of death in patients with malignant lymphoma. *Am J Med Sci* 1974;268:97–106.
6. Chang HY, Rodriguez V, Narboni G, et al. Causes of death in adults with acute leukemia. *Medicine (Baltimore)* 1976;55:259–268.
7. Balducci L, Halbrook JC, Chapman SW, et al. Acute leukemia and infections: perspectives from a general hospital. *Am J Hematol* 1983;15:57–63.
8. Bodey GP, Rodriguez V, Chang HY, et al. Fever and infection in leukemic patients: a study of 494 consecutive patients. *Cancer* 1978;41:1610–1622.
9. Pizzo PA, Robichaud KJ, Gill FA, et al. Duration of empiric antibiotic therapy in granulocytopenic patients with cancer. *Am J Med* 1979;67:194–200.
10. Pizzo PA, Robichaud KJ, Gill FA, et al. Empiric antibiotic and antifungal therapy for cancer patients with prolonged fever and granulocytopenia. *Am J Med* 1982;72:101–111.
11. Bodey GP, Fainstein V, Elting LS, et al. Beta-lactam regimens for the febrile neutropenic patient. *Cancer* 1990;65:9–16.
12. Jones PG, Rolston KV, Fainstein V, et al. Aztreonam therapy in neutropenic patients with cancer. *Am J Med* 1986;81:243–248.
13. Rolston KV, Berkley P, Bodey GP, et al. A comparison of imipenem to ceftazidime with or without amikacin as empiric therapy in febrile neutropenic patients. *Arch Intern Med* 1992;152:283–291.
14. Rubin M, Hathorn JW, Pizzo PA. Controversies in the management of febrile neutropenic cancer patients. *Cancer Invest* 1988;6:167–184.
15. Dale DC, Guerry IVD, Wewerka JR, et al. Chronic neutropenia. *Medicine (Baltimore)* 1979;58:128–144.
16. Shenep JL. Combination and single-agent empirical antibacterial therapy for febrile cancer patients with neutropenia and mucositis. *National Cancer Institute Monograph* 1990;9:117–122.
17. Kern W, Kurrle E, Schmeiser T. Streptococcal bacteremia in adult patients with leukemia undergoing aggressive chemotherapy: a review of 55 cases. *Infection* 1990;18:138–145.
18. Weisman SJ, Scoopo FJ, Johnson GM, et al. Septicemia in pediatric oncology patients: the significance of viridans streptococcal infections. *J Clin Oncol* 1990;8:453–459.
19. Bochud PY, Eggiman P, Calandra T, et al. Bacteremia due to viridans streptococcus in neutropenic patients with cancer: clinical spectrum and risk factors. *Clin Infect Dis* 1994;18:25–31.
20. Rossetti F, Cesaro S, Putti MC, et al. High-dose cytosine arabinoside and viridans streptococcus sepsis in children with leukemia. *Pediatr Hematol Oncol* 1995;12:387–392.
21. Schimpff SC, Young VM, Greene WH, et al. Origin of infection in acute nonlymphocytic leukemia: significance of hospital acquisition of potential pathogens. *Ann Intern Med* 1972;77:707–714.
22. Keusch GT. Nutrition and infections. *Compative Therapy* 1982;8:7–15.
23. Rubin M, Hathorn JW, Marshall D, et al. Gram-positive infections and the use of vancomycin in 550 episodes of fever and neutropenia. *Ann Intern Med* 1988;108:30–35.
24. Whitecar JPJ, Luna M, Bodey GP. *Pseudomonas* bacteremia in patients with malignant diseases. *Am J Med Sci* 1970;60:216–223.
25. Rodriguez V, Bodey GP. Antibacterial therapy—special considerations in neutropenic patients. *Clinical Haematology* 1976;5:347–360.
26. Bodey GP, Jadeja L, Elting L. *Pseudomonas* bacteremia: retrospective analysis of 410 episodes. *Arch Intern Med* 1985;145:1621–1629.
27. Pizzo PA, Hathorn JW, Hiemenz J, et al. A randomized trial comparing ceftazidime alone with combination antibiotic therapy in cancer patients with fever and neutropenia. *N Engl J Med* 1986;315:552–558.
28. Klastersky J, Glauser MP, Schimpff SC, et al. Prospective randomized comparison of three antibiotic regimens for empirical therapy of suspected bacteremic infection in febrile granulocytopenic patients. *Antimicrob Agents Chemother* 1986;29: 263–270.
29. Mortimer J, Miller S, Black D, et al. Comparison of cefoperazone and mezlocillin with imipenem as empiric therapy in febrile neutropenic cancer patients. *Am J Med* 1988;85:17–20.
30. Pizzo PA, Robichaud KJ, Wesley R, et al. Fever in the pediatric and young adult patient with cancer: a prospective study of 1001 episodes. *Medicine (Baltimore)* 1982;61:153–165.
31. Bodey GP. Infection in cancer patients: a continuing association. *Am J Med* 1986;81:11–26.
32. Hughes WT, Armstrong D, Bodey GP, et al. 1997 Guidelines for the use of antimicrobial agents in neutropenic patients with unexplained fever. Infectious Diseases Society of America. *Clin Infect Dis* 1997;25: 551–573.
33. Shenep JL, Adair JR, Hughes WT, et al. Infrared, ther-

mistor, and glass-mercury thermometry for measurement of body temperature in children with cancer. *Clin Pediatr* 1991;30(Suppl):36–41.

34. Hughes WT. Fatal infections in childhood leukemia. *Amer J Dis Child* 1971;122:283–287.

35. Schimpff SC. Empiric antibiotic therapy for granulocytopenic cancer patients. *Am J Med* 1986;80:13–20.

36. Sickles EA, Greene WH, Wiernik PH. Clinical presentation of infection in granulocytopenic patients. *Arch Intern Med* 1975;135:715–719.

37. Schimpff SC. Diagnosis of infection in patients with cancer. *Eur J Cancer* 1975;11(Suppl):29–38.

38. Schimpff SC, Wiernik PH, Block JB. Rectal abscesses in cancer patients. *Lancet* 1972;2:844–847.

39. Valdivieso M, Gil-extremera B, Zornoza J, et al. Gramnegative bacillary pneumonia in the compromised host. *Medicine (Baltimore)* 1977;56:241–254.

40. Berger AM, Kilroy TJ. Oral complications of cancer therapy. In: DeVita VT, Hellman S, Rosenberg SA, eds. *Cancer*: principles and practices of oncology. Philadelphia: Lippincott-Raven, 1997:2714–2725.

41. Eras P, Goldstein MJ, Sherlock P. *Candida* infection of the gastrointestinal tract. *Medicine (Baltimore)* 1972; 51:367–379.

42. Meyer RD, Young LS, Armstrong D, Yu B. *Aspergillosis* complicating neoplastic disease. *Am J Med* 1973; 54:6–15.

43. Gerson SL, Talbot GH, Lusk E, Hurwitz S, et al. Invasive pulmonary aspergillosis in adult acute leukemia: clinical clues to its diagnosis. *J Clin Oncol* 1985;3: 1109–1116.

44. Gerson SL, Talbot GH, Hurwitz S, et al. Discriminant scorecard for diagnosis of invasive pulmonary aspergillosis in patients with acute leukemia. *Am J Med* 1985;79:57–64.

45. Glenn J, Cotton D, Wesley R, et al. Anorectal infections in patients with malignant diseases. *Rev Infect Dis* 1988;10:42–52.

46. Venditti M, Micozzi A, Gentile G, et al. Invasive *Fusarium solani* infections in patients with acute leukemia. *Rev Infect Dis* 1988;10:653–660.

47. Jarowski CI, Fialk MA, Murray HW, et al. Fever, rash, and muscle tenderness: a distinctive clinical presentation of disseminated candidiasis. *Arch Intern Med* 1978;138:544–546.

48. Arena FP, Perlin M, Brahman H, et al. Fever, rash, and myalgias of disseminated candidiasis during antifungal therapy. *Arch Intern Med* 1981;141:1233.

49. Henrickson KJ, Shenep JL. Fulminating *Staphylococcus epidermidis* bacteremia. *South Med J* 1990;83: 231–234.

50. Shenep JL, Kalwinsky DK, Feldman S, et al. Mycotic cervical lymphadenitis following oral mucositis in children with leukemia. *J Pediatr* 1985;106:243–246.

51. Bodey GP. Infections in cancer patients. *Cancer Treat Rev* 1975;2:89–128.

52. Weber DJ, Gammon WR, Cohen MS. The acutely ill patient with fever and rash. In: Mandell GL, Douglas RG, Bennett JE, eds. *Principles and practices of infectious diseases*. New York: Churchill Livingstone, 1990;479–489.

53. Fine JD, Miller JA, Harrist TJ, et al. Cutaneous lesions in disseminated candidiasis mimicking ecthyma gangrenosum. *Am J Med* 1981;70:1133–1135.

54. Bodey GP, Bolivar R, Fainstein V, et al. Infections

caused by *Pseudomonas aeruginosa. Rev Infect Dis* 1983;5:279–313.

55. Meyer RD, Kaplan MH, Ong M, et al. Cutaneous lesions in disseminated mucormycosis. *JAMA* 1973;225: 737–738.

56. Kramer BS, Hernandez AD, Reddick RL, et al. Cutaneous infarction: manifestation of disseminated mucormycosis. *Arch Dermatol* 1977;113:1075–1076.

57. Bodey GP, Luna M. Skin lesions associated with disseminated candidiasis. *JAMA* 1974;229:1466–1468.

58. Kressel B, Szewczyk C, Tuazon CU. Early clinical recognition of disseminated candidiasis by muscle and skin biopsy. *Arch Intern Med* 1978;138:429–433.

59. Allen U, Smith CR, Prober CG. The value of skin biopsies in febrile, neutropenic, immunocompromised children. *Am J Dis Child* 1986;140:459–461.

60. Arrese JE, Pierard-Franchimont C, Pierard GE. Fatal hyalohyphomycosis following *Fusarium onychomycosis* in an immunocompromised patient. *Am J Dermatopathol* 1996;18:196–198.

61. Aly R, Berger T. Common superficial fungal infections in patients with AIDS. *Clin Infect Dis* 1996; 22(Suppl 2):S128–S132.

62. Flynn PM, Van Hooser B, Gigliotti F. Atypical mycobacterial infections of Hickman catheter exit sites. *Pediatr Infect Dis J* 1988;7:510–513.

63. Engler HD, Hass A, Hodes DS, et al. *Mycobacterium chelonei* infection of a Broviac catheter insertion site. *Eur J Clin Microbiol Infect Dis* 1989;8:521–523.

64. Flynn PM, Shenep JL, Barrett FF. Differential quantitation with a commercial blood culture tube for diagnosis of catheter-related infection. *J Clin Microbiol* 1988;26:1045–1046.

65. Benezra D, Kiehn TE, Gold JW, et al. Prospective study of infections in indwelling central venous catheters using quantitative blood cultures. *Am J Med* 1988;85:495–498.

66. Newman KA, Schimpff SC. Hospital hotel services as risk factors for infection among immunocompromised patients. *Rev Infect Dis* 1987;9:206–213.

67. Kramer BS, Pizzo PA, Robichaud KJ, et al. Role of serial microbiologic surveillance and clinical evaluation in the management of cancer patients with fever and granulocytopenia. *Am J Med* 1982;72:561–568.

68. Marina NM, Flynn PM, Rivera GK, et al. *Candida tropicalis* and *Candida albicans* fungemia in children with leukemia. *Cancer* 1991;68:594–599.

69. Flynn PM, Marina NM, Rivera GK, et al. *Candida tropicalis* infections in children with leukemia. *Leuk Lymphoma* 1993;10:369–376.

70. Wingard JR, Merz WG, Saral R. *Candida tropicalis*: a major pathogen in immunocompromised patients. Ann Intern Med 1979;91:539–543.

71. Wingard JR, Dick JD, Merz WG, et al. Pathogenicity of *Candida tropicalis* and *Candida albicans* after gastrointestinal inoculation in mice. *Infect Immun* 1980;29:808–813.

72. Wingard JR, Dick JD, Merz WG, et al. Differences in virulence of clinical isolates of *Candida tropicalis* and *Candida albicans* in mice. *Infect Immun* 1982;37: 833–836.

73. McCullers JA, Vargas SL, Flynn PM, et al. *Candida meningitis* in children with cancer. *Clin Infect Dis* 2000 (*in press*).

74. McCullers JA, Flynn PM. *Candida tropicalis* osteo-

myelitis: case report and review. *Clin Infect Dis* 1998;26:1000–1001.

75. Wingard JR, Merz WG, Rinaldi MG, et al. Increase in *Candida krusei* infections among patients with bone marrow transplantation and neutropenia treated prophylactically with fluconazole. *N Engl J Med* 1991; 325:1274–1277.

76. Anonymous. Surveillance cultures in neutropenia [Editorial]. *Lancet* 1989;1:1238–1239.

77. Aisner J, Murillo J, Schimpff SC, et al. Invasive aspergillosis in acute leukemia: correlation with nose cultures and antibiotic use. *Ann Intern Med* 1979;90: 4–9.

78. Yu VL, Muder RR, Poorsattar A. Significance of isolation of Aspergillus from the respiratory tract in diagnosis of invasive pulmonary aspergillosis: results from a three-year prospective study. *Am J Med* 1986;81: 249–254.

79. Korones DN, Hussong MR, Gullace MA. Routine chest radiography of children with cancer hospitalized for fever and neutropenia. *Cancer* 1997;80;6: 1160–1164.

80. Donowitz GR, Harman C, Pope T, et al. The role of the chest roentgenogram in febrile neutropenic patients. *Arch Intern Med* 1991:151;701–704.

81. Katz JA, Bash R, Rollins N, et al. The yield of routine chest radiography in children with cancer hospitalized for fever and neutropenia. *Cancer* 1991;68:940–943.

82. Jochelson M, Altschuler J, Stomper PC. The yield of chest radiography in febrile and neutropenic patients. *Ann Intern Med* 1986;105;5:708–709.

83. Feusner J, Cohen R, O'Leary M, et al. Use of routine chest radiography in the evaluation of fever in neutropenic pediatric oncology patients. *J Clin Oncol* 1988;6:1699–1702.

84. Bartley DL, Hughes WT, Parvey LS, et al. Computed tomography of hepatic and splenic fungal abscesses in leukemic children. *Pediatr Infect Dis* 1982;1:317–321.

85. Flynn PM, Shenep JL, Crawford R, et al. Use of abdominal computed tomography for identifying disseminated fungal infection in pediatric cancer patients. *Clin Infect Dis* 1995;20:964–970.

86. Feld R, Bodey GP. Infections in patients with malignant lymphoma treated with combination chemotherapy. *Cancer* 1977;39:1018–1025.

87. Weinberger M, Pizzo PA. The evaluation and management of neutropenic patients with unexplained fever. In: Patrick CC, ed. *Infections in immunocompromised infants and children.* New York: Churchill-Livingstone, 1992:335–356.

88. Love LJ, Schimpff SC, Hahn DM, et al. Randomized trial of empiric antibiotic therapy with ticarcillin in combination with gentamicin, amikacin or netilmicin in febrile patients with granulocytopenia and cancer. *Am J Med* 1979;66:603–610.

89. Martino P, Girmenia C, Raccah R, et al. Ceftriaxone and amikacin as single daily dose in the empiric therapy for febrile episodes in neutropenic patients. *Haematologica* 1990;75:69–74.

90. Meunier F, Snoeck R, Lagast H, et al. Empirical antimicrobial therapy with timentin plus amikacin in febrile granulocytopenic cancer patients. *J Antimicrob Chemother* 1986;17(Suppl C):195–201.

91. Mackie MJ, Reilly JT, Purohit S, et al. A randomized trial of timentin and tobramycin versus piperacillin and tobramycin in febrile neutropenic patients. *J Antimicrob Chemother* 1986;17(Suppl C):219–224.

92. Kramer BS, Ramphal R, Rand KH. Randomized comparison between two ceftazidime-containing regimens and cephalothin-gentamicin-carbenicillin in febrile granulocytopenic cancer patients. *Antimicrob Agents Chemother* 1986;30:64–68.

93. Rotstein C, Cimino M, Winkey K, et al. Cefoperazone plus piperacillin versus mezlocillin plus tobramycin as empiric therapy for febrile episodes in neutropenic patients. *Am J Med* 1988;85:36–43.

94. de Jongh CA, Joshi JH, Thompson BW, et al. A double beta-lactam combination versus an aminoglycoside-containing regimen as empiric antibiotic therapy for febrile granulocytopenic cancer patients. *Am J Med* 1986;80:101–111.

95. The EORTC International Antimicrobial Therapy Cooperative Group. Ceftazidime combined with a short or long course of amikacin for empirical therapy of gram-negative bacteremia in cancer patients with granulocytopenia. *N Engl J Med* 1987;317:1692–1698.

96. Winston DJ, Ho WG, Bruckner DA, et al. Controlled trials of double beta-lactam therapy with cefoperazone plus piperacillin in febrile granulocytopenic patients. *Am J Med* 1988;85:21–30.

97. Clough JV, Farrell ID, Wood MJ, et al. Ceftazidime plus mezlocillin as initial antibiotic therapy in febrile neutropenic patients with haematological malignancy. *J Antimicrob Chemother* 1985;15:353–363.

98. Menichetti F, Del Favero A, Guerciolini R, et al. Empiric antimicrobial therapy in febrile granulocytopenic patients: randomized prospective comparison of amikacin plus piperacillin with or without parenteral trimethoprim/sulfamethoxazole. *Infection* 1986;14: 261–267.

99. Rhodes EG, Harris RI, Welch RS, et al. Empirical treatment of febrile, neutropenic patients with tobramycin and latamoxef. *J Hosp Infect* 1987;9:278–284.

100. Smith GM, Leyland MJ, Farrell ID, et al. A clinical, microbiological and pharmacokinetic study of ciprofloxacin plus vancomycin as initial therapy of febrile episodes in neutropenic patients. *J Antimicrob Chemother* 1988;21:647–655.

101. Bru JP, Michallet M, Legrand C, et al. A prospective randomized study comparing the efficacy of timentin alone or in combination with amikacin in the treatment of febrile neutropenic patients. *J Antimicrob Chemother* 1986;17(Suppl C):203–209.

102. Granowetter L, Wells H, Lange BJ. Ceftazidime with or without vancomycin vs. cephalothin, carbenicillin and gentamicin as the initial therapy of the febrile neutropenic pediatric cancer patient. *Pediatr Infect Dis J* 1988;7:165–170.

103. Shenep JL, Hughes WT, Roberson PK, et al. Vancomycin, ticarcillin, and amikacin compared with ticarcillin-clavulanate and amikacin in the empirical treatment of febrile, neutropenic children with cancer. *N Engl J Med* 1988;319:1053–1058.

104. Lau WK, Young LS, Black RE, et al. Comparative efficacy and toxicity of amikacin/carbenicillin versus gentamicin/carbenicillin in leukopenic patients: a randomized prospective trail. *Am J Med* 1977;62:959–966.

105. Schimpff SC, Gaya H, Klastersky J, et al. Three antibiotic regimens in the treatment of infection in febrile granulocytopenic patients with cancer: the EORTC In-

ternational Antimicrobial Therapy Project Group. *J Infect Dis* 1978;137:14–29.

106. Schaison G, Reinert P, Leverger G, et al. Timentin (ticarcillin and clavulanic acid) in combination with aminoglycosides in the treatment of febrile episodes in neutropenic children. *J Antimicrob Chemother* 1986; 17(Suppl C):177–181.

107. Palmblad J, Lonnqvist B. Combination of amikacin and either ampicillin or cephalothin as initial treatment of febrile neutropenic patients. *Acta Med Scand* 1982; 212:379–384.

108. Ramphal R, Kramer BS, Rand KH, et al. Early results of a comparative trial of ceftazidime versus cephalothin, carbenicillin and gentamicin in the treatment of febrile granulocytopenic patients. *J Antimicrob Chemother* 1983;12(Suppl A):81–88.

109. Morgan G, Duerden BI, Lilleyman JS. Ceftazidime as a single agent in the management of children with fever and neutropenia. *J Antimicrob Chemother* 1983; 12(Suppl A):347–351.

110. The International Antimicrobial Therapy Project Group of the European Organization for Research and Treatment of Cancer. Combination of amikacin and carbenicillin with or without cefazolin as empirical treatment of febrile neutropenic patients. *J Clin Oncol* 1983;1:597–603.

111. Winston DJ, Barnes RC, Ho WG, et al. Moxalactam plus piperacillin versus moxalactam plus amikacin in febrile granulocytopenic patients. *Am J Med* 1984;77: 442–450.

112. Feld R, Louie TJ, Mandell L, et al. A multicenter comparative trial of tobramycin and ticarcillin vs moxalactam and ticarcillin in febrile neutropenic patients. *Arch Intern Med* 1985;145:1083–1088.

113. Huijgens PC, Ossenkoppele GJ, Weijers TF, et al. Imipenem-cilastatin for empirical therapy in neutropenic patients with fever: an open study in patients with hematologic malignancies. *Eur J Haematol* 1991; 46:42–46.

114. Viscoli C, Moroni C, Boni L, et al. Ceftazidime plus amikacin versus ceftazidime plus vancomycin as empiric therapy in febrile neutropenic children with cancer. *Rev Infect Dis* 1991;13:397–404.

115. European Organization for Research and Treatment of Cancer (EORTC) International Antimicrobial Therapy Cooperative Group and the National Cancer Institute of Canada—Clinical Trials Group. Vancomycin added to empirical combination antibiotic therapy for fever in granulocytopenic cancer patients. *J Infect Dis* 1991; 163:951–958.

116. Winston DJ, Ho WG, Bruckner DA, et al. Beta-lactam antibiotic therapy in febrile granulocytopenic patients: a randomized trial comparing cefoperazone plus piperacillin, ceftazidime plus piperacillin, and imipenem alone. *Ann Intern Med* 1991;115:849–859.

117. Feliu J, Artal A, Gonzalez Baron M, et al. Comparison of two antibiotic regimens (piperacillin plus amikacin versus ceftazidime plus amikacin) as empiric therapy for febrile neutropenic patients with cancer. *Antimicrob Agents Chemother* 1992;36:2816–2820.

118. Micozzi A, Nucci M, Venditti M, et al. Piperacillin/tazobactam/amikacin versus piperacillin/amikacin/teicoplanin in the empirical treatment of neutropenic patients. *Eur J Clin Microbiol Infect Dis* 1993;12:1–8.

119. Petrilli AS, Melaragno R, Barros KV, et al. Fever and

neutropenia in children with cancer: a therapeutic approach related to the underlying disease. *Pediatr Infect Dis J* 1993;12:916–921.

120. Petrilli AS, Bianchi A, Kusano E, et al. Fever and granulocytopenia in children with cancer: a study of 299 episodes with two treatment protocols in Brazil. *Med Pediatr Oncol* 1993;21:356–361.

121. Link H, Maschmeyer G, Meyer P, et al. Interventional antimicrobial therapy in febrile neutropenic patients: Study Group of the Paul Ehrlich Society for Chemotherapy. *Ann Hematol* 1994;69:231–243.

122. Freifeld AG, Walsh T, Marshall D, et al. Monotherapy for fever and neutropenia in cancer patients: a randomized comparison of ceftazidime versus imipenem. *J Clin Oncol* 1995;13:165–176.

123. Del Favero A, Menichetti F, Bucaneve G, et al. Septicaemia due to gram-positive cocci in cancer patients. *J Antimicrob Chemother* 1988;21(Suppl C):157–165.

124. Wade JC, Schimpff SC, Newman KA, et al. *Staphylococcus epidermidis:* an increasing cause of infection in patients with granulocytopenia. *Ann Intern Med* 1982;97:503–508.

125. Winston DJ, Dudnick DV, Chapin M, et al. Coagulase-negative staphylococcal bacteremia in patients receiving immunosuppressive therapy. *Arch Intern Med* 1983;143:32–36.

126. Langley J, Gold R. Sepsis in febrile neutropenic children with cancer. *Pediatr Infect Dis J* 1988;7:34–37.

127. Viscoli C, Garaventa A, Boni L, et al. Role of Broviac catheters in infections in children with cancer. *Pediatr Infect Dis J* 1988;7:556–560.

128. Lowder JN, Lazarus HM, Herzig RH. Bacteremias and fungemias in oncologic patients with central venous catheters: changing spectrum of infection. *Arch Intern Med* 1982;142:1456–1459.

129. Karp JE, Dick JD, Angelopulos C, et al. Empiric use of vancomycin during prolonged treatment-induced granulocytopenia: randomized, double-blind, placebo-controlled clinical trial in patients with acute leukemia. *Am J Med* 1986;81:237–242.

130. Donowitz GR. Third generation cephalosporins. *Infect Dis Clin North Am* 1989;3:595–612.

131. Martin MA, Pfaller MA, Wenzel RP. Coagulase-negative staphylococcal bacteremia: mortality and hospital stay. *Ann Intern Med* 1989;110:9–16.

132. Archer GL. *Staphylococcus epidermidis* and other coagulase-negative staphylococci. In: Mandell GL, Douglas RG, Bennett JE, eds. *Principles and practices of infectious diseases* New York: John Wiley, 1990:1511–1518.

133. Haley RW, Hightower AW, Khabbaz RF, et al. The emergence of methicillin-resistant *Staphylococcus aureus* infections in United States hospitals: possible role of the house staff-patient transfer circuit. *Ann Intern Med* 1982;97:297–308.

134. Myers JP, Linnemann CCJ. Bacteremia due to methicillin-resistant *Staphylococcus aureus. J Infect Dis* 1982;145:532–536.

135. Leblanc T, Leverger G, Arlet G, et al. Frequency and severity of systemic infections caused by *Streptococcus mitis* and *sanguis II* in neutropenic children. *Pathol Biol (Paris)* 1989;37:459–464.

136. Dybedal I, Lamvik J. Respiratory insufficiency in acute leukemia following treatment with cytosine arabinoside and septicemia with streptococcus viridans [Letter]. *Eur J Haematol* 1989;42:405–406.

137. Villablanca JG, Steiner M, Kersey J, et al. The clinical spectrum of infections with viridans streptococci in bone marrow transplant patients. *Bone Marrow Transplant* 1990;5:387–393.

138. Ruescher TJ, Sodeifi A, Scrivani SJ, et al. The impact of mucositis on alpha-hemolytic streptococcal infection in patients undergoing autologous bone marrow transplantation for hematologic malignancies. *Cancer* 1998;82:2275–2281.

139. Ringden O, Heimdahl A, Lonnqvist B, et al. Decreased incidence of viridans streptococcal septicaemia in allogeneic bone marrow transplant recipients after the introduction of acyclovir [Letter]. *Lancet* 1984;1:744.

140. Uttley AH, Woodford N, Johnson AP, et al. Vancomycin-resistant enterococci [Letter]. *Lancet* 1993;342:615–616.

141. Leclercq R, Derlot E, Duval J, Courvalin P. Plasmid-mediated resistance to vancomycin and teicoplanin in *Enterococcus faecium. N Engl J Med* 1988;319:157–161.

142. Henning KJ, Delencastre H, Eagan J, et al. Vancomycin-resistant *Enterococcus faecium* on a pediatric oncology ward: duration of stool shedding and incidence of clinical infection. *Pediatr Infect Dis J* 1996;15:848–854.

143. Anglim AM, Klym B, Byers KE, et al. Effect of a vancomycin restriction policy on ordering practices during an outbreak of vancomycin-resistant *Enterococcus faecium. Arch Intern Med* 1997;157:1132–1136.

144. Centers for Disease Control and Prevention. Recommendations for preventing the spread of vancomycin resistance: recommendations of the Hospital Infection Control Practices Advisory Committee (HICPAC), *MMWR Morb Mortal Wkly Rep* 1995;44(RR-12):1–13.

145. Hande KR, Witebsky FG, Brown MS, et al. Sepsis with a new species of Corynebacterium. *Ann Intern Med* 1976;85:423–426.

146. Young VM, Meyers WF, Moody MR, et al. The emergence of coryneform bacteria as a cause of nosocomial infections in compromised hosts. *Am J Med* 1981;70:646–650.

147. Van Etta LL, Filice GA, Ferguson RM, et al. *Corynebacterium equi:* a review of 12 cases of human infection. *Rev Infect Dis* 1983;5:1012–1018.

148. McWhinney PH, Kibbler CC, Gillespie SH, et al. *Stomatococcus mucilaginosus:* an emerging pathogen in neutropenic patients. *Clin Infect Dis* 1992;14:641–646.

149. Henwick S, Koehler M, Patrick CC. Complications of bacteremia due to *Stomatococcus mucilaginosus* in neutropenic children. *Clin Infect Dis* 1993;17:667–671.

150. Brown EA, Talbot GH, Provencher M, et al. Anaerobic bacteremia in patients with acute leukemia. *Infect Control Hosp Epidemiol* 1989;10:65–69.

151. Fainstein V, Elting LS, Bodey GP. Bacteremia caused by non-sporulating anaerobes in cancer patients: a 12-year experience. *Medicine (Baltimore)* 1989;68:151–162.

152. Cotton DJ, Gill VJ, Marshall DJ, et al. Clinical features and therapeutic interventions in 17 cases of *Bacillus* bacteremia in an immunosuppressed patient population. *J Clin Microbiol* 1987;25:672–674.

153. Bodey GP, Rodriguez S, Fainstein V, et al. *Clostridium*

bacteremia in cancer patients: a 12-year experience. *Cancer* 1991;67:1928–1942.

154. Anonymous. *Clostridium septicum* and neutropenic enterocolitis [Editorial]. *Lancet* 1987;2:608.

155. Thaler M, Gill V, Pizzo PA. Emergence of *Clostridium tertium* as a pathogen in neutropenic patients. *Am J Med* 1986;81:596–600.

156. Henrickson KJ, Shenep JL, Flynn PM, et al. Primary cutaneous bacillus cereus infection in neutropenic children. *Lancet* 1989;1:601–603.

157. Parenti DM, Snydman DR. *Capnocytophaga* species: infections in nonimmunocompromised and immunocompromised hosts. *J Infect Dis* 1985;151:140–147.

158. Weinberger M, Wu T, Rubin M, et al. *Leptotrichia buccalis* bacteremia in patients with cancer: report of four cases and review. *Rev Infect Dis* 1991;13:201–206.

159. Bartlett JG. Pseudomembranous enterocolitis and antibiotic-associated colitis. In: Feldman M, Scharschmidt BF, Sleisenger MH, eds. *Sleisenger & Fordtran's gastrointestinal and liver disease, 6th disease,* 6th ed. Philadelphia. W.B. Saunders Co., 1998:1633–1647.

160. Chiesa C, Gianfrilli P, Occhionero M, et al. *Clostridium difficile* isolation in leukemic children on maintenance cancer chemotherapy. A preliminary study. *Clin Pediatr* 1985;24:252–255.

161. Gerard M, Defresne N, Daneau D, et al. Incidence and significance of *Clostridium difficile* in hospitalized cancer patients. *Eur J Clin Microbiol Infect Dis* 1988;7:274–278.

162. Milligan DW, Kelly JK. Pseudomembranous colitis in a leukemia unit: report of five fatal cases. *J Clin Pathol* 1979;32:1237–1243.

163. Rampling A, Warren RE, Bevan PC, et al. *Clostridium difficile* in haematological malignancy. *J Clin Pathol* 1985;38:445–451.

164. Delmee M, Vandercam B, Avesani V, et al. Epidemiology and prevention of *Clostridium difficile* infections in a leukemia unit. *Eur J Clin Microbiol* 1987;6:623–627.

165. Brunetto AL, Pearson AD, Craft AW, et al. *Clostridium difficile* in an oncology unit. *Arch Dis Child* 1988;63:979–981.

166. Roghmann MC, McCarter RJJ, Brewrink J, et al. *Clostridium difficile* infection is a risk factor for bacteremia due to vancomycin-resistant enterococci (VRE) in VRE-colonized patients with acute leukemia. *Clin Infect Dis* 1997;25:1056–1059.

167. Climo MW, Israel DS, Wong ES, et al. Hospital-wide restriction of clindamycin: effect on the incidence of *Clostridium difficile*-associated diarrhea and cost. *Ann Intern Med* 1998;128:989–995.

168. Horn R, Wong B, Kiehn TE, et al. Fungemia in a cancer hospital: changing frequency, earlier onset, and results of therapy. *Rev Infect Dis* 1985;7:646–655.

169. Bodey GP. Fungal infection and fever of unknown origin in neutropenic patients. *Am J Med* 1986;80:112–119.

170. Bodey GP. The emergence of fungi as major hospital pathogens. *J Hosp Infect* 1988;11(Suppl A):411–426.

171. Anaissie EJ, Bodey GP, Rinaldi MG. Emerging fungal pathogens. *Eur J Clin Microbiol Infect Dis* 1989;8:323–330.

172. Vartivarian SE, Anaissie EJ, Bodey GP. Emerging fungal pathogens in immunocompromised patients: classification, diagnosis, and management. *Clin Infect Dis* 1993;17(Suppl 2):S487–S491.

173. Walsh TJ, Pizzo PA. Nosocomial fungal infections: a classification for hospital-acquired fungal infections and mycoses arising from endogenous flora or reactivation. *Annu Rev Microbiol* 1988;42:517–545.

174. Kaplan MH, Rosen PP, Armstrong D. Cryptococcosis in a cancer hospital: clinical and pathological correlates in forty-six patients. *Cancer* 1977;39:2265–2274.

175. Reubush TK II, Weinstein RA, Baehner RL. An outbreak of *Pneumocystis* pneumonia in children with acute lymphocytic leukemia. *Am J Dis Child* 1978;132:143–148.

176. Hughes WT. Hematogenous histoplasmosis in the immunocompromised child. *J Pediatr* 1984;105:569–575.

177. Edman JC, Kovacs JA, Masur H, et al. Ribosomal RNA sequence shows *Pneumocystis carinii* to be a member of the fungi. *Nature* 1988;334:519–522.

178. Hughes WT, Rivera GK, Schell MJ, et al. Successful intermittent chemoprophylaxis for Pneumocystis carinii pneumonitis. *N Engl J Med* 1987;316:1623–1627.

179. Meunier F. Candidiasis. *Eur J Clin Microbiol Infect Dis* 1989;8:438–447.

180. Komshian SV, Uwaydah AK, Sobel JD, et al. Fungemia caused by *Candida* species and *Torulopsis glabrata* in the hospitalized patient: frequency, characteristics, and evaluation of factors influencing outcome. *Rev Infect Dis* 1989;11:379–390.

181. Girmenia C, Martino P, De Bernardis F, et al. Rising incidence of *Candida parapsilosis* fungemia in patients with hematologic malignancies: clinical aspects, predisposing factors, and differential pathogenicity of the causative strains. *Clin Infect Dis* 1996;23:506–514.

182. Dupont B. Clinical manifestations and management of candidosis in the compromised patient. In: Warnock DW, Richardson MD, eds. *Fungal infection in the compromised patient*, 2nd ed. Chichester: John Wiley & Sons, Ltd., 1991:55–83.

183. Walsh TJ, Dixon DM. Nosocomial aspergillosis: environmental microbiology, hospital epidemiology, diagnosis and treatment. *Eur J Epidemiol* 1989;5:131–142.

184. Abbasi S, Shenep JL, Hughes WT, et al. Aspergillosis in children with cancer: a 34-year experience. *Clin Infect Dis* 1999;29:1210–1219.

185. Perfect JR, Schell WA. The new fungal opportunists are coming. *Clin Infect Dis* 1996;22(Suppl 2):S112–S118.

186. Anaissie E, Kantarjian H, Ro J, et al. The emerging role of *Fusarium* infections in patients with cancer. *Medicine (Baltimore)* 1988;67:77–83.

187. Antony SJ. Disseminated *Fusarium* infection in an immunocompromised host. *Int J Dermatol* 1996;35:815–816.

188. Walsh TJ, Gonzalez C, Lyman CA, et al. Invasive fungal infections in children: recent advances in diagnosis and treatment. *Adv Pediatr Infect Dis* 1996:11:187–290.

189. Anonymous. Mucormycosis. *Ann Intern Med* 1980;93:93–108.

190. Halpin TCJ, Dahms BB. Complications associated with intravenous lipids in infants and children. *Acta Chir Scand Suppl* 1983;517:169–177.

191. Grigg AP, Phillips P, Durham S, et al. Recurrent *Pseudallescheria boydii* sinusitis in acute leukemia. *Scand J Infect Dis* 1993;25:263–267.

192. Feldman S, Hughes WT, Daniel CB. Varicella in children with cancer: seventy-seven cases. *Pediatrics* 1975;56:388–397.

193. Morgan ER, Smalley LA. Varicella in immunocompromised children: incidence of abdominal pain and organ involvement. *Am J Dis Child* 1983;137:883–885.

194. Miliauskas JR, Webber BL. Disseminated varicella at autopsy in children with cancer. *Cancer* 1984;53:1518–1525.

195. Feldman S, Hughes WT, Kim HY. Herpes zoster in children with cancer. *Am J Dis Child* 1973;126:178–184.

196. Goodman R, Jaffe N, Filler R, et al. Herpes zoster in children with stage I–III Hodgkin's disease. *Radiology* 1976;118:429–431.

197. Schucter LM, Wingard JR, Piantadosi S, et al. Herpes zoster infection after autologous bone marrow transplantation. *Blood* 1989;74:1424–1427.

198. Saral R. Management of mucocutaneous herpes simplex virus infections in immunocompromised patients. *Am J Med* 1988;85:57–60.

199. Montgomery MT, Redding SW, Le Maistre CF. The incidence of oral herpes simplex virus infection in patients undergoing cancer chemotherapy. *Oral Surg Oral Med Oral Pathol* 1986;61:238–242.

200. Rand KH, Kramer B, Johnson AC. Cancer chemotherapy associated symptomatic stomatitis: role of herpes simplex virus. *Cancer* 1982;50:1262–1265.

201. Buss DH, Scharyj M. Herpesvirus infection of the esophagus and other visceral organs in adults: incidence and clinical significance. *Am J Med* 1979;66:457–462.

202. Ramsey PG, Fife KH, Hackman RC, et al. Herpes simplex virus pneumonia: clinical, virologic, and pathologic features in 20 patients. *Ann Intern Med* 1982;97:813–820.

203. Saral R, Ambinder RF, Burns WH, et al. Acyclovir prophylaxis against herpes simplex virus infections in patients with cancer. *Ann Intern Med* 1983;99:773–776.

204. Burns WH, Saral R, Santos GW, et al. Isolation and characterization of resistant herpes simplex virus after acyclovir therapy. *Lancet* 1982;1:421–423.

205. Henson D, Siegel SE, Fuccillo DA, et al. Cytomegalovirus infections during acute childhood leukemia. *J Infect Dis* 1972;126:469–481.

206. Meyers JD, Flournoy N, Thomas ED. Risk factors for cytomegalovirus infection after human marrow transplantation. *J Infect Dis* 1986;153:478–488.

207. Schmidt GM, Horak DA, Forman SJ, et al. A randomized, controlled trial of prophylactic ganciclovir for cytomegalovirus pulmonary infection in recipients of allogeneic bone marrow transplants. *N Engl J Med* 1991;324:1005–1011.

208. Emmanuel D, Cunningham I, Jules-Elysee K, et al. Cytomegalovirus pneumonia after bone marrow transplantation successfully treated with the combination of ganciclovir and high-dose intravenous immune globulin. *Ann Intern Med* 1988;109:777–782.

209. Reed EC, Bowden RA, Dandliker PS, et al. Treatment of cytomegalovirus pneumonia with ganciclovir and intravenous cytomegalovirus immunoglobulin in patients with bone marrow transplants. *Ann Intern Med* 1988;109:783–788.

210. Hall CB, Powell KR, MacDonald NE, et al. Respiratory syncytial viral infection in children with compromised immune function. *N Engl J Med* 1986;315:77–81.

211. Ruuskanen O, Meurman O, Akusjavvi G. Adenoviruses. In: Richman DD, Whitley RJ, Hayden FG. *Clinical virology.* New York: Churchill Livingstone, 1997:525–547.

212. Schooley RS. Morbidity in compromised patients related to viruses other than herpes group and hepatitis viruses. In: Rubin RH, Young LS, eds. *Clinical approach to infection in the compromised host.* New York: Plenum, 1994:397–410.

213. Miyamura K, Minami S, Matsuyama T, et al. Adenovirus-induced late onset hemorrhagic cystitis following allogeneic bone marrow transplant. *Bone Marrow Transplant* 1987;2:109–110.

214. Wendt CH, Weisdorf DJ, Jordan MC, et al. Parainfluenza virus respiratory infection after bone marrow transplantation. *N Engl J Med* 1992;326:921–926.

215. Feldman S, Webster RG, Sugg M. Influenza in children and young adults with cancer: 20 cases. *Cancer* 1977;39:350–353.

216. Lewis IJ, Hart CA, Baxby P. Diarrhea due to *Cryptosporidium* in acute lymphoblastic leukemia. *Arch Dis Child* 1985;60:60–62.

217. Wells GM, Gajjar A, Pearson TA, et al. Pulmonary cryptosporidiosis and *Cryptococcal albidus* fungemia in a child with acute lymphocytic leukemia. *Med Pediatr Oncol* 1988;31:544–546.

218. Chandrasekar PH, Momin F, and the Bone Marrow Transplant Team. Disseminated toxoplasmosis in marrow recipients: a report of three cases and a review of the literature. *Bone Marrow Transplant* 1997:19;685–689.

219. Igra-Siegman Y, Kapila R, Sen P, et al. Syndrome of hyperinfection with *Strongyloides stercoralis. Rev Infect Dis* 1981;3:397–407.

220. Fishman JA. *Pneumocystis carinii* and parasitic infections in the immunocompromised host. In: Rubin RH, Young LS, eds. *Clinical approach to infection in the compromised host.* New York: Plenum, 1994:275–334.

221. Shenep JL. Antimicrobial therapy in the immunocompromised host. *Semin Pediatr Infect Dis* 1998;9: 330–338.

222. Pizzo PA, Ladisch S, Ribichaud K. Treatment of gram-positive septicemia in cancer patients. *Cancer* 1980; 45:206–207.

223. Pizzo PA, Meyers J. Supportive care of the cancer patient: infections in the cancer patient. In: DeVita VT Jr, et al., eds. *Cancer: principles and practice of oncology,* 3rd ed. Philadelphia: JB Lippincott, 1989:2088–2133.

224. Pizzo PA, Thaler M, Hathorn J, et al. New beta-lactam antibiotics in granulocytopenic patients. New options and new questions. *Am J Med* 1985;79:75–82.

225. Bizette GA, Brooks BJ Jr, Alvarez S. Ceftazidime as monotherapy for fever and neutropenia: experience in a community hospital. *J La State Med Soc* 1994;146: 448–452.

226. de Pauw BE, Deresinski SC, Feld R, et al. Ceftazidime compared with piperacillin and tobramycin for the empiric treatment of fever in neutropenic patients with cancer: a multicenter randomized trial. The Intercontinental Antimicrobial Study Group. *Ann Intern Med* 1994;120:834–844.

227. Jacobs RF, Vats TS, Pappa KA, et al. Ceftazidime versus ceftazidime plus tobramycin in febrile neutropenic children. *Infection* 1993;21:223–228.

228. Liang R, Yung R, Chiu E, et al. Ceftazidime versus imipenem-cilastatin as initial monotherapy for febrile neutropenic patients. *Antimicrob Agents Chemother* 1990;34:1336–1341.

229. Novakova I, Donnelly P, De Pauw B. Amikacin plus piperacillin versus ceftazidime as initial therapy in granulocytopenic patients with presumed bacteremia. *Scand J Infect Dis* 1990;22:705–711.

230. Novakova I, Donnelly JP, De Pauw B. Ceftazidime as monotherapy or combined with teicoplanin for initial empiric treatment of presumed bacteremia in febrile granulocytopenic patients. *Antimicrob Agents Chemother* 1991;35:672–678.

231. Novakova IR, Donnelly JP, de Pauw BE. Ceftazidime with or without amikacin for the empiric treatment of localized infections in febrile, granulocytopenic patients. *Ann Hematol* 1991;63:195–200.

232. Rubinstein E, Lode H, Grassi C. Ceftazidime monotherapy vs. ceftriaxone/tobramycin for serious hospital-acquired gram-negative infections. Antibiotic Study Group. *Clin Infect Dis* 1995;20:1217–1228.

233. Sanders JW, Powe NR, Moore RD. Ceftazidime monotherapy for empiric treatment of febrile neutropenic patients: a meta-analysis. *J Infect Dis* 1991; 164:907–916.

234. Au E, Tow A, Allen DM, et al. Randomised study comparing imipenem/cilastatin to ceftriaxone plus gentamicin in cancer chemotherapy-induced neutropenic fever. *Ann Acad Med Singapore* 1994;23:819–822.

235. Bodey GP, Elting L, Jones P, et al. Imipenem/cilastatin therapy of infections in cancer patients. *Cancer* 1987;60:255–262.

236. Hauer C, Urban C, Slavc I, et al. Imipenem-antibiotic monotherapy in juvenile cancer patients with neutropenia. *Pediatr Hematol Oncol* 1990;7:229–241.

237. Leyland MJ, Bayston KF, Cohen J, et al. A comparative study of imipenem versus piperacillin plus gentamicin in the initial management of febrile neutropenic patients with haematological malignancies. *J Antimicrob Chemother* 1992;30:843–854.

238. Miller JA, Butler T, Beveridge RA, et al. Efficacy and tolerability of imipenem-cilastatin versus ceftazidime plus tobramycin as empiric therapy of presumed bacterial infection in neutropenic cancer patients. *Clin Ther* 1993;15:486–499.

239. Riikonen P. Imipenem compared with ceftazidime plus vancomycin as initial therapy for fever in neutropenic children with cancer. *Pediatr Infect Dis J* 1991;10: 918–923.

240. Rolston KV, Berkey P, Bodey GP, et al. A comparison of imipenem to ceftazidime with or without amikacin as empiric therapy in febrile neutropenic patients. *Arch Intern Med* 1992;152:283–291.

241. Cometta A, Calandra T, Gaya H, et al. Monotherapy with meropenem versus combination therapy with ceftazidime plus amikacin as empiric therapy for fever in granulocytopenic patients with cancer. *Antimicrob Agents Chemother* 1996;40:1108–1115.

242. Lindblad R, Rodjer S, Adriansson M, et al. Empiric monotherapy for febrile neutropenia—a randomized study comparing meropenem with ceftazidime. *Scand J Infect Dis* 1998;30:237–243.

243. Equivalent efficacies of meropenem and ceftazidime as empirical monotherapy of febrile neutropenic patients. The Meropenem Study Group of Leuven, London and Nijmegen. *J Antimicrob Chemother* 1995;36: 185–200.

244. Wiseman LR Lamb HM. Cefpirome. A review of its antibacterial activity, pharmacokinetic properties and clinical efficacy in the treatment of severe nosocomial infections and febrile neutropenia. *Drugs* 1997;54: 117–140.

245. Bodey GP, Elting LS, Narro J, et al. An open trial of cefoperazone plus sulbactam for the treatment of fever in cancer patients. *J Antimicrob Chemother* 1993;32: 141–152.

246. Eggimann P, Glauser MP, Aoun M, et al. Cefepime monotherapy for the empirical treatment of fever in granulocytopenic cancer patients. *J Antimicrob Chemother* 1993;32(Suppl B):151–163.

247. Yamamura D, Gucalp R, Carlisle P, et al. Open randomized study of cefepime versus piperacillin-gentamicin for treatment of febrile neutropenic cancer patients. *Antimicrobial Agents Chemother* 1997;41: 1704–1708.

248. Kieft H, Hoepelman AI, Rozenberg-Arska M, et al. Cefepime compared with ceftazidime as initial therapy for serious bacterial infections and sepsis syndrome. *Antimicrob Agents Chemother* 1994;38:415–421.

249. Ramphal R, Gucalp R, Rotstein C, et al. Clinical experience with single agent and combination regimens in the management of infection in the febrile neutropenic patient. *Amer J Med* 1996;100:83S–89S.

250. Elting LS, Bodey GP, Keefe BH. Septicemia and shock syndrome due to viridans streptococci: a case–control study of predisposing factors. *Clin Infect Dis* 1992;14: 1201–1207.

251. Martino R, Subira M, Manteiga R, et al. Viridans streptococcal bacteremia and viridans streptococcal shock syndrome in neutropenic patients: comparison between children and adults receiving chemotherapy or undergoing bone marrow transplantation [Letter]. *Clin Infect Dis* 1995;20:476–477.

252. Steiner M, Villablanca J, Kersey J, et al. Viridans streptococcal shock in bone marrow transplantation patients. *Am J Hematol* 1993;42:354–358.

253. Young LS. Neutropenia: antibiotic combinations for empiric therapy. *Eur J Clin Microbiol Infect Dis* 1989; 8:118–122.

254. Gibson J, Johnson L, Snowdon L, et al. A randomised dosage study of ceftazidime with single daily tobramycin for the empirical management of febrile neutropenia in patients with hematological diseases. *Int J Hematol* 1994;60:119–127.

255. Klastersky J, Vamecq G, Cappel R, et al. Effects of the combination of gentamicin and carbenicillin on the bactericidal activity of serum. *J Infect Dis* 1972;125: 183–186.

256. Sepkowitz KA, Brown AE, Armstrong D. Empirical therapy for febrile, neutropenic patients: persistence of susceptibility of gram-negative bacilli to aminoglycoside antibiotics. *Clin Infect Dis* 1994;19:810–811.

257. Brown AE, Kiehn TE, Armstrong D. Bacterial resistance in the patient with neoplastic disease. *Infect Dis Clin Pract* 1995;4:136–144.

258. Ramphal R, Bolger M, Oblon DJ, et al. Vancomycin is not an essential component of the initial empiric treatment regimen for febrile neutropenic patients receiving ceftazidime: a randomized prospective study. *Antimicrob Agents Chemother* 1992;36:1062–1067.

259. Cony-Makhoul P, Brossard G, Marit G, et al. A prospective study comparing vancomycin and teicoplanin as second-line empiric therapy for infection in neutropenic patients. *Br J Haematol* 1990;76 (Suppl 2):35–40.

260. Pico JL, Marie JP, Chiche D, et al. Should vancomycin be used empirically in febrile patients with prolonged and profound neutropenia? Results of a randomized trial. *Eur J Med* 1993;2:275–280.

261. Bodey GP, Fainstein V, Elting LS, et al. Beta-lactam regimens for the febrile neutropenic patient. *Cancer* 1990;65:9–16.

262. Kelsey SM, Shaw E, Newland AC. Aztreonam plus vancomycin versus gentamicin plus piperacillin as empirical therapy for the treatment of fever in neutropenic patients: a randomised controlled study. *J Chemother* 1992;4:107–113.

263. Harvey WH, Harvey JH, Moskowitz MJ. Ciprofloxacin/vancomycin (C/V) as initial empiric therapy in febrile neutropenic leukemia/lymphoma patients (pts) with indwelling venous access devices: preliminary results of an effective regimen with reduced hospital stay. *Proceedings of the Annual Meeting of the American Society of Clinical Oncology* 1994;13:A1639.

264. Kureishi A, Jewesson PJ, Rubinger M, et al. Double-blind comparison of teicoplanin versus vancomycin in febrile neutropenic patients receiving concomitant tobramycin and piperacillin: effect on cyclosporin A-associated nephrotoxicity. *Antimicrob Agents Chemother* 1991;35:2246–2252.

265. Raad II, Whimbey EE, Rolston KV, et al. A comparison of aztreonam plus vancomycin and imipenem plus vancomycin as initial therapy for febrile neutropenic cancer patients. *Cancer* 1996;77:1386–1394.

266. Traub WH, Spohr M, Bauer D. *In vitro* additive effect of imipenem combined with vancomycin against multiple-drug resistant, coagulase-negative staphylococci. *Zentralbl Bakteriol* 1986;262:361–369.

267. Chow AW, Jewesson PJ, Kureishi A, et al. Teicoplanin versus vancomycin in the empirical treatment of febrile neutropenic patients. *Eur J Haematol Suppl* 1993;54:18–24.

268. de Pauw BE, Novakova IR, Donnelly JP. Options and limitations of teicoplanin in febrile granulocytopenic patients. *Br J Haematol* 1990;76(Suppl 2):1–5.

269. Kelsey SM, Collins PW, Delord C, et al. A randomized study of teicoplanin plus ciprofloxacin versus gentamicin plus piperacillin for the empirical treatment of fever in neutropenic patients. *Br J Haematol* 1990;76 (Suppl 2):10–13.

270. Kelsey SM, Weinhardt B, Collins PW, et al. Teicoplanin plus ciprofloxacin versus gentamicin plus piperacillin in the treatment of febrile neutropenic patients. *Eur J Clin Microbiol Infect Dis* 1992;11:509–514.

271. Lim SH, Smith MP, Goldstone AH, et al. A randomized prospective study of ceftazidime and ciprofloxacin with or without teicoplanin as an empiric antibiotic regimen for febrile neutropenic patients. *Br J Haematol* 1990;76(Suppl 2):41–44.

272. Shenep JL, Flynn PM, Baker DK, et al. Oral cefixime is comparable to continued intravenous antibiotics in the empirical treatment of febrile, neutropenic children with cancer. *Clin Infect Dis* (in press).

273. Karp JE, Burch PA, Merz WG. An approach to intensive antileukemia therapy in patients with previous invasive aspergillosis. *Am J Med* 1988;85:203.

274. Robertson MJ, Larson RA. Recurrent fungal pneumonias in patients with acute nonlymphocytic leukemia

undergoing multiple courses of intensive chemotherapy. *Am J Med* 1988;84:233–239.

275. Ng TT, Denning DW. Liposomal amphotericin B (AmBisome) in invasive fungal infections: evaluation of United Kingdom compassionate use data. *Arch Intern Med* 1995;155:1093–1098.

276. Bodey GP. Azole antifungal agents. *Clin Infect Dis* 1992;14(Suppl 1):S161–169.

277. Talbot GH, Provencher M, Cassileth PA. Persistent fever after recovery from granulocytopenia in acute leukemia. *Arch Intern Med* 1988;148:129–135.

278. Joshi JH, Schimpff SC, Tenney JH, et al. Can antibacterial therapy be discontinued in persistently febrile granulocytopenic cancer patients? *Am J Med* 1984;76:450–457.

279. Glaspy JA, Golde DW. Clinical applications of the myeloid growth factors. *Semin Hematol* 1989;26:14–17.

280. Gabrilove JL. Introduction and overview of hematopoietic growth factors. *Semin Hematol* 1989;26:1–4.

281. Peters WP. The effects of recombinant human colony-stimulating factors on hematopoietic reconstitution following autologous bone marrow transplantation. *Semin Hematol* 1989;26:18–23.

282. Shepro DS, Sullivan R. Clinical use of hematopoietic recombinant colony-stimulating factors. *Adv Intern Med* 1991;36:329–362.

283. Groopman JE, Molina J-M, Scadden DT. Hematopoietic growth factors: biology and clinical implications. *N Engl J Med* 1989;321:329.

284. Strauss RG, Connett JE, Gale RP, et al . A controlled trial of prophylactic granulocyte transfusions during initial induction chemotherapy for acute myelogenous leukemia. *N Engl J Med* 1981;305:597–603.

285. Bhatia S, McCullough J, Perry EH, Clay M, Ramsay NKC, Neglia JP. Granulocyte transfusions: efficacy in treating fungal infections in neutropenic patients following bone marrow transplantation. *Transfusion* 1994;34:226–232.

286. Hersman J, Meyer JD, Thomas ED, et al. The effect of granulocyte transfusion on the incidence of cytomegalovirus infection after allogeneic marrow transplantation. *Ann Intern Med* 1982;96:149–152.

287. Wright DG. Leukocyte transfusion: thinking twice. *Am J Med* 1984;76:637–644.

288. Kern W, Kurrle E. Ofloxacin versus trimethoprim-sulfamethoxazole for prevention of infection in patients with acute leukemia and granulocytopenia. *Infection* 1991;19:73–80.

18

Sinopulmonary Infections in Immunocompromised Infants and Children

Dennis C. Stokes

Department of Pediatrics, Division of Pediatric Pulmonary Medicine, Vanderbilt University School of Medicine, Nashville, Tennessee 37232

The clinical approach to sinopulmonary infections in immunocompromised pediatric patients is difficult because of the number of potentially infectious and the myriad of noninfectious processes (1–11). The list of organisms associated with sinopulmonary infections in the immunocompromised host is extensive, and this chapter focuses on common sinopulmonary infections. The use of diagnostic tools such as needle aspiration, flexible bronchoscopy and bronchoalveolar lavage (BAL) are important in providing a specific diagnosis.

COMMON CAUSES OF PULMONARY DISORDERS IN THE IMMUNOCOMPROMISED HOST

Noninfectious Pulmonary Disorders

Immunocompromised patients are at risk for a variety of noninfectious complications that simulate infection and complicate the diagnostic workup. These disorders are not discussed extensively, but the common noninfectious processes associated with clinical scenarios such as pulmonary hemorrhage post bone marrow transplantation (BMT) are addressed (Table 18.1).

Infectious Pneumonias

Viral

Cytomegalovirus

Cytomegalovirus (CMV) is a herpes virus that causes infections in both neonates and immunocompromised children. The age and immune status of the infected individual determine whether an infection by CMV will lead to disease. The organism is transmitted through an infected birth canal, by breast milk, saliva, and blood (through infected white cells). Both humoral and cellular immune mechanisms are important in establishing protection against CMV. Persons who are CMV negative before immunosuppression as a result of organ or marrow transplantation and acquire the virus by transfusion are at high risk for disease. CMV-positive persons who then are immunosuppressed also possess a significant risk for "reactivation" of the virus.

Most infants who acquire the virus are asymptomatic, although occasional cases of protracted pneumonia have been reported. The major risk groups for CMV pneumonia include patients with acquired immunodeficiency syndrome (AIDS), congenital immunodeficiencies, and organ-transplant pa-

TABLE 18.1. *Noninfectious processes complicating or simulating pneumonia*

Process	Associated with
Chemical pneumonitis	Aspiration syndromes, smoke inhalation
Immune-mediated	Hypersensitivity pneumonitis, collagen vascular disease
Atelectasis	Reactive airways disease, endobronchial obstruction
Hemorrhage	Hemosiderosis, thrombocytopenia, coagulopathy, *Aspergillus*
Pulmonary edema	
Cardiogenic	Anthracycline cardiotoxicity, sepsis, myocarditis
Noncardiogenic	ARDS, pancreatitis, fluid overload
Drug-induced lung injury	Chemotherapy, azathioprine
Radiation pneumonitis	Radiation, 6–8 wk previously
Leukostasis	Hyperleukocytosis, amphotericin B, WBC transfusions
Leukemia, lymphoma	Active disease
Lymphocytic interstitial pneumonitis	HIV infection in children
"Idiopathic pneumonitis"	Allogeneic bone marrow transplantation
Other	Thymus, sequestration, tumor

ARDS, acute respiratory disease syndrome; HIV, human immunodeficiency virus; WBC, white blood cell count.

tients, particularly kidney, bone marrow, and heart-lung recipients (12–17). The radiographic pattern of the pneumonia is usually a diffuse reticulonodular pattern that is less alveolar involvement than *Pneumocystis carinii* pneumonia (PCP). Pathology varies from small hemorrhagic nodules scattered throughout the lung surrounded by relatively normal lung to diffuse alveolar damage to chronic interstitial pneumonia. Approximately 50% of patients with aplastic anemia or hematologic malignancy treated by allogeneic BMT develop CMV infection. In this setting, CMV pneumonia had a 90% mortality before the advent of effective antiviral therapy. CMV frequently is found as a copathogen with other opportunistic organisms, including *P. carinii* and *Aspergillus* spp., particularly in AIDS patients.

The diagnosis of CMV pneumonia usually is made by the demonstration of typical inclusions in lung tissue. Isolation of CMV from urine is not sufficient evidence that CMV is the cause of the pneumonia. Diagnostic methods using immunofluorescence (IF), DNA hybridization, or shell vial culture provide rapid diagnosis of CMV from BAL. Such techniques, although highly sensitive, must be interpreted cautiously because CMV can be detected in the lungs of asymptomatic persons.

Varicella Zoster Virus and Herpes Simplex Virus

These DNA viruses typically cause lesions of the skin and mucous membranes; however, in certain groups, including neonates, cancer, and BMT and solid-organ transplant patients, AIDS and congenital defects of cell-mediated immunity, varicella zoster virus (VZV) and herpes simplex virus (HSV) can lead to visceral dissemination and pneumonia. In cancer patients, VZV pneumonitis occurs in 85% of cases of visceral dissemination and is the principal cause of death (18,19). Before specific antiviral therapy was available, mortality secondary to VZV pneumonitis was 85%. Pneumonitis is much less common with reactivation of herpes zoster, but it is a potentially serious infection in BMT. HSV is a less common cause of dissemination in oncology patients, but it is a significant infection in neonates.

The clinical presentation of pneumonia in both HSV and VZV infections is nonspecific and includes fever, cough, dyspnea, and chest pain. Patients with an increasing number of skin lesions from VZV, abdominal or back pain, or persistent fevers and are at high risk for dissemination and pneumonia. HSV pneumonitis may be more subtle in its presentation, and pneumonitis can occur in the

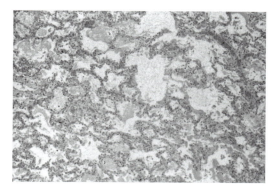

FIG. 18.1. Open lung biopsy from an immuno-compromised patient with varicella-zoster pneumonia.

absence of mucocutaneous lesions in new-borns and BMT patients. Chest radiographs of herpesvirus pneumonia typically show ill-defined nodular densities scattered through both lung fields, often beginning at the periphery. These nodules progress and coalesce into extensive infiltrates. Secondary infections such as staphylococcal pneumonia were seen more commonly in the preantibiotic era. Microscopically, these infections involve alveolar walls, blood vessels, and small bronchioles. Electron microscopy shows intranuclear inclusions of herpesvirus. Hemorrhage, necrosis, and extensive alveolar edema are seen in severe areas of involvement (Fig. 18.1). The trachea and large bronchi are often involved.

Varicella zoster immune globulin (VZIG) can modify or prevent varicella in high-risk hosts exposed to the infection if it is given within 48 to 72 hours of exposure. Acyclovir and VZIG have been major factors in the reduced incidence of serious VZV pneumonias in immunocompromised hosts. Acyclovir is the antiviral drug of choice to treat HSV. Foscarnet is a secondary drug for both viruses if acyclovir resistance occurs.

Human Herpesvirus 6

Human herpesvirus 6 (HHV-6) is a DNA virus that is the etiologic agent for roseola. It persists in normal hosts and can be isolated from lymphocytes and other sites. In the abnormal host, reactivation can lead to fever, hepatitis, bone marrow suppression and pneumonia.

Cone et al. described the identification of HHV-6 by using the polymerase chain reaction (PCR) in 15 of 15 lung biopsy specimens from patients with idiopathic pneumonitis following BMT (20). Serologic studies also supported its role in pneumonitis after transplant (20,21). Further studies documented other clinical situations where HHV-6 caused disease in immunocompromised populations, including renal transplant and AIDS (22–24). At present, effective therapy for HHV-6 is available.

Adenovirus

Adenovirus, a DNA virus, is a common cause of community-acquired lower respiratory disease. Serotypes 1, 2, and 5 are common causes of sporadic respiratory disease, and types 3 and 7 are associated with epidemics of bronchiolitis and pneumonia in the general population. In immunocompromised patients, adenovirus is one of the most important viral pneumonia etiologies, one that results in serious morbidity and mortality (25–30). Respiratory infections caused by adenoviruses in immunocompromised patients often are nosocomial infections acquired from hospital staff or family members. Adenovirus typically causes fever, pharyngitis, cough, and conjunctivitis. Pneumonia, which is usually mild in normal hosts, may progress rapidly in the immunocompromised patient with a necrotizing bronchitis and bronchiolitis (25,26). The radiographic picture is nonspecific and resembles other causes of diffuse pneumonia.

The diagnosis usually is made by lung biopsy or BAL brushings demonstrating typical adenoviral inclusions by microscopic examination or by cell culture. The diagnosis may be delayed by a misdiagnosis of a bacterial or fungal etiology, leading to the institution of empiric antibiotic and antifungal therapy. Serology may provide a diagnosis, but there is a delay. Failure of pneumonia to respond despite therapy, particularly when there have been epidemics of typical acute respiratory disease in the community or hospital staff, should raise the strong possibility of adenovirus.

Although there is no approved antiviral therapy for adenovirus, ribavirin has *in vitro* activity against it and has been used in anecdotal cases by the intravenous and inhaled route in immuncompromised patients. Supportive therapy includes oxygen, treatment of bacterial superinfections, IVIG, and assisted ventilation. The main concern for hospitalized immunocompromised patients is prevention by means of careful handwashing and other isolation procedures and segregation of staff with respiratory illnesses.

Respiratory Synctial Virus

Respiratory synctial virus (RSV) is an RNA virus with a seasonal predilection to cause respiratory diseases (31–33).

Fungal

Aspergillus *Species*

Aspergillus spp. are a group of ubiquitous fungal organisms found in soil and other settings, including the hospital environment. *Aspergillus fumigatus* is the most common cause of pneumonia in immunocompromised hosts, but other pathogenic species include *A. flavus, A. terreus,* and *A. niger* (34). In tissue, the organisms form septate hyphae with regular 45-degree dichotomous branching, best seen with methenamine silver staining (Fig. 18.2).

Aspergillus causes both acute invasive pulmonary aspergillosis and a more chronic necrotizing form (34,35). The former occurs most commonly in patients undergoing cancer therapy as well as in other immunocompromised patients, such as those with aplastic anemia. *Aspergillus* infection of the lung often is

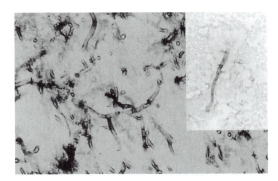

FIG. 18.2. GMS stain of *Aspergillus* spp. from a open lung biopsy; insert shows hyhal fragment from a bronchoscopy (BAL).

preceded or accompanied by invasion of the nose and paranasal sinuses in susceptible hosts. The major risk factors for Aspergillus include prolonged neutropenia, concurrent chemotherapy, and steroid therapy as well as broad-spectrum antibiotic therapy. The common occurrence of cutaneous aspergillosis often helps provide the diagnosis. In the lungs, *Aspergillus* infection can cause tracheobronchitis, pneumonia, abscesses and cavity formation, and diffuse interstitial pneumonia. The organisms often extend along blood vessels, and nodular lesions of necrosis surrounded by air often develop within an area of pneumonia, leading to the typical air crescent sign.

Diagnosis of *Aspergillus* pneumonia generally is made by pathologic examination of the infected tissue. *Aspergillus* can be isolated from BAL lavage in about 50% of cases, and needle-aspiration biopsy of suspected lesions also can demonstrate typical fungal elements. Isolation of *Aspergillus* from a nasal culture in a patient with typical clinical risk features (prolonged neutropenia, steroid therapy, progressive nodular infiltrates, cavitary lung lesion) may be helpful, but negative cultures do not exclude *Aspergillus*.

The treatment of *Aspergillus* pneumonia is amphotericin B, given at a dose of 1 to 1.5 mg/kg. Amphotericin B–lipid complex formulations are less nephrotoxic than amphotericin and are preferred for patients whose tolerance for amphotericin is limited by nephrotoxity. The addition of flucytosine or rifampin is a consideration; however, controlled studies have not been performed. Surgical excision of *Aspergillus* lesions is generally recommended whenever possible. Invasive pulmonary aspergillosis during treatment of hematologic malignancy generally is considered a contraindication to subsequent BMT, but adult patients treated with amphotericin B and surgery have survived disease-free and without reactivation of *Aspergillus* following BMT. The outcome of *Aspergillus* pneumonia depends primarily on such host factors as degree of immunosuppression and recovery of neutrophil counts as well as early diagnosis and treatment (36).

Mucormycosis

Mucormycosis includes fungal disease caused by a variety of species in the class Zygomycetes, including *Mucoraceae* and *Cunninghamellacaeae.* In tissues, they are differentiated from *Aspergillus* by their broad, nonseptate hyphae that branch at angles up to 90 degrees and have an appearance of "twisted ribbons" (Fig. 18.3). Zygomycete organisms cause disease only in patients with underlying disease (37). In adults, this is associated with chronic acidosis states, such as ketoacidosis in diabetes mellitus. Most pediatric cases of pneumonia occur in the oncol-

ogy population, and this organism is found in the same patient risk groups as *Aspergillus.*

Pneumonia due to the Zygomycetes is usually an insidious segmental pneumonia that is slowly progressive despite antifungal therapy (Fig. 18.4). Persistent fever, chest pain, hemoptysis, and weight loss are typical. Cavitation may occur, and dissemination to the brain and other sites occurs as a result of the propensity of the organism to invade blood vessels. Death may occur suddenly with massive pulmonary hemorrhage, mediastinitis, or airway obstruction.

Specific diagnosis usually depends on demonstration of the organism in open, transbronchial, or needle-aspiration lung biopsy specimens.

As with *Aspergillus,* treatment with amphotericin B and possibly surgical resection as early as possible is critical to achieving a

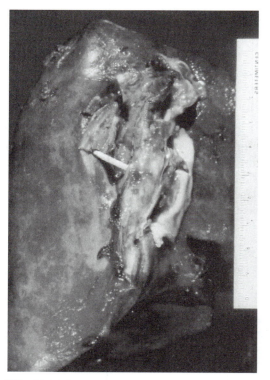

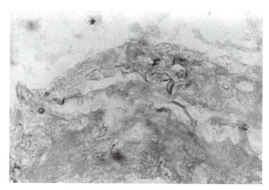

FIG. 18.3. GMS stain of *Mucor* sp. in infected tissue. Note the "twisted ribbon" morphology.

FIG. 18.4. Autopsy specimen showing invasion and necrosis of lung hilar and mediastinal structures by *Mucor* sp.

cure. Correction of chronic acidosis, if present, is also important in some forms.

Candida *Species*

Candida spp. are an important cause of fungal sepsis and secondary hematogenous pulmonary involvement, but primary *Candida* pneumonia is unusual (38). *C. albicans* and *C. tropicalis* are the most important causes of fungal sepsis and secondary pulmonary involvement (39,40). Patients with HIV infection, primary immunodeficiencies, and prolonged neutropenia are at greatest risk, but other predisposing conditions include diabetes, corticosteroid administration, broad-spectrum antibiotic treatment, intravenous hyperalimentation, and venous access devices.

In tissue, silver stains show oval budding yeasts 2 to 6 μ in diameter with pseudohyphae. In a series of 31 patients with primary *Candida* pneumonia from M.D. Anderson, the prominent histologic features included bronchopneumonia, intraalveolar exudates, and hemorrhage.

Amphotericin B is usually the treatment of choice for invasive *Candida* infections, along with flucytosine if synergism is desired. The imidazole antifungal agents, including ketoconazole, fluconazole, and itraconazole, have activity against some *Candida* species and have been used successfully in small series. Use of the imidazole antifungal agents for prophylaxis may select more resistant fungal organisms in high-risk populations.

Histoplasma capsulatum *and* Blastomyces dermatitidis *Infections*

Histoplasma capsulatum and *Blastomyces dermatitidis* are ubiquitous soil fungi endemic to the eastern and southeastern United States. Histoplasmosis is a common infection, and it may be asymptomatic or lead to an acute pneumonia with fever, hilar adenopathy, and pulmonary infiltrates (41). Blastomycosis is a less common, more serious infection (Fig. 18.5) (42). Both can cause chronic granulo-

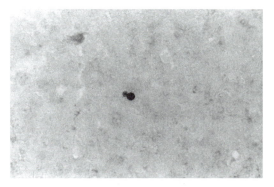

FIG. 18.5. Microscopic examination of Blastomycoses dermatitidis showing large, double refractile cell with a single bud that is connected by a broad base.

matous pulmonary disease as well as disseminated disease.

In the immunocompromised patient, including patients with AIDS, the major risk for both organisms is dissemination with pulmonary infiltrates, hepatosplenomegaly, fevers, and adenopathy. Histoplasmosis is much more common in the immunocompromised host than is blastomycosis.

Amphotericin B is indicated for both histoplasmosis and blastomycosis in immunocompromised hosts. Itraconazole is also effective for histoplasmosis and moderate blastomycosis without central nervous system involvement.

Crytococcus neoformans *Infection*

Crytococcus neoformans is a yeast that causes protean clinical manifestations in immunocompromised patients, particularly those with AIDS (43). Meningitis is the most common presentation, but endocarditis, pneumonia, and involvement of the skin and lymph nodes often occur (44). The lungs are the portal of entry for *C. neoformans*, and pulmonary involvement may be minimal if dissemination occurs quickly. Pneumonia typically is accompanied by chest pain, fever, and cough. Pulmonary disease with *Cryptococcus* is rarer in pediatric AIDS patients than in adults. Treatment is with intravenous amphotericin B and oral flucytosine.

TABLE 18.2. *Unusual fungal infections with potential pulmonary involvement*

Primary primary *Candida* pneumonia (as opposed to secondary pneumonia following septicemia) is rare
Increased importance of non-*albicans Candida*:
    primarily fungemia with secondary pulmonary involvement
    Candida tropicalis
    Candida parapilosis
    Candida kruzei
    Torulopis gabrata
Emerging pathogens
    Phaeohyphomycoses
        Curvularia: sinusitis
        Bipolaris, Exserohilum, Alternaria: similar in clinical presentation to *Aspergillus*
    Hyalohyphomycoses
        Fusarium: sinusitis or rhinocerebral disease
        Scopulariopsis
        Pseudallesheria boydii: sinusitis, pneumonia
    Trichosporon: risk factors similar to Candida, primarily hematogenous
    Malessizia furfur type h

With the expansion of the immunocompromised population, several recent trends have noted the emergence of rarer fungal pathogens, including saprophytic fungi (Table 18.2) These fungi cause skin and soft-tissue infections and occasionally invade the lungs and sinuses. They are often difficult to diagnose, and their response to therapy with amphotericin B may be very poor. Fungal infections associated with a high mortality include *Chrysosporium, Fusarium,* and *Scopulriosis.*

Bacterial

The bacterial pathogens most commonly associated with pneumonia in immunocompromised hosts include those pathogens typically associated with pneumonia, including *Staphylococcus aureus, Haemophilus influenzae,* and *Streptococcus pneumoniae.* More unusual bacterial causes of pneumonia are discussed later.

Pseudomonas aeruginosa is an important cause of pneumonia in immunocompromised children, particularly hospitalized patients. In a large series of 98 immunocompromised children with bacteremia due to *P. aeruginosa,* 21% had evidence of pneumonia; overall mortality from this infection was 27% (45). Significant risk factors included neutropenia and perineal skin lesions.

Other gram-negative organisms that cause pneumonia include *Legionella pneumophila* and *Capnocytophagia* sp.

Listeria monocytogenes is a gram-positive rod that causes primarily septicemia in immunocompromised patients, with subsequent pulmonary involvement. Antibiotic coverage for *Listeria* is ampicillin plus an aminoglycoside. Significantly, cephalosporins are not active against *Listeria.*

Corynebacteria (commonly called diphtheroids) are gram-positive bacilli or coccobacilli that exist as saprophytes on mucous membranes and skin. *Corynebacterium jeikeium* is a strain from this group that causes sepsis and pneumonia in oncology and BMT patients (46). *C. jeikeium* is resistant to most antibiotics except vancomycin; all immunocompromised patients with pneumonia should have vancomycin included in their treatment regimen if *C. jeikeium* is suspected.

Bordetella bronchiseptica is a bacterial infection acquired from pets and can cause pneumonia in the immunocompromised host (47).

Until the 1980s, pulmonary disease due to *Mycobacterium tuberculosis* had been declining (48). With the onset of the AIDS epidemic, disease attributable to both *M. tuberculosis* and atypical strains such as *Mycobacterium avium-intracellulare* has been increasing. Detailed discussion of mycobacterial infections in AIDS patients is beyond the scope of this chapter but is covered in Chapter 3.

Parasites

Pneumocystis carinii *Infection*

Pneumocystis carinii has been an organism of uncertain taxonomy and was regarded as a parasite because of its resemblance to cystic spore-forming protozoa. More recent studies using DNA hybridization methods classify *P. carinii* as a fungus (49,50). The organism exists in three forms in tissues: the trophozoite, the sporozoite, and the cyst. The trophozoites measure 2 to 5 μm and stain best with Giemsa stain; they are not visible with Gomori's methenamine silver nitrate (GMS) or toluidine blue O stains, which stain the 5- to 8-μm cyst forms (Fig. 18.6). The cysts are spherical or cup-shaped and often appear to contain up to eight 1- to 2-μm sporozoites within the cyst wall. The organism cannot be cultured from routine clinical specimens and must be identified in tissue, sputum, or alveolar lavage.

The organism is found primarily within the alveoli, although extrapulmonary occurrence of organisms has been reported commonly in AIDS patients. The trophozoites appear to attach to type I cells through surface glycoproteins that resemble lectins and there to undergo encystation (51–53). This interaction directly or through soluble factors leads to cell injury. The alveoli of lungs infected with *P. carinii* are filled with trophozoites and protein-rich debris, and the altered permeability produced by the organism contributes to the development of pulmonary edema and surfactant abnormalities, which lead to stiff lungs (54) (Fig. 18.6).

Whereas the earliest reports of PCP were in epidemics occurring in severely malnourished infants, most cases of PCP occur in infants and children with congenital or acquired immunodeficiencies. Latent infection with *P. carinii* was once thought to be common, but more recent studies using sensitive PCR and fluorescent antibody tests have failed to demonstrate *P. carinii* in autopsy or BAL specimens from normal lungs, making it more likely that disease in immunocompromised persons originates from an environmental source, including other infected patients.

The clinical features of PCP are nonspecific and include dyspnea, tachypnea, fever, and cough (54–58). Cyanosis occurs later, but hypoxemia with a mild respiratory alkalosis is common (59). The most common chest radiographic finding is diffuse bilateral infiltrates (Fig. 18.7).

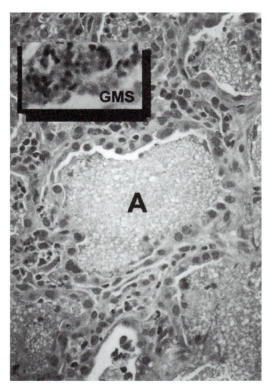

FIG. 18.6. Microscopic examination of hematoxylin and eosin stain of *Pneumocystis carinii* pneumonia. Insert shows a Gomori's methanamine silver stain (GMS) showing lung *P. carinii* cysts.

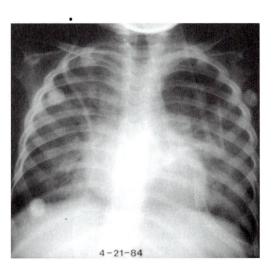

FIG. 18.7. Chest radiograph of a patient with *Pneumocysitis carinii* pneumonia showing diffuse bilateral infiltrates.

Since 1980, the most common underlying host disease in patients with *P. carinii* is AIDS. The clinical features of *P. carinii* pneumonia in the pediatric AIDS population differs from the pneumonias seen in other immunocompromised populations (60). Patients typically have a longer duration of symptoms, a more insidious presentation, and often less intense hypoxemia. Organisms appear to be abundant in AIDS patients and usually can be identified in sputum, lavage, or even gastric lavage samples. Other superinfections (such as CMV) and pulmonary complications are often present in AIDS patients, however, and it is often difficult to know what role these infections play in the AIDS patient's symptoms. AIDS patients are more likely to have spread *P. carinii* to nodes, spleen, bone marrow, and other sites. They are more likely to have atypical radiographic pictures, including lobar pneumonias, unilateral disease, and solitary nodules, although atypical radiographic presentations also can occur in other host disorders.

Several drugs are used in the treatment of PCP. The earliest drug available was pentamidine, an inhibitor of dihydrofolate reductase. Pentamidine at doses of 4.0 mg/kg daily administered intravenously is as safe as it is administered intramuscularly, although both routes are associated with a high rate of immediate reactions, such as hypotension, tachycardia, and nausea. Hypoglycemia and nephrotoxicity are serious side effects of parenteral pentamidine. Pentamidine is also given by the aerosol route for the treatment of mild to moderate pulmonary disease in AIDS patients, but its effectiveness is highly dependent on the delivery system used and the aerosol route may predispose AIDS patients to extrapulmonary disease with *P. carinii*.

Trimethoprim–sulfamethoxazole (co-trimazole, TMP-SM) is as effective as pentamidine (about 70%) with fewer side effects. Of non-AIDS patients for whom TMP-SMZ fails to be effective, 60% will respond to treatment with pentamidine. In addition to pentamidine and TMP-SM, several other drugs have been identified that are effective in PCP, including dapsone and trimetrexate. AIDS patients have a high incidence of reactions to many types of drugs, including TMP-SM. Atovaquone is a newly released hydroxynaphthoquinone for patients with mild to moderate PCP. Atovaquone has fewer side effects than TMP-SMX, but it has more treatment failures.

Supportive therapy is still a major component of therapy for PCP. Oxygen, continuous positive airway pressure, continuous negative pressure, and assisted ventilation all have been used effectively in PCP. Trials of corticosteroids in AIDS patients indicate that corticosteroid administration during therapy improves outcome in HIV-infected patients with PCP, but this is not clear for non-HIV immunosuppressed patients. Typically, patients require 4 to 6 days before showing improvement with either pentamidine or TMP-SM, and failure to improve warrants consideration of other infections and a change to another antipneumocystis drug.

All patients at known risk for *P. carinii* receive prophylaxis. For pediatric oncology and immunocompromised patients, oral TMP-SM given 3 times weekly is effective (61–63). If patients or parents are noncompliant, however, there is a risk of breakthrough pneumonias on this schedule. For most patients, TMP-SM remains the drug of choice, but other prophylactic regimens have been used, particularly in AIDS patients, including aerosolized and intravenous pentamidine and dapsone. Intravenous pentamidine may be associated with a higher risk of failure.

T. gondii *and* C. parvum *Infections*

Both *T. gondii* and *C. parvum* are parasitic infections that cause infections in the immunocompromised host; the usual symptoms are extrapulmonary. *T. gondii* infects cats and other animals and secondarily infects humans, causing congenital toxoplasmosis during intrauterine infection; primary infection later in life usually causes only lymphadenopathy and mild systemic symptoms. In AIDS patients, toxoplasma primarily causes central nervous system disease but also causes disseminated disease with secondary pulmonary involvement. Treatment of *T. gondii* is with pyrimethamine-sulfadiazine.

C. parvum infects a variety of hosts and often occurs in waterborne outbreaks. It causes severe diarrhea, but disseminated disease with pulmonary involvement can occur. Treatment of *C. parvum* is with azithromycin.

CLINICAL PRESENTATIONS OF SINOPULMONARY INFECTIONS

Unusual or Opportunistic Pulmonary Pathogens

The opportunistic pathogens are those typically not seen except in the patient with altered host defense. PCP is probably the best example of infection from an opportunistic pathogen and occurs in a variety of immunocompromised patients, including those with AIDS, T-cell disorders, agammaglobulinemia, pediatric oncology patients, and patients on high-dose corticosteroids.

The clinical course of opportunistic infections is varied and may be altered by the degree of residual host immunity. For example, corticosteroid therapy accelerates the resolution of *P. carinii* in AIDS patients, suggesting that residual host inflammatory response to this organism is important in the pathogenesis of respiratory dysfunction with PCP, even in these profoundly immunosuppressed patients. Fungal pulmonary infections in patients with chemotherapy-induced neutropenia often result in mild clinical symptoms and radiographic findings until return of their neutrophil counts results in significant inflammation, lung destruction and cavitation, and clinical deterioration.

Childhood cancer therapy, BMT and organ transplantation, primary immunodeficiencies, and AIDS are each associated with specific pathogen groups (Table 18.3).

TABLE 18.3. *Pulmonary infections in patients with specific host defense deficits*

Host defense deficit	Etiologic agents
Oral and tracheobronchial	Oral fluid
Ulceration and obstruction	Enterobacteriaceae
Neutropenia	Oral flora
	Enterobacteriaceae
	Pseudomonas aeruginosa
Hypogammaglobulinemia	*Streptococcus pneumoniae*
	Haemophilus influenza type b
	Pneumocystis carinii
Cell-mediated immunity	Mycobacteria
	Fungi
	Viruses (e.g., CMV, VZV, HSV)
	Pneumocystis carinii
	Toxoplasma gondii
	Strongyloides stercoralis
Complement	*Streptococcus pneumoniae*
	Haemophilus influenza type b

CMV, cytomegalovirus; HSV, herpes simplex virus; VZV, varicella zoster virus.

Childhood Cancer

Patients with childhood cancer are at high risk for respiratory infections for a variety of reasons in addition to the immunosuppressive effects of chemotherapy and radiation (Table 18.4) Among childhood cancer groups, there are differing risks for various pulmonary pathogens.

TABLE 18.4. *Predisposition to pneumonia in childhood malignancy*

Granulocytopenia
Mucosal disruption: skin, gut, lung
Cellular immune dysfunction
Humoral defects
Splenectomy
Mechanical catheters
Malnutrition
Radiation
Graft-versus-host disease
Corticosteroids

Childhood Leukemia (Leukemia and Acyte Lymphoblastic Leukemia)

The major risk factor for pneumonia in patients with leukemia is chemotherapy-induced neutropenia (64) (Table 18.4). Because patients with nonlymphocytic leukemia undergo the most intensive chemotherapy, they are at greatest risk for developing pneumonia. Bacterial pneumonias are most common, but RSV, adenovirus, and enteroviruses are also significant causes of pneumonia in patients with leukemia (65). Fungal pneumonias occur in patients with prolonged neutropenia, hospitalization, and broad-spectrum antibiotic therapy. *Aspergillus* and *Zygomyces* (*Mucor, Rhizopus, Cunninghamella*) are the two most common fungal pulmonary pathogens. *Candida* spp. frequently cause disseminated fungal infection, but their role in pulmonary disease is difficult to determine because it frequently contaminates sputum and bronchial washings of patients without *Candida* pneumonia, and primary isolated *Candida* pneumonia is relatively uncommon. *P. carinii* and varicella were major causes of pneumonia in leukemia patients in the 1970s, but the use of prophylaxis and effective thera-pies has reduced their impact as causes of pneumonitis in oncology patients, although both still occur in this population.

Lymphomas (Hodgkin's Disease, Non-Hodgkin's Lymphoma)

Patients with lymphoma are at risk for pneumonia because of neutropenia during therapy and from a variety of nonspecific immunologic defects, including anergy (66,67). Hodgkin's disease patients are often infected with *T. gondii* and fungi such as *C. neoformans*. The mediastinal adenopathy and lung nodules commonly seen in these children at diagnosis often require extensive evaluation to differentiate lymphoma from granulomatous pulmonary infection such as tuberculosis and histoplasmosis.

Tissue Transplantation: Bone Marrow and Solid Organ

Hematopoietic Stem Cell Transplantation

The types of pulmonary complications seen in allogeneic hematopoietic stem cell transplantation (HSCT) vary with the period following transplantation (68,69). Immedi-

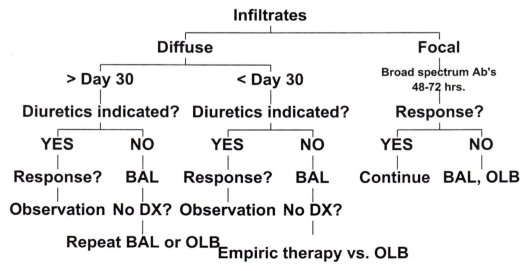

FIG. 18.8. Diagnostic approach to bone marrow transplant patient with pneumonia. (From Dichter JR, Levine SJ, Shelhamer JH. Approach to the immunocompromised host with pulmonary symptoms. *Hematol Oncol Clin North Am* 1993;7:887, with permission.)

ately following the BMT, patients are neutropenic and at risk for bacterial pneumonias with *P. aeruginosa* and *S. aureus* (70). As the transplant becomes established and neutrophils return, acute graft versus host pulmonary disease (GVHD) becomes a serious concern. Immunosuppressive therapy for GVHD with corticosteroids or cyclosporine adds to the risk of pneumonia with viral pathogens (CMV, HSV, adenovirus) as well as *P. carinii* and fungi (71). If engraftment fails and prolonged neutropenia occurs, the risk of fungal pneumonia increases significantly. Idiopathic interstitial pneumonias also occur during this later period, possibly related to radiation or chemotherapy (72,73). Late (>4–6 months posttransplant) causes of pneumonia include *H. influenzae* and *S. pneumoniae* and are associated with persistent immune deficits to these encapsulated organisms. A frequent cause of morbidity in the late transplant period is bronchiolitis obliterans, thought to be an immunologic disorder related to chronic GVHD (74–77). The frequency of this complication in pediatric BMT patients is not clear, and it may be less common than in adult BMT patients. Infection may play a role in provoking or exacerbating chronic lung damage resulting from bronchiolitis obliterans.

Cytomegalovirus infection remains a major cause of morbidity and mortality in pediatric BMT. CMV occurs more frequently in allogenic than autologous BMT patients (12.4% vs. 3.3%) and in patients who are seropositive prior to transplant or who receive marrow from seropositive donors. Incidence increases with age and is 1.3% and 2.1% in the age groups of 0 to 9 years and 10 to 19 years. Mortality from CMV pneumonitis was greater than 90% prior to use of ganciclovir and immunoglobulin therapy, which must be begun early for it to be effective. In one series, only 10 of 75 BMT patients with CMV pneumonitis survived long-term, and of these nine were all ventilator independent at the initiation of therapy with ganciclovir and immunoglobulin. Studies of risk groups for CMV pneumonitis in a group of 62 allogeneic pediatric and adult transplant patients confirmed a low incidence in those seronegative recipients who received grafts from seronegative donors and screened blood products. T-cell depletion to prevent GVH in a CMV-seropositive recipient grafted from a nonimmune donor was associated with a high risk of developing CMV interstitial pneumonia; overall, the incidence of CMV interstitial pneumonia was 31% in the high-risk group.

Fungal infections, including invasive pulmonary disease, are another major cause of morbidity and mortality in the BMT population (78). Prolonged neutropenia is a major risk factor for development of fungal infections. Recombinant cytokines to stimulate bone marrow recovery offer promise in reducing fungal infection. Adult and pediatric BMT patients treated with recombinant human macrophage colony-stimulating factor (rhM-CSF) had greater overall survival (27% vs. 5%, due entirely to a 50% survival in *Candida* infections), although survival in patients who developed *Aspergillus* infection remained poor.

A diagnostic approach to the BMT patient with pneumonia is shown in Fig. 18.8.

Renal and Other Solid-Organ Transplant

The development of pulmonary infections following transplant is attributable to chronic immunosuppression with cyclosporine A and corticosteroid therapy (79,80). CMV is the most significant pulmonary infection in all transplant patients; in heart and lung transplant patients, *P. carinii* and toxoplasmosis are also quite common (81,82). The highest risk for CMV infection occurs in the first 12 weeks posttransplant and donor CMV seropositivity, regardless of recipient CMV serostatus, is significantly associated with CMV infection (83). Gram-negative and fungal infections are the most common pulmonary complications in liver transplant patients and occur primarily in the first month after transplant (84).

Primary Immunodeficiency

Agammaglobulinemia and Hypogammaglobulinemia

In patients with common variable immunodeficiency and x-linked agammaglobulinemia, repeated bacterial pneumonias are most common with *P. carinii,* occasionally being seen in patients with hypogammaglobulinemia (85–92).

Congentital T-Cell Disorders

These disorders include severe combined immunodeficiency. Patients with this disorder are at risk for most of the same opportunistic pathogens as AIDS patients, including PCP (93,94).

Chronic Granulomatous Disease

Fungi, primarily *Aspergillus* sp. and *S. aureus,* are the most common lung infections in children with chronic granulomatous disease. Extensive lung destruction and hilar adenopathy are common in these patents (95).

Chronic Mucocutaneous Candidiasis

Although persistent and recurrent *C. albicans* infection of the mucous membranes and skin are associated with this T-cell disorder, 50% have recurrent bacterial pneumonias, and they are at risk for other opportunistic pathogens, including *P. carinii, Nocardia,* and varicella virus pneumonias. Pulmonary complications, including bronchiectasis, empyema, and lung abscess, frequently occur (96).

Acquired Immunodeficiency Syndrome

The extensive list of pulmonary infections associated with AIDS includes *P. carinii,* CMV, bacterial pneumonias, and atypical mycobacteria as major causes of pneumonia in this group (97,98).

A diagnostic approach to pulmonary infections in the AIDS population is shown in Fig. 18.9.

Recurrent or Persistent Pneumonia

Often the first clue to an abnormal host disorder is the development of recurrent or persistent pneumonia (99). Patients usually present with persistent or recurrent radiologic evidence of pneumonia, associated with typical signs of infection such as fever and tachypnea. It is important to note whether these infiltrates clear completely after therapy, whether they involve

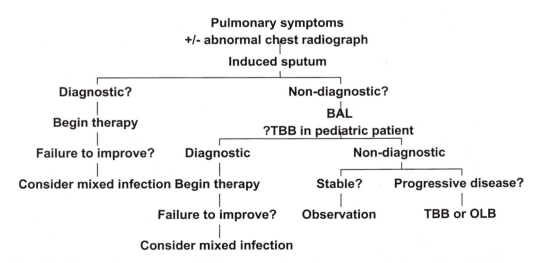

FIG. 18.9. Diagnostic approach to HIV-infected patient with pneumonia. (From Dichter JR, Levine SJ, Shelhamer JH. Approach to the immunocompromised host with pulmonary symptoms. *Hematol Oncol Clin North Am* 1993;7:887, with permission.)

one lobe or more than one lobe, and whether they are associated with other radiologic findings such as hyperinflation, situs inversus, hyperinflation, and other conditions. The differential diagnosis of recurrent or persistent pneumonia is extensive and includes many causes other than immunodeficiency.

Atypical Presentations of Common Respiratory Infections

The patient with an abnormal ability to deal with infection will often have an atypical course when infected with a "usual" childhood respiratory pathogen. For example, RSV leads to more serious disease in immunocompromised patients. VZV, influenza and parainfluenza, and measles are all potentially devastating pulmonary infections in immunocompromised hosts. Although adenovirus is capable of causing severe pneumonia in any child, it is particularly devastating in immunocompromised hosts and possibly exceeds VZV and *P. carinii* as a cause of fatal pneumonias in high-risk populations, such as BMT.

Infections of the Larynx and Airway, Including Trachea

Infections of the upper airway in immunocompromised patients can affect any of the structures of the upper respiratory tract, including the larynx, supraglottic structures, and trachea (99). Bacterial infections can lead to abscesses or invasive disease with bacteremia and sepsis.

Less common upper-airway involvement includes laryngeal involvement with *Candida* (100). *Aspergillus* also can lead to an extensive necrotizing bronchitis or tracheitis that causes physical obstruction of the trachea or large airways by pseudomembranes composed of pseudohyphae and inflammatory exudates (Fig. 18.10).

Rhinocerebral mucormycosis attributable to fungi of the class Zygomycetes occurs primarily in diabetic ketoacidosis but is also associated with neutropenia, neutrophil dysfunction disorders, malignancy, and transplantation

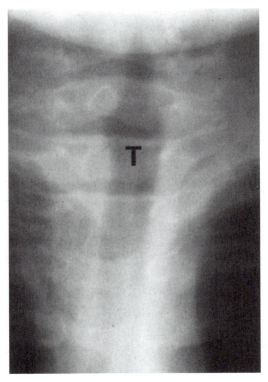

FIG. 18.10. Radiograph of necrotizing tracheitis caused by *Aspergillus*. Note the edema and narrowing of the subglottic trachea with visible exudates in the tracheal lumen.

(101,102). Pain and swelling of the face, headaches, and altered mental status and bloody nasal discharge are the classic symptoms, but suspicion should be high to make the diagnosis early before complications such as cavernous sinus thrombosis occur. Diagnosis requires a tissue biopsy because these fungi also can cause superficial colonization of the upper respiratory tract. Treatment includes systemic antifungal therapy with amphotericin B, aggressive debridement, and control of underlying metabolic abnormalities, such as acidosis. Overall survival of rhinocerebral mucormycosis ranges from 21% to 70%.

Infections of the Sinuses

Infections of the sinuses in immunocompromised hosts can be due to a variety of pathogens, including the usual bacterial pathogens associated with acute and chronic sinusitis (103–105). Immunocompromised patients are at increased risk for the complications of sinusitis, including meningitis, septicemia, cavernous venous thrombosis, and brain abscess.

Aspergillus spp. are the most common fungal infections of the nose and sinuses. Invasive sinus aspergillosis can be indolent or fulminate, leading to bone destruction and extension into the cranial fossa, orbit, and brain. Like invasive aspergillosis at other sites, infection in the sinuses is associated with prolonged immunosuppression or neutropenia, with or without broad-spectrum antibiotic therapy. Clinically, the presentation may be relatively silent or present with facial pain, swelling, headache, and erythema. Diagnosis generally requires computed tomography (CT) scans and biopsy because plain sinus radiographs are often nondiagnostic.

DIAGNOSTIC STUDIES

General Approach

Although clinical factors such as types of pulmonary pathogens associated with certain at-risk groups and general radiographic patterns may be useful, both approaches have limitations in the immunocompromised patient with pneumonia (106). Many noninfectious pulmonary processes also occur in this group (Table 18.1), and the list of organisms causing pneumonia is extensive (107–118). Generally, empiric broad-spectrum antibiotic therapy must be started in patients with known immunodeficiency at the first sign of fever and often before the development of overt pneumonia. This necessity often complicates subsequent diagnostic studies.

Indirect Diagnostic Tests

Radiography

Pneumonias in this population can be classified by their general radiologic appearance, including (a) diffuse alveolar or interstitial

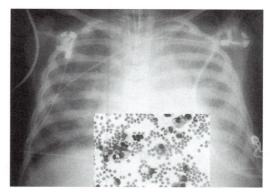

FIG. 18.11. Chest radiograph showing pulmonary leukemic infiltrates. The blood smear from a bronchoalveolar lavage revealed myelomonocytic leukemia, as depicted in the insert.

pneumonias, (b) localized alveolar lobar or lobular pneumonias (which may involve more than one lobe), and (c) nodular infiltrates, which may be cavitary or may progress to frank lung abscess (Figs. 18.11 and 18.12). The common causes of these general radiographic patterns are shown in Fig. 18.13, but it must be emphasized that radiographic appearances are often deceptive in immunocompromised hosts and usually are not helpful in making a specific etiologic diagnosis.

Diffuse Interstitial or Alveolar Pneumonias

Pneumocystis carinii is the prototypical organism associated with this radiographic

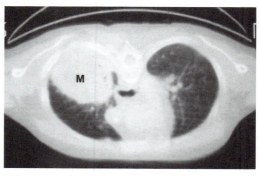

FIG. 18.12. Computed tomography of the chest in a patient with Mucor.

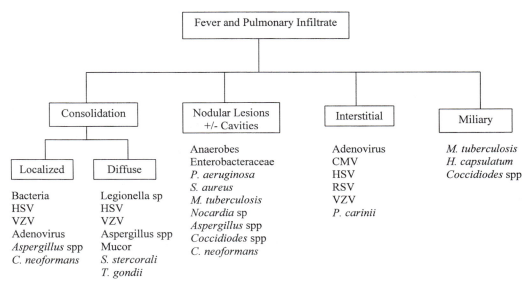

FIG. 18.13. Algorithm for etiologic agent causing a pulmonary infiltrate and fever in an immunocompromised host.

pattern. Although *P. carinii* has declined significantly in patient populations receiving prophylaxis, PCP remains the major pathogen associated with AIDS. Atypical radiographic appearances of *P. carinii* are common and include normal radiographs and cystic, unilateral, and granulomatous radiographic changes and associated pleural disease. The use of aerosolized pentamidine for prophylaxis of PCP in AIDS may alter the radiographic presentation toward more upper-lobe disease. This was thought to occur because of preferential distribution of the drug to the lower lobes, but studies of drug levels suggested that other factors may be involved because drug levels are similar in both upper and lower lung zones, despite larger numbers of organisms in the upper lung zones. CMV also is associated with diffuse pneumonia in immunocompromised patients and is frequently seen as a co-pathogen with other infectious agents. Viral infections, including adenovirus, and influenza are also important causes of diffuse pneumonia.

Localized Alveolar Lobar or Lobular (Bronchopneumonia) Pneumonias

Bronchopneumonias and lobar consolidation can occur in immunocompromised patients caused by the usual pathogens, such as *S. pneumoniae, H. influenzae,* and *S. aureus.* The radiographic changes are dependent on the host's inflammatory response to the organism, and patients with abnormal host defenses often show an altered initial radiographic pattern that underestimates the true extent of disease.

Nodular, Cavitary, and Lung Abscess Lesions

Solitary pulmonary nodules, either unilateral or bilateral, are a less common presentation of infection in most immunocompromised patients, but they do occur frequently in pediatric oncology patients. Although most often these represent fungal pneumonias, other organisms, including *Nocardia* also can present as pulmonary nodules. The development of a lung abscess generally indicates some degree of host immunity sufficient to localize an infection. The most common causes of cavitary lesions in pediatric cancer patients are fungi, especially *Aspergillus* spp. PCP and mycobacterial infections are associated with cavitary disease in AIDS patients. CT of the chest is often helpful in patients with disseminated fungal disease from *Aspergillus* and other fungal pathogens. In a review of chest CT findings in 14 pediatric patients with malignancy and pulmonary fungal disease due to *Aspergillus,* two basic types of involvement were seen: multiple nodules or fluffy masses. Cavitation occurred in 6 of 14 patients. CT is much more sensitive than plain radiographs and can reveal early evidence of cavitation, including the typical air crescent sign of aspergillus.

Clinical Laboratory Studies

Sputum Examination and Culture

Sputum samples are difficult to obtain in children under 10 years of age and, when obtained, must be interpreted cautiously (119, 120). Sputum produced by cough induced with inhalation of hypertonic saline aerosols has been useful in older children with AIDS and PCP. Gastric aspirates can be used in the younger child and are particularly helpful when the pathogen being considered is not a usual colonizing organism of the upper airway, such as tuberculosis.

Endotracheal Tube Aspirates

If the child requires endotracheal intubation for respiratory distress, endotracheal aspirates are easy to obtain. Diagnostic yield in complex immunocompromised patients is improved by using wax-protected microbiologic brushes or nonbronchoscopic BAL.

Blood Cultures

Although blood culture should be obtained in all immunocompromised children in whom a bacterial or fungal pneumonia is suspected, positive cultures are unusual; if positive, they are usually highly specific.

Antigen and Antibody Detection Methods

The ability to detect capsular polysaccharide antigens of bacterial pathogens even after antibiotics have been administered is occasionally helpful in hospitalized patients. Most hospitals routinely test for group B streptococcus, *N. meningitidis, S. pneumoniae,* and *H. influenzae* type b using latex agglutination or counterimmunoelectrophoresis. Concentrated urine samples are superior to serum samples. Antibiotic treatment does not affect the sensitivity of the test, which is between 30% and 45%, depending on the study. Numerous tests for direct detection of fungal antigens have been described, but none is in widespread clinical use. Direct IF used to detect *Legionella* sp. has a sensitivity of 50% and a specificity of 94%.

Rapid diagnosis of respiratory syncytial virus, influenza A virus, parainfluenza viruses, and *Chlamydia* infections by enzyme-linked immunosorbent assay and direct IF is now available. The sensitivities of these tests depend partly on the adequacy of the sample provided to the laboratory. Viral cultures are generally available, and the shell vial technique for rapid identification of respiratory viral pathogens such as CMV is extremely useful. Although *Mycoplasma pneumoniae* can be cultured on enriched media, this usually takes several weeks, and the diagnosis usually is based on serologic conversion. Genetic probes for detecting *Legionella, Mycobacteria,* and *M. pneumoniae* are now commercially available.

Flexible Bronchoscopy

Flexible bronchoscopy is safe in experienced hands and provides excellent culture material in the immunocompromised child with pneumonia (121–152). Indications for bronchoscopy in children with pneumonia include (a) failure of pneumonia or fever to clear with appropriate antibiotic therapy; (b) suspicion of endobronchial obstruction by infection or tumor; (c) recurrent pneumonia in a lobe or segment; and (d) suspicion of unusual organisms such as PCP, fungi, or tuberculosis. Although the yield of gastric aspiration is probably superior to bronchoscopy for tuberculosis, bronchoscopy also can evaluate for endobronchial disease or bronchial compression.

The bronchoscope suction channel is contaminated by upper-airway organisms, and simple washings obtained through the bronchoscope channel are generally useless (Figs. 18.14 and 18.15). Several techniques have been developed to circumvent this problem, and these include the use of a double-sheath, wax-protected sterile brush and quantitative cultures of BAL, which is the most useful technique in the immunocompromised host. A variety of infectious and noninfectious diagnoses can be made by BAL, including hemorrhage and pulmonary involvement with leukemia (Fig. 18.11). BAL is generally safe even in patients with reduced platelets. Brushings obtained through the bronchoscope can be used for cytologic examination and viral cultures, but the yield is usually low and adds little to BAL.

Although the usefulness of bronchoscopy is well documented in this population, it is important to recognize the limitations of bronchoscopy. In patients on empiric broad-spectrum antibiotic therapy, the yield of bacterial pathogens is likely to be low. In oncology patients and other non-AIDS immunocompromised patients, the number of PCP organisms is usually low compared with AIDS patients, and BAL may be falsely negative. In populations receiving prophylaxis for this infection the yield for PCP is likely to be low. CMV also can be diagnosed rapidly by bronchoscopy, but patients may have other complicating infections, such as fungi, in addition to CMV that are missed more easily by bronchoscopy. *Aspergillus* and other fungi are often difficult to diagnose by bronchoscopy, particularly early in the infection when therapy is most likely to be effective.

Transbronchial biopsies (TBBs) also can be taken through the bronchoscope. Although

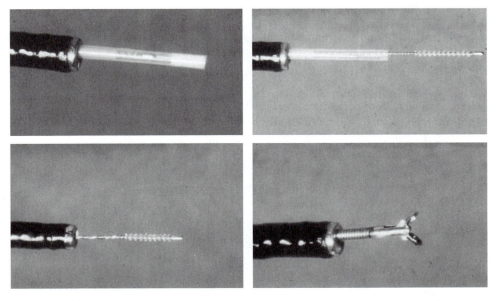

FIG. 18.14. Flexible bronchoscopy instrumentation: *1,* **left upper panel:** Wax-protected microbiologic brush; *2,* **Right upper panel:** Wax-protected microbiologic brush extended; *3,* **Left lower panel:** Cytology brush, pediatric bronchoscope; *4,* **Right lower panel:** Transbronchial biopsy forceps, open.

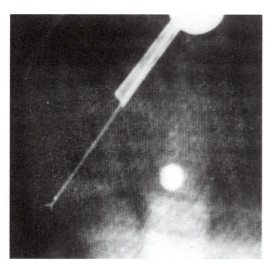

FIG. 18.15. Radiograph showing transbronchial biopsy forceps extended via rigid bronchoscope, open for lower lobe biopsy.

safe in older patients, transbronchial lung biopsies yield an unacceptable number of false-negative results in immunosuppressed patients and is most useful when organisms such as *P. carinii* or granulomatous lesions are likely. Reported experience with TBB in pediatric patients is limited, but TBB has a significant role in monitoring rejection and infections in the pediatric lung transplant patient.

Transthoracic Needle Aspiration Biopsy

Needle aspiration of the lung has been used in the diagnosis of PCP in pediatric cancer patients and for the diagnosis of localized infections in other immunosuppressed patients (153,154). Pneumothoraces complicated 37% of the needle aspirates done for PCP, and this risk must be considered. Use of CT or fluoroscopic guidance greatly improves the yield and safety of this procedure, and it is the procedure of choice for many children with suspected peripheral fungal lesions that can safely be aspirated.

Open-Lung Biopsy

Open-lung biopsy (OLB) is the "gold standard" by which other diagnostic modalities

are judged (155–157). Using current surgical techniques, OLB is generally a procedure with a low morbidity that can be done rapidly and that allows the surgeon to obtain the optimal tissue for culture and microscopic examination. "Minithoracotomy" and lingular biopsy may be all that is necessary in patients with diffuse pulmonary processes. Biopsy using fiberoptic thoracoscopy may be adequate for pleural-based lesions and reduces the morbidity associated with open biopsy (158,159).

In immunocompromised patients, it is difficult to make generalizations about OLB, and much depends on local factors such as the availability of flexible bronchoscopy, age of the child, underlying conditions, complications such as thrombocytopenia or coagulopathies, and prior antibiotic or antifungal therapy. Recent studies of OLB have questioned how often OLB results will lead to a change in therapy if one excludes patients with organisms covered by empiric therapy such as *P. carinii* and nonspecific histologic findings. A randomized trial of open biopsy versus empiric antibiotic therapy in a small series of nonneutropenic adult oncology patients tended to support the idea that broad-spectrum antibiotic therapy, including erythromycin and TMZ-SM, was equivalent to early OLB in outcome. Similar data are needed for immunocompromised pediatric patients, and one must be careful about generalizing results in adults. Published results in OLB in immunocompromised pediatric patients indicated yields that ranged from 36% to 94% for a specific diagnosis.

Although OLB is the procedure of choice for obtaining definitive diagnostic information in immunosuppressed patients with pulmonary infiltrates, the timing of the biopsy is difficult. The clinician does not want to commit the patient too early, especially if empirical therapy appears to be working and the patient is in good condition. On the other hand, in the face of marginally successful therapy, the surgeon does not want to wait so long that the patient deteriorates and the risk of biopsy significantly increases. We generally suggest relatively early biopsy in immunosuppressed patients with pneumonia. Any patient who is not clearly responding to therapy chosen on the basis of other diagnostic techniques (including bronchoscopy) or therapy chosen empirically usually would benefit from a specific diagnosis by biopsy. In most medical centers, this is a relatively safe procedure, especially when performed before the patient has the need for respiratory support. The risks only increase when the biopsy is delayed until the patient has become critically ill. When used for diagnosis of diffuse disease, only a limited thoracotomy with a superficial subsegmental resection is necessary. In localized disease, which is typical of fungal infections, a more extensive procedure may be required to obtain an adequate specimen.

In specific patient groups, such as BMT and AIDS patients, the utility and timing of OLB may be different. In AIDS patients, OLB is rarely necessary because a specific diagnosis usually can be made by BAL or transbronchial lung biopsy. If the disease process is progressing despite apparently adequate therapy or bronchoscopy is nondiagnostic, then OLB should be considered to rule out other co-pathogens. In BMT patients, the approach may be modified to allow therapy of common non-infectious complications, such as pulmonary edema, before embarking on invasive diagnostic studies (Figs. 18.8 and 18.9).

TREATMENT

Early treatment is necessary for the immunocompromised patient, with pneumonia and empiric antibiotic therapy generally is started at the first sign of clinical pneumonia. In many patients, such as febrile, neutropenic patients, empiric antibiotic therapy already may have started before the pneumonia becomes clinically or radiographically apparent. Antibiotic therapy is typically broad spectrum, aimed at both gram-positive and gram-negative bacterial infections, such as vancomycin-aminoglycoside/semisynthetic penicillin. If a patient presents with a new diffuse, bilateral pneumonia with respiratory distress and hypoxemia, a rapid decision must be made as to whether to proceed to bronchoscopy or to OLB before the patient progresses to respiratory failure and any procedure becomes more hazardous. Empiric therapy usually is guided by the underlying disorder and the radiographic and clinical features of the pneumonia and would usually include TMP-SM for PCP as well as erythromycin for *Mycoplasma* and *Legionella* infections. Amphotericin B often is started in the febrile neutropenic patient who develops a new pulmonary infiltrate while on antibiotics. Empiric viral therapy with acyclovir for HSV is sometimes necessary, but the treatment of CMV pneumonitis with ganciclovir/immunoglobulin usually requires a histologic diagnosis of CMV pneumonitis (160,161). PCP therapy involves aggressive antibiotic therapy with consideration of steroids (162–175). Because of its low morbidity, flexible bronchoscopy should be considered early in the course of the pneumonia. If bronchoscopy is negative, the risks and benefits of open lung biopsy must be weighed for each patient, particularly if the pneumonia progresses despite appropriate antimicrobial therapy. If the patient shows a good response to empiric antibiotic therapy, it should be continued for a minimum of 2 weeks, and in the case of suspected fungal pneumonia, antifungal therapy may be required for much longer periods.

REFERENCES

1. Armstrong D. History of opportunistic infection in the immunocompromised host. *Clin Infect Dis* 1993;17:S318–S321.
2. Fishman JA, Rubin RH. Infection in organ-transplant-recipients. *N Engl J Med* 1998;338:1741–1751.
3. Mayaund C, Cadranel J. A persistent challenge: the diagnosis of respiratory disease in the non-AIDS immunocompromised host. *Thorax* 2000;55:511–517.
4. Wilson G, Dermody T. Respiratory infections in the immunocompromised host. *Seminars in Pediatric Infectious Diseases* 1995;
5. Stokes DC. Pulmonary complications of tissue transplantation in children. *Curr Opin Pediatr* 1994;6:272–279.
6. Robbins RA, Floreani AA, Buchalter SE, et al. Pulmonary complications of transplantation. *Ann Rev Med* 1992;43:425–435.
7. Sable CA, Donowitz GR. Infections in bone marrow transplant recipients. *Clin Infect Dis* 1994;18:273–284.
8. White DA, Zaman MK. Management of AIDS pa-

tients: pulmonary disease. *Med Clin North Am* 1992; 76:19–44.

9. Murray JF, Mills J. Pulmonary infectious complications of human immunodeficiency virus infection. *American Review of Respiratory Diseases* 1992;141: 1356–1372.

10. Afessa B, Gay PC, Plevak DJ, et al. Pulmonary complications of orthotopic liver transplantation. *Mayo Clin Proc* 1993;68:427–434.

11. Walsh TJ, Gonzalez C, Lyman CA, et al. Invasive fungal infections in children: recent advances in diagnosis and therapy. *Adv Pediatr Infect Dis* 1996; 11:189–290.

12. Enright H, Haake R, Weisdorf D, et al. Cytomegalovirus pneumonia after bone marrow transplantation: risk factors and response to therapy. *Transplantation* 1993;55:1339–1346.

13. Goodrich JM, Bowden RA, Fisher L, et al. Ganciclovir prophylaxis to prevent cytomegalovirus disease after allogenic marrow transplant. *Ann Intern Med* 1993 118:173–178.

14. Foot ABM, Caul EO, Roome AP, et al. Cytomegalovirus pneumonitis and bone marrow transplantation: identification of a specific high risk group. *J Clin Pathol* 1993;46:415–419.

15. Salomon N, Perlman DC. Cytomegalovirus pneumonia. *Semin Respir Infect* 1999;14:353–358.

16. Kitchen BJ, Engler HD, Gill VJ, et al. Cytomegalovirus infection in the child with human immunodeficiency virus infection. *Pediatr Infect Dis J* 1997;16:358–363.

17. Einsele H, Ehninger G, Steidle M, et al. Lymphopenia as an unfavorable prognostic factor in patients with cytomegalovirus infection after bone marrow transplantation. *Blood* 1993;82:1672–1678.

18. Feldman S, Hughes WT, Daniel CB. Varicella in children with cancer: Seventy seven cases. *Pediatrics* 1985;56:388–397.

19. Feldman S, Stokes DC. Varicella zoster and herpes simplex virus pneumonias. *Semin Respir Infect* 1987; 2:84–94.

20. Cone RW, Hackman RC, Huang MI, et al. Human herpesvirus 6 in lung tissue from patients with pneumonitis after bone marrow transplantation. *N Engl J Med* 1993;329:156–161.

21. Wilborn F, Brinkman V, Schmidt C, et al. Herpesvirus type 6 in patients undergoing bone marrow transplantation: serologic features and detection by PCR. *Blood* 1994;83:3052–3058.

22. Robinson WS. Human herpes virus 6. *Curr Clin Top Infect Dis* 1994;14:159–169.

23. Knox KK, Petryga D, Harrington DJ, et al. Progressive immunodeficiency and fatal pneumonitis associated with human herpesvirus 6 in an infant. *Clin Infect Dis* 1995;20:406–413.

24. Herbein G, Strasswimmer J, Altieri M, et al. Longitudinal study of human herpesvirus 6 infection in organ transplant recipients. *Clin Infect Dis* 1996;22:171–173.

25. Flomenberg P, Babbitt J, Drobyski WR, et al. Increasing incidence of adenovirus disease in bone marrow transplant recipients. *J Infect Dis* 1994;169:775–781.

26. Morris DJ, Corbitt G, Bailey AS, et al. Fatal disseminated adenovirus type 2 infection after bone marrow transplantation for Hurler's syndrome: a primary infection *J Infect* 1993;26:181–184.

27. Shields AF, Hackman RC, Fife KH, et al. Adenovirus infections in patients undergoing bone marrow transplantation. *N Engl J Med* 1985;312:529–533.

28. Zahradnik JM, Spencer JM, Porter DD. Adenovirus infection in the immunocompromised patient. *Am J Med* 1980;68:725–732.

29. Michaels MG, Green M, Wal ER, et al. Adenovirus infection in pediatric liver transplant recipients. *J Infect Dis* 1992;165:170–174.

30. Hale GA, Heslop HE, Krance RA, et al. Adenovirus infections after pediatric bone marrow transplantation. *Bone Marrow Transplant* 1999;23:277–282.

31. Hall CB, Powell KR, MacDonald NE, et al. Respiratory syncytial virus infection in children with compromised immune function. *N Engl J Med* 1986;315:77–81.

32. Hertz MI, Englund JA, Stover D, et al. Respiratory virus-induced acute lung injury in adult patients with bone marrow transplants: a clinical approach and review of the literature. *Medicine* 1989;68:269.

33. Parham DM, Bozeman P, Killian C, et al. Cytologic diagnosis of respiratory syncytial virus infection in a bronchoalveolar lavage specimen from a bone marrow transplant recipient. *Am J Clin Pathol* 1993;99:588–592.

34. Walmsley S, Devi S, King S, et al. Invasive *Aspergillus* infections in a pediatric hospital: a ten-year review. *Pediatr Infect Dis J* 1993;12:673–682.

35. Iwen PC, Rupp ME, Langnas AN, et al. Invasive pulmonary aspergillosis due to *Aspergillus terreus*: 12 year experience and review of the literature. *Clin Infect Dis* 1998;26:1092–1097.

36. Denning DW. Therapeutic outcome in invasive *Aspergillus*. *Clin Infect Dis* 1996;23:608–615.

37. Kline MW. Mucormycosis and children: review of the literature and report of cases. *Pediatr Infect Dis* 1985; 4:672–678.

38. Haron E, Vartivarian S, Anaissie E, et al. Primary *Candida* pneumonia. *Medicine* 1993;72:137–142.

39. Hughes WT. Systemic candidiasis: a study of 109 fatal cases. *Pediatr Infect Dis* 1982;1:11–18.

40. Flynn PM, Marina NM, Rivera GK, et al. *Candida tropicalis* infections in children with leukemia. *Leuk Lymphoma* 1993;10:369–376.

41. Maxson S, Jacobs RF. Community-acquired fungal pneumonia in children. *Semin Respir Infect* 1996;11: 191–200.

42. Pappas PG. Blastomycosis in the immunocompromised patient. *Semin Respir Infect* 1997;12:243–251.

43. Newman TG, Soni A, Acaron S, et al. Pleural cryptococcosis in the acquired immune deficiency syndrome. *Chest* 1987;91:459–461.

44. Katz AS, Niesenbaum L, Mass B. Pleural effusion as the initial manifestation of disseminated cryptococcosis in acquired immune deficiency syndrome: diagnosis by pleural biopsy. *Chest* 1989;96:440–441.

45. Fergie JE, Shema SJ, Lott L, et al. *Pseudomonas aeruginosa* bacteremia in immunocompromised children: analysis of factors associated with a poor outcome. *Clin Infect Dis* 1994;18:390–394.

46. Water BL. Pathology of culture-proven JK corynebacterium pneumonia: an autopsy case report. *Am J Clin Pathol* 1989;91:616.

47. Dworkin MS, Sullivan PS, Buskin SE, et al. *Bordetella bronchiseptica* in human immunodeficiency virus infected patients. *Clin Infect Dis* 1999;28:1095–1099.

48. Schneider RF. Bacterial pneumonia [in HIV]. *Semin Respir Infect* 1999;14:327–332.

49. Walzer PD. *Pneumocystis carinii: recent advances in basic biology and their clinical application.* AIDS 1993;7:1293–1305.

50. Edman J, Kovacs J, Masur H, et al. Ribosomal RNA sequence shows *Pneumocystis carinii* to be a member of the fungi. *Nature* 1988;334:517–522.

51. Pottratz ST, Paulsrud J, Smith JS, et al. *Pneumocystis carinii* attachment to cultured lung cells by pneumocystis gp120, a fibronectin binding protein. *J Clin Invest* 1991;88:403–407.

52. Su TH, Martin WJ. Pathogenesis and host response in *Pneumocystis carinii* pneumonia. *Annu Rev Med* 1994;45:261–272.

53. Wisniowski P, Pasula R, Martin WJ. Isolation of *Pneumocystis carinii* gp120 by fibronectin affinity: evidence for manganese affinity. *Am J Respir Cell Moll Biol* 1994;11:262–269.

54. Sheehan PM, Stokes DC, Yeh YY, et al. Surfactant phospholipid and lavage phospholipase A2 in experimental *Pneumocystis carinii* pneumonia. *Am Rev Respir Dis* 1986;134:526–531.

55. Schliep TL, Yarrish RL. *Pneumocystis carinii* pneumonia. *Semin Respir Infect* 1999;14:333–343.

56. Nuesch R, Belini C, Zimmerli W. *Pneumocystis carinii* pneumonia in human immunodeficiency virus (HIV) positive and HIV-negative immunocompromised patients. *Clin Infect Dis* 1999;29:1519–1523.

57. Sapkowitz KA. *Pneumocystis carinii* pneumonia in patients without AIDS. *Clin Infect Dis* 1993;17:S416–S422.

58. Hughes WT. *Pneumocystis carinii* pneumonitis (vols. 1 and 2). Boca Raton, FL: CRC Press, 1987.

59. Sanyal SK, Chebib FS, Gilbert JR, et al. Sequential changes in vital signs and acid-base and blood-gas profiles in *Pneumocystis carinii* pneumonitis in children with cancer. *Am J Respir Crit Care Med* 1994;149:1092–1098.

60. Rose RM, Catalano PJ, Koziel H, et al. Abnormal lipid composition of bronchoalveolar lavage fluid obtained from individuals with AIDS-related lung disease. *Am J Respir Crit Care Med* 1994;149:332–338.

61. Hughes WT, Kuhn S, Chaudary S, et al. Successful chemoprophylaxis for *Pneumocystis carinii* pneumonia. *N Engl J Med* 1977;297:419–426.

62. Hughes WT. Successful intermittent chemoprophylaxis for *Pneumocystis carinii* pneumonia. *N Engl J Med* 1987;316:1627–1632.

63. Hughes WT. Five year absence of *Pneumocystic carinii* pneumonitis in a pediatric oncology center. *J Infect Dis* 1984;150:305.

64. Lehrnbecher T, Foster C, Vazquez N, et al. Therapy-induced alterations in host defenses in children receiving therapy for cancer. *J Pediatr Hematol Oncol* 1997;19:399–417.

65. Aroia M, Ruuskanen O, Ziegler T, et al. Respiratory virus infections during anticancer treatment in children. *Pediatr Infect Dis J* 1995;14:690–694.

66. Young RC, Corder NP, Haynes HA, et al. Delayed hypersensitivity in Hodgkin's disease: a study of 103 untreated patients. *Am J Med* 1972;52:63–72.

67. Fisher RI, DeVita VT, Bostick F. Persistent immunologic abnormalities in long term survivors of advanced Hodgkin's disease. *Ann Intern Med* 1980;92:595–599.

68. Johnson FL, Stokes DC, Ruggiero M, et al. Chronic obstructive airways disease after bone marrow transplantation. *J Pediatr* 1984;105:370–376.

69. Peterson PK, McGlave P, Ramsay NK, et al. A prospective study of infectious diseases following bone marrow transplantation: emergence of *Aspergillus* and cytomegalovirus as the major causes or mortality. *Infect Control* 1983;4:81–89.

70. Johnson FL, Schofer O. Pulmonary complications of bone marrow transplantation. In: Laraya-Cuasay LR, Hughes WT, eds. *Interstitial lung diseases in children,* vol. 2. Boca Raton, FL: CRC Press, 1988.

71. Gonzalez Y, Martino R, Badell I, et al. Pulmonary enterovirus infections in stem cell transplant recipients. *Bone Marrow Transplant* 1999;23:511–513.

72. Clark JG, Hansen JA, Hertz MI, et al. Idiopathic pneumonia syndrome after bone marrow transplantation. *Am Rev Respir Dis* 1993;147:1601–1606.

73. Chan CK, Hyland RH, Hucheon MA, et al. Small-airways disease in recipients of allogenic bone marrow transplants. *Medicine* 1987;66:327–340.

74. Schwarer AP, Hughes JM, Trotman-Dickenson B, et al. A chronic pulmonary syndrome associated with graft-versus-host disease after allogeneic marrow transplantation. *Transplantation* 1992;54:1002–1008.

75. Kaplan EB, Wodell RA, Wilmott RW, et al. Chronic graft-versus-host disease and pulmonary function. *Pediatr Pulmonol* 1992;14:141–148.

76. Clark JG, Schwartz DA, Flournoy N, et al. Risk factors for airflow obstruction in recipients of bone marrow transplants. *Ann Intern Med* 1987;107:648–656.

77. Roca J, Granena A, Rodriquez-Roisin R, et al. Fatal airway disease in an adult with chronic graft-versus-host disease. *Thorax* 1982;37:77–78.

78. Morrison VA, Haake RJ, Weisdorf DJ. The spectrum of *non-Candida* fungal infections following bone marrow transplantation. *Medicine* 1993;72:78–89.

79. Rubin RH. Infectious disease complications of renal transplantation. *Kidney Int* 1993;44:221–236.

80. Rubin RH. Infectious disease complications of renal tranplantation. *Kidney Int* 1993;44:221–236.

81. Gryzan S, Paradis IL, Zeevi A, et al. Unexpectedly high incidence of *Pneumocystis carinii* infection after lung-heart transplantation: implications for lung defense and allograft survival. *Am Rev Respir Dis* 1988;137:1268–1274.

82. Hertzler GL, Bryan JA, Perlino C, et al. Diagnosis of pulmonary toxoplasmosis by bronchoalveolar lavage in cardiac transplant recipients. *Diagn Cytopathol* 1993;9:650–654.

83. Igagorri S, Pillay D, Scrine M, et al. Prospective cytomegalovirus surveillance in pediatric renal transplant patients. *Pediatr Nephrol* 1993;7:55–60.

84. O'Brien JD, Ettinger NA. Pulmonary complications of liver transplantation. *Clin Chest Med* 1996;17:99–114.

85. Oxelius VA, Lavrall AB, Lindquist B, et al. IgG subclasses in selective IgA deficiency: importance of IgG2-IgA deficiency. *N Engl J Med* 1981;304:1476–1477.

86. Smith TF, Morris EC, Bain RP. IgG subclasses in nonallergic children with chronic chest symptoms. *J Pediatr* 1981;105:896–900.

87. Herrod HG, Gross S, Insel R. Selective antibody deficiency to Hemophilus influenza type B capsular polysaccharide vaccination in children with recurrent respiratory tract. *Infect J Clin Immunol* 1989;9:429–434.

88. Wald ER. Recurrent pneumonia in children. *Adv Pediatr Infect Dis* 1990;5:183–203.

89. Rubin BK. The evaluation of the child with recurrent chest infections. *Pediatr Infect Dis* 1985;4:88–98.

90. Stiehm ER, Chin TW, Haas A, et al. Infectious complications of the primary immunodeficiencies. *Clin Immunol Immunopathol* 1986;40:69–86.

91. Dukes RJ, Rosenow EC III, Hermans PE. Pulmonary manifestations of hypogammaglobulinemia. *Thorax* 1978;33:603–607.

92. Saulsbury FT, Bernstein MT, Winkelstein JA. *Pneumocystis carinii* pneumonia as the presenting infection in congenital hypogammaglobulinemia. *J Pediatr* 1979;95:559–561.

93. Conley ME, Park CL, Douglas SD. Childhood common variable immunodeficiency with autoimmune disease. *J Pediatr* 1986;108:915–922.

94. Leggiadro RJ, Winkelstein JA, Hughes WT. Prevalence of *Pneumocystis carinii* pneumonitis in severe combined immunodeficiency. *J Pediatr* 1981;99:96–98.

95. Caldicott WJH, Baehner RL. Chronic granulomations disease of childhood. *AJR Am J Roentgenol* 1968;103:133–139.

96. Chipps BE, Saulsbury FT, Hsu SH, et al. Non-candidal infections in children with chronic mucocutaneous candidiasis. *The Johns Hopkins Medical Journal* 1979;144:175–179.

97. McSherry GD. Human immunodeficiency-virus-related pulmonary infections in children. *Semin Infect Dis* 1996;11:173–183.

98. Rubenstein A, Morechi R, Silverman B, et al. Pulmonary disease in children with acquired immune deficiency syndrome and AIDS-related complex. *J Pediatr* 1986;108:498–503.

99. Morrison VA, Pomeroy C. Upper respiratory infections in the immunocompromised host. *Semin Respir Infect* 1995;10:37–50.

100. Fisher EW, Richards A, Anderson G, et al. Laryngeal candidiasis: a cause of airway obstruction in the immuncompromised child. *J Laryngol Otol* 1992;106:168–170.

101. Peterson KL, Wang M, Canalis RF, et al. Rhinocerebral mucormycosis: evolution of the disease and treatment options. *Laryngoscope* 1997;107:855–862.

102. Gillespie MB, O'Malley BW, Francis HW. An approach to fulminant invasive fungal rhinosinusitis in the immunocompromised host. *Arch Otololaryngol Head Neck Surg* 1998;124:520–526.

103. Kennedy CA, Adams GL, Neglia JP, et al. Impact of surgical treatment on paranasal fungal infections in bone marrow transplant patients. *Otolaryngol Head Neck Surg* 1997;116:610–616.

104. Vierschraegen CF, Besien KWV, Dignani C, et al. Invasive aspergillosis sinusitis during bone marrow transplantation. *Scand J Infect Dis* 1997;29:436–438.

105. Iwen PC, Rupp ME, Hinrichs SH. Invasive mold sinusitis: 17 cases in immunocompromised patients and review of the literature. *Clin Infect Dis* 1997;24:1178–1784.

106. Stokes DC, Shenep JL, Horowitz ME, et al. WT Presentation of *Pneumocystis carinii* pneumonia as unilateral hyperlucent lung. *Chest* 1988;94:201–212.

107. Goodman PC. Pulmonary disease in children with acquired immunodeficiency syndrome. *J Thorac Imaging* 1991;6:60–64.

108. Gratton-Smith D, Harrison LF, Singleton EB. Radiology of acquired immunodeficiency syndrome in the pediatric patient. *Curr Prob Diagn Radiol* 1992;21:79–109.

109. Chechani V, Zaman MK, Finch PJP. Chronic cavitary *Pneumocystis carinii* pneumonia in a patient with AIDS. *Chest* 1989;95:1347–1348.

110. Klein JS, Warnock M, Webb WR, et al. Cavitating and noncavitating granulomas in AIDS patients with *Pneumocystis pneumonitis*. *AJR Am J Roentgenol* 1989;152:753–754.

111. Scannell KA. Atypical presentation of *Pneumocystis carinii* in a patient receiving inhalational pentamidine *Am J Med* 1988;85:881–884.

112. Horowitz ML, Schiff M, Samuels J, et al. *Pneumocystis carinii* pleural effusion: pathogenesis and pleural fluid analysis. *Am Rev Respir Dis* 1993;148:232–234.

113. Chow P, Templeton PA, White CS. Lung cysts associated with *Pneumocystis carinii* pneumonia: radiographic characteristics, natural history and complications. *AJR Am J Roentgenol* 1993;161:527–531.

114. Taccone A, Occhi M, Garaventa A, et al. CT of invasive pulmonary aspergillosis in children with cancer. *Pediatr Radiol* 1993;23:177–180.

115. Lubat E, Megibow AJ, Balthazar EJ, et al. Extrapulmonary *Pneumocystis carinii* infection in AIDS: CT findings. *Radiology* 1990;174:157–160.

116. McLoud TC, Naidich DP. Thoracic disease in the immunocompromised patient. *Radiol Clin North Am* 1992;30:525–554.

117. Matar LD, McAdams HP, Palmer SM, et al. Respiratory viral infections in lung transplant recipients: radiologic findings with clinical correlation. *Radiology* 1999;213:735–742.

118. Barloon TJ, Galvin JR, Mori M, et al. High resolution ultrafast chest CT in the clinical management of febrile bone marrow transplant patients with normal or nonspecific roentgenograms. *Chest* 1991;99:928–933.

119. Kirsch CM, Jensen WA, Kagawa FT, et al. Analysis of induced sputum for the diagnosis of recurrent *Pneumocystis carinii* pneumonia. *Chest* 1992;102:1152–1154.

120. Rabella N, Rodriquez P, Labega R. Conventional respiratory viruses recovered from immunocompromised patients: clinical considerations. *Clin Infect Dis* 1999;28:1043–1048.

121. Delvenne P, Arrese JE, Thiry A, et al. Detection of cytomegalovirus, *Pneumocystis carinii,* and *Aspergillus* species in bronchoalveolar lavage fluid: a comparison of techniques. *Am J Clin Pathol* 1993;100:414–418.

122. Honda J, Hoshino T, Natori H, et al. Rapid and sensitive diagnosis of cytomegalovirus and *Pneumocystis carinii* pneumonia in patients with hematological neoplasia by using capillary polymerase chain reaction. *Br J Haematol* 1994;86:138–142.

123. Wolf DG, Spector S. Early diagnosis of human cytomegalovirus disease in transplant recipients by DNA amplification in plasma. *Transplantation* 1993;56:330–334.

124. Storch GA, Ettinger NA, Ockner D, et al. Quantitative cultures of the cell fraction and supernatant of bronchoalveolar lavage fluid for the diagnosis of cytomegalovirus pneumonitis in lung transplant recipients. *J Infect Dis* 1993;168:1502–1506.

125. Crawford SW, Bowden RA, Hackman RC, et al. Rapid detection of cytomegalovirus pulmonary infection by

bronchoalveolar lavage. *Ann Intern Med* 1988;108:180–185.

126. Wehner JH, Jensen WA, Kirsch CM, et al. Controlled utilization of induced sputum analysis in the diagnosis of *Pneumocystis carinii* pneumonia. *Chest* 1994;105:1770–1774.

127. Tang CM, Holden DW, Aufuvre-Brown A, et al. The detection of Aspergillus spp by the PCR reaction and its elevation in bronchoalveolar lavage fluid. *Am Rev Respir Dis* 1993;148:1313–1317.

128. Ramsey BW, Marcuse EK, Roy HM, et al. Use of bacterial antigen detection in the diagnosis of pediatric lower respiratory tract infections. *Pediatrics* 1986;78:1–9.

129. Kan VL. Polymerase chain reaction for the diagnosis of candidemia. *J Infect Dis* 1993;168:779–831.

130. Edelstein PH. The laboratory diagnosis of Legionnaire's disease. *Semin Respir Infect* 1987;2:235–241.

131. Berenguer J, Buck M, Witebsky F, et al. Lysis-centrifugation blood cultures in the detection of tissue-proven invasive candidiasis: disseminated versus single-organ infection *Diagn Mircobiol Infect Dis* 1993;17:103–109.

132. Pattishall EN, Noyes BE, Orenstein DM. Use of bronchoalveolar lavage in immunocompromised children with pneumonia. *Pediatr Pulmonol* 1988;5:1–5.

133. Wood RE. The diagnostic effectiveness of the flexible bronchoscope in children. *Pediatr Pulmonol* 1985;1:188–192.

134. Wood RE, Leigh MW, Retsch-Bogart G. Diagnosis of pneumonia in immunocompromised patients. *J Pediatr* 1990;116:836–837.

135. Stokes DC, Shenep JL, Parham D, et al. Role of flexible bronchoscopy in the diagnosis of pulmonary infiltrates in pediatric patients with cancer. *J Pediatr* 1989;115:561–567.

136. deBlic J, McKelvie P, leBourgeois M, et al. Value of bronchoalveolar lavage in the mangement of severe acute pneumonia and interstitial pneumonias in the immunocompromised child. *Thorax* 1987;42:759–765.

137. Abadco DL, Amaro-Galvez R, Rao M, et al. Experience with flexible bronchoscopy with bronchoalveolar lavage as a diagnostic tool in children with AIDS. *Am J Dis Child* 1992;146:1056–1059.

138. Mattey JE, Fitzpatrick SB, Josephs SH, et al. Bronchoalveolar lavage for pneumocystis pneumonia in HIV-infected children. *Ann Allergy* 1990;64:393–397.

139. Rodriguez de Castro F, Sole Violan J, Lafarga Capuz BM, et al. Reliability of the bronchoscopic protected catheter brush in the diagnosis of pneumonia in mechanically ventilated patients. *Crit Care Med* 1991;19:171–175.

140. Grigg J, van den Borre C, Malfroot A, et al. Bilateral fiberoptic bronchoalveolar lavage in acute unilateral lobar pneumonia. *J Pediatr* 1993;122:606–608.

141. Birriel JA Jr, Adams JA, Saldana MA, et al. Role of flexible bronchoscopy and bronchoalveolar lavage in the diagnosis of pediatric acquired immunodeficiency syndrome-related pulmonary disease. *Pediatrics* 1991;87:897–899.

142. Winthrop AL, Waddell T, Superina RA. The diagnosis of pneumonia in the immunocompromised child: use of bronchoalveolar lavage. *J Pediatr Surg* 1990;25:878–880.

143. McCubbin MM, Trigg ME, Hendricker CM, et al. Bronchoscopy with bronchoalveolar lavage in the evaluation of pulmonary complications of bone marrow transplantation in children. *Pediatr Pulmonol* 1992;12:43–47.

144. Breuer R, Lossos IS, Lafair JS, et al. Utility of bronchoalveolar lavage in the assessment of diffuse pulmonary infiltrates in non-AIDS immunocompromised patients. *Respir Med* 1990;84:313–316.

145. Stokes DC. Is there room for another bronchoscope? *Pediatr Pulmonol* 1992;12:201.

146. Whitehead B, Scott JP, Helms P, et al. Technique and use of transbronchial lung biopsy in children and adolescents. *Pediatr Pulmonol* 1992;12:240–246.

147. Rigal E, Roze JC, Villers D, et al. Prospective evaluation of the protected specimen brush for the diagnosis of pulmonary infections in ventilated newborns. *Pediatr Pulmonol* 1990;8:268–272.

148. Koumbourlis AC, Kurland G. Nonbronchoscopic bronchoalveolar lavage in mechanically ventilated infants: technique, efficacy and applications. *Pediatr Pulmonol* 1993;15:257–262.

149. Godfrey S, Avital A, Maayan C, et al. Yield for flexible bronchoscopy in children. *Pediatr Pulmonol* 1997;23:261–269.

150. Salzman SH. Bronchoscopic techniques for the diagnosis of pulmonary complications of HIV infection. *Semin Respir Infect* 1999;14:318–326.

151. Tu JV, Biem HJ, Detsky AS. Bronchoscopy versus empirical therapy in HIV-infected patients with presumptive *Pneumocystis carinii* pneumonia: a decision analysis. *Am Rev Respir Dis* 1993;148:370–377.

152. Chaudhary S, Hughes WT, Feldman S, et al. Percutaneous transthoracic needle aspiration of the lung. Diagnosing *Pneumocystic carinii* pneumonitis. *Am J Dis Child* 1977;131:902–907.

153. Sokolowski JW Jr, Burgher LW, Jones FL Jr., et al. Guidelines for percutaneous transthoracic needle biopsy. *Am Rev Respir Dis* 1989;140:255–256.

154. Imoke E, Dudgeon DL, Colombani P, et al. Open lung biopsy in the immunocompromised pediatric patient. *J Pediatr Surg* 1983;18:816.

155. Doolin EJ, Luck SR, Sherman JO, et al. Emergency lung biopsy: friend or foe of the immunosuppressed child. *J Pediatr Surg* 1986;21:485.

156. Shorter NA, Ross AJ III, August C, et al. The usefulness of open lung biopsy in the pediatric bone marrow transplant population. *J Pediatr Surg* 1988;23:533.

157. Feins RH. The role of thoracoscopy in the AIDS/immunocompromised patient. *Ann Thorac Surg* 1993;56:649–650.

158. Daniel TM, Kern JA, Tribble CG, et al. Thoracoscopic surgery for diseases of the lung and pleura: effectiveness, changing indications, and limitations. *Ann Surg* 1993;217:566–574.

159. Schmidt GM, Kovacs A, Zaia JA, et al. Ganciclovir/immunoglobulin combination therapy for the treatment of human cytomegalovirus-associated interstitial pneumonia in bone marrow allograft recipients. *Transplantation* 1988;46:905–907.

160. Goodrich JM, Mori M, Gleaves CA, et al. Early treatment with ganciclovir to prevent cytomegalovirus disease after allogeneic bone marrow transplantation. *N Engl J Med* 1991;325:1601–1607.

161. Schmidt GM, Horak DA, Niland JC, et al. A randomized controlled trial of prophylactic ganciclovir for cy-

tomegalovirus pulmonary infection in recipients of bone marrow transplants. *N Engl J Med* 1991;324:1005–1011.

162. Bye MR, Cairns-Bazarian AM, Ewig JM. Markedly reduced mortality associated with corticosteroid therapy of *Pneumocystis carinii* in children with acquired immunodeficiency syndrome. *Arch Pediatr Adolesc Med* 1994;148:638–641.

163. Sleasman JW, Hemenway C, Klein AS, et al. Corticosteroids improve survival of children with AIDS and *Pneumocystis carinii* pneumonia. *Am J Dis Child* 1993;147:30–34.

164. Rankin JA, Pella JA. Radiographic resolution of *Pneumocystis carinii* pneumonia in response to corticosteroid therapy. *Am Rev Respir Dis* 1987;136:182–183.

165. Gallacher BP, Gallacher WN, MacFadden DK. Treatment of acute *Pneumocystis carinii* pneumonia with corticosteroids in a patient with acquired immunodeficiency syndrome. *Crit Care Med* 19899;17:104–105.

166. Bozette SA, Sattler FR, Chiu J, et al. A controlled trial of adjunctive treatment with corticosteroids for *Pneumocystis carinii* pneumonia in acquired immunodeficiency syndrome. *N Engl J Med* 1990;323:1451–1457.

167. NIH Expert Panel for Corticosteroids as Adjunctive Therapy for *Pneumocystis carinii*. Concensus statement on the use of corticosteroids as adjunctive therapy for *Pneumocystis carinii* pneumonia in the ac-

quired immunodeficiency syndrome. *N Engl J Med* 1990;323:1500–1504.

168. Nemunaitis J, Shannon Dorcy K, Appelbaum FR, et al. Long-term follow-up of patients with invasive fungal disease who received adjunctive therapy with recombinant human macrophage colony-stimulating factor. *Blood* 1993;82:1422–1427.

169. Lupinetti FM, Behrendt DM, Giller RH, et al. Pulmonary resection for fungal infection in children undergoing bone marrow transplantation. *J Thorac Cardiovasc Surg* 1992;10:684–687.

170. Denning DW, Stevens DA. Antifungal and surgical treatment of invasive aspergillosis: review of 2121 published cases. *Rev Infect Dis* 1990;12:1147–1201.

171. Richard C, Romon I, Baro J, et al. Invasive pulmonary aspergillosis prior to BMT in acute leukemia patients does not predict a poor outcome. *Bone Marrow Transplant* 1993;12:237–241.

172. Weintrub PS, Wara DW, Duliege A-M. Failure of intravenous pentamidine prophylaxis for *Pneumocystis carinii* pneumonia. *J Pediatr* 1993;122:163–164.

173. Schuval SJ, Bonagura VR. Failure of pentamidine as prophylaxis for Pneumocystis carinii in HIV-infected children. *Arch Pediatr Adolesc Med* 1994;148:876–879.

174. Doherry MJ, Thomas SHL, Gibb D, et al. Lung deposition of nebulized pentamidine in children. *Thorax* 1993;48:220–226.

19

Enteric Infections

Douglas K. Mitchell and Larry K. Pickering

Center for Pediatric Research, Eastern Virginia Medical School, Norfolk, Virginia 23510

The gastrointestinal tract is exposed constantly to a variety of pathogenic and nonpathogenic organisms. A network of physical, chemical, and immunologic mechanisms protects this environment. Disruption of local or systemic host defense mechanisms can result in an increase in frequency, severity, and duration of enteric infectious diseases. Altered morphology or function of the gastrointestinal tract of an immunocompromised patient can be produced by a variety of infectious agents including bacteria, viruses, parasites, and fungi. Immunocompromised children are exposed to an array of enteropathogens similar to those that infect immunocompetent children. In contrast to diseases that occur in children with intact immune systems, disease in immunocompromised children often is characterized by the presence of more than one pathogen, a propensity for invasion, chronicity, and relapse. Gastrointestinal tract manifestations that occur in immunocompromised persons include diarrhea, anorexia, abdominal pain, malabsorption, weight loss, vomiting, dysphagia, odynophagia, and death (1). In general, clinical manifestations may be acute or chronic, with failure to gain weight or significant weight loss and debilitation depending on the specific cause of infection and the nutritional and immunologic status of the patient. Diagnosis and therapy are often frustrating and difficult because of the diversity of agents that produce infection, the frequent finding of more than one potential cause, and the compromised immune system that makes

resolution difficult. The cause of diarrhea is not always infectious, and the mechanism for diarrhea is not always clear (2,3). Enteropathogens that infect the gastrointestinal tract are generally similar worldwide, but the frequency of infection depends on the age of the patient, the underlying immune deficit, and the geographic location and exposure of the individual.

Patients receiving chemotherapy for malignancies and those whose immune systems are suppressed after bone marrow or solid organ transplantation are at an increased risk for infection by organisms that involve the gastrointestinal tract. Serious infections of the gastrointestinal tract have been reported in patients undergoing heart, lung, kidney, liver, and bone marrow transplantation (4–8). Although any enteric pathogen may infect an immunocompromised host, organisms that are more frequent in transplant recipients include *Listeria monocytogenes*, Salmonella, *Clostridium difficile*, cytomegalovirus (CMV), adenovirus, herpes simplex virus (HSV), Candida, Aspergillus, Strongyloides, and Cryptosporidium (Table 19.1). The frequency of infection by a particular organism depends in part on the immune status of the host.

Prolonged hospital stay is a risk factor for nosocomial gastroenteritis. Hospitalized children are at risk both because of their underlying medical condition and because of their continued exposure to a variety of enteropathogens. Children in long-term care fa-

TABLE 19.1. *Organisms of greater importance in selected immunocompromised hosts compared with immunocompetent hosts*

| Condition | Organisms | | | |
	Bacteria	Viruses	Fungi	Parasites
Transplantation	*Listeria*	CMV	*Candida*	*Cryptosporidium*
	Salmonella	HSV	*Aspergillus*	*Strongyloides*
	Clostridium difficile	Adenovirus		
AIDS[a]	*Salmonella*	CMV	*Candida*	*Cryptosporidium*
	MAC	HSV	*Histoplasma*	*Isospora*
	C. difficile			
Neutropenia	Gram-negative bacilli	HSV	*Candida*	—
	C. difficile			

AIDS, acquired immunodeficiency syndrome; CMV, cytomegalovirus; HSV, herpes simplex virus; MAC, *Mycobacterium avium* complex.
[a]The listed organisms are AIDS-defining gastrointestinal tract opportunistic infections, except for *C. difficile*.

cilities have an increased risk of foodborne and waterborne disease as well as person-to-person transmission of enteropathogens (9–12). In one study, 10% of children with an infected roommate developed nosocomial diarrhea. The risk was directly proportional to the number of roommates. Younger hospitalized children were at greater risk: 10% of diapered children developed nosocomial diarrhea, compared with only 2% of nondiapered children (13). The rate of viral nosocomial diarrhea decreases with the age of the patient: 9% at 0 to 11 months; 4% at 12 to 35 months; and 0.6% at 36 months or older (13–17).

Many primary and secondary immunodeficiency syndromes manifest with chronic diarrhea (18). Other common clinical findings that occur in children with primary immunodeficiencies include recurrent respiratory tract infections, severe bacterial infections, and failure to thrive. In some patients there may be exudative diarrhea with loss of serum proteins and lymphocytes. The use of antimicrobial agents and the presence of concomitant respiratory tract infection often aggravate these gastrointestinal tract symptoms. Patients with T-lymphocyte immunodeficiency are particularly likely to have chronic diarrhea. In any person with an immune deficiency, recognition and treatment of enteropathogens associated with gastrointestinal tract disease may result in a cure or in prevention of the disease process. For some organisms, particularly the protozoa, therapeutic avenues have not been developed, and the morbidity caused by these organisms has provided a strong impetus for research.

NORMAL DEFENSE MECHANISMS OF THE GASTROINTESTINAL TRACT

A combination of host factors determines who develops illness after ingestion of infectious enteric pathogens. The majority of ingested pathogens fail to cause disease when host factors are intact. The gastrointestinal tract factors that influence growth or suppression of organisms include gastric acid, bile salts, gastrointestinal tract transport time, competitive indigenous flora, nonimmune host factors including glycoconjugates and oligosaccharides, composition of the mucous layer (e.g., viscosity, barrier, lubrication), secretory immunoglobulin A (IgA), and accessible cell receptors (19–22). Most enteric pathogens are transmitted by the fecal-oral route, so they must survive the acid environment of the stomach to cause disease. Hypoacidic states caused by use of antacids, achlorhydria, or gastric resection may increase the likelihood of disease caused by some enteropathogens. The indigenous flora of the gastrointestinal tract compete for nutrients, exchange plasmids, release antimicrobial agents and toxins, release iron-binding compounds, and release other factors that influence their growth. Interference with this biologic equilibrium through alteration of peristalsis, administration of antibiotics, bowel surgery, inflammatory bowel disease, or dietary changes increases the opportunities for a pathogen to become established (23,24).

Mucous secretions regulate access of organisms to the intestinal surface. The mucus contains receptor analogs that bind toxin and serve as a scaffold to hold secretory IgA (25). The functions of this specialized immunoglobulin are to prevent attachment, neutralize toxins and viruses, and prevent uptake of antigens (26,27). The systemic immune system becomes involved when gastrointestinal tract cells become infected or damaged and when the mucosal barrier is breached.

TABLE 19.2. *Immunodeficiencies and conditions associated with gastrointestinal tract infections or chronic diarrhea*

Acquired conditions
  Human immunodeficiency virus/acquired
    immunodeficiency syndrome
  Antimicrobial therapy
  Malnutrition
  Hematologic malignancy
  Chemotherapy
  Radiation
  Protein-losing enteropathies
  Bone marrow transplantation
  Solid organ transplantation
  Intestinal tract surgery
  Inflammatory bowel disease
Primary conditions
  T-cell defects
    Severe combined immunodeficiency (SCID)
      Adenosine deaminase deficiency
      Purine nucleoside phosphorylase deficiency
    T-cell activitation deficiencies
      MHC class I deficiency (bare lymphocyte
        syndrome)
      MHC class II deficiency
    Other
      DiGeorge's syndrome
  B-cell defects
    Common variable immunodeficiency
    Bruton's X-linked agammaglobulinemia
    Immunoglobulin A deficiency
  Complement deficiencies
Miscellaneous conditions
  Immaturity
    Transient hypogammaglobulinemia of infancy
  Genetic predisposition (race, sex, HLA type, blood
    group)

HLA, human leukocyte antigen; MHC, major histocompatibility complex.

Other factors may account for susceptibility of the gastrointestinal tract to enteropathogens. They can be grouped under the headings of genetic factors, maturational factors, and exogenously mediated factors (such as those that occur with chemotherapy or irradiation). Alteration of various parts of the immune system through genetic abnormalities or as a result of an exogenous or environmental cause can directly influence the response of the gastrointestinal tract to an enteropathogen. Chronic diarrhea and failure to thrive are common in children with various immunodeficiency syndromes, including children infected with the human immunodeficiency virus (HIV). A list of described diseases or conditions associated with inadequate responses to gastrointestinal tract infection is shown in Table 19.2.

In summary, any perturbation of the host-defense system can permit a diarrheal pathogen to become established in its own preferred niche in the intestine. In addition, some pathogens are sufficiently virulent to override the intact system of host intestinal defense mechanisms. Other substances, specifically human milk, contain compounds that protect suckling infants from diarrheal disease (28,29).

PATHOPHYSIOLOGY

Enteropathogens produce disease in the gastrointestinal tract by several mechanisms, including enterotoxin production, cytotoxin production, epithelial cell invasion, adherence, and translocation (30–33). Various host factors, such as gastric hypoacidity and decreased intestinal motility, have been associated with quantitative bacterial overgrowth and opportunistic enteric infections (34). In addition, decreased acid production may interfere with absorption of some medications. Enterotoxin-producing *Escherichia coli* (ETEC) and some other enteric organisms produce one or more enterotoxins that induce sodium and water secretion by enterocytes of the small intestine through activation of adenylate cyclase (in a manner similar to that of heat-labile cholera enterotoxin) or through activation of guanylate cyclase by a heat-stable toxin (31). There is laboratory evidence that *Cryptosporidium* also acts through the effect of an enterotoxin (35). Studies report that a rotavirus nonstructural protein, NSP4, acts as an enterotoxin to induce Ca^{2+}-dependent fluid secretion (36,37). Cytotoxins do not cause active fluid secretion, but they bind to globotriaosylceramide and act by inhibiting protein synthesis. Several organisms, including *Shigella dysenteriae* type 1, *C. difficile,* and *E. coli* O157:H7, produce cytotoxins (31). The enteric viruses, *Giardia lamblia, Cryptosporidium parvum, Isospora belli,* and *Enterocytozoon bieneusi* produce a noninflammatory insult to absorptive surfaces of the small intestine that results in watery diarrhea and carbohydrate malabsorption (32). A study of *Cyclospora cayetanensis* demonstrated abnormalities characterized by an inflammatory reaction in small bowel mucosa, surface epithelial disarray, and evidence of villous atrophy and crypt hyperplasia (32). For most enteric pathogens, the ability to colonize a relevant region of the intestine is as important in causing disease as is production of a toxin. An inflammatory response of the distal small and large intestine can be produced by organisms that invade the epithelial cells of the intestine, including *Salmonella, Shigella, Campylobacter jejuni, Yersinia enterocolitica,* and enteroinvasive *E. coli* (EIEC).

For clinical consideration, these pathophysiologic mechanisms can be grouped into one of three categories. The first consists of episodes of diarrhea that are noninflammatory and result from the action of an enterotoxin or another process that specifically alters the absorptive function of the villous tip in the upper small intestine, such as occurs with enteropathogenic *E. coli* (EPEC) and most enteric viruses and protozoa. The second manifestation of disease is inflammatory and usually occurs in the large intestine after an invasive process and/or cytotoxin production, such as occurs with *Shigella, Salmonella, C. jejuni, E. coli* O157: H7 (EHEC), and *Entamoeba histolytica.* A third manifestation of infection occurs when organisms enter Peyer's patches and translocate to regional lymph nodes and blood, resulting in a systemic infection such as occurs with *Salmonella typhi,* other *Salmonella* species, *Campylobacter fetus,* and *Y. enterocolitica.* Al-

though most enteropathogens are generally restricted to the intestine, many cause extraintestinal and/or systemic manifestations, especially in patients who have certain immunodeficiencies.

Noninfectious pathophysiologic mechanisms for gastrointestinal tract dysfunction may occur. For example, patients with primary hypogammaglobulinemia and diarrhea but no known enteropathogen had histologic evidence of inflammation in the stomach and jejunum (38). Granulomatous enteropathy is a gastrointestinal tract manifestation of common variable immune deficiency (CVID), as demonstrated in three adult females with CVID and protracted diarrhea (39). Diarrhea is a common occurrence after bone marrow transplantation; it occurred in 57% of patients at a median of 9.5 days after transplantation (40). Protein-losing enteropathy complicated 91% of diarrhea episodes and was more severe in those patients with graft-versus-host disease (40). The cause of many previously described diarrheal episodes in immunocompromised patients was not detected owing to a lack of appropriate diagnostic tests which are now available (41).

EPIDEMIOLOGY

The rate of gastrointestinal tract infection by a specific enteropathogen varies by geographic location, mode of transmission, age and sex of infected individuals, degree and type of immune suppression, complexity of the laboratory evaluation of patients studied, and the presence of continuing risk factors (Table 19.1). The occurrence of chronic diarrhea and perhaps malabsorption depends on the immune status of the host as well as the virulence properties of the enteropathogen. There are several general concepts that can be applied to the epidemiology of organisms that infect the gastrointestinal tract: (a) most infections of the intestine occur via the fecal-oral route; (b) the infectious dose of organisms varies, but it generally is lower in patients with immune deficiency; (c) there is often overlap in the clinical manifestations of infection by various enteropathogens; (d) enteropathogens may be acquired from animals or from contaminated food or water, and some are transmitted easily from person to person or may be hospital acquired; and (e) the severity of defects in host defense influences the clinical course, diagnosis, treatment, and prognosis (42).

The risk of infection in patients with acquired immunodeficiency syndrome (AIDS) increases over time, and the potential infecting agents increase according to potential exposures. In contrast, the risk for enteric infection of patients who have undergone transplantation is greatest in the early postoperative period when the degree of immune deficiency is greatest. The risk declines with time, but it still remains higher than in immunocompetent patients. The number of potential enteropathogens also decreases over time. During the first 3 to 4 weeks after transplantation, infections result from the transplant procedure or its complications. In solid organ transplantations, the procedure, intubation, anesthesia, and catheter placements are the main contributors to infection. Nosocomially acquired bacteria, including endogenous gastrointestinal tract flora, are the common pathogens. HSV infection reactivates in the early posttransplantation period. During the next interval, from 1 to 6 months after transplantation, there is increased risk from opportunistic infections such as CMV, adenovirus, and nonenteric infections. Beyond 6 months after transplantation, there is a chronic increased risk of infection with community-acquired enteric pathogens.

The principal reservoirs for bacterial enteropathogens are animals (poultry, livestock, reptiles, pets), contaminated animal and meat products, contaminated water, and infected humans. Infected humans are the only known reservoir for *Shigella* species and *S. typhi*. Modes of transmission of enteric pathogens include ingestion of contaminated food or water, contact with infected animals, person-to-person transmission via the fecal-oral route, and contact with a contaminated environment, including contaminated inanimate objects.

Most human infections with enteric viruses result from contact with infected humans via the fecal-oral route. Transmission via contaminated food and water also has been reported, especially for caliciviruses. Rotavirus infections

universally occur in the first 2 years of life (43). All enteric viruses have been implicated in nosocomial infections. Rotavirus, adenovirus, and astrovirus infections have been documented in recipients of bone marrow transplants. Case reports have documented chronic diarrhea with excretion of rotaviruses, caliciviruses, and astroviruses among children with other immunodeficiencies (4,8,44). In all of these scenarios including varied immunodeficiencies and enteropathogens, these infections are associated with increased morbidity and mortality.

The primary parasitic causes of enteric infection in the United States include several protozoa. Since the onset of the AIDS epidemic, the number of parasitic pathogens recognized and the frequency with which they are encountered in humans have increased. The four intestinal protozoa that have been increasingly identified in patients with AIDS are cryptosporidia, isospora, microsporidia, and cyclospora (32). *Cryptosporidium* has been identified throughout the world in a variety of hosts, including birds, reptiles, and mammals. Infection occurs after ingestion and possibly after inhalation of oocysts (45). Person-to-person and animal-to-human transmission have been documented and can result in outbreaks of disease, such as in child care centers where person-to-person transmission occurs. In addition, spread can occur via water or food substances that are fecally contaminated (46). The parasite is resistant to chlorine; therefore, water filtration systems are important for public water supplies. Humans are the only known host for *I. belli*. The organism is acquired through ingestion of sporulated oocysts, but the infective dose for humans is unknown. *G. lamblia* is a common cause of enteritis and is found with increased frequency in children in child care centers, travelers to endemic areas, and male homosexuals. Transmission occurs via the fecal-oral route by passage of infectious cysts from one person to another or by ingestion of fecally contaminated food or water (47). Microsporidia (*E. bieneusi* and *Encephalitozoon intestinalis*) are obligate intracellular spore-forming protozoan parasites that have been recognized in a variety of animals, particularly invertebrates (48). *C. cayetanensis* has been associated with large foodborne outbreaks and with waterborne transmission (49,50); direct animal-to-animal or person-to-person transmission has not been documented (51). *Strongyloides stercoralis* transmission occurs via contaminated soil. The worm burden depends on the size of larval inoculation and the degree of autoinfection. People with compromised immune systems may have enhanced autoinoculation and develop overwhelming infection that can be fatal (52).

Waterborne disease may be difficult to identify and investigate. The Centers for Disease Control and Prevention (CDC) surveillance system for waterborne disease outbreaks identified 30 such outbreaks in a 2-year period (1993–1994). One outbreak of cryptosporidiosis was first recognized among persons infected with HIV due to their more severe symptoms. Many other waterborne enteropathogens have been identified, including caliciviruses, hepatitis A virus, *Aeromonas* spp., and *Vibrio* spp. (53–57). The association of diarrheal disease with contaminated food and water is a major problem for persons with immune deficiencies. Education regarding prevention of infection by enteropathogens through improved hygiene, improved water supply, and careful preparation of food is critical.

Immunosuppressed patients frequently are hospitalized, and nosocomial diarrhea is a significant problem. Nosocomial diarrhea rates among immunocompetent children vary with age and have been reported as follows: 0 to 11 months, 9%; 12 to 35 months, 4%; 36 months and older, 1%. The rate by length of hospital stay was 3 to 7 days, 8%; 8 to 14 days, 10%; 15 to 21 days, 8%; longer than 21 days, 9% (13). The risk of nosocomial diarrhea was greatest among diapered children and increased with prolonged length of hospital stay. The nosocomially acquired enteropathogens identified in this study included rotavirus (43%), calicivirus (16%), astrovirus (14%), minireovirus (12%), adenovirus (8%), *Salmonella* spp. (4%), and parvovirus/picornavirus (3%) (13).

The HIV/AIDS epidemic has resulted in a large population of immunodeficient children and adults as subjects for the study and identification of new enteropathogens. Acute and chronic diarrhea are common complications of AIDS. A case-controlled cross-sectional study demonstrated an increased prevalence of enteric pathogens in HIV-infected children (57%), compared with healthy controls (17%) (58). Eight organisms that infect the gastrointestinal tract fulfill the CDC revised classification system for HIV infection and expanded AIDS surveillance case definition for adolescents and adults and for children younger than 13 years of age: *Candida, Cryptosporidium,* CMV, HSV, *Histoplasma capsulatum, Isospora, Mycobacterium avium* complex (MAC), and *Salmonella* (59,60). Although only these gastrointestinal tract organisms currently are listed in the CDC case definition, many other organisms can produce enteric disease in children with HIV infection. Children attending a child care center specifically for children with AIDS were investigated for parasitic enteric infections. In almost 700 child-months of surveillance, only one infection with *G. lamblia* and one infection with *E. histolytica* were identified (61). Therefore, care of children with AIDS by well-educated child care providers in a group care setting does not present an unnecessary risk.

CLINICAL PRESENTATION

Most episodes of diarrhea that occur during infancy and childhood are acute and self-limited. However, in children with immunodeficiency, infection with any enteropathogen can result in prolonged diarrhea and malabsorption with subsequent malnutrition, recurrence of infection after a course of appropriate antimicrobial therapy, and bacteremia associated with diarrhea (62). Children with small bowel disease generally have abdominal pain, weight loss, and watery diarrhea of large volume. Large bowel disease is manifested by small-volume stools, lower quadrant pain, tenesmus, bloody diarrhea containing mucus, and fever. The differential diagnosis of prolonged diarrhea is similar to that of chronic diarrhea of childhood; it usually occurs because of persistence of an enteropathogen or because of damage to the gastrointestinal tract that persists after the organism cannot be detected (63). Enteric infection may manifest differently in transplant recipients compared with immunocompetent patients.

Symptoms are often milder in immunosuppressed patients, possibly as a result of the use of antiinflammatory corticosteroids. Because of the altered response to infection and altered perception by the patient, presentations of infection may occur at a relatively advanced stage. Fever accompanies most, but not all, enteric infections.

Complications of intestinal infection, including intestinal perforation or hemorrhage, peritonitis, and bacteremia, have been associated with amebiasis, shigellosis, salmonellosis, *C. difficile, E. coli* O157:H7, and CMV infection of the ileocecal region. These complications need to be recognized and appropriately diagnosed so that correct therapy can be administered.

Neutropenic enterocolitis (typhlitis) is a clinical entity that occurs most commonly among patients with hematologic malignancies and chemotherapy-induced neutropenia. It also has been described in patients with AIDS (64).

Manifestations include fever, abdominal pain, and diarrhea, usually occurring in a granulocytopenic host. Patients with neutropenia also may have gram-negative sepsis, stomatitis, or necrotizing typhlitis (characterized by fever, abdominal pain, cecal edema, cecal necrosis, and bloody or watery diarrhea) (65).

DIFFERENTIAL DIAGNOSIS

Infectious causes of gastrointestinal tract diseases can be divided into several major categories based on the microbiologic classification of infectious agents (bacteria, viruses, parasites, fungi); the region of the digestive tract involved (esophagus, stomach, small intestine, colon); the pathophysiology of disease produced; and the host response to individual agents. For the purposes of this discussion the microbiologic classification is considered. The infectious agents and their most frequent modes of transmission are shown in Table 19.3.

TABLE 19.3. *Differential diagnosis of enteropathogens causing diarrhea in immunocompromised children and their most frequent modes of transmission*

Organism	Foodborne	Waterborne	Nosocomial	Person-to-person	Zoonotic
Bacteria					
Aeromonas hydrophila	X	X			
Campylobacter spp.	X				X
Clostridium difficile			X		
Escherichia coli	X	X		X	X
Plesiomonas shigelloides		X	X		
Pseudomonas aeruginosa		X	X		
Salmonella spp.	X			X	X
Shigella spp.	X			X	
Vibrio spp.	X	X			
Yersinia enterocolitica	X				
Viruses					
Enteric adenovirus			X	X	
Astrovirus	X		X	X	
Calicivirus	X	X	X	X	
Rotavirus			X	X	
Herpes simplex virus			X	X	
Cytomegalovirus			X	X	
Parasitic agents					
Blastocystis hominis		X			X
Cryptosporidium parvum	X	X		X	X
Cyclospora cayetanensis	X	X			
Entamoeba histolytica	X	X		X	
Giardia lamblia	X	X		X	X
Isospora belli	X			X	
Microsporidia		X			
Strongyloides stercoralis[a]					

[a]Organism acquired by penetration of skin by infective larvae.

Bacteria

The major bacterial enteric pathogens associated with acute infectious diarrhea are *Aeromonas* spp., *Campylobacter* spp., *C. difficile, E. coli, Plesiomonas shigelloides, Salmonella* spp., *Shigella* spp., *Vibrio* spp. including *Vibrio cholerae*, and *Y. enterocolitica*. Each of these enteropathogens is addressed briefly.

Aeromonas *Species*

Species of *Aeromonas,* including *Aeromonas caviae, Aeromonas hydrophila,* and *Aeromonas sobria,* have been associated with acute gastroenteritis (66–71), but other studies do not support this finding (72). *Aeromonas* was identified in the stool specimens of 25% of children during an outbreak of diarrheal illness in child care centers (56). These outbreaks of diarrhea were unusual in that several different *Aeromonas* species were involved in each center. In another study, *Aeromonas* spp. were recovered from stool specimens of 15 hospitalized children but all were community acquired (73). Surveillance in a French hospital revealed a seasonal variation in nosocomial *A. hydrophila* infection that was correlated with the number of *Aeromonas* organisms in the hospital water supply (74,75). Studies have revealed a predominance of Aeromonas-*associated diarrhea in very young children (6 months to 5 years), but cytotoxigenic strains appeared to be more commonly* recovered from older individuals (more than 50 years of age) (55). The incidence of diarrhea due to *Aeromonas* strains does not appear to be increased among immunocompromised persons.

Campylobacter *Species*

Campylobacter organisms are small, spiral or curved, motile, microaerophilic gram-negative bacilli. *Campylobacter* species considered to be human enteric pathogens include *C. fetus, Campylobacter coli, Campylobacter lari, C. jejuni, Campylobacter concisus, Campylobacter sputorum, Campylobacter hyointestinalis,* and *Campylobacter upsaliensis* (76–80). The most common cause of diarrhea is *C. jejuni.*

Transmission of *Campylobacter* occurs by ingestion, most often of contaminated water or food. The most common sources are unpasteurized milk, raw or partially cooked poultry, and contaminated water. Disease due to *Campylobacter* infection is most commonly gastrointestinal in nature, but 25% of persons with culture-proven infection acquired in large outbreaks report no symptoms. The diarrhea may be quite severe, with eight or more stools occurring on at least one day of the illness. In addition to diarrhea, most patients have fever, abdominal pain, nausea, and malaise. Fecal leukocytes and gross or occult fecal blood are found in persons infected with invasive strains of *Campylobacter* (76). Extraintestinal complications include bacteremia, meningitis, cholecystitis, and urinary tract infection (76–80). The incubation period is 1 to 7 days, and diarrhea usually is self-limited, lasting 2 to 7 days, although persistent and relapsing symptoms are well described. The duration of excretion of the organisms varies from 2 weeks to 3 months in immunocompetent hosts not treated with antibiotics. The clinical features of *C. jejuni* infections range from an absence of symptoms to fulminant sepsis and death (76).

The incidence of *C. jejuni* infection among patients with AIDS (mean annual incidence, 519 cases per 100,000 patients) is higher than that in the healthy population (13.3 cases per 100,000) (81). This excess of *C. jejuni* infections affects only patients in the later stages of HIV disease; patients with early HIV infection and relatively high CD4 counts usually are not prone to either *C. jejuni* infections or relapses of such infections (76). *C. jejuni, C. upsaliensis,* and *C. coli* also can cause prolonged diarrhea in HIV-infected patients (77). A study of stool samples from 204 HIV-infected adults isolated 12 *Campylobacter* strains from 7 (16%) patients with diarrhea and from 5 (3%) patients without diarrhea (81). *Campylobacter* was the most frequently isolated enteropathogenic bacteria. Eleven of the 12 *Campylobacter* strains isolated grew only on nonselective agars when a membrane filter technique was performed at an incubation temperature of 37°C for 5 days; therefore it appears that cultures performed with only selective enrichment medium for *Campylobacter* isolation miss many significant *Campylobacter* pathogens.

C. jejuni is the most common species of *Campylobacter* causing bacteremia worldwide; *C. upsaliensis* and *C. fetus* are infrequently described (76,78,79). Most of the infected children were younger than 2 years of age. Forty percent of children with *Campylobacter* bacteremia were malnourished, supporting the likelihood that malnutrition is a risk factor for *Campylobacter* bacteremia (82). A recent history of diarrhea is not a prerequisite for the development of *Campylobacter* bacteremia (82).

Patients with hypogammaglobulinemia develop severe, persistent, and relapsing infections due to *C. jejuni*. A lack of opsonizing activity also predisposes individuals to bacteremia and other extraintestinal manifestations, including osteomyelitis, cellulitis, and meningitis. Therefore, early intervention with antimicrobial therapy is warranted in this population (76).

Clostridium difficile *Infection*

Clostridium difficile is recognized as the etiologic agent of pseudomembranous colitis and has been implicated as the cause of many of the episodes of antibiotic-associated diarrhea. A specific chain of events results in *C. difficile* colitis: disruption of the normal bacterial flora of the colon, colonization with *C. difficile,* and release of toxins that cause mucosal damage and inflammation (31,83). Antibiotic therapy is the key factor that alters colonic flora and allows *C. difficile* to flourish. Cytotoxic chemotherapy, for example with methotrexate, doxorubicin, cyclophosphamide, or fluorouracil, also may predispose to cytotoxigenic *C. difficile* colitis.

Environmental contamination by *C. difficile* is particularly common in hospitals, including oncology wards and facilities providing long-term care (84). The organism can be cultured from hospital floors, toilets, bedpans, bedding, mops, scales, and furniture. When established in the colon, pathogenic strains of *C. difficile*

produce toxins that cause diarrhea and colitis; strains that do not produce toxins are not pathogenic. Both toxin genes have been cloned and sequenced, revealing that they encode two large protein exotoxins. These exotoxins are toxin A, a 308-kD enterotoxin, and toxin B, a 250- to 270-kD cytotoxin. Toxin A causes fluid secretion, mucosal damage, and intestinal inflammation when injected into rodent intestine. Toxin B is more potent than toxin A as a cytotoxin in tissue culture, but it is not enterotoxic in animals (31). Hospitalized patients are the primary target of *C. difficile,* because they receive antimicrobial therapy in a setting in which environmental contamination with *C. difficile* spores is commonplace (83). Clinical features that distinguish infection with *C. difficile* antibiotic-associated diarrhea from that caused by many other enteric pathogens are hyperpyrexia, leukemoid reactions, toxic megacolon, pseudomembranous colitis, hypoalbuminemia, and chronic diarrhea (85).

C. difficile has been isolated frequently from patients in chronic care facilities. In this population of debilitated persons, the organism may cause greater morbidity and mortality than in other settings (86,87). *C. difficile* has been associated with significant morbidity and mortality among patients with immunosuppression (83). In a study of adults with AIDS, *C. difficile* was the most prevalent pathogen and was associated with increased mortality (88,89). Infections with *C. difficile* are commonly reported after liver or bone marrow transplantation, owing to the greater use of antibiotics in patients with these transplants (4,5,7,90,91) and to nosocomial spread (84–87). Infection with *C. difficile* is less widely reported among renal and heart transplant patients. One study failed to associate *C. difficile* toxin and diarrhea in pediatric oncology patients (92); another showed that *C. difficile* infection was a risk factor for bacteremia caused by vancomycin-resistant enterococci in adult patients with acute leukemia (93).

Escherichia coli *Infection*

Several clinical syndromes may result from infection with *E. coli,* including urinary tract infection, sepsis/meningitis, and enteric/diarrheal disease. *E. coli* strains that cause acute diarrheal disease may be classified into six groups: enterotoxigenic (ETEC), enteroaggregative (EAEC), enteroinvasive (EIEC), enteropathogenic (EPEC), enterohemorrhagic (EHEC), and diffusely adherent (DAEC) (30). The incidence of nosocomial gastroenteritis caused by these groups of *E. coli* is low (94). This may be a reflection of detection methods that are not available in most clinical microbiology laboratories.

ETEC usually infects infants and children in developing countries or adults who have traveled in developing countries. Nosocomial ETEC-associated diarrheal outbreaks in special care nurseries, caused by strains producing heat-stable enterotoxin, have been reported, with ETEC cultured from infants, nurses, family members, infant formula, and surfaces in the nursery (95). ETEC frequently is associated with traveler's diarrhea, food and water being the most common vehicles for transmission (96). Some reports implicate person-to-person transmission and foodborne transmission via formula. *E. coli* also has been reported as a contaminant of expressed human milk, which caused both asymptomatic infections and gastroenteritis in a nursery (97).

EAEC produces acute or chronic diarrhea in all age groups, but predominantly in infants, through attachment to and effacement of the intestinal mucosa. EAEC is associated with diarrhea in developing countries, most prominently with persistent diarrhea (longer than 14 days). EAEC has been linked to diarrhea in patients with HIV infection, but its precise role in AIDS diarrhea is unknown (98,99).

EIEC infects individuals of all ages and causes diarrhea containing blood and mucus as a result of tissue invasion. These infections may occasionally be foodborne or occur as the result of travel to developing countries. The pathogenesis of EIEC is similar to that of *Shigella* spp. EIEC has been associated with foodborne and waterborne outbreaks.

EPEC produces acute and chronic diarrhea, usually in infants younger than 2 years of age in developing countries (100). EPEC is the strain most commonly associated with nosocomial infections. Many studies of outbreaks of diarrhea in neonatal intensive care units have demonstrated person-to-person transmission on the hands of hospital personnel. Premature infants are the most susceptible to severe morbidity and to mortality resulting from these infections (30,101). Detection of EPEC requires a high level of suspicion. Colonies of *E. coli* from a routine bacterial culture must be screened by type-specific antisera. Research methods for identifying related serotypes include adherence of organisms in HEp-2 human laryngeal tumor cells, DNA probes, and polymerase chain reaction (PCR) to detect EPEC strains with the enteroadherence plasmid. EPEC strains have been isolated from patients with AIDS and chronic diarrhea (98).

EHEC causes abdominal pain and bloody diarrhea in children and adults, mostly in developed countries. Hemolytic-uremic syndrome in children and thrombotic thrombocytopenic purpura in adults may complicate the illness. EHEC is most frequently spread by undercooked contaminated meat, but many other vehicles of transmission have been described (102,103). Community-acquired foodborne outbreaks of EHEC serotype O157:H7 are well documented. Many outbreaks have occurred in nursing homes, and a report of an outbreak in an institution for mentally retarded children and adults demonstrated the devastating effects of this organism in an outbreak (103,104). Twenty-nine children with *E. coli* O157:H7 were identified in nine child care centers. There was evidence of person-to-person transmission in all nine facilities (105). Spread of *E. coli* O157:H7 from a patient to a nurse in the hospital setting has been reported (106). Immunocompromised persons may be more susceptible to infections with EHEC and to sequelae once infected, but data are limited.

Listeria *Infection*

Listeria is one of the classic infections occurring in patients with defects in cell-mediated immunity. Transplantation patients account for 10% to 15% of cases of *Listeria* infection. The rate of infection in transplantation patients is increased at least 1000-fold over that in immunocompetent populations (107). The greatest risk of listeriosis occurs during the first year after transplantation. *Listeria* are susceptible to trimethoprim-sulfamethoxazole (TMP/SMX), and the use of this antibiotic agent for *Pneumocystis carinii* prophylaxis may decrease the risk of listeriosis among transplant recipients. *L. monocytogenes* has a high case-fatality rate, particularly among immunocompromised hosts, neonates, and pregnant women. The annual incidence of invasive listeriosis was 7.4 cases per 1 million population, and 23% of cases were fatal (108). Of cases occurring in nonpregnant adults, 69% involved patients with cancer, persons with AIDS, organ transplant recipients, or patients receiving corticosteroid therapy. Infection of a pregnant woman frequently resulted in loss of the pregnancy. The risk of infection was related to eating soft cheeses, food from delicatessens, hot dogs, prepackaged meat products, or undercooked chicken (109–111). Fever, gastrointestinal tract manifestations, and flu-like symptoms may precede invasive listeriosis. A median incubation period for invasive illness of 31 days (range, 2 to 8 weeks) has been proposed.

Plesiomonas *Infection*

P. shigelloides is primarily a freshwater organism, with isolation rates increasing during warm months. Fish and shellfish frequently harbor plesiomonads. *Plesiomonas* can be isolated from the feces of asymptomatic cold-blooded animals and warm-blooded animals such as cats and dogs. Plesiomonads are facultatively anaerobic gram-negative rods. The organism grows on a variety of common differential or selective agars. A pathogenic role of this organism is supported by evidence of a lessening of symptoms with appropriate antibiotic therapy, a low asymptomatic carriage rate, and outbreaks of diarrheal disease (112). Symptoms usually occur 24 to 48 hours after exposure. The symptoms and severity are quite diverse. The gastrointestinal tract symptoms last 2 to 14 days and include severe abdominal pain or cramping, vomiting, fever, and headaches.

Salmonella *Species*

The genus *Salmonella* is now considered to comprise a single species, named *Salmonella enterica,* based on DNA structure and biochemical properties. Within this species are seven subspecies, with almost all serotypes pathogenic for humans classified into subgroup I (*S. enterica* subspecies *enterica*). The subspecies can be divided into serotypes based on O (somatic) and H (flagellar) antigens. Two main clinical syndromes are associated with *Salmonella.* The first syndrome includes some *Salmonella* serotypes, especially *S. typhi* and *Salmonella paratyphi,* that are adapted to humans, have no other natural hosts, and cause the protracted bacteremia of typhoid fever (*S. typhi*) and paratyphoid fever (*S. paratyphi*). The second includes non-*typhi Salmonella* organisms that cause predominantly gastrointestinal tract illness. Non-*typhi Salmonella* strains are distributed widely in nature in the gastrointestinal tracts of wild and domestic mammals, birds, reptiles, and insects (113–119). *Salmonella typhimurium* is the serotype most commonly reported as the cause of human *Salmonella* infections in the United States. Sources of transmission include contaminated animal products (meat, milk, eggs), contaminated water, medications and dyes (120,121), medical equipment (122–127), and even blood transfusions. *S. typhi* infects only humans, and *S. paratyphi* has a reservoir primarily in humans, so direct contact with fecally contaminated food, water, or other sources results in infection.

Outbreaks of *Salmonella* infection have been reported in nurseries. The organism usually is introduced into the nursery by an infant recently born to a mother with either clinical or asymptomatic salmonellosis (128) or by a child with community-acquired *Salmonella* infection. *Salmonella* may be transmitted among staff and patients by person-to-person contact. Acquisition of multiply resistant organisms by premature infants in special care nurseries results in increased rates of morbidity and mortality (129,130). In general, neonates who acquire *Salmonella* from their mothers are at high risk for severe bacteremia and meningitis.

Host susceptibility to salmonellosis is influenced by a variety of anatomic, pharmacologic, and immunologic factors. *Salmonella* infections occur more frequently in persons with HIV infection than in the general population (131–133), and recurrent *Salmonella* bacteremia is an AIDS-defining illness (59). Patients with AIDS may have severe salmonellosis with fulminant and persistent diarrhea, enterocolitis, recurrent bacteremia, and death. The incidence and severity of *Salmonella* infections may have decreased with the use of current effective antiretroviral therapy. There is an increased severity of salmonellosis among patients with organ transplantation and lymphoproliferative disease due to dysfunction of cell-mediated immunity. Risk factors for extraintestinal salmonellosis in children have been studied: 72% of patients with extraintestinal salmonellosis had underlying risk factors, the most common being age younger than 3 months, sickle cell anemia, and gastrointestinal tract surgery (134,135).

Shigella *Species*

Shigellosis occurs worldwide, although its prevalence differs by location. It is largely a disease associated with poverty, crowding, poor levels of personal hygiene, inadequate water supplies, and malnutrition (136). There are four species of *Shigella*—*S. dysenteriae*, *Shigella flexneri*, *Shigella boydii*, and *Shigella sonnei*—which are differentiated by group-specific polysaccharide antigens of lipopolysaccharides (designated A, B, C, and D, respectively), biochemical properties, and phage or colicin susceptibility. *S. sonnei* is the most common cause of bacillary dysentery in the United States, and *S. flexneri* is responsible for most of the remaining cases. *S. dysenteriae* type 1 and *S. flexneri* are the most common species causing disease in developing countries. Direct fecal-oral transmission can con-

tribute to endemic shigellosis in institutional environments such as mental hospitals, child care centers, nursing homes, prisons, and outdoor gatherings (137,138). The incubation period is 1 to 7 days. Nosocomial outbreaks have seldom been reported despite the low inoculum necessary to cause infection (139).

Both *S. flexneri* and *S. sonnei* have been reported in newborn infants who acquired the organism from an infected mother during labor and delivery, but in general bacteremia in neonates is uncommon (140–142). Among HIV-infected patients, *Shigella* spp. can cause recurrent or chronic diarrhea or bacteremia associated with fever and abdominal cramps (143–146). Reports of *Shigella* infection in transplantation patients are uncommon (147–149).

Vibrio *Species*

V. cholerae O1, the etiologic agent of cholera, and *V. cholerae* non-O1 strains, including *V. cholerae* O139, are recognized as important causes of acute, often severe, diarrheal disease in developing countries (150). A number of other *Vibrio* species have been identified and associated with gastroenteritis, including (151–153): *Vibrio parahaemolyticus, Vibrio mimicus, Vibrio fluvialis, Vibrio furnissii, Vibrio vulnificus,* and *Vibrio hollisae.* In the United States, virtually all cases of non-O1 *V. cholerae* gastroenteritis, including *V. parahaemolyticus* and *V. vulnificus,* are associated with eating raw or undercooked shellfish, particularly raw oysters (151,152, 154,155). However, transmission may occur through other routes, including water and a variety of other foods. Foodborne outbreaks have been reported in the United States, primarily in coastal areas (151,152). In countries with endemic cholera, all ages are affected, although children older than 1 year of age are disproportionately involved. The incubation period of cholera is usually 1 to 3 days.

Cholera may affect immunocompromised individuals similarly to immunocompetent hosts. There are no reports of an increased incidence or severity of infection in immunocompromised hosts. A single case of severe cholera has been reported in an HIV-infected adult (156). In Guatemala, 48% of HIV-infected patients had acute or chronic diarrhea during follow-up, 11% had cryptosporidiosis, and 6% had cholera. In fact, the HIV-infected individuals had mild diseases associated with *V. cholerae* serogroup O1 infection (157).

V. vulnificus is a gram-negative bacterium that can cause serious illness and death in persons with preexisting liver disease or compromised immune systems (158,159). Persons with compromised immune systems (e.g., chronic renal insufficiency, cancer, diabetes, steroid-dependent asthma, chronic intestinal disease) or iron-overload states (e.g., thalassemia, hemochromatosis) may be at increased risk for infection with *V. vulnificus* and death (160). It is not known whether the risk is increased in persons with HIV infection.

Yersinia *Infection*

Y. enterocolitica is associated with a wide spectrum of clinical and immunologic manifestations depending in part on the age and physical state of the host (161). The clinical illness caused by this pathogen ranges from self-limited enterocolitis to potentially fatal systemic infection; postinfection manifestations include erythema nodosum and reactive arthritis. *Y. enterocolitica* enterocolitis is characterized by diarrhea with blood-streaked stools, fever, vomiting, and abdominal pain (161,162). The clinical course of *Y. enterocolitica* septicemia in immunocompetent or immunocompromised hosts may include abscess formation in the liver and spleen, pneumonia, septic arthritis, meningitis, cellulitis, empyema, and osteomyelitis (162). Serogroups 0:3, 0:8, and 0:9 are most commonly implicated as a cause of enterocolitis in the United States. *Y. enterocolitica* has been isolated from a variety of animate reservoirs, including birds, frogs, fish, flies, fleas, snails, crabs, oysters, and a wide array of mammals, with swine the major reservoir for human pathogens (161). Acquisition and excretion of *Yersinia* spp. has been associated with consumption of pasteurized milk on a pediatric ward (163). The same serotype of *Y. enterocolitica* was isolated from the patients and from the pasteurized milk. Animal products, including raw milk, whipped cream, ice cream, beef, lamb, and poultry, also may harbor the organism. Inanimate reservoirs include lakes, streams, well water, soil, and vegetables (164). Outbreaks in the United States have most frequently been associated with preparation of chitterlings for holiday meals in the south (165–167). Virulent *Y. enterocolitica* localize to the distal small intestine (terminal ileum) and proximal colon after penetration through the mucous layer (161). Septicemia is typically a severe illness, with case-fatality rates of 7% to 50% (168). Pathologic conditions associated with an iron-overloaded state are well-recognized predisposing factors for severe systemic *Yersinia* infection.

Transfusion-related yersiniosis has been reported in several countries, including the United States and in Europe (169). Blood donors apparently had low-grade *Y. enterocolitica* bacteremia at the time of donation, and the organism replicated under the storage conditions provided for units of red blood cells (170,171). Children and adults with hematologic conditions resulting in iron overload are at greater risk of yersiniosis (161,172).

Viruses

Acute infectious diarrhea of viral origin is usually a self-limited disease associated with an enteric adenovirus, astrovirus, calicivirus, or rotavirus (173). These viruses usually infect infants and young children but may involve the gastrointestinal tracts of older children and adults. Case reports have documented chronic diarrhea associated with excretion of adenovirus, astrovirus, calicivirus, rotavirus, and other viruses among children with immunodeficiencies, most notably severe combined immunodeficiency (SCID) syndrome. Rotavirus, astrovirus, and adenovirus infections have been documented in recipients of bone marrow transplants, and such infections are associated with increased morbidity and mortality (4,8,174–176).

Enteric Adenoviruses

Enteric adenovirus types 40 and 41 are the recognized enteropathogens of the adenovirus group. Symptoms of enteric adenovirus infection typically last 5 to 12 days and occasionally can linger for more than 2 weeks; enteric adenovirus diarrhea appears to last longer than other forms of viral gastroenteritis. Watery diarrhea is most prominent, usually followed by 1 to 2 days of vomiting (177). Most infants and young children have low-grade fever for 2 to 3 days. Severe dehydration is less common than with rotavirus in some series, but as common in others. Diarrhea due to enteric adenoviruses is not necessarily recognized as being particularly severe or persistent in immunocompromised children with cancer (178,179). However, infection with these adenoviruses has been tentatively linked with chronic diarrhea in patients with AIDS, a child who received a bone marrow transplant, and an adult with chronic lymphocytic leukemia (179,180). In addition, enteric adenoviruses are a common cause of nosocomial diarrhea. In one report, 44% of infections were hospital acquired, and 35% of those patients had underlying immune defects. Children with immune defects appear to have prolonged fever associated with this infection (181,182).

Adenovirus type 5 is known to cause life-threatening pneumonia in immunocompromised patients, including those undergoing bone marrow transplantation. This strain also was implicated as the probable cause of severe gastroenteritis in an immunocompromised child undergoing cytostatic therapy for acute lymphocytic leukemia (183).

Astroviruses

Eight antigenic types of human astrovirus have been identified. Gastroenteritis due to astrovirus occurs worldwide and has been associated with outbreaks of mild diarrhea in schools, child care centers, nursing homes, and pediatric hospital wards (184). Astroviruses are responsible for approximately 3% to 5% of hospital admissions for gastroenteritis. Illness occurs mainly in children younger than 2 years of age and frequently causes asymptomatic infection (185). The illness lasts 1 to 4 days after an incubation period of 24 to 36 hours. Gastrointestinal tract symptoms are nonspecific, consisting of vomiting, diarrhea, fever, and abdominal pain. Transmission is person-to-person among children. Astrovirus has been reported to be responsible for 5% to 7% of nosocomial gastroenteritis in children's hospitals (186–188). Astrovirus caused a prolonged outbreak of diarrhea among immunocompromised patients in a pediatric bone marrow transplantation unit, with excretion occurring for 60 to 90 days (8). Astrovirus was reported as a cause of prolonged diarrhea in two children with SCID. One patient was coinfected with rotavirus, and the other was coinfected with enteric adenovirus (8,189,190).

Caliciviruses

Four genera of calicivirus have been described (191). Two of these genera, the Norwalk-like viruses and the Sapporo-like viruses, infect humans. Many of the Norwalk-like viruses are known only from a single outbreak and were named after the site at which the outbreak occurred. They include Norwalk, Hawaii, Snow Mountain, MX (Mexico), and Lordsdale (191–193). Norwalk virus is the best studied member of the genus. Human calicivirus infections occur year-round, although some studies suggest a seasonal predominance. Norwalk virus illness occurs after an incubation period of 18 to 48 hours and is characterized by vomiting, diarrhea, abdominal pain, and low-grade fever lasting 1 to 2 days (194). Serologic studies indicate that 50% to 70% of residents in the United States have antibodies to Norwalk agent by 30 years of age (195), but these serum antibodies do not necessarily confer immunity. Symptoms caused by caliciviruses are indistinguishable from those caused by other enteric viruses (196,197). Persistent excretion of caliciviruses may occur in immunocompromised hosts. Caliciviruses have been identified in stools for up to 2 weeks after the onset of symptoms (198). Illness due to Norwalk virus is reported most commonly among persons of school age and older. Epidemics of Norwalk-like viruses have been reported in nursing homes, schools, recreational areas, and hospitals (199–205). Waterborne (206), foodborne (207,208), and person-to-person transmission have all been implicated in epidemics (192,209,210), and results of volunteer studies suggest fecal-oral transmission. In an outbreak in a children's ward, 15 children had Norwalk virus in stool specimens, and the ward had to be closed to control the outbreak (199). Calicivirus can be detected in stool specimens from 0.2% to 6% of children hospitalized for gastroenteritis. Calicivirus was detected in stool specimens from 4 of 10 children with nosocomial diarrhea and from 3 of 8 asymptomatic contacts in the same room (197,211). The role of caliciviruses in causing disease in immunocompromised children is unknown.

Coxsackievirus

Coxsackievirus A1 generally has not been associated with diarrhea in immunocompetent hosts, but in an outbreak in one bone marrow transplantation unit diarrhea and mortality were associated with this virus. During this outbreak there were seven cases of diarrhea and six deaths (212). There have been no other studies or reports to confirm this association.

Rotaviruses

Rotavirus infection occurs seasonally in North America. In the United States a yearly wave of rotavirus illness spreads across North America, originating in Mexico in November and ending in New England. Rotavirus infection occurs year-round in countries within 10° latitude of the equator. Rotavirus infection is rapidly lytic to enterocytes, leading to microscopic alterations, including mild shortening of villi and crypt hyperplasia, as well as moderate round-cell infiltration of the lamina propria. Rotavirus infection is frequently asymptomatic. In symptomatic infection, the incubation period is 1 to 3 days and illness usually lasts 5 to 7 days. In an immunocompromised host the period may be prolonged substantially (177). Rotavirus gastroenteritis is characterized by frequent vomiting, which starts early in the illness, and commonly is associated with mild-to-moderate dehydration with normal serum sodium concentrations and mild acidosis. Fever is common, but signs or symptoms of dysentery, such as bloody diarrhea and tenesmus, indicate concurrent bacterial infection.

Rotaviruses are ubiquitous; 95% of children worldwide are infected by 3 to 5 years of age. Rotavirus infections of adults are usually subclinical but occasionally cause illness in parents of children with rotavirus diarrhea, immunocompromised patients (including person infected with HIV), the elderly, and travelers to developing countries (213).

Although rotavirus infection generally is restricted to the small bowel, investigations in mice with combined immunodeficiency and in immunocompromised children indicate that rotavirus can infect the liver and kidneys under some circumstances (177). Antigen has been detected in liver, kidney, and serum in children with immunodeficiency, suggesting that viremia may occur (44,214). The unique genomic rearrangements of rotavirus have been noted among patients with T-cell deficiency (44,190). Rotavirus has been associated with prolonged diarrhea in HIV-infected patients (215). One study in Zambia demonstrated that HIV and rotavirus commonly coexist, but the rotavirus infection was not more common nor was the illness more severe in HIV-positive infants (216). The full extent of rotavirus disease in immunocompromised children and adolescents is unknown.

Parasites

With the advent of HIV, there has been a renewed interest in protozoan organisms that involve the gastrointestinal tract. Organisms in this category that are associated with diarrhea in patients with HIV infection include *Blastocystis hominis, C. parvum, C. cayetanensis, G. lamblia, I. belli,* microsporidia (*E. bieneusi* and *E. intestinalis*), and *S. stercoralis* (32,45,51,217–219).

Cryptosporidium *Infection*

C. parvum is a protozoan parasite transmitted via the ingestion of oocysts that have been excreted in feces of humans or animals. Infection can be transmitted through person-to-person or animal-to-person contact, ingestion of fecally contaminated water or food, or contact with fecally contaminated environmental surfaces. The risk of household transmission is low (5%) if the index case is an adult. The clinical presentation of cryptosporidiosis includes, in order of decreasing frequency, diarrhea (100% of patients), abdominal cramps, fatigue, anorexia, nausea, fever, chills, sweats, headache, and vomiting (220). Persistent disease due to *Cryptosporidium* has been associated with CD4-positive T-lymphocyte counts of less than 200 cells per microliter (221).

C. parvum causes a mild to moderately severe diarrhea in immunocompetent individuals and profuse watery diarrhea in immunocompromised persons, particularly in patients with AIDS (42,222). Stools in patients with cryptosporidiosis usually contain mucus but no blood or leukocytes. The severity and duration of illness depend on the degree of immune suppression (223). A similar clinical presentation occurs in individuals with other defects of cell-mediated or humoral immunity. From 0.3% to 4% of all diarrheal illness in the United States is estimated to be caused by *C. parvum*. A study in Oklahoma demonstrated a seroprevalence of 38% in persons 5 to 13 years of age, increasing to 58% in those 14 to 21 years of age. African-Americans and Native Americans had higher seropositivity rates than did white Americans (224). The seroprevalence is higher in children attending child care centers than in children not in child care. *Cryptosporidium* transmission can occur from children in child care centers to adults, and the risk is related to changing diapers (225). Outbreaks of *Cryptosporidium* occur in child care centers. *Cryptosporidium* is shed for a prolonged period by immunocompromised individuals.

One report of a child with acute lymphocytic leukemia and cryptosporidiosis implicated contact with a dog with a diarrheal illness. The child also had two siblings with diarrhea. An intestinal biopsy revealed slight blunting and distortion of the villi, with lengthening of the crypts and modest mononuclear infiltration of the lamina propria in the proximal jejunum (226). There also have been case reports of cryptosporidiosis in children with a renal transplant and IgA deficiency, with IgA deficiency, or with congenital hypogammaglobulinemia (227,228).

The prevalence of *Cryptosporidium* infection varies widely but appears to be highest among young children and immunocompromised persons (229). Among patients with AIDS who have diarrhea, cross-sectional studies indicate that approximately 16% are positive for *C. parvum*; however up to 50% of patients with AIDS may acquire the parasite at some point during their illness.

Cyclospora *Infection*

C. cayetanensis has been recognized as a cause of prolonged diarrhea in both immunocompetent and immunocompromised patients. *C. cayetanensis* infection causes profuse watery diarrhea after an incubation period of 2 to 11 days. Cyclosporiasis is clinically indistinguishable from cryptosporidiosis or isosporiasis (230). Various fresh fruit and vegetable sources have been incriminated as the source of outbreaks in the United States (50). *Cyclospora* is in the subclass Coccidia, phylum Apicomplexa. This genus is taxonomically related to four other coccidian genera that have been described as pathogens in humans: *Cryptosporidium, Isospora, Toxoplasma,* and *Sarcocystis. Cyclospora* resembles *Isospora* in that oocysts are excreted unsporulated and require a period of time outside the host for maturation to occur (51). *Cyclospora* is widely distributed throughout the world, and persons of all ages have been infected. Most of the current knowledge of the epidemiology of *Cyclospora* spp. is derived primarily from Nepal, Haiti, and Peru; the parasite appears to be endemic in these countries, where there is an annual surge of cyclosporiasis that coincides with the rainy season. Prevalence rates of 11% have been documented among nonnative adults and children during the rainy season in endemic areas (51). Symptomatic infection is more common in children older than 18 months, but younger children may have asymptomatic infection. The rates of infection are lower among native compared with nonnative residents.

The incubation period for *Cyclospora* infection ranges from 2 to 11 days. Cyclosporiasis is said to be clinically indistinguishable from cryptosporidiosis and isosporiasis, but diarrhea may not be the presenting or predominant symptom for patients who have *Cyclospora* infection. Clinical manifestations of cyclosporiasis include watery diarrhea that occurs in a relapsing, cyclic pattern, sometimes alternating with constipation. Important associated symptoms include profound fatigue, "indigestion"-like or "heartburn"-like symptoms, nausea, abdominal cramps, anorexia, weight loss, and vomiting. A flulike prodrome with accompanying myalgias and arthralgias may precede the onset of diarrhea. Although the illness is self-limited, it may be prolonged and last for weeks; progressive fatigue, anorexia, and weight loss may overshadow the presenting diarrheal symptoms (51).

Among immunocompromised hosts, *Cyclospora* infection has occurred primarily in HIV-infected individuals. Clinical illness caused by *Cyclospora* in HIV-infected persons, like that caused by *Cryptosporidium*, is prolonged and severe and is associated with a high rate of recurrence that can be attenuated with long-term suppressive therapy. In immunocompromised patients, specifically individuals with HIV infection, the reported duration of diarrhea has been highly variable, ranging from several days to many months (231, 232). Diarrhea is less severe in terms of frequency in HIV-infected patients than in patients without HIV infection (mean number of stools passed per day, 5 versus 11, respectively) (233). However, the illness was more prolonged in HIV-infected patients, who also lost more weight than did infected persons without HIV infection. Two patients with AIDS had evidence of an extra-intestinal infection; both had acalculous cholecystitis that responded to TMP/SMX treatment at the same time that *Cyclospora* oocysts disappeared from their stools (233). The mechanism by which *Cyclospora* causes diarrhea has not yet been defined. *Cyclospora* infection is known to be associated with an inflammatory process in the small bowel that results in villus fusion and atrophy, which may reduce the surface area available for absorption and thus cause diarrhea (233).

Entamoeba *Infection*

Entamoeba infects 10% of the world's population but causes disease in fewer than 1% (234). This is best explained by the finding of two species of *Entamoeba* that infect humans: invasive *E. histolytica*, which is associated with disease in humans, and noninvasive *Entamoeba dispar*, which does not cause disease in humans (234). In most infected patients, the trophozoites exist as harmless commensals in the lumen of the large bowel. To initiate symptomatic infection, trophozoites must penetrate the mucous layer and adhere to the underlying mucosa. Four major intestinal syndromes caused by infection with *E. histolytica* are asymptomatic colonization, acute amebic colitis, fulminant colitis, and ameboma (235). The risk of amebiasis is related to traveling or living in endemic areas of developing countries. Most infections in developed countries occur in male homosexuals. Children have a greater risk for fulminant colitis than adults, but there are no data for increased risk of amebiasis in immunodeficiency syndromes. Patients with AIDS do not appear to be at increased risk for invasive disease.

Giardia *Infection*

G. lamblia infection may result in acute or chronic diarrhea or asymptomatic excretion. The acute illness typically includes watery, foul-smelling stools, nausea, abdominal distention, and flatulence with no fever and no blood in the stools. Chronic giardiasis may result in abdominal pain and distention; greasy, foul-smelling stools; and weight loss (47,236). Prolonged infection with the parasite is uncommon if the infection is diagnosed and appropriately treated. Severe giardiasis may occur among immunocompetent individuals, with the highest rates among children younger than 5 years of age and women of child-bearing age. Severe giardiasis caused failure to thrive in 19% of children younger than 5 years of age (237).

G. lamblia is transmitted directly from person to person by fecal-oral transmission of cysts or indirectly by transmission in water and occasionally in food (238). *G. lamblia* is the leading known cause of reported outbreaks of waterborne disease in the United States. Travellers often become infected when they ingest contaminated ground water or surface water. The cyst is highly infectious for humans, and infections can occur after ingestion of as few as 10 to 100 cysts (239). Outbreaks of infection and endemic infections occur in child care centers and other institutional settings and among family members of infected children (237,240). The incubation period is usually 1 to 4 weeks. Immunodeficiency predisposes to infection and appears to be a major contributor to the persistence of symptoms (241). Giardiasis has been described in patients with CVID, primarily those with hypogammaglobulinemia or agammaglobulinemia (242–244). Chronic *Giardia* infection is associated with chronic diarrhea and malnutrition in children.

Isospora *Infection*

I. belli is most common in tropical and subtropical climates. *I. belli* is an opportunistic enteric pathogen reported to cause severe diarrhea in patients with AIDS. The organism was found in the stools of 60% of Haitians with AIDS and chronic diarrhea, whereas *G. lamblia* and *E. histolytica* were noted in only 7%. The clinical symptoms of isosporiasis are indistinguishable from those of cryptosporidiosis or cyclosporiasis. Infection with *I. belli* is characterized by profuse, watery diarrhea without blood or polymorphonuclear leukocytes in stools; crampy abdominal pain; weight loss; malaise; and flatulence. Fever and leukocytosis are uncommon. Diarrhea usually is self-limited, but chronic, relapsing infection also has been reported in patients with AIDS (245,246). The role of *I. belli* as a cause of disease in persons with other immune deficiencies is unknown.

Microsporidia

Microsporidia are ubiquitous, spore-forming, intracellular protozoal parasites that cause disease in a wide range of vertebrate and invertebrate animals. Manifestations of disease in humans range from asymptomatic infections to fulminant cerebritis and/or nephritis; ocular infections are recognized infrequently (247–249). Since 1985, enteric microsporidial infections have been reported with increasing frequency in patients with AIDS and chronic diarrhea (247,250). *E. bieneusi* and *E. intestinalis* are the species associated with diarrhea (48). The link between infection with *E. bienuesi* or *E. intestinalis* and clinically apparent disease is strong, although asymptomatic excretion has been reported. Diarrhea in immunocompetent hosts is uncommon. Infection in immunodeficient persons, especially those with AIDS, can range from mild diarrhea to severe, life-threatening diarrhea, dehydration, and malabsorption (217,251). Clinical manifestations associated with gastrointestinal tract involvement include chronic diarrhea and weight loss. The role of microsporidia in other immunocompromised patients is not clear, but it was associated with chronic diarrhea and weight loss in a heart-lung transplant recipient (252,253). Common epidemiologic characteristics have not been identified, and the mode of transmission in humans is not known for certain. Fecal-oral transmission is the likely route of infection in humans with intestinal microsporidiosis, but the source of ocular infections is not clear.

Strongyloides *Infection*

S. stercoralis is a nematode that infects humans and sometimes other animals worldwide. It has a complicated life cycle that may have both parasitic and free-living phases. The prevalence of infection varies inversely with socioeconomic level and is highest in warm, moist regions where sanitary practices are poor. The parasite is endemic in certain southern areas of the United States. Most human infections are acquired outdoors when polluted soil containing filariform larvae comes in contact with skin. The filariform larvae penetrate intact skin of the new host, travel through blood vessels to the lungs, penetrate alveoli, are coughed up and swallowed, and then establish infection in the mucosa of the small intestine (254,255). Human-to-human transmission of *S. stercoralis* has been reported in residents of homes for the mentally retarded (256–258). The incubation period is not known.

Clinical manifestations can range from asymptomatic infection (in one third of patients) to death. The type of symptomatology depends on the stage of infection. Skin and pulmonary disease consists of pruritus, an erythematous maculopapular rash, and a Loffler-like syndrome with eosinophilia (259). Signs and symptoms associated with the intestinal phase of disease include abdominal pain, diarrhea containing mucus, and occasionally nausea, vomiting, weight loss, and malabsorption. When infection occurs, particularly in immunocompromised individuals, signs and symptoms include generalized abdominal pain, diffuse pulmonary infiltrates, ileus, and meningitis or sepsis from gram-negative bacilli.

Disseminated strongyloidiasis was reported in two recipients of kidney allografts from a single cadaver donor (260). Neither recipient had previous evidence of parasitic infection or risk factors for strongyloidiasis. Disseminated strongyloidiasis also has been reported as a complication of immunosuppression. Patients with a history of exposure to *S. stercoralis* many years previously have experienced hyperinfection with the parasite during immunosuppression after renal transplantation (259,261–263). These individuals may have mild eosinophilia.

Other Infectious Agents

Candida spp. have been associated with gastroenteritis in two settings: noninvasive enteritis in healthy persons (264) and invasive enteritis in patients with underlying diseases (265). *Candida* is a saprophyte in healthy humans and is present in approximately 60% of stool specimens (266). Because *Candida* spp. frequently can be isolated from the gastrointestinal tract of immunocompetent individuals, its presence does not necessarily signify disease. Gastroenteritis associated with *Candida* is characterized by intermittent, watery, explosive diarrhea that is not bloody and rarely is accompanied by fever, nausea, anorexia, or vomiting. These symptoms can be chronic and have been reported for up to 3 months (267). Immunocompetent individuals who develop *Candida* gastroenteritis usually do not develop candidemia and usually respond to either nystatin or clotrimazole within 72 hours (267). Nosocomial diarrhea associated with *Candida albicans* is especially prevalent in immunocompromised or malnourished patients (268,269) and in patients receiving antibiotic or antineoplastic drugs (270,271).

DIAGNOSIS

Immunodeficient persons who have either acute or chronic diarrhea should be thoroughly evaluated to determine the cause of the diarrhea. A specific pathogen can be identified in most cases, and specific therapy can often reduce the volume and/or frequency of diarrhea (62,272,273). In addition, nutritional assessment should be performed on a routine basis to identify and treat new problems that may arise (3). In many children with AIDS and gastrointestinal tract disease, the causative agent is no longer present by the time the child is evaluated, but residual damage to the intestine persists. In children with AIDS, a subset of the causes of chronic diarrhea should be considered in the differential diagnosis (63). The history and physical examination should provide information that helps direct the laboratory evaluation. The history should emphasize stool frequency and characteristics, duration of illness, and whether abdominal pain, nausea, vomiting, fever, or weight loss has occurred or is occurring. The physical examination should include evaluation for signs of dehydration and emphasis on the oral cavity, abdomen, and rectum. In addition, an evaluation of the patient's nutritional status should be performed. Laboratory diagnosis should be approached in a stepwise manner, with the initial evaluation including stool culture and microscopy and further evaluation including more invasive procedures (Table 19.4).

Current guidelines advocate a limited, cost-effective approach to the diagnosis of enteric pathogens (274–276). These guidelines are intended for the immunocompetent individual with acute diarrhea that is either community acquired or nosocomially acquired. This same logical, stepwise approach may be applied to immunocompromised individuals, but additional testing and flexibility are required. For example, organisms such as *Salmonella, Campylobacter, Shigella,* and the protozoa, which are common causes of sporadic diarrheal disease in the United States, are for the most part community acquired and rarely cause nosocomial infections. Therefore, routine stool cultures and examination for ova and parasites for the hospitalized immunocompetent individual with diarrhea manifesting longer than 3 to 4 days after admission results in a low yield. Severely immunocompromised patients may have other bacterial pathogens present in the stool, so bacterial cultures for evaluation of nosocomial diarrhea may be warranted. One study identified bacterial enteropathogens in eight immunocompromised patients more than 3 days after admission, but seven of the eight were symptomatic at the time of admission (275). *C. difficile* causes both community-acquired and nosocomial diarrhea in immunocompetent and immunocompromised children, so testing for this enteropathogen is an important part of the evaluation.

TABLE 19.4. *Diagnostic approach to immunocompromised children and adolescents with gastrointestinal tract infection*

Phase I
  Standard stool culture for *Campylobacter jejuni/coli, Salmonella* species, *Shigella* species, and *Escherichia coli* O157:H7
  Other stool cultures for *Vibrio* species, other *Campylobacter* species, *Yersinia enterocolitica,* and *Aeromonas* species
  Enzyme immunoassay for rotavirus (if winter season) and *Clostridium difficile* toxins
  Occult blood and fecal leukocyte examination of stool sample
  Microscopy using direct and concentration techniques for *Giardia lamblia, Cryptosporidium, Cyclospora,* and *Isospora* (enzyme immunoassay is an alternative method of detection for *Giardia* and *Cryptosporidium*)
Phase II
  Microscopy for microsporidium and *Mycobacterium avium* complex using concentration techniques and acid–fast stain
  Gastroduodenoscopy for observation of intestinal mucosa and to obtain duodenal fluid and biopsy material for staining for histology, parasites, mycobacteria, herpes viruses, fungi, and bacterial culture (including mycobacteria)
  Colonoscopy to view intestinal mucosa and to obtain fluid and biopsy material for stains and cultures
Phase III
  Consider evaluation of hepatobiliary tract or operative procedure depending on noninvasive evaluation of the abdominal contents

Current guidelines recommend that routine stool cultures and ova and parasite examination be limited to outpatients or inpatients who have been hospitalized for less than 3 or 4 days. The microbiology laboratory of each hospital should routinely culture for *Campylobacter, Salmonella, Shigella,* and *E. coli* O157:H7; other agents to be included on the routine culture panel (e.g., *Yersinia, Vibrio*) should be determined on the basis of regional data. In any case, direct communication with the microbiology laboratory may be necessary to guide testing for unusual enteropathogens in immunocompromised patients. Additional culture samples for less common bacteriologic agents may be submitted after the common agents have been ruled out. For optimal sensitivity, up to two stool samples should be submitted for bacteriologic culture and three samples for examination for ova and parasites. The existence of rapid laboratory tests for *G. lamblia, E. histolytica,* and *Cryptosporidium* should prompt testing for these agents specifically, rather than a request for routine "ova and parasite" examination in situations where other parasitic agents are unlikely (274).

Specific strategies for the evaluation and management of diarrhea in children with AIDS have been proposed (221,277,278). A logical approach consists of obtaining at least two stool cultures for *Salmonella, Shigella, C. jejuni,* and *E. coli* O157:H7 as well as organisms that require special laboratory techniques (42). Commercially available enzyme immunoassays (EIAs) can detect rotavirus, enteric adenovirus, *G. lamblia, Cryptosporidium,* and the toxins of *C. difficile.* EIAs for *C. difficile* toxin A are rapid but do not detect disease caused by toxin A–negative, toxin B–positive strains (279). Microscopy should be performed to detect fecal leukocytes and parasites. Stools should be prepared using saline, iodine, trichrome, and acid-fast stains. If the patient is febrile, blood cultures for bacteria, mycobacteria, and CMV should be ordered. If a diagnosis is not established and a response to symptomatic treatment is not achieved, then esophagogastroduodenoscopy and/or colonoscopy could be performed to vi-

sualize the mucosa and to obtain biopsy specimens and luminal fluid (Table 19.4) (280).

Acute Diarrhea

The causes of acute diarrhea are numerous and include infectious and noninfectious etiologies. Identification of the cause of diarrhea depends on many factors, including availability of laboratory technology. In several studies, microscopic examination and culture of stool and duodenal fluid, followed by duodenal and/or colonic biopsy, led to a diagnosis in 85% of patients studied. Blood cultures should be obtained from febrile patients for bacteria, mycobacteria, and CMV. Other tests that should be reserved for patients with more persistent episodes in which a diagnosis is not established include sigmoidoscopy, barium enema, intestinal biopsy, and tests for malabsorption. Children with persistent diarrhea need periodic reevaluation of stool specimens.

Chronic Diarrhea

Children with immunodeficiencies often develop chronic diarrhea or are recognized as having failure to thrive. The impact of the illness on the health and development of the child should be reassessed continually. Important aspects of the care of children with immunodeficiency and chronic diarrhea, malabsorption, and failure to thrive are observation of weight gain, status of the height and weight curves, and stool pattern. Infectious causes of diarrhea should be evaluated. These initial tests should include evaluation of stool specimens and blood. Stool cultures, ova and parasite examination, and fecal leukocyte testing may yield an infectious cause of the episode (277). More invasive tests may be necessary (Table 19.4).

Bacterial Causes

Most bacterial enteropathogens can be identified by standard diagnostic or modified diagnostic stool cultures, although other detection methods (e.g., serotyping, tissue culture assays, EIA, gene probes) are available. Standard microbiologic cultures detect *Shigella* spp., *Salmonella* spp., *Campylobacter jejuni,* and *E. coli* O157:H7. If other bacterial agents are suspected, laboratory personnel must be notified so that modified laboratory procedures can be used for identification. Bacterial enteropathogens in this category include pathogenic *E. coli, Vibrio* spp., non-*jejuni* species of *Campylobacter, Y. enterocolitica,* and *Aeromonas.*

For isolation of *Campylobacter* spp. from feces, two methods are used: a selective enrichment medium containing antibiotics to suppress the colonic microflora and a filtration method using cellulose membranes. The filtration method allows for isolation of species that are inhibited by antibiotics, such as *C. upsaliensis, C. fetus,* and *C. hyointestinalis.*

C. difficile antibiotic-associated colitis or pseudomembranous colitis is diagnosed by the detection of *C. difficile* toxins A or B (or both) in feces. The cytotoxin assay performed by tissue culture detects only toxin B. Commercial EIAs are available to detect either or both toxins; assays to detect both toxins are preferred.

Diarrheagenic *E. coli* strains are differentiated from other Enterobacteriaceae by standard biochemical reactions. Specific phenotypic assays such as the HEp-2 adherence assay are used to identify EAEC. DNA probes for heat-labile and heat stable enterotoxins in EIEC have revolutionized the identification of pathogenic *E. coli.* DNA probes can now be used for most pathogenic *E. coli,* but they are generally available only in reference or research laboratories (30). It is recommended that bloody diarrhea stools be cultured on sorbitol MacConkey agar plates as a screening test for *E. coli* O157:H7.

Vibrio spp. may be isolated from stool specimens on thiosulfate-citrate-bile salts-sucrose agar (TCBS). Serotyping is performed to distinguish O1 from non-O1 strains. Enterotoxins may be detected by animal or tissue culture assays, EIA, or DNA probes (151).

The detection of *Y. enterocolitica* requires isolation on selective media. Cold enrichment techniques may increase the rate of recovery from stool cultures. Serotyping is performed to identify the most common serotypes in human disease and may be used for outbreak evaluation. Chromosomal DNA restriction fragment length polymorphism (RFLP) (166), plasmid profile analysis, and phage typing have been used to evaluate the relatedness of serotypes during outbreaks.

Viral Causes

Commercially available assays can be used to detect rotavirus and enteric adenoviruses. Diagnostic methods that are used to detect other enteric virus are less suitable for routine use and include gel electrophoresis, PCR, electron microscopy, EIA, radioimmunoassay, and viral culture (1). Rotaviruses are detected by commercially available rapid assays including EIAs. Electron microscopy (EM) and reverse transcription–polymerase chain reaction (RT-PCR) are available in research laboratories. Type-specific EIAs also are available for epidemiologic studies. Astrovirus-associated gastroenteritis is diagnosed by examination of a stool specimen by EM, EIA, or RT-PCR (8,173,184,281). There are no commercially available methods for the detection of astroviruses. Caliciviruses can be detected in stool specimens by EM, immune EM, EIA, or RT-PCR, but these tests are available only in research laboratories (282).

In patients with CMV colitis, sigmoidoscopy reveals areas that range from diffuse or focal mucosal erythema to extensive, deep, friable ulcerations with clearly defined borders and non-purulent bases, although 10% of patients with histologic evidence of CMV colitis may have a grossly normal appearing mucosa (283,284). Barium radiographs may demonstrate diffuse abnormalities ranging from edema, mucosal fold thickening, and superficial erosions to deep ulcerations (283). When the disease occurs in the antrum of the stomach, lack of distensibility of the stomach may occur; terminal ileal involvement may appear indistinguishable from Crohn's disease. Focal mass lesions are rare and must be distinguished from malignancy. Computed tomography may reveal diffuse bowel-wall thickening, luminal narrowing, and inflammatory changes in the surrounding mesenteric and pericolonic fat. The presence of CMV inclusions in a biopsy is the most important evidence to support the diagnosis of CMV colitis. The presence of CMV antigen, a positive culture of biopsy tissue, or genome detection by PCR can help substantiate the diagnosis.

Parasitic Causes

Diagnosis of parasitic causes of diarrhea generally depends on microscopy, although rapid diagnostic tests are available for several of the parasitic enteropathogens. Diagnosis of infection with *Cryptosporidium* is made by identification of the 4- to 6-µm oocyst form of the parasite by microscopic examination of stool, histologic examination of tissue sections, or EIA testing of stool (285,286). For microscopic diagnosis, stool specimens are concentrated and then stained with a modified Kinyoun acid-fast stain, which permits differentiation of acid-fast cryptosporidial oocysts from yeast. The auramine O fluorescent stain is a rapid, sensitive screening procedure used to detect oocysts. Patients with AIDS and diarrhea due to *Cryptosporidium* often excrete high numbers of oocysts, frequently making concentration of stool unnecessary to establish a diagnosis (287). Organisms also may be identified in jejunal or rectal biopsy specimens and in aspirated duodenal contents. Cryptosporidial oocysts also can be detected by an indirect immunofluorescent detection procedure in which monoclonal antibody binds to the cell wall of the oocysts (Merifluor-Cryptosporidium, Meridian Diagnostics, Cincinnati, OH). Although not helpful in rapid diagnosis, an EIA technique that detects IgG and IgM antibodies in serum has been used (288). Radiographic studies show barium flocculation, mucosal thickening, and small bowel dilatation.

The diagnosis of *C. cayetanensis* infection is based on microscopic detection of oocysts in fecal specimens. Examination of wet mounts of fresh, unpreserved stool by means of bright-field microscopy reveals nonrefractile spheres that are 8 to 10 µm in diameter and contain numerous refractive lobules enclosed within membranes. Like the oocysts of *Cryptosporidium* and *Isospora,* the oocysts of *Cyclospora* are acid-fast and therefore can be seen with the use of one of the many acid-fast staining techniques (e.g., modified Ziehl-Nielsen stain, Kinyoun acid-fast stain). Despite their distinct characteristics, *Cyclospora* oocysts may be confused with *Cryptosporidium* oocysts unless their diameter is measured with a micrometer. *Cyclospora* oocysts are autofluorescent and appear as neon-blue circles when examined with an ultraviolet fluorescence microscope fitted with a 365-nm excitation filter.

Oocysts of *I. belli* are acid-fast and can easily be distinguished from cryptosporidia by their ellipsoidal shape and larger size (20 to 30 µm by 10 to 20 µm, compared with 4- to 6-µm diameter cryptosporidial oocysts). The oocysts appear in the stool for as long as 120 days after infection, but they are few in number or are shed intermittently. Because of the low number of organisms shed, use of concentration methods may improve the yield. Oocysts of *Isospora* do not stain well with methods frequently used for diagnosis of other intestinal protozoa. Oocysts are easily seen in duodenal aspirate and in small bowel biopsy material by routine light microscopy.

Confirmation of infection by *Giardia* depends on demonstration of cysts or trophozoites by microscopic examination of stool, duodenal aspirate, or biopsy material. The merthiolate-iodine-formalin concentration technique improves the sensitivity of stool examination when compared with Lugol's iodine and methylene blue wet mounts. Rapid diagnostic tests that detect *Giardia* antigens in stool specimens also are available (286,289). Specific DNA probes for *Giardia* may assist in the diagnosis in the future.

Diagnosis of microsporidial infection is difficult because the parasites are easily overlooked in routine tissue examinations owing to their 2- to 3-µm size, poor staining characteristics, and lack of tissue response. Proper identification requires careful attention to the preparative technique. Identification of intracellular and luminal *E. bieneusi* spores can facilitate diagnosis and can best be accomplished with the use of Brown-Brenn and acid-fast stains (217). A method whereby microsporidial spores can be identified using modified trichrome staining of stool specimens has been developed (250,290). This method simplifies the diagnosis of intestinal microsporidiosis and reduces the need for biopsies of the small intestine. A comparison of methods to detect *E. intestinalis* found Calcofluor staining to be the most sensitive; modified trichrome blue staining was slightly more specific (291). Microsporidia have been detected from formalin-fixed stool specimens after staining by a chromotrope-based technique and examination by light microscopy (290). EM can be used to detail the presence of the organism, which permits appropriate classification. Newer diagnostic methods include PCR to detect microsporidial ribosomal RNA or DNA from stool samples or small intestine biopsy material (251,292). Routine histopathologic studies can provide presumptive identification, but diagnostic confirmation requires EM visualization of the organism's characteristic ultrastructure (218).

Diagnosis of *Strongyloides* depends on demonstration of rhabditiform larvae in feces or duodenal fluid. Rhabditiform larvae are the products of ova produced by the parasitic females in the small intestine of infected persons. The eggs hatch deep in the mucosa of the duodenum and are almost never identified in stool. Stool should be examined after being subjected to a concentration technique such as zinc sulfate. Repeat examinations of concentrated stool specimens are often necessary. The method of placing stool in an agar plate and observing worms and worm tracks on the agar is an efficient means of detecting the parasite (293,294). Several immunoassays for detection of serum antibodies against filarial larvae or larval antigens are available (295). Serodiagnosis can be useful but is limited in availability, and cross-reaction with antigens of filarial worms occurs, limiting the sensitivity.

MANAGEMENT AND THERAPY

Treatment of patients with acute diarrhea includes replacement and maintenance of fluid and electrolytes and early reintroduction of normal nutrients (296,297). Specific causes of fever, diarrhea, decreased intake, and feeding problems should be sought and treated. Infectious and noninfectious agents or diseases that involve the gastrointestinal tract or other organ systems (e.g., pneumonia) may contribute to decreased intake and malnutrition. In patients in whom no specific cause can be identified, symptomatic treatment is the mainstay of therapy. In general, nutritional support is an essential component of long-term management in all children (3). Specific therapy is available for treatment of infections with certain enteropathogens. Infections in patients with defects in their host defense mechanisms are often severe, commonly disseminate, require prolonged therapy, and frequently relapse when therapy is stopped.

Most nonprescription and prescription antidiarrheal compounds are not approved for children younger than 2 or 3 years of age. These compounds may be classified by their mechanisms of action, which include alteration of intestinal motility, adsorption, alteration of intestinal microflora, and alteration of fluid and electrolyte secretion. Drugs that alter intestinal motility should be avoided in patients with high fever, toxemia, or bloody mucoid stools, because they may worsen the clinical course of shigellosis and perhaps that of infections with other invasive bacteria as well. The condition of patients with shigellosis, *E. coli* O157:H7, or antimicrobial-associated colitis reportedly became worse when diphenoxylate with atropine (Lomotil) was given; therefore, the use of opiates and other antiperistaltic agents should be avoided in such patients (298).

Currently no antimicrobial agents are effective for the treatment of gastroenteritis caused by the viral enteropathogens including astroviruses, rotaviruses, enteric adenoviruses, and caliciviruses.

Bacteria

Antimicrobial therapy is administered to selected patients with bacterial gastroenteritis to abbreviate the gastrointestinal tract illness or decrease fecal shedding of the causative organism, or both (1,298). Stool cultures should be obtained to identify the enteropathogen and provide an organism on which antimicrobial susceptibility testing can be performed. Table 19.5 outlines recommended antimicrobial therapy for commonly encountered bacterial enteropathogens (299). Considerations of therapy should include whether dissemination has occurred and whether coinfection with another enteropathogen is present. Therapy may need to be administered for a longer period than what is recommended for immunocompetent persons. Resistance to antimicrobial agents among enteric bacteria follows widespread antibiotic use, such as occurs in immunocompromised patients. Therefore constant monitoring of the susceptibility of bacterial isolates is critical for selection of appropriate antimicrobial agents for therapy. Drug resistance may develop during therapy,

causing relapse, as has been reported with *C. jejuni* gastroenteritis.

The most important aspect of therapy for antimicrobial-associated colitis caused by *C. difficile* toxins is discontinuation of the antimicrobial agent. Almost all antimicrobial agents have been reported to produce this condition, with ampicillin, clindamycin, lincomycin, the cephalosporins, erythromycin, and TMP/SMX most frequently implicated. Patients with mild disease may respond to discontinuation of the precipitating antibiotic and provision of fluid and electrolyte therapy. If symptoms persist or worsen, or if the disease is severe, specific therapy with metronidazole or vancomycin should be administered. Oral metronidazole is the treatment of choice for patients with severe antimicrobial-associated colitis. Oral vancomycin may be given but is avoided in accordance with guidelines for judicious use of vancomycin (300). Patients who are unable to take oral medications should be treated with intravenous metronidazole or vancomycin.

In general, antibiotics are not used in the treatment of nontyphoidal *Salmonella* infections with mild gastroenteritis in immuno-

TABLE 19.5. *Treatment of bacterial enteropathogens*

Organism	Antimicrobial agent	Alternative antimicrobial agent	Days of therapy
Aeromonas spp.	TMP/SMX	Gentamicin, imipenem, ciprofloxacin[a]	3–5
Campylobacter fetus	Imipenem, meropenem	Gentamicin, ampicillin	5–7
Campylobacter jejuni	Ciprofloxacin[a] or erythromycin	Tetracycline[a], gentamicin	5–7
Clostridium difficile[b]	Metronidazole	Vancomycin	7–14
Enterotoxigenic *Escherichia coli*	Cefotaxime	TMP/SMX, ciprofloxacin[a]	3–5
Enteroinvasive *E. coli*	TMP/SMX	Ampicillin, ciprofloxacin, ceftriaxone	3–5
Plesiomonas shigelloides	TMP/SMX	Ciprofloxacin[a]	3–5
Salmonella			
Colitis	Ampicillin, cefotaxime, or ceftriaxone	Chloramphenicol, TMP/SMX	14
Systemic	Same as for colitis		>14
Shigella	TMP/SMX, ciprofloxacin[a]	Ceftriaxone, cefotaxime, cefixime	5
Vibrio cholerae	Tetracycline[a], doxycycline[a]	Ciprofloxacin[a], TMP/SMX	3
Vibrio vulnificus	Tetracycline[a]	Cefotaxime	—[c]
Yersinia	TMP/SMX	Ciprofloxacin[a], gentamicin, cefotaxime, chloramphenicol	—[c]

TMP/SMX, trimethoprim-sulfamethoxazole.
[a]Not approved by the U.S. Food and Drug Administration for patients younger than 17 years of age.
[b]If possible, discontinue or change other antimicrobial agents.
[c]No recommended duration of therapy.

competent persons. Antimicrobial therapy should be provided in newborn infants and in patients with enterocolitis who have an underlying condition or disease that impairs host resistance, such as AIDS, hemoglobinopathy (including sickle cell anemia), lymphoma, or leukemia. Immunocompromised patients should be treated with ampicillin or a third-generation cephalosporin.

Shigella strains have become increasingly resistant to multiple antimicrobial agents. Third-generation cephalosporins have been used successfully in the treatment of shigellosis in children. Ciprofloxacin has been used successfully in patients with multidrug-resistant *Shigella* (301,302). Five days of therapy should be sufficient in immunocompetent children.

C. jejuni strains are generally susceptible to erythromycin in addition to a wide variety of other antimicrobial agents, but penicillin, ampicillin, and the cephalosporins are relatively inactive. *C. fetus* strains are susceptible to ampicillin, gentamicin, imipenem, and meropenem (303). The role of antimicrobial therapy in patients with colitis caused by *E. coli* O157:H7 is uncertain. The organisms are usually susceptible to antimicrobial agents typically used for *E. coli*, but treatment does not appear to influence either the duration of symptoms or the risk of progression to hemolytic-uremic syndrome.

Antimicrobial therapy shortens the duration of cholera and reduces fluid losses. Tetracycline and doxycycline are the drugs of choice, but they are not recommended for children younger than 9 years of age. However, in severe cholera infections, the benefits of therapy with tetracycline may offset the risk of tooth staining.

Parasites

Enteric infections caused by protozoal organisms are not always self-limiting in children with immunodeficiency, do not always respond to specific therapy if available, and frequently cause relapse after an appropriate therapeutic course. Nonspecific therapy and careful attention to dietary intake and nutrition can provide relief for some patients and help prevent the malnutrition and wasting that so frequently occur. Reconstitution of the immune system has resulted in dramatic resolution of chronic disease. This has been seen most dramatically in patients with AIDS who have diarrhea caused by cryptosporidiosis that resolves after initiation of highly active antiretroviral therapy (HAART). Recovery after bone marrow transplant engraftment would lead to similar resolution of diarrheal symptoms (8).

Specific antimicrobial therapy for *Cryptosporidium* is not available. Paromomycin and azithromycin have been used with varied response in AIDS patients. Paromomycin generally is thought to be ineffective; azithromycin has led to a decrease in symptoms and oocyst excretion in a few patients (Table 19.6) (304). The combination of both medications was used with clinical benefit in a small study of patients with AIDS (305). Orally administered bovine transfer factor, hyperimmune bovine colostrum, and cow's milk immunoglobulin have been evaluated. Bovine immunoglobulin concentrate has been shown to neutralize *C. parvum* sporozoites and to partially decrease stool volume. Management includes fluid therapy, nutritional support, and use of antidiarrheal agents.

Unlike *Cryptosporidium, Isospora* responds to treatment with oral TMP/SMX; however, recurrent symptomatic disease occurs in 50% of patients. Recurrent disease may be prevented by the use of prophylaxis with TMP/SMX, which in immunocompromised patients may need to be continued indefinitely (304). In sulfonamide-sensitive patients, daily pyrimethamine has been effective in adults. The U.S. Food and Drug Administration considers both of these compounds investigational for isosporiasis. Patients receiving either compound should be monitored carefully for bone marrow suppression, skin reactions, and allergic manifestations (304). Metronidazole and pyrimethamine also have been reported to be effective in a limited number of patients, and

TABLE 19.6. *Treatment of enteric parasites*

Organism	Antiparasitic	Alternative
Blastocystis hominis	Metronidazole, 15 mg/kg/dose t.i.d. × 10 d	Iodoquinol, 10 mg/kg/dose t.i.d. × 10 d
Cryptosporidium parvum	Azithromycin, 5–12 mg/kg/d	Paromomycin, 25–35 mg/kg/dose t.i.d.–q.i.d.
Cyclospora cayetanensis	TMP/SMX, TMP 5 mg/kg/dose b.i.d. × 7 d	
Entamoeba histolyticus[a]	Metronidazole, 35–50 mg/kg/d divided t.i.d. × 10 d	Tinidazole,[b] 50 mg/kg/d × 5 d
Giardia lamblia	Metronidazole, 15 mg/kg/d divided t.i.d. × 7 d	Furazolidone, 6 mg/kg/d divided q.i.d. × 10 d
Isospora belli	TMP/SMX, TMP 5 mg/kg/dose q.i.d. × 10 d, then b.i.d. × 3 wk	
Microsporidia	Albendazole, 400 mg b.i.d.	
Strongyloides	Ivermectin, 200 µg/kg/d × 1–2 d	Thiabendazole, 50 mg/kg/d divided b.i.d. × 2 d

TMP, trimethoprim; TMP/SMX, trimethoprim-sulfamethoxazole.
[a]Treatment should be followed by a course of iodoquinol 30–40 mg/kg/d (maximum 2 g) divided t.i.d. × 20 d.
[b]Not available in the United States.

they may be considered as alternative therapies in sulfa-allergic individuals.

Metronidazole and furazolidone are recommended therapies for patients with *G. lamblia*. Furazolidone is the only drug available in liquid suspension for use in young children. Metronidazole is not approved for treatment of patients with giardiasis in the United States, but it is used widely. Tinidazole and ornidazole are as effective as and better tolerated than metronidazole but are not available for use in the United States. Metronidazole has an unpleasant taste that may preclude ingestion by children. Relapse is common in immunocompromised patients, and therapy in these individuals may need to be prolonged.

There is no known effective therapy for microsporidiosis, although albendazole alleviated symptoms and parasite excretion in some patients, as reported in small, uncontrolled studies (306–312).

Cyclospora infection may be treated with TMP/SMX for 7 days, but immunocompromised persons may need a higher dosage and prolonged therapy (230,304).

Individuals infected with *S. stercoralis* should be treated with ivermectin or thiabendazole. Patients with the hyperinfection syndrome should receive therapy for at least 5 days, but mortality is high despite treatment.

Fungi

Thrush or esophagitis caused by *C. albicans* usually responds to a 7- to 14-day course of ketoconazole or fluconazole. If this therapy fails, other causes should be sought before considering therapy with amphotericin B (313). Esophageal lesions may not completely resolve in patients who have a favorable clinical response, despite months of therapy. An oral solution of itraconazole is equally effective as fluconazole in the treatment of esophageal candidiasis. For oropharyngeal candidiasis refractory to other antifungal drugs, amphotericin B oral suspension may be effective.

Esophagitis or colitis caused by CMV may improve with ganciclovir, foscarnet, or cidofovir therapy. Neutropenia is a dose-limiting adverse effect of ganciclovir. Relapses and recurrences are common, and maintenance therapy is often necessary. Herpes esophagitis usually responds to acyclovir, but maintenance therapy often is needed to prevent relapses.

PREVENTION

Hospital isolation procedures are crucial for the prevention of nosocomial enteric infections in high-risk patients (314). The current guidelines recommend "contact precautions" for children with diarrhea. These isolation procedures should be used in cases of gastrointestinal tract infection with "epidemiologically important" organisms, enteric infection with a low infectious dose (*Shigella*) or prolonged environmental survival (*C. difficile*), or enterohemorrhagic *E. coli* O157:H7, *Shigella,* hepatitis A, or rotavirus in children in diapers and incontinent patients (315). Contact precautions include the use of hand washing for all patient contacts, a single room for the patient, and the use of gowns and gloves for patient contact. Children under isolation precautions should be excluded from general use areas such as playrooms and schoolrooms. Spread of enteropathogens to contacts of infected persons can be prevented through the use of contact precautions in the hospital and home environments. To ensure protection of health care professionals and patients, standard precautions must be practiced together with appropriate disinfection or sterilization of equipment used on all patients.

The CDC has published detailed guidelines for prevention of opportunistic infections in patients with AIDS or other immunocompromised conditions (316,317). The Food and Drug Administration and the CDC have prepared a pamphlet and videotape on safe food guidelines for HIV-infected persons entitled "Eating Defensively: Food Safety Advice for Persons with AIDS" (318). These publications and the video contain practical advice for any immunocompromised patient.

Limiting exposure prevents bacterial enteric infections. Chemoprophylaxis is not recommended. Patients should be advised to avoid raw or undercooked eggs, poultry, meat, and seafood. The public health measures of improved water supply and sanitation facilities are important for control of most enteric infections. Use of appropriate hygiene measures, especially hand washing, and careful preparation of food further decrease the occurrence of enteric infection. Attention to nutritional status helps to offset the debilitation that frequently occurs in children with immune deficiencies. Table 19.7 lists recommendations that minimize exposure to foodborne and waterborne pathogens.

TABLE 19.7. *Recommendations for immunocompromised patients to minimize foodborne and waterborne exposures to pathogens*

Avoid raw and undercooked eggs, poultry, and meat.
Avoid raw fish or shellfish.
Avoid unpasteurized milk and cheese and foods made from unpasteurized milk.
Avoid soft cheeses and some ready-to-eat foods (hot dogs and cold cuts from delicatessen counters).
Avoid unpasteurized fruit juices.
Avoid raw alfalfa sprouts.
Keep uncooked meats separate from vegetables, cooked foods, and ready-to-eat foods.
Wash raw vegetables before eating.
Wash hands, knives, and cutting boards after handling uncooked foods.
Avoid drinking water from lakes or rivers, and boil tap water for consumption during community outbreaks.

No current data indicate that immunocompromised persons are more likely than immunocompetent persons to acquire cryptosporidiosis during waterborne or foodborne outbreaks. However, immunocompromised persons who have HIV/AIDS, patients receiving treatment for cancer, recipients of organ or bone marrow transplants, and persons who have congenital immunodeficiencies are at greater risk than are immunocompetent persons for development of severe, life-threatening cryptosporidiosis if they become infected. Therefore, all immunocompromised persons should be educated and counseled about the ways that *Cryptosporidium* can be transmitted. These mechanisms of transmission include sexual practices involving fecal exposure, contact with infected adults or with infected children who wear diapers, contact with infected animals, drinking or eating contaminated water or food, and exposure to contaminated recreational water (319). All persons, especially immunocompromised persons, should avoid drinking water directly from lakes or rivers. Because water can be ingested unintentionally, immunocompromised persons should be advised that swimming in lakes, rivers, or public swimming pools also could place them at increased risk for infections. Current data are inadequate to make a general recommendation that immunocompromised persons in the United States boil or avoid drinking tap water in nonoutbreak settings (319).

Patients should avoid pets with diarrhea and wash their hands after handling pets. Routine prevention measures should be taken for foreign travel (316,320). Persons at increased risk for infection or serious complications of salmonellosis (e.g., children younger than 5 years of age and immunocompromised persons) should avoid contact with reptiles. Reptiles should not be in the same household with children younger than 1 year of age or with immunocompromised persons (113).

There is increasing evidence that probiotics and prebiotics may be useful in the prevention and treatment of diarrheal diseases. Probiotics consist of organisms that are considered normal intestinal flora, such as *Lactobacillus* spp., that may be supplemented in the diet. Intake of fermented milk products containing *Lactobacillus* and *Bifidobacterium* is effective in the treatment of acute diarrhea and rotavirus-associated diarrhea (321). There are preliminary data that probiotics also may reduce the risk of diarrhea in young children when given prophylactically. There is no specific information on the use of probiotics (live bacteria) or prebiotics (bacterial nutritional supplements) in immunocompromised patients, but this is a fertile field for investigation and intervention.

Vaccines against *Shigella* and diarrhea-producing *E. coli* strains are being tested but are not commercially available. The rotavirus vaccine is not recommended for use in immunodeficient infants or in older individuals, because it is a live vaccine that has not been studied in these populations (43). There are no effective vaccines against parasitic enteric infections. Pharmacologic antagonists to microbial adherence or toxin action are being evaluated.

Three typhoid vaccines are commercially available for persons traveling to areas in which *S. typhi* is endemic. The live attenuated typhoid vaccine is not recommended in young children or immunocompromised persons (322,323).

REFERENCES

1. Pickering LK. Approach to diagnosis and management of gastrointestinal tract infections. In: Long SS, Pickering LK, Prober CG, eds. *Principles and practice of pediatric infectious diseases.* New York: Churchill-Livingstone, 1997;410–418.
2. Finlay BB, Falkow S. Common themes in microbial pathogenicity revisited. *Microbiol Mol Biol Rev* 1997; 61:136–169.
3. Miller TL, Garg S. Gastrointestinal and nutritional problems in pediatric HIV disease. In: Pizzo PA, Wilfert CM, eds. *Pediatric AIDS: the challenge of HIV infection in infants, children, and adolescents,* 3rd ed. Baltimore: William & Wilkins, 1998;363–382.
4. Blakey JL, Barnes GL, Bishop RF, et al. Infectious diarrhea in children undergoing bone-marrow transplantation. *Aust N Z J Med* 1989;19:31–36.
5. George DL, Arnow PM, Fox AS, et al. Bacterial infection as a complication of liver transplantation: epidemiology and risk factors. *Rev Infect Dis* 1991;13: 387–396.
6. Sternbach GL, Varon J, Hunt SA. Emergency department presentation and care of heart and heart/lung transplant recipients. *Ann Emerg Med* 1992;21: 1140–1144.
7. Yolken RH, Bishop CA, Townsend TR, et al. Infectious gastroenteritis in bone-marrow-transplant recipients. *N Engl J Med* 1982;306:1010–1012.
8. Cubitt WD, Mitchell DK, Carter MJ, et al. Application of electronmicroscopy, enzyme immunoassay, and RT-PCR to monitor an outbreak of astrovirus type 1 in a paediatric bone marrow transplant unit. *J Med Virol* 1999;57:313–321.
9. Josephson A, Karanfil L, Alonso H, et al. Risk-specific nosocomial infection rates. *Am J Med* 1991;91: 131s–137s.
10. Jarvis WR, Edwards JR, Culver DH, et al. Nosocomial infection rates in adult and pediatric intensive care units in the United States. National Nosocomial Infections Surveillance System. *Am J Med* 1991;91: 185s–191s.
11. Brown RB, Stechenberg B, Sands M, et al. Infections in a pediatric intensive care unit. *Am J Dis Child* 1987; 141:267–270.
12. Gaynes RP, Martone WJ, Culver DH, et al. Comparison of rates of nosocomial infections in neonatal intensive care units in the United States. National Nosocomial Infections Surveillance System. *Am J Med* 1991;91:192s–196s.
13. Ford Jones EL, Mindorff CM, Gold R, et al. The incidence of viral-associated diarrhea after admission to a pediatric hospital. *Am J Epidemiol* 1990;131:711–718.
14. Lam BC, Tam J, Ng MH, et al. Nosocomial gastroenteritis in paediatric patients. *J Hosp Infect* 1989;14: 351–355.
15. Ford Jones EL, Mindorff CM, Langley JM, et al. Epidemiologic study of 4684 hospital-acquired infections in pediatric patients. *Pediatr Infect Dis J* 1989;8: 668–675.
16. Anderson LJ. Major trends in nosocomial viral infections. *Am J Med* 1991;91:107–111.
17. Brady MT, Pacini DL, Budde CT, et al. Diagnostic studies of nosocomial diarrhea in children: assessing their use and value. *Am J Infect Control* 1989;17:77–82.
18. Rosen FS, Cooper MD, Wedgwood RJ. The primary immunodeficiencies. *N Engl J Med* 1995;333: 431–440.
19. Vollaard EJ, Clasener HA. Colonization resistance. *Antimicrob Agents Chemother* 1994;38:409–414.
20. Newburg DS. Oligosaccharides and glycoconjugates

in human milk: their role in host defense. *J Mamm Gland Biol Neoplas* 1996;1:271–283.

21. Zopf D, Roth S. Oligosaccharide anti-infective agents. *Lancet* 1996;347:1017–1021.

22. Reid G, Bruce AW, McGroarty JA, et al. Is there a role for lactobacilli in prevention of urogenital and intestinal infections? *Clin Microbiol Rev* 1990;3:335–344.

23. King CE, Toskes PP. Small intestine bacterial overgrowth. *Gastroenterology* 1979;76:1035–1055.

24. Lonnroth I, Lange S. Intake of monosaccharides or amino acids induces pituitary gland synthesis of proteins regulating intestinal fluid transport. *Biochim Biophys Acta* 1987;925:117–123.

25. Strombeck DR, Harrold D. Binding of cholera toxin to mucins and inhibition by gastric mucin. *Infect Immun* 1974;10:1266–1272.

26. Lim PL, Rowley D. The effect of antibody on the intestinal absorption of macromolecules and on intestinal permeability in adult mice. *Int Arch Allergy Appl Immunol* 1982;68:41–46.

27. Cunningham Rundles C, Brandeis WE, Good RA, et al. Bovine antigens and the formation of circulating immune complexes in selective immunoglobulin A deficiency. *J Clin Invest* 1979;64:272–279.

28. Morrow AL, Pickering LK. Human milk and infectious diseases. In: Long SS, Pickering LK, Prober CG, eds. *Principles and practice of pediatric infectious diseases.* New York: Churchill-Livingstone, 1997;87–95.

29. Morrow AL, Pickering LK. Human milk protection against diarrheal disease. *Semin Pediatr Infect Dis* 1994;5:236–242.

30. Nataro JP, Kaper JB. Diarrheagenic *Escherichia coli. Clin Microbiol Rev* 1998;11:142–201.

31. Sears CL, Kaper JB. Enteric bacterial toxins: mechanisms of action and linkage to intestinal secretion. *Microbiol Rev* 1996;60:167–215.

32. Goodgame RW. Understanding intestinal spore-forming protozoa: cryptosporidia, microsporidia, isospora, and cyclospora. *Ann Intern Med* 1996;124:429–441.

33. Kapikian AZ. Overview of viral gastroenteritis. *Arch Virol Suppl* 1996;12:7–19.

34. Belitsos PC, Greenson JK, Yardley JH, et al. Association of gastric hypoacidity with opportunistic enteric infections in patients with AIDS. *J Infect Dis* 1992; 166:277–284.

35. Guarino A, Canani RB, Casola A, et al. Human intestinal cryptosporidiosis: secretory diarrhea and enterotoxic activity in Caco-2 cells. *J Infect Dis* 1995; 171:976–983.

36. Dong Y, Zeng CQY, Ball JM, et al. The rotavirus enterotoxin NSP4 mobilizes intracellular calcium in human intestinal cells by stimulating phospholipase C-mediated inositol 1,4,5-trisphosphate production. *Proc Natl Acad Sci U S A* 1997;94:3960–3965.

37. Ball JM, Tian P, Zeng CQY, et al. Age-dependent diarrhea induced by a rotaviral nonstructural glycoprotein. *Science* 1996;272:101–104.

38. Teahon K, Webster AD, Price AB, et al. Studies on the enteropathy associated with primary hypogammaglobulinaemia. *Gut* 1994;35:1244–1249.

39. Mike N, Hansel TT, Newman J, et al. Granulomatous enteropathy in common variable immunodeficiency: a cause of chronic diarrhoea. *Postgrad Med J* 1991;67: 446–449.

40. Papadopoulou A, Lloyd DR, Williams MD, et al. Gas-trointestinal and nutritional sequelae of bone marrow transplantation. *Arch Dis Child* 1996;75:208–213.

41. Hines J, Nachamkin I. Effective use of the clinical microbiology laboratory for diagnosing diarrheal diseases. *Clin Infect Dis* 1996;23:1292–1301.

42. Mitchell DK, Snyder J, Pickering LK. Gastrointestinal Infections. In: Pizzo PA, Wilfert CM, eds. *Pediatric AIDS: the challenge of HIV infection in infants, children, and adolescents,* 3rd ed. Baltimore: William & Wilkins, 1998;267–291.

43. American Academy of Pediatrics. Prevention of rotavirus disease: guidelines for use of rotavirus vaccine. *Pediatrics* 1998;102:1483–1491.

44. LeBaron CW, Furutan NP, Lew JF, et al. Viral agents of gastroenteritis: public health importance and outbreak management. *MMWR Morb Mortal Wkly Rep* 1990; 39:1–24.

45. Janoff EN, Reller LB. *Cryptosporidium* species, a protean protozoan. *J Clin Microbiol* 1987;25:967–975.

46. Hoxie NJ, Davis JP, Vergeront JM, et al. Cryptosporidiosis-associated mortality following a massive waterborne outbreak in Milwaukee, Wisconsin. *Am J Public Health* 1997;87:2032–2035.

47. Pickering LK, Engelkirk PG. *Giardia lamblia. Pediatr Clin North Am* 1988;35:565–567.

48. Didier ES. Microsporidiosis. *Clin Infect Dis* 1998;27: 1–8.

49. Update: outbreaks of cyclosporiasis—United States and Canada, 1997. *MMWR Morb Mortal Wkly Rep* 1997;46:521–523.

50. Herwaldt BL, Beach MJ. The return of *Cyclospora* in 1997: another outbreak of cyclosporiasis in North America associated with imported raspberries. Cyclospora Working Group. *Ann Intern Med* 1999;130: 210–220.

51. Soave R. *Cyclospora:* An overview. *Clin Infect Dis* 1996;23:429–437.

52. Neva FA. Biology and immunology of human strongyloidiasis. *J Infect Dis* 1986;153:397–406.

53. Kramer MH, Herwaldt BL, Craun GF, et al. Surveillance for waterborne-disease outbreaks—United States, 1993–1994. *MMWR Morb Mortal Wkly Rep* 1996;45:1–33.

54. Goldstein ST, Juranek DD, Ravenholt O, et al. Cryptosporidiosis: an outbreak associated with drinking water despite state-of-the-art water treatment. *Ann Intern Med* 1996;124:459–468.

55. Janda JM. Recent advances in the study of the taxonomy, pathogenicity, and infectious syndromes associated with the genus *Aeromonas. Clin Microbiol Rev* 1991;4:397–410.

56. de la Morena ML, Van R, Singh K, et al. Diarrhea associated with *Aeromonas* species in children in day care centers. *J Infect Dis* 1993;168:215–218.

57. Centers for Disease Control and Prevention. Outbreak of *Vibrio parahaemolyticus* infection associated with eating raw oysters and clams harvested from Long Island Sound—Connecticut, New Jersey, and New York, 1998. *JAMA* 1999;281:603–604.

58. Intestinal malabsorption of HIV-infected children: relationship to diarrhoea, failure to thrive, enteric microorganisms and immune impairment. The Italian Paediatric Intestinal/HIV Study Group. *AIDS* 1993;7: 1435–1440.

59. 1993 Revised classification system for HIV infection

and expanded surveillance case definition for AIDS among adolescents and adults. *MMWR Morb Mortal Wkly Rep* 1992;41:1–19.

60. 1994 Revised classification system for human immunodeficiency virus infection in children less than 13 years of age. *MMWR Morb Mortal Wkly Rep* 1994; 43:1–10.

61. Stoller JS, Adam HM, Weiss B, et al. Incidence of intestinal parasitic disease in an acquired immunodeficiency syndrome day-care center. *Pediatr Infect Dis J* 1991;10:654–658.

62. Sharpstone D, Gazzard B. Gastrointestinal manifestations of HIV infection. *Lancet* 1996;348:379–383.

63. Lo CW, Walker WA. Chronic protracted diarrhea of infancy: a nutritional disease. *Pediatrics* 1983;72: 786–800.

64. Cutrona AF, Blinkhorn RJ, Crass J, et al. Probable neutropenic enterocolitis in patients with AIDS. *Rev Infect Dis* 1991;13:828–831.

65. Gomez L, Martino R, Rolston KV. Neutropenic enterocolitis: spectrum of the disease and comparison of definite and possible cases. *Clin Infect Dis* 1998;27: 695–699.

66. Deodhar LP, Saraswathi K, Varudkar A. *Aeromonas* spp. and their association with human diarrheal disease. *J Clin Microbiol* 1991;29:853–856.

67. Namdari H, Bottone EJ. Microbiologic and clinical evidence supporting the role of *Aeromonas caviae* as a pediatric enteric pathogen. *J Clin Microbiol* 1990;28: 837–840.

68. San Joaquin VHS, Pickett DA. *Aeromonas*-associated gastroenteritis in children. *Pediatr Infect Dis J* 1988;7:53–57.

69. Challapalli M, Tess BR, Cunningham DG, et al. *Aeromonas*-associated diarrhea in children. *Pediatr Infect Dis J* 1988;7:693–698.

70. Burke V, Gracey M, Robinson J, et al. The microbiology of childhood gastroenteritis: *Aeromonas* species and other infective agents. *J Infect Dis* 1983;148:68–74.

71. Janda JM, Abbott SL. Evolving concepts regarding the genus *Aeromonas*: an expanding panorama of species, disease presentations, and unanswered questions. *Clin Infect Dis* 1998;27:332–344.

72. Figura N, Marri L, Verdiani S, et al. Prevalence, species differentiation, and toxigenicity of *Aeromonas* strains in cases of childhood gastroenteritis and in controls. *J Clin Microbiol* 1986;23:595–599.

73. Janda JM, Bottone EJ, Reitano M. *Aeromonas* species in clinical microbiology: significance, epidemiology, and speciation. *Diagn Microbiol Infect Dis* 1983;1: 221–228.

74. Picard B, Goullet P. Seasonal prevalence of nosocomial *Aeromonas hydrophila* infection related to aeromonas in hospital water. *J Hosp Infect* 1987;10: 152–155.

75. Picard B, Goullet P. Epidemiological complexity of hospital aeromonas infections revealed by electrophoretic typing of esterases. *Epidemiol Infect* 1987; 98:5–14.

76. Allos BM, Blaser MJ. *Campylobacter jejuni* and the expanding spectrum of related infections. *Clin Infect Dis* 1995;20:1092–1099.

77. Jenkin GA, Tee W. *Campylobacter upsaliensis*-associated diarrhea in human immunodeficiency virus-infected patients. *Clin Infect Dis* 1998;27:816–821.

78. Ichiyama S, Hirai S, Minami T, et al. *Campylobacter fetus* subspecies *fetus* cellulitis associated with bacteremia in debilitated hosts. *Clin Infect Dis* 1998; 27:252–255.

79. Bourke B, Chan VL, Sherman P. *Campylobacter upsaliensis: waiting in the wings.* Clin Microbiol Rev 1998;11:440–449.

80. Pigrau C, Bartolome R, Almirante B, et al. Bacteremia due to *Campylobacter* species: clinical findings and antimicrobial susceptibility patterns. *Clin Infect Dis* 1997;25:1414–1420.

81. Snijders F, Kuijper EJ, de Wever B, et al. Prevalence of *Campylobacter*-associated diarrhea among patients infected with human immunodeficiency virus. *Clin Infect Dis* 1997;24:1107–1113.

82. Reed RP, Friedland IR, Wegerhoff FO, et al. *Campylobacter* bacteremia in children. *Pediatr Infect Dis J* 1996;15:345–348.

83. Kelly CP, Pothoulakis C, LaMont JT. *Clostridium difficile* colitis. *N Engl J Med* 1994;380:256–261.

84. Cohen SH, Tang YJ, Muenzer J, et al. Isolation of various genotypes of *Clostridium difficile* from patients and the environment in an oncology ward. *Clin Infect Dis* 1997;24:889–893.

85. Bartlett JG. *Clostridium difficile: history of its role as an enteric pathogen and the current state of knowledge about the organism.* Clin Infect Dis 1994;18: S265–S272.

86. Gerding DN, Johnson S, Peterson LR, et al. *Clostridium difficile*-associated diarrhea and colitis. *Infect Control Hosp Epidemiol* 1995;16:459–477.

87. Johnson S, Gerding DN. *Clostridium difficile*-associated diarrhea. *Clin Infect Dis* 1998;26:1027–1036.

88. Willingham FF, Ticona Chavez E, Taylor DN, et al. Diarrhea and *Clostridium difficile* infection in Latin American patients with AIDS. Working Group on AIDS in Peru. *Clin Infect Dis* 1998;27:487–493.

89. Mastroianni A, Coronado O, Nanetti A, et al. Nosocomial *Clostridium difficile*-associated diarrhea in patients with AIDS: a three-year survey and review. *Clin Infect Dis* 1997;25[Suppl 2]:S204–S205.

90. Gerding DN, Olson MM, Peterson LR, et al. *Clostridium difficile*-associated diarrhea and colitis in adults: a prospective case-controlled epidemiologic study. *Arch Intern Med* 1986;146:95–100.

91. Kusne S, Dummer JS, Singh N, et al. Infections after liver transplantation: an analysis of 101 consecutive cases. *Medicine (Baltimore)* 1988;67:132–143.

92. Burgner D, Siarakas S, Eagles G, et al. A prospective study of *Clostridium difficile* infection and colonization in pediatric oncology patients. *Pediatr Infect Dis J* 1997;16:1131–1134.

93. Roghmann MC, McCarter RJ Jr, Brewrink J, et al. *Clostridium difficile* infection is a risk factor for bacteremia due to vancomycin-resistant enterococci (VRE) in VRE-colonized patients with acute leukemia. *Clin Infect Dis* 1997;25:1056–1059.

94. Mitchell DK, Pickering LK. Nosocomial gastrointestinal tract infections in pediatric patients. In: Mayhall CG, ed. *Hospital epidemiology and infection control,* 2nd ed. Philadelphia: Lippincott Williams & Wilkins, 1999;629–647.

95. Ryder RW, Wachsmuth IK, Buxton AE, et al. Infantile diarrhea produced by heat-stable enterotoxigenic *Escherichia coli. N Engl J Med* 1976;295:849–853.

96. DuPont HL, Ericsson CD. Prevention and treatment of traveler's diarrhea. *N Engl J Med* 1993;328:1821–1827.

97. Stiver HG, Albritton WL, Clark J, et al. Nosocomial colonization and infection due to *E. coli* 0125:K70 epidemiologically linked to expressed breast-milk feedings. *Can J Public Health* 1977;68:479–482.

98. Polotsky Y, Nataro JP, Kotler D, et al. HEp-2 cell adherence patterns, serotyping, and DNA analysis of *Escherichia coli* isolates from eight patients with AIDS and chronic diarrhea. *J Clin Microbiol* 1997;35:1952–1958.

99. Wanke CA, Gerrior J, Blais V, et al. Successful treatment of diarrheal disease associated with enteroaggregative *Escherichia coli* in adults infected with human immunodeficiency virus. *J Infect Dis* 1998;178:1369–1372.

100. Robins-Browne RM. Traditional enteropathogenic *Escherichia coli* of infantile diarrhea. *Rev Infect Dis* 1987;9:28–53.

101. Levine MM, Ferreccio C, Prado V, et al. Epidemiologic studies of *Escherichia coli* diarrheal infections in a low socioeconomic level peri-urban community in Santiago, Chile. *Am J Epidemiol* 1993;138:849–869.

102. Cody SH, Glynn MK, Farrar JA, et al. An outbreak of *Escherichia coli* O157:H7 infection from unpasteurized commercial apple juice. *Ann Intern Med* 1999;130:202–209.

103. Mead PS, Griffin PM. *Escherichia coli* O157:H7. *Lancet* 1998;352:1207–1212.

104. Pavia AT, Nichols CR, Green DP, et al. Hemolytic-uremic syndrome during an outbreak of *Escherichia coli* O157:H7 infections in institutions for mentally retarded persons: clinical and epidemiologic observations. *J Pediatr* 1990;116:544–551.

105. Belongia EA, Osterholm MT, Soler JT, et al. Transmission of *Escherichia coli* O157:H7 infection in Minnesota child day-care facilities. *JAMA* 1993;269:883–888.

106. Karmali MA, Arbus GS, Petric M, et al. Hospital-acquired *Escherichia coli* O157:H7 associated haemolytic uraemic syndrome in a nurse. *Lancet* 1988;1:526.

107. Dummer JS, Allos BM. Gastrointestinal infections in transplant recipients. In: Blaser MJ, Smith PD, Ravdin JI, et al. eds. *Infections of the gastrointestinal tract.* New York: Raven Press, 1995;511–525.

108. Schuchat A, Deaver KA, Wenger JD, et al. Role of foods in sporadic listeriosis: I. Case-control study of dietary risk factors. The Listeria Study Group. *JAMA* 1992;267:2041–2045.

109. Pinner RW, Schuchat A, Swaminathan B, et al. Role of foods in sporadic listeriosis: II. Microbiologic and epidemiologic investigation. The Listeria Study Group. *JAMA* 1992;267:2046–2050.

110. Update: multistate outbreak of listeriosis—United States, 1998–1999. *MMWR Morb Mortal Wkly Rep* 1999;47:1117–1118.

111. Centers for Disease Control and Prevention. Update: multistate outbreak of listeriosis—United States, 1998–1999. *JAMA* 1999;281:317–318.

112. Janda JM, Abbott SL, Morris JG. *Aeromonas, Plesiomonas,* and *Edwardsiella.* In: Blaser MJ, Smith PD, Ravdin JI, et al., eds. *Infections of the gastrointestinal tract.* New York: Raven Press, 1995;905–917.

113. Mermin J, Hoar B, Angulo FJ. Iguanas and *Salmonella marina* infection in children: a reflection of the increasing incidence of reptile-associated salmonellosis in the United States. *Pediatrics* 1997;99:399–402.

114. Telzak EE, Budnick LD, Greenberg MS, et al. A nosocomial outbreak of *Salmonella enteritidis* infection due to the consumption of raw eggs. *N Engl J Med* 1990;323:394–397.

115. Mishu B, Koehler J, Lee LA, et al. Outbreaks of *Salmonella enteritidis* infections in the United States, 1985–1991. *J Infect Dis* 1994;169:547–552.

116. Hennessy TW, Hedberg CW, Slutsker L, et al. A national outbreak of *Salmonella enteritidis* infections from ice cream. *N Engl J Med* 1996;334:1281–1286.

117. L'Ecuyer PB, Diego J, Murphy D, et al. Nosocomial outbreak of gastroenteritis due to *Salmonella senftenberg. Clin Infect Dis* 1996;23:734–742.

118. Cook KA, Dobbs TE, Hlady WG, et al. Outbreak of *Salmonella* serotype Hartford infections associated with unpasteurized orange juice. *JAMA* 1998;280:1504–1509.

119. Van Beneden CA, Keene WE, Strang RA, et al. Multinational outbreak of *Salmonella enterica* serotype Newport infections due to contaminated alfalfa sprouts. *JAMA* 1999;281:158–162.

120. Lang DJ, Kunz LJ, Martin AR, et al. Carmine as a source of nosocomial salmonellosis. *N Engl J Med* 1967;276:829–832.

121. Komarmy LE, Oxley ME, Brecher G. Hospital-acquired salmonellosis traced to carmine dye capsules. *N Engl J Med* 1967;276:850–852.

122. Chmel H, Armstrong D. *Salmonella oslo*: a focal outbreak in a hospital. *Am J Med* 1976;60:203–208.

123. Dwyer DM, Klein EG, Istre GR, et al. *Salmonella newport* infections transmitted by fiberoptic colonoscopy. *Gastrointest Endosc* 1987;33:84–87.

124. Ip HMH, Sin WK, Chau PY, et al. Neonatal infection due to *Salmonella worthington* transmitted by a delivery room suction apparatus. *J Hyg* 1976;77:307–314.

125. Khan MA, Abdur Rab M, Israr N, et al. Transmission of *Salmonella worthington* by oropharyngeal suction in hospital neonatal unit. *Pediatr Infect Dis J* 1991;10:668–672.

126. Aber RC, Banks WV. An outbreak of nosocomial *Salmonella typhimurium* infection linked to environmental reservoir. *Infect Control* 1980;1:386–390.

127. McAllister TA, Roud JA, Marshall A, et al. Outbreak of *Salmonella eimsbuettel* in newborn infants spread by rectal thermometers. *Lancet* 1986;1:1262–1264.

128. Kostiala AA, Westerstrahle M, Muttilainen M. Neonatal *Salmonella panama* infection with meningitis. *Acta Paediatr* 1992;81:856–858.

129. Lamb VA, Mayhall CG, Spadora AC, et al. Outbreak of *Salmonella typhimurium* gastroenteritis due to an imported strain resistant to ampicillin, chloramphenicol, and trimethoprim-sulfamethoxazole in a nursery. *J Clin Microbiol* 1984;20:1076–1079.

130. Smith SM, Palumbo PE, Edelson PJ. *Salmonella* strains resistant to multiple antibiotics: therapeutic implications. *Pediatr Infect Dis J* 1984;3:455–460.

131. Ramos JM, Garcia-Corbeira P, Aguado JM, et al. Clinical significance of primary vs. secondary bacteremia due to nontyphoid *Salmonella* in patients without AIDS. *Clin Infect Dis* 1994;19:777–780.

132. Aliaga L, Mediavilla JD, Lopez de la Osa A, et al. Nontyphoidal *salmonella* intracranial infections in HIV-infected patients. *Clin Infect Dis* 1997;25:1118–1120.

133. Fernandez Guerrero ML, Ramos JM, Nunez A, et al.

Focal infections due to non-*typhi Salmonella* in patients with AIDS: report of 10 cases and review. *Clin Infect Dis* 1997;25:690–697.

134. Schutze GE, Schutze SE, Kirby RS. Extraintestinal salmonellosis in a children's hospital. *Pediatr Infect Dis J* 1997;16:482–485.

135. Wright J, Thomas P, Serjeant GR. Septicemia caused by *Salmonella* infection: an overlooked complication of sickle cell disease. *J Pediatr* 1997;130:394–399.

136. Keusch GT, Bennish ML. Shigellosis: recent progress, persisting problems and research issues. *Pediatr Infect Dis J* 1989;8:713–719.

137. Pillay DG, Karas JA, Pillay A, et al. Nosocomial transmission of *Shigella dysenteriae* type 1. *J Hosp Infect* 1997;37:199–205.

138. Brian MJ, Van R, Townsend I, et al. Evaluation of the molecular epidemiology of an outbreak of multiply resistant *Shigella sonnei* in a day-care center by using pulsed-field gel electrophoresis and plasmid DNA analysis. *J Clin Microbiol* 1993;31:2152–2156.

139. Hale TL. Genetic basis of virulence in *Shigella* species. *Microbiol Rev* 1991;55:206–224.

140. Ruderman JW, Stoller KP, Pomerance JJ. Bloodstream invasion with *Shigella sonnei* in an asymptomatic newborn infant. *Pediatr Infect Dis J* 1986;5:379–380.

141. Starke JR, Baker CJ. Neonatal shigellosis with bowel perforation. *Pediatr Infect Dis J* 1985;4:405–407.

142. Huskins WC, Griffiths JK, Faruque AS, et al. Shigellosis in neonates and young infants. *J Pediatr* 1994;125:14–22.

143. Baskin DH, Lax JD, Barenberg D. *Shigella* bacteremia in patients with the acquired immune deficiency syndrome. *Am J Gastroenterol* 1987;82:338–341.

144. Blaser MJ, Hale TL, Formal SB. Recurrent shigellosis complicating human immunodeficiency virus infection: failure of pre-existing antibodies to confer protection. *Am J Med* 1989;86:105–107.

145. Mandell W, Neu H. *Shigella* bacteremia in adults. *JAMA* 1986;255:3116–3117.

146. Gander RM, LaRocco MT. Multiple drug-resistance in *Shigella flexneri* isolated from a patient with human immunodeficiency virus. *Diagn Microbiol Infect Dis* 1987;8:193–196.

147. Severn M, Michael J. *Shigella* septicaemia following renal transplantation. *Postgrad Med J* 1980;56:852–853.

148. Gueco I, Saniel M, Mendoza M, et al. Tropical infections after renal transplantation. *Transplant Proc* 1989;21:2105–2107.

149. Neter E, Merrin C, Surgalla MJ, et al. *Shigella sonnei* bacteremia: unusual antibody response from immunosuppressive therapy following renal transplantation. *Urology* 1974;4:198–200.

150. Faruque SM, Albert MJ, Mekalanos JJ. Epidemiology, genetics, and ecology of toxigenic *Vibrio cholerae*. *Microbiol Mol Biol Rev* 1998;62:1301–1314.

151. Janda JM, Powers C, Bryant RG, et al. Current perspectives on the epidemiology and pathogenesis of clinically significant *Vibrio* spp. *Clin Microbiol Rev* 1988;1:245–267.

152. Morris JG Jr, Black RE. Cholera and other vibrioses in the United States. *N Engl J Med* 1985;312:343–350.

153. Hlady WG, Klontz KC. The epidemiology of *Vibrio* infections in Florida, 1981–1993. *J Infect Dis* 1996;173:1176–1183.

154. Outbreak of *Vibrio parahaemolyticus* infection associated with eating raw oysters and clams harvested from Long Island Sound—Connecticut, New Jersey, and New York, 1998. *MMWR Morb Mortal Wkly Rep* 1999;48:48–51.

155. Shapiro RL, Altekruse S, Hutwagner L, et al. The role of Gulf Coast oysters harvested in warmer months in *Vibrio vulnificus* infections in the United States, 1988–1996. Vibrio Working Group. *J Infect Dis* 1998;178:752–759.

156. Dahdouh MA, Ismail A, Berger JJ. Cholera in a patient infected with human immunodeficiency virus. *Clin Infect Dis* 1995;21:689–690.

157. Estrada y Martin RM, Samayoa B, Arathoon E, et al. Atypical infection due to *Vibrio cholerae* in patients infected with human immunodeficiency virus. *Clin Infect Dis* 1995;21:1516–1517.

158. Hor LI, Chang TT, Wang ST. Survival of *Vibrio vulnificus* in whole blood from patients with chronic liver diseases: association with phagocytosis by neutrophils and serum ferritin levels. *J Infect Dis* 1999;179:275–278.

159. Ko WC, Chuang YC, Huang GC, et al. Infections due to non-O1 *Vibrio cholerae* in southern Taiwan: predominance in cirrhotic patients. *Clin Infect Dis* 1998;27:774–780.

160. *Vibrio vulnificus* infections associated with raw oyster consumption—Florida, 1981–1992. *MMWR Morb Mortal Wkly Rep* 1993;42:405–407.

161. Bottone EJ. *Yersinia enterocolitica: the charisma continues*. Clin Microbiol Rev 1997;10:257–276.

162. Hoogkamp-Korstanje JA, Stolk-Engelaar VM. *Yersinia enterocolitica* infection in children. *Pediatr Infect Dis J* 1995;14:771–775.

163. Greenwood MH, Hooper WL. Excretion of *Yersinia* spp. associated with consumption of pasteurized milk. *Epidemiol Infect* 1990;104:345–350.

164. Cover TL, Aber RC. *Yersinia enterocolitica*. *N Engl J Med* 1989;321:16–24.

165. Metchock B, Lonsway DR, Carter GP, et al. *Yersinia enterocolitica: a frequent seasonal stool isolate from children at an urban hospital in the southeast United States.* J Clin Microbiol 1991;29:2868–2869.

166. Blumberg HM, Kiehlbauch JA, Wachsmuth IK. Molecular epidemiology of *Yersinia enterocolitica* O:3 infections: use of chromosomal DNA restriction fragment length polymorphisms of rRNA genes. *J Clin Microbiol* 1991;29:2368–2374.

167. Lee LA, Taylor J, Carter GP, et al. *Yersinia enterocolitica* O:3: an emerging cause of pediatric gastroenteritis in the United States. The *Yersinia enterocolitica* Collaborative Study Group. *J Infect Dis* 1991;163:660–663.

168. Cover TL. *Yersinia enterocolitica* and *Yersinia pseudotuberculosis*. In: Blaser MJ, Smith PD, Ravdin JI, et al. eds. *Infections of the gastrointestinal tract*. New York: Raven Press, 1995;811–823.

169. Update: *Yersinia enterocolitica* bacteremia and endotoxin shock associated with red blood cell transfusions—United States, 1991. *MMWR Morb Mortal Wkly Rep* 1991;40:176–178.

170. Jacobs J, Jamaer D, Vandeven J, et al. *Yersinia enterocolitica* in donor blood: a case report and review. *J Clin Microbiol* 1989;27:1119–1121.

171. Wright DC, Selss IF, Vinton KJ, et al. Fatal *Yersinia enterocolitica* sepsis after blood transfusion. *Arch Pathol Lab Med* 1985;109:1040–1042.

172. Cherchi GB, Pacifico L, Cossellu S, et al. Prospective study of *Yersinia enterocolitica* infection in thalassemic patients. *Pediatr Infect Dis J* 1995;14:579–584.

173. Grohmann GS, Glass RI, Pereira HG, et al. Enteric viruses and diarrhea in HIV-infected patients. Enteric Opportunistic Infections Working Group. *N Engl J Med* 1993;329:14–20.

174. Yuen KY, Woo PC, Liang RH, et al. Clinical significance of alimentary tract microbes in bone marrow transplant recipients. *Diagn Microbiol Infect Dis* 1998; 30:75–81.

175. Cox GJ, Matsui SM, Lo RS, et al. Etiology and outcome of diarrhea after marrow transplantation: a prospective study. *Gastroenterology* 1994;107:1398–1407.

176. Kapelushnik J, Or R, Delukina M, et al. Intravenous ribavirin therapy for adenovirus gastroenteritis after bone marrow transplantation. *J Pediatr Gastroenterol Nutr* 1995;21:110–112.

177. Blacklow NR, Greenberg HB. Viral gastroenteritis. *N Engl J Med* 1991;325:252–264.

178. Morris DJ. Virus infections in children with cancer. *Rev Med Microbiol* 1990;1:49–57.

179. Schofield KP, Morris DJ, Bailey AS, et al. Gastroenteritis due to adenovirus type 41 in an adult with chronic lymphocytic leukemia. *Clin Infect Dis* 1994; 19:311–312.

180. Cunningham AL, Grohman GS, Harkness J, et al. Gastrointestinal viral infections in homosexual men who were symptomatic and seropositive for human immunodeficiency virus. *J Infect Dis* 1988;158:386–391.

181. Krajden M, Brown M, Petrasek A, et al. Clinical features of adenovirus enteritis: a review of 127 cases. *Pediatr Infect Dis J* 1990;9:636–641.

182. Harville TO, Tang ML, Garcia-Turner AM, et al. Gastrointestinal (GI) adenovirus treated with oral ribavirin in severe combined immunodeficiency (SCID). *Pediatr Res* 1998(abst).

183. Johansson ME, Wirgart BZ, Grillner L, et al. Severe gastroenteritis in an immunocompromised child caused by adenovirus type 5. *Pediatr Infect Dis J* 1990;9:449–450.

184. Glass RI, Noel J, Mitchell D, et al. The changing epidemiology of astrovirus-associated gastroenteritis: a review. *Arch Virol Suppl* 1996;12:287–300.

185. Mitchell DK, Van R, Morrow AL, et al. Outbreaks of astrovirus gastroenteritis in day care centers. *J Pediatr* 1993;123:725–732.

186. Esahli H, Breback K, Bennet R, et al. Astroviruses as a cause of nosocomial outbreaks of infant diarrhea. *Pediatr Infect Dis J* 1991;10:511–515.

187. Kotloff KL, Herrmann JE, Blacklow NR, et al. The frequency of astrovirus as a cause of diarrhea in Baltimore children. *Pediatr Infect Dis J* 1992;11:587–589.

188. Kurtz JB, Lee TW, Pickering D. Astrovirus associated gastroenteritis in a children's ward. *J Clin Pathol* 1977;30:948–952.

189. Noel J, Cubitt D. Identification of astrovirus serotypes from children treated at the Hospitals for Sick Children, London 1981–1993. *Epidemiol Infect* 1994;113: 153–159.

190. Wood DJ, David TJ, Chrystie IL, et al. Chronic enteric virus infection in two T-cell immunodeficient children. *J Med Virol* 1988;24:435–444.

191. Berke T, Golding B, Jiang X, et al. Phylogenetic analysis of the caliciviruses. *J Med Virol* 1997;52:419–424.

192. Lewis DC, Hale A, Jiang X, et al. Epidemiology of Mexico virus, a small round-structured virus in Yorkshire, United Kingdom, between January 1992 and March 1995. *J Infect Dis* 1997;175:951–954.

193. Jiang X, Cubitt D, Hu J, et al. Development of an ELISA to detect MX virus, a human calicivirus in the Snow Mountain Agent genogroup. *J Gen Virol* 1995; 76:2739–2747.

194. Kaplan JE, Gary GW, Baron RC, et al. Epidemiology of Norwalk gastroenteritis and the role of Norwalk virus in outbreaks of acute nonbacterial gastroenteritis. *Ann Intern Med* 1982;96:756–761.

195. Blacklow NR, Cukor G, Bedigian MK, et al. Immune response and prevalence of antibody to Norwalk enteritis virus as determined by radioimmunoassay. *J Clin Microbiol* 1979;10:903–909.

196. Cubitt WD, McSwiggan DA, Moore W. Winter vomiting disease caused by calicivirus. *J Clin Pathol* 1979; 32:786–793.

197. Cubitt WD, McSwiggan DA. Calicivirus gastroenteritis in North West London. *Lancet* 1981;2:975–977.

198. Matson DO, Estes MK, Tanaka T, et al. Asymptomatic human calicivirus infection in a day care center. *Pediatr Infect Dis J* 1990;9:190–196.

199. Spender QW, Lewis D, Price EH. Norwalk like viruses: study of an outbreak. *Arch Dis Child* 1986;61: 142–147.

200. Storr J, Rice S, Phillips AD, et al. Clinical associations of Norwalk-like virus in the stools of children. *J Pediatr Gastroenterol Nutr* 1986;5:576–580.

201. Riordan T, Wills A. An outbreak of gastroenteritis in a psycho-geriatric hospital associated with a small round structured virus. *J Hosp Infect* 1986;8:296–299.

202. Vinje J, Altena SA, Koopmans MPG. The incidence and genetic variability of small round-structured viruses in outbreaks of gastroenteritis in The Netherlands. *J Infect Dis* 1997;176:1374–1378.

203. Russo PL, Spelman DW, Harrington GA, et al. Hospital outbreak of Norwalk-like virus. *Infect Control Hosp Epidemiol* 1997;18:576–579.

204. Jiang X, Turf E, Hu J, et al. Outbreaks of gastroenteritis in elderly nursing homes and retirement facilities associated with human caliciviruses. *J Med Virol* 1996; 50:335–341.

205. Cubitt WD, Jiang X. Study on occurrence of human calicivirus (Mexico strain) as cause of sporadic cases and outbreaks of calicivirus-associated diarrhoea in the United Kingdom, 1983–1995. *J Med Virol* 1996; 48:273–277.

206. Khan AS, Moe CL, Glass RI, et al. Norwalk virus-associated gastroenteritis traced to ice consumption aboard a cruise ship in Hawaii: comparison and application of molecular method-based assays. *J Clin Microbiol* 1994;32:318–322.

207. Pether JV, Caul EO. An outbreak of food-borne gastroenteritis in two hospitals associated with a Norwalk-like virus. *J Hyg Lond* 1983;91:343–350.

208. Kilgore PE, Belay ED, Hamlin DM, et al. A university outbreak of gastroenteritis due to a small round-structured virus: application of molecular diagnostics to identify the etiologic agent and patterns of transmission. *J Infect Dis* 1996;173:787–793.

209. Morse DL, Guzewich JJ, Hanrahan JP, et al. Widespread outbreaks of clam- and oyster-associated gastroenteritis: role of Norwalk virus. *N Engl J Med* 1986; 314:678–681.

210. Sharp TW, Hyams KC, Watts D, et al. Epidemiology of Norwalk virus during an outbreak of acute gastroenteritis aboard a US aircraft carrier. *J Med Virol* 1995; 45:61–67.

211. Spratt HC, Marks MI, Gomersall M, et al. Nosocomial infantile gastroenteritis associated with minirotavirus and calicivirus. *J Pediatr* 1978;93:922–926.

212. Townsend TR, Bolyard EA, Yolken RH, et al. Outbreak of coxsackie A1 gastroenteritis: a complication of bone-marrow transplantation. *Lancet* 1982;1:820–823.

213. Parashar UD, Bresee JS, Gentsch JR, et al. Rotavirus. *Emerg Infect Dis* 1998;4:561–570.

214. Gilger MA, Matson DO, Conner ME, et al. Extraintestinal rotavirus infections in children with immunodeficiency. *J Pediatr* 1992;120:912–917.

215. Albrecht H, Stellbrink HJ, Fenske S, et al. Rotavirus antigen detection in patients with HIV infection and diarrhea. *Scand J Gastroenterol* 1993;28:307–310.

216. Oshitani H, Kasolo FC, Mpabalwani M, et al. Association of rotavirus and human immunodeficiency virus infection in children hospitalized with acute diarrhea, Lusaka, Zambia. *J Infect Dis* 1994;169:897–900.

217. Weber R, Bryan RT. Microsporidial infections in immunodeficient and immunocompetent patients. *Clin Infect Dis* 1994;19:517–521.

218. Rijpstra AC, Canning EU, Van Ketel RJ, et al. Use of light microscopy to diagnose small-intestinal microsporidiosis in patients with AIDS. *J Infect Dis* 1988;157:827–831.

219. Garcia LS. Classification of human parasites. *Clin Infect Dis* 1997;25:21–23.

220. MacKenzie WR, Schell WL, Blair KA, et al. Massive outbreak of waterborne *Cryptosporidium* infection in Milwaukee, Wisconsin: recurrence of illness and risk of secondary transmission. *Clin Infect Dis* 1995;21: 57–62.

221. Smith PD, Quinn TC, Strober W. Gastrointestinal infection with AIDS. *Ann Intern Med* 1992;116:63–77.

222. McLoughlin LC, Nord KS, Joshi VV, et al. Severe gastrointestinal involvement in children with the acquired immunodeficiency syndrome. *J Pediatr Gastroenterol Nutr* 1987;6:517–524.

223. Flanigan T, Whalen C, Turner J, et al. *Cryptosporidium* infection and CD4 counts. *Ann Intern Med* 1992;116: 840–842.

224. Kuhls TL, Mosier DA, Crawford DL, et al. Seroprevalence of cryptosporidial antibodies during infancy, childhood, and adolescence. *Clin Infect Dis* 1994;18: 731–735.

225. Cordell RL, Addiss DG. Cryptosporidiosis in child care settings: a review of the literature and recommendations for prevention and control. *Pediatr Infect Dis J* 1994;13:310–317.

226. Miller RA, Holmberg RE Jr, Clausen CR. Life-threatening diarrhea caused by *Cryptosporidium* in a child undergoing therapy for acute lymphocytic leukemia. *J Pediatr* 1983;103:256–259.

227. Ok UZ, Cirit M, Uner A, et al. Cryptosporidiosis and blastocystosis in renal transplant recipients. *Nephron* 1997;75:171–174.

228. Chieffi PP, Sens YA, Paschoalotti MA, et al. Infection by *Cryptosporidium parvum* in renal patients submitted to renal transplant or hemodialysis. *Rev Soc Bras Med Trop* 1998;31:333–337.

229. Chappell CL, Okhuysen PC, Sterling CR, et al. *Cryp-*

tosporidium parvum: intensity of infection and oocyst excretion patterns in healthy volunteers. *J Infect Dis* 1996;173:232–236.

230. Pape JW, Verdier RI, Boncy M, et al. *Cyclospora* infection in adults infected with HIV: clinical manifestations, treatment, and prophylaxis. *Ann Intern Med* 1994;121:654–657.

231. Wurtz RM, Kocka FE, Peters CS, et al. Clinical characteristics of seven cases of diarrhea associated with a novel acid-fast organism in the stool. *Clin Infect Dis* 1993;16:136–138.

232. Wurtz R. *Cyclospora*: a newly identified intestinal pathogen of humans. *Clin Infect Dis* 1994;18:620–623.

233. Sifuentes Osornio J, Porras Cortes G, Bendall RP, et al. *Cyclospora cayetanensis* infection in patients with and without AIDS: biliary disease as another clinical manifestation. *Clin Infect Dis* 1995;21:1092–1097.

234. Reed SL. New concepts regarding the pathogenesis of amebiasis. *Clin Infect Dis* 1995;21[Suppl 2]:S182–185.

235. Reed SL. Amebiasis: an update. *Clin Infect Dis* 1992; 14:385–393.

236. Hopkins RS, Juranek DD. Acute giardiasis: an improved clinical case definition for epidemiologic studies. *Am J Epidemiol* 1991;133:402–407.

237. Lengerich EJ, Addiss DG, Juranek DD. Severe giardiasis in the United States. *Clin Infect Dis* 1994;18: 760–763.

238. Petersen LR, Carter ML, Hadler JL. A foodborne outbreak of *Giardia lamblia*. *J Infect Dis* 1988;157:846–848.

239. Adam RD. The biology of *Giardia* spp. *Microbiol Rev* 1991;55:706–732.

240. Wolfe MS. Giardiasis. *Clin Microbiol Rev* 1992;5: 93–100.

241. Webster AD. Giardiasis and immunodeficiency diseases. *Trans R Soc Trop Med Hyg* 1980;74:440–443.

242. Herbst EW, Armbruster M, Rump JA, et al. Intestinal B cell defects in common variable immunodeficiency. *Clin Exp Immunol* 1994;95:215–221.

243. Cruz I, Ricardo JL, Nunes JF, et al. *Giardia* and immune deficiency. *Am J Gastroenterol* 1991;86:1554–1555.

244. Washington K, Stenzel TT, Buckley RH, et al. Gastrointestinal pathology in patients with common variable immunodeficiency and X-linked agammaglobulinemia. *Am J Surg Pathol* 1996;20:1240–1252.

245. Pape JW, Verdier RI, Johnson WD Jr. Treatment and prophylaxis of *Isospora belli* infection in patients with the acquired immunodeficiency syndrome. *N Engl J Med* 1989;320:1044–1047.

246. Sorvillo FJ, Lieb LE, Seidel J, et al. Epidemiology of isosporiasis among persons with acquired immunodeficiency syndrome in Los Angeles County. *Am J Trop Med Hyg* 1995;53:656–659.

247. Bryan RT, Cali A, Owen RL, et al. Microsporidia: opportunistic pathogens in patients with AIDS. In: Sun T, ed. *Progress in clinical parasitology*. Philadelphia: Field and Wood, 1991;21–26.

248. Gunnarsson G, Hurlbut D, DeGirolami PC, et al. Multiorgan microsporidiosis: report of five cases and review. *Clin Infect Dis* 1995;21:37–44.

249. Enriquez FJ, Taren D, Cruz-Lopez A, et al. Prevalence of intestinal encephalitozoonosis in Mexico. *Clin Infect Dis* 1998;26:1227–1229.

250. Asmuth DM, DeGirolami PC, Federman M, et al. Clinical features of microsporidiosis in patients with AIDS. *Clin Infect Dis* 1994;18:819–825.

251. Coyle CM, Wittner M, Kotler DP, et al. Prevalence of microsporidiosis due to *Enterocytozoon bieneusi* and *Encephalitozoon (Septata) intestinalis* among patients with AIDS-related diarrhea: determination by polymerase chain reaction to the microsporidian small-subunit rRNA gene. *Clin Infect Dis* 1996;23:1002–1006.

252. Rabodonirina M, Bertocchi M, Desportes Livage I, et al. *Enterocytozoon bieneusi* as a cause of chronic diarrhea in a heart-lung transplant recipient who was seronegative for human immunodeficiency virus. *Clin Infect Dis* 1996;23:114–117.

253. Wanke CA, DeGirolami P, Federman M. *Enterocytozoon bieneusi* infection and diarrheal disease in patients who were not infected with human immunodeficiency virus: case report and review. *Clin Infect Dis* 1996;23:816–818.

254. Burke JA. Strongyloidiasis in childhood. *Am J Dis Child* 1978;132:1130–1136.

255. Smith SB, Schwartzman M, Mencia LF, et al. Fatal disseminated strongyloidiasis presenting as acute abdominal distress in an urban child. *J Pediatr* 1977;91:607–609.

256. Yoeli M, Most H, Berman HH, et al. The problem of strongyloidiasis among the mentally retarded in institutions. *Trans R Soc Trop Med Hyg* 1963;57:336–345.

257. Proctor EM, Muth HA, Proudfoot DL, et al. Endemic institutional strongyloidiasis in British Columbia. *Can Med Assoc J* 1987;136:1173–1176.

258. Braun TI, Fekete T, Lynch A. Strongyloidiasis in an institution for mentally retarded adults. *Arch Intern Med* 1988;148:634–636.

259. DeVault GA Jr, King JW, Rohr MS, et al. Opportunistic infections with *Strongyloides stercoralis* in renal transplantation. *Rev Infect Dis* 1990;12:653–671.

260. Hoy WE, Roberts NJ Jr, Bryson MF, et al. Transmission of strongyloidiasis by kidney transplant? Disseminated strongyloidiasis in both recipients of kidney allografts from a single cadaver donor. *JAMA* 1981;246:1937–1939.

261. Liepman M. Disseminated *Strongyloides stercoralis*: a complication of immunosuppression. *JAMA* 1975;231:387–388.

262. Purtilo DT, Meyers WM, Connor DH. Fatal strongyloidiasis in immunosuppressed patients. *Am J Med* 1974;56:488–493.

263. Igra Siegman Y, Kapila R, Sen P, et al. Syndrome of hyperinfection with *Strongyloides stercoralis*. *Rev Infect Dis* 1981;3:397–407.

264. Talwar P, Chakrabarti A, Chawla A, et al. Fungal diarrhoea: association of different fungi and seasonal variation in their incidence. *Mycopathologia* 1990;110:101–105.

265. Guerrant RL, Bobak DA. Bacterial and protozoal gastroenteritis. *N Engl J Med* 1991;325:327–340.

266. Cohen R, Roth FJ, Delgado E, et al. Fungal flora of the normal human small and large intestine. *N Engl J Med* 1989;280:638–641.

267. Kane JG, Chretien JH, Garagusi VF. Diarrhoea caused by *Candida*. *Lancet* 1976;1:335–336.

268. Gupta TP, Ehrinpreis MN. *Candida*-associated diarrhea in hospitalized patients. *Gastroenterology* 1990;98:780–785.

269. Ullrich R, Heise W, Bergs C, et al. Gastrointestinal symptoms in patients infected with human immunodeficiency virus: relevance of infective agents isolated from gastrointestinal tract. *Gut* 1992;33:1080–1084.

270. Danna PL, Urban C, Bellin E, et al. Role of candida in pathogenesis of antibiotic-associated diarrhoea in elderly inpatients. *Lancet* 1991;337:511–514.

271. Zaidi M, Ponce de Leon S, Ortiz RM, et al. Hospital-acquired diarrhea in adults: a prospective case-controlled study in Mexico. *Infect Control Hosp Epidemiol* 1991;12:349–355.

272. Smith PD, Lane HC, Gill VJ, et al. Intestinal infections in patients with the acquired immunodeficiency syndrome (AIDS): etiology and response to therapy. *Ann Intern Med* 1988;108:328–333.

273. Laughon BE, Druckman DA, Vernon A, et al. Prevalence of enteric pathogens in homosexual men with and without acquired immunodeficiency syndrome. *Gastroenterology* 1988;94:984–993.

274. Hines J, Nachamkin I. Effective use of the clinical microbiology laboratory for diagnosing diarrheal diseases. *Clin Infect Dis* 1996;23:1291–1301.

275. Rohner P, Pittet D, Pepey B, et al. Etiological agents of infectious diarrhea: implications for requests for microbial culture. *J Clin Microbiol* 1997;35:1427–1432.

276. Chitkara YK, McCasland KA, Kenefic L. Development and implementation of cost-effective guidelines in the laboratory investigation of diarrhea in a community hospital. *Arch Intern Med* 1996;156:1445–1448.

277. Powell KR. Guidelines for the care of children and adolescents with HIV infection: approach to gastrointestinal manifestations in infants and children with HIV infection. *J Pediatr* 1991;119:S34–40.

278. Johanson JF, Sonnenberg A. Efficient management of diarrhea in the acquired immunodeficiency syndrome (AIDS): a medical decision analysis. *Ann Intern Med* 1990;112:942–948.

279. Wilcox CM, Schwartz DA, Cotsonis G, et al. Chronic unexplained diarrhea in human immunodeficiency virus infection: determination of the best diagnostic approach. *Gastroenterology* 1996;110:30–37.

280. Kato H, Kato N, Watanabe K, et al. Identification of toxin A-negative, toxin B-positive *Clostridium difficile* by PCR. *J Clin Microbiol* 1998;36:2178–2182.

281. Mitchell DK, Monroe SS, Jiang X, et al. Virologic features of an astrovirus diarrhea outbreak in a day care center revealed by reverse transcriptase-polymerase chain reaction. *J Infect Dis* 1995;172:1437–1444.

282. Jiang X, Matson DO, Cubitt WD, et al. Genetic and antigenic diversity of human caliciviruses (HuCVs) using RT-PCR and new EIAs. *Arch Virol Suppl* 1996;12:251–262.

283. Edwards P, Wodak A, Cooper DA, et al. The gastrointestinal manifestations of AIDS. *Aust N Z J Med* 1990;20:141–148.

284. Frager DH, Frager JD, Wolf EL, et al. Cytomegalovirus colitis in acquired immune deficiency syndrome: radiologic spectrum. *Gastrointest Radiol* 1986;11:241–246.

285. Dagan R, Fraser D, El-On J, et al. Evaluation of an enzyme immunoassay for the detection of *Cryptosporidium* spp. in stool specimens from infants and young children in field studies. *Am J Trop Med Hyg* 1995;52:134–138.

286. Garcia LS, Shimizu RY. Evaluation of nine immunoassay kits (enzyme immunoassay and direct fluorescence) for detection of *Giardia lamblia* and *Cryptosporidium parvum* in human fecal specimens. *J Clin Microbiol* 1997;35:1526–1529.

287. Blackman E, Binder S, Gaultier C, et al. Cryp-

tosporidiosis in HIV-infected patients: diagnostic sensitivity of stool examination, based on number of specimens submitted. *Am J Gastroenterol* 1997;92:451–453.

288. Ungar BL, Soave R, Fayer R, et al. Enzyme immunoassay detection of immunoglobulin M and G antibodies to *Cryptosporidium* in immunocompetent and immunocompromised persons. *J Infect Dis* 1986;153:570–578.

289. Knisley CV, Engelkirk PG, Pickering LK, et al. Rapid detection of giardia antigen in stool with the use of enzyme immunoassays. *Am J Clin Pathol* 1989;91:704–708.

290. Weber R, Bryan RT, Owen RL, et al. Improved light-microscopical detection of microsporidia spores in stool and duodenal aspirates. The Enteric Opportunistic Infections Working Group. *N Engl J Med* 1992; 326:161–166.

291. Didier ES, Orenstein JM, Aldras A, et al. Comparison of three staining methods for detecting microsporidia in fluids. *J Clin Microbiol* 1995;33:3138–3145.

292. David F, Schuitema ARJ, Sarfati C, et al. Detection and species identification of intestinal microsporidia by polymerase chain reaction in duodenal biopsies from human immunodeficiency virus-infected patients. *J Infect Dis* 1996;174:874–877.

293. Koga K, Kasuya S, Khamboonruang C, et al. A modified agar plate method for detection of *Strongyloides stercoralis*. *Am J Trop Med Hyg* 1991;45:518–521.

294. Liu LX, Weller PF. Strongyloidiasis and other intestinal nematode infections. *Infect Dis Clin North Am* 1993;7:655–682.

295. Mahmoud AA. Strongyloidiasis. *Clin Infect Dis* 1996; 23:949–952.

296. American Academy of Pediatrics, Provisional Committee on Quality Improvement, Subcommittee on Acute Gastroenteritis. Practice parameter: the management of acute gastroenteritis in young children. *Pediatrics* 1996;97:424–435.

297. Duggan C, Santosham M, Glass RI. The management of acute diarrhea in children: oral rehydration, maintenance, and nutritional therapy. Centers for Disease Control and Prevention. *MMWR Morb Mortal Wkly Rep* 1992;41:1–20.

298. Pickering LK, Matson DO. Therapy for diarrheal disease in children. In: Blaser MJ, Smith PD, Ravdin JI, et al., eds. *Infections of the gastrointestinal tract.* New York: Raven Press, 1995;1401–1415.

299. The choice of antibacterial drugs. *Med Lett Drugs Ther* 1998;40:33–42.

300. Recommendations for preventing the spread of vancomycin resistance: Recommendations of the Hospital Infection Control Practices Advisory Committee (HICPAC). *MMWR Morb Mortal Wkly Rep* 1995;44:1–13.

301. Khan WA, Seas C, Dhar U, et al. Treatment of shigellosis: V. Comparison of azithromycin and ciprofloxacin. A double-blind, randomized, controlled trial. *Ann Intern Med* 1997;126:697–703.

302. Salam MA, Dhar U, Khan WA, et al. Randomised comparison of ciprofloxacin suspension and pivmecillinam for childhood shigellosis. *Lancet* 1998;352:522–527.

303. Tremblay C, Gaudreau C. Antimicrobial susceptibility testing of 59 strains of *Campylobacter fetus* subsp. *fetus*. *Antimicrob Agents Chemother* 1998;42:1847–1849.

304. Drugs for parasitic infections. *Med Lett Drugs Ther* 1998;40:1–12.

305. Smith NH, Cron S, Valdez LM, et al. Combination drug therapy for cryptosporidiosis in AIDS. *J Infect Dis* 1998;178:900–903.

306. Franzen C, Fatkenheuer G, Salzberger B, et al. Intestinal microsporidiosis in patients with acquired immunodeficiency syndrome—report of three more German cases. *Infection* 1994;22:417–419.

307. Dore GJ, Marriott DJ, Hing MC, et al. Disseminated microsporidiosis due to *Septata intestinalis* in nine patients infected with the human immunodeficiency virus: response to therapy with albendazole. *Clin Infect Dis* 1995;21:70–76.

308. Lecuit M, Oksenhendler E, Sarfati C. Use of albendazole for disseminated microsporidian infection in a patient with AIDS. *Clin Infect Dis* 1994;19:332–333.

309. Weber R, Sauer B, Spycher MA, et al. Detection of *Septata intestinalis* in stool specimens and coprodiagnostic monitoring of successful treatment with albendazole. *Clin Infect Dis* 1994;19:342–345.

310. Blanshard C, Ellis DS, Tovey DG, et al. Treatment of intestinal microsporidiosis with albendazole in patients with AIDS. *AIDS* 1992;6:311–313.

311. Dieterich DT, Lew EA, Kotler DP, et al. Treatment with albendazole for intestinal disease due to *Enterocytozoon bieneusi* in patients with AIDS. *J Infect Dis* 1994;169:178–183.

312. Molina JM, Chastang C, Goguel J, et al. Albendazole for treatment and prophylaxis of microsporidiosis due to *Encephalitozoon intestinalis* in patients with AIDS: a randomized double-blind controlled trial. *J Infect Dis* 1998;177:1373–1377.

313. Systemic antifungal drugs. *Med Lett Drugs Ther* 1997; 39:86–88.

314. Garner JS. Guideline for isolation precautions in hospitals. *Infect Control Hosp Epidemiol* 1996;17:53–80.

315. The revised CDC guidelines for isolation precautions in hospitals: implications for pediatrics. *Pediatrics* 1998;101:e13.

316. 1997 USPHS/IDSA guidelines for the prevention of opportunistic infections in persons infected with human immunodeficiency virus. USPHS/IDSA Prevention of Opportunistic Infections Working Group. *MMWR Morb Mortal Wkly Rep* 1997;46:1–46.

317. Update: foodborne listeriosis—United States, 1988–1990. *MMWR Morb Mortal Wkly Rep* 1992;41: 251, 257–258.

318. Angulo FJ, Swerdlow DL. Bacterial enteric infections in persons infected with human immunodeficiency virus. *Clin Infect Dis* 1995;21[Suppl 1]:S84–S93.

319. Assessing the public health threat associated with waterborne cryptosporidiosis: report of a workshop. *MMWR Morb Mortal Wkly Rep* 1995;44:1–19.

320. Advice for travelers. *Med Lett Drugs Ther* 1998;40: 47–50.

321. Shornikova AV, Casas IA, Mykkanen H, et al. Bacteriotherapy with *Lactobacillus reuteri* in rotavirus gastroenteritis. *Pediatr Infect Dis J* 1997;16:1103–1107.

322. Typhoid immunization: recommendations of the Immunization Practices Advisory Committee (ACIP). *MMWR Morb Mortal Wkly Rep* 1990;39:1–5.

323. Woodruff BA, Pavia AT, Blake PA. A new look at typhoid vaccination: information for the practicing physician. *JAMA* 1991;265:756–759.

20

Central Nervous System Infections in the Immunocompromised Host

Ram Yogev

Department of Infectious Diseases, Northwestern University Medical School, Chicago, Illinois 60614

Infections of the central nervous system (CNS) in the immunocompromised child are infrequent. Although in recent years there has been an increase in CNS infections in adults with human immunodeficiency virus (HIV) infection related to reactivation of a latent disease, such infections are uncommon in HIV-infected children who have not yet been exposed to these pathogens (1). It is commonly thought that the immunocompromised patient is typically infected with different organisms than the normal host. Although this is true in many cases, these patients also may acquire infections with those organisms that commonly cause CNS infections in the general population. Therefore, an immunocompromised patient presenting with signs and symptoms suggestive of CNS involvement should be evaluated rapidly not only for organisms that exploit the immune defect but also for common pathogens. It may be difficult to appreciate a CNS infection in an immunocompromised patient, because some patients have multiple organ involvement that can mask the CNS manifestations. In addition, the reduced inflammatory response due to immunosuppression may greatly diminish the clinical manifestations of a disease, resulting in subtle signs and symptoms. The diagnosis can be difficult, so the slightest suspicion of CNS involvement—as suggested by headache, focal neurologic signs, or altered mental state—should prompt a full diagnostic workup. After an appropriate physical examination, laboratory studies should include cerebrospinal fluid (CSF) cell count, differential count, and cytology; protein and glucose levels; Gram, India ink, and acid-fast stains; aerobic and anaerobic cultures as well as fungal and acid-fast cultures; and various antigen determinations (e.g., common pathogens, Cryptococcus). In addition, radiographic examinations can be invaluable in reaching the diagnosis without a brain biopsy, as when the ring-enhancing lesions of *Toxoplasma gondii* are seen on computed tomography (CT) scans.

The spectrum of CNS infections in an immunocompromised child depends to a large extent on the nature of the underlying disease (Table 20.1) For example, patients with Hodgkin's disease have a cell-mediated immune defect and are especially susceptible to infections caused by intracellular organisms such as *Listeria monocytogenes, Cryptococcus neoformans,* and *T. gondii.* Splenectomy for staging in Hodgkin's patients decreases the phagocytic mass and impairs the humoral response to capsular antigens, making these patients more vulnerable to infections with encapsulated bacteria such as *Streptococcus pneumoniae* and *Haemophilus influenzae.* In contrast, patients with leukemia who develop neutropenia, either as part of their malignancy or in response to chemotherapy, are more

TABLE 20.1. *Common opportunistic pathogens in various immunocompromised hosts*

Predisposing factors	Most common isolated opportunistic pathogens
T-cell defect (e.g., lymphoma, HIV)	*Listeria monocytogenes, Candida, Toxoplasma, Cryptococcus, Nocardia*, mycobacteria
Neutropenia	*Pseudomonas, Escherichia coli, Serratia, Candida, Staphylococcus epidermidis, Aspergillus*
Splenectomy, sickle-cell disease, asplenia, *Streptococcus pneumoniae, Haemophilus influenzae, Neisseria meningitidis, Salmonella*	*Streptococcus pneumoniae, Haemophilus influenzae, Neisseria meningitidis, Salmonella*
Indwelling catheters, *Corynebacterium,* intraventricular shunt or reservoir	*Staphylococcus epidermidis, Staphylococcus,*
Hypogammaglobulinemia, *Staphylococcus*	*Candida, Serratia, Enterobacter*
nephrotic syndrome	*S. pneumoniae, H. influenzae,* Enteric bacteria,
Transplantation	*aureus, N. meningitidis*
Immunosuppression (e.g., steroid therapy)	*Pseudomonas, Candida, Aspergillus*
	Staphylococci, *Klebsiella cytomegalovirus,* hepatitis viruses

HIV, human immunodeficiency virus.

likely to develop a CNS infection with an organism that is usually removed from the blood by neutrophils. Such organisms include *Pseudomonas aeruginosa, Escherichia coli,* and *Staphylococcus aureus.* In addition, the enhanced susceptibility of leukemic patients to certain organisms (e.g., *P. aeruginosa*) may be partly related to their inability to develop specific opsonins (2). The development of lymphopenia may predispose to infection with viruses and fungi. Another example is patients with cancer who receive indwelling intravenous or urinary catheters, CNS intraventricular shunts or reservoirs, parenteral alimentation, and/or broad-spectrum antibiotics. These therapeutic maneuvers facilitate access of opportunistic organisms to sterile body fluids. Representative pathogens of this group are *Enterobacter cloacae, Candida albicans,* coagulase-negative staphylococci, and group D streptococci. Table 20.1 lists other immune defects or predisposing factors for CNS infections and the most common pathogens expected in the various situations.

The spectrum of potential CNS infections includes meningitis, meningoencephalitis, encephalitis, and brain abscess. Because the list of likely opportunistic pathogens is very long, only the more common or unique offenders are discussed here.

MENINGITIS AND MENINGOENCEPHALITIS

The common underlying conditions causing meningitis or meningoencephalitis in the immunocompromised patient are impaired cell-mediated and/or humoral immunity, bacteremia or sepsis, nosocomial infection after administration of intrathecal chemotherapy, and complications of intraventricular shunts or reservoirs. As can be seen from Table 20.1, *C. neoformans* and *L. monocytogenes* are the typical pathogens in patients with defects in cell-mediated immunity, whereas gram-negative bacteria are more common in patients with humoral defects. *Staphylococcus epidermidis, Candida,* and other pathogens commonly colonizing the skin are expected in patients with neutropenia, indwelling catheters, or intraventricular devices.

Bacterial Infections

Listeria monocytogenes *Infection*

L. monocytogenes is widespread and has been isolated from water, soil, sewage, and various animals. Epidemiologic data suggest that food may be a major source of transmission of the bacteria from animals to humans, as illustrated by several foodborne outbreaks

(3). The bacteria probably enter the body via the gastrointestinal tract, and decreased immune resistance predisposes to infection. This explains why *L. monocytogenes* infections are increasingly observed in newborns, elderly individuals, and immunocompromised patients. Coinfection with other organisms of the gastrointestinal tract may precipitate dissemination of the bacteria to other organs (4). Cellular immune impairment (T cell–mediated) plays an important role in enhancing susceptibility to this infection, which explains the increased incidence of listeriosis in patients with lymphoreticular malignances, transplantation (5), or acquired immunodeficiency syndrome (AIDS) (6).

L. monocytogenes has a particular tropism for the CNS, and meningitis is the most commonly reported infection with this bacteria (3), although brain abscess is rarely reported (7). In adults, a rare brain-stem encephalitis (rhombencephalitis) is also rarely reported (8). The ratio of immunocompromised to normal patients with severe *Listeria* infections is probably higher than that for any other bacteria. For example, it has been estimated that the risk of listeriosis in patients with AIDS is hundreds of times that in the general population (6). Therefore, if *L. monocytogenes* is isolated in a patient who is not a neonate, the possibility of an immunocompromised condition should be considered.

L. monocytogenes is a gram-positive rod that can be seen in a Gram stain of the CSF as residing intracellularly or extracellularly. Because of its diphtheroid-like shape and possible variable morphology, it can be confused with other bacteria. The rod shape is indistinguishable from that of *Corynebacterium* or *Erysipelothrix,* and only the characteristic tumbling motility at 25°C (77°F) of *Listeria* is helpful in distinguishing among them. The coccobacillary forms may resemble *S. pneumoniae,* and an overdecolorized gram stain may cause confusion with gram-negative rods. The hemolysis that *Listeria* produces on subculturing may lead to confusion with group A streptococci. The ability of *Listeria* to grow at relatively low temperatures can be used to increase its isolation rate (9).

The mode of transmission in most immunocompromised patients is unknown, but foodborne infection is probably the most common route (6). Hospital-associated clustering in these patients has been described (10).

Listeria meningitis usually manifests with symptoms and signs commonly seen with many other CNS infections. No significant difference in clinical presentation (i.e., signs and symptoms) was found between immunocompromised and previously healthy patients (11). Because listeriosis is high on the list of possible pathogens in the immunocompromised host with T-cell and/or mononuclear phagocyte impairment, and because the mortality rate with late treatment is high, a lumbar puncture should be performed promptly in any patient who shows even minimal signs of CNS involvement (e.g., irritability, headaches, mental changes). The CSF often reveals an elevated white blood cell (WBC) count, ranging between 150 and 3,000 cells per microliter with a predominance of neutrophils. Sometimes monocytes and macrophages are seen and can be characteristic for *L. monocytogenes.* Protein concentration, although usually high, can be in the normal range, and the glucose level can range from normal to undetectable. Gram stains of the CSF are positive in fewer than 50% of cases (12), because the number of organisms in the CSF is lower than the number needed for a positive stain (i.e., 5×10^5 per microliter). If the Gram stain is positive, short gram-positive rods are seen extracellularly or intracellularly. To increase the yield of the Gram stain, inspection of the sediment from centrifuged CSF (at least 5 to 10 mL) maybe considered. In addition, incubation of the CSF for 12 hours at 22° to 35°C causes the bacteria to multiply rapidly and increases the yield of the Gram stain. Several serologic tests have been developed, but none of them should be routinely used (13). Cultivation of the organism is the only reliable means for definitive diagnosis. If the patient received antibiotics before the lumbar puncture, a portion of the CSF specimen should be cultured using an antibiotic-removing device. The addition of nalidixic acid, polymyxin B, sodium thiosulfate, and potassium tellurate to the appropriate basic medium increases the yield of positive cultures.

In vitro studies suggest that, although *L. monocytogenes* is susceptible *in vitro* to ampicillin, penicillin, and chloramphenicol (14), these drugs are only bacteriostatic in levels achievable in the CSF. In addition, none of the second- and third-generation cephalosporins commonly used to treat meningitis (e.g., cefuroxime, cefotaxime, ceftriaxone) is active against *L. monocytogenes*. Furthermore, the concentration of these antibiotics needed to kill the bacteria (e.g., the minimal bactericidal concentration) is often higher than the levels attained in the CSF, making them even less effective in eradicating the bacteria, especially in immunocompromised hosts. There is evidence both *in vitro* and from studies of immunodeficient animals that the combination of ampicillin and an aminoglycoside (e.g., gentamicin) acts synergistically against *L. monocytogenes* (15). The combination of trimethoprim and sulfamethoxazole (TMP/SMX) was also effective in an animal model (16), but the role of rifampin treatment in such infections is controversial (16,17). Newer antibiotics such as macrolides and quinolones are only moderately effective against *Listeria* and should not be considered for therapy.

The treatment of choice for *L. monocytogenes* meningitis in the immunocompromised patient is the combination of ampicillin (400 mg per kilogram per day given every 6 hours) and an aminoglycoside (e.g., gentamicin, 7 .5 mg per kilogram per day, or amikacin, 22.5 mg per kilogram per day given every 8 hours). If the patient is allergic to penicillin, desensitization should be attempted. Alternative therapy with TMP/SMX was reported to be successful in *L. monocytogenes* meningitis (18,19) and should be offered to patients for whom initial therapy with ampicillin and an aminoglycoside has failed. Chloramphenicol is less effective than ampicillin, and the combination of the two drugs appeared to be inferior to ampicillin alone. Therefore, chloramphenicol—as well as erythromycin, tetracycline, and vancomycin—should be avoided, if possible.

Delayed bacterial clearance of the CSF has been observed in some immunocompromised patients despite seemingly appropriate therapy (19a). A lumbar puncture is suggested every other day until eradication is documented. If the organism is still present after the second lumbar puncture, the possibility of cerebritis or brain abscess should be investigated. In some such cases, CT has revealed not only cerebritis but also cerebellar atrophy and development of hydrocephalus (20). If the patient responds to therapy with prompt clinical improvement (defervescence within 72 hours) and the culture of the second lumbar puncture (48 hours after initiation of therapy) is negative, 10 to 14 days of treatment is adequate. However, if the response is slower, a longer period of therapy is needed (e.g., 21 days).

Other Bacterial Agents

Bacterial meningitis due to encapsulated bacteria (e.g., *S. pneumoniae*, *Neisseria meningitidis*) remains a relatively common disease in children and may also affect the immunocompromised child. In general, the incidence of meningitis caused by these organisms is not increased in most immunocompromised hosts (e.g., cancer patients). However, in patients with congenital deficiency (e.g., hypogammaglobulinemia) or acquired deficiency (e.g., Hodgkin's disease after chemotherapy) of humoral immunity or defects in thymic-dependent function, an increased incidence of bacterial meningitis has been reported. Congenital asplenia or splenectomy also has been associated with increased incidences of *S. pneumoniae* and *H. influenzae* meningitis (20a). Children with hemoglobinopathies (e.g., sickle cell disease) are more prone to meningitis with these bacteria or with *Salmonella*, and deficiencies in various components of the complement system predispose to an increased risk of *N. meningitidis* or *S. pneumoniae* meningitis (21,22). The diagnosis rests on CSF examination, which should include specific tests (e.g., latex particle agglutination) to detect bacterial antigens. If an encapsulated bacterium is suspected as the cause of the meningitis, the initial treatment, before the etiologic agent is verified, should include a third-generation cephalosporin (i.e., ceftriaxone or cefotaxime) combined with vancomycin (because of the recent rapid increase in resistance of *S. pneumoniae* to penicillin). The choice of antibiotics if other bacteria are suspected should be based on the type of underlying immune abnormality; for example, in patients with neutropenia, one should also treat for *Pseudomonas* (Table 20.2).

Gram-negative bacteria are not a rare cause of meningitis in the immunocompromised host. *E. coli* and *P. aeruginosa* are two of the most common etiologic agents in patients with neutropenia. Other, less common bacteria include *Klebsiella pneumoniae, Proteus mirabilis, Enterobacter* sp., and *Acinetobacter* sp. Most of these bacteria are found in the gastrointestinal tract and may invade the bloodstream through rectal fissures or inapparent ulcers resulting from chemotherapy and thrombocytopenia. They reach the CNS by the hematogenous route. In a few patients, colonization of the nasopharynx with gram-negative bacteria during broad-spectrum antibiotic therapy, chronic suppurative otitis media, or intubation may lead to CNS spread via anatomic defects or by extension of local infections such as sinusitis or otitis media. *P. aeruginosa* is also commonly found in sinks, humidifiers, water, and vegetables, which facilitate its colonization of the gastrointestinal tract of immunocompromised patients admitted to the hospital and may explain its role as a cause of sepsis and meningitis in this population.

Usually, meningitis caused by a gram-negative bacterium manifests with acute signs and symptoms of meningeal irritation, including high fever, headaches, vomiting, neck stiffness and irritability, or mental changes. The CSF is

TABLE 20.2. *Common in vitro antibiotic susceptibility of gram-negative bacteria*

Bacteria	Common resistances	Suggested therapy
Pseudomonas aeruginosa	Ceftriaxone Cefotaxime Cefuroxime	Ceftazidime or Aztreonam or Aminoglycoside[a] + antipseudomonal penicillin
Escherichia coli	Ampicillin	Third-generation cephalosporin + antipseudomonal penicillin or Meropenem or Aztreonam or Trimethoprim-sulfamethoxazole
Klebsiella pneumoniae	Ampicillin	Third-generation cephalosporin ± aminoglycoside or
	Carbenicillin Ticarcillin	Aztreonam or Trimethoprim-sulfamethoxazole
Proteus mirabilis Acinetobacter spp.	Ampicillin	As for E. coli
Haemophilus influenzae	Ampicillin Chloramphenicol	Third-generation cephalosporin or Meropenem
Neisseria meningitidis		Penicillin or Third-generation cephalosporin

[a]In each geographic area, the particular aminoglycoside should depend on the *in vitro* sensitivity of isolates in that area.

usually purulent with a predominance of polymorphonuclear leukocytes. Especially in neutropenic patients, the clinical presentation may be subtle as a result of the reduced ability of the host to mount a vigorous inflammatory response, and few WBCs may be found in the CSF. This is also true for patients with severe sepsis and leukopenia. Therefore, a peripheral blood count is important to help in the evaluation of the CSF WBC count. The CSF protein is commonly elevated and the CSF glucose is decreased. Usually a Gram stain reveals many gram-negative bacilli.

The definitive identification of the offending gram-negative species is important because the various bacteria have important differences in their susceptibility to antibiotics (Table 20.2). As can be seen from Table 20.2, the third-generation cephalosporins (e.g., cefotaxime, ceftriaxone) are the drugs of choice to treat gram-negative bacillary meningitis. Although aminoglycosides played a major role in the treatment of gram-negative bacterial meningitis in the past, their penetration into the CSF was erratic and their track records were relatively poor (40% to 80% mortality). Ceftazidime is recommended for treatment of *P. aeruginosa* meningitis because it is the only cephalosporin that sufficiently penetrates the blood-brain barrier to reach concentrations within the CSF required to kill susceptible strains (23). If the patient does not respond to the initial therapy, an alternative regimen should be considered; or, on rare occasions, intraventricular administration of an aminoglycoside without preservatives may be indicated. *K. pneumoniae* strains are almost always resistant to carbenicillin and ticarcillin; therefore, an aminoglycoside and a third-generation cephalosporin are recommended, instead of the more traditional therapy of an aminoglycoside and an antipseudomonal penicillin. Aztreonam (a monobactam antibiotic) is effective against most gram-negative bacteria, including *P. aeruginosa*, and may be used in selected patients (24). Meropenem (a carbapenem) is another antibiotic that is effective in the treatment of bacterial meningitis; it should be

considered in cases caused by organisms resistant to the third-generation cephalosporins (25). Although the fluoroquinolones seem to be effective against gram-negative bacterial meningitis, the limited available data and the restricted use of these drugs in children in the United States suggest that they should be considered only for patients infected with multidrug-resistant strains who fail to respond to standard therapy.

Coagulase-Negative Staphylococcus

This is a rare cause of meningitis in immunocompromised hosts, despite the fact that it is one of the most common causes of bacteremia and sepsis in this population (26). Coagulase-negative *Staphylococcus* is a gram-positive bacterium that can be differentiated from *S. aureus* by its colonial morphology and by its fermentation of mannitol and production of nucleases. There are at least 29 coagulase-negative species that can be differentiated by their biochemical characteristics (27), but *S. epidermidis* is by far the most common isolate from CNS infections. The introduction of intraventricular devices such as ventriculoperitoneal shunts and Ommaya reservoirs to facilitate the administration of chemotherapy to leukemic patients has increased the incidence of CNS infection with *S. epidermidis*, which is the most common organism to colonize these devices. Many other bacteria can cause CNS infections of the intraventricular device. *S. aureus*, group D streptococci, *Corynebacterium*, *Propionibacterium acnes*, and gram-negative enteric bacteria are only few of the more commonly isolated pathogens (28,29). The ability of *S. epidermidis* to produce a polysaccharide substance (slime), particularly when a foreign body is present (30), may explain why this agent is so prevalent in foreign body infections. Slime production seems to interfere with polymorphonuclear function; it also increases the ability of the organism to erode the surface of the device and to adhere to it. In the immunocompromised host, the interruption of skin integrity combined with neutropenia or neutrophil dysfunction and impairment of other facets of the cellular immune mechanism involved in staphylococcal immunity contribute to the increase in staphylococcal infections including meningitis in this population.

Most patients with intraventricular device infection are asymptomatic. However, some present with fever, local cellulitis (along the shunt or around the device), headache, loss of appetite, vomiting, and, rarely, meningismus. A major dilemma, especially in the asymptomatic patient, is how to interpret a positive culture result from a routine CSF sample obtained when chemotherapy is given through the intraventricular device. The possible options include contamination from the skin, colonization of the device, and infection (e.g., ventriculitis, meningitis). Extra care in cleansing the skin before the intraventricular reservoir is punctured eliminates many cases of skin contamination. Because many patients are asymptomatic, close follow-up without antibiotics is appropriate. Repeat cultures may be helpful in reaching a decision. If the cultures continue to be positive and an increase in the WBC count (with an increase in neutrophils) is noted, the patient should receive antibiotics. On the other hand, if the patient remains asymptomatic and no change in the CSF parameters (i.e., WBC, glucose, or protein) is noted, the patient may be observed closely for development of signs or symptoms of meningeal irritation. If the decision is made to treat the patient with antibiotics and the patient is asymptomatic, it is not always necessary to remove the intraventricular device in order to eradicate the infection. The intraventricular reservoir should be removed only if CSF cultures continue to be positive despite antibiotic therapy, the patient develops signs and symptoms suggestive of meningitis, or there is local cellulitis around the device.

Most *S. epidermidis* isolates are resistant to penicillin and ampicillin, and frequently they are also resistant to the semisynthetic penicillins, such as nafcillin, oxacillin, and methicillin. If the staphylococcus is resistant to the semisynthetic penicillins, it should be considered resistant to all β-lactam antibiotics, including cephalosporins, even if *in vitro* data suggest that it is sensitive (31). For treatment of *S. epidermidis* (*S. aureus*) ventriculitis or meningitis in areas where less than 10% to 15% of the isolates are resistant to methicillin, nafcillin (200 mg per kilogram per day, given intravenously every 6 hours) is the drug of choice. If the staphylococcus is resistant to methicillin or there is a high prevalence of methicillin-resistant strains (more than 15%), intravenous vancomycin (50 to 60 mg per kilogram per day, given every 6 hours) is the drug of choice. Vancomycin should be used sparingly, because widespread use may result in the emergence of vancomycin-resistant organisms. Reports of *S. epidermidis* relatively resistant to vancomycin suggest that coagulase-negative staphylococci have the ability to acquire vancomycin resistance (32). A change in therapy may be needed if there is no clinical or bacteriologic response. Gentamicin or rifampin may be added if *in vitro* tests show synergism and no antagonism between these antibiotics and vancomycin (33).

Fungal Infections

Cryptococcus neoformans *Infection*

This fungus is probably the most common cause of fungal meningitis in immunosuppressed hosts such as children with leukemia, lymphoma, congenital or acquired immunodeficiency, organ transplantation, or extended steroid therapy. Infection with *C. neoformans* probably occurs through the respiratory tract after inhalation of the fungus, although the gastrointestinal tract may also be the initial portal of entry. Dissemination occurs via the bloodstream with a predilection to the CNS. In one study that included both immunocompetent and immunodeficient patients, 76% of patients had CNS involvement (34). Meningitis is the most common event, with development of subarachnoid exudates. The cellular reaction in the CSF is usually mild. Rarely, with more extensive infection, the fungus moves along blood vessels into various areas of the brain substance, producing small cysts in the gray or white matter; the reaction of the host (i.e., production of granuloma) may result in a presentation like that of space-occupying lesions.

The most common presenting complaints are headache and low-grade fever. Lethargy, vomiting, altered mentation, and visual deficits are less common. Rarely, stiff neck, seizures, or focal neurologic symptoms are the presenting symptoms. The symptoms can be very subtle, and their duration before diagnosis varies from a few days to months. On physical examination papilledema may be present, but nuchal rigidity, cranial nerve involvement including diplopia, and cerebellar signs are infrequent findings. Examination of the CSF reveals fewer than 500 WBCs per microliter, mostly mononuclear leukocytes, with minimal changes in glucose and protein. Gram stain is sometimes helpful in showing a gramnegative capsule with a bluish center, but India ink preparation is very helpful, with more than 50% of the cases giving positive results (35). With an India ink preparation, a defined halo around the organism or budding must be seen for the diagnosis to be made. Red blood cells, WBCs, or granular contaminants (e.g., talcum, starch) may be confused with the organism. Cultures of CSF yield the organism in approximately 90% of patients (depending on the collection and processing of the specimen), although sometimes the organism can be diagnosed only by detection of cryptococcal antigen in serum or CSF. The latex agglutination test for the cryptococcal polysaccharide antigen is specific, sensitive, simple, and rapid. Titers equal to or greater than 1:4 suggest the diagnosis of cryptococcal infection, if the appropriate controls (to rule out the presence of rheumatoid factor or other nonspecific agglutinins) are negative. However, smallcapsule *Cryptococcus* strains do not produce much antigen and the latex agglutination test can be negative. Enzyme immunoassays using monoclinal or polyclonal antibody to detect this antigen are also available, and their results correlate well with those obtained with latex agglutination (36).

In vitro studies indicate that almost all cryptococcal strains are sensitive to amphotericin B and that amphotericin B and flucytosine are additive in their effects (36a). Clinical studies showed only a trend in favor of the combination, and therefore treatment can be with amphotericin alone or in combination with flucytosine. It has been reported that use of fluorocytosine during the first 2 weeks of therapy is associated with a much lower risk of relapse (37). The recommended dose is intravenous amphotericin B, 0.5 to 0.7 mg per kilogram per day if amphotericin is used alone, or 0.3 to 0.5 mg per kilogram per day if it is used in combination with oral 5-fluorocytosine (100 to 150 mg per kilogram per day given every 6 hours). The duration of therapy should be 6 weeks. A 4-week course should be reserved only for patients who have meningitis without neurologic complications, a pretreatment CSF WBC count higher than 20 cells per microliter, and a serum cryptococcal antigen titer below 1:32. A negative CSF India ink staining and serum and CSF cryptococcal antigen below 1:8 is also required (38). Repeat weekly lumbar punctures to document a decrease in cryptococcal antigen and sterility of culture are useful in evaluating the response to treatment. Serum antigen titers are not helpful for this purpose (39). Even with 6 weeks of therapy, the relapse rate is high (about 20%) and the toxicity of the combination is approximately 40%, suggesting that combination therapy is far from ideal (38).

Oral fluconazole (8 to 12 mg per kilogram per day twice daily) is an acceptable alternative (at least in AIDS patients) for maintenance treatment of this infection. Initial therapy with fluconazole alone is not recommended because it is associated with more failures (compared with amphotericin B therapy) in the first few weeks. However, after initial amphotericin B therapy for 2 weeks, switching to fluconazole has been very successful (39a). Itraconazole (100 mg per day once or twice daily for children 3 to 16 years of age) may be considered as an alternative treatment in some cases. Yet, its poor penetration into the CSF suggests that it should be used cautiously (40). In patients who are intolerant of amphotericin B, liposomal amphotericin B (5 mg per kilogram per day as a starting dose) may be considered (41).

A serum cryptococcal antigen titer greater than 1:32 before therapy and CSF titers greater than 1:8 at the end of therapy are more likely to be associated with failure or relapse. However, pretreatment CSF titers are not predictive of the outcome. Clinical parameters, such as headache and diagnosis of AIDS, were predictive of better survival (42).

The high relapse rate after cessation of therapy favors maintenance therapy for as long as immunosuppression continues. The drug of choice is fluconazole (6 mg per kilogram per day once daily) (43). Neither itraconazole nor weekly doses of amphotericin B seems to be better in reducing the recurrence rate (43a).

Candida *Species*

C. albicans is part of the normal human flora and is the most commonly isolated fungus from the normal flora of the mouth and the gastrointestinal tract. Rarely, *C. albicans* causes CNS infections in immunocompromised hosts. Other *Candida* species, such as *Candida tropicalis, Candida krusei,* and *Candida parapsilosis,* can also cause infection in these patients. *Candida* species can be found in two morphologic forms, yeast about 3 to 5 μm in diameter and hyphae, which are filamentous structures. The presence of hyphae in a biologic specimen signifies tissue invasion. The increased frequency of *C. albicans* (compared with other *Candida* species) as a cause of disease in humans is a result of its increased virulence and abundance during exposure of the immunocompromised host.

Many defects in host defense can facilitate a candidal CNS infection (44,45). Patients with impaired neutrophil function are particularly susceptible to infection with *C. albicans.* Indwelling intravascular catheters or catheterization of the bladder may provide a portal of entry for the fungus. Another major source for *Candida* dissemination is the gastrointestinal tract. Therapy with antibiotics, steroids, and immunosuppressive drugs also predisposes the patient to *Candida* infections. With the widespread use of these drugs, there is an increase in candidemia. The increased prevalence of candidemia in the immunocompromised host is a major risk factor for spread to the meninges to cause meningitis. Direct inoculation into the CSF through intraventricular devices or via intrathecal chemotherapy is another source of the infection.

The clinical course of candidal meningitis is frequently indolent, with low-grade fever and lack of signs and symptoms of meningeal irritation (44,45). This mild symptomatology contributes, in many cases, to the interpretation of a *Candida* isolate from the CSF as a contaminant. The CSF usually reveals only mild to moderate pleocytosis with predominance of either mononuclear or polymorphonuclear cells. In more than one third of the patients, no pleocytosis is found. The protein levels range from normal to mildly elevated, and the glucose concentrations may be normal or depressed. Hypoglycorrhachia is present in fewer than 50% of the cases (46). Gram stain may be helpful in the diagnosis, showing a gram-positive yeast and sometime hyphae budding from the yeast cells. However, isolation of *Candida* species from the CSF is not always achievable. A partial explanation for this observation may be that, in many cases of CNS candidiasis, the infection affects the parenchyma of the brain without meningeal involvement, and unless the infection encroaches on the subarachnoid space, the CSF findings are negative or inconspicuous. The CNS lesions caused by *Candida* include parenchymal microabscesses, vasculitis from invasion of the vessel wall, mycotic aneurysm, demyelination, and transverse myelitis. CT is very helpful in revealing these infections.

Several available serologic tests, such as complement fixation, indirect fluorescent antibodies, and agglutinins, have been shown to be of little value in diagnosing systemic *Candida* infection, at least in part because colonization alone can result in a rise of antibody titers. The detection of *Candida* antibodies in the CSF may be helpful in the diagnosis and should be used more often (47). Detection of *Candida* antigenemia in patients with disseminated disease by counterimmunoelectrophoresis or enzyme-linked immunosorbent assay (ELISA) seems to be better for early detection of the infection. In addition, the application of antigen detection (e.g., mannan, D-arabinitol) in the CSF of patients with candidal CNS infection may be helpful in establishing the diagnosis when other laboratory tests have failed. Studies using polymerase chain reaction (PCR) for the identification of *Candida* in clinical specimens are encouraging (48).

In vitro studies of *Candida* sensitivity to various antifungal agents are difficult to perform and to interpret. In addition, amphotericin B, the basic therapeutic agent available today for invasive *Candida* disease, penetrates poorly through the blood-brain barrier, and its concentration in the CSF is usually undetectable by bioassay. In contrast, 5-fluorocytosine achieves high concentrations in the CSF (greater than 50% of the serum concentration). Clinical experience with the combination of amphotericin B and 5-fluorocytosine suggests that it is effective and may be better than amphotericin B alone (49). Therefore, the combination of amphotericin B (1 mg per kilogram per day in one dose) and 5-fluorocytosine (100 to 150 mg per kilogram per day every 6 hours) should be the treatment of choice. Treatment should be given for 4 to 6 weeks, and in complicated cases a longer period should be considered. With appropriate therapy, mortality can be reduced to 10% or less.

Other Fungal Agents

Rarely, fungi other than *Candida* cause meningitis. *Coccidioides immitis* is one example. This fungus is usually spread to the CNS from the lung. A unique feature of *Coccidioides* meningitis is the frequent occurrence of eosinophilia (more than 10 eosinophils per microliter) in the CSF (50). However, fewer than one third of patients have a positive CSF culture, and direct examination is usually negative. In these patients,

only the presence of complement-fixing antibodies in the CSF may suggest the diagnosis. However, only 75% of patients with active meningitis demonstrated this antibody (51), and an even lower percentage is expected in immunocompromised hosts. The treatment of choice is amphotericin B, which should be given for several months. Treatment with fluconazole or itraconazole demonstrated clinical improvement in up to 80% of the patients (52,53), but the relapse rate is high, suggesting that these drugs are effective in suppressing the disease but not in eradicating the fungus (54). If they are used, a very prolonged therapy (i.e., years) will be needed.

Viral Infections

Herpesviruses (e.g., herpes simplex virus [HSV], varicella-zoster virus [VZV], human herpesvirus-6) are unusual causes of meningitis without apparent involvement of the brain (i.e., encephalitis, discussed later) (55,56). The clinical course is indistinguishable from other cases of aseptic meningitis, and the outcome is usually good. PCR testing of the CSF may be useful in identifying the etiologic agent when viral cultures are negative.

Although most seasonal cases of aseptic meningitis without serious morbidity in immunocompromised hosts are probably caused by enteroviruses (as in the general population), these viruses can cause a severe and chronic CNS infection in children with antibody deficiencies (e.g., hypogammaglobulinemia). Most reported patients with chronic enteroviral meningoencephalitis (CEM) had X-linked agammaglobulinemia (X-LA), and some had common variable immunodeficiency (CVID) (57). Severe deficiency of mature B cells, a distinctive feature of X-LA, predisposes to CEM. The echoviruses (especially echovirus 11) cause most cases of CEM. The clinical presentation includes (a) total absence of CNS symptoms in patients who present with edema or a dermatomyositis-like syndrome and subsequently develop neurologic symptoms; (b) acute onset of aseptic meningitis with fever, headache, and altered mental status that fails to resolve within 7 to 10 days; or (c) the more typical presentation of slow and progressive development of neurologic symptoms. Because of the diversity in the clinical presentation of CEM, any patient with hypogammaglobulinemia who develops a neurologic symptoms should be investigated for this disease. The CSF in most patients reveals a mild lymphocytic pleocytosis (fewer than 1,000 cells per microliter), elevated protein (50 to 500 mg/dL) and mild hypoglycorrhachia (15 to 40 mg/dL). Confirmation of CEM requires isolation of an enterovirus from the CSF, which is more easily achieved during the onset or exacerbation of the CNS symptoms. Treatment with intravenous gammaglobulin has been shown to improve and stabilize the infection but relapses are reported (57).

ENCEPHALITIS

The prevalence of viral encephalitis in immunocompromised hosts is higher than in the general population. Patients with humoral immune defects more commonly develop meningoencephalitis due to enteroviruses (see previous discussion), whereas patients with impaired T-lymphocyte or mononuclear phagocyte function are more susceptible to the herpesviruses (e.g., HSV, cytomegalovirus [CMV], and Epstein-Barr virus [EBV]), measles, and adenovirus. In addition, these patients have a higher prevalence of *T. gondii* encephalitis.

The common clinical presentation of patients with early encephalitis is sometimes indistinguishable from meningitis because in many cases both the brain and the meninges are involved (e.g., meningoencephalitis). The meningeal irritation causes fever, headache, photophobia, and nuchal rigidity, while brain involvement is evidenced by altered mentation, confusion, behavioral and speech disturbances, focal neurologic signs, and seizures. With progression of the infection, stupor and coma develop. The specific diagnosis of encephalitis in the immunocompromised patient is difficult for several reasons: (a) many other conditions such as toxins, metabolic changes, or spread of a neoplastic process may imitate infectious encephalitis; (b) routine examination of the CSF is not very helpful because in most instances it shows a mild to moderate pleocytosis with mostly mononuclear cells, mild (if any) elevation of protein, and normal to decreased glucose; and (c) in many cases serology is not very helpful because a rise in antibody titer may not develop. However, it is important to pursue a specific diagnosis (even with a brain biopsy), because increasingly specific treatments are available to improve the outcome in these patients.

Parasitic Infections: *Toxoplasma gondii*

CNS toxoplasmosis can occur rarely in a variety of immunocompromised hosts. These include patients with malignancies (58) and those with heart or heart-lung transplants (59), bone marrow transplants (60), or renal transplants (61). In addition, patients receiving immunosuppressive therapy (e.g., prolonged corticosteroids) and those with a collagen vascular disorder (e.g., systemic lupus erythematosus) may also develop this complication. In recent years the incidence of CNS toxoplasmosis increased dramatically among adult AIDS patients. Yet, *Toxoplasma* encephalitis is rare in HIV-infected children (fewer than 1% of children with AIDS).

The parasite exists in three forms: the oocyst, which is found in cat feces; the tachyzoite, which is seen in the acute phase of infection in humans; and the cyst, which develops when the infection reaches the latent or chronic stage. Transmission is usually from contaminated material (soil, meat) to humans. Transmission from human to human is very rare and may occur via blood or leukocyte transfusion or organ transplantation.

The acute infection (tachyzoite stage) is usually asymptomatic. After local invasion of the tissues, termination of the infection depends both on cell-mediated immunity and humoral antibodies. If the host is able to maintain a good cell-mediated response, recrudescence of a latent infection will not occur (62). In the immunocompromised host, the development of *T. gondii* infection may occur as a result of acquisition of new infection; reactivation of cysts with release of tachyzoites, which then invade contiguous brain cells causing tissue destruction; or hematogenous spread of the parasite with specific tropism to the CNS. In the brain, necrosis of the parenchyma occurs because of vascular involvement. The necrosis may progress to form cysts with calcifications.

The clinical manifestations of the disease vary from slowly progressing neurologic impairment to acute mental deterioration with or without focal neurologic signs such as seizures, hemiparesis or hemiplegia, visual field defects, or cranial nerve palsies.

Because the routine CSF examination in suspected patients is not contributory to the diagnosis, the diagnosis of *T. gondii* infection is established by isolation of the parasite from body fluids or by serology. However, isolation of the parasite takes too long to permit early diagnosis. Most laboratories use the indirect fluorescent antibody test, the ELISA, or the immunoglobulin M (IgM) or IgE immunosorbent agglutination assay to make the diagnosis. Antibody response to *T. gondii* may be impaired in immunocompromised hosts, and therefore a negative serology result does not exclude the diagnosis. Determination of CSF *Toxoplasma* antibody, produced intrathecally, may be useful in the diagnosis of *Toxoplasma* encephalitis (63). Serologic changes may occur during an asymptomatic infection that does not involve the CNS, and an immunocompromised patient with asymptomatic toxoplasmosis may develop a CNS infection with another agent. Demonstration of the tachyzoite form of the parasite in tissue (e.g., brain biopsy) or in the CSF in tissue culture (64) or by use of PCR (65) may be the only way to establish the diagnosis. CT and magnetic resonance imaging (MRI) are almost always positive in patients with *Toxoplasma* encephalitis.

The treatment of active toxoplasmosis should include the combination of pyrimethamine (1 mg per kilogram per day every day) and sulfadiazine (50 mg per kilogram per day every 12 hours). Both drugs achieve acceptable CSF levels and have been shown to be effective. The combination of clindamycin (30 to 40 mg per kilogram per day divided every 16 hours) and pyrimethamine, which was shown to be beneficial in patients with CNS toxoplasmosis, should be used for patients who are allergic to sulfadiazine. Folinic acid (5 to 10 mg 2 to 3 times per week) should be added to both combinations. Therapy should be continued for at least 6 weeks, and prednisone (2 mg per kilogram per day in divided doses) can be added in cases of cerebral edema or chorioretinitis. Although the combined therapy is very effective in suppressing the acute episode, the relapse rate is high in patients who remained severely immunocompromised (e.g., AIDS patients). Therefore, maintenance therapy is required and pyrimethamine (0.25 to 0.5 mg per kilogram per day) with sulfadiazine (30 to 35 mg per kilogram per day) should be considered. The optimal length of the maintenance phase is undetermined.

Viral Infections: Herpesviruses

Herpesviruses are large DNA viruses with a similar structural element arranged in concentric layers. This family of viruses includes HSV, VZV, CMV, and EBV. For more details about the molecular, antigenic, and epidemiologic characteristics of herpesviruses, the reader is referred to other publications (66). Approximately one third of the cases of HSV encephalitis are the result of primary infection; in the remaining two thirds, preexisting antibodies against HSV suggest that the encephalitis is a consequence of reactivation of latent virus. One of the most characteristic properties of herpesviruses is their ability to establish latency. After replication at the site of primary infection, the virus is transported to the dorsal root ganglia, where the viral genome persists in the host for life. The mechanism for reactivation is not clear, but it occurs despite the presence of both cell-mediated and humoral immunity. Primary infection of the

CNS with HSV is unusual in the normal host. If the cause of the infection is HSV-2, the infection is usually mild and self-limited. In contrast, infection with HSV-1 can be rapidly progressive, with death occurring within 1 to 2 weeks in two thirds of untreated patients. In the immunocompromised host with depressed T-lymphocyte function, a primary infection with herpes may become disseminated from dermal and mucosal areas to visceral involvement, but not necessarily involving the CNS. Recurrent HSV infections, which are usually mild in the normal host, can cause an atypical CNS infection with subacute and slowly progressive disease. Except for the rare patient with visual/auditory hallucinations, there are no historical or clinical findings in HSV encephalitis that differentiate this infection from other causes of encephalitis. Most patients present with fever, mental changes, and focal neurologic findings. Seizures, either focal or generalized, occur in 75% of patients. A variety of other diseases—such as brain abscess, subdural hematoma or empyema, tumors, vascular diseases and other viral infections (e.g., EBV, togaviruses, influenza, enteroviruses, mumps)—can mimic HSV encephalitis. In one study, 432 patients with clinical features indicative of HSV encephalitis underwent brain biopsy. HSV was isolated from only 193 patients (45%). Therefore, in many cases the initial impression of HSV encephalitis was incorrect (67).

Neurodiagnostic evaluation may be helpful in cases of localized brain involvement. Electroencephalography (EEG) may be as useful as a brain scan or CT or MRI scans in demonstrating localized disease. MRI seems to be more sensitive than CT for detecting focal changes. However, neither a normal CT scan or EEG nor absence of CSF findings excludes the diagnosis. HSV sometimes can be cultivated from the CSF, but results are usually available only after 48 hours. Rising HSV titers from the acute to the convalescent phase can help in the diagnosis but are not particularly helpful at the onset. Furthermore, high titers in the acute stage do not always indicate an acute infection; they may occur as a result of a previous asymptomatic infection. CSF PCR, which detects HSV DNA, is the method of choice for diagnosing HSV encephalitis. In patients with HSV encephalitis who had a brain biopsy to confirm the diagnosis, the sensitivity and specificity of PCR were found to be 91% and 92%, respectively (68).

Acyclovir (30 mg per kilogram day divided every 8 hours) is the drug of choice for the management of HSV encephalitis. Because prompt therapy in proven HSV cases does improve the outcome, empiric administration of acyclovir is justified in an immunocompromised patient with signs and symptoms of encephalitis for whom PCR results are not yet available. Therapy should be given for 14 days. With such therapy, relapses are rare.

CMV can cause life-threatening encephalitis in the immunocompromised host (69–71). The virus is very common, but even most severely immunocompromised hosts remain asymptomatic. CMV can be found in the saliva and urine of these patients for many weeks or months without causing an infection. Although the patient is asymptomatic, a rise in antibody titers may occur that makes the serologic test difficult to interpret when a CMV-like disease occurs. Even isolation of the virus from blood in an asymptomatic patient may not indicate an active infection. The presentation and clinical and laboratory findings in patients with CMV encephalitis do not differ from those resulting from other causes of encephalitis. Although isolation of CMV from the CSF and/or brain tissue or identification of the typical inclusion bodies and giant cells in a histologic preparation are accepted as confirming the diagnosis, these tests are too insensitive to detect small amounts of CMV. PCR has become the method of choice, and several investigators have shown it to be highly sensitive and specific (72,73). There is no known effective therapy, although a few studies suggest that ganciclovir or foscarnet may have some efficacy. Neither of these drugs penetrates well into the CSF.

Cidofavir, a new anti-CMV drug, has not been studied as therapy for CMV encephalitis.

Herpes zoster encephalitis is very rare and usually occurs as an extension from a cranial nerve dermatome (74). Rarely, dissemination from a distant dermatome (usually involving the lung and the liver) results in spread to the brain. VZV encephalitis is more common and more severe in patients with cell-mediated immunodeficiency. A multifocal leukoencephalitis has been described in cancer patients (75). The diagnosis is usually obvious because of the skin involvement. Culture of the base of a vesicle or of CSF verifies the diagnosis. Although no studies to evaluate the efficacy of acyclovir in VZV encephalitis have been done, treatment with this drug should be offered, because one case of rapid response with resolution of CNS symptoms has been reported (76).

Viral Infections: Measles Virus

Measles virus, which causes acute meningoencephalitis and postinfectious measles encephalitis in the normal host, also can produce measles inclusion-body encephalitis in the immunocompromised host (77). Most patients with this disease have leukemia or are receiving immunosuppressive drugs. The incubation period is up to 6 months. Brain biopsy demonstrates intranuclear inclusion bodies with cortical necrosis and a relatively mild inflammatory reaction. Although measles antigen is often found, viable virus is rarely isolated. Subacute measles encephalitis may be the result of an opportunistic defective, nonproductive measles virus that infects certain neural cells (78). No specific therapy for this disease is currently available, although neurologic improvement was observed with ribavirin treatment in two cases (79).

BRAIN ABSCESS

Brain abscess is not a common event in immunocompromised hosts, but it is an important part of the differential diagnosis of a focal CNS lesion or mass. Predisposing factors for the development of brain abscess can be divided into two categories. Factors that predispose to this infection in the normal host include contiguous infected sites (e.g., sinusitis, otitis media, dental abscess); cyanotic congenital heart disease or bacterial endocarditis; hematogenous spread from distant sites (e.g., pneumonia, osteomyelitis); penetrating head trauma or head surgery; and burns. Viridans streptococcal strains (especially members of the *Streptococcus intermedius* group) and *S. aureus* are the most commonly isolated bacteria. With the use of proper techniques, anaerobic bacteria are increasingly isolated from brain abscesses. Enteric gram-negative bacilli are also isolated from 15% to 20% of patients. Because the bacterial flora of the immunocompromised patient may be different from that of the normal host, several opportunistic pathogens should also be considered (see later discussion). Factors unique to the immunocompromised host include impaired neutrophil killing, prolonged use of broad-spectrum antibiotics, T-lymphocyte–mononuclear phagocyte deficient states, and the presence of intraventricular devices. Fungi such as *Candida, Mucor,* and *Aspergillus* and bacteria such as *Nocardia asteroides, Bacillus cereus,* and, rarely, mycobacteria are particularly likely to cause a brain abscess in the immunocompromised host.

Early evaluation is important, because brain abscesses must be differentiated from other mass-producing lesions in the brain. The differential diagnosis includes primary brain tumor, metastatic malignancy, brain infarct, and necrotizing viral encephalitis. In addition, the specific diagnosis allows effective antimicrobial therapy and/or neurosurgical intervention, which greatly improves the outcome.

Nocardia asteroides Infection

N. asteroides usually causes brain abscess in patients with T-lymphocyte or mononuclear phagocyte defects, such as those with organ transplants (80), immunosuppressive therapy, cancer (81), or AIDS (82). A review of 131 cases of nocardial brain abscess revealed that fewer than 40% occurred in immunocompromised hosts, with an increasing number of cases in patients with HIV infection (83). It is possible that the incidence of this infection might have been higher in HIV-infected patients but for the common use of TMP/SMX for *Pneumocystis carinii* prophylaxis, which is also effective in preventing nocardial infections. *Nocardia* enter the host through the respiratory system and can be isolated from the respiratory secretions of asymptomatic normal hosts. In the immunocompromised host, dissemination of *N. asteroides* can cause pneumonia, skin abscess, and liver, kidney, and CNS involvement. In the brain the most common manifestation is an abscess, but meningitis can occur rarely (84). If the abscess is close to the brain surface, meningeal irritation or rupture of the abscess with meningeal spillover can occur. The clinical manifestations vary with the stage of the infection and the affected site. In the initial stages, fever, generalized malaise, vomiting, and headache may be the presenting symptoms. Papilledema and nuchal rigidity are relatively rare (fewer than 25% of cases). In later stages, focal neurologic signs and seizures develop in almost half of the patients. A change in mental status occurs in most patients. The first stage may be inconspicuous for weeks until the sudden development of focal signs. Frontal lobe abscesses may result in few symptoms for weeks or months, whereas abscesses developing in sensory or motor portions of the brain cause neurologic deficits early in the infection. A sudden worsening in the patient's condition with development of shock, stupor, and meningismus should alert the physician to the possibility of rupture of an abscess into the subarachnoid or ventricular space.

When a brain abscess is suspected, lumbar puncture is contraindicated because the procedure could cause herniation and in most cases the nonspecific results of the CSF examination do not help in the diagnosis. Humoral antibodies against *Nocardia* are not specific, and they cross-react with *Strepto-myces* and *Mycobacterium* species; therefore, serologic tests are not helpful in the diagnosis (85). However, an enzyme immunoassay, using a common immunodominant protein (55 kD) for *Nocardia,* has shown greater specificity (85). Diagnosis is commonly made by demonstrating on CT or MRI scans, especially when contrast material is used to produce ring enhancement of the abscess in patients who are not neutropenic. In some cases, the appearance of brain abscess manifestations in a patient with involvement of other organs from which *N. asteroides* was isolated may be the only clue to the diagnosis. EEG is also valuable in localizing the abscess and is characterized by unilateral slow delta waves. CSF examination may show mild to moderate leukocytosis—except in rupture of the abscess into the ventricle, in which case 10,000 or more WBCs per microliter are found—with either a polymorphonuclear or mononuclear response. The protein level is mildly increased or normal, and glucose is mildly decreased or normal. Gram stain is usually negative, but when it is positive branching rods are seen. If the Gram stain is not done quickly after the sample is available, the branching can be fragmented and resemble chains of gram-positive cocci. If a modified Ziehl-Nielsen stain is used, *Nocardia* organisms appear as acid-fast bacteria (86). The bacteria sometimes grow very slowly, and more than 4 to 5 days is needed before the typical colonies are seen. Because of this slow growth, the microbiology laboratory should be alerted to the possibility of *Nocardia* so that the specimen is not discarded prematurely.

In vitro studies demonstrate that susceptibility to many antibiotics is variable among clinical isolates of *N. asteroides.* The most active agents are the sulfonamides (100%). Ninety percent of the isolates are sensitive to amikacin or imipenem, and 80% are sensitive to cefotaxime and ceftriaxone (87). Only 40% are sensitive to ampicillin. Sulfonamides should be used for treatment of *N. asteroides.* Use of any other drug must be supported by *in vitro* susceptibility testing. The intravenous combination of TMP/SMX (20 and 100 mg per kilogram per day divided every 6 to 8 hours, respectively) has been used successfully to treat CNS *Nocardia* infections in children (88). Other drugs (for patients intolerant to sulfa), such as amikacin or the combination of cefotaxime with amikacin, have shown to be successful in experimental cerebral nocardiosis, but their efficacy in human disease is unknown. Minocycline is another alternative that has been used successfully in a few cases (89). In general, if the brain abscess diameter is less than 2 cm, an antibiotic trial alone may be successful. If the patient's condition deteriorates or there is no decrease in size after 4 weeks of therapy, stereotactic aspiration or surgical excision is recommended. Because of the tendency for relapse, antibiotic therapy should be given for 3 months or longer.

Bacillus cereus Infection

B. cereus is a very rare cause of brain abscess in the immunocompromised host. The major risk for infection with this bacterium is impaired neutrophil killing, including neutropenia. *B. cereus* is ubiquitous in nature and may be found in the gastrointestinal tract as part of the normal flora. It reaches the brain via hematogenous spread and produces localized tissue necrosis due to the production of a potent exotoxin (90). On Gram stain, the bacteria are easily recognized as large gram-positive rods with spores. Antimicrobial sensitivity of *B. cereus* is variable. It is usually sensitive *in vitro* to vancomycin and gentamicin. It is also sensitive to rifampin and imipenem, but there is very little clinical experience in using these antibiotics for this infection. When planning antimicrobial therapy, it is important to consider not only the *in vitro* activity of the antibiotic but also its ability to achieve bactericidal levels in the brain. A combination of vancomycin with gentamicin should be considered. Rifampin may be added or alternated with gentamicin when CNS inflammation decreases, because penetration of the aminoglycoside is minimal. Although surgical excision of the abscess is usually neces-

sary, in some cases the location of the abscess precludes surgery and antibiotic therapy alone may be successful (91).

Aspergillus fumigatus Infection

The *Aspergillus* genus has more than 200 species, but only 9 have been shown to cause infections in humans, the most common being *A. fumigatus*. Aspergillosis is the second most common fungal infection in the immunocompromised host (92), and the CNS may be involved secondary to hematogenous spread. Predisposing risk factors include neutropenia, hematologic neoplasms with chemotherapy, transplantation (e.g., solid organ, bone marrow), and chronic steroid treatment. Brain abscess (or abscesses) is the most common presentation of CNS involvement with this fungus. *A. fumigatus* has been found to colonize the respiratory and gastrointestinal tracts, and usually it disseminates to the brain via the blood from another infected organ (most often the lung). Direct extension from the nasopharynx through the cribiform plate can also occur, leading to single or multiple abscesses that may imitate mucormycosis. Depending on the area of the brain involved, the presentation of *A. fumigatus* abscess varies from mild symptoms to cranial nerve involvement, focal seizures, hemiparesis, and coma. Because premortem diagnosis in the immunocompromised host is difficult, this infection should be suspected in any immunocompromised host who develops a focal brain lesion. The CSF findings are not specific; usually there is a moderate increase in WBCs (100 to 500 cells per microliter) with either polymorphonuclear leukocytes or monocytes, and normal glucose and protein levels. If the Gram stain is positive, it shows acutely branching septated hyphae. Isolation of the fungus from the CSF rarely occurs. Serologic assays are usually unreliable, especially in the immunocompromised host, and should not be used. Antigen detection methods (e.g., radioimmunoassay, immunoblotting, ELISA) have been more reliable but are not yet recommended for routine use for early detection

(93). CT scanning may be disappointing, because in many cases the CNS lesion appears as a poorly circumscribed, low-density area without capsule formation. This appearance makes the diagnosis of a brain abscess very difficult (94). MRI appears to be more sensitive, and often more than one lesion is seen that was not clinically suspected (95). Brain biopsy and/or culture may be the only way to reach the diagnosis.

The treatment of choice is amphotericin B and surgical drainage of the abscess. The recommended dose of amphotericin B is 1.0 mg per kilogram once a day, but doses up to 1.5 mg per kilogram once a day are recommended for patients who do not respond to more conventional doses (96). The use of liposomal amphotericin B is preferred by some because there are fewer side effects with this product. *In vitro* data suggest that rifampin is often synergistic with amphotericin B. Therefore, this combination, or the combination of amphotericin B and 5-fluorocytosine (100 to 150 mg per kilogram per day divided every 6 hours), should be considered. Itraconazole, which has a good *in vitro* activity against *Aspergillus,* may be considered as an alternative drug. Limited experience suggests that high doses of itraconazole (800 mg per day in adults; 10 to 15 mg per kilogram per day in children) are effective in treating cerebral aspergillosis (97). The prognosis is guarded, and only 50% to 70% of patients survive. Only the combination of a high index of suspicion, surgical drainage, recovery of granulocytes, and early administration antifungal therapy may lead to improved success in combating this fungal infection.

CENTRAL NERVOUS SYSTEM INFECTIONS IN HIV-INFECTED PATIENTS

The most common CNS manifestations of HIV infection are caused by HIV itself (98). Primary and persistent HIV infection of the CNS is responsible for the progressive encephalopathy seen in children, which is manifested as loss of developmental milestones, microcephaly, hypertonia or hypotonia, ataxia, and seizures. Opportunistic CNS infections, which are seen in about 10% of adults with AIDS, are relatively rare in children (99), probably because the young child has had a relatively short time in which to become exposed to these pathogens. The observations that children with AIDS have few opportunistic CNS infections but frequently suffer from encephalopathy, combined with reports of HIV isolation from CSF and brain tissue, suggest that HIV itself is the major cause for the neurologic manifestations in this population. The most commonly reported opportunistic CNS infections in adults and children are listed in Table 20.3. Many opportunistic infections reported in adults are not yet reported in the pediatric patients. The main reason for this observation is the relatively small number of pediatric patients with AIDS (less than 2% of the total known AIDS cases). With the increase in the life expectancy of HIV-infected children in the next decade that is anticipated because of the availability of more potent antiretroviral drugs, more cases of opportunistic infections including CNS infections can be expected in children.

TABLE 20.3. *Opportunistic CNS infections in patients with HIV infection*

Organisms	Adults	Children
Viruses		
HIV	3+	4+
Cytomegalovirus	2+	1+
Epstein-Barr virus	1+	NR
Varicella-zoster virus	1+	NR
Papovavirus-JC virus	1+	NR
Parasites		
Toxoplasma	4+	1+
Fungi		
Cryptococcus neoformans	4+	1+
Candida	UK	1+
Bacteria		
Nocardia asteroides	1+	NR
Gram-negative enteric	UK	1+
Treponema pallidum	1+	1+

4+, very common; 3+, common; 2+, uncommon; 1+, rare; CNS, central nervous system; HIV, human immunodeficiency virus, NR, not reported, UK, unknown.

Recurrent serious bacterial infections are common in HIV-infected children. Probably the alteration in B-cell function is more severe in children than in adults with AIDS. Therefore, CNS infections with encapsulated bacteria (e.g., *H. influenzae, S. pneumoniae, Salmonella*) are relatively common in HIV-infected children and cause significant mortality. Awareness of this possibility should initiate a complete workup of the febrile HIV-infected child who has even minimal CNS signs and symptoms. Prompt diagnosis and therapy decrease the morbidity and mortality of these children.

REFERENCES

1. Civitello LA, Brouwers P, Pizzo PA. Neurological and neuropsychological manifestations in 120 children with symptomatic human immunodeficiency virus infection. *Ann Neurol* 1993;34;481.
2. Wollman RR, Young LS, Armstrong D, et al. Anti-*Pseudomonas* heat-stabile opsonins in acute lymphoblastic leukemia. *J Pediatr* 1975;86:376.
3. Gellin BG, Broome CV. Listeriosis. *JAMA* 1989;261;1313.
4. Schwartz B, Hexter D, Broome CV, et al. Investigation of an outbreak of listeriosis: new hypotheses for the etiology of epidemic *Listeria monocytogenes* infection. *J Infect Dis* 1989;159:680.
5. Stamm AM, Dismukes WE, Simmons BP, et al. Listeriosis in renal transplant recipients: report of an outbreak and review of 102 cases. *Rev Infect Dis* 1982;4:665.
6. Jurado RL, Farley MM, Pereira E, et al. Increased risk of meningitis and bacteremia due to *Listeria monocytogenes* in patients with human immunodeficiency virus infection. *Clin Infect Dis* 1993;17:224.
7. Dee RR, Lorber B. Brain abscess due to *Listeria monocytogenes:* case report and literature review. *Rev Infect Dis* 1986;8:968.
8. Armstrong RW, Fung PC. Brainstem encephalitis (rhombencephalitis) due to *Listeria monocytogenes:* case report and review. *Clin Infect Dis* 1993;16:689.
9. Schuchat A, Swaminathan B, Broome CV. Epidemiology of human listeriosis. *Clin Microbiol Rev* 1991;4:169.
10. Gantz NM, Myerwitz RL, Medieros AA, et al. Listeriosis in immunosuppressed patients, a cluster of eight cases. *Am J Med* 1975;58:637.
11. Skogberg K, Syrjanen J, Jahkola M, et al. Clinical presentation and outcome of listeriosis in patients with and without immunosuppressive therapy. *Clin Infect Dis* 1992;14:815.
12. Kessler SL, Dajani AS. *Listeria* meningitis in infants and children. *Pediatr Infect Dis J* 1990;9:61.
13. Hudak AP, Lee SH, Issekutz AC, et al. Comparison of three serological methods—enzyme-linked immunoabsorbent assay, complement fixation, and microagglutination—in the diagnosis of human perinatal *Listeria monocytogenes* infection. *Clin Invest Med* 1984;7:349.
14. Espaze EP, Reynaud AE. Antibiotic susceptibilities of *Listeria:* In vitro studies. *Infection* 1988;16[Suppl. 2]:S160.
15. Bakker-Woundenberg IAJM, de Bos P, van Leeuwen WB, et al. Efficacy of ampicillin therapy in experimental listeriosis in mice with impaired T-cell mediated immune response. *Antimicrob Agents Chemother* 1981;19:76.
16. Hawkins AE, Bortolussi R, Issekutz AC. *In vitro* and *in vivo* activity of various antibiotics against *Listeria monocytogenes* type 4b. *Clin Invest Med* 1984;7:335.
17. Scheld WM. Evaluation of rifampin and other antibiotics against *Listeria monocytogenes in vitro* and *in vivo. Rev Infect Dis* 1983;5:S593.
18. Spitzer PG, Hammer SM, Karchmer AW. Treatment of *Listeria monocytogenes* infection with trimethoprim-sulfamethoxazole: case report and review of the literature. *Rev Infect Dis* 1986;8:427.
19. Levitz RE, Quintiliani R. Trimethoprim-sulfamethoxazole for bacterial meningitis. *Ann Intern Med* 1984;100:881.
19a. Bortolussi R, Schlech W, III. Listeriosis. In: Remington JS, Klein JO, eds. *Infectious diseases of the fetus and newborn infant.* Philadelphia: WB Saunders, 1995:1055–1073.
20. Marrie TJ, Riding M, Grant B. Computed tomographic scanning in *Listeria monocytogenes* meningitis. *Clin Invest Med* 1984;7:335.
20a. Eraklis AJ, Kevy SV, Diamond LK, et al. Hazard of overwhelming infection after splenectomy in childhood. *N Engl J Med* 1967;276:1225–1229.
21. Ross SC, Densen P. Complement deficiency states and infection: epidemiology, pathogenesis and consequences of neisserial and other infections in an immune deficiency. *Medicine (Baltimore)* 1984;63:243.
22. Zoppi M, Weiss M, Nydegger UE, et al. Recurrent meningitis in a patient with congenital deficiency of the C9 component of complement. *Arch Intern Med* 1990;150:2395.
23. Rodriguez WJ, Khan WN, Cocchetto DM, et al. Treatment of *Pseudomonas* meningitis with ceftazidime with or without concurrent therapy. *Pediatr Infect Dis J* 1990;9:83.
24. Kilpatrick M, Girgis N, Farid Z, et al. Aztreonam for treating meningitis caused by gram-negative rods. *Scand J Infect Dis* 1991;23:125.
25. Klugman KP, Dagan R, The Meropenem Meningitis Study Group. Randomized comparison of meropenem with cefotaxime for treatment of bacterial meningitis. *Antimicrob Agents Chemother* 1995;39:1140.
26. Patrick CC. Coagulase-negative staphylococci: pathogens with increasing clinical significance. *J Pediatr* 1990;116:497.
27. Kloos WE, Bannerman TL. Update of clinical significance of coagulase-negative staphylococci. *Clin Microbiol Rev* 1994;7:117.
28. Browne MJ, Dinndorf PA, Perek D, et al. Infectious complications of intraventricular reservoirs in cancer patients. *Pediatr Infect Dis J* 1987;6:182.
29. Hanekom W, Yogev R. Diagnosis and management of CSF shunt infections. *Adv Pediatr Infect Dis* 1995;11:29.
30. Younger JJ, Christensen GD, Bartley DL, et al. Coagulase-negative staphylococci isolated from cerebrospinal fluid shunts: importance of slime production, species identification and shunt removal to clinical outcome. *J Infect Dis* 1987;156:548.
31. John JF, McNeill WF. Activity of cephalosporins against

methicilin-susceptible and methicillin-resistant, coagulase-negative staphylococci: minimal effect of beta-lactamases. *Antimicrob Agents Chemother* 1980;17:179.

32. Schwalbe RS, Stapleton JT, Gilligan PH. Emergence of varicomycin resistance in coagulase-negative staphylococci. *N Engl J Med* 1987;316:927.

33. Lowy FD, Chang DS, Lash PR. Synergy of combinations of vancomycin, gentamicin, and rifampin against methicillin-resistant, coagulase-negative staphylococci. *Antimicrob Agents Chemother* 1983;23:932.

34. Rozenbaum R, Rios Goncalves AJ. Clinical epidemiological study of 171 cases of cryptococcosis. *Clin Infect Dis* 1994;18:369.

35. Diamond RD, Bennet JE. Prognostic factors in cryptococcal meningitis: a study of 111 cases. *Ann Intern Med* 1974;80:176.

36. Frank UK, Nishimura SL, Li NC, et al. Evaluation of an enzyme immunoassay for detection of cryptococcal capsular polysaccharide antigen in serum and cerebrospinal fluid. *Clin Microbiol* 1993;31:97.

36a. Medoff G, Comfort M, Kobayashi GS. Synergistic action of amphotericin B and 5-fluorocytosine against yeast-like organisms. *Proc Soc Exp Biol Med* 1971;138:571–574.

37. Saag MS, Cloud GA, Graybill JR, et al. A comparison of itraconazole versus fluconazole as maintenance therapy for AIDS-associated cryptococcal meningitis. *Clin Infect Dis* 1999;28:291.

38. Dismukes WE, Cloud G, Gallis HA, et al. Treatment of cryptococcal meningitis with combination amphotericin B and flucytosine for four as compared with six weeks. *N Engl J Med* 1987;317:334.

39. Powderly WG, Cloud GA, Dismukes WE, et al. Measurement of cryptococcal antigen in serum and cerebrospinal fluid: value in the management of AIDS-associated cryptococcal meningitis. *Clin Infect Dis* 1994;18:789.

39a. van der Horst CM, Saag MS, Cloud GA, et al. Treatment of cryptococcal meningitis associated with the acquired immunodeficiency syndrome. NIAID Mycoses Study Group and ACTG. *N Engl J Med* 1997;337:15–21.

40. De Gans G, Portegies P, Tiessens G, et al. Itraconazole compared with amphotericin B plus flucytosine in AIDS patients with cryptococcal meningitis. *AIDS* 1992;6:185.

41. Leenders AC, Reiss P, Portegies P, et al. Liposomal amphotericin B (AmBisome) compared with amphotericin B followed by oral fluconazole in the treatment of AIDS-associated cryptococcal meningitis. *AIDS* 1997;11:1463.

42. White M, Cirrincione C, Blevins A, et al. Cryptococcal meningitis: outcome in patients with AIDS and patients with neoplastic disease. *J Infect Dis* 1992;165:960.

43. Larsen RA. Editorial response: a comparison of itraconazole versus fluconazole as maintenance therapy for AIDS-associated cryptococcal meningitis. *Clin Infect Dis* 1999;28:297.

43a. Powderly WG, Saag MS, Cloud GA, et al. A controlled trial of fluconazole or amphotericin B to prevent relapse of crytococcal meningitis in patients with the acquired immunodeficiency syndrome. The NIAID ACTG and Mycoses Study Group. *N Engl J Med* 1992;326:793–798.

44. Lipton SA, Hickey WF, Morris JH, et al. Candidal infection in the central nervous system. *Am J Med* 1984; 76:101.

45. Walsh TJ, Hier DB, Caplan LP. Fungal infections of the central nervous system: comparative analysis of risk factors and clinical signs in 57 patients. *Neurology* 1985;35:1654.

46. Smego RA, Devoe PW, Sampson HA, et al. *Candida* meningitis in two children with severe combined immunodeficiency. *J Pediatr* 1984;104:902.

47. Iwashita H, Araki K, Kuroiwa Y, et al. Occurrence of *Candida*-specific oligoclonal IgG antibodies in CSF with *Candida* meningoencephalitis. *Ann Neurol* 1978;64:579.

48. Burgener-Kairuz P, Zuber JP, Jaunin P, et al. Rapid detection and identification of *Candida albicans* and *Torulopsis (Candida) glabrata* in clinical specimens by species-specific nested PCR amplification of a cytochrome P-450 lanosterol-alpha-demethylase (L1A1) gene fragment. *J Clin Microbiol* 1994;32:1902.

49. Smego RA, Perfect JR, Durack DT. Combined therapy with amphotericin B and 5-flucytosine for *Candida* meningitis. *Rev Infect Dis* 1984;6:791.

50. Ragland AS, Arusa E, Ismail Y, et al. Eosinophilic pleocytosis in coccidioidal meningitis: frequency and significance. *Am J Med* 1993;195:254.

51. Smith CE, Saito MT, Simons SA. Pattern of 39,500 serologic tests in coccidioidomycosis. *JAMA* 1956;160:546.

52. Galgiani JN, Catanzaro A, Cloud GA, et al. Fluconazole therapy for coccidioidal meningitis: The NIAID-Mycoses Study Group. *Ann Intern Med* 1993;119:28.

53. Tucker RM, Denning DW, Dupont B, et al. Itraconazole therapy for chronic coccidioidal meningitis. *Ann Intern Med* 1990;112:108.

54. Dewsnup DH, Galgiani JN, Graybill JR, et al. Is it ever safe to stop azole therapy for *Coccidioides immitis* meningitis? *Ann Intern Med* 1996;124:305.

55. Schlesinger Y, Storch GA. Herpes simplex meningitis in infancy. *Pediatr Infect Dis J* 1994;13:141.

56. Huang LM, Lee CY, Lee PI, et al. Meningitis caused by human herpesvirus-6. *Arch Dis Child* 1991;66:1443.

57. McKinney RE, Katz SL, Wilfert CM. Chronic enteroviral meningoencephalitis in agammaglobulinemic patients. *Rev Infect Dis* 1987;9:334.

58. Hakes TB, Armstrong D. Toxoplasmosis: problems in diagnosis and treatment. *Cancer* 1983;52:1535.

59. Hall WA, Martinez AJ, Dummer JS, et al. Central nervous system infections in heart and heart-lung transplant recipients. *Arch Neurol* 1989;46:173.

60. Fisher MA, Levy J, Helfrich M, et al. Detection of *Toxoplasma gondii* in the spinal fluid of a bone marrow transplant recipient. *Pediatr Infect Dis J* 1987;6:81.

61. Reynolds ES, Walls KW, Pfeiffer RI. Generalized toxoplasmosis following renal transplantation: report of a case. *Arch Intern Med* 1966;118:401.

62. Subauste CS, Remington JS. Immunity to *Toxoplasma gondii*. *Curr Opin Immunol* 1993;5:532.

63. Potsman I, Resnick L, Luft BJ, et al. Intrathecal production of antibodies against *Toxoplasma gondii* in patients with toxoplasmic encephalitis and the acquired immunodeficiency syndrome (AIDS). *Ann Intern Med* 1988;108:49.

64. Derouin F, Mazeron MC, Garin YJF. Comparative study of tissue culture and mouse inoculation methods for demonstration of *Toxoplasma gondii*. *J Clin Microbiol* 1987;25:1597.

65. Holliman RE, Johnson JD, Savra D. Diagnosis of cerebral toxoplasmosis in association with AIDS using the polymerase chain reaction. *Scand J Infect Dis* 1990;22:240.

66. Whitley RJ. Herpes simplex virus. In: Scheld WA, Whitley RJ, Durack DT, eds. *Infections of the central nervous system*, 2nd ed. New York: Lippincott-Raven, 1997:73.

67. Whitley RJ, Cobbs CG, Alford CA Jr, et al. Diseases

that mimic herpes simplex encephalitis: diagnosis, presentation and outcome. *JAMA* 1989;262:234.

68. Lakeman FD, Whitley RJ, CASG NIAID. Diagnosis of herpes simplex encephalitis: application of polymerase chain reaction to cerebrospinal fluid from brain biopsied patients and correlation with disease. *J Infect Dis* 1995;171:857.

69. Glenn J. Cytomegalovirus infections following renal transplantation. *Rev Infect Dis* 1981;3:1151.

70. Winston DJ, Gale RP, Meyer DV, et al. Infectious complications of human bone marrow transplantation. *Medicine (Baltimore)* 1979;58:1.

71. Jacobson MA, Mills J. Serious cytomegalovirus disease in the acquired immunodeficiency syndrome (AIDS): clinical findings, diagnosis, and treatment. *Ann Intern Med* 1988;108:585.

72. Clifford DB, Buller RS, Mohammed S, et al. Use of polymerase chain reaction to demonstrate cytomegalovirus DNA in CSF of patients with human immunodeficiency virus infection. *Neurology* 1993;43:75.

73. Fox JD, Brink NS, Zuckerman MA, et al. Detection of herpesvirus DNA by nested polymerase chain reaction in cerebrospinal fluid of human immunodeficiency virus-infected persons with neurologic disease: a prospective evaluation. *J Infect Dis* 1995;172:1087.

74. Jemsek J, Greenberg S, Taber L, et al. Herpes zoster-associated encephalitis: clinicopathologic report of 12 cases and review of the literature. *Medicine (Baltimore)* 1983;62:81.

75. Horton B, Price RW, Jimenez D. Multifocal varicella-zoster virus leukoencephalitis temporally remote from herpes zoster. *Ann Neurol* 1981;9:251.

76. Johns DR, Gress DR. Rapid response to acyclovir in herpes zoster-associated encephalitis. *Am J Med* 1987;82:560.

77. Ohuchi M, Ohuchi R, Mifune K, et al. Characterization of the measles virus isolated from the brain of a patient with immunosuppressive measles encephalitis. *J Infect Dis* 1987;156:436.

78. Roos RP, Graves MC, Wollmann RL, et al. Immunologic and virologic studies of measles inclusion body encephalitis in an immunosuppressed host: the relationship to subacute sclerosing panencephalitis. *Neurology* 1981;31:1263.

79. Mustafa MM, Weitman SD, Winick NJ, et al. Subacute measles encephalitis in the young immunocompromised host: report of two cases diagnosed by polymerase chain reaction and treated with ribavirin and review of the literature. *Clin Infect Dis* 1993;16:654.

80. Wilson JP, Turner HR, Kirchner KA, et al. Nocardial infections in renal transplant recipients. *Medicine (Baltimore)* 1989;68:38.

81. Berkey P, Bodey GP. Nocardial infection in patients with neoplastic disease. *Rev Infect Dis* 1989;11:407.

82. Lechtenberg R, Sierra MF, Pringle GF, et al. *Listeria monocytogenes*: brain abscess or meningoencephalitis? *Neurology* 1979;29:86.

83. Mamelak AN, Obana WG, Flaherty JF, et al. Nocardial brain abscess: treatment strategies and factors influencing outcome. *Neurosurgery* 1994;35:622.

84. Bross JE, Gordon G. Nocardial meningitis: case reports and review. *Rev Infect Dis* 1991;13:160.

85. Boiron P, Stynen D. Immunodiagnosis of nocardiosis. *Gene* 1992;115:219.

86. Palmer DL, Harvey RL, Wheeler JK. Diagnostic and therapeutic considerations in *Nocardia asteroides* infection. *Medicine (Baltimore)* 1974;53:391.

87. Wallace RJ Jr, Steele L, Sumter G, et al. Antimicrobial susceptibility patterns of *Nocardia asteroides*. *Antimicrob Agents Chemother* 1988;32:1776.

88. Mills VA, Cleary TG, Frankel L, et al. Central nervous system *Nocardia* infection. *Clin Pediatr (Phila)* 1982;21:248.

89. Wren MV, Savage AM, Alford RH. Apparent cure of intracranial *Nocardia asteroides* infection with minocycline. *Arch Intern Med* 1979;139:249.

90. Thrubull PCB, Kramer JM. Non-gastrointestinal *Bacillus cereus* infections: an analysis of exotoxin production by strains isolated over a two-year period. *J Clin Pathol* 1983;36:1091.

91. Jenson HB, Levy SR, Duncan C, et al. Treatment of multiple brain abscesses caused by *Bacillus cereus*. *Pediatr Infect Dis J* 1989;8:795.

92. Walsh TJ, Hier DB, Caplan LR. Aspergillosis of the central nervous system: clinicopathological analysis of 17 patients. *Ann Neurol* 1985;18:574.

93. Andriole VT. Infections with *Aspergillus* species. *Clin Infect Dis* 1993;17[Suppl. 2]:S481.

94. Grossman RI, Davis KR, Taveras JM, et al. Computed tomography of intracranial aspergillosis. *Comput Assist Tomogr* 1981;5:646.

95. Mikhael MA, Rushovich AM, Ciric I. Magnetic resonance imaging of cerebral aspergillosis. *Comput Radiol* 1985;9:85.

96. Denning DW, Stevens DA. Antifungal and surgical treatment of invasive aspergillosis: review of 2,121 published cases. *Rev Infect Dis* 1990;12:1147.

97. Sanchez C, Mauri E, Dalmau D, et al. Treatment of cerebral aspergillosis with itraconazole: do high doses improve prognosis? *Clin Infect Dis* 1995;21:1485.

98. Lobato MN, Caldwell MB, Ng P, et al. Encephalopathy in children with perinatally acquired human immunodeficiency virus infection. *J Pediatr* 1995;126:710.

99. Kozlowski PB, Sher JH, Dickson DW, et al. Central nervous system in pediatric HIV infection: a multicenter study. In: Kozlowski PB, Snider PM, Vietze PM, et al., eds. *Brain in Pediatric AIDS*. Basel, Switzerland: Karger, 1990:132

21

Dermatologic Findings with Infection

Deanna Soloway-Simon and *Moise Levy

*Departments of Pediatrics and *Dermatology, Texas Children's Hospital, Houston, Texas 77030*

The skin plays a critical role in prevention and evaluation of infection in the immunocompromised host. The mucous membrane and skin surfaces shield the body from invasion by exogenous microorganisms and yet may be a portal of entry for bacteria, fungi, and viruses, enabling local or disseminated infection. It is essential in the patient with an immunologic defect to protect the skin and prevent maceration or trauma as much as possible. If an organism is allowed to trespass the skin's surface and enter the bloodstream, a weakened host may be incapable of preventing its spread and the development of septicemia. Initially the spread of disseminated disease may not provide any physical signs or symptoms. Dermatologic manifestations may be the first evidence of a latent systemic infection. In the immunocompromised host diagnosis of infection can be especially challenging, because patients often have an altered inflammatory response and an uncharacteristic morphologic appearance of dermatologic disease. Because the skin is so readily accessible, it often serves as a diagnostic aid. Biopsy and culture of skin lesions allows for rapid diagnosis, early initiation of treatment, and prevention of systemic disease.

In this chapter, the various causes of skin disease, together with their clinical appearance, manner of diagnosis, treatment options, and prognosis, are described. One theme will become apparent: the immunocompromised host is particularly susceptible to infections involving the skin and mucous membranes. Although these infections are often caused by the same etiologic agents that lead to infection in immunocompetent hosts and may have a similar appearance, they may be more extensive, have an atypical morphology, or be more resistant to standard therapies. Opportunistic diseases are also seen in the immunocompromised patient. The need to biopsy the lesions is especially important in these cases to allow for rapid diagnosis and a more expeditious treatment and resolution.

THE SKIN AS AN IMMUNOLOGIC ORGAN

The skin possesses a distinct network of cells that operate to protect it as a distinct organ and to prevent its being a portal of entry for disseminated infection. The skin and mucous membranes create an unfavorable environment for microorganism invasion by maintaining an intact keratinized layer of epidermis, by providing a dry environment that prevents the growth of organisms nurtured by moisture (e.g., *Candida,* gram-positive bacilli), and by hosting a population of normal skin flora which retard colonization of pathogenic bacteria through "bacterial interference" (1). One would expect to encounter an infection when the keratinized layer of the skin is compromised by the use of intravenous devices, when the skin remains moist beneath plastic occlusive dressings, or when broad-spectrum antibiotics alter the normal flora of the skin.

At the mucous membrane level, lysozyme and lactoferrin are produced, both of which act as physiologic antimicrobials. Lysozyme induces lysis by disrupting the architecture of the mucopeptides within the cell membrane of gram-positive bacteria. Lactoferrin binds iron and therefore competes for this substance with aerobic bacteria, which require iron for their metabolism (2).

In the skin, lymphocytes travel throughout the dermal layer in search of antigens. The unique antigen-presenting cell of the skin is the Langerhans cell. This cell of the monocyte-macrophage lineage is located in the epidermis and is derived from precursor cells in the bone marrow (3). Like other monocyte cells, Langerhans cells possess both class I and class II major histocompatibility (MHC) antigens, which when joined with processed antigen on the cell surface can be identified by the surface receptor on the T lymphocyte. The proliferation of these T-helper lymphocytes and the production of various lymphokines mediate the inflammatory response. An example of one such cytokine is interferon-γ (IFN-γ). IFN-γ interacts with epidermal cells, causing chemotaxis of the Langerhans cells and their precursors and enhancing antigen processing (3).

After the Langerhans cell has presented its antigen, it secretes interleukin-1 (IL-1), which, along with the products of the lymphocyte, induces an immunologic reaction to the antigen. IL-1 specifically stimulates additional lymphokine production, B-cell proliferation, and antibody production; enhanced phagocytosis; and T-lymphocyte proliferation. These unique epidermal cells also play a vital role in the surveillance of the skin for potentially harmful environmental antigens and in delayed hypersensitivity reactions in the skin (e.g., Mantoux test).

Although antigen-presenting cells may present antigens within the dermis, often these cells migrate through the lymphatic channels within the skin to regional lymph nodes. Here they interact with T cells and present the antigens. Through cell division stimulated by IL-2 (a cytokine that functions as a T-cell growth factor), several clones or subsets of the particular T cell are produced. One subset comprises the memory T cells, which provide long-lasting immunity against any antigen presented. The other subset consists of effector T lymphocytes, which return to the site of infection (in this case the dermis) via a complex homing system in which proteins on the surface of the T cells interact with other proteins on the surface of epidermal cells (3). Once within the epidermis, the effector lymphocytes produce lymphokines that attract other cells of the immune system, which orchestrate an inflammatory response.

In the skin the immune system works to contact and fight infection, to exhibit signs of inflammation, and to initiate allergic and hypersensitive responses in the skin (3). The armamentarium of immunologic defense in other areas of the body, such as complement, B and T lymphocytes, monocytes, and plasma cells, are also active in the skin.

Children possess an immune system identical to that in adults. However, unlike their adult counterparts, children have been exposed to fewer antigens and possess fewer developed antibodies to common antigens; they are therefore more susceptible to acquiring infections by common organisms that they have previously never encountered. This situation becomes further magnified in children with primary or acquired immunologic disorders, who are unable to protect themselves from the onslaught of infectious organisms.

Examples can be seen in pediatric diseases such as X-linked agammaglobulinemia (X-LA), human immunodeficiency virus (HIV) infection, and malignancies. X-LA is a primary immunodeficiency that affects the B lymphocytes and results in a defective capacity to produce an antibody response to bacteria. Children with X-LA are susceptible to recurrent bacterial infections of the gastrointestinal and respiratory tracts and skin (4). In children with HIV infection, there is an inversion in the normal ratio of CD4+ helper cells to CD8+ suppressor cells. When antigens are presented to lymphocytes, there is a diminished proliferative response of the T cells. Although many of these children show hypergammaglobulinemia, thought to be caused by stimulation of B cells by the retrovirus, they have an inadequate ability to produce specific antibodies to bacteria (4). Therefore, both the cell-mediated and the humoral arms of the immune system are affected, leaving the child vulnerable.

Children with cancer have similar physiologic handicaps. Many of the infections seen in cancer patients are similar to those diseases that plague the child with HIV: mucocutaneous *Candida*, recurrent herpes simplex virus (HSV), *Pneumocystis carinii,* and varicella-zoster virus (VZV) (5). These children may also have both quantitative and qualitative defects of granulocytes, which instrumental in preventing bacterial and fungal infections. A decreased number of neutrophils and band forms may occur secondary to the malignancy or as an effect of the treatment. In either case, the degree and duration of granulocytopenia is inversely related to the risk for infection. Cancer patients also have qualitative defects in their granulocytes involving chemotaxis, bactericidal capacity, and phagocytosis. For example, corticosteroids, which cause a decrease in the migratory and phagocytotic capabilities of granulocytes, put these children at increased risk for bacteremia from sources in the lungs, skin, and intestines, as well as indwelling devices such as Port-a-Cath and intravenous lines (4).

It is clear that the skin plays an important role both in preventing infection and in displaying the signs and symptoms of inflammation. Having a crippled defense mechanism exposes a patient to infectious antigens. This is what occurs in the immunocompromised host. Infections from both common and atypical organisms become more severe and more numerous. The skin becomes a window into the immune status of the individual. As the patient loses the ability to fight off infection, the visible cutaneous signs of disease herald the vulnerability within.

BACTERIAL INFECTIONS

Gram-Positive Cocci

Etiology

Coagulase-positive *Staphylococcus*, or *Staphylococcus aureus,* are part of normal human flora as well as being ubiquitous in the environment. Occasionally these organisms can be found on the skin, but, unlike its coagulase-negative counterparts (*Staphylococcus epidermidis*), they are not universally present. Because coagulase-positive *Staphylococcus* can be cultured from the nares and fingernails of 30% of the general population, they readily infect small wounds on the body (6). These organisms are sturdy when exposed to environmental factors such as dryness and warm temperatures and therefore can survive for long periods on clothing and fomites (7). In addition, they cause a wide variety of superficial skin infections: folliculitis, furunculosis, cellulitis, and wound infections.

Group A β-hemolytic *Streptococcus* (GABHS, *Streptococcus pyogenes*) is one of the most common pathogenic bacteria isolated from the pediatric population. These organisms can cause skin infections, but they do so only if the skin is traumatized in some manner and the epithelial surface is no longer intact. Although the bacteria can be found on normal skin, in general the skin provides an unwelcome environment for these organisms because of the competitive bacterial flora and lipids on its surface. Skin infections caused by GABHS, such as impetigo, are more common in children below school age and occur with greater frequency in tropical climates (8).

Streptococci are identified in the nonbullous form of impetigo, but studies prove that staphylococci remain the organisms more frequently isolated. *S. aureus* is cultured with a much higher frequency from both bullous and crusted impetigo. For this reason resistance is often encountered when penicillin is used as the sole treatment for impetigo (9). Examples of study data include the figures compiled in Florida from more than 100 children with impetigo: 77%

of the lesions, when cultured, exhibited pure growth of *S. aureus*. In only 1% was there pure growth of GABHS, and in 9% both organisms were isolated.

Skin infections caused by staphylococci and streptococci can be primary or secondary. Primary diseases (pyodermas) are those superficial infections that involve only the epidermis, such as impetigo, folliculitis, or cellulitis. Secondary infections occur when the bacteria are invaders into skin already damaged by preexisting dermatoses (i.e., atopic dermatitis).

Course in the Immunocompromised Patient

S. aureus is the bacterial pathogen that is isolated most frequently in both cutaneous and systemic disease in the immunocompromised population. In one report, up to 83% of patients with acquired immunodeficiency syndrome (AIDS) had some type of *S. aureus* infection during their disease course (10). *Staphylococcus* has a 50% nasal carriage rate in immunocompromised patients, which is twice that in their immunocompetent counterparts (10). The increased nasal carriage rate is significant because the immune system is unable to protect the host from developing skin infections from these bacteria. These infections have a tendency to become more invasive if not treated in an expedient manner with systemic β-lactamase–resistant antibiotics. Deep infections such as ecthyma, abscesses, and pyomyositis are more common sequelae. Topical treatment is not an effective substitute.

Clinical Manifestations

Impetigo remains one of the more common and easily diagnosed skin infections observed in children. There are two distinct variants of impetigo—crusted and bullous—each with a distinct clinical appearance. This form of superficial infection comprises 10% of the skin diseases seen by pediatricians (11). Primary infections are most common in children younger than 6 years of age, whereas secondary infections occur at any age.

Bullous Impetigo

Bullous impetigo occurs on previously normal skin. Initially it appears as small vesicles with minimal surrounding erythema that later develop into larger, fluid-filled bullae. The fluid within the bullae is clear at the onset but may later become turbid and pustular. These bullae are fragile; when they are unroofed, a clear shiny appearance on the skin remains. With bullous impetigo, children rarely complain of discomfort and tenderness or systemic symptoms (e.g., fever). Regional lymphadenopathy is also an uncommon observation on physical examination.

Pathogenesis. Bullous impetigo is most often caused by an *S. aureus* that releases an exfoliative toxin similar to that identified in staphylococcal scalded skin infection. Eighty percent of the *S. aureus* in bullous impetigo are phage 2 staphylococci; 60% of these are type 71 (12). In the skin infection with type 71, however, the toxin is released locally and its effect remains locally mediated.

Management. Diagnosis of bullous impetigo can often be made solely on the basis of its clinical appearance. Cultures can be useful, however, if there is any doubt to the pathogenesis of the skin infection. Cultures are also useful in identifying the antimicrobial sensitivities, expediting the choice of treatment, and enhancing the probability of cure. Because these infections spread quickly, topical antimicrobial therapy alone is often not sufficient. The treatment of choice is systemic antibiotics, and the drug of choice is a penicillinase-resistant penicillin (13). Examples include cloxacillin (orally at 50 to 100 mg per kilogram per day divided every 4 hours) or dicloxacillin (orally at 25 to 50 mg per kilogram per day divided every 6 hours). Cephalexin is also a popular antibiotic; it is given orally at a dose of 50 mg per kilogram per day. Treatment is often continued for 7 to 10 days (14).

Nonbullous or Crusted Impetigo

Nonbullous impetigo is often caused by staphylococci but, in contrast to bullous impetigo, streptococci are cultured as well. Although this infection may be seen on previously normal skin, it often occurs on diseased skin previously weakened by other dermatoses, such as atopic or contact dermatitis, scabies, or insect bites.

Lesions begin as small vesicles or pustules that quickly rupture and spontaneously form a golden, honey-colored crust. An area of erythema surrounding the expanding crusted lesion is often seen. As in the bullous variety, these lesions are typically asymptomatic. Local lymphadenopathy is rarely seen if staphylococci are the etiologic organisms but more commonly characterizes streptococcal impetigo. The disease is often spread from one area of the body to another by autoinoculation. If treatment is not instituted, lesions may resolve within about 10 days to 2 weeks, only to be replaced on other areas of the body.

In the immunocompromised host, impetigo often begins as localized or widespread erythematous, painful macules that quickly develop into vesicles that rupture and ooze serous and pustular material. A characteristic yellow crust subsequently forms (Fig. 21.1). In these patients the areas most commonly affected are the axillary, inguinal, and other intertriginous areas, whereas in immunocompetent patients the face is most commonly affected. Satellite lesions are often found as well.

The prognosis with impetigo is excellent. Local scarring is rare, although postinflamma-

tory hypopigmentation can occur in dark-skinned children once the local lesions have cleared. More serious complications are associated frequently with streptococcal impetigo. If left untreated, this form of impetigo can become invasive, resulting in cellulitis and lymphadenopathy. Another well-recognized nonsuppurative complication of streptococcal infection is acute glomerulonephritis. There are specific nephrogenic strains of streptococci associated with this sequela. Patients with streptococcal disease produce antibodies against various enzymes within the streptococcus organism. The antibodies usually can be detected 1 month after exposure to the organism. Antibodies against antistreptolysin O are present. This is not true after streptococcal pyoderma infections. It is theorized that the lipids present on the skin inactivate streptolysin (7). Antideoxyribonuclease B titers are most commonly increased; streptozyme and antistreptolysin O are increased in only 50% of cases (9).

Management. The initial treatment for non-bullous impetigo is with an antibiotic that covers both GABHS and *S. aureus*, such as a cephalosporin, erythromycin, or a penicillinase-resistant penicillin. Some studies have compared systemic antibiotic therapy with the use of a topical antibiotic such as mupirocin (Bactroban) (15,16). It was concluded that the efficacy of mupirocin is comparable to that of oral therapy when used in a 2% concentration. Drawbacks to this therapy include its expense and its weakness in accessing the diaper area, the perioral area, and the nares. The use of topical therapy may be impractical for young children because it is difficult to keep them from removing the ointment from the affected areas.

Secondary Infections

S. aureus commonly invades skin affected by other dermatoses, such as atopic dermatitis, contact dermatitis, and ichthyosis. In 90% of children with atopic dermatitis *S. aureus* can be isolated from the affected areas. Adding cloxacillin, specifically for the underlying cutaneous disease, to the treatment regimen eradicates the superinfection (11).

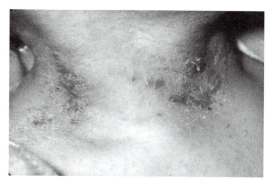

FIG. 21.1. Golden crusts overlying erythematous skin in the typical appearance of impetigo. Culture was positive for *Staphylococcus aureus*.

Cellulitis

Etiology. Cellulitis is an infection of the subcutaneous tissue with occasional extension into the dermis. It usually occurs after trauma to the skin or disruption of the epidermal barrier. Predisposing factors include insect bites, tinea pedis, or an immunodeficient state. GABHS and *S. aureus* are the most common bacterial pathogens in pediatric populations. In children younger than 5 years of age and when the cellulitis appears on the periorbital, buccal, or other facial areas, *Haemophilus influenzae* may be the cause. Gram-negative rods such as *Pseudomonas aeruginosa* can cause these superficial infections as well—often after trauma to the soles of the feet. Fungi (e.g., *Cryptococcus*), *Proteus mirabilis, Escherichia coli, Acinetobacter, P. aeruginosa,* and *Mycobacterium spp.* can cause cellulitis in patients who are immunocompromised.

Clinical Manifestations. In patients with cellulitis, the involved skin is often erythematous, edematous, warm, and tender (Fig. 21.2). The erythema and warmth are caused by the small numbers of bacteria and bacterial fragments that remain in the affected area and are enhanced by the release of lymphokines. There is no clearly identifiable border, as is seen with more superficial erysipelas. Affected children often complain of associated

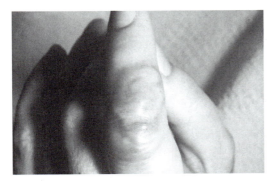

FIG. 21.2. An annular area of erythema is seen over the dorsal aspect of the left index finger. This is a case of cellulitis occurring at the site of a prior injury.

systemic symptoms such as fever and malaise, which, like the cutaneous infection are acute at onset. Tender regional lymphadenopathy is a common finding on physical examination. A history of antecedent trauma may or may not be elicited, and a portal of entry (e.g., insect bite, puncture wound) may not be identifiable. A suppurative wound may be the presentation; in this case, the likely etiologic agent is *S. aureus.* Infections are often limited to the subcutaneous and dermal areas, but occasionally there is extension of infection. In these instances, osteomyelitis and septic arthritis may be complications.

Periorbital (preseptal) cellulitis is a superficial eye infection involving the eyelid anterior to the orbital septum. There is no proptosis of the eye or pain and limitation associated with extraocular movements. *S. aureus,* GABHS, type b *H. influenzae,* and *Streptococcus pneumoniae* may cause this subtype of facial cellulitis. Lid gangrene can occur as a result of streptococcal periorbital cellulitis. GABHS releases proteolytic enzymes that cause local edema with eventual compression of the small vasculature and ischemia. This is more commonly seen in elderly or immunocompromised patients (9).

H. influenzae produces a characteristic cellulitis and occurs almost exclusively in children younger than 5 years of age (17). The cheek is most commonly involved, the neck and periorbital area less frequently. The infected skin is violaceous in color. An ipsilateral otitis media is a typical concurrent finding on physical examination. These children are usually ill and require a blood culture and lumbar puncture as part of their workup, because 10% to 15% have a secondary focus of infection (17). It is important to remember that *S. pneumoniae* can manifest similarly, often causing the skin to appear violaceous and the child to be bacteremic.

Management. The management of cellulitis depends on the presentation of the patient. Outpatient treatment of cellulitis is appropriate for adolescents and children with minimal systemic symptoms (i.e., fever, chills) and a white blood cell count lower than 15,000 cells per microliter. If the child appears toxic and has an elevated leukocyte count (15,000 cells per microliter or higher), a blood culture and complete blood count with differential may be indicated. Initial hospitalization with intravenous antibiotic therapy is often necessary until improvement is apparent. Antibiotic therapy should be initiated with drugs that cover both staphylococci and streptococci, such as a penicillinase-resistant penicillin or cephalosporin. In a child younger than 4 years of age, and in all patients with facial and periorbital cellulitis, *H. influenzae* should be a consideration. Additional supportive care, such as the use of warm compresses and elevation of the affected area, are also helpful treatment conjuncts. Aspiration of the affected areas to determine the organism is often of low yield (5% to 12%) (18). In the immunocompromised patient population, the physician should attempt to identify the causative organism by aspiration, and empiric antibiotic therapy should include coverage of *P. aeruginosa* and gram-negative enteric organisms as well as staphylococci and streptococci. Examples of such empiric antibiotics in these patients are an aminoglycoside, along with an antistaphylococcal penicillin, or a third-generation cephalosporin such as ceftazidime (17).

Erysipelas

This is a specific superficial cellulitis caused by GABHS that involves the dermis, the uppermost portion of the subcutaneous tissue, and the superficial lymphatics. Decreased host resistance is one predisposing factor for development of this streptococcal skin infection.

Clinical Manifestations. Erysipelas is a rapidly enlarging, erythematous plaque that has a demarcated, elevated, and advancing margin. The margin of erythema is distinct in comparison with the less-defined border seen in cellulitis. The involved skin is painful, indurated, and warm and may take on a peau d'orange appearance. In addition, there may be an area of central clearing surrounded by the erythematous advancing area. With erysipelas, there may be a prodrome of malaise or myalgias and associated systemic toxicity including fever, chills, headache, nausea, and vomiting.

Management. Diagnosis is often based on the clinical appearance. Aspiration from the advancing margin or from the central wound may yield streptococci. Biopsy of the area illustrates edema and vascular dilatation within the dermal layer and neutrophil infiltration in the upper subcutaneous tissue. Intravenous antibiotic therapy with penicillin V, cephalosporins, or erythromycin for 24 to 48 hours is necessary for severe infections until defervescence and a decrease in the progression of the erythema are seen. Bed rest, warm compresses, and elevation of the involved area are helpful adjuncts. Once an initial response is seen, a 10-day regimen of oral antibiotics is possible. Complications of hematogenous spread resulting in mediastinitis or subacute bacterial endocarditis may ensue. Postinfectious glomerulonephritis is also a possibility.

Folliculitis/Furunculosis

Etiology. Folliculitis is a superficial infection in which the inflammation is limited to the orifice of the hair follicle. It is most commonly caused by *S. aureus* (17). It occurs after skin colonized with *S. aureus* is occluded by emollients (as used for atopic eczema) or occlusive dressings. Furunculosis describes cutaneous abscesses that are centered on the hair follicle and are caused by certain strains of coagulase-positive *Staphylococcus*, most commonly phage type 80 or 81 (17). These organisms are able to penetrate previously normal or damaged skin through the hair follicle. Once within the follicle, the bacteria multiply and attract neutrophils. The tiny vessels within the area become thrombosed, resulting in central necrosis.

Differential Diagnosis. Many bacteria can produce lesions morphologically similar to those of folliculitis or furunculosis. Pityrosporum folliculitis, seen most commonly in tropical areas, consists of erythematous papules that are pruritic and occur on the back and upper arms. *P. aeruginosa* produces papules and pustules on the lower extremities and buttocks. Often there is a precedent history of bathing in a communal "hot tub." Gram-negative bacteria cause folliculitis in individuals with acne vulgaris and appear as pustules and abscesses on the face and upper trunk. Dermatophytes may also initiate infections involving the hair follicle. The clinical appearance of *Microsporum canis*, "gray patch" tinea capitis, is an alopecia associated with scaling of the scalp that leaves behind a round, hyperkeratotic plaque. "Black dot" tinea capitis is caused by *Tricophyton tonsurans*, which causes hairs to break off near the scalp, leaving multiple block dots surrounded by scale. *Candida albicans* produces large follicular pustules and occurs on surface areas occluded by bandages or on the back of febrile patients who are hospitalized. Eosinophilic folliculitis occurs in children with HIV and is very pruritic. Lesions are typically small, edematous papules and pustules that occur on the upper trunk, face, neck, and proximal extremities and number in the hundreds.

Clinical Manifestations. The lesions of folliculitis are typically small, round, and purulent and occur in crops. There is a halo of erythema surrounding the lesions. They are tender but otherwise asymptomatic. The lesions usually resolve without intervention within days after their appearance without scar formation; they only rarely progress into deeper follicular infections such as furunculosis.

Furuncles begin as tender papules that subsequently enlarge to form firm nodules around the hair follicle (Fig. 21.3). These nodules eventually become fluctuant and form a central area of necrosis. Spontaneous rupture and drainage usually follows and the area heals, forming a depressed scar. These lesions can occur once and resolve without recurrence, or they may relapse multiple times and involve various areas of the body. Recurrent cases may take longer than 1 year to resolve completely and are found more commonly in the warm, humid months of the year.

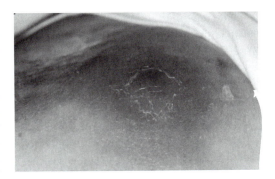

FIG. 21.3. This photograph illustrates a deep seated inflammation around a hair follicle, typical of furunculosis.

In the immunocompromised host, folliculitis manifests as papules and pustules widely distributed over the skin. They may be pruritic with evidence of excoriation. Often they is confined to the skin, but, if the bacterial density increases secondary to the underlying immunodepression, a more deep-seated infection may arise (e.g., botryomycosis). Botryomycosis, most commonly caused by *S. aureus*, represents bacterial colonization of the dermis; it is clinically seen as papules or plaques on the skin's surface surrounded by pustules on the trunk, extremities, or neck area (Fig. 21.4) (12).

Management. Most cases of folliculitis resolve with removal of predisposing factors

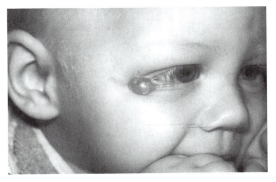

FIG. 21.4. A solitary nodule is seen at the lateral margin of the right eye of this child. It proved to be a case of botryomycosis caused by *Staphylococcus aureus*.

and cleansing of the skin with antibacterial cleansers such as chlorhexidine or with benzoyl peroxide. Topical antibiotic ointment (e.g., mupirocin), applied to lesions twice daily, facilitates rapid recovery. Ointment should be applied to the nares also, because they are the site of staphylococcal carriage. Oral antibiotics should be reserved for those cases that are resistant to topical therapy. Antistaphylococcal antibiotics, such as dicloxacillin or cephalexin, are first-line treatment choices (11). Erythromycin can be used, although the incidence of resistance of *S. aureus* is high in many areas.

The therapeutic options for furuncles depends on the appearance of the lesions at the time treatment is initiated. If the lesions are papular without a pustular core, warm compresses and oral antibiotics, such as dicloxacillin, cloxacillin, or a first-generation cephalosporin, are the preferred treatments. In these early lesions, incision and drainage is avoided to prevent inoculation of the bacteria deeper into the skin. Once a central pustular core has formed, incision and drainage along with oral antibiotics is the appropriate treatment regimen. If the furuncles involve the central eyebrow, the nares, or the lip, incision and drainage is dangerous and should be avoided to prevent cavernous venous thrombosis caused by an uncontrolled infection. Warm compresses should also be used.

Recurrent furunculosis and folliculitis must be treated with a prolonged antibiotic course as well as elimination of the carrier state in the patient. Reduction of bacterial load can be accomplished by cleansing the hands, axillae, and groin areas with antibacterial soaps. Instillation of antibacterial ointment (e.g., mupirocin) into the nares has been shown to eradicate *S. aureus* after 5 days of application in 100% of patients, and 50% of patients are free from carriage for 5 months after treatment (9).

Erythromycin-resistant *S. aureus* is even more common in immunocompromised persons than in normal hosts. β-Lactamase–resistant antibiotics should be initiated from the outset (12). Therapy is continued until total elimination of infection is apparent, which

may take several weeks in these patients. Chlorhexidine gluconate washes and mupirocin application to the nares are useful for eradication of bacterial colonization. Some physicians advocate the use of rifampin (300 mg twice daily for 3 days) to facilitate elimination of the chronic carrier state (19).

Necrotizing Fasciitis

Etiology. This rapidly progressive soft tissue infection can be caused by GABHS, *S. aureus*, *P. aeruginosa*, *S. epidermidis*, anaerobes, or gram-negative enterics. Although it is rare in children, the pediatric cases that do exist are seen mostly in neonatal patients. Predisposing factors for fasciitis include immunodeficiencies such as leukemia, aplastic anemia, trauma, varicella, and recent surgery.

Clinical Manifestations. Necrotizing fasciitis is a rapidly progressive extensive cellulitis that involves subcutaneous tissue including fascia. It can be rapidly fatal unless diagnosed early and treated with early surgical intervention. Its initial appearance is similar to that of cellulitis, but it quickly develops purpura, blistering, necrosis, and systemic toxicity. The pain is excruciating and seems out of proportion to the erythema present. The tissues become hard and dusky secondary to poor perfusion and may exude a thin, brown liquid. Crepitation of the skin and subcutis is a possible but not essential finding. There is loss of sensation to deep pinprick as cutaneous nerves are involved in the necrotic process. Lymphadenopathy or lymphangitis is rare. Systemic symptoms may dominate the clinical picture and include fever, tachycardia, lethargy, disorientation, and even frank shock.

Management. If necrotizing fasciitis is suspected, surgical consultation is imperative. If surgery is postponed for longer than 24 hours, mortality rates approach 50% (9). The diagnosis usually is made solely on clinical grounds and visualization of the fascia. Radiographically gas may be visualized, but this is an inconsistent finding. Cultures should be taken from the exudate as well as from the blood, because bacteremia is a common associated finding. Necrotizing fasciitis may be associated with hypocalcemia secondary to calcium deposition in the necrotic tissue. Supportive care such as intravenous fluids and calcium, if necessary, should not be overlooked to maintain hemodynamic stability. Immediate surgical debridement is essential for survival, and total resection of all involved tissue must be ensured. Because of the limited blood supply to the area, antibiotics alone, even at high doses, are not curative. Postoperative intravenous antibiotics, including penicillinase-resistant penicillins and an aminoglycoside, must be instituted until results of cultures and bacterial sensitivity studies return. Repair of the wound should not be attempted until the infection is completely resolved.

Other Gram-Positive Bacteria

Nocardiosis

Nocardia are aerobic actinomycetes that are ubiquitous in the environment. They are gram-positive filamentous and branched organisms that are variably acid-fast and fragment into pleomorphic rod-shaped or coccoid elements which, to an inexperienced eye, may be mistaken for hyphae (19). They are slow growers and must be placed in media such as blood agar, brain-heart infusion agar, or fungal or mycobacterial media such as Sabourad dextrose or Lowenstein-Jensen agar. Antibiotics inhibit the growth of these organisms in culture, and the addition of 10% carbon dioxide to culture media may speed their growth and therefore, ultimately the diagnosis of nocardial infection. These organisms grow well at temperatures between 25° and 45°C. The characteristic morphology of *Nocardia* in culture are small, chalky-white heaped, wrinkled, or verrucose colonies that may take up to 4 weeks to be identified within culture (20).

In humans, virulent *Nocardia* are facultative intracellular pathogens that are able to evade bactericidal defenses requiring an intact cell-mediated immune response to clear the organisms. Neutrophils are mobilized early that are capable of delaying or retarding nocardial cell growth. Later a mixed lymphocyte and phagocyte phase dominates. A lymphocytic response is necessary to eradicate these organisms by signalling phagocytes. The predominant species causing infection within humans are *Nocardia asteroides, Nocardia brasiliensis,* and *Nocardia otitidiscavarium (caviae). N. asteroides* is responsible for more than 90% of all reported cases of pulmonary and disseminated disease.

Clinical Manifestations

The incidence of nocardiosis in the United States is about 1,000 new cases annually (20). Infections with *Nocardia* have been seen in patients of all ages and are more common in patients with underlying immunodeficiency; those at special risk include children with chronic granulomatous disease, prior transplantation, current cytotoxic chemotherapy (especially steroids), lymphoreticular neoplasms, or AIDS. Seventy percent of all patients with such infections are immunosuppressed, resulting in the labelling of *Nocardia* as an opportunistic organism (20). The most common presentation of *Nocardia* infection, occurring in 75% of cases, is a pulmonary infection caused by inhalation of these soil-dwelling bacteria; person-to-person communicability is not possible (9). Predisposing factors to lung infection include bronchial obstruction and decreased bronchociliary clearance. Common symptoms include anorexia, weight loss, productive cough, dyspnea, pleuritic pain, and hemoptysis. If untreated, these infections may take a chronic course or resolve spontaneously.

Primary *Nocardia* infections may remain localized to the lung, or the infection may erode into blood vessels, leading to hematogenous spread and disseminated disease. Systemic disease is diagnosed by the presence of infection in two or more noncontiguous organs. The most common site of metastatic disease (one third of all cases) is the central nervous system (CNS). Other sites include the skin and soft tissues, the eye (especially the retina), bone, and heart.

Cutaneous nocardiosis occurs in three distinct patterns. The first and most common type occurs as a result of hematogenous spread from primary pulmonary infection. This is the most ominous type of infection. Lesions characteristically seen with disseminated disease include single or multiple abscesses, cellulitis, subcutaneous nodules, and draining sinuses (Fig. 21.5). The second type of infection is called actinomycoma or chronic cutaneous nocardiosis. Tropical and subtropical climates are more conducive to this form of infection. These lesions, most commonly seen on the trunk and extremities, are chronic, deep, penetrating, progressively destructive skin lesions with multiple draining sinuses with purulent drainage or granules. The grains that may exude from these lesions are granules containing multiple filaments of bacteria. These lesions may be difficult to distinguish from cutaneous mycetomas secondary to infections by other actinomycetes, streptomycetes, or true fungi. Culture is necessary to make the ultimate differentiation. The third type of infection is acute primary cutaneous nocardiosis. Direct inoculation of bacteria through a traumatic puncture, insect bite, or cat scratch causes this type of infection, which is characterized by cellulitis, subcutaneous abscesses, or lymphocutaneous disease (cutaneous lesions associated with regional lymphadenopathy or lymphadenitis). A cervicofacial lymphocutaneous presentation may make the diagnosis more difficult, because infections by many other organisms have a similar appearance, including infections by *S. aureus*, GABHS, *Bartonella henselaii*, and atypical mycobacteria, as well as brucellosis, tularemia, or sporotrichosis (9). Any *Nocardia* species may cause subcutaneous or cutaneous lesions, but *N. brasiliensis* most commonly evolves into locally progressive or invasive infection (19).

Diagnosis

Multiple specimens should be obtained to increase the yield of cultures. Skin lesions should be biopsied, because smears or cultures obtained by means other than biopsy are often negative. Gram stain shows delicate branching filaments less than 1 μm in diameter.

Chest radiographs show a wide range of patterns, including bronchopneumonia, lobar pneumonia, necrotizing pneumonia, and pleural empyema. One third of all sputum analyses and cultures are positive for *Nocardia*. These figures may be misleading because the organisms are respiratory saprophytes. If the patient is immunocompromised, however, growth of *Nocardia* on culture cannot be considered lightly; treatment must be initiated in all vulnerable hosts. If sputum culture remains negative, bronchoalveolar lavage or biopsy may be needed to make the diagnosis. Blood may be sent for culture, but the results are not commonly positive except in cases of an immunocompromised host.

Serologic diagnostic methods lack specificity secondary to a high incidence of cross-reactivity among the *Nocardia,* streptomycetes, and mycobacteria. An enzyme immunoassay using a 55-kD protein specific for *Nocardia* holds promise for earlier diagnosis of this serious infection than other materials (20). A high suspicion for *Nocardia* infection should be maintained with any pyoderma unresponsive to penicillinase-resistant penicillins or erythromycin, cutaneous disease with underlying pulmonary infection,

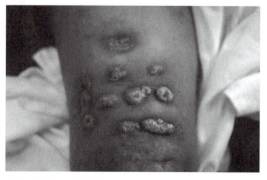

FIG. 21.5. Multiple crusted nodules over the extremity of a patient with culture-proven nocardiosis.

or cutaneous lesions characterized by draining sinuses.

Treatment

Sulfonamides are the treatment of choice, and high-dose, prolonged therapy is often required. Sulfisoxazole (150 mg per kilogram per day divided into four to six doses) or trimethoprim-sulfamethoxazole (15 mg per kilogram per day of trimethoprim and 75 mg per kilogram per day of sulfamethoxazole) is commonly prescribed (20). Minor infections require 3 to 4 months of treatment secondary to a high incidence of relapse and late-appearing metastatic disease. Systemic disease or infection may require up to 1 year of treatment to cure. AIDS patients may need to be treated indefinitely. Abscesses should be surgically drained to ensure resolution.

Even when specific treatment is initiated, the mortality rate of this infection is 25% to 40%. CNS infection is associated with an especially poor prognosis. Other poor prognostic factors include prior treatment with steroids or antineoplastics, disseminated disease, and symptoms present for less than 3 months before presentation (20).

MYCOBACTERIAL INFECTIONS

Mycobacterium tuberculosis Infection

Etiology

Mycobacterium tuberculosis is classified within the family Mycobacteriaceae and in the order Actinomycetales, along with *Nocardia* and *Corynebacterium*. These organisms are nonmotile, slender, pleomorphic, weakly gram-positive rods 1 to 5 μm long (21). Their walls are composed of lipid and mycolic acid, which explains their ability to stain with Ziehl-Neelson stain and to resist discoloration with alcohol or hydrochloric acid and therefore remain acid-fast (9). *Mycobacteria* can grow in "classic" media such as Loewenstein-Jensen medium, and their isolation from solid media may take anywhere from 3 to 6 weeks (21). Improvements

have been made in laboratory technology that enable culture results and drug sensitivities to be achieved more rapidly.

The tubercle bacilli most commonly enter the body and cause infection by inhalation. In rare cases the bacilli may inoculate the skin through wounds or bites. The incubation period may be as short as 1 day and as long as 3 months. It takes about 3 months for delayed hypersensitivity to tuberculin to develop, as illustrated by a positive Mantoux test result. The end of the incubation period is heralded by the onset of tuberculin hypersensitivity; there may be an associated fever initially that may last from 1 to 3 weeks (21).

There are three stages of tuberculosis. The first stage is exposure, which occurs when a child is in close contact with an adult with infectious pulmonary tuberculosis. Transmission of disease is through droplets of mucus containing tubercle bacilli that are later inhaled. It may take only one single droplet containing one to three organisms to initiate infection in another person. This most commonly occurs in a household but may occur in a school or day care setting (21). While the child remains in this stage the chest radiograph is within normal limits, the tuberculin skin test is negative, and there are no signs or symptoms of illness.

The second stage occurs after inhalation of tubercle bacilli that become established within pulmonary tissues and associated lymphoid tissue. Detection of infection is possible with the tuberculin skin test. There still are no signs or symptoms, and the chest radiograph remains negative during this stage.

The third stage is defined by the onset of signs or symptoms of tuberculosis: night sweats, cough, weight loss, and the development of an abnormal chest radiograph. The lifetime risk of developing tubercular disease in an immunocompetent adult once infected is 5% to 10%; disease usually occurs within the first 2 to 3 years after infection. In immunocompetent infants, the risk of developing disease is about 40% (21). The rate of disease within the pediatric population is highest in children younger than 5 years of age (21).

Clinical Manifestations

The primary complex of disease was first described by Ghon and encompasses three parts: the primary focus of parenchymal infection, lymphangitis, and regional lymphadenitis (21). Pulmonary, CNS, cutaneous, renal, ocular, and skeletal manifestations of tuberculosis are possible in children. Extrapulmonary disease had been decreasing, but a resurgence with the increase in AIDS cases has occurred in recent years (22).

The first description of a cutaneous form of tuberculosis was by Laennec in 1826, who described his own "prosecutor wart" (22). Cutaneous tuberculosis has remained rare in the United States, as was documented in the past by Lincoln and Sewell, who studied tuberculosis at Bellevue Hospital in New York City and found that only 3% of patients initially had skin lesions (23). A more recent study by Farina et al. in Madrid (22) reported an incidence of 2.4%. The manifestations of tuberculosis in the skin can be classified accordingly: lesions caused by inoculation from an exogenous source in a previously uninfected or infected child, including inoculation with the bacille Calmette-Guérin (BCG) vaccine; lesions caused by hematogenous dissemination; lesions arising from an endogenous source; and erythema nodosum (9).

Infection of the skin may arise from direct contact with mycobacteria. Because the skin is relatively resistant to the bacilli, infection tends to occur in traumatized skin, such as abrasions, bites, or a circumcision site. The initial lesion is a reddish-brown, small, painless nodule, occasionally with satellite lesions, that may ulcerate in the center. There may be a silvery scale in the central depression, which has been described as having an "apple jelly translucence" with diascopy (Fig. 21.6) (9). A lymphangitis may be associated with the clusters of lesions along its path. It takes 3 to 4 weeks for regional lymphadenopathy to develop; with time, lymphadenopathy becomes quite large and persists for months. This feature is often the most

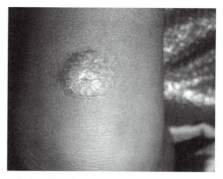

FIG. 21.6. *Mycobacterium tuberculosis* was cultured from this scaling of plaque on the knee of a child.

striking symptom and incites a visit to the physician. There are often few systemic symptoms such as fever or malaise. These lymph nodes are firm initially but may eventually soften and develop a sinus extending and draining to the overlying skin. This lesion, which represents extension from an underlying lymphadenitis or adjacent tuberculous bone or joint process, is termed scrofula or scrofuloderma. Cervical lymph nodes are most commonly infected. If the material draining from the center of these lesions is cultured early in the course of the disease, the tubercle bacilli can often be identified. Histologic examination reveals ulceration of the epidermis and superficial abscesses in the dermis in the center of the lesion with epithelioid granulomas and areas of caseation necrosis and acid-fast bacilli (9,22). This lesion is analogous to the Ghon complex or primary complex, with the portal of entry being the skin versus the lung.

People already infected with tuberculosis who are inoculated with *M. tuberculosis* develop skin lesions that can be termed "reinfection" tuberculosis. These cases are quite rare in the United States among the pediatric population. The lesions are localized to the site of inoculation and appear as a purplish "wart" 2 to 5 cm in diameter unassociated with lymphadenitis or lymphangitis (9).

BCG vaccination may produce a small papule 2 weeks after administration. This papule enlarges slowly over the following months and may reach 10 mm in diameter. Eventually there is a breakdown of the lesion to form an ulcer. This occurs in 1 of every 100,000 vaccine administrations (9).

In the early phase of hematogenous dissemination of tuberculosis, skin lesions may develop which are termed papulonecrotic tuberculids. They are rarely seen in the United States but are the most common dermatologic manifestation of tuberculosis in children worldwide. These are small nodules, often with a central area of "apple jelly" translucence or scale. They often occur on the face, thighs, and abdomen and resemble chickenpox in appearance; they heal with the formation of small, deep pits. On histologic examination, a vasculitis is seen, followed by a mononuclear infiltrate or giant cells with scattered bacilli visible (9).

Lupus vulgaris is a skin manifestation of chronic, indolent tuberculosis. It is often difficult to demonstrate bacilli on histologic examination, and the condition responds quite slowly to antituberculosis medications. It often results from reinfection of a person who has a high degree of tuberculin sensitivity, frequently after hematogenous, lymphatic, or contiguous spread from visceral disease (22). Cultures are often negative. One study demonstrated that only 6% of cutaneous cultures were positive with lupus vulgaris (24,25).

Erythema nodosum has multiple causes, one of which is tuberculosis. Others include streptococcal, meningococcal, and *Histoplasma* infections along with sensitivity reactions to medications such as sulfonamides. They are large indurated, tender, subcutaneous nodules that occur most commonly on the shins and other extensor areas of the body. Biopsy of the lesions fails to illustrate the organisms. In patients infected with tuberculosis, a purified protein derivative (PPD) test should be positive.

Diagnosis and Treatment

The differential diagnosis of cutaneous tuberculosis includes lesions caused by environmental mycobacteria including *Mycobacterium kansasii* or *Mycobacterium marinum*. Other diagnoses that may need to be considered are impetigo, cat-scratch disease, and sporotrichosis (9). Obtaining material for appropriate stains, smears, and cultures by biopsy, aspiration, or swabbings may aid in diagnosis. Patients with underlying immunosuppression (e.g., AIDS) often have lesions with an atypical appearance or multiple, widespread lesions. The Mantoux test is also useful in documenting tuberculin sensitivity and is often positive in children with cutaneous disease. Patients with overwhelming infection, concurrent viral infection, or an immunocompromised state and those taking immunosuppressive drugs may be anergic and have no reaction to the PPD. The treatment for tuberculous cutaneous disease is similar to that for pulmonary disease. Isoniazid at a dose of 10 to 15 mg per kilogram per day given once daily is used along with rifampin 10 to 20 mg per kilogram per day daily (9). The usual practice is to begin treatment with three drugs, the third being either pyrazinamide, streptomycin, or ethambutol. The third drug is used for the first 2 months of therapy or until a resistant organism can be ruled out. In the United States about 10% of *M. tuberculosis* organisms are resistant to at least one drug, and resistance is especially high in certain populations including Hispanics and Asians (21). Resistance to isoniazid and streptomycin is most prevalent, whereas resistance to rifampin remains relatively rare (21). Treatment should be initiated when the clinical suspicion for infection is high. A thorough history, physical examination, and Mantoux test should be sufficient to identify patients when this diagnosis is suspected. The diagnosis of environmental mycobacteria (as opposed to tuberculosis) may be difficult based on presentation. If such debate in diagnosis exists, one should begin empiric therapy with isoniazid and rifampin plus erythromycin, clarithromycin, and a sulfonamide so that coverage is achieved for both (9).

Other Mycobacteria

The incidence of infections by nontuberculous *Mycobacteria* has risen steadily as the prevalence of AIDS has increased. These organisms, which include *M. kansasii, M. marinum, Mycobacterium avium-intracellulare,* and *Mycobacterium ulcerans,* are not transmitted person-to-person, unlike *M. tuberculosis.*

M. marinum is an opportunistic pathogen that affects aquatic animals and humans. The organism can be found in water within heated swimming pools as well as in the open sea and in natural pools. These slow-growing organisms grow well in most media, producing whitish, shiny colonies when grown in the dark. Once they are exposed to light, a yellow pigment develops within a few days (9).

Lesions are often found on exposed areas of the body where the skin has been injured previously. Initially there are multiple purplish-pink papules or nodules that eventually become keratotic, then suppurative, and then ulcerate (Fig. 21.7) (10). Biopsy with culture allows one to make the diagnosis and to differentiate this disease from primary inoculation tuberculosis, sporotrichosis, or lupus vulgaris. Microscopic examination reveals a granulomatous dermatitis with a diffuse epithelioid cell reaction, fibrinoid changes, and tubercle formation. Acid-fast organisms are rarely seen (9). If organisms are visualized, they are larger and longer acid-fast bacilli than their mycobacterial counterparts. PPD may or may not be positive.

Excision of lesions is suggested to debulk the infection. Local care may include warm compresses or a heating pad, because the growth of the causative organisms is inhibited at temperatures higher than 35°C. Treatment includes one of the following: tetracycline (25 to 50 mg per kilogram per day; maximum, 3 g); minocycline (50 to 100 mg daily to three times daily); doxycycline (2.5 to 5.0 mg per kilogram per day; maximum, 200 mg); rifampin (10 to 20 mg per kilogram per day; maximum, 600 mg); or ethambutol (15 to 25 mg per kilogram per day). Antibiotics should be continued for 2 to 3 months (9).

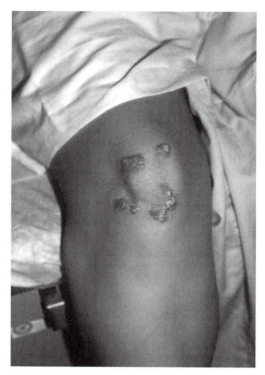

FIG. 21.7. Multiple crusted nodules are seen over the knee of this patient. Culture was positive for *Mycobacterium marinum.*

M. avium-intracellulare is an opportunistic pathogen that can be isolated from the soil, water, animals, or foods. In the immunosuppressed patient it can be aggressive, causing pulmonary disease in adults and lymphadenitis in children. Skin lesions can also be a manifestation of *M. avium-intracellulare.* A disseminated maculopapular rash is most commonly seen; it may appear quite similar to the papular rash of miliary tuberculosis. The treatment for this infection is clarithromycin or azithromycin continued for weeks to months.

GRAM-NEGATIVE INFECTIONS

Pseudomonas Infection

Etiology

Pseudomonas and related species are aerobic, motile, gram-negative bacilli that can be found in the soil, in water, on plants, and on animals. Most of these organisms are rarely pathogenic to humans, and if they do cause disease they are opportunists seen in patients with underlying burns, cystic fibrosis, malignancy, immunodeficiencies, immunosuppressive therapy, or malnourished state. The member of the *Pseudomonas* family most commonly found to cause such opportunistic infections is *P. aeruginosa*. These organisms grow easily on standard laboratory media at 37°C. Their name comes from the characteristic blue-green pigment they produce, termed pyocyanin (26).

P. aeruginosa contains many virulence factors, including multiple extracellular enzymes, an endotoxin, and an exotoxin. The extracellular enzymes include elastases, lipases, and collagenase, among others, and are believed to be responsible for the localized necrosis seen in the cutaneous and pulmonary infections caused by this bacterium. The pili and fimbriae they possess enhance adherence to mucosal surfaces (26).

Epidemiology

Although 5% to 30% of normal hosts have *P. aeruginosa* in their gastrointestinal tract, it is usually not found as part of the normal microflora in the human body (26). The organism frequently colonizes the hospital environment by entering on clothes, skin, and shoes of patients and staff. It grows in moist environments within the hospital and often can be identified in distilled water, kitchen facilities, whirlpools, irrigation and dialysis fluids, and respiratory care and dialysis equipment. The likelihood of developing an infection from *P. aeruginosa* increases proportionally to the length of the hospital stay (26). Outside the hospital, sources for infection include swimming pools, hot tubs, contact lens solution, and soles of sneakers.

Clinical Manifestations

P. aeruginosa can produce infection in normal, healthy pediatric hosts. This typically occurs as the bacteria is introduced into a wound through contamination by water or soil. A cellulitis develops that initially appears as an erythematous macule and later progresses to small hemorrhagic nodules with areas of necrosis and eschar formation surrounded by an erythematous halo.

Otitis externa occurs secondary to maceration of the skin of the external auditory canal from a perforated otitis media or from failure to dry the ear canal after swimming and showering. Pain is followed by drainage and swelling around the orifice of the external ear canal. Characteristically, patients complain of extreme pain with movement of the pinna. Treatment should be initiated quickly. In the immunocompromised patient a specific type of otitis externa, termed malignant otitis externa, occurs that is not limited to dermal involvement. There is invasion of the cartilage, bones, and nerves; patients have high fever and may develop cranial nerve palsies, necrosis of parts of the external ear, osteomyelitis of the temporal bone or basilar skull, or mastoiditis. With this severe form there is a small risk of meningitis, which primarily occurs in patients with underlying malnutrition, malignancy, or leukopenia. The mortality rate in malignant otitis externa can be as high as 50% (9). There have been multiple reports of *Pseudomonas* otitis externa in infants with HIV infection (27).

Hot tub folliculitis consists of superficial pruritic papules, pustules, or erythematous nodules that manifest 8 to 48 hours after use of a hot tub or swimming pool and are the most dense in areas covered by bathing suits. These lesions typically resolve without intervention, although topical treatment may be employed in certain instances. Steroids should be avoided, because they exacerbate the condition and may lead to spread of the lesions. In the immunosuppressed host these lesions may progress to ecthyma gangrenosum. This condition may be prevented by cleaning the pool or hot tub every 6 to 8 weeks, maintaining a water pH of 7.2 to 7.4, and keeping the chlorine concentration at an appropriate level (9).

P. aeruginosa may produce a secondary pyoderma in an area affected by another dermatitis or previously traumatized. There is a characteristic blue-green exudate that seeps from the wound, and a sweet, grape-like odor exudes from the area. Treatment of the underlying skin condition along with the *Pseudomonas* allows for a more rapid resolution. This bacterium may also cause a blastomycosis-like pyoderma which appears as large, verrucous plaques with multiple pustules and elevated borders (28). Histologically they can be differentiated from blastomycosis by the presence of pseudoepitheliomatous hyperplasia with abscesses that lack giant cells or fungal elements (9).

Thirty percent of cases of *Pseudomonas* sepsis are associated with cutaneous lesions (29). The most typical of these lesions is ecthyma gangrenosum. This begins as an area of erythema and edema that quickly develops into a hemorrhagic bulla that ruptures (Fig. 21.8). This progresses into an area of

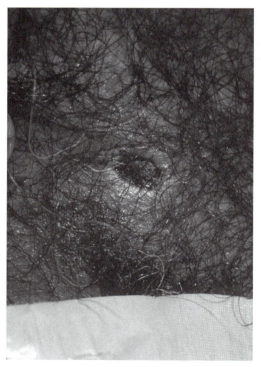

FIG. 21.8. A dark eschar is seen overlying an area of ulceration on the skin of a patient with *Pseudomonas* septicemia. This lesion is typical of ecthyma gangrenosum.

central necrosis surrounded by an erythematous halo. These lesions evolve over 12 to 24 hours. Histologically they are characterized by a vasculitis without thrombosis. Gram-negative bacilli can be detected in the adventitia and media of the veins deep within the dermis but sparing the intima and lumen. There is minimal inflammation, with few neutrophils seen. Diagnosis is made by a suggestive, painful lesion leading to aspiration biopsy and Gram stain demonstrating gram-negative rods. Cultures of fluid from the lesions and blood cultures are usually positive. Underlying immunosuppression secondary to malignancy, chemotherapy, malnutrition, or diabetes mellitus is a predisposing factor for the development of *Pseudomonas* septicemia and ecthyma gangrenosum. Patients with granulocytopenia are prone to life-threatening *Pseudomonas,* sepsis with the portal of entry of the organisms being the gastrointestinal tract (30). Any patient with this underlying condition who has suspicious cutaneous lesions should rapidly undergo aspiration biopsy of a lesion with blood culture and initiation of appropriate treatment. Other lesions also may be seen with bacteremia, including painful vesicles or erythematous maculopapules or nodules.

Children with leukemia, especially if they are receiving chemotherapy and are neutropenic, are at high risk for development of *Pseudomonas* septicemia. Infection results from invasion of the bloodstream by the bacteria present within the gastrointestinal tract. Those at highest risk are patients with an absolute neutrophil count lower than 100 cells per microliter. Patients with a higher mortality rate are those who have an absolute neutrophil count lower than 100 cells per microliter, perineal skin lesions, and bacteremia during remission or induction therapy versus relapse of disease (30). The single factor that places these children at such high risk is granulocytopenia. The presence of indwelling intravenous lines or Foley catheters places a patient at increased risk for *Pseudomonas* infection.

Treatment

Otitis externa is frequently treated with topical gentamicin or Neosporin, or tobramycin otic solution is applied with a cotton wick four times daily. If these infections recur frequently, 2% acetic acid solution is applied to the external auditory canal for weeks to months. With malignant otitis externa, intravenous antibiotics are added, such as tobramycin 6 mg per kilogram per day divided into three doses for 10 to 14 days (9). Minor skin infections (e.g., local cellulitis, pyodermas) may be treated with topical treatment such as acetic acid, Neosporin, or gentamicin creams. An intravenous aminoglycoside and a semisynthetic penicillin should be added as well. With older teens, oral ciprofloxacin at 500 mg twice daily or ofloxacin 400 mg twice daily can be used. Hot tub folliculitis may resolve without medical intervention. If treatment is desired, topical acetic acid or gentamicin cream can be used until the lesions improve. Any cutaneous abscesses or abscesses in other locations should be surgically incised and drained; failure to do this may result in a failure of intravenous antibiotics. Osteomyelitis of the foot must be surgically debrided and treated with a 10- to 14-day course of intravenous antibiotics.

For *Pseudomonas* septicemia and ecthyma gangrenosum, intravenous antibiotic therapy should be initiated quickly. Intravenous aminoglycosides such as tobramycin, gentamicin, or amikacin, along with a β-lactam antibiotic such as an antipseudomonal penicillin or third- or fourth-generation cephalosporin, should be the treatment of choice. This combination is synergistic against this organism (26).

FUNGAL INFECTIONS

Cutaneous infections caused by fungi are among the most common type of infections seen among immunocompromised patients. Although many of these infections are not life-threatening, they can cause considerable morbidity because they are difficult to eradicate and tend to recur. The presence of these infections also predisposes patients to further infections, such as bacterial superinfection. Infection of the skin and the subcutaneous tissue may be the initial manifestation of fungal disease in the immunocompromised patient (31). In patients with HIV infection, fungal infection involving the skin and mucous membranes may be the first warning sign of an underlying immunodeficiency. Early diagnosis, therefore, is important to identify any comorbid condition in the host, such as overwhelming infection or immunodeficiency, for which early intervention may improve the ultimate prognosis.

There are two mechanisms by which the body defends itself against fungal infection: the nonimmune or natural resistance and the immune or acquired resistance. Nonimmune defense protects the skin from colonization and local invasion by fungi. The skin and mucous membranes possess normal bacterial flora that prevent colonization by pathogenic bacteria and fungi. This defense is weakened by the use of broad-spectrum antibiotics, which alter the normal flora and thereby make the patient vulnerable to fungal infection (32). An intact skin or membrane barrier makes colonization by pathogenic fungi more difficult. The breakdown of this barrier by the insertion of catheters or the presence of wounds or burns facilitates local invasion of the skin by fungi (32). The last mechanism of natural resistance that can be used if local defenses are disrupted involves the stimulation of polymorphonuclear leukocytes. Intracellular killing of yeast forms by phagocytosis and extracellular killing of hyphae are involved in this phase of defense. Neutropenia with neutrophil function defects, as is seen in chronic granulomatous disease or after chemotherapy, is the most important neutrophil defect resulting in fungal infections, particularly those due to *Aspergillus* and *Candida* (32).

The immune response against fungal infection involves primarily the cellular immune system carried out by T lymphocytes, macrophages, and cytokines. Patients with defective cellular immune systems, such as patients taking high-dose corticosteroids, undergoing cytotoxic chemotherapy, struggling with lymphoma or AIDS, or recovering from transplantation, are very susceptible to the development of recurrent fungal infections localized to the skin and mucous membranes. Because the cellular immune system is the principal defense against fungal infection, these patients are also at increased risk for development of disseminated disease once colonization has occurred (32).

Fungal skin infections occur by two mechanisms. Primary skin infection occurs when direct contact with the organism results in symptoms. Secondary infection results from hematogenous spread of the organism to the skin from an underlying visceral site. Exceptions to this rule are *Candida* and *Malessezia furfur,* which are part of the normal human flora. Ordinarily these organisms do not cause cutaneous infection, but if host resistance is lowered or the local environment becomes favorable they can cause clinical infection. Risk factors include diabetes mellitus; the use of occlusive dressings, broad-spectrum antibiotics, or steroids; and increased humidity (32).

The environment itself can be a source of fungal infection. Dermatophyte infections are acquired by coming in contact with these organisms present in the soil or on animals. Other infections result from inoculation of infected material into a wound. Most disseminated fungal infections are exogenously acquired, and skin manifestations occur as a result of hematogenous dissemination from an internal primary source, most often the lungs.

The diagnosis of superficial fungal infection is usually suspected based on appearance. If a systemic infection is suspected and, for that reason, systemic antifungal therapy is to be administered, diagnosis should be made based on microscopic examination and culture of tissue. A more in-depth diagnostic workup should also be performed in patients for whom topical treatments have failed and in immunosuppressed hosts (32). Microscopic examination of collected scrapings from various lesions after preparation with potassium hydroxide (KOH) allows for identification of any hyphae, pseudohyphae, or yeast forms. A presumptive diagnosis may be made based on the morphology of the organisms observed under the microscope with wet preparation techniques, allowing for a more appropriate choice of empiric antifungal therapy. Culture does provide the definitive diagnosis. Materials may be attained from scrapings alone, but if superficial specimens are not diagnostic a biopsy should be performed. This is especially important in the immunocompromised patient, in whom the clinical appearance of many fungal infections may be atypical and in whom biopsy may provide an early diagnosis of disseminated infection. Various media may be used (e.g., Sabouraud's agar) to isolate the organisms. It may take 1 week for yeast to grow and as long as 4 to 6 weeks for any hyphal growth.

Superficial Cutaneous Fungal Infections

Dermatophytes

There are three genera that compose the dermatophytes: *Microsporum, Trichophyton,* and *Epidermophyton.* The species that are most commonly responsible for disease vary with the geographic area. In the United States the predominant organisms isolated are *Trichophyton rubrum* (55%), *T. tonsurans* (31%), *Trichophyton mentagrophytes* (6%), *M. canis* (4%), and *Epidermophyton floccosum* (2%) (33,34). The incidence of dermatophyte infections in immunocompromised persons is similar to that in immunocompetent individuals. Referral centers have reported a 15% to 40% incidence of dermatophyte infections among their HIV-infected populations (35). The severity of symptoms and the difficulty of eradication make this disease process more challenging in the host with a compromised immune system (36).

These organisms are able to digest and invade keratin, including the stratum corneum of the skin, hair, and nails (37). It is the host's inflammatory response and active keratin destruction that are responsible for the clinical appearance of disease (32).

Infections caused by dermatophytes are classified by the involved body site. During childhood the hair and general body surface are more commonly involved; infections of the nails are often seen after puberty (37).

Tinea Pedis

This infection affects the feet and is the most common dermatophyte infection seen in patients with AIDS. In one study this infection was identified as the third most common cutaneous fungal infection in HIV-positive patients (38). It is most commonly caused by *T. rubrum*; *T. mentagrophytes* and *E. floccosum* are also isolated (39,40). This infection is found most commonly after the age of puberty. Occlusion of the feet, which results in an increase of heat and moisture to the area, results in infection. There are three patterns of clinical symptoms. The first and most common is the interdigital form in which the web spaces between the toes, the lateral toes affected first, become erythematous, cracked, and scaly. Fissures develop in the stratum corneum which may serve as a portal of entry for bacteria (37). Secondary cellulitis, lymphangitis, or lymphadenitis may result. The "moccasin" type of infection involves the plantar surface of the foot. Erythematous, dry, and hyperkeratotic plaques develop on the plantar or lateral surface of the foot (37). A third form is characterized by the presence of vesicles on any part of the foot. The lesions are intensely pruritic and often cause large, denuded areas of skin along the foot. This type of infection is often caused by *T. mentagrophytes* (32). Bullae, wart-like papules, and involvement of both hands and feet with such lesions are atypical appearances of infection seen in the context of immunodeficiency (35).

Examination of the scale or contents of the vesicles under the microscope after KOH preparation allows one to visualize multiple branching septate hyphae. Topical antifungals, such as an azole or one of the fungicidal allylamines, are often the first line of treatment, along with maintenance of a cool, dry environment for the affected skin. If resolu-

tion fails to occur, oral griseofulvin, itraconazole, or terbinafine is given for 3 to 4 weeks. One study suggested that itraconazole be given twice daily as the treatment of choice, followed by maintenance therapy with ketoconazole cream (38).

Tinea Capitis

Tinea capitis is an infection of the scalp and hair. It is more often seen in children before the onset of puberty. Although *Microsporum* species were more often isolated in the past, *T. tonsurans* is currently the predominant species responsible for these infections in the United States (32,41). This organism causes infection most commonly in children in the first decade of life, but infection may persist into the adult years if not adequately treated. It is transmitted from person to person by direct contact. There are many different patterns of infection, and pruritus may or may not be an associated symptom. *Trichophyton* species cause an infection characterized by scaling of the scalp, occasionally associated with erythema and alopecia (Fig. 21.9). An associated inflammatory response with papules and pustules may accompany *Trichophyton* infections and was seen in 60% of patients in one series (42). Occipital and cervical lymphadenopathy, leukocytosis, and fever are occasionally associated complaints. The affected hairs may break close to the scalp,

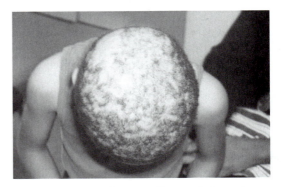

FIG. 21.9. The diffuse scaling and alopecia on the scalp of this child is characteristic of *Trichophyton tonsurans* infection.

leaving a pattern labeled as "black dot" alopecia. This is not a common finding, and in one series by Bronson et al. (42) it was seen in only 10% of cases. Its most dramatic form is termed kerion, which is a large, boggy, tender, raised area of the scalp with pustules, scaling, erythema, or alopecia.

Microsporum species may also cause tinea capitis in young children. The hairs are often gray-tinged secondary to the growth of the spores outside the hair shaft. There is moderate scale, and the hairs break further from the scalp surface. There is only a small inflammatory response, demonstrated by small papules at the base of the hair shafts along the periphery of the lesions, resulting in the clinical picture known as "ringworm." The hyphae can be found within the hair shaft, whereas spores are located outside the hair (37). When viewed with a Wood's lamp, the hair fluoresces a yellow-green color.

Another manifestation of tinea capitis is an immune reaction to the fungus seen in an area distant from the scalp. This dermatophytid, or "id" reaction is a result of the interaction between the fungal antigen and the host's immune system (43). Although these reactions may occur with any type of dermatophyte infection, they are most commonly associated with inflammatory tinea capitis (e.g., kerion) (37). The proximal extremities and trunk are most often involved, but the forehead and postauricular areas are not uncommonly affected. Clinically, the reaction appears as a papular rash or a dermatitis similar in appearance to pityriasis rosea. The rash may become follicular as well. This id reaction typically occurs shortly after initiation of treatment and therefore can be mistakenly identified as a drug reaction (37).

Diagnosis of tinea capitis requires identification of the causative organism. The most common differential diagnosis includes seborrheic dermatitis, contact dermatitis, trichtillomania, impetigo, and primary bacterial folliculitis. Wood's lamp evaluation can be used, but most cases of tinea capitis are caused by organisms that do not fluoresce (*Trichophyton*). Observation of a hair prepared initially with KOH under the microscope is another means of tentative and more rapid diagnosis. Definitive diagnosis requires culture on a medium such as Sabourad's agar, the standard mycologic medium. Short hairs that have previously broken off can be removed for culture by gently rubbing the area of the scalp with a dull surface such as a tongue depressor. One should avoid plucking the hair forcefully, because this may cause the hair to break, leaving the infected portion of the hair attached to the scalp and therefore leading to a false-negative culture result. Another medium that may be used is dermatophyte test medium, which consists of phytone dextrose agar along with chlortetracycline, cycloheximide, gentamicin, and buffered phenol red. This medium is selective for dermatophytes and visibly turns from its original brown appearance to red in the presence of dermatophyte growth. This color change can be seen within 14 days (37).

Because of the high risk of contagious spread, treatment of tinea capitis should begin quickly in any child with an inflammatory condition of the scalp associated with hair loss. Tinea capitis is less likely to resolve without treatment than are other dermatophyte infections. Griseofulvin remains the drug of choice because of its low cost and relatively few adverse effects. It functions by interfering with microtubular structure and function, resulting in the production of defective DNA, and inhibiting cell wall synthesis (44,45). It is begun at a dose of 15 mg per kilogram per day (ultramicrosized form) or 20 mg per kilogram per day (microsized form) and should be taken with milk or a fatty meal for at least 2 weeks after resolution of visible lesions (45,46). The minimum length of treatment depends on the site of infection: tinea capitis, 6 to 12 weeks; tinea pedis, 4 to 6 months; and tinea unguium, 6 to 12 months. The cure rate is 95% for any lesions of the body or scalp but 50% for lesions of the feet and 20% for infections of the toenails (47). If compliance is good, there are few cases refractive to this therapy. Liver enzymes and blood counts should be monitored monthly during courses lasting longer than 2 months in healthy children. Side effects include headache, nausea, diarrhea, abdominal cramping, hepatic dysfunction, leukopenia, and neutropenia (45,48).

Itraconazole is a triazole with a similar mechanism of action to ketoconazole. It has shown to be effective when given as continuous or pulse therapy. For continuous therapy, 5 mg per kilogram per day is given for 4 weeks. As a pulse regimen, the dose is 5 mg per kilogram per day for 1 week, followed by a second week of therapy, if necessary, after 2 to 3 weeks off therapy (45). Adverse effects include headache, skin rashes, and gastrointestinal complaints (49). Another option is terbinafine, an allylamine that inhibits fungal squalene epoxidase, leading to the accumulation of squalene (50). The dose used is 62.5 mg once daily for patients weighing less than 20 kg, 125 mg for those weighing between 20 and 40 kg, and 250 mg for those weighing more than 40 kg (51). In one study by Krafchik and Pelletier (51), administration of terbinafine once daily for 2 weeks led to a mycologic cure in 86% of patients (51). Adverse effects are few and include taste impairment and gastrointestinal complaints (50). Efficacy of all these treatments is less against *Microsporum* species, and longer duration of treatment is often required.

Prednisone in a dose of 1 mg per kilogram given once daily for 1 to 2 weeks is usually sufficient for the treatment of very tender kerions, along with antifungal therapy (37).

Onychomycosis

Onychomycosis describes a fungal infection of the nail. Tinea unguium specifically describes infection of the nail by a dermatophyte. This infection is rarely seen in children before the onset of puberty, and its incidence steadily increases with increasing age. One study found a prevalence of 1.3% in persons 16 to 34 years of age, 2.4% in those between 35 and 50 years, and 4.7% in those older than 55 years of age (52). *T. rubrum* is the organism most commonly isolated in fungal infections of the nails, but other fungi, such as *Candida* species, *Scopulariopsis brevicaulis,*

Hendersonula toruloidea, and *Scytalidium hyalinum,* may also cause similar infections (32). Because of the variety of etiologic organisms, cultures should be taken before therapy is begun.

There are three forms of onychomycosis. Distal subungual disease is the most common presentation. Infection begins at the distal and lateral margins and progressively extends onto the nail centripetally. The fungus may infect a previously healthy nail, or it may colonize an already diseased nail (53). A white patch initially appears on the most distal and lateral edge of the nail, with progressive involvement occurring over a matter of weeks in the immunocompromised patient. Eventually the nail becomes opaque, thickened, friable, and raised by the underlying debris. The toenails are more often involved, and when the hands are infected it is usually unilateral disease. *T. rubrum, T. mentagrophytes,* and *E. floccosum* are the most common etiologic agents of this subtype of onychomycosis (37).

The second form is superficial white onychomycosis, or leukonychia trichophyta, which is seen almost exclusively on the toenails. It is most commonly caused by *T. mentagrophytes* (32). In an article published by Ploysangam and Lucky (54), samples from a small series of pediatric patients with white superficial onychomycosis were cultured and all grew *T. rubrum.* Most of the patients had an associated tinea pedis. Onychomycosis is rare in prepubertal children, and white superficial onychomycosis is even more unusual (55,56). This article illustrates the possibility of a different pathogen's being responsible for white superficial onychomycosis in the pediatric population compared with the adult population. Owing to the presence of tinea pedis in association with the nail findings, it was hypothesized that childhood onychomycosis could be acquired from a concomitant tinea pedis (54). Here the pathogenic fungus affects only the superior, outer aspect of the nail plate.

The last type is proximal subungual onychomycosis, which is similar to the distal form except that the infection begins in the cuticle and appears as a white plaque extending distally. The pathogen enters by way of the cuticle and then migrates along the proximal nail groove to involve the matrix, the nail bed, and ultimately the nail plate. It is less common than the distal subtype but has become increasingly common with the increasing incidence of HIV infection. It often occurs on the fingernails in association with chronic paronychia (53). *T. rubrum, T. tonsurans, Trichophyton schoenleinii,* and *Trichophyton megninii* are the most common offenders. Dystrophic nails may eventually arise as a complication of distal or proximal onychomycosis or secondary to chronic mucocutaneous candidiasis.

Because dystrophic nail changes can be misdiagnosed as tinea, KOH or periodic acid–Schiff examination or culture should be performed on a nail sample before treatment is begun to accurately establish a diagnosis. In immunocompromised patients, such as those with HIV infection and those receiving cytotoxic chemotherapy, *Candida* species may infect nails, yielding onychomycosis indistinguishable from that of dermatophyte-infested nails. If one fails to obtain appropriate cultures before initiating therapy, therefore, a candidal infection that is unresponsive to griseofulvin may be missed.

Tinea unguium is the most resistant dermatophyte to treatment. Topical therapy does not clear the infection, and systemic antifungals often fail. Cure rates of 70% are often reported with griseofulvin treatment of fingernail infection, but cure rates are merely 20% to 30% when the same agent is used for toenail infection (32). Four to 6 months of therapy is required for tinea unguium of the fingernails to resolve, and 6 to 12 months for tinea unguium of the toenails. The introduction of itraconazole has allowed more effective and shorter courses of therapy. The use of pulse itraconazole was shown by Hay (57) to work well in the immunosuppressed patient. Total length of therapy may be only 12 weeks. Liver functions should be monitored if itraconazole is used, although true risk of hepatotoxicity in children is low.

Candidiasis

Candida species are members of the phylum Dikaryomycota, which also includes *Malessezia,* the dermatophytes, *Trichosporon,* and *Cryptococcus* (37). *C. albicans* is part of the normal flora of the alimentary canal and mucocutaneous surfaces of humans. Normally this organism is noninvasive; infection results from disruption of local barriers or functional compromise and remains limited to mucocutaneous surfaces. With the increase in the immunocompromised population, the incidence of systemic disease associated with *Candida* species is increasing; it is now listed as a presenting sign of HIV infection (58). There are numerous factors that may affect whether this organism's presence within the body results in disease secondary to overgrowth and invasion of mucous membranes or cutaneous surfaces: age, endocrine dysfunction (e.g., diabetes mellitus), use of systemic antimicrobials, resident flora, malnutrition, trauma, and prematurity (37). The great majority of infections are caused by *C. albicans* but there are about 20 species that may be isolated.

Oral Candidiasis

C. albicans is present in the mouths of most newborn infants by the second week of life, and the organism may be cultured from the oropharyngeal cavity of 80% of infants by 4 weeks (37). In most of these culture-positive babies, clinical infection does not result. It is not uncommon or alarming, however, for infants to present to their pediatrician's office with acute proliferation of the organism, an infection termed acute pseudomembranous candidiasis or thrush. It has been estimated that 0.5% to 20% of healthy infants will have thrush; the persistence or repeated occurrence of this disease beyond 6 months of life should raise suspicion of an underlying immunocompromised state such as congenital HIV infection (59). It is also frequently seen in patients receiving chronic corticosteroid therapy or cytotoxic chemotherapy for malignancy. Oral candidiasis is by far the most common oral opportunistic infection seen in the HIV population, occurring in more than 90% of HIV patients at some time during their illness (60). It can occur during acute retroviral disease, but it is seen more commonly with disease progression, especially in the pseudomembranous and erythematous forms (37).

There are three presentations of oral candidiasis: pseudomembranous, erythematous, and angular cheilitis. The pseudomembranous form manifests as a removable white to gray plaque that may occur on any mucosal surface. When the superficial surface of the plaque is gently removed, an erythematous base is left behind. KOH preparation reveals abundant pseudohyphae mixed with yeast forms. These lesions should be distinguished from other oral white plaques caused by lichen planus, squamous cell carcinoma, secondary syphilis, or leukoplakia—all of which do not normally occur in the healthy neonate (37).

Erythematous candidiasis appears as an erythematous "thumbprint-like" patch on the hard or soft palate or as an area on the tongue with papillary loss. A local burning sensation and a metallic taste may result.

Angular cheilitis, or perleche, is a cracking or fissuring of the commissures of the mouth. It is an inflammatory reaction that stems from dryness or irritation of the skin at the corners of the mouth that subsequently become superinfected with *Candida.*

Oropharyngeal candidiasis can be diagnosed clinically or by examination of smears from the lesions with a KOH preparation. Culture is used only if identification of the specific strain of fungus is necessary.

A variety of agents that may be used in the treatment of oral candidiasis, including the polyene antifungals, the azoles, gentian violet, and chlorhexidine. There are also numerous forms of topical treatments: oral troches, vaginal tablets, rinses, creams, slow-release preparations, and pastilles. These available topical therapies allow the avoidance of systemic therapy and its associated adverse effects. For topical therapy to be effective, the medication must have sufficient time in contact with the oral mucosa.

Nystatin is the only polyene antifungal available for topical use for oropharyngeal candidiasis, and its efficacy varies with the formulation and dose used. It is available as an unflavored 100,000-unit vaginal tablet, a 200,000-unit licorice-flavored oral pastille, a 50% oral rinse, and a slow-release preparation. The vaginal troches are very effective, although the medication has an unpleasant taste and causes mild nausea or other gastrointestinal disturbance. It does not contain sucrose, so the risk of dental caries with prolonged use is minimized. The rinse is expensive and is prepared with sucrose to make it more palatable. It often cannot provide adequate contact time with the oral mucosa and therefore is often ineffective. Oral pastilles must be used five times daily; they are licorice-flavored to camouflage any unpleasant taste (60).

Clotrimazole has a pleasant taste and is an effective antifungal agent. It is used as a oral troche that is dissolved in the mouth five times daily. As an ointment, it can be applied to the commissures of the mouth to treat angular cheilitis. Clotrimazole troches taken daily have proved to be as effective as systemic therapy as prophylaxis in cancer patients undergoing chemotherapy (61).

Systemic therapy with fluconazole is another option. In studies comparing the efficacy of clotrimazole five times daily with that of once-daily fluconzole, fluconazole was more effective in clearing the candidiasis and in providing a longer disease-free interval (62). However, one article reported a fluconazole resistance among *Candida* species (60).

If there is no response to initial fluconazole therapy, resistance should be assumed, and a change in therapy should immediately occur.

Cutaneous Candidiasis

Candida species cannot be cultured from most areas of the skin in healthy individuals. Superficial yeast infections may often be attributed to local factors such as heat, moisture, and maceration. These factors are found in the diaper area of the healthy infant, which accounts for the candidal diaper dermatitis commonly encountered by pediatricians. Infected skin appears very erythematous (often described as "beefy red") and edematous, with areas of erosion and weeping. Tiny pustules with a rim of scale are often present along the periphery of infected areas as "satellite" lesions. Erythematous plaques resembling psoriasis can also be seen on occasion. The most commonly affected sites are intertriginous areas such as the groin, axilla, inframammary, and perianal areas. Balanitis and vaginitis may be seen as well. Pruritus is a common associated symptom. Paronychia, inflammation of the skin surrounding the nail, can be caused by *Candida*. It is commonly seen in persons whose hands or feet are exposed to moisture repeatedly throughout the day, resulting in skin maceration. It manifests with erythema and edema of the skin and separation of the skin from the surrounding nail. Dystrophic nails can be a complication of this often chronic infection. Diagnosis is made by examination of a KOH preparation and observation of mycelial forms. Culture may be necessary to make the diagnosis; however, the results can be misleading, because *Candida* can be occasionally cultured from noninfected skin.

The first goal in treatment of candidal infections is to avoid moisture, occlusion, and maceration of the skin. Drying of affected areas quickly leads to a reduction in the swelling and pain. Burow's soaks used twice daily can expedite the drying process. Topical nystatin or another antifungal cream or ointment can be used (37). Other topical agents, such as clotrimazole and miconazole, have proved to be very effective. It is the rare patient who requires systemic antifungal therapy with ketoconazole or fluconazole to clear cutaneous infections; however, oral agents are often necessary for nail and paronychial infections.

Cryptococcosis

Cryptococcus neoformans is a fungus that is distributed in the soil worldwide and is spread by pigeon droppings. Primary infection occurs through inhalation of aerosolized soil particles containing the yeast forms into the lungs. The skin and nasal mucosa can also serve as portals of entry for the yeast. Subclinical infection occurs in the majority of the cases, with patients occasionally complaining of flu-like symptoms. In the healthy individual, transient symptoms may be localized to the lung, bone, genitourinary tract, CNS, or other organs. In the immunocompromised patient, hematogenous spread of the organism often results in disseminated disease. Those patients at highest risk for disseminated disease are patients with AIDS, lymphoma, transplantation, or corticosteroid use. It is an encapsulated yeast form, unlike other fungi, and it has a propensity for attacking the CNS. Mucocutaneous findings are present in 10% to 15% of cases of disseminated disease (35). After the CNS and lungs, the skin is the third most common site of cryptococcal infection (35). In children with AIDS it is one of the most common opportunistic infections, along with *Candida*. In a series of almost 200 patients who had undergone renal transplantation, cryptococcosis was the most common deep fungal infection (63).

Primary skin infection due to *Cryptococcus* has been reported but is extremely rare. Patients with isolated cutaneous disease have a favorable prognosis, whereas disseminated disease is fatal if treatment is not instituted immediately. Cutaneous manifestations of infection with this encapsulated yeast are multiple and may include erythematous papules, nodules, pustules, acneiform lesions, ulcers, abscesses, verrucous papules, granulomas, or tumor-like swellings (10). Lesions may be located on any area of the body but have a tendency to occur on the face and neck. Because their appearance is polymorphous and may mimic that of many other cutaneous diseases, differential diagnosis must be made via skin biopsy to distinguish cryptococcal disease from molluscum contagiosum, HSV infection, pyoderma gangrenosum, and cellulitis. In AIDS patients, umbilicated papules resembling molluscum contagiosum are a common presentation.

The possibility of cutaneous *Cryptococcus* infection must be considered in any im-

munocompromised individual with lesions resembling molluscum. A quick diagnosis can be made by performing a scraping of a papule with a scalpel blade and examining the material microscopically after staining with Giemsa stain. One should look for the characteristic molluscum bodies or fungal elements; if they are not identified, additional material should be obtained for fungal stain and culture for histologic examination. Stains such as methenamine stain and periodic acid–Schiff stain allow better visualization of the organism but are not taken up by the capsule. India ink stain can be used on tissue specimens to allow the fungal capsules to be identified (37). *C. neoformans* colonies can be grown in culture on Sabouraud's glucose agar at 37°C within 24 to 48 hours, although the culture should be held for about 1 month (37). A serum cryptococcal antigen level can be obtained as well to confirm the diagnosis.

Histoplasmosis

Mild, self-limited disease in persons living in the central and southeastern United States is the usual course with *Histoplasma capsulatum* infection. The incidence of new cases has been reported to be 200,000 annually, making it the most common endemic mycosis in the country (64). It is often a disseminated disease in immunocompromised patients with AIDS, a transplant, or malignancy, as well as in the very old and the very young. In reports from studies done in endemic areas, the incidence of disseminated disease among the AIDS population was reported to be 5% to 60% (35). The infection with *H. capsulatum* occurs through inhalation. Pulmonary disease may be associated with erythema nodosum, erythema multiforme, or exfoliative dermatitis. In 1997 reports, 10% of patients presented with myalgias, arthralgias, and erythema nodosum (64). Cutaneous manifestations of disseminated disease occurred in 10% to 17% of AIDS patients and in 4% to 6% of transplant patients (10). Skin involvement may take a variety of forms, including erythematous macules or patches, fistulas, papules, nodules, pustules, acneiform lesions, abscesses, herpetiform lesions, and verrucous plaques. These lesions occur most commonly on the face, arms, and trunk (10). Papular and papulonecrotic lesions are the most common presentation. They must be differentiated from the lesions of molluscum contagiosum and acne vulgaris. Mucous membrane involvement, in the form of ulcers, nodules, and vegetating plaques, is also commonly seen and often produces pain. Primary cutaneous histoplasmosis is extremely rare and occurs only from direct inoculation of the fungus into the skin of an immunocompromised patient or from a laboratory accident.

A histoplasmosis skin test can be performed; it becomes positive within 2 weeks after exposure but remains positive for years and therefore is nonspecific and of little diagnostic value (64). Culture confirms the diagnosis, with the marrow producing the highest yield, followed by blood, sputum, lung, and skin. Peripheral blood smears also demonstrate the fungi within phagocytes (65). Biopsy of the skin confirms the diagnosis in 80% of cases and should be performed on any immunocompromised patient with nonspecific skin lesions to rule out disseminated histoplasmosis (35). Material for biopsy should be stained with methenamine silver to illustrate the budding yeasts within phagocytic cells. These yeast forms can be difficult to differentiate from *Coccidioides immitis, Cryptococcus neoformans,* and *Blastomyces dermatitidis*; for definitive diagnosis, culture must be performed on Sabourad's or blood agar at 37°C and kept for at least 3 months (37).

Amphotericin B has had disappointing results and has been replaced by itraconazole for the treatment of histoplasmosis. Itraconazole is used at a dose of 5 mg per kilogram per day. In a report by Denning et al. (66), 92% of patients responded well to itraconazole; the one failure was caused to a shortened course of therapy. As with treatment for cryptococcosis, maintenance therapy is required to prevent relapse.

Aspergillosis

Aspergillus species are ubiquitous and can be found in the soil, amidst decaying vegetation, and in the air. More than 900 species exist, but disease is most commonly caused by *Aspergillus fumigatus,* followed by *Aspergillus flavus* and *Aspergillus niger.* Defects in neutrophil function or quantity and macrophage defects predispose to the development of aspergillosis, because the neutrophil and the macrophage are the body's primary defense mechanisms to prevent clinical disease from this fungus. Animal studies have shown that the macrophage defends against the *Aspergillus* spores while the neutrophil protects the body from the mycelia (67). Therefore, aspergillosis is seen primarily in patients with neutropenia or impaired neutrophil function and in patients receiving corticosteroids. These organisms are respiratory pathogens, so the major sites of infection are the lungs and sinuses. Most cases result from inhalation of the conidia into the lungs or sinuses. In 30% of cases, dissemination to other organs occurs, and cutaneous involvement is seen in 5% of these patients (67). *Aspergillus* can infect many sites of the body, including the sinuses, lungs, eye, ear, CNS, genitourinary tract, bone, skin, and nails.

Aspergillus species have a propensity to invade small or large blood vessels, allowing the organism to disseminate and causing thrombosis and infarction. The lesions of the skin represent areas of infarcted tissue, which explains the well-circumscribed lesions separated from apparently normal skin (68). Skin disease is rare and can occur as a primary infection from direct inoculation or secondary to hematogenous spread of the organism to the skin. Primary cutaneous infection with *Aspergillus* species has been reported in immunosuppressed patients, most commonly in children with leukemia (69). Intravenous sites where the skin is covered by an arm board or tape and other points where the skin is covered by an occlusive dressing are most likely to be involved (70). The lesion that results is characteristic: it begins as a well-circumscribed red or violaceous papule that soon becomes pustular. The pustule then becomes larger and is transformed into an ulcer with a punched-out center and an elevated margin. The center is covered by a dark eschar; the margin is surrounded by an erythematous halo.

Other, rarer types of skin lesions are associated with disseminated aspergillosis. Subcutaneous granulomas or abscesses may be seen, as may erythematous dermal macropapules with indistinct margins that can eventually become vegetating or pustular (71). Lesions associated with sinus disease appear as black eschars located on the nasal septum, nasal bridge, anterior nares, or palate. These lesions can cause tissue destruction which can eventually result in facial disfigurement.

Rapid diagnosis and treatment are essential for patient survival. Biopsy of cutaneous lesions stained with methenamine silver often illustrates the broad, septate, branching hyphae. In a study evaluating the skin lesions of more than 40 febrile, neutropenic patients with biopsy, *Aspergillus* species accounted for 22% of the lesions for which a diagnosis could be established, making it the most frequently identified organism (72). The organism can be cultured on Sabourad's agar and grows rapidly. It has been reported that serodiagnosis via radioimmunoassay has a sensitivity of 70% to 80% (73).

Treatment of aspergillosis in the neutropenic patient is still not always satisfactory. Amphotericin B, which is used as the first-line agent, is ineffective unless the neutrophil count recovers (74). Itraconazole is now being explored as an alternative treatment for invasive disease, but its role in treatment in the neutropenic patient has yet to be defined. The elimination of risk factors—such as use of broad-spectrum antibiotic therapy, immunosuppressive agents, contaminated occlusive dressings, or contaminated intravenous catheters—is crucial in helping prevent disease occurrence. With bone marrow recovery, surgical excision of skin lesions and postoperative skin grafting may be necessary. If the patient remains neutropenic, surgery often fails to control the infection.

VIRAL DISEASE

Human Papillomavirus

Human papillomaviruses (HPV) are DNA viruses that make up a subgroup of the family Papovaviridae. More than 70 subtypes of this virus have been identified, each associated with a specific clinical entity or location of cutaneous manifestations. In all types, transmission occurs by direct contact. In infants, condyloma acuminata and laryngeal papillomas can arise from delivery through an infected birth canal (75).

The common wart can be found on healthy individuals on any body surface and is caused by HPV types 1, 2, 4, or 7 (75). They are typically flesh-colored and sessile, occasionally appearing as filiform papules with numerous projections. They may be solitary or grouped (Fig. 21.10). Their appearance is usually sufficient to make a diagnosis, and laboratory confirmation rarely necessary. Biopsy, if performed, would show hyperkeratosis, koilocytosis, papillomatosis, benign acanthosis, and vertical parakeratosis (75). Plantar warts are lesions found on the foot. They can cause substantial discomfort as pressure is put on their surface with ambulation.

Flat warts, or verruca plana, are caused by infection with HPV types 3, 10, or 28 (75). They are broad based with a flat surface and occasionally with a small amount of scale. They can be found on any body surface and, in older chil-

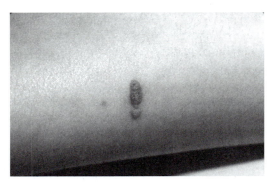

FIG. 21.10. Typical verrucous papules on the extremity of an individual with verruca vulgaris.

dren and adolescents, autoinoculation can arise from the trauma of shaving. These lesions may be difficult to distinguish from molluscum contagiosum, folliculitis, granuloma annulare, juvenile xanthogranuloma, or benign cephalic histiocytosis (75).

Condyloma acuminatum is caused by HPV types 6, 11, 16, 18, and 30. Genital warts have been on the rise in the United States and now account for more consultations than does herpes simplex (76). The serious complication of these types of papillomas is their association with subsequent intraepithelial neoplasia and carcinoma of the vulva, cervix, penis, and rectum. Cervical and vulvar dysplasia associated with HPV types 16 and 18 have been reported in adolescent girls (77). The lesions are often soft, sessile papules with surfaces that range from smooth to rough with multiple projections. They are located on the anogenital region, the external genitalia, and mucous membranes. Warts have also been found in the oral cavity (78), in the nasal cavity (79), and on the conjunctiva (80), making the transmission from one mucous membrane to another likely. In the immunosuppressed individual, the condylomata can progress to cover a large surface of the body, and each lesion can become quite large. Sexual transmission is often the mode of acquisition in persons older than 3 years of age (81). Vertical transmission or direct contact can be the source of transmission in younger children. When faced with a child with condyloma acuminatum, the physician must obtain an in-depth history from both the parents and the child, together with a thorough physical examination, because of the possibility of sexual abuse (82).

Children with HIV infection can present with multiple verruca vulgaris lesions, extensive flat warts, or multiple plantar warts. Patients with a weakened immune system often have a larger number of common warts than the general population (35). Children with HIV infection have been reported to present with multiple condylomata acuminata involving the perineal area (83). These warts are often difficult to eradicate and fail to respond to numerous treatments. Transplantation patients are often infected with HPV, and clinical manifestations are frequently seen after the graft has survived 1 year. In one study the incidence of verruca vulgaris was greater than 75% in patients more than 5 years after grafting (63).

HPV cannot be cultured directly. Identification of the virus is achieved through electron microscopy, DNA probe analysis, and enzymatic restriction methods. Skin biopsy show the dermatologic features described earlier and allows for a presumptive diagnosis. With condyloma acuminatum, serologic tests can be performed to exclude condyloma lata. The histologic appearance is crucial in condyloma acuminatum, because the presence of atypical nuclei or other signs of dysplasia identifies this lesion as having future oncogenic potential. The term Bowenoid papulosis is used for genital lesions that show features of squamous cell carcinoma *in situ*.

The treatment of these lesions can be challenging, especially in the immunocompromised patient, in whom conventional treatments often fail to provide resolution of clinical disease. There is currently no treatment that completely eradicates HPV infection. An intact cell-mediated immune system is required for clearing these warts, so treatment regimens are often prolonged in children with weakened immunity. There is a high rate of recurrence in these individuals as well, probably because of reactivation of latent infection. Common and plantar warts are treated by conventional cryotherapy, keratolytics, intralesional injections of bleomycin, electrodesiccation, and laser cautery. For children with few warts, none of which presents a cosmetic problem, the therapy options should be limited to topical treatments and local care, because spontaneous regression of lesions can occur with time. Topical treatments include salicylic acid applied repeatedly along with the use of local abrasion. Cryotherapy or electrodesiccation is used for more resilient lesions. Topical 5-fluorouracil or intralesional injection of dilute concentrations of bleomycin are other options

(75). Flat warts are treated similarly to common warts or with topical tretinoin.

The treatment of condyloma acuminatum consists of weekly destructive therapy using liquid nitrogen, cautery, or trichloroacetic acid. Podophyllin 10% to 25% in tincture of benzoin, alone or after the application of trichloroacetic acid 25% to 35%, can be administered in the office (84). Podofilox, or podophyllotoxin, a substance derived from podophyllin, is an option. The 0.5% concentration, applied twice daily for 3 days alternating with four drug-free days, is a home regimen (75). It does have a high relapse rate. In children the use of podophyllin can be hazardous because of its ability to be systemically absorbed, its production of an inflammatory response, and its carcinogenic properties. Injection of 1 to 1.5 million IU of IFN-α2b into the warts three times a week for 3 weeks has shown some success (75). Surgical excision, cryotherapy with liquid nitrogen, topical or intralesional injection 5-fluorouracil, and topical trichloroacetic acid 80% to 90% are other options. In a study by Beutner et al. (86), the use of 5% imiquimod cream applied to external warts three times weekly for 8 weeks was found to produce complete clearance in 40%. Imiquimod is an immune-response modifier that is able to induce IFN-α, tumor necrosis factor-α, and IL-6 (85). Sixty-two percent of patients experienced an 80% or greater reduction in baseline wart area, and 76% experienced a reduction of more than 50% in wart surface area (86). Local reactions were reported as mild or moderate and included erythema, burning, tenderness, and itching. Persistent or atypical appearing lesions should be biopsied looking for dysplastic characteristics.

Cytomegalovirus

Cytomegalovirus (CMV), a DNA virus, is a member of the herpesvirus family. Twenty percent to 80% of healthy adults in the United States have antibodies to CMV. Transmission of the virus is most common through respiratory droplets, but fecal-oral and urine-oral transmission have also been described (87). Infection with CMV in the healthy individual is most commonly self-limited. A mononucleosis-like presentation with fever, malaise, mild hepatitis, and atypical lymphocytosis is typically seen. An exudative pharyngitis with cervical lymphadenopathy are seen less often than with Epstein-Barr virus (EBV) (87). Reactivation of CMV can be seen in transplant recipients as a mononucleosis-type syndrome.

Cutaneous manifestations of acquired CMV are rarely seen; in contrast, the cutaneous lesions seen with congenital infection are quite characteristic. In the immunosuppressed patient, dermatologic manifestations of CMV have been reported and include erythematous morbilliform eruption, nodular lesions, verrucous plaques, ulcers, palpable purpuric papules bullae, and vesicles (88). Perineal ulcerations often result from spread of the virus involved in a concurrent colitis to contiguous mucous membranes. Therefore, there are no consistently observed lesions associated with CMV, and often other infectious agents can be isolated in skin biopsy specimens or cultures. The question arises whether CMV is actually the cause of these lesions or merely a silent organism present in skin already infected by another agent.

In the immunocompromised child, CMV causes retinitis, colitis, esophagitis, and pneumonitis. CMV is the most common cause of serious opportunistic viral infection in patients with AIDS. One report stated that 90% of AIDS patients develop active CMV infection at some time during the course of their disease (35). CMV retinitis occurs in 5% to 10% of AIDS patients, as does gastrointestinal disease (35).

Another study found 96% of renal transplantation patients to have some form of active CMV infection (63). In these patients CMV infection is much more serious than infection with other herpesviruses because it can result in graft rejection.

Isolation of viral particles is the best way to diagnose CMV infection. Urine specimens are easily obtained and identify active infection, since systemic infections are frequently associated with viruria. The virus can also be isolated from the throat, sputum, and cerebrospinal fluid. An atypical lymphocytosis and elevation of liver function tests may be seen. If blood for serology is sent, one must demonstrate virus-specific immunoglobulin M (IgM) or document a fourfold rise in complement fixation titers over time (75).

The first-line drug for disseminated CMV infection in the immunocompromised host is ganciclovir. It is associated with myelosuppression, which can be a dose-limiting side effect and may necessitate the use of an alternative therapy, commonly foscarnet. Ganciclovir has activity against both CMV and HIV viruses, which is an additional advantage in the HIV-infected patient. It can cause renal toxicity as well as ulcerations of the oral cavity or genital region. The long-term safety of these therapies in the pediatric population is still being investigated.

Varicella-Zoster Virus

VZV, or herpesvirus-3, belongs to the subfamily of α-herpesviridae along with herpesvirus types 1 and 2 (89). It is an enveloped virus that contains a double-stranded DNA genome, the smallest genome of all herpesviruses. The term herpes zoster comes from the Greek words *herpein,* meaning "to creep or spread," and *zoster,* meaning "girdle" (90). This virus causes two distinct clinical entities: primary varicella (chickenpox) and herpes zoster (shingles).

Varicella is a common infectious disease seen in children. More than 90% of cases of varicella are seen in persons between the ages of 1 and 14 years. Most cases occur between the ages of 5 and 9 years; only 3% of patients are younger than 1 year or older than 19 years of age (91). The virus tends to occur in late winter and early spring. The disease is spread via inhalation of infected respiratory droplets or direct contact with skin lesions. After inhalation of infected droplets, viral replication takes place within regional lymph nodes on days 2 through 4 after initial exposure, with dissemination of the virus throughout the body on days 4 through 6. Further replication of virus particles occurs within the liver or spleen, and a subsequent viremic phase allows seeding of the endothelial cells of the capillaries and spread into the epidermis by days 14 though 16. The rash is seen about 5 days after this second viremia (Fig. 21.11) (90). The incubation period ranges from 10 to 23 days; 99% of children develop symptomatic disease within 20 days after exposure to an index case (92). Chickenpox is considered infectious for up to 4 days before and 5 days after the development of the rash.

Typically in children the onset of the illness is marked by simultaneous development of a rash, low-grade fever, and malaise. Lesions typically begin on the face and trunk as erythematous macules that quickly transform into papules, pustules, and ultimately crusts. These lesions develop in crops, and groups of lesions in different phases of development are often observed on the body at the same time. The number of lesions varies from a handful to hundreds. Pruritus is characteristic, and its severity is variable. Mucous membrane involvement can be seen. Vesicles break down into shallow ulcers that are often painful. The hard palate, uvula, and tonsillar pillars are the most common areas of mucosal involvement (75). Fever is usually mild, ranging from 37.1° to 39.5°C and lasting 3 to 6 days. The height of the fever parallels the severity of the eruption, and the length of the febrile illness often corre-

lates with the duration of new lesion formation (90). Differential diagnosis includes other viral infections that cause vesicular lesions, such as herpesvirus, coxsackievirus (hand-foot-and-mouth disease), and enterovirus.

Complications of varicella are atypical in the immunocompetent child. One study found the incidence of complications from varicella to be 5.2% (93). The most common complication is scarring. Repeated scratching of lesions allows inoculation of bacteria beneath the epidermis, with resulting bacterial superinfection. Impetigo, cellulitis, folliculitis, erysipelas, or bullae are evidence of bacterial involvement, as is the presence of edematous lesions or prolonged fever. *Staphylococcus* and β-hemolytic *Streptococcus* are the most frequent causes of secondary skin infection.

Pneumonia is a significant complication of adult-onset primary varicella, occurring in 1 of every 400 cases. Patients present with dyspnea, cough, hemoptysis, pleuritic chest pain, tachypnea, and high fever. One survey found the incidence of pneumonia in children with varicella to be 7% (94). Other manifestations of progressive varicella are hepatitis and CNS infection. CNS complications of varicella include encephalitis, meningitis, cerebellar ataxia, transverse myelitis, Reye syndrome, and Guillain-Barré syndrome (95). Reye syndrome usually occurs during the recovery period and is associated with the uses of aspirin or other salicylates. It is marked by an acute onset of vomiting, delirium, and confusion associated with abnormal liver function tests and an increased ammonia level. The mortality rate of progressive varicella is 20% (96).

The immunocompromised child often has a higher rate of morbidity and mortality associated with varicella infections. This is particularly true among those with a defect in cell-mediated immunity, such as children with lymphoproliferative or solid organ malignancies who are receiving cytotoxic chemotherapy, those with immune suppression after bone marrow or other organ transplantation, those chronically dependent on corticosteroids, and those with HIV infection. The virus has a prolonged replication time within

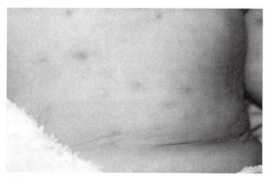

FIG. 21.11. Discrete vesicle overlying an erythematous base on the trunk of a child with varicella.

these patients, resulting in prolonged fever, a high-level viremia, new lesions for 2 or more weeks, a more extensive rash with hemorrhagic lesions, and frequent involvement of the lungs, CNS, and liver. The individual lesions are often larger, more deep-seated, and umbilicated, and they may affect the palms and soles (75).

Herpes zoster is the second clinical entity caused by the varicella virus. The incidence of zoster increases with age. It is rare in children, the incidence in those younger than 9 years of age being reported in one study as 0.74 per 1,000 (97). It has been reported to be more than 100 times higher in children with leukemia than in those without malignancies. Herpes zoster often occurs in healthy children who had a primary infection (varicella) when younger than 6 to 12 months of age. Reactivation of this latent virus occurs when there is suppression of the cell-mediated immunity that is responsible for keeping the virus in its dormant state. On reactivation, the virus initially replicates within the dorsal ganglion, causing ganglionitis. There is extensive monocytic and lymphocytic infiltration within the ganglion cells, with evidence of nerve cell destruction (90). The inflammation and necrosis cause what is clinically perceived as neuralgia. The virus then travels down the nerve fiber to the skin, where the lesions become evident.

The initial complaint of patients with herpes zoster infection is pain within the area of the involved dermatome. This pain is usually present 2 to 3 days before the onset of the rash. This pain has often been misdiagnosed as pleurisy, myocardial infarction, cholecystitis, peptic ulcer disease, or a herniated intervertebral disc. Children often experience a prodromal illness consisting of fever, malaise, and headache. The eruption is typically unilateral; it occurs in a dermatomal distribution and can affect one to three dermatomes. The ophthalmic branch of the trigeminal nerve and the thoracic nerve dermatomes are those most commonly affected. The initial cutaneous findings are erythematous macules or papules within the area of the affected dermatome. They evolve into vesicles within 24 hours, into pustules within 2 to 3 days, and into crusts within 10 days. The entire process often resolves within 2 to 3 weeks.

Seven percent of all cases of zoster involve the ophthalmic branch of the trigeminal nerve (89). If the nasociliary branch of the ophthalmic branch is affected, a clinical entity known as Hutchinson's triad may occur, with vesicles on the side and tip of the nose. This entity should be promptly recognized, because it may be associated with ocular findings such as keratitis, conjunctivitis, and other manifestations. Ocular disease occurs in 20% to 70% of patients who have involvement of the ophthalmic branch (90). An ophthalmologist should be consulted immediately. Another clinical entity associated with zoster is the Ramsay Hunt syndrome. The facial and auditory nerves can be affected, and lesions may occur on the external ear and anterior two thirds of the tongue. Bell's palsy, otalgia, tinnitus, vertigo, and loss of hearing and taste may result. One of the most dreaded sequelae of herpes zoster infection is postherpetic neuralgia. This is pain that lasts for longer than 1 month after regression of skin lesions. Ten percent to 15% of patients with zoster develop this distressing symptom; it is seen more commonly in adults.

The pain and rash are more intense in the immunocompromised patient. Recurrence is not uncommon; in one study 5% to 23% of AIDS patients had a second episode of zoster during their illness (35). Disseminated infection occurs in up to 40% of immunocompromised patients. Cutaneous dissemination may be followed by involvement of the CNS, lungs, and liver in up to 10%. The lesions may be atypical in this population. Erythematous, punched-out ulcerations, which can be covered by a dark eschar, may last for many months. These lesions are often concentrated on the lower extremities and buttocks. A second atypical pattern is the verrucous lesions that are chronic and are often associated with resistance to acyclovir therapy (98).

Diagnosis can be made by scraping a vesicle and applying the Tzanck preparation to identify the characteristic balloon cells and multinucleated giant cells. The test is not specific for the varicella virus, however. Cultures of vesicular fluid early in the course of the illness may provide a specific diagnosis. Methods of detecting antibodies in the serum have been developed, including fluorescent antibody to VZV membrane antigen, radioimmunoassay, and enzyme-linked immunosorbent assay. VZV DNA can be identified in skin lesions by polymerase chain reaction and dot-blot hybridization. Direct immunofluorescence staining of cellular material obtained from skin lesions is often used to detect virus antigens and infected cells (90).

Treatment of both primary varicella and herpes zoster in the immunocompetent individual mainly involves supportive care. In healthy children, topical lotions such as calamine or menthol may alleviate some of the pruritus. Oral antihistamines such as hydroxyzine or diphenhydramine may also be used to control the urge to scratch. Oral antibiotics may be necessary if any evidence of bacterial superinfection develops. In the immunocompromised child, acyclovir should be initiated early in the course of infection to prevent any complications or dissemination. The dosage is 10 mg per kilogram given intravenously every 8 hours. If there is no evidence of visceral disease, oral acyclovir can be used at a dosage of 20 mg per kilogram per dose every 6 hours. All patients with herpes zoster ophthalmicus should also receive intravenous acyclovir, because without treatment the rate of ocular complications is high. If chronic verrucous lesions are observed and treatment with acyclovir fails to lead to regression, resistance should be assumed, and a switch to intravenous foscarnet should follow. Passive immunization with varicella immune globulin has been shown to be effective in preventing infection in high-risk patients if administered within 72 hours of exposure. It is recommended for use especially in children who have a malignancy, are receiving immunosuppressive agents, or have HIV infection or AIDS.

Herpes Simplex Virus

Herpesvirus types I and II are viruses within the herpesvirus family which includes VZV, CMV, and EBV. Infection is transmitted from person to person via sexual or other close contact. The incubation period in humans varies from 1 to 26 days (99). The virus is absorbed across the epithelium of mucous membranes, the eye, the lung, or skin and travels down contiguous nerve endings to the nerve ganglion cells, where it remains for life. The virus remains dormant within the nerve ganglion cells, protected from the body's immune system and therefore not accessible for eradication. Periodically the virus reactivates as a result of temporary immune suppression, exposure to ultraviolet radiation, or local trauma, and the viral particles travel back down the nerve fibers to the skin or mucous membrane, where they cause clinical disease. The immune mechanisms involved in this reactivation process have not been fully explained. However, patients with defects in cell-mediated immunity are more likely to have more severe and prolonged episodes than are those with defects in humoral immunity (75).

HSV can cause a variety of clinical entities in children. Patients with primary herpes may be asymptomatic, or they may have a mild, flu-like illness. Herpetic gingivostomatitis caused by HSV type I manifests with erythema, edema, and ulcerations of the mucous membranes of the buccal mucosa, tongue, or palate. Patients have a sore mouth and are quite irritable. Dehydration resulting from the inability to eat or drink can occur in severe cases. Regional lymphadenopathy is often present. Primary herpetic lesions of the skin appear as a group of vesicles on an erythematous base (Fig. 21.12). They are often more painful and associated with more systemic symptoms than are the lesions of recurrent disease. Genital herpetic infection can be caused by type I or type II. Ulcerations are present on the external genitalia or perirectal areas. Cystitis, cervicitis, urethritis, and dysuria are common associated complaints. If a patient was previously exposed to herpes type

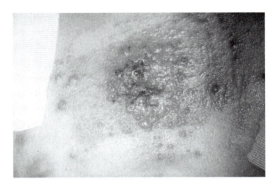

FIG. 21.12. Grouped vessels overlying an erythematous base at a central line site. Culture was positive for herpes simplex virus.

I infection, primary infection with herpes type II in the genital area may be less severe (75). Herpetic infection of the eye causes pain, blurred vision, and conjunctivitis. Examination of the cornea reveals dendritic ulcerations, a characteristic pattern for herpes (99). Early evaluation and intervention is necessary to prevent blindness.

Recurrent lesions can occur at any location previously affected by primary herpes infection. The most common location is the vermilion border of the lip. The appearance of discrete lesions is preceded by a sensation in the area of eruption such as tingling or burning. A small vesicle initially forms and rapidly breaks down into a superficial ulceration. Within a week to 10 days new epithelium covers the area.

Superinfection by herpesvirus of skin affected by other dermatoses can occur. This is most commonly seen as a complication of severe atopic dermatitis, a condition known as eczema herpeticum. Other conditions susceptible to herpes superinfection include ichthyosis, Darier's disease, and pemphigus vulgaris. In contrast to primary herpes infection, the lesions are not found in groups but rather are disseminated, involving all the skin affected by the underlying dermatosis. The ulcerations may become confluent and form large areas of denuded skin.

These lesions are found more commonly in immunocompromised patients. A patient with

ulcerative mucocutaneous HSV present on the body for longer than 1 month has AIDS unless another source of immune deficiency is known (35). Infants with AIDS may present with severe herpetic gingivostomatitis. If this infection becomes chronic, it can interfere with oral intake and lead to dehydration or failure to thrive (100). Mucocutaneous lesions are the most common manifestation of HSV infection in the immunocompromised patient, but chorioretinitis, herpetic whitlow (infection of the periungual area), and follicular lesions (herpetic folliculitis) can also be seen. Other epithelial surfaces that can be affected by ulcerative lesions include the cornea, bronchial tree, and esophagus. HSV infections are also common among transplantation patients and in children with acute lymphocytic leukemia. The risk for infection in bone marrow transplantation patients who are seropositive for infection is greater than 70% (67). The disease is seen in about 25% of patients with acute lymphocytic leukemia, with oral lesions being the most common manifestation. Healing normally takes up to 1 week in a host with an intact immune system, but it may take 5 or 6 weeks in immunocompromised patients. In one study, HSV was recovered from up to 85% of patients with chemotherapy-induced mucositis, compared with only 30% of patients who did not develop mucositis (67). The overall risk of bacteremia was found to be lower in patients who were treated prophylactically with acyclovir during chemotherapy.

Diagnosis of herpes infection can be made by using a Tzanck smear, viral culture, or direct fluorescent antibody staining. If the diagnosis is still unclear, a skin biopsy will demonstrate herpetic infection of the epithelium. In the normal host, the lesions are self-limited and require no treatment. Oral acyclovir seems to reduce the frequency of infections, and topical acyclovir works to decrease the duration of cutaneous lesions. The dose is 10 mg per kilogram per day by mouth divided every 6 hours for 5 days for mucocutaneous infection. Intravenous acyclovir is reserved for the immunocompromised patient or the patient with extensive eczema herpeticum. The dose is 10 mg per kilogram per dose every 8 hours for 5 to 7 days. Any lesion that fails to respond to treatment should be biopsied and sent for evaluation for acyclovir resistance. Foscarnet is the second-line drug used in cases of acyclovir-resistant viruses.

Molluscum Contagiosum

Molluscum contagiosum is caused by a poxvirus (MCV), a brick-shaped particle containing a genome of double-stranded DNA (103). There are two molecular subtypes, MCV I and MCV II. In several studies, MCV I was more commonly isolated, identified in up to 95% of patients sampled (101). The two produce identical-appearing lesions, but MCV II is not found in children younger than 15 years of age. The virus is found worldwide and mainly affects children, sexually active adults, and immunocompromised persons. Although it can be encountered in any of these populations, it is most common in children younger than 5 years old (102). The virus is spread by direct contact, via fomites, or by sexual contact.

The incubation period is between 14 and 50 days (103). Lesions are typically 2- to 5-mm smooth-surfaced, dome-shaped, flesh-colored, firm papules with central umbilications (Fig. 21.13). A white, thick material can be ex-

pressed from the core if pressure is applied. There are usually fewer than 20 lesions present on the body. In children, lesions appear on the face, extremities, and trunk; in sexually active adults they occur on the genitalia, thighs, and lower abdomen (104,105). In rare cases lesions develop intraorally, periocularly, or intraocularly. If lesions are present near the lid margin, there is an increased association with the development of toxic conjunctivitis (106). Ten percent of patients with molluscum develop an eczematous reaction around the molluscum papules, termed molluscum dermatitis. This inflammatory condition clears once the molluscum is treated. Erythema annulare centrifugum has also been associated with the virus (107). The lesions of molluscum are usually asymptomatic, although some patients complain of tenderness or pruritus. In the healthy individual lesions resolve spontaneously within months if left untreated. In the immunocompromised patient, lesions may remain for several years if no therapy is initiated.

The papular lesions of molluscum can have an appearance similar to lesions of other dermatologic conditions. The differential diagnosis includes basal cell carcinoma, histiocytoma, keratoacanthoma, sebaceous adenoma, Darier's disease, and intradermal nevus. In the immunocompromised patient, the cutaneous manifestations of disseminated cryptococcosis or histoplasmosis can be misdiagnosed as molluscum contagiosum.

In the immunocompromised patient, molluscum contagiosum can have an atypical appearance, have a chronic course, and be resistant to conventional therapies. These lesions are encountered frequently in patients receiving chronic corticosteroid or immunosuppressive therapies and in patients with congenital or acquired immunodeficiency states. The disease is estimated to occur in 5% to 18% of patients with HIV infection (107). Giant papules as large as 8 cm have been reported (108). Hundreds of lesions may be present at once, or coalescence of multiple lesions to form a large plaque may been seen. The distribution of the papules is different from that

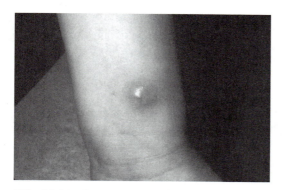

FIG. 21.13. A giant molluscum nodule is illustrated. Such presentations are unusual but may be seen in both normal and immunocompromised individuals.

seen in healthy adults, with lesions concentrated on the face, neck, and trunk rather than on the genital region or thighs. Sexual contact as the mode of transmission of the virus in these patients can therefore be called into question. It has been theorized that this may be yet another example of reactivation of a latent viral infection, as is seen with herpes simplex or herpes zoster (109). Along with a reduction in the CD4+ T-lymphocyte count, a decrease in the number of Langerhans cells within the affected epidermis is another finding in patients with HIV infection. These cells play a role in immunosurveillance within the skin, and their paucity may provide one explanation of the increased incidence and severity of molluscum infection in this population (109).

This viral infection proved in retrospective studies of immunocompromised patients to provide an estimate of the degree of immunodeficiency. There exists an inverse relation between the degree of immunocompromise in AIDS patients, as quantified by the CD4 count, and the extent of infection. The mean CD4 count of patients with molluscum was found to be 86 cells per microliter. An association between lower counts and more extensive disease was proven (110). Therefore, molluscum contagiosum serves as a marker for a decline in the immune status in patients with HIV infection.

Under microscopic examination, the papules of molluscum consist of lobules of epidermis extending into the dermis and opening onto the skin's surface though a central pore. The central core is filled with fragments of keratin and material known as molluscum bodies. The molluscum bodies are large intracytoplasmic inclusion bodies within keratinocytes, termed Henderson-Patterson bodies (111). Within the stratum malpighii of the epidermis, the virus induces a transformation of cells resulting in the formation of the molluscum body. It appears as an aggregate of small, ovoid, eosinophilic material within the infected epidermal cell (112). As it moves up the layers of the epidermis, the molluscum body enlarges and becomes more basophilic.

With atypical-appearing lesions, skin biopsy should be used to diagnose molluscum contagiosum or to exclude the possibility of disseminated fungal disease (e.g., histoplasmosis, cryptococcosis). The presence of molluscum bodies within the cells is diagnostic. Serologic tests are not used regularly, although low titers of antibody can be demonstrated in some patients. The lack of substantial humoral response may be explained by the superficial nature of the infection.

Although the lesions are self-limited and asymptomatic in most healthy patients, treatment is often given to prevent spread of the virus from one part of the body to another or from person to person. In the immunosuppressed individual, infection is often more chronic and more extensive, and removal of lesions becomes essential for cosmesis. The application of caustic agents such as cantharidin 0.9%, tincture of iodine, 25% podophyllin resin in tincture of benzoin, tretinoin cream 0.05 to 0.1%, or trichloroacetic acid is often the first-line therapy (75). These materials cause blistering of the epidermis and sufficient inflammation to eradicate the organisms. More aggressive techniques include curettage, cryotherapy with liquid nitrogen, and incision with a small blade to remove the central plug. In children, topical application of EMLA cream 1 hour before the procedure provided pain relief in more than 90% of patients (109). The lesions of the immunocompromised patient are often refractory to many of these conventional therapies. Griseofulvin has been tried in several patients with molluscum. Treatment is continued for 4 to 6 weeks at a dosage used of 500 mg in children older than 14 years of age and 250 mg in younger children. Lesions resolved within 6 weeks after therapy was begun, and there was no recurrence within an 8 months after to treatment completion (109). There is no consistently effective systemic therapy, although zidovudine was found to improve the course of infection in one patient (113). The use of IFN-α failed to result in cure in several studies. Imiquimod has also been used successfully. In one study by Meadows et al. (114), cidofivir, a nucleotide analog of deoxycytidine monophosphate, used intravenously or topically, cleared advanced cases of molluscum contagiosum.

Patients with periocular molluscum contagiosum should be referred to an ophthalmologist. When molluscum is present around the eye, it can induce a toxic conjunctivitis that can be associated with extreme discomfort (115). However, because of its location it is more difficult to treat than lesions elsewhere on the body. Because this is often a self-limited disease, a choice arises between close observation with eventual spontaneous resolution of the lesions, with intervention only if conjunctivitis occurs, and immediate intervention with the risks that the procedures entail. In 1 study by Margo and Katz (116), the majority of ophthalmologists treated periocular molluscum even if it was not associated with conjunctivitis. Only 11% of the cases studied were allowed to spontaneously regress. Ocular complications of molluscum (e.g., corneal ulceration) are very rare. Conjunctivitis, which occurs in fewer than 50% of cases, resolves once the lesions are excised.

REFERENCES

1. Wolfson JS, Sober AJ, Rubin RH. Dermatologic manifestations of infection in the compromised host. *Annu Rev Med* 1983;34:205–217.
2. Murray PR, Kobayashi GS, Pfaller MA, et al., eds. Host-parasite interactions. In: *Medical microbiology,* 2nd ed. St. Louis: Mosby–Year Book, 1994:78–116.
3. Dahl MV. Basic immunology. In: Schachner LA, Hansen RC, eds. *Pediatric dermatology,* 2nd ed. New York: Churchill Livingstone, 1995:71.
4. Tosi MF, Cates KL. Immunologic and phagocytic responses to infection. In: Feigin RD, Cherry JD, eds. *Textbook of pediatric infectious diseases,* 4th ed. Philadelphia: WB Saunders, 1998:14.
5. Pizzo PA. Infectious complications in the child with cancer: pathophysiology of the compromised host and the initial evaluation and management of the febrile cancer patient. *J Pediatr* 1981;98:341–354.
6. Melish ME, Campbell KA. Coagulase-positive staphylococcus. In: Feigin RD, Cherry JD, eds. *Textbook of pediatric infectious diseases,* 4th ed. Philadelphia: WB Saunders, 1998:1039.
7. Murray PR, Kobayashi GS, Pfaller MA, et al., eds. Bacteriology. In: *Medical microbiology,* 2nd ed. St. Louis: Mosby–Year Book, 1994:160–400.
8. Kaplan EL, Gerber MA. Group A, group C, and group G beta-hemolytic streptococcal infections. In: Feigin RD, Cherry JD, eds. *Textbook of pediatric infectious diseases,* 4th ed. Philadelphia: WB Saunders, 1998:1076.
9. Galen WK, Rogers M, Cohen I, et al. Bacterial infec-

tions. In: Schachner LA, Hansen RC, eds. *Pediatric dermatology,* 2nd ed. New York: Churchill Livingstone, 1995:1169.
10. Castano-Molina C, Cockerell CJ. Diagnosis and treatment of infectious diseases in HIV-infected hosts. *Infect Dis Dermatol* 1997;15:267–283.
11. Tunnessen WW Jr. A survey of skin disorders seen in pediatric general and dermatology clinics. *Pediatr Dermatol* 1984;1:218–222.
12. Melish ME, Glasgow LA. Staphylococcal scalded skin syndrome: the expanded clinical syndrome. *J Pediatr* 1971;78:958–967.
13. Dagan R, Bar-David Y. Comparison of amoxicillin and clavalonic acid (Augmentin) for the treatment of nonbullous impetigo. *Am J Dis Child* 1989;143:916–918.
14. Schachner LA, Taplin D, Scott GB, et al. A therapeutic update of superficial skin infections. *Pediatr Clin North Am* 1983;30:397–404.
15. Esterly NB, Nelson DB, Dunne WM Jr. Impetigo. *Am J Dis Child* 1991;145:125–126.
16. Britton J, Fajardo E, Krafte-Jacobs B. Comparison of mupirocin and erythromycin in the therapy of impetigo. *J Pediatr* 1990;117:827–829.
17. Buchness MR. Treatment of skin diseases in HIV-infected patients. *Dermatol Clin* 1995;13:231–238.
18. Sachs M. Cutaneous cellulitis. *Arch Dermatol* 1991;127:493–496.
19. Lerner PI. Nocardiosis. *Clin Infect Dis* 1996;22:891–903.
20. Darville T, Jacobs RF. *Nocardia.* In: Feigin RD, Cherry JD, eds. *Textbook of pediatric infectious diseases,* 4th ed. Philadelphia: WB Saunders, 1998:1266.
21. Starke JR, Smith MHD. Tuberculosis. In: Feigin RD, Cherry JD, eds. *Textbook of pediatric infectious diseases,* 4th ed. Philadelphia: WB Saunders, 1998:1196.
22. del Carmen Farina M, Gegundez MI, Pique E, et al. Cutaneous tuberculosis: a clinical, histopathologic, and bacteriologic study. *J Am Acad Dermatol* 1995;33:433–440.
23. Lincoln EM, Sewell EM. *Tuberculosis in children.* New York: McGraw-Hill, 1963.
24. Duhra P, Grattan LEH, Ryatt KS. Lupus vulgaris with numerous tubercle bacilli. *Clin Exp Dermatol* 1988;13:31–33.
25. Serfling U, Penneys NS, Leonardi CL. Identification of *Mycobacterium tuberculosis* DNA in a case of lupus vulgaris. *J Am Acad Dermatol* 1993;28:318–322.
26. Brady MT, Feigin RD. *Pseudomonas* and related species. In: Feigin RD, Cherry JD, eds. *Textbook of pediatric infectious diseases,* 4th ed. Philadelphia: WB Saunders, 1998:1401.
27. Prose NS. Cutaneous manifestations of HIV infection in children. *Dermatol Clin* 1991;9:543–550.
28. Su WP, Duncan SC, Perry HO. Blastomycosis-like pyoderma. *Arch Dermatol* 1979;115:170–173.
29. Bodey GP. Dermatologic manifestations of infections in neutropenic patients. *Infect Dis Clin North Am* 1994;8:655–675.
30. Weinberg AN, Swartz MN. Gram-negative coccal and bacillary infections. In: Fitzpatrick TB, Eisen AZ, Wolff K, et al., eds. *Dermatology in general medicine.* New York: McGraw-Hill, 1979:1445.
31. Benedict LM, Kusne S, Tone-Cisneros J, et al. Primary cutaneous fungal infection after solid-organ transplantation: report of five cases and review. *Clin Infect Dis* 1992;15:17–21.

32. Chapman SW, Daniel CR. Cutaneous manifestations of fungal infection. *Infect Dis Clin North Am* 1994;8:879–910.

33. Sinski JT, Flouras K. A survey of dermatophytes isolated from human patients in the United States from 1985 to 1987. *Mycopathologia* 1991;114:117–126.

34. Sinski JT, Flouras K. A survey of dermatophytes isolated from human patients in the united states from 1979 to 1981 with chronological listings of worldwide incidence of 5 dermatophytes often isolated in the United States. *Mycopathologia* 1984;86:97–120.

35. Berger TG, Greene I. Bacterial, viral, fungal, and parasitic infections in HIV disease and AIDS. *Dermatol Clin* 1991;9:465–492.

36. Lowinger-Seoane M, Torres-Rodriguez JM, Madrenys-Brunet N, et al. Extensive dermatophytosis caused by *Trichophyton mentagrophytes* and *Microsporum canis* in a patient with AIDS. *Mycopathologia* 1992;120:143–146.

37. Stein DH. Fungal, protozoan, and helminth infections. In: Schachner LA, Hansen RC, eds. *Pediatric dermatology*, 2nd ed. New York: Churchill Livingstone, 1995:1295.

38. Conant MA. The AIDS epidemic. *J Am Acad Dermatol* 1994;31:S47–50.

39. Terragni L, Buzzetti I, Lasagni A, et al. Tinea pedis in children. *Mycoses* 1991;34:273–276.

40. Cohen B. Tinea pedis in children. *Am J Dis Child* 1992;146:844–847.

41. Rosenthal JR. Pediatric fungal infections from head to toe: what's new? *Curr Opin Pediatr* 1994;6:435–441.

42. Bronson DM, Desai DR, Barsky S, et al. An epidemic of infection with *T. tonsurans* revealed in a twenty year survey of fungal infections in Chicago. *J Am Acad Dermatol* 1983;8:322–330.

43. Kaaman T, Torssander J. Dermatophytid: a misdiagnosed entity? *Acta Derm Venereol* 1983;63:404–408.

44. Degreef H, DeDoncker PR. Current treatment of dermatophytosis. *J Am Acad Dermatol* 1994;31:S25–30.

45. Gupta AK, Hufstader SLR, Adam P, et al. Tinea capitis: an overview with emphasis on management. *Pediatr Dermatol* 1999;16:171–189.

46. Buchness MR. Treatment of skin diseases in HIV-infected patients. *Dermatol Clin North Am* 1995;13:31–38.

47. Rasmussen JE. Cutaneous fungus infections in children. *Pediatr Rev* 1992;13:152–156.

48. Gan VN, Petruska M, Ginsburg CM. Epidemiology and treatment of tinea capitis: ketoconazole versus griseofulvin. *Pediatr Infect Dis J* 1987;6:46–49.

49. Nolting S, Gupta AK, de Prost Y, et al. *Itraconazole for the treatment of dermatophytoses in children.* Poster presented at the 54th Annual Meeting of the American Academy of Dermatology, Washington, DC, February, 1996.

50. Gupta AK, Shear NH. Terbinafine: an update. *J Am Acad Dermatol* 1997;37:979–988.

51. Krafchik B, Pelletier J. An open study of tinea capitis in fifty children treated with a two-week course of oral terbinafine. *J Am Acad Dermatol* 1999;41:60–63.

52. Roberts DT. Prevalence of dermatophyte onychomycosis in the United Kingdom: results of an omnibus survey. *Br J Dermatol* 1992;126:23–27.

53. Fitzpatrick TB, Johnson RA, Wolff K, et al. *Color atlas and synopsis of clinical dermatology.* New York: McGraw-Hill, 1997.

54. Ploysangam T, Lucky AW. Childhood white superficial onychomycosis caused by *Trichophyton rubrum*: report of seven cases and review of the literature. *J Am Acad Dermatol* 1997;36:29–32.

55. Hancke E. Fungal infections of the nail. *Semin Dermatol* 1991;10:41–48.

56. Chang P, Logemann H. Onychomycosis in children. *Infect J Dermatol* 1994;33:550–551.

57. Hay RJ. Antifungal treatment of yeast infections. *J Am Acad Dermatol* 1994;31:S6–9.

58. McCarthy GM. Host factors associated with HIV-related oral candidiasis: a review. *Oral Surg Oral Med Oral Pathol* 1992;73:181–186.

59. Samaranayake LP, Holmstrup P. Oral candidiasis and human immunodeficiency virus infection. *J Oral Pathol Med* 1989;18:554–564.

60. Greenspan D. Treatment of oropharyngeal candidiasis in HIV-positive patients. *J Am Acad Dermatol* 1994;31:S1–5.

61. Cuttner J, Trey KM, Furano L, et al. Clotrimazole treatment for prevention of oral candidiasis in with acute leukemia undergoing chemotherapy: results of a double-blind study. *Am J Med* 1986;81:771–774.

62. Pons V, Greenspan D, Debruin M. Therapy for oropharyngeal candidiasis in HIV-infected patients: a randomized, prospective multicenter study of oral fluconazole versus clotrimazole troches. *J Acquir Immun Defic Syndr* 1993;6:1311–1316.

63. Parker C. Skin lesions in transplant patients. *Dermatol Clin North Am* 1990;8:313–325.

64. Wheat LJ. Histoplasmosis in Indianapolis. *Clin Infect Dis* 1992;14:S91–99.

65. Stevens DA. Management of systemic manifestations of fungal disease in patients with AIDS. *J Am Acad Dermatol* 1994;31:S64–67.

66. Denning DW, Tucker RM, Hostetler JS. Itraconazole treatment of cryptococcal meningitis and cryptococcosis in patients with AIDS. In: Vanden BE, Mackenzie DWR, Cauwenbergh G, et al., eds. *Mycoses in AIDS patients.* Dienum Press, 1990:305.

67. Allo MD, Miller J, Townsend T, et al. Primary cutaneous aspergillosis associated with Hickman intravenous catheters. *N Engl J Med* 1987;317:1105–1108.

68. Findlay GH, Roux HF, Simson IW. Skin manifestations in disseminated aspergillosis. *Br J Dermatol* 1971;85:94–98.

69. Grossman ME, Fithian EC, Behrens C, et al. Primary cutaneous aspergillosis in six leukemic children. *J Am Acad Dermatol* 1985;12:313–318.

70. Estes SA, Hendricks AA, Merz WG. Primary cutaneous aspergillosis. *J Am Acad Dermatol* 1980;3:397–400.

71. Prystowsky SD, Vogelstein B, Ettinger DS. Invasive aspergillosis. *N Engl J Med* 1976;295:655–658.

72. Allen U, Smith CR, Prober CG. The value of skin biopsies in febrile, neutropenic, immunocompromised children. *Am J Dis Child* 1986;140:459–461.

73. Repentigny L. Serodiagnosis of candidiasis, aspergillosis, and cryptococcosis. *Clin Infect Dis* 1992;14:S11–22.

74. Bodey GP, Vartivarian S. Aspergillosis. *Eur J Clin Microbiol Infect Dis* 1989;8:413–437.

75. Frieden IJ, Penneys IS. Viral infections. In: Schachner LA, Hansen RC, eds. *Pediatric dermatology*, 2nd ed. New York: Churchill Livingstone, 1995:1257.

76. Centers for Disease Control and Prevention. Condy-

loma acuminatum—United States, 1966–1981. *MMWR Morb Mortal Wkly Rep* 1983;23:206.

77. Lister UM, Akinla O. Carcinoma of the vulva in childhood. *Br J Obstet Gynaecol* 1972;79:470–473.

78. Naghashfar Z, Sawada E, Kutchen MJ, et al. Identification of genital tract papillomavirus HPV-6 and HPV-16 in warts of the oral cavity. *J Med Virol* 1985;17:313–324.

79. Wu TC, Trujillo JM, Kashima HK,, et al. Association of human papillomavirus with nasal neoplasia. *Lancet* 1993;341:522–524.

80. Lass JH, Grove AS, Papale JJ, et al. Detection of human papillomavirus DNA sequences in conjunctival papilloma. *Am J Ophthalmol* 1983;96:670–674.

81. Gutman LT, Herman-Giddens ME, Phelps WC. Transmission of human genital papillomavirus disease: comparison of data from adults and children. *Pediatrics* 1993;91:31–38.

82. Schachner L, Hankin DE. Assessing child abuse in childhood condyloma acuminatum. *J Am Acad Dermatol* 1985;12:157–160

83. Forman A, Prendiville J. Association of human immunodeficiency virus seropositivity and extensive perineal condylomata acuminata in a child. *Arch Dermatol* 1988;124:1010–1011.

84. Buchness MR. Treatment of skin diseases in HIV-infected patients. *Dermatol Clin* 1995;13:231–238.

85. Kono T, Kondo S, Pastore S, et al. Effects of a novel topical immunomodulator, imiquimod, on keratinocyte cytokine gene expression. *Lymph Cytokine Res* 1994;13:71–76.

86. Beutner KR, Spruance SL, Hougham AJ, et al. Treatment of genital warts with an immune-response modifier (imiquimod). *J Am Acad Dermatol* 1998;38:230–239.

87. Demmler GJ. Acquired cytomegalovirus infections. In: Feigin RD, Cherry JD, eds. *Textbook of pediatric infectious diseases,* 4th ed. Philadelphia: WB Saunders, 1998:1532.

88. Bournerias I, Boisnic S, Patey O, et al. Unusual cutaneous cytomegalovirus involvement in patients with acquired immunodeficiency syndrome. *Arch Dermatol* 1989;125:1243–1246.

89. Roizman B, Carmichael LE, Deinhardt F, et al. Herpesviridae: definition, provisional nomenclature, and taxonomy. *Intervirology* 1981;16:201–217.

90. Rockley PF, Tyring SK. Pathophysiology and clinical manifestations of varicella zoster virus infections. *Int J Dermatol* 1994;33:227–232.

91. Preblud SR, Orenstein WA, Bart KJ. Varicella: clinical manifestations, epidemiology, and health impact in children. *Pediatr Infect Dis* 1984;3:505–509.

92. Grose C. Variation on a theme by Fenner: the pathogenesis of chickenpox. *Pediatrics* 1981;68:735–737.

93. Bullona JGM, Wishik SM. Complications of varicella: their occurrence among 2534 patients. *Am J Dis Child* 1935;49:923–932.

94. Fleisher G, Henry W, McSorley M, et al. Life-threatening complications of varicella. *Am J Dis Child* 1981;135:896–899.

95. Brunnell PA. Varicella-zoster virus. In: Mandell GL, Douglas RG, Bennett JE, eds. *Principles and practice of infectious diseases,* 2nd ed. New York: John Wiley & Sons, 1985.

96. Brunnell PA. Varicella-zoster infections. In: Feigin RD, Cherry JD, eds. *Textbook of pediatric infectious diseases,* 4th ed. Philadelphia: WB Saunders, 1992:1206.

97. Hope-Simpson RE. The nature of herpes zoster: a long-term study and a new hypothesis. *Proc R Soc Med* 1969;62:1138–1142.

98. Alessi E, Cusini M, Zerboni R, et al. Unusual varicella-zoster virus infection in patients with acquired immunodeficiency syndrome. *Arch Dermatol* 1988;124:1011–1013.

99. Corey L, Spear PG. Infections with herpes simplex viruses. *N Engl J Med* 1986;314:686–691.

100. Prose NS. Cutaneous manifestations of HIV infection in children. *Dermatol Clin* 1991;9:543–550.

101. Porter CD, Blake NW, Archard LC, et al. Moluscum contagiosum virus types in genital and non-genital lesions. *Br J Dermatol* 1989;120:37–41.

102. Brown ST, Nalley JF, Krause SJ. Molluscum contagiosum. *Sex Transm Dis.* 1981;8:227–234.

103. Fenner F. Poxviruses. In: Fields BN, Knipe DM, eds. *Virology,* 2nd ed. New York: Raven Press, 1990.

104. Sholtz J, Rosen-Wolff A, Bugert J, et al. Molecular epidemiology of molluscum contagiosum. *J Infect Dis* 1988;158:898–900.

105. Wilkin JK. Molluscum contagiosum venereum in a women's outpatient clinic: a venereally transmitted disease. *Am J Obstet Gynecol* 1977;128:531–535.

106. Margo C, Katz NNK. Management of periocular molluscum contagiosum in children. *J Pediatr Ophthalmol Strabismus* 1983;20:19–21.

107. Vasily DB, Bhatia AG. Erythema annulare centrifugum and molluscum contagiosum. *Arch Dermatol* 1978;114:1853.

108. Izu R, Manzano D, Gardeazabal J, et al. Giant molluscum contagiosum presenting as a tumor in an HIV-infected patient. *J Dermatol* 1994;33:266–267.

109. Gottlieb SL, Myskowski PL. Molluscum contagiosum. *Int J Dermatol* 1994;33:453–461.

110. Schwartz JJ, Myskowski PL. Molluscum contagiosum in patients with human immunodeficiency virus infection: a review of 27 patients. *J Am Acad Dermatol* 1992;27:583–588.

111. Shelley WB, Burkmeister V. Demonstration of a unique viral structure: the molluscum viral colony sac. *Br J Dermatol* 1986;115:557–562.

112. Lever WF, Schaumberg-Lever G. Diseases caused by viruses. In: *Histopathology of the skin.* Philadelphia: JB Lippincott, 1983.

113. Betlloch I, Pinazo I, Mestre F, et al. Molluscum contagiosum in HIV infection: response to zidovudine. *Int J Dermatol* 1989;28:351–352.

114. Meadows KP, Tyring SK, Pavia AT, et al. Resolution of recalcitrant molluscum contagiosum virus lesions in human immunodeficiency virus-infected patients treated with cidofovir. *Arch Dermatol* 1997;133:987–990.

115. Curtin BJ, Theodore FH. Ocular molluscum contagiosum. *Am J Ophthalmol* 1955;39:302–310.

116. Margo C, Katz NNK. Management of periocular molluscum contagiosum. *J Pediatr Ophthalmol Strabismus* 1983;20:19–21.

PART IV

Prevention and Therapy

22

Immunizations in the Immunocompromised Host

William C. Gruber

Department of Clinical Research, Wyeth-Lederle Vaccines, Pearl River, New York 10990

During the twentieth century, dramatic advances were made in the prevention of infection. Progress in public health and sanitation was responsible for early reductions, and the broad application of antimicrobials and vaccines, beginning in the 1930s, contributed significantly to further decreases in infections. In the face of such improvements in health, new populations with impaired immunity have emerged in increasing numbers. Patients with congenital or acquired immunodeficiency, human immunodeficiency virus (HIV) infection, bone marrow transplant (BMT), solid-organ transplant, autoimmune diseases, and other conditions requiring immunosuppressive therapy present formidable challenges to immunization strategies.

For purposes of decision making regarding vaccine use, persons with immunocompromising conditions can be divided into three groups as outlined by the Advisory Committee on Immunization Practices (ACIP) of the Centers for Disease Control and Prevention (CDC): (a) persons who are severely immunocompromised, not as a result of HIV infection; (b) persons with HIV infection; and (c) persons with conditions that cause limited immune deficits (e.g., asplenia, renal failure) that may require the use of special vaccines or higher doses of vaccines but do not contraindicate the use of any particular vaccine (1). Live vaccines are contraindicated in all persons in the first group, for some vaccines and some persons in the second group, and are not contraindicated in the third group (1). In addition to safety issues, attention must be paid to the level of immunosuppression and its role in affecting immune response. For example, when cancer chemotherapy (including radiation) or immunosuppressive therapy is being contemplated, indicated vaccines that can be safely administered should precede this therapy by 2 weeks or longer. Patients inadvertently vaccinated proximate to or during therapy should be considered unimmunized; these patients should be reimmunized at least 3 months after discontinuing therapy.

The specific defect in immune response provides clues to the type of vaccine that may put the patient at risk as well as the likelihood of inadequate immune response. For example, persons who have defects in T-cell mediated cytotoxicity can be at risk for unchecked replication of live vaccines and concomitant disease. In fact, live bacterial and live virus vaccines are contraindicated in patients with congenital disorders of immune function (1). Patients with congenital or acquired humoral immunodeficiency and

TABLE 22.1. *Recommendations for use of common vaccines in immunocompromised children*

Vaccine	Type	Use in immunocompromised patients
BCG	Live bacteria	Contraindicated
Diphteria, pertussis or acellular pertussis, tetanus	Subunit and toxic[a]	Recommended
Haemophilus influenza b	Polysaccharide	Recommended
Hepatitis A	Inactivated virus	Not contraindicated
Hepatitis B	Subunit (HBsAg)	Recommended
Influenza	Inactivated virus	Recommended
Lyme disease	Outer surface protein	Recommendations pending[b]
Meningococcal	Polysaccharide	Specific indications[c]
MMR		
Measles	Live virus	Contraindicated in congenital immunodeficiency; special indications in acquired immunodeficiency and HIV[d]
Mumps	Live virus	
Rubella	Live virus	
Polio	OPV live virus	Contraindicated
	IPV inactivated virus	Recommended
Pneumococcal	Polysaccharide	Special indications[e]
Rotavirus	Live reassortant virus	Contraindicated
Varicella	Live virus	Special indications[f]

Note: Live oral poliovirus vaccine (OPV) is contraindicated, but other live vaccines listed may be given to children for whom vaccine is otherwise indicated in households with contacts who are immunocompromised (see text).

BCG, bacille Calmette-Guérin; HBsAG, hepatitis B surface antigen; HIV, human immunodeficiency virus; IPV, inactivated polio vaccine; MMR, measles mumps rubella; OPV, oral poliovirus vaccine.

[a]Acellular pertussis vaccines contain inactivated pertussis toxin (PT) and one or more pertussis subunit antigens, for example, filamentous hemagglutinin (FHA), a 69-KD outer-membrane protein—pertactin (Pn), and fimbriae (Fim) types 2 and 3.

[b]Licensed for use in persons 15 to 70 years of age. Advisory Committee on Immunization Practices (ACTPs) recommendations pending.

[c]Indicated for persons who have terminal complement deficiencies and persons who have anatomic or functional asplenia (see text for other indications).

[d]Persons with leukemia in remission who were not immune to measles, rubella, or mumps when diagnosed with leukemia may receive MMR or its component vaccines. Vaccine should be considered in those for whom it is indicated at least 2 weeks before or at least 3 months after immunosuppressive therapy is completed but is contraindicated in congenital immunodeficiency and those with severe acquired immunodeficiency. Newly diagnosed HIV-infected children and adults without acceptable evidence of measles immunity should receive MMR vaccine as soon as possible after diagnosis, unless severely immunocompromised. Measles vaccine is not recommended for HIV-infected persons with severe immunosuppression as defined by age specific CD4 count criteria.

[e]Pneumococcal vaccine is currently recommended for patients with asplenia, splenic dysfunction (including sickle hemoglobinopathies), HIV infection, leukemia, lymphoma, Hodgkin's disease, multiple myeloma, generalized malignancy, chronic renal failure, or nephrotic syndrome, those receiving immunosuppressive chemotherapy (including corticosteroids), and those who have received an organ or bone marrow transplant (see text for dosing recommendations). The advent of protein conjugated pneumococcal vaccines will likely alter recommendations.

[f]Contaminated in congenital immunodeficiency. Available under special protocol for patients with leukemia (see text). Currently contraindicated in children with HIV infection, but this recommendation is subject to change for individuals without severe immunocompromise.

complement disorders can be expected to respond poorly to polysaccharide antigens. Persons with splenic dysfunction or asplenia may respond poorly to polysaccharide antigens that are not conjugated to a carrier protein but respond adequately to some conjugated antigens. Premature infants may fail to receive the full measure of passively transferred maternal antibody that is their due, and young infants in general lack maturity in response to some antigens (e.g. polysaccharides). Other than a diminished response to polysaccharide-containing antigens and possibly poliovirus type 3, however, responses to routine vaccines administered at appropriate chronological age are remarkably similar to those of full-term infants (2). Although not commonly recognized as an "immunocompromised host," the elderly patient clearly demonstrates reduced protective responses to vaccines directed against targeted pathogens. Both cell-mediated and humoral deficits abound in aged persons. As the "baby-boomers" of the 1940s and 1950s age, the geriatric population will continue to grow, and infections in the elderly population will increase in prominence. (This trend may have already begun, as evidenced by an increasing rate of influenza and pneumonia in the geriatric age group [3]). Immunocompromised children may reap the rewards of the development of vaccines for geriatrics; strategies that prove successful in augmenting immune response in elderly persons may prove applicable in young infants and immunocompromised children.

The successful application of current and future vaccines for the immunocompromised patient requires a clear understanding of safety limitations and potency of each candidate vaccine. Recommendations for use of common vaccines are given in Table 22.1. This chapter addresses the safety, immunogenicity, and use of vaccines in children with impaired immunity. Live vaccines, inactivated vaccines, polysaccharide vaccines, and subunit vaccines will be addressed.

LIVE VACCINES

General Considerations

Licensed live virus vaccines recommended routinely in the United States include vaccines for the prevention of measles, mumps, rubella, rotavirus, and varicella zoster. Vaccinia virus vaccine is no longer routinely recommended and is contraindicated in immunocompromised children (1). Live influenza, parainfluenza, and respiratory syncytial virus vaccines are currently in development for routine use in children and adults and ultimately may have indications in persons with impaired immunity. Although not routinely recommended in the United States, bacillus Calmette–Guerin (BCG) vaccine for prevention of *Mycobacterium tuberculosis* disease is recommended at birth in more than 100 countries by the Expanded Program on Immunization (EPI) of the World Health Organization (WHO). A live attenuated oral *Salmonella typhi* is available for prevention of typhoid fever. It is not recommended for routine general use in the United States, is contraindicated in immunocompromised persons, and alternative protective inactivated preparations exist. Adenovirus vaccines originally approved to prevent epidemics of adenovirus type 4 and 7 in military recruits are no longer produced, and yellow fever vaccine has specific indications for persons traveling to endemic areas. Typhoid, adenovirus and yellow fever vaccines will not be discussed further; the use of these vaccines in immunocompromised patients is included in the comprehensive review by Pirofski and Casadevall (4).

Although methods vary for producing an attenuated pathogenic agent, all live vaccines share a common feature: The vaccine agent produces a mild infection without disease. Live vaccines elicit protective immune responses in otherwise healthy persons, and mucosally delivered live vaccines offer the additional advantage of inducing local pathogen specific immunity. In immunocompromised patients, the timing of vaccine administration and the degree of immune deficiency can be critical determinants of protective immune response.

Live vaccines by their nature raise safety concerns because of the potential loss of attenuation and unbridled virus or bacterial replication leading to disease. Because live vaccines may be transmitted to susceptibles, the risk of disease often extends to immunocompromised household contacts of otherwise healthy vaccinees. The risk of this complication varies with the degree of immunocompromise and the type of vaccine. Hence, some vaccines may be contraindicated in certain types of immunocompromised patients, whereas other vaccines may not be contraindicated. Also, the degree of immunocompromise may be variable for an individual patient. For example, persons with leukemia in remission who have not received chemotherapy for at least 3 months are not considered severely immunocompromised for the purpose of receiving live vaccines (5). Each recommendation surrounding the use of these vaccines must carefully weigh the risks of vaccination versus the potential benefit of preventing disease that could prove life threatening.

Specific Live Virus Vaccines

Measles, Mumps, Rubella Vaccine

Live attenuated parenteral measles vaccines have been used in the United States since 1963 to protect against the morbidity of this exanthem-associated respiratory illness and complications including pneumonia, encephalopathy, and death. Mumps vaccine followed in 1967 to prevent mumps parotitis, orchitis, meningitis, meningoencephalitis, and sequelae, such as neurologic deficits and sensorineural deafness. Rubella vaccine came next in 1969, and infant vaccination in the United States is recommended primarily to prevent miscarriages and congenital anomalies associated with infection later in life during pregnancy. These vaccines were com-

bined as the measles, mumps, rubella (MMR) vaccine in routine use today. Immunization is recommended for infants 12 to 15 months old and 4 to 6 years of age. Each of the components of MMR is contraindicated in severely immunocompromised patients; however, policy is focused on the measles component of the vaccine. Natural measles infection poses the greatest risk of morbidity and death, but measles vaccine poses the greatest risk of vaccine-associated disease for the severely immunocompromised patient. Measles-containing vaccine is contraindicated in persons with congenital disorders of immunity, but it is recommended for some children with HIV infection. This disparity is due to differences in risks based on level of immunocompromise.

Risk of death from natural measles infection in oncology patients and patients with HIV have been reported to exceed 40% and 70%, respectively (6,7); however, disseminated infections after measles vaccination in children with congenital immunodeficiency and hematologic malignancy are also described (8,9). This has tempered consideration of measles immunization in these populations. Rather, the focus has been placed on immunization of household contacts of immunocompromised patients to reduce the likelihood of exposure. This is practical because vaccinated persons do not transmit vaccine virus. Measles vaccine has been safely administered after brief chemotherapy and 2 years after BMT in patients without evidence of acute rejection (10,11). Chemotherapy or immunosuppressive therapy may reduce antibody response to measles vaccine; however, satisfactory responses (50%–75%) have been seen in leukemic, organ transplant, and BMT patients to MMR vaccine, when it is administered appropriately (10–14). Persistent T-cell response to measles antigen after transplant may correlate with reduced humoral response (15). MMR should not be administered to persons who are judged to be severely immunocompromised; however, persons with leukemia in remission who were not immune to measles, rubella, or mumps when diagnosed with leukemia may receive MMR or its component vaccines. Vaccine should be considered in those for whom it is indicated at least 2 weeks before or at least 3 months after immunosuppressive therapy is completed.

The use of measles-containing vaccines in patients on steroids is not well studied; the minimum dose associated with immunosuppression sufficient to increase the risk of vaccine-associated disease or diminish immune response is undefined. A steroid dose equivalent to or greater than 2 mg/kg or 20 mg/day of prednisone may increase the risk of vaccine-associated disease. Delay of measles-containing vaccine for 1 month is recommended for persons who have received steroids in these doses for 14 days or longer. For patients who receive this regimen for less than 14 days, MMR may be administered immediately, although some experts prefer to wait 2 weeks (5).

A large amount of data demonstrated the safety of measles vaccine administered to children with HIV infection in the United States and Africa (16–19). Adverse events generally have been infrequent, although case reports exist of disseminated infection in persons with severe depressions in CD4 counts (20). In addition, immunization of HIV-infected persons early in the course of infection has been associated with acceptable antibody response, but responses decrease with progressive immunodeficiency (19,21). Rubella and mumps vaccines have not been associated with serious illness in HIV-infected patients. Based on these experiences, measles-containing vaccine is recommended for infants at 1 year of age (or earlier if at risk for exposure) (5). The second dose of measles vaccine may be given as soon as 1 month after the first (rather than at 4 to 6 years of age) to enhance the likelihood of good immune response prior to the onset of significant immunodeficiency (5). Newly diagnosed HIV-infected children and adults without acceptable evidence of measles immunity should receive MMR vaccine as soon as possible after diagnosis, unless they are severely immunocompromised. Measles vaccine is not recommended for HIV-infected persons with severe immunosuppression as defined by age-specific CD4 count criteria (5).

Occasionally, a person for whom measles vaccine is contraindicated may be exposed to natural measles virus. In this circumstance, intramuscular immunoglobulin can prevent or modify illness if it is administered within 6 days of exposure (22). Protection is transient because of the loss of this passive antibody over time. The dosage for immunocompromised persons is 0.5 mL/kg of body weight (maximum dose 15 mL), administered intramuscularly. If the patient is already receiving intravenous immunoglobulin, administration of at least 100 mg/kg within the preceding 3 weeks is likely to be protective. Immunoglobulin preparations do not prevent rubella or mumps infection (5).

The use of high-dose immunoglobulin preparations can reduce the response to measles and rubella vaccine (23). The effect of immunoglobulin administration on mumps immunity is unknown. The duration of antibody inhibition after immunoglobulin administration is related to type of preparation and dose. Hence different delays have been recommended for administration of MMR after receipt of preparations likely to contain antibody (Table 22.2) (5).

Poliovirus Vaccine

Until recently, live attenuated oral poliovirus vaccine (OPV) was used routinely for all immunizations against poliomyelitis for healthy infants and children in the United States. This vaccine is contraindicated in patients with congenital immunodeficiency, HIV infection, and acquired immunodeficiency. The alternative vaccine, inactivated polio vaccine (IPV), is administered intramuscularly and is widely used for primary immunization against polio in developed coun-

TABLE 22.2. *Suggested intervals between administration of (IG) preparation for various indications and vaccines containing live-measles virus*[a]

Indications	Dose (mg IgG/kg)	Interval (mo) before measles vaccination
TIG prophylaxis	250 U (10 mg IgG/kg) i.m.	3
Hepatitis A IG prophylaxis		
Contact prophylaxis	0.02 mL/kg (3.3 mg IgG/kg) i.m.	3
International travel	0.06 mL/kg (10 mg IgG/kg) i.m.	3
HBIG prophylaxis	0.06 mL/kg (10 mg IgG/kg) i.m.	3
HRIG prophylaxis	21 IU/kg (22 mg IgG/kg) i.m.	4
VZIG prophylaxis	125 units/10 kg (20–40 mg IgG/kg) i.m.	5
Measles IG prophylaxis		
Standard (i.e. nonimmunocompromised) contact	0.25 mL/kg (40 mg IgG/kg) i.m.	5
Immunocompromised contact	0.50 mL/kg (80 mg IgG/kg) i.m.	6
Blood transfusion:		
RBCs	10 mL/kg (negligible IgG/kg) i.v.	0
RBCs, adenine-saline added	10 mL/kg (10 mg IgG/kg) i.v.	3
Packed RBCs (Hct 65%)	10 mL/kg (60 mg IgG/kg) i.v.	6
Whole blood (Hct 35%–50%)[b]	10 mL/kg (80–100 mg IgG/kg) i.v.	6
Plasma/platelet products	10 mL/kg (160 mg IgG/kg) i.v.	7
Replacement therapy for immune deficiencies[c]	300–400 mg/kg i.v. (as IVIG)	8
Respiratory syncytial virus prophylaxis	750 mg/kg i.v. (as RSV-IGIV)	9
ITP	400 mg/kg i.v. (as IVIG)	8
	1,000 mg/kg i.v. (as IVIG)	10
Kawasaki disease	2 g/kg i.v. (as IVIG)	11

HBIG, hepatitis B immune globulin; Hct, hematocrit; HIV, human immunodeficiency virus; HRIG, human rabies immune globulin; IgG, immunoglobulin G; IG, immune globulin; IGIV, immunoglobulin, intravenous; IM, intramuscular; ITP, immune thrombocytopenic purpura; IV, intravenous; RBCs, red blood cells; RSV-IGIV, respiratory syncytial virus immune globulin, intravenous; TIG, tetanus immune globulin; VZIG, varicella zoster immune globulin.

[a]This table is not intended for determining the correct indications and dosage for the use of immune globulin (IG) preparations. Unvaccinated persons may not be fully protected against measles during the entire suggested time interval, and additional doses of immune globulin or measles vaccine may be indicated after measles exposure. The concentration of measles antibody in a particular immune globulin preparation can vary by lot, and the rate of antibody clearance after receipt of an immune globulin preparation can vary. The recommended intervals are extrapolated from an estimated half-life of 30 days for passively acquired antibody and an observed interference with the immune response to measles vaccine for 5 months after a dose of 80 mg IgG/kg.

[b]Assumes a serum immunoglobulin G (IgG) concentration of 16 mg/mL.

[c]Measles vaccination is recommended for human immunodeficiency virus (HIV)-infected children aged 36 months who do not have evidence of severe immunosuppression but is contraindicated for patients who have congenital disorders of the immune system.

Adapted from Krupova I, Kaiserova E, Foltinova A, et al. Bacteremia and fungemia in pediatric versus adult cancer patients after chemotherapy: comparison of etiology risk factors and outcome. *J Chemother* 1998;10: 236–242, with permission.

tries of Europe. A more immunogenic IPV introduced in 1987 had been shown to produce protective levels of antibody against types 1, 2, and 3 poliovirus in 99% to 100% of children by 6 months of age after the second dose that was comparable or better than those produced by OPV (24). Recent studies showed the persistence of antibody after sequential dosing of IPV for two doses followed by OPV (25).

Recommendations in the United States changed recently in response to the eradication of poliovirus from the Western Hemisphere (26) and the low risk of vaccine-associated disease. The American Academy of Pediatrics now recommends a 4-dose all IPV vaccine schedule for immunization of all infants and children in the United States (27). However, OPV still is widely used internationally as part of the efforts of the EPI for polio eradication of WHO.

In children and adults with severe immunodeficiency, OPV has been associated with paralytic disease (VAPP). Most cases have included some degree of dygammaglobulinemia or agammaglobulinemia (28). Manifestations have varied from mild meningoencephalitis to severe paralytic disease and death (28–35). The risk for VAPP is low (approximately one case to 2.4 million doses), but the greatest burden appears to be seen with infants receiving their first doses (one case in 750,000 children receiving their first dose of OPV) (36). Because congenital immunodeficiencies and HIV disease often are not detected prior to routine poliovirus immunization at age 2 months, it is understandable that this age group faces the greatest risk of VAPP. Paralytic polio may be the first manifestation of immunocompromise (30, 32,34). The CDC estimates that 30 to 40 cases of vaccine-associated paralysis would have occurred in the United States during 1997 through 2000 if the previously recommended poliovirus vaccination practices had not changed (36). Prolonged replication of poliovirus accompanied by significant changes in surface proteins can be seen in immunodeficient persons after OPV, which may have implications for the polio eradication effort (37). Retrospective surveys have indicated that HIV-infected infants have received OPV without ill effect; nevertheless, IPV is recommended because of the theoretic risk and acceptable tolerance and immunogenicity of IPV (38).

It also should be remembered that 40 of 125 VAPP cases in 1980 through 1994 were seen in immunocompromised family contacts of healthy vaccinated individuals (36). Hence IPV is the only poliovirus vaccine recommended for immunocompromised persons and their family contacts (27,36). This recommendation extends to persons living in households with patients receiving steroids or chemotherapy. Poliovirus is excreted in maximum titers from secretions and stool for approximately 4 weeks after administration. If poliovirus vaccine is inadvertently administered to a household contact of an immunocompromised person, the vaccine recipient should avoid contact with the immunocompromised person for 4 to 6 weeks. When this is impractical, avoidance of contact with secretions or stool and good handwashing practices is acceptable but less effective.

Varicella Virus Vaccine

Live attenuated varicella virus vaccine is recommended in the United States for protection against varicella (chicken pox) for use in susceptible healthy children aged 12 months to 12 years and is given as 0.5-mL dose, subcutaneously (39). For persons aged 13 years and older, two doses are administered 4 to 8 weeks apart. The live vaccine is composed of the Oka strain of live, attenuated varicella zoster virus (VZV), which was derived from virus isolated in the early 1970s from vesicular fluid in a healthy child with natural varicella (40). The vaccine virus was attenuated through multiple passages in tissue culture.

The vaccine was first licensed for use among high-risk children in Europe, Japan, and Korea and extended to healthy children in 1989. Efficacy has been estimated to be as high as 95% after seven years (41).

The vaccine is not currently licensed for use in immunocompromised children in the United States (42). Factors leading to this decision include an increased risk of rash in vaccinee, transmission to household contacts, and the success of early administration of the antiviral acyclovir in reducing the morbidity of varicella in children with hematologic malignancy. Varicella virus vaccine should not be administered to persons who have primary immunodeficiency, cellular immunodeficiencies, hypogammaglobulinemia, or dysgammaglobulinemia. Varicella vaccine is also contraindicated in persons with a family history of congenital or hereditary immunodeficiency in first-degree relatives unless immunocompetence is confirmed by appropriate laboratory tests (42). Varicella vaccine is recommended for healthy household contacts of immunocompromised patients, based on low risk of transmission from healthy individuals and the likelihood of reducing household exposure to wild-type virus (42). Family members who receive varicella vaccine and develop a rash should avoid contact with immuncompromised patients until lesions have crusted. For purposes of deciding the merits of immunization, both healthy and immunocompromised children and adults who have positive histories of varicella (except for BMT recipients) can be considered immune.

Varicella vaccine has been studied extensively in pediatric patients with hematologic malignancy. Approximately 5% and 40% of patients with acute lymphocytic leukemia (ALL) who have completed or are on maintenance chemotherapy, respectively, may experience a mild to moderate varicella-like rash of 2 to 200 lesions after receiving varicella vaccine (43). Although healthy children and adults are unlikely to transmit vaccine virus to susceptible contacts (4%–6% after the first dose), the risk for transmission from vaccinees with leukemia is higher (17%) and may be associated with the occurrence of rash (12.5%) and tertiary spread ($\leq$1% or less) following vaccination (44,45). Cases of varicella in the index case and siblings were associated with mild rash and few lesions. Varicella vaccine is not licensed for use in children with hematologic malignancies but is available to any physician free of charge from the manufacturer through a research protocol (46) for use in patients who have ALL who (a) are aged 12 months to 17 years, (b) have disease that has been in remission for at least 12 continuous months, (c) have a negative history of varicella disease, (d) have a peripheral blood-lymphocyte count greater than 700 cells/mm^3, and (e) have a platelet count greater than 100,000 cells/mm^3 within 24 hours of vaccination. Vaccine has been shown to be well tolerated, immunogenic, and protective in children who meet these criteria (43,47–51). Administration of heat-inactivated vaccine virus has been reported to reduce the incidence of zoster after BMT in persons who have been previously infected with wild-type virus (52), but an inactivated vaccine is currently not available for routine use. A multicenter trial of live varicella vaccine is currently under way in elderly subjects to evaluate the effectiveness of boosting cell mediated immunity in reducing shingles. The results of this study may have implications for immunosuppressed persons at risk for zoster.

Varicella virus vaccine should not be administered to persons who are receiving immunosuppressive therapy. Pharmacologic doses of systemic steroids can be associated with extensive rash and systemic disease (53). For children who have been receiving less than 2 mg/kg daily of prednisone for less than 2 weeks, vaccine may be administered, but evidence of serologic immunity should be confirmed after 6 weeks; patients without immunity should be revaccinated (42). For patients receiving higher doses for more prolonged periods, immunization should be performed 1 to 3 months after the completion of therapy. There are no data on the use of vaccine in patients receiving inhaled steroids, but most experts believe that vaccine can be administered safely to such patients. In circumstances where immunosuppression can be anticipated (such as solid-organ transplantation), varicella immunization prior to immunosuppression should be considered in susceptible patients (54).

Routine screening for HIV is not indicated prior to varicella vaccine administration (46). Epidemiologic studies suggest that in children with HIV infection, primary varicella infection is often not a serious problem, although low CD4 counts are associated with a subsequent risk of zoster (shingles) as high as 70%. There is speculation that, as with other immunocompromised patients, the risk of zoster following immunization may be less than that observed after natural wild-type infection (55). The incidence of zoster was lower in persons with vaccine or natural exposure to varicella after their initial exposure to live vaccine (55). After weighing the potential risks and benefits, varicella vaccine should be considered for HIV-infected children in CDC Class I with a CD4+ T-lymphocyte percentage of 25% or greater. Two doses of vaccine separated by 3 months should be administered and the child should return for evaluation of any post-immunization varicella-like rash (46). If inadvertent vaccination of HIV-infected persons results in clinical disease, the use of acyclovir may modify the severity of disease.

The effect of prior administration of blood products or immunoglobulin administration on immunity to live varicella vaccine is unknown. Experience based on immunity to measles vaccine after immunoglobulin administration has been used to formulate recommendations (23, 39,42). Five months or longer should elapse after blood products are received before vari-cella vaccine is administered. Immunoglobulin products should not be received for 3 weeks after vaccination unless the benefits exceed those of vaccination.

Varicella zoster immune globulin (VZIG) is a preparation of human immunoglobulin from human donors that has high titers of antibody to varicella. After effectiveness in preventing severe varicella infection was demonstrated when given within 96 hours of natural varicella exposure, the product was licensed in 1978 for this use. The recommended dose is 125 U/10 kg of body weight, up to a maximum of 625 U. The minimum dose is 125 U. Preexisting immunity, level of immunocompromise, and type of exposure are all important when assessing the indications for receipt of VZIG varicella. For example, VZIG is commonly indicated for children and adults without documented historical immunity to varicella who (a) have primary and acquired immune-deficiency disorders, (b) have neoplastic diseases, and (c) are receiving immunosuppressive treatment (39,42). BMT should not be considered immune regardless of history unless they have had varicella subsequent to transplantation. *Direct contact exposure* is defined as more than 1 hour of direct contact with an infectious person while indoors. For children routinely receiving intravenous immunoglobulin, antibody titers against varicella may be insufficient to provide protection, and patients at risk for severe disease should be given VZIG (56).

Bacillus Calmette–Guerin Vaccine

The BCG vaccine is derived from an attenuated strain of *Mycobacterium bovis* and is used for the prevention of tuberculosis. Although used extensively worldwide, it is not used routinely in the United States and is contraindicated in most persons with immunodeficiency (57). Disseminated infection has been observed in patients with primary and acquired immunodeficiency and symptomatic HIV infection (58,59); however, no significant adverse events were seen in a population of Brazilian children with HIV infection vaccinated at birth (60). Recently, defects in interferon-gamma receptors have been described that have been associated with disseminated myobacterial infection, including disseminated BCG (61). The immunogenicity and protection afforded by BCG are variable, even in immunocompetent persons, and even less information is available about protection in immunocompromised subjects. There is evidence that tuberculin skin test reactivity is weaker in HIV-infected persons, suggesting diminished immunogenicity in this population (57).

INACTIVATED AND SUBUNIT VACCINES

General Considerations

In contrast to issues of safety that are prominent in assessing the role of live attenuated vaccines, inactivated and subunit vaccines are generally as free of adverse effects in immunocompromised persons as in healthy children. There are some possible exceptions. Investigations of the relationship between immunization and subsequent changes in virus load have yielded mixed results in HIV patients. Recent studies usually indicated nonspecific increases in circulating virus populations, with some exceptions; tetanus immunization disproportionately increases nonsyncytial forming virus compared with virus prone to form syncytia (62,63). The increase in viremia is typically brief. The clinical significance of this is unclear and does not preclude immunization of HIV-infected patients; the benefits of immunization are believed to outweigh any potential hazard of transient increase in virus load.

The immunogenicity of a vaccine is related to both the vaccine and the level of immunocompromise. For example, inactivated and subunit vaccines can be immunogenic in many types of immunocompromised pa-

tients, but dialysis alone can interfere with immunogenicity of tetanus and hepatitis B vaccine in renal patients (64). This section focuses on inactivated and subunit vaccines that are routinely recommended for immunocompetent or immunocompromised hosts. These include vaccines against diphtheria, pertussis, tetanus, *Haemophilus influenzae* type b, meningococcus, pneumococcus, hepatitis A, hepatitis B, and influenza. Rabies vaccine, which has specific indications based on exposure to a potentially rapid animal, is not discussed, but the reader is referred to the comprehensive ACIP review and recommendations on rabies immunization (65). Recently, a vaccine containing outer surface protein A of *Borrelia burgdorferi,* the cause of Lyme disease, has been licensed in the United States (LYMErix, SmithKline Beecham Biologicals, Philadelphia, PA, U.S.A.). It is approved for use in individuals aged 15 to 70 years of age, but data are lacking on the safety and efficacy of the vaccine in individuals with immunodeficiencies. General guidelines for administration of inactivated or subunit vaccines are recommended (66). Other vaccines containing killed antigens, including cholera, plague, and anthrax, are not recommended for general routine use in the United States, but they do not pose a risk to immunocompromised persons. They may be used for the same indications as for immunologically normal persons and are not discussed further in this chapter (1).

Diphtheria, Pertussis, Tetanus Vaccines

Formulations of vaccines against diphtheria, pertussis, and tetanus (DPT) contain inactivated bacterial products of the respective antigens. These "toxoid" vaccines have been licensed and in extensive use since the 1940s. The standard DPT vaccine contains "whole-cell" pertussis antigen, which was prepared from suspensions of *Bordetella pertussis* organisms. Since 1996, a formula-

tion labeled DaPT is recommended for the series of four infant immunizations and the booster dose at 4 to 6 years of age. This vaccine includes inactivated pertussis toxin (PT) and one or more pertussis subunit antigens (e.g., filamentous hemagglutinin [FHA], a 69-kD outer-membrane protein-pertactin [Pn], and fimbriae [Fim] types 2 and 3). The formulations and manufacturers of acellular vaccines licensed in the United States are described in detail in the ACIP recommendations issued by the CDC (67).

Newly licensed DaPT vaccines have been shown in comparison trials to be safe and immunogenic for pertussis (68,69). A series of trials demonstrated the efficacy of acellular pertussis vaccine, but serologic correlates of immunity require further definition (70). Whole-cell pertussis containing DPT remains an acceptable alternative for healthy children. Vaccination against diphtheria, pertussis, and tetanus is recommended for all children, including those with immunocompromising conditions. Recommendations for acellular pertussis vaccine do not exclude immunocompromised children for whom DPT vaccine is otherwise indicated (71). An adult formulation, dT, is recommended for immunization every 10 years beyond the last pediatric dose.

Tetanus, diphtheria, and pertussis immunizations have been shown to be immunogenic in persons who have underlying malignancy while they undergo chemotherapy (72–74). In one study, more than 95% of pediatric renal transplant patients ranging from 8 to 19 years of age and who had received primary infant vaccination were successfully boosted with tetanus using standard toxoid vaccines. Responses to diphtheria toxoid have been more variable in children, and poor responses in adult dialysis patients paralleled poor responses to hepatitis B vaccine (64,75,76).

In BMT recipients in whom responses to some types of vaccine antigens can be particularly poor, tetanus toxoid vaccines can be immunogenic when they are administered 12 and 24 months after transplantation (77,78). Additional doses administered in children younger than 12 months of age do not appear to confer significant advantages over the two-dose regimen 24 months after transplant (79).

Immunization with tetanus and diphtheria toxoid has been evaluated in HIV-infected patients. Responses correlate with CD4 cell counts but generally are diminished compared with responses in healthy controls (80–82). Limited information exists on immunogenicity of acellular pertussis-containing vaccines in immunocompromised patients, but responses to this vaccine also have been shown to correlate with CD4 counts in infants with HIV infection (83).

Haemophilus influenza Type B

Since the mid-1980s, the licensure of a polysaccharide vaccine followed by protein-conjugated vaccines against *H. influenzae* type B (HiB) dramatically reduced the incidence of invasive HiB disease. The original vaccine contained the purified polysaccharide polyribosylribitol phosphate (PRP), which proved to be insufficiently immunogenic in children younger than 2 years of age. Conjugation of the PRP polysaccharide with protein carriers conferred T-cell-dependent characteristics to the vaccine and substantially enhanced the immunologic response to the PRP antigen. Conjugation was a necessary step to provide protection for young infants at highest risk for invasive HiB disease. Conjugated vaccines now are recommended for routine use in infants and children to provide protection against HiB disease. Carrier proteins used in conjugated preparations include diphtheria toxoid (PRP-D, ProHIBiT, Aventis Pasteur Inc., Swiftwater, PA, U.S.A.), altered diphtheria toxoid (CRM197, HbOC,-HibTITER, Wyeth-Lederle Vaccines, Pearl River, NY, U.S.A.), *Neisseria meningitidis* outer-membrane protein complex (PRP-OMP, Pedvax-HIB, Merck & Company, Inc., West Point, PA, U.S.A.), and tetanus toxoid (PRP-T, ActHIB,

OmniHIB, Aventis Pasteur). The precise level of antibody required for protection against invasive disease is not clearly established, but a 1 µg/mL geometric mean titer (GMT) 3 weeks after vaccination has been associated with protection from invasive disease (84,85). Currently licensed vaccines include monovalent preparations and multivalent preparations that also contain other vaccine antigens recommended for children. Because studies in infants demonstrated that using one of these combination products may induce a lower immune response to the HiB component (86), DTaP/HiB combination products should not be used for primary vaccination in infants aged 2, 4, or 6 months (87). Licensed combination Dtap/Hib vaccines may be given for the 15- to 18-month booster dose.

The HiB vaccine can be immunogenic in patients with increased risk for invasive disease, such as those with sickle cell disease (88), leukemia (89), HIV infection (90), and in those who have had splenectomies (91). Not all conjugated HiB vaccine preparations have been tested in each of these types of immunocompromised patients, but it is presumed that protection afforded by each vaccine will be comparable when administered as recommended. Efficacy studies have not been performed in immunocompromised populations with increased risk of invasive disease (1).

Recent studies indicated that polysaccharide HiB vaccines produce an immunoglobulin G (IgG) response in splenectomized patients comparable to healthy subjects. It is speculated that confusion surrounding prior studies may be due to relative deficiency in IgM response accounting for a lower total antibody response (91). Children with decreased or absent splenic function and who have received a primary series of HiB immunizations followed by a booster at 12 months of age or older do not require additional doses (92); however, patients who have completed their primary series and are undergoing elective splenectomy may benefit from an additional

dose of licensed conjugate vaccine, best given at least 7 to 10 days prior to the procedure (92,93).

Children with leukemia have been shown to respond well to conjugated HiB if it is administered within 1 year of onset of chemotherapy, but they show reduced responses if it is administered after prolonged chemotherapy (89). The durability of antibody response is not yet known, and it is not yet clear whether these groups of patients will benefit from additional doses after receiving the primary series. Immunization in patients undergoing BMT or solid-organ transplantation is consistently associated with defects in T- and B-cell responses to polysaccharide and protein antigens (94,95). Recently, a strategy of immunizing autologous and allogenic BMT patients with conjugated HiB vaccine prior to transplantation has shown promise as a means of priming subsequently transplanted cells against the polysaccharide of *H. influenzae* type B. After a dose prior to harvest and four successive doses after transplantation, bone marrow cell recipients have responded to booster doses with an anamnestic response that reaches higher levels than patients immunized only after transplantation (96,97).

In persons with HIV infection, IgG_2 subclass deficiency and in those receiving chemotherapy for malignancies, immunogenicity varies with the stage of infection and the degree of immunocompromise (98). After receiving the primary series of conjugated HiB vaccine, geometric mean titers of PRP antibody at 9 and 24 months in HIV-infected children with mild to moderate disease did not differ significantly from uninfected children (99). In children with clinical acquired immunodeficiency syndrome (AIDS), antibody titers at 1 year are inadequate in nearly half of immunized children (100). Older children with IgG_2 deficiencies fail to respond to HiB polysaccharide alone, and some require booster doses when given protein-conjugated HiB vaccine, a pattern of response like that in infants less than 6 months of age (101).

Meningococcal Vaccines

Consequent to the success of HiB vaccination, *N. meningitidis* now supersedes HiB as a cause of bacterial meningitis in children and young adults in the United States, with an estimated 2,600 cases each year (102). The quadrivalent A,C,Y,W-135 vaccine (Menomune-A,C,Y,W-135, Aventis Pasteur) is the formulation currently available in the United States for prevention of common serotypes of menigococcus causing disease. Serotype B, a common serotype of sporadic meningococcal disease, is not included in the vaccine. This preparation has shown good immunogenicity in children as young as 3 months of age against serotype A, but it is generally poorly immunogenic against type C in children less than 18 to 20 months of age (103,104). Routine vaccination of civilians is not recommended because of its relative ineffectiveness in children younger than 2 years of age, who represent the highest risk group for invasive disease (105). Rather, the meningococcal vaccine is recommended for control of serogroup C meningococcal disease outbreaks and for persons at increased risk for meningococcal infections, including (a) persons who have terminal complement deficiencies, (b) persons who have anatomic or functional asplenia, and, (c) laboratory personnel who routinely are exposed to *N. meningitidis* in solutions that may be aerosolized (105). Recently, meningococcal C protein-conjugated vaccines have been licensed in the United Kingdom for use in children, but these vaccines are not licensed in the United States. Military recruits also routinely receive the quadrivalent meningococcal vaccine. The need for revaccination of older children and adults has not been determined, but antibody levels decline rapidly over 2 to 3 years. Hence, if indications still exist for immunization, revaccination may be considered within 3 to 5 years.

Asplenic persons and those with terminal complement deficiencies (C3, C5–C9) are at particular risk for severe meningococcal infection and death (106,107); however, it is not clear whether most such patients will be adequately protected after vaccination. Some persons who are homozygous for complement deficiency have been reported to show good responses to polysaccharide meningococcal antigens (108). For persons who have undergone splenectomy for trauma, vaccination with A and C meningococcal polysaccharide produced seroconversion rates commensurate with those of control subjects, but subjects with prior chemotherapy for lymphoma did not responded so well (109). Although IgM responses may be diminished, IgG responses appear to be comparable to controls (91). Responses often were less durable in patients on chemotherapy for Hodgkin's disease and were most diminished in those on intensive regimens (110). These patients also failed to demonstrate a booster response to vaccine. When possible, it is recommended that vaccination be performed 2 weeks before splenectomy (1). Given the general lack of studies demonstrating the efficacy of vaccine in these populations, discerning physicians should remain alert to the possibility of invasive meningococcal disease in asplenic and complement-deficient patients, even when they have been immunized.

Immunologic responses to meningococcal vaccine in other immunocompromised populations has not been as well described. Children with leukemia have responses to meningococcal A and C serotypes approaching those observed in controls (111). Responses to meningococcal vaccine in BMT patients were reportedly poor according to one article (112), but the success of conjugated HiB vaccine regimens in this population suggested that a similar approach to meningococcal vaccination may prove effective (97). Patients with HIV infection may be at some increased risk of meningococcal infection (108), but reports of vaccine immunogenicity in this population are sparse (113). Tetravalent meningococcal vaccine efficacy has yet to be evaluated in immunocompromised adults and children (74).

Pneumococcal Vaccines

Pneumococcal vaccines (Pneumovax 23, Merck & Company, Inc.; Pnu-Immune 23, Wyeth-Lederle Vaccines) include 23 purified capsular polysaccharide antigens of *Streptococcus pneumoniae* (serotypes 1, 2, 3, 4, 5, 6B, 7F, 8, 9N, 9V, 10A, 11A, 12F, 14, 15B, 17F, 18C, 19A, 19F, 20, 22F, 23F, and 33F). In 1983, these vaccines replaced an earlier 14-valent formulation that was licensed in 1977. The current vaccine includes nearly 90% of the serotypes that cause invasive pneumococcal infections among children and adults in the United States. Pneumococcal capsular polysaccharide antigens induce type-specific antibodies by 2 to 3 weeks in more than 80% of healthy young adults (114), but there is variability in the induction of antibody to individual serotypes contained in the vaccine. The levels of antibodies that correlate with protection against pneumococcal disease have not been completely defined. Pneumococcal capsular polysaccharides induce antibodies primarily by T-cell-independent mechanisms, and antibody responses to most pneumococcal capsular types are poor in children younger than 2 years whose immune systems are immature (115,116).

Currently licensed pneumococcal polysaccharide vaccine is recommended for the protection of children and adults aged 2 years and older with underlying cardiopulmonary disease and persons with splenic dysfunction or asplenia. Routine vaccination also is recommended for adults aged 65 years and older. There is strong epidemiologic and clinical evidence to support the recommendation for vaccine use in these populations (117). The effectiveness of pneumococcal

vaccine is less clearly established in immunocompromised persons aged 2 years and older, but the potential benefits and safety are believed to justify vaccination. Pneumococcal vaccine is currently recommended for patients with HIV infection, leukemia, lymphoma, Hodgkin's disease, multiple myeloma, generalized malignancy, chronic renal failure, or nephrotic syndrome; those receiving immunosuppressive chemotherapy (including corticosteroids); and those who have received an organ transplant or BMT. A single repeat vaccination is recommended for persons with splenic dysfunction or immunodeficiency if 5 years or longer elapsed since receipt of first dose. If the patient is 10 years of age or younger, revaccination should be reconsidered 3 years after the previous dose (117). Revaccination after a second dose is not routinely recommended.

The risk for pneumococcal infection is highest for persons who are asplenic or experience splenic dysfunction. It is also high for those with decreased responsiveness to polysaccharide antigens or an increased rate of decline in serum antibody concentrations as a result of immunocompromising conditions. Unfortunately, this means that in the very patients for whom protection is indicated, a pneumococcal polysaccharide vaccine is likely to perform less well than in healthy individuals. Persons aged 2 to 64 years who have functional or anatomic asplenia (e.g., sickle cell disease or splenectomy) should be vaccinated. Penicillin prophylaxis should be initiated in children with sickle cell anemia or asplenia beginning at 4 months of age. Although recently immunologic responses have been shown to be adequate in many of these patients (118), anyone with such a condition should be informed that vaccination does not guarantee protection against fulminant pneumococcal disease, for which the case fatality rate is 50% to 80% (117). Failures to poorly immunogenic serotypes 6b, 14, 18, 19F, and 23F have been reported in sickle cell patients

(119). Even if vaccinated, asplenic patients with fever and signs consistent with pneumococcal infection should receive prompt medical attention. In patients scheduled for splenectomy, antibody responses are greater if immunization is performed 2 weeks or longer before surgery rather than after removal of the spleen (110).

In patients with congenital immunodeficiencies, hematologic malignancies, and nephrotic syndrome, antibody response to pneumococcal vaccination is often lower, and antibody levels decrease more rapidly than response among patients who are immunocompetent (111,120–122). Patients undergoing transplantation present a particularly formidable challenge to successful immunization against pneumococcus. Fewer than 20% of BMT patients demonstrated antibody titers likely to provide protection against six common pneumococcal serotypes after two successive immunizations with polysaccharide vaccine following transplantation (94). In a population of BMT subjects vaccinated within 6 months of transplantation, pneumococcal infection developed in nearly 13% of 39 patients; preinfection antibody levels were lower than the protective level in two of three cases in which a vaccine serotype was identified as the infecting organism (123). In a pediatric population, IgG$_2$ antibody responses were reduced independent of age or time of measurement after immunization when immunized with pneumococcal polysaccharide vaccine 1 year or longer after transplantation. Donor immunization with protein-conjugated *H. influenzae* type B vaccine followed by booster immunization in the recipient produced levels of HiB-specific antibody associated with protection. These observations may herald future success with a similar approach using conjugated pneumococcal polysaccharide vaccines (97).

Streptococcus pneumoniae is the most commonly identified bacterial pathogen that causes pneumonia in HIV-infected persons and is often the first clinical manifestation in children (124).

Transient increases in virus load after immunization of HIV-infected patients against pneumococcus have been variably observed but are not considered to be a contraindication to vaccination against this life-threatening pathogen (125,126). Children who have HIV infection may have a diminished antibody response to pneumococcal vaccine, but they respond better to vaccination when it is performed earlier in the course of their infection (98,127); however, it should be remembered that healthy infants younger than 2 years of age fail to make a comprehensive antibody response to serotypes contained in the pneumococcal polysaccharide vaccine. In children with HIV infection or congenital or acquired immunodeficiency diseases who experience recurrent serious pneumococcal infections (i.e., two or more serious bacterial infections, including bacteremia, pneumonia, or meningitis) in a 1-year period, intramuscular or intravenous immunoglobulin administration may be useful for preventing pneumococcal infection (128).

Following the success of HiB-conjugated vaccines in inducing antibody responses, conjugated pneumococcal vaccines are now being investigated. Recently, a heptavalent protein conjugated pneumococcal vaccine was reported to protect infants younger than 2 years of age against invasive disease (129). This vaccine (Prevnar, Wyeth-Lederle Vaccines), has now been licensed and recommended for routine use in infants and children to prevent invasive pneumococcal infection. Conjugated pneumococcal vaccines offer promise of improved immunogenicity in immunocompromised patients and possibly the elderly. Studies are being planned to evaluate their potential.

Hepatitis A

Until recently, passive immunization with standard commercial immunoglobulin administered intramuscularly (IG) was the standard prophylaxis against hepatitis A virus (HAV) disease. Now two vaccines are currently licensed in the United States (HAVRIX, SmithKline Beecham Biologicals, Philadelphia, PA, U.S.A.; and VAQTA, Merck & Company, Inc.). These vaccines contain inactivated HAV and are prepared in much the same way that inactivated polio vaccine virus vaccines are made. The highest rates of hepatitis A are among children 5 to 14 years of age; these children represent almost 30% of all cases (130). It is anticipated that HAV vaccines ultimately will be licensed for general use among children under 2 years of age, but dosing and immunogenicity in young children are incompletely defined. In the interim, a strategy to prevent and control hepatitis A has been developed that focuses on preexposure vaccination of the following persons: (a) those at increased risk for HAV infection or its consequences (e.g., travelers and persons who have chronic liver disease, intravenous drug users, men who have sex with men); (b) children living in communities that have high rates of hepatitis A to help prevent recurrent epidemics; and, if indicated, (c) children and young adults in communities that have intermediate rates of hepatitis A to help control ongoing and prevent future epidemics (130). Susceptible contacts of persons with hepatitis A should be administered postexposure prophylaxis (i.e., IG or, when appropriate, IG and hepatitis A vaccine [130]).

Immune globulin does not interfere with the immune response to oral poliovirus vaccine or, in general, to inactivated vaccines (including hepatitis A vaccine); however, it can interfere with the response to live, attenuated vaccines (e.g., measles, mumps, rubella, and varicella) when vaccines are administered either individually or as combination vaccines. Administration of these vaccines should be delayed for at least 5 months after administration of IG for hepatitis A prophylaxis, and IG should not be administered within 2 to 3 weeks after the administration of live, attenuated vaccines unless the benefits of IG administration exceed the benefits of vaccination (1).

Both licensed HAV vaccines are highly immunogenic in children over 2 years of age and in adults (131–134). Immunogenicity in infants is less clear, although studies to date that have included young children are encouraging (134,135). Infants with passively transferred maternal anti-HAV had a reduced anti-HAV GMT after vaccination (135). The efficacy of both vaccines has been demonstrated in children 1 to 16 years of age (136,137).

Efficacy of HAV vaccine in immunocompromised populations has not been demonstrated, but safety and immunogenicity have been demonstrated in patients with chronic liver disease and HIV infection (138,139). In men with HIV who responded to vaccine, mean CD4 counts were higher than in nonresponders (140). Nonresponders may fail to respond to booster doses (141). Recommendations do not yet encompass these populations, and no experience to date with hepatitis A vaccine in immunocompromised children has been published.

Hepatitis B

Two types of hepatitis B vaccines (Recombivax HB, Merck & Company, Inc.; Engerix-B, SmithKline Beecham Biologicals) made by recombinant DNA technology are now licensed in the United States for immunization against hepatitis B virus (HBV) infection. These vaccines contain only a portion of the outer protein of HBV or hepatitis B surface antigen (HBsAg). An earlier vaccine made from plasma containing HbsAg is no longer produced in the United States, but plasma-derived vaccines still are used in other countries. Because previous strategies targeting high-risk populations have failed to prevent the significant morbidity and mortality of HBV infection, universal immunization of infants and "catch-up" immunization of older children and adolescents is now recommended (142–144). The 5 μg/0.5 mL dose of Recombivax HB is now indicated for all vaccinees aged 0 to 19 years, regardless of the mother's HBsAg status. The change was made to simplify the dosing of Recombivax HB and to eliminate potential confusion when determining the correct dose of hepatitis B vaccine. A series of three doses is recommended for most children and adults, and vaccine can be safely administered to immunocompromised children. An immune globulin preparation (HBIG) is prepared from hyperimmunized donors with high titers of anti-HBsAg antibody. It provides temporary protection against hepatitis B and is used in conjunction with vaccine in infants born of HBsAg-positive mothers and in those with exposure to blood or body fluid associated with risk for acquisition of infection.

Vaccine has been shown to be 90% to 95% effective in preventing HBV infection in otherwise healthy susceptible children and adults (145–149). Unfortunately, vaccine is less reliably immunogenic in patients on hemodialysis or in those with immunocompromising conditions. Patients on hemodialysis often respond poorly to hepatitis B vaccine, and efficacy is reduced in adults on hemodialysis (150). Substantially higher doses of hepatitis B vaccine (40 μg/mL) are recommended for immunization of pediatric and adult dialysis patients, and specially formulated preparations are available for this purpose. Repeat serologic testing for immunity is not recommended after routine vaccination of infants, children, or adolescents. Testing for immunity is advised only for persons whose subsequent clinical management depends on knowledge of their immune status. For example, testing after immunoprophylaxis of infants born to HBsAg-positive mothers should be performed from 3 to 9 months after completion of the vaccination.

Response of patients with immunocompromising conditions is less well studied, but antibody responses are often reduced. Responses of children and adults undergoing chemotherapy for malignancy are often poor, but protective antibody levels are achieved in nearly 90% of children after chemotherapy

has been discontinued (151–153). Responses to hepatitis B vaccine prior to solid-organ transplantation are often better than after transplant, but the underlying cause of disease requiring transplantation may itself have adverse effects on antibody response (154–156). More than half of children vaccinated prior to liver transplantation for biliary atresia have protective levels of antibody 1 to 15 months after transplantation, but the durability of response and the relationship to the level of immunosuppression are incompletely explored (157).

Nearly half of HIV-infected adults demonstrate antibody responses below the level associated with protection after vaccination with hepatitis B vaccine (158). Antibody responses to hepatitis B vaccine are also poor in HIV-infected children (159–161). In infants immunized after birth to HIV-infected mothers, seroconversion occurred in 100% of 13 infants whose HIV antibody disappeared, compared with one of five HIV-infected children (162). Satisfactory responses to booster doses occurred in only 14% of HIV-infected children who failed to respond to primary immunization (160). Until additional data on responses to booster immunizations using more frequent or higher doses are available, specific recommendations are not available on advisability of booster doses for immunocompromised children (144,163).

Influenza Vaccine

Influenza vaccines currently contain three virus strains (influenza A strains H1N1 and H3N2 and influenza B). Several vaccines are available in the United States (Fluzone whole or split, Aventis Pasteur Inc.; Fluvirin purified surface antigen vaccine, Evans Medical Ltd., Leatherhead, Surrey, UK; Fluogen Split, Parkedale Pharmaceuticals, Inc., Bristol, TN, U.S.A.; Flushield Split, Wyeth-Lederle Vaccines). The vaccine antigens are changed yearly to reflect changes in circulating influenza viruses. The vaccine is made from highly purified egg-grown viruses that have been made noninfectious (inactivated). Although whole virus and purified detergent treated vaccine (split product) are available, split-product vaccines are recommended for children younger than 12 years of age because of their reduced reactogenicity (164). Two doses administered at least 1 month apart are recommended for children younger than 9 years of age who have not been vaccinated previously (164). In circumstances described subsequently herein, in which antibody responses to influenza vaccine are likely to be inadequate, use of rimantadine or amantadine prophylaxis may be considered an alternative for prevention of influenza A but not influenza B infection (165).

Influenza vaccine is licensed and approved for use in persons aged 6 months and older. It is targeted primarily for patients whose underlying conditions place them at risk for severe influenza infection, primarily children with cardiopulmonary disease; however, influenza has been associated with severe disease in children and adults with immunocompromising conditions including BMT and solid-organ transplants (166,167). It is clear that shedding of influenza virus can be prolonged in immunodeficient children; shedding of amantadine-resistant virus for prolonged periods may occur in children with leukemia and severe combined immunodeficiency, as identified by the polymerase chain reaction (168). Sustained virus shedding may have implications for the spread of drug-resistant influenza to susceptible persons in a family or hospital setting. The efficacy of influenza vaccine in immunocompromised children has not been established by clinical trials, but safety and immmuogenicity studies have been performed and efficacy has been inferred from these results of these investigations. Hence, inactivated influenza vaccine is recommended for children with underlying immunocompromise (164).

The safety of these vaccines has been demonstrated in transplant patients because of concern that influenza vaccines might promote rejection; a controlled trial in a small population of heart-transplant patients showed no increase in biopsy evidence of rejection after two doses of influenza vaccine compared with placebo recipients (169). Influenza immunization in children with HIV infection has not been associated with significant increases in viral load (170), but temporary increases in virus load have been noted occasionally in adults (171,172).

Poor immunogenicity after yearly dosing has been observed in some solid-organ transplant patients (173), but responses in a small number of renal transplant recipients have been satisfactory, and one study demonstrated good antibody responses in pediatric solid-organ transplants who had preexisting antibody (174,175). Two doses have been boosted successfully by a third dose of vaccine in one trial of heart-transplant recipients (176), but additional doses have not always been reported to be beneficial in transplant populations (173).

Immunogenicity of vaccine varies with the level of immunodeficiency. In children with leukemia, up to 68% of previously vaccinated children and 100% of previously unvaccinated children have been observed to develop antibody levels (≥1:40) associated with protection against influenza. Prior experience with the swine influenza vaccine in hematologic and solid tumor cancer patients indicated that responses were diminished during active chemotherapy but were comparable to controls as soon as 30 days after completing chemotherapy (177).

As with other vaccine antigens, the adequacy of antibody responses to influenza antigens after inactivated vaccine in HIV-infected patients reflects the stage of disease; antibody responses of seroconverters approach those of healthy controls, but patients with AIDS have a significantly reduced likelihood of protective response (178). In adults, CD4 count has been a stronger predictor of antibody response than was HIV

RNA level (172). Correlation of responses in children is more closely associated with clinical status than CD4 count; children with clinically defined AIDS have the lowest responses (179). Prolonged use of high-dose steroids (e.g., ≥2 mg/kg or 20 mg/day as used in persons with rheumatologic disease) may have a deleterious effect on response to influenza vaccines (180), but pulse steroid therapy as used in children for the treatment of asthma exacerbations does not appear to blunt response (181,182). Hence brief or intermittent use of high-dose steroids, particularly in children with asthma who are at increased risk for influenza complications, does not necessitate deferring administration of influenza vaccine (165).

FUTURE VACCINES

Although significant advances have been made in our ability to protect children from severe disease by use of vaccines, challenges remain. Currently, work is proceeding on a number of fronts: development of live and subunit vaccines for respiratory syncytial virus (RSV), influenza virus, parainfluenza virus, and cytomegalovirus; further development of protein-conjugated vaccines or vaccines against other surface antigens of pneumococcus and meningococcus; exploration of subunit vaccines against tuberculosis; use of new adjuvants and novel delivery schemes to boost the immunogenicity of vaccine antigens; use of DNA vaccines to promote cell-associated antigen presentation and cell-mediated immune response; reassortant and recombinant technologies to provide novel ways for attenuating live vaccines, presenting immunogenic epitopes, or coproducing cytokines to direct immune response (183,184).

Many of these vaccines may have application in healthy and immunocompromised patients. For example, live attenuated influenza vaccines have shown 85% or greater efficacy in protecting young children from influenza illness (185) and may prove sufficiently atten-

uated for some immunocompromised populations. The young infant is the primary target for routine administration of a protective vaccine against RSV disease. Live attenuated RSV vaccines are beginning to show promise of safety and immunogenicity in young infants, and purified RSV fusion protein vaccines have demonstrated protection against RSV in a limited number of patients with cystic fibrosis (186,187). Recent trials of antibody preparations containing high titers of polyclonal or monoclonal antibody to RSV have demonstrated prophylactic but not therapeutic efficacy against RSV disease in at-risk infants (188–190). BMT patients also represent an important target group to consider for immunization because they are at risk for severe or fatal RSV infection; whether active immunization or passive antibody is best suited for providing protection in such high-risk populations remains to be determined. An experimental heptavalent conjugated pneumococcal vaccine was shown to prime successfully for polysaccharide vaccine 1 year later in Hodgkin's disease patients. The attenuated Towne strain of cytomegalovirus has shown promise in renal transplant patients and healthy women in producing humoral and cell-mediated immune response (191,192).

CONCLUSIONS

The success of intervention strategies against chronic diseases, malignancies, and HIV infections can be expected to increase steadily the ranks of children with immunocompromising conditions whose responses to vaccines will pose challenges. Live vaccines can pose special risks. Live poliovirus vaccine is contraindicated in all immunocompromising conditions. Live measles and varicella may have specific indications in some immunodeficient persons, but caution should be exercised in their use. Future live virus vaccines against respiratory viruses may see use in compromised persons if they are sufficiently attenuated. Passively administered specific monoclonal antibody may prove effective, although expensive, prophylaxis for RSV and other pathogens.

Inactivated vaccines generally can be regarded as safe in immunocompromised individuals, but immunogenicity and the potential for protection vary with the condition and severity of disease. Immunization appears to succeed best when vaccines can be administered prior to anticipated immunocompromise or after immunosuppression has ended. Booster doses of vaccine may be indicated in some circumstances where failure of response occurs. The advent of conjugated and adjuvanted vaccines may circumvent some of the shortcomings of currently available agents. In addition to strategies directed specifically at the immunocompromised patient, it should be remembered that household exposure to vaccine-preventable diseases poses a risk. Strategies that encourage immunization of susceptible household contacts against *H. influenzae* type B, measles, polio (IPV only!), and varicella may compensate partially for poor response to vaccines in the immunodeficient child. The advances of the past decade herald future success.

REFERENCES

1. ACIP. Recommendations of the Advisory Committee on Immunization Practices (ACIP): use of vaccines and immune globulins for persons with altered immunocompetence. *MMWR Morb Mortal Wkly Rep* 1993;42:1–18.
2. Khalak R, Pichichero ME, D'Angio CT. Three-year follow-up of vaccine response in extremely preterm infants. *Pediatrics* 1998;101:597–603.
3. Armstrong GL, Conn LA, Pinner RW. Trends in infectious disease mortality in the United States during the 20th century. *JAMA* 1999;281:61–66.
4. Pirofski LA, Casadevall A. Use of licensed vaccines for active immunization of the immunocompromised host. *Clin Microbiol Rev* 1998;11:1–26.
5. Watson JC, Hadler SC, Dykewicz CA, et al. Measles, mumps, and rubella—vaccine use and strategies for elimination of measles, rubella, and congenital rubella syndrome and control of mumps: recommendations of the Advisory Committee on Immunization Practices (ACIP). *MMWR Morb Mortal Wkly Rep* 1998;47:1–57.
6. Breitfeld V, Hashida Y, Sherman FE, et al. Fatal measles infection in children with leukemia. *Lab Invest* 1973;28:279–291.
7. Kaplan LJ, Daum RS, Smaron M, et al. Severe measles in immunocompromised patients. *JAMA* 1992;267:1237–1241.
8. Mitus A, Holoway A, Evans AE, et al. Attenuated measles vaccine in children with acute leukemia. *Am J Dis Child* 1962;103:242–248.
9. Monafo WJ, Haslam DB, Roberts RL, et al. Disseminated measles infection after vaccination in a child with a congenital immunodeficiency. *J Pediatr* 1994;124:273–276.
10. Torigoe S, Hirai S, Oitani K, et al. Application of live attenuated measles and mumps vaccines in children with acute leukemia. *Biken Journal* 1981;24:147–151.
11. Ljungman P, Fridell E, Lonnqvist B, et al. Efficacy and safety of vaccination of marrow transplant recipients with a live attenuated measles, mumps, and rubella vaccine. *J Infect Dis* 1989;159:610–615.
12. Hisano S, Miyazaki C, Hatae K, et al. Immune status of children on continuous ambulatory peritoneal dialysis. *Pediatr Nephrol* 1992;6:179–181.
13. Schulman SL, Deforest A, Kaiser BA, et al. Response to measles-mumps-rubella vaccine in children on dialysis. *Pediatr Nephrol* 1992;6:187–189.
14. King SM, Saunders EF, Petric M, et al. Response to measles, mumps and rubella vaccine in paediatric bone marrow transplant recipients. *Bone Marrow Transplant* 1996;17:633–636.
15. Pauksen K, Linde A, Lonnerholm G, et al. Influence of the specific T cell response on seroconversion after measles vaccination in autologous bone marrow transplant patients. *Bone Marrow Transplant* 1996;18:969–973.
16. McLaughlin M, Thomas P, Onorato I, et al. Live virus vaccines in human immunodeficiency virus-infected children: a retrospective survey. *Pediatrics* 1988;82:229–233.
17. Cutts FT, Mandala K, St Louis M, et al. Immunogenicity of high-titer Edmonston-Zagreb measles vaccine in human immunodeficiency virus-infected children in Kinshasa, Zaire. *J Infect Dis* 1993;167:1418–1421.
18. Lepage P, Dabis F, Msellati P, et al. Safety and immunogenicity of high-dose Edmonston-Zagreb measles vaccine in children with HIV-1 infection. A cohort study in Kigali, Rwanda. *Am J Dis Child* 1992;146:550–555.
19. Frenkel LM, Nielsen K, Garakian A, et al. A search for persistent measles, mumps, and rubella vaccine virus in children with human immunodeficiency virus type 1 infection. *Arch Pediatr Adolesc Med* 1994;148:57–60.
20. Measles pneumonitis following measles-mumps-rubella vaccination of a patient with HIV infection, 1993. *MMWR Morb Mortal Wkly Rep* 1996;45:603–606.
21. Arpadi SM, Markowitz LE, Baughman AL, et al. Measles antibody in vaccinated human immunodeficiency virus type 1-infected children. *Pediatrics* 1996;97:653–657.
22. Markowitz LE, Katz SL. Measles vaccine. In: Plotkin S, Morimer, eds. *Vaccines.* Philadelphia: WB Saunders, 1994:252–253.
23. Siber GR, Werner BG, Halsey NA, et al. Interference of immune globulin with measles and rubella immunization. *J Pediatr* 1993;122:204–211.

24. McBean AM, Thoms ML, Albrecht P, et al. Serologic response to oral polio vaccine and enhanced-potency inactivated polio vaccines. *Am J Epidemiol* 1988;128: 615–628.

25. Modlin JF, Halsey NA, Thoms ML, et al. Humoral and mucosal immunity in infants induced by three sequential inactivated poliovirus vaccine-live attenuated oral poliovirus vaccine immunization schedules. Baltimore Area Polio Vaccine Study Group. *J Infect Dis* 1997; 175(Suppl 1):S228–S234.

26. Hull HF, Ward NA. Progress towards the global eradication of poliomyelitis. *World Health Stat Q* 1992; 45:280–284.

27. Poliovirus infections. In: Pickering LK, ed. *Red book 2000: report of the Committee on Infectious Diseases*, 25th ed. Elk Grove Village, IL: American Academy of Pediatrics, 2000:468.

28. Sutter RW, Prevots DR. Vaccine-associated paralytic poliomyelitis among immunodeficient persons. *Infect Med* 1994;11:426,429–430,435–438.

29. Chang TW, Weinstein L, MacMahon HE. Paralytic poliomyelitis in a child with hypogammaglobulinemia: probable implication of type I vaccine strain. *Pediatrics* 1966;37:630–636.

30. Feigin RD, Guggenheim MA, Johnsen SD. Vaccine-related paralytic poliomyelitis in an immunodeficient child. *J Pediatr* 1971;79:642–647.

31. Lopez C, Biggar WD, Park BH, et al. Nonparalytic poliovirus infections in patients with severe combined immunodeficiency disease. *J Pediatr* 1974;84:497–502.

32. Saulsbury FT, Winkelstein JA, Davis LE, et al. Combined immunodeficiency and vaccine-related poliomyelitis in a child with cartilage-hair hypoplasia. *J Pediatr* 1975;86:868–872.

33. Davis LE, Bodian D, Price D, et al. Chronic progressive poliomyelitis secondary to vaccination of an immunodeficient child. *N Engl J Med* 1977;297:241–245.

34. Wright PF, Hatch MH, Kasselberg AG, et al. Vaccine-associated poliomyelitis in a child with sex-linked agammaglobulinemia. *J Pediatr* 1977;91:408–412.

35. Gaebler JW, Kleiman MB, French ML, et al. Neurologic complications in oral polio vaccine recipients. *J Pediatr* 1986;108:878–881.

36. ACIP. Poliomyelitis prevention in the United States: introduction of a sequential vaccination schedule of inactivated poliovirus vaccine followed by oral poliovirus vaccine. Recommendations of the Advisory Committee on Immunization Practices (ACIP) *MMWR Morb Mortal Wkly Rep* 1997;46:1–25.[Published erratum appears in *MMWR Morb Mortal Wkly Rep* 1997;46:183.]

37. Kew OM, Sutter RW, Nottay BK, et al. Prolonged replication of a type 1 vaccine-derived poliovirus in an immunodeficient patient. *J Clin Microbiol* 1998;36: 2893–2899.

38. Barbi M, Biffi MR, Binda S, et al. Immunization in children with HIV seropositivity at birth: antibody response to polio vaccine and tetanus toxoid. *AIDS* 1992;6:1465–1469.

39. American Academy of Pediatrics Committee on Infectious Diseases. Recommendations for the use of live attenuated varicella vaccine. *Pediatrics* 1995;95: 791–796. [Published erratum appears in *Pediatrics* 1995;96(1 Pt 1):preceding 151 and following 171.]

40. Takahashi M, Kamiya H, Baba K, et al. Clinical experience with Oka live varicella vaccine in Japan. *Postgrad Med J* 1985;61:61–67.

41. Kuter BJ, Weibel RE, Guess HA, et al. Oka/Merck varicella vaccine in healthy children: final report of a 2-year efficacy study and 7-year follow-up studies. *Vaccine* 1991;9:643–647.

42. ACIP. Prevention of varicella: recommendations of the Advisory Committee on Immunization Practices (ACIP). Centers for Disease Control and Prevention. *MMWR Morb Mortal Wkly Rep* 1996;45:1–36.

43. Gershon AA, Steinberg SP, Gelb L, et al. Live attenuated varicella vaccine: efficacy for children with leukemia in remission. *JAMA* 1984;252:355–362.

44. Tsolia M, Gershon AA, Steinberg SP, et al. Live attenuated varicella vaccine: evidence that the virus is attenuated and the importance of skin lesions in transmission of varicella-zoster virus: National Institute of Allergy and Infectious Diseases Varicella Vaccine Collaborative Study Group. *J Pediatr* 1990;116: 184–189.

45. Weibel RE, Neff BJ, Kuter BJ, et al. Live attenuated varicella virus vaccine: Efficacy trial in healthy children. *N Engl J Med* 1984;310:1409–1415.

46. Varicella-Zoster infections. In: Pickering LK, ed. *Red book 2000: report of the Committee on Infectious Diseases*, 25th ed. Elk Grove Village, IL: American Academy of Pediatrics, 2000:636.

47. Brunell PA, Shehab Z, Geiser C, et al. Administration of live varicella vaccine to children wtih leukaemia. *Lancet* 1982;2:1069–1073.

48. Brunell PA, Geiser CF, Novelli V, et al. Varicella-like illness caused by live varicella vaccine in children with acute lymphocytic leukemia. *Pediatrics* 1987;79: 922–927.

49. Gershon AA, Steinberg SP. Persistence of immunity to varicella in children with leukemia immunized with live attenuated varicella vaccine. *N Engl J Med* 1989; 320:892–897.

50. Gershon AA, Steinberg S, Gelb L, et al. A multicentre trial of live attenuated varicella vaccine in children with leukaemia in remission. *Postgrad Med J* 1985; 61:73–78.

51. Arbeter AM, Granowetter L, Starr SE, et al. Immunization of children with acute lymphoblastic leukemia with live attenuated varicella vaccine without complete suspension of chemotherapy. *Pediatrics* 1990;85:338–44.

52. Redman RL, Nader S, Zerboni L, et al. Early reconstitution of immunity and decreased severity of herpes zoster in bone marrow transplant recipients immunized with inactivated varicella vaccine. *J Infect Dis* 1997;176:578–585.

53. Lydick E, Kuter BJ, Zajac BA, et al. Association of steroid therapy with vaccine-associated rashes in children with acute lymphocytic leukaemia who received Oka/Merck varicella vaccine. NIAID Varicella Vaccine Collaborative Study Group. *Vaccine* 1989;7: 549–553.

54. Fivush BA, Neu AM. Immunization guidelines for pediatric renal disease [Review]. *Semin Nephrol* 1998; 18:256–263.

55. Gershon AA, LaRussa P, Steinberg S, et al. The protective effect of immunologic boosting against zoster:

an analysis in leukemic children who were vaccinated against chickenpox. *J Infect Dis* 1996;173:450–453.

56. ACIP issues recommendations on the prevention of varicella. *Am Fam Physician* 1996;54:2578, 2581.

57. CDC issues recommendations on the role of BCG vaccine in the prevention and control of tuberculosis. *Am Fam Physician* 1996;54:1115–1118.

58. O'Brien KL, Ruff AJ, Louis MA, et al. Bacillus Calmette-Guerin complications in children born to HIV-1-infected women with a review of the literature. *Pediatrics* 1995;95:414–418.

59. Jacob CM, Pastorino AC, Azevedo AM, et al. *Mycobacterium bovis* dissemination (BCG strain) among immunodeficient Brazilian infants. *J Investig Allergol Clin Immunol* 1996;6:202–206.

60. Ryder RW, Oxtoby MJ, Mvula M, et al. Safety and immunogenicity of bacille Calmette-Guerin, diphtheria-tetanus-pertussis, and oral polio vaccines in newborn children in Zaire infected with human immunodeficiency virus type 1. *J Pediatr* 1993;122:697–702.

61. Altare F, Jouanguy E, Lamhamedi S, et al. Mendelian susceptibility to mycobacterial infection in man. *Curr Opin Immunol* 1998;10:413–417.

62. Stanley S, Ostrowski MA, Justement JS, et al. Effect of immunization with a common recall antigen on viral expression in patients infected with human immunodeficiency virus type 1. *N Engl J Med* 1996;334:1222–1230.

63. Ostrowski MA, Krakauer DC, Li Y, et al. Effect of immune activation on the dynamics of human immunodeficiency virus replication and on the distribution of viral quasispecies. *J Virol* 1998;72:7772–7784.

64. Girndt M, Pietsch M, Kohler H. Tetanus immunization and its association to hepatitis B vaccination in patients with chronic renal failure. *Am J Kidney Dis* 1995;26:454–460.

65. ACIP. Human rabies prevention, United States—1999: recommendations of the Advisory Committee on Immunization Practices (ACIP). *MMWR Morb Mortal Wkly Rep* 1999;48:1–24.

66. Lyme disease. In: Pickering LK, ed. *Red book 2000: report of the Committee on Infectious Diseases*, 25th ed. Elk Grove Village, IL: American Academy of Pediatrics, 2000:379.

67. ACIP. Pertussis vaccination: use of acellular pertussis vaccines among infants and young children: recommendations of the Advisory Committee on Immunization Practices (ACIP) *MMWR Morb Mortal Wkly Rep* 1997;46:1–25. [Published erratum appears in *MMWR Morb Mortal Wkly Rep* 1997;46:706.]

68. Decker MD, Edwards KM, Steinhoff MC, et al. Comparison of 13 acellular pertussis vaccines: adverse reactions. *Pediatrics* 1995;96:557–566.

69. Edwards KM, Meade BD, Decker MD, et al. Comparison of 13 acellular pertussis vaccines: overview and serologic response. *Pediatrics* 1995;96:548–557.

70. Edwards KM, Decker MD. Comparison of serological results in the NIAID Multicenter Acellular Pertussis Trial with recent efficacy trials. *Dev Biol Stand* 1997;89:265–273.

71. American Academy of Pediatrics Committee on Infectious Diseases. Acellular pertussis vaccine: recommendations for use as the initial series in infants and children. *Pediatrics* 1997;99:282-288.

72. Orgel HA, Hamburger RN, Mendelson LM, et al. An-

tibody responses in normal infants and in infants receiving chemotherapy for congenital neuroblastoma. *Cancer* 1977;40:994-997.

73. Kung FH, Orgel HA, Wallace WW, et al. Antibody production following immunization with diphtheria and tetanus toxoids in children receiving chemotherapy during remission of malignant disease. *Pediatrics* 1984;74:86–89.

74. Ambrosino DM, Molrine DC. Critical appraisal of immunization strategies for prevention of infection in the compromised host. *Hematol Oncol Clin North Am* 1993;7:1027–1050.

75. Ghio L, Pedrazzi C, Assael BM, et al. Immunity to diphtheria and tetanus in a young population on a dialysis regimen or with a renal transplant [see comments]. *J Pediatr* 1997;130:987–989.

76. Enke BU, Bokenkamp A, Offner G, et al. Response to diphtheria and tetanus booster vaccination in pediatric renal transplant recipients. *Transplantation* 1997;64:237–241.

77. Vance E, George S, Guinan EC, et al. Comparison of multiple immunization schedules for *Haemophilus influenzae* type b-conjugate and tetanus toxoid vaccines following bone marrow transplantation [In Process Citation]. *Bone Marrow Transplant* 1998;22:735–41.

78. Ljungman P, Wiklund-Hammarsten M, Duraj V, et al. Response to tetanus toxoid immunization after allogeneic bone marrow transplantation. *J Infect Dis* 1990;162:496–500.

79. Vance E, George S, Guinan EC, et al. Comparison of multiple immunization schedules for *Haemophilus influenzae* type b-conjugate and tetanus toxoid vaccines following bone marrow transplantation. *Bone Marrow Transplant* 1998;22:735–741.

80. Kroon FP, van Dissel JT, Labadie J, et al. Antibody response to diphtheria, tetanus, and poliomyelitis vaccines in relation to the number of CD4+ T lymphocytes in adults infected with human immunodeficiency virus. *Clin Infect Dis* 1995;21:1197–1203.

81. Kroon FP, Van Furth R, Bruisten SM. The effects of immunization in human immunodeficiency virus type 1 infection [Letter; Comment]. *N Engl J Med* 1996;335:817–819.

82. Opravil M, Fierz W, Matter L, et al. Poor antibody response after tetanus and pneumococcal vaccination in immunocompromised, HIV-infected patients. *Clin Exp Immunol* 1991;84:185–189.

83. de Martino M, Podda A, Galli L, et al. Acellular pertussis vaccine in children with perinatal human immunodeficiency virus-type 1 infection. *Vaccine* 1997;15:1235–1238.

84. Peltola H, Kayhty H, Virtanen M, et al. Prevention of *Hemophilus influenzae* type b bacteremic infections with the capsular polysaccharide vaccine. *N Engl J Med* 1984;310:1561–1566.

85. Kayhty H, Peltola H, Karanko V, et al. The protective level of serum antibodies to the capsular polysaccharide of *Haemophilus influenzae* type b. *J Infect Dis* 1983;147:1100.

86. Edwards KM, Decker MD. Combination vaccines consisting of acellular pertussis vaccines. *Pediatr Infect Dis J* 1997;16:S97–S102.

87. Unlicensed use of combination of *Haemophilus influenzae* type b conjugate vaccine and diphtheria and

tetanus toxoid and acellular pertussis vaccine for infant. *MMWR Morb Mortal Wkly Rep* 1998;47:787.

88. Frank AL, Labotka RJ, Rao S, et al. *Haemophilus influenzae* type b immunization of children with sickle cell diseases. *Pediatrics* 1988;82:571–575.

89. Feldman S, Gigliotti F, Shenep JL, et al. Risk of *Haemophilus influenzae* type b disease in children with cancer and response of immunocompromised leukemic children to a conjugate vaccine. *J Infect Dis* 1990;161:926–931.

90. Kroon FP, van Dissel JT, Rijkers GT, et al. Antibody response to *Haemophilus influenzae* type b vaccine in relation to the number of CD4+ T lymphocytes in adults infected with human immunodeficiency virus. *Clin Infect Dis* 1997;25:600–606.

91. Molrine DC, Siber GR, Samra Y, et al. Normal IgG and impaired IgM responses to polysaccharide vaccines in asplenic patients. *J Infect Dis* 1999;179:513–517.

92. *Haemophilus Influenza* infections. In: Peter G, ed. *1997 Red book:* report of the Committee on Infectious Diseases. Vol. 24. Elk Grove Village, IL: American Academy of Pediatrics, 1997:229.

93. Jakacki R, Luery N, McVerry P, Lange B. *Haemophilus influenzae* diphtheria protein conjugate immunization after therapy in splenectomized patients with Hodgkin disease. *Ann Intern Med* 1990;112: 143–144.

94. Guinan EC, Molrine DC, Antin JH, et al. Polysaccharide conjugate vaccine responses in bone marrow transplant patients. *Transplantation* 1994;57:677–684.

95. Barra A, Cordonnier C, Preziosi MP, et al. Immunogenicity of Haemophilus influenzae type b conjugate vaccine in allogeneic bone marrow recipients. *J Infect Dis* 1992;166:1021–1028.

96. Molrine DC, Guinan EC, Antin JH, et al. *Haemophilus influenzae* type b (HIB)-conjugate immunization before bone marrow harvest in autologous bone marrow transplantation. *Bone Marrow Transplant* 1996;17: 1149–1155.

97. Molrine DC, Guinan EC, Antin JH, et al. Donor immunization with *Haemophilus influenzae* type b (HIB)-conjugate vaccine in allogeneic bone marrow transplantation. *Blood* 1996;87:3012–3018.

98. Weiss PJ, Wallace MR, Oldfield EC III, et al. Response of recent human immunodeficiency virus seroconverters to the pneumococcal polysaccharide vaccine and *Haemophilus influenzae* type b conjugate vaccine. *J Infect Dis* 1995;171:1217–1222.

99. Read JS, Frasch CE, Rich K, et al. The immunogenicity of *Haemophilus influenzae* type b conjugate vaccines in children born to human immunodeficiency virus-infected women. Women and Infants Transmission Study Group. *Pediatr Infect Dis J* 1998;17: 391–397.

100. Gibb D, Giacomelli A, Masters J, et al. Persistence of antibody responses to Haemophilus influenzae type b polysaccharide conjugate vaccine in children with vertically acquired human immunodeficiency virus infection. *Pediatr Infect Dis J* 1996;15:1097–1101.

101. Shackelford PG, Granoff DM, Polmar SH, et al. Subnormal serum concentrations of IgG2 in children with frequent infections associated with varied patterns of immunologic dysfunction. *J Pediatr* 1990;116: 529–538.

102. Surveillance for diabetes mellitus—United States, 1980–1989, and laboratory-based surveillance for meningococcal disease in selected areas—United States, 1989–1991. *MMWR Morb Mortal Wkly Rep* 1993;42:21–30.

103. Peltola H, Kayhty H, Kuronen T, et al. Meningococcus group A vaccine in children three months to five years of age: adverse reactions and immunogenicity related to endotoxin content and molecular weight of the polysaccharide. *J Pediatr* 1978;92:818–822.

104. Gold R, Lepow ML, Goldschneider I, et al. Kinetics of antibody production to group A and group C meningococcal polysaccharide vaccines administered during the first six years of life: prospects for routine immunization of infants and children. *J Infect Dis* 1979;140: 690–697.

105. ACIP. Control and prevention of meningococcal disease: recommendations of the Advisory Committee on Immunization Practices (ACIP). *MMWR Morb Mortal Wkly Rep* 1997;46:1–10.

106. Francke EL, Neu HC. Postsplenectomy infection. *Surg Clin North Am* 1981;61:135–155.

107. Figueroa JE, Densen P. Infectious diseases associated with complement deficiencies. *Clin Microbiol Rev* 1991;4:359–395.

108. Stephens DS, Hajjeh RA, Baughman WS, et al. Sporadic meningococcal disease in adults: results of a 5-year population-based study. *Ann Intern Med* 1995;123:937–940.

109. Ruben FL, Hankins WA, Zeigler Z, et al. Antibody responses to meningococcal polysaccharide vaccine in adults without a spleen. *Am J Med* 1984;76:115–121.

110. Siber GR, Gorham C, Martin P, et al. Antibody response to pretreatment immunization and post-treatment boosting with bacterial polysaccharide vaccines in patients with Hodgkin's disease. *Ann Intern Med* 1986;104:467–475.

111. Rautonen J, Siimes MA, Lundstrom U, et al. Vaccination of children during treatment for leukemia. *Acta Paediatr Scand* 1986;75:579–585.

112. Quinti I, Velardi A, Le Moli S, et al. Antibacterial polysaccharide antibody deficiency after allogeneic bone marrow transplantation. *J Clin Immunol* 1990; 10:160–166.

113. Rhoads JL, Birx DL, Wright DC, et al. Safety and immunogenicity of multiple conventional immunizations administered during early HIV infection. *J Acquir Immune Defic Syndr Hum Retrovirol* 1991;4:724–731.

114. Musher DM, Luchi MJ, Watson DA, et al. Pneumococcal polysaccharide vaccine in young adults and older bronchitics: determination of IgG responses by ELISA and the effect of adsorption of serum with nontype-specific cell wall polysaccharide. *J Infect Dis* 1990;161:728–735.

115. Koskela M, Leinonen M, Haiva VM, et al. First and second dose antibody responses to pneumococcal polysaccharide vaccine in infants. *Pediatr Infect Dis* 1986;5:45–50.

116. Leinonen M, Sakkinen A, Kalliokoski R, et al. Antibody response to 14-valent pneumococcal capsular polysaccharide vaccine in pre-school age children. *Pediatr Infect Dis* 1986;5:39–44.

117. ACIP. Prevention of pneumococcal disease: recommendations of the Advisory Committee on Immuniza-

tion Practices (ACIP). *MMWR Morb Mortal Wkly Rep* 1997;46:1–24.

118. Jackson LA, Benson P, Sneller VP, et al. Safety of re-vaccination with pneumococcal polysaccharide vaccine. *JAMA* 1999;281:243–248.

119. Wong WY, Overturf GD, Powars DR. Infection caused by *Streptococcus pneumoniae* in children with sickle cell disease: epidemiology, immunologic mechanisms, prophylaxis, and vaccination. *Clin Infect Dis* 1992;14:1124–1136.

120. Weintrub PS, Schiffman G, Addiego JE Jr, et al. Long-term follow-up and booster immunization with poly-valent pneumococcal polysaccharide in patients with sickle cell anemia. *J Pediatr* 1984;105:261–263.

121. Spika JS, Halsey NA, Le CT, et al. Decline of vaccine-induced antipneumococcal antibody in children with nephrotic syndrome. *Am J Kidney Dis* 1986;7:466–470.

122. Giebink GS, Le CT, Schiffman G. Decline of serum antibody in splenectomized children after vaccination with pneumococcal capsular polysaccharides. *J Pediatr* 1984;105:576–582.

123. Winston DJ, Ho WG, Schiffman G, et al. Pneumococcal vaccination of recipients of bone marrow trans-plants. *Arch Intern Med* 1983;143:1735–1737.

124. Keller DW, Breiman RF. Preventing bacterial respiratory tract infections among persons infected with human immunodeficiency virus. *Clin Infect Dis* 1995;21 (Suppl 1):S77–S83.

125. Katzenstein TL, Gerstoft J, Nielsen H. Assessments of plasma HIV RNA and CD4 cell counts after combined Pneumovax and tetanus toxoid vaccination: no detectable increase in HIV replication 6 weeks after immunization. *Scand J Infect Dis* 1996;28:239–241.

126. Brichacek B, Swindells S, Janoff EN, et al. Increased plasma human immunodeficiency virus type 1 burden following antigenic challenge with pneumococcal vaccine. *J Infect Dis* 1996;174:1191–1199.

127. Gibb D, Spoulou V, Giacomelli A, et al. Antibody responses to *Haemophilus influenzae* type b and *Streptococcus pneumoniae* vaccines in children with human immunodeficiency virus infection. *Pediatr Infect Dis J* 1995;14:129–135.

128. Mofenson LM, Moye J Jr, Bethel J, et al. Prophylactic intravenous immunoglobulin in HIV-infected children with CD4+ counts of $0.20 \times 10(9)/L$ or more: effect on viral, opportunistic, and bacterial infections. The National Institute of Child Health and Human Development Intravenous Immunoglobulin Clinical Trial Study Group. *JAMA* 1992;268:483–488.

129. Black S, Shinefield H, Fireman B, et al. Efficacy, safety, and immunogenicity of heptavalent pneumococcal conjugate vaccine in children. *Pediatr Infect Dis J* 2000;19:187–195.

130. American Academy of Pediatrics Committee on Infectious Diseases. Prevention of hepatitis A infections: guidelines for use of hepatitis A vaccine and immune globulin. *Pediatrics* 1996;98:1207–1215.

131. Clemens R, Safary A, Hepburn A, et al. Clinical experience with an inactivated hepatitis A vaccine. *J Infect Dis* 1995;171(Suppl 1):S44–S49.

132. McMahon BJ, Williams J, Bulkow L, et al. Immunogenicity of an inactivated hepatitis A vaccine in Alaska Native children and Native and non-Native adults. *J Infect Dis* 1995;171:676–679.

133. Balcarek KB, Bagley MR, Pass RF, et al. Safety and immunogenicity of an inactivated hepatitis A vaccine in preschool children. *J Infect Dis* 1995;171(Suppl 1):S70–S72.

134. Horng YC, Chang MH, Lee CY, et al. Safety and immunogenicity of hepatitis A vaccine in healthy children. *Pediatr Infect Dis J* 1993;12:359–362.

135. Effect of maternal antibody on immunogenicity of hepatitis A vaccine in infants. Presented at: *Interscience Conference on Antimicrobial Agents and Chemotherapy (ICAAC)*. American Society for Microbiology, 1995:190(abst H61).

136. Werzberger A, Mensch B, Kuter B, et al. A controlled trial of a formalin-inactivated hepatitis A vaccine in healthy children. *N Engl J Med* 1992;327:453–457.

137. Innis BL, Snitbhan R, Kunasol P, et al. Protection against hepatitis A by an inactivated vaccine. *JAMA* 1994;271:1328–1334.

138. Keeffe EB, Iwarson S, McMahon BJ, et al. Safety and immunogenicity of hepatitis A vaccine in patients with chronic liver disease [see comments]. *Hepatology* 1998;27:881–886.

139. Bodsworth NJ, Neilsen GA, Donovan B. The effect of immunization with inactivated hepatitis A vaccine on the clinical course of HIV-1 infection: 1-year follow-up. *AIDS* 1997;11:747–749.

140. Neilsen GA, Bodsworth NJ, Watts N. Response to hepatitis A vaccination in human immunodeficiency virus- infected and -uninfected homosexual men. *J Infect Dis* 1997;176:1064-1067.

141. Tilzey AJ, Palmer SJ, Harrington C, et al. Hepatitis A vaccine responses in HIV-positive persons with haemophilia. *Vaccine* 1996;14:1039–1041.

142. Immunization of adolescents: recommendations of the Advisory Committee on Immunization Practices, the American Academy of Pediatrics, the American Academy of Family Physicians, and the American Medical Association. *MMWR Morb Mortal Wkly Rep* 1996;45:1–16.

143. Halsey NA. Discussion of Immunization Practices Advisory Committee/American Academy of Pediatrics recommendations for universal infant hepatitis B vaccination. *Pediatr Infect Dis J* 1993;12:446–449.

144. Hepatitis B virus: a comprehensive strategy for eliminating transmission in the United States through universal childhood vaccination: recommendations of the Immunization Practices Advisory Committee (ACIP). *MMWR Morb Mortal Wkly Rep* 1991;40:1–25.

145. Andre FE. Summary of safety and efficacy data on a yeast-derived hepatitis B vaccine. *Am J Med* 1989;87:14S–20S.

146. Szmuness W, Stevens CE, Harley EJ, et al. Hepatitis B vaccine: demonstration of efficacy in a controlled clinical trial in a high-risk population in the United States. *N Engl J Med* 1980;303:833–41.

147. Zajac BA, West DJ, McAleer WJ, et al. Overview of clinical studies with hepatitis B vaccine made by recombinant DNA. *J Infect* 1986;13(Suppl A):39–45.

148. Stevens CE, Taylor PE, Tong MJ, et al. Yeast-recombinant hepatitis B vaccine: efficacy with hepatitis B im-

mune globulin in prevention of perinatal hepatitis B virus transmission. *JAMA* 1987;257:2612–2616.

149. Hilleman MR. Yeast recombinant hepatitis B vaccine. *Infection* 1987;15:3–7.

150. Stevens CE, Alter HJ, Taylor PE, et al. Hepatitis B vaccine in patients receiving hemodialysis. Immunogenicity and efficacy. *N Engl J Med* 1984;311:496–501.

151. Ridgway D, Wolff LJ. Active immunization of children with leukemia and other malignancies. *Leuk Lymphoma* 1993;9:177–192.

152. Goyal S, Pai SK, Kelkar R, et al. Hepatitis B vaccination in acute lymphoblastic leukemia. *Leuk Res* 1998; 22:193–195.

153. Rokicka-Milewska R, Jackowska T, Sopylo B, et al. Active immunization of children with leukemias and lymphomas against infection by hepatitis B virus. *Acta Paediatr Jpn* 1993;35:400–403.

154. Jacobson IM, Jaffers G, Dienstag JL, et al. Immunogenicity of hepatitis B vaccine in renal transplant recipients. *Transplantation* 1985;39:393–395.

155. Lefebure AF, Verpooten GA, Couttenye MM, et al. Immunogenicity of a recombinant DNA hepatitis B vaccine in renal transplant patients. *Vaccine* 1993;11: 397–399.

156. Chalasani N, Smallwood G, Halcomb J, et al. Is vaccination against hepatitis B infection indicated in patients waiting for or after orthotopic liver transplantation? *Liver Transpl Surg* 1998;4:128–132.

157. Sokal EM, Ulla L, Otte JB. Hepatitis B vaccine response before and after transplantation in 55 extrahepatic biliary atresia children. *Dig Dis Sci* 1992;37: 1250–1252.

158. Collier AC, Corey L, Murphy VL, et al. Antibody to human immunodeficiency virus (HIV) and suboptimal response to hepatitis B vaccination. *Ann Intern Med* 1988;109:101–105.

159. Diamant EP, Schechter C, Hodes DS, et al. Immunogenicity of hepatitis B vaccine in human immunodeficiency virus-infected children. *Pediatr Infect Dis J* 1993;12:877–878.

160. Choudhury SA, Peters VB. Responses to hepatitis B vaccine boosters in human immunodeficiency virus-infected children. *Pediatr Infect Dis J* 1995;14: 65–67.

161. Zuin G, Principi N, Tornaghi R, et al. Impaired response to hepatitis B vaccine in HIV infected children. *Vaccine* 1992;10:857–860.

162. Zuccotti GV, Riva E, Flumine P, et al. Hepatitis B vaccination in infants of mothers infected with human immunodeficiency virus. *J Pediatr* 1994;125:70–72.

163. Hepatitis B. In: Peter G, ed. *1997 Red book:* report of the Committee on Infectious Diseases. Vol 24. Elk Grove Village, IL: American Academy of Pediatrics, 1997:253.

164. Anonymous. Prevention and control of influenza: recommendations of the Advisory Committee on Immunization Practices (ACIP). Centers for Disease Control and Prevention. *MMWR Morb Mortal Wkly Rep* 1998;47:1–26.

165. Influenza. In: Peter G, ed. *1997 Red book:* report of the Committee on Infectious Diseases. Vol 24. Elk Grove Village, IL: American Academy of Pediatrics, 1997: 307–315.

166. Whimbey E, Champlin RE, Couch RB, et al. Commu-nity respiratory virus infections among hospitalized adult bone marrow transplant recipients. *Clin Infect Dis* 1996;22:778–782.

167. Apalsch AM, Green M, Ledesma-Medina J, et al. Parainfluenza and influenza virus infections in pediatric organ transplant recipients. *Clin Infect Dis* 1995; 20:394–399.

168. Klimov AI, Rocha E, Hayden FG, et al. Prolonged shedding of amantadine-resistant influenzae A viruses by immunodeficient patients: detection by polymerase chain reaction-restriction analysis. *J Infect Dis* 1995; 172:1352–1355.

169. Blumberg EA, Fitzpatrick J, Stutman PC, et al. Safety of influenza vaccine in heart transplant recipients. *J Heart Lung Transplant* 1998;17:1075–1080.

170. Jackson CR, Vavro CL, Valentine ME, et al. Effect of influenza immunization on immunologic and virologic characteristics of pediatric patients infected with human immunodeficiency virus. *Pediatr Infect Dis J* 1997;16:200-204.

171. Staprans SI, Hamilton BL, Follansbee SE, et al. Activation of virus replication after vaccination of HIV-1-infected individuals. *J Exp Med* 1995;182: 1727–1737.

172. Fuller JD, Craven DE, Steger KA, et al. Influenza vaccination of human immunodeficiency virus (HIV)-infected adults: impact of plasma levels of HIV type 1 RNA and determinants of antibody response. *Clin Infect Dis* 1999;28:541–547.

173. Blumberg EA, Albano C, Pruett T, et al. The immunogenicity of influenza virus vaccine in solid organ transplant recipients. *Clin Infect Dis* 1996;22:295–302.

174. Furth SL, Neu AM, McColley SA, et al. Immune response to influenza vaccination in children with renal disease. *Pediatric Nephrol* 1995;9:566–568.

175. Mauch TJ, Bratton S, Myers T, et al. Influenza B virus infection in pediatric solid organ transplant recipients. *Pediatrics* 1994;94:225–229.

176. Admon D, Engelhard D, Strauss N, et al. Antibody response to influenza immunization in patients after heart transplantation. *Vaccine* 1997;15:1518–1522.

177. Steinherz PG, Brown AE, Gross PA, et al. Influenza immunization of children with neoplastic diseases. *Cancer* 1980;45:750–756.

178. Nelson KE, Clements ML, Miotti P, et al. The influence of human immunodeficiency virus (HIV) infection on antibody responses to influenza vaccines. *Ann Intern Med* 1988;109:383–388.

179. Chadwick EG, Chang G, Decker MD, et al. Serologic response to standard inactivated influenza vaccine in human immunodeficiency virus-infected children. *Pediatr Infect Dis J* 1994;13:206–211.

180. Herron A, Dettleff G, Hixon B, et al. Influenza vaccination in patients with rheumatic diseases. Safety and efficacy. *JAMA* 1979;242:53–56.

181. Park CL, Frank AL, Sullivan M, et al. Influenza vaccination of children during acute asthma exacerbation and concurrent prednisone therapy. *Pediatrics* 1996; 98:196–200.

182. Fairchok MP, Trementozzi DP, Carter PS, et al. Effect of prednisone on response to influenza virus vaccine in asthmatic children. *Arch Pediatr Adolesc Med* 1998; 152:1191–1195.

183. O'Hagan DT. Recent advances in vaccine adjuvants

for systemic and mucosal administration. *J Pharm Pharmacol* 1998;50:1–10.

184. Liu MA. Vaccine developments. *Nat Med* 1998;4: 515–519.

185. Belshe RB, Mendelman PM, Treanor J, et al. The efficacy of live attenuated, cold-adapted, trivalent, intranasal influenzavirus vaccine in children. *N Engl J Med* 1998;338:1405–1412.

186. Karron RA, Wright PF, Crowe JE Jr, et al. Evaluation of two live, cold-passaged, temperature-sensitive respiratory syncytial virus vaccines in chimpanzees and in human adults, infants, and children. *J Infect Dis* 1997;176:1428–1436.

187. Piedra PA, Grace S, Jewell A, et al. Sequential annual administration of purified fusion protein vaccine against respiratory syncytial virus in children with cystic fibrosis. *Pediatr Infect Dis J* 1998;17:217–224.

188. Rodriguez WJ, Gruber WC, Groothuis JR, et al. Respiratory syncytial virus immune globulin treatment of RSV lower respiratory tract infection in previously healthy children. *Pediatrics* 1997;100:937–942.

189. The PREVENT Study Group. Reduction of respiratory syncytial virus hospitalization among premature infants and infants with bronchopulmonary dysplasia using respiratory syncytial virus immune globulin prophylaxis. *Pediatrics* 1997;99:93–99.

190. The IMpact-RSV Study Group. Palivizumab, a humanized respiratory syncytial virus monoclonal antibody, reduces hospitalization from respiratory syncytial virus infection in high-risk infants. *Pediatrics* 1998;102:531–537.

191. Plotkin SA, Higgins R, Kurtz JB, et al. Multicenter trial of Towne strain attenuated virus vaccine in seronegative renal transplant recipients. *Transplantation* 1994;58:1176–1178.

192. Adler SP, Hempfling SH, Starr SE, et al. Safety and immunogenicity of the Towne strain cytomegalovirus vaccine. *Pediatr Infect Dis J* 1998;17:200–206.

23

Prevention of Infection

James H. Conway

Department of Pediatric Infectious Diseases, James Whitcomb Riley Hospital for Children, Indianapolis, Indiana 46202

Immunodeficient patients are predisposed to infections by common organisms with greater severity and frequency than healthy persons. Opportunistic pathogens that uncommonly afflict healthy persons also infect these patients with some regularity. Children with congenital immunodeficiency syndromes constitute a small and relatively stable portion of these at-risk patients. The numbers of children with transient and permanent acquired immunodeficiencies, however, are growing; these immunodeficiencies include children who are transplant recipients, those who are infected with the human immunodeficiency virus (HIV), and those receiving chemotherapy; periods of resulting immunosuppression are variable.

Opportunistic pathogens in immunodeficient patients may originate from endogenous flora or from the surrounding environment. Infections may be prevented by interventions in personal hygiene and changes to the surrounding environment. The structural integrity of the integument is critical protection from invasion because translocation of potentially pathogenic organisms is facilitated by indwelling transcutaneous central venous access catheters and chemotherapy-induced mucositis of the alimentary tract. Antiinfective prevention strategies involve managing such risk factors for infection, including microbial colonization and exposure to potential pathogens.

The healthy child has a carefully balanced immune system that is dependent on both function and signaling between the various components. Disruption of any component can put patients at some risk for infection. The ability of the immune system to protect from invasion by most pathogens depends primarily on the presence and activity of granulocytes, as seen in states of neutropenia. Other cell-mediated, humoral, and cytokine defects also can contribute significantly to the risk of infection. Some protection from colonization and infection may be provided by active and passive immunization. Reconstitution of immunity and modulation of these underlying immunodeficiencies is an evolving science.

When the risk for particular infections is determined to be significant, preemptive therapy or chemoprophylaxis is one strategy used to minimize infections, but it carries the risk of inducing microbial resistance. Such prophylaxis may impact significantly the effectiveness of empiric antibiotic selections during acute illness. Besides bacterial chemoprophylaxis, trials have evaluated antimicrobial strategies against fungi, viruses, and protozoa with varying degrees of success.

CAUSES OF INFECTION

A variety of opportunistic organisms can infect immunodeficient patients. Bacteria account for most such infections in neutropenic patients and frequently in patients with other immunodeficiencies. Most strategies for prevention and empiric therapy of infections focus on these pathogens (1). Table 23.1 lists the relative frequency of bacterial etiologies of infection.

Agents selected for antibacterial chemoprophylaxis and empiric therapy require broad-spectrum activity against these disparate organisms. Such patterns of antibiotic use have contributed to shifting the infection patterns in neutropenic patients over the past three decades. Whereas approximately 70% of bacteremia in such patients was caused by gram-negative organisms in the 1970s, data from the last decade show that more than two thirds of bacteremic episodes were caused by gram-positive organisms (2). The expanding use of indwelling central venous access catheters and the duration of neutropenic episodes also appear to contribute to the increased incidence of gram-positive bacteremias (3,4). Interestingly, Krupova et al. (5) reported significantly more gram-positive infections in neutropenic adults than in children, suggesting that the disparate use of chemoprophylactic fluoroquinolones in adults may be important.

The increased incidence of antibiotic resistant gram-positive organisms selected with the routine use of prophylactic and empiric antibiotic therapy gives cause for concern. Significant increases in methicillin-resistant staphyloccal infections and penicillin-resistant viridans streptococcal infections, and subsequently increased mortality and morbidity, are seen in patients receiving antibacterial prophylaxis with quinolones and penicillin (6–8). Recent beta-lactam antibiotic use for empiric therapy has increased the incidence of penicillin-resistant viridans streptococcal infections (9). Finally, the emergence of vancomycin-resistant enterococci in the late 1980s has been cause for some alarm. Data suggest that prolonged vancomycin administration, as is commonly used in some settings for empiric therapy of fever with neutropenia, may be involved in the selection of endogenously vancomycin-resistant strains of enterococci (10).

Although the prevalence of gram-negative infections in neutropenic patients has decreased over time, empiric and preventive broad-spectrum antibiotic administration appears to be associated with an increasing incidence of antibiotic resistant gram-negative organisms. A significant increase in the incidence

TABLE 23.1. *Bacterial causes of infection in neutropenic patients*

Frequent
  Gram positive
    Staphylococcus coagulase-negative, *Staphylococcus aureus*, Viridans streptococcus group,
      Streptococcus pneumoniae, Streptococcus pyogenes, Enterococcus faecalis/faecium
  Gram negative
    Escherichia coli, Klebsiella sp., *Pseudomonas aeruginosa*
Less frequent
  Gram positive
    Listeria monocytogenes, Stomatococcus mucilagnosus, Micrococcus, Corynebacterium, and
      Leuconostoc sp.
  Gram negative
    Haemophilus influenzae, Serratia marcescens, Yersinia, Enterobacter, Proteus, Salmonella, Actinobacillus,
      Aeromonas, Acinetobacter, Alcaligenes, Capnocytophagia, Citrobacter, Chromobacterium, Eikenella,
      Erwinia, Edwardsiella, Flavobacterium, Gardnerella, Hafnia, Kingella, Legionella, Moraxella, Morganella,
      Neisseria, Providencia, Shigella, Stenotrophomonas, Aeromonas, and *Xanthomonas* sp.
  Anaerobic bacteria
    Bacteroides, Clostridium, Propionibacterium, Actinomyces, Proprionobacterium, Lactobacillus, Bacillus,
      Fusobacterium, Peptococcus, Peptostreptococcus, and *Veillonella* sp.
  Acid-fast organisms
    Nocardia, Myobacterium sp.

of multidrug-resistant gram-negative bacteremia has been documented in neutropenic patients receiving fluoroquinolone chemoprophylaxis or empiric broad-spectrum antibiotics compared with the incidence in control patients with bacteremia. Such resistant species include *Pseudomonas, Enterobacter, Klebsiella* species, and *Escherichia coli* (11,12). Martina et al. (13) showed that discontinuation of routine fluoroquinolone prophylaxis during neutropenic episodes at one Spanish institution resulted in an increase in susceptible gram-negative bacteremias with no significant change in infectious morbidity, suggesting that selection of colonizing flora may be reversible.

As increasing attention has been directed to chemoprophylaxis and empiric therapy against bacterial organisms, fungal organisms have emerged as a significant cause of infectious mortality and morbidity in the neutropenic patient. Invasive fungal infections generally occur in children with prolonged immunosuppressed states who are treated with intensive broad-spectrum antibiotics and most likely result from fungal overgrowth and secondary mycotic infection. Table 23.2 summarizes the frequency of fungal pathogens seen in the neutropenic patient.

In recent years, the number of invasive fungal infections in immunocompromised patients has increased substantially (1). With the availability of many new antifungal compounds, attention has turned toward the diagnosis, prevention, and role of preventive and empiric therapy for fungal infections. Similar to the shift in resistance patterns and organisms isolated from bacteremic patients in the past three decades, there has been an increasing incidence of non-albicans *Candida* and other fungal infections, such as *Aspergillus* (14–16). Recent administration of broad-spectrum antibiotics and antifungal prophylaxis appears to contribute to the incidence and types of infection that occur (14,15).

Neutropenic patients occasionally are infected with other opportunistic organisms, including viruses (e.g., cytomegalovirus [CMV], herpes simplex, varicella), protozoa (e.g., *Toxoplasma gondii, Pneumocystis carinii)*, and unusual bacteria including intracellular (e.g., *Bartonella, Chlamydia, Rickettsia* sp.), cell-wall defective (*Mycoplasmataceae*), spirochetes, and acid-fast organisms. Patients with disruption of cellular-mediated immunity—either acquired, as in those infected with HIV, or congenital, with T-lymphocytopenias and severe combined immunodeficiencies—are most susceptible to such opportunistic infections. Risk for such opportunistic infections is estimated by CD4+ T-lymphocyte counts (absolute counts and percentage of circulating lymphocytes) and by lymphocyte function. Function of T-lymphocytes is assessed *in vivo* by a history of prior opportunistic infections and intradermal skin testing and *in vitro* using mitogen stimulation and proliferation assays (17,18). Patients with immunodeficiencies involving humoral immunity, complement defects, and asplenia have a variety of problems, depending on severity, but they tend to have difficulty with viral and common bacterial pathogens, especially encapsulated organisms (e.g., *Streptococcus pneumoniae, Neisseria, Haemophilus,* and *Salmonella* sp.).

TABLE 23.2. *Fungal causes of infection in neutropenic patients*

Frequent
  Candida albicans
  Non-albicans *Candida (Candida parapsilosis, Candida tropicalis, Torulopsis glabrata, Candida lusitania, Candida krusei)*
  Aspergillus spp.
Less Frequent
  Rhizopus, Mucor, Absida, Fusarium, Coccidioides, Acremonium, Cryptococcus, Histoplasma, Trichosporum, Pseudoallescheria, Penicillium, Saccharomyces, Dreschlera and Rhodotorula spp.

NONMEDICINAL INTERVENTIONS

Hygiene and Mechanical Techniques

A significant impact in preventing infections can be made with simple educational and hygienic measures because most organisms that cause infections in the immunocompromised patient are present as flora in the surrounding environment. Careful handwashing remains the single most effective procedure for preventing infection (19). It is essential that patients, families, and health care staff be instructed and frequently reminded of proper technique and required repetition. Printed material combined with verbal instructions to reinforce strategies may be useful.

A totally protective environment for immunocompromised patients during hospitalization is more controversial, largely because of the expense involved. Because most infections arise from the individual patient's endogenous flora, the routine use of reverse isolation techniques (e.g., single rooms; visitors wearing gowns, masks, and gloves; patients wearing masks) and food sterilization do little to prevent infection (20). High-efficiency particulate air (HEPA) filtration systems do offer some benefit, especially in relation to pulmonary aspergillosis (21). Special considerations and interventions are required during times of construction activity contiguous to areas with immunosuppressed patients because aerosolized fungi are a well-documented problem during such activity (22,23).

The care of patient mucocutaneous surfaces should receive special attention, especially during periods of predictable neutropenia, because skin and mucous membrane integrity will minimize the risk of infection by endogenous flora. Skin-care hygiene using gentle soaps and inspection for lesions that may serve as portals of entry should be encouraged. Sites of venipuncture, lumbar puncture, bone marrow aspiration, lacerations, surgical incisions, and catheter sites should be examined regularly. Dental consultation before immunosuppression and careful oral hygiene will prevent some complications of mucositis. Published guidelines should be implemented for preventing indwelling vascular access device-related infections during both hospitalization and outpatient care (24).

Hospital infection-control programs offer an effective, centralized monitoring system for nosocomial events. Health care personnel caring for patients with immunodeficiencies should serve an active role in reporting events and utilizing hospital policy regarding issues of visitation, plants, gifts, equipment use and sterilization, and common areas (19,25,26). Policies regarding immunization of health care workers (27) and exclusion of health care workers with transmissible diseases (28) should be clearly delineated and available. Typical requirements for employee screening include documentation of immunization or past infection for measles, mumps, rubella, hepatitis B, varicella, influenza, tetanus and diphtheria, and tuberculosis Mantoux skin testing.

Careful screening of visitors to hospitalized patients should be performed routinely for potentially infectious conditions or recent exposures to communicable diseases. Persons with possibly transmissible diseases should be excluded from contact with severely immunocompromised patients. Disease-appropriate isolation precautions can be used for less compromised patients, for example, wearing masks and handwashing for close contacts with respiratory illnesses, especially on an outpatient basis where complete avoidance is impractical.

Infection-control practices for preventing the spread of specific nosocomial infections must be followed strictly. New isolation guidelines from the U.S. Centers for Disease Control and Prevention (CDC) attempted to simplify practice by dividing precautions into *standard* for the management of all patients regardless of diagnosis and *transmission-based* for organisms identified as colonizing or infecting patients (29). Standard precautions attempt to reduce transmission risk from unrecognized sources of infections in hospitals. Transmission-based precautions are designed specifically to interrupt transmission from suspected sources and are subdivided by mode of transmission into *airborne, droplet,* and *contact.* These precautions are combined, when necessary, for pathogens with multiple routes of transmission and always are used in addition to the standard precautions (30).

Parents, patients, families, visitors, and health care workers should be taught and reminded frequently that they can take measures to avoid exposures to infectious agents. Education for patients and families should include risks for exposure and evidence of infection. Principles of good personal hygiene should be urged as a means to empower the patient and family to be active participants in preventive measures.

Some specific recommendations for avoiding the acquisition of certain opportunistic pathogens are especially important for HIV-infected patients and transplant recipients. Sexually active patients should be advised to continue using latex condoms to prevent further transmission but also the acquisition of other sexually transmitted diseases, including herpes simplex virus, CMV, and papillomaviruses (31). Sexual practices that result in oral exposure to feces should be avoided (17).

Risks involved in pet ownership and animal contact should be discussed with the patient and family, and contact between immunocompromised patients and animals needs to be minimized because of the risk of zoonotic infections (32). Any pet with a diarrheal illness as well as all new pets present a risk for contracting enteric pathogens, including *Cryptosporidium, Salmonella,* and *Campylobacter.*

Handwashing should be encouraged and supervised in small HIV-infected children. Cats present further risks related to toxoplasmosis and *Bartonella* infections. Only ownership of older indoor cats should be accepted. Such pets are less likely to acquire most pathogens, and biting and scratching behavior are less frequent. Litter boxes, cages, and aquariums should be cleaned by healthy persons when possible and with disposable gloves and careful handwashing by patients when necessary. Contacts with all reptiles, ducklings, chicks, and exotic pets should be avoided because of the risk of salmonellosis (17).

Occupational and recreational exposures in some patients also represent a risk for opportunistic infections. Employees in health care settings, prisons, and homeless shelters are at risk for tuberculosis exposure. Patients involved in gardening and agriculture are exposed to pathogens including *T. gondii, Nocardia* sp., and fungi, especially *Aspergillus* spp.

Recommendations for food preparation are similar to those for the general public and are largely related to cross-contamination and proper cooking. Raw, unpasteurized, and undercooked foods carry the highest risk for enteric pathogen contamination. Table 23.3 lists high-risk foods. Meat and poultry should be cooked thoroughly. Fruits and vegetables should be thoroughly cleaned, and uncooked meats should not be allowed to contact prepared food directly or indirectly (33). Un-

TABLE 23.3. *Food items presenting high-risk of contamination and subsequent infection in immunocompromised patients*

Food type	Highest risk
Raw and undercooked eggs	Salad dressings, egg nog, puddings, omelettes
Unpasteurized dairy products	Moldy, aged, and soft cheeses; milk, cream, butter
Unpasteurized fruits and vegetables	Fresh, squeezed juices
Undercooked meats	Rare–medium rare hamburgers, steak tartare
Undercooked poultry	Contaminates cutting boards
Undercooked fish and seafood	Sushi, ceviche, raw bars
Raw fruits, vegetables, nuts	Cannot be peeled, especially those grown at ground level, i.e., berries, herbs, lettuce
Ice cream/yogurt	Soft-serve products
Tofu	Raw or undercooked
Honey	Raw or unpasteurized
Spices	Variable contaminants

treated water should be avoided for swimming or drinking because contamination with *Cryptosporidium* and other protozoa may occur. Boiling water, filtration systems, bottled water, or other packaged beverages represent alternatives (17).

Travel presents magnified versions of the same issues related to animals and food, especially when travel destinations are within developing countries. Exposure to pathogens that are regionally endemic must be managed expectantly. Even within the confines of North America, travel to and residence in particular areas may place immunodeficient patients at risk for infection. Examples of geographic illness affecting the immunocompromised host include histoplasmosis in the midwestern United States, coccidioidomycosis in the southwestern United States extending into Central and South America, and strongyloidiasis in the Appalachian Mountain region. Consultation with a university-based travel clinic and the CDC may be useful, along with reviewing pertinent sections in the most current *Red Book:* Report of the Committee on Infectious Diseases (18).

Immunologic Interventions

Active Immunization

Routine immunization against viral and bacterial pathogens plays an important role in protecting the immunocompromised patient. Immunization of household contacts and health care workers, as discussed earlier, can help minimize infection or carriage of many pathogens in this population and therefore decrease exposure of the immunodeficient patient. Caution must be exercised with routine administration of varicella or oral polio vaccines to healthy persons because these can be transmitted to immunodeficient household members (17,34–36). Mild varicella has been transmitted from immunized persons developing vesicular rash, and both polio and rotavirus are shed in the stool of immunized persons (34–36). In addition to routine childhood immunizations for young contacts, older house-

hold contacts should be up to date with vaccination against measles–mumps–rubella (MMR) and tetanus-diphtheria toxoids, and they should receive yearly influenza boosters (37).

The impact of required routine immunizations for preventing infections in the individual immunocompromised patient is less well defined and requires special consideration. Whereas such patients may be at increased risk of serious complications from primary infection, they also may be at increased risk for complications from vaccination or of inadequate protective response to the vaccination. Patients with altered immunocompetence can be vaccinated safely with killed vaccines given in the same doses and according to the same schedule as immunocompetent persons (38). Live vaccines (bacterial or viral) are contraindicated in children with congenital immunodeficiencies and in most other immunodeficient states because vaccine-strain poliomyelitis, measles, and varicella infections have been reported (39). Whenever possible, inactivated vaccines should be substituted, such as inactivated polio vaccine (34). Exceptions include asymptomatic HIV-infected children who can be immunized against measles, mumps, and rubella (17) and the judicious use of varicella vaccine in patients with acute lymphocytic leukemia (39). The oral tetravalent rotavirus vaccine was the most recently licensed live viral vaccine but was contraindicated in immunocompromised persons because safety and efficacy was never established in clinical trials (40). The vaccine has since been recalled due to an association with intussusception.

Some specific populations of immunodeficient patients merit special immunizations. Asplenic patients are specifically at risk for serious infections from the encapsulated organisms *S. pneumoniae* and *Haemophilus influenzae* and, less commonly, *Neisseria meningitidis* as well as a variety of other gram-positive and gram-negative organisms (39). Besides chemoprophylaxis with antimicrobial agents and routine childhood immunizations, pneumococcal and meningococcal vaccines should be given to these children after 2 years of age to maximize the potential immunologic response (38). Revaccination with pneumococcal vaccine after 3 to 5 years is recommended for asplenic children under 10 years of age (41). The duration of protection from meningococcal vaccine is less well established. Revaccination should be considered after 1 year in children first vaccinated before 4 years of age and after 5 years for children who were first vaccinated when older than 4 years (42,43).

Other patients also should receive pneumococcal immunization if they are at increased risk of acquiring pneumococcal infection or of experiencing severe disease if infected. This includes patients with any chronic immunosuppressive state, sickle cell disease, nephrotic syndrome, renal failure, cerebrospinal fluid leaks, or chronic pulmonary, hepatic, or cardiovascular disease (41). Whereas the currently available 23-valent polysaccharide pneumococcal vaccine has limited immunogenicity in children younger than 2 years, newer conjugate pneumococcal vaccines have undergone trials, are immunogenic in young infants (44) and were recently licensed for routine administration to all children under 2 years and high-risk children 24 to 59 months of age (41). Besides asplenic patients, meningococcal vaccine is indicated for select populations during outbreaks, for travelers to endemic areas, and for persons with terminal complement and properdin deficiencies (42,43).

Children who are infected with HIV should be immunized according to the recommended childhood immunization schedule, excluding varicella, and using inactivated polio rather than oral polio vaccine (17). Asymptomatic patients should receive MMR vaccine immediately after their first birthday, and the second dose should be considered earlier than school age but at least 28 days after the first dose (17,39). HIV-infected children should routinely receive pneumococcal vaccination at 24 months and yearly influenza vaccines after 6 months of age (17,37). Response to vaccination is variable and largely dependent on CD4+ T-lymphocyte counts and function. Data suggest that HIV patients with a longer duration of infection and more severe disruption in immune function display diminished immunity after pneumococcal, influenza, tetanus, and *H. influenzae* vaccinations (44–47). The immunologic stimulation provided by such vaccinations does appear to affect HIV homeostasis temporarily because some vaccines have been shown to lead to transiently increased HIV circulating viral loads (48). Generally, the benefit of vaccine protection outweighs this transient disruption of the immune system.

Hematopoietic cell transplant recipients offer an unusual challenge. Many factors influence immunity after transplant in such patients, including the source of transplanted cells (e.g., autologous or allogeneic), the type and dosage of immunosuppressive agents, graft-versus-host disease (GVHD), time elapsed since transplant, and donor immunity (49). Immunity from donor cells may be acquired but often without serologic immunity (39). Immunization of donors prior to transplant and reimmunization of recipients after transplantation may stimulate donor immune memory with specific antigen and has been demonstrated with diphtheria and tetanus (50). Given this information, it seems prudent to vaccinate transplant recipients posttransplantation. Protocols suggest beginning a schedule of vaccination 12 months after transplant with inactivated vaccines for diphtheria–tetanus and acellular pertussis (for children younger than 7 years), *H. influenza* type B, hepatitis B, and inactivated polio, with boosters at 14 and 24 months (38,39,51). Pneumococcal vaccine should be administered at 12 and 24 months (41). Influenza vaccine must be given to patients and family contacts yearly in fall (37). MMR vaccine can be given at 24 months after transplant and should be administered again a month later except to patients with GVHD (38,39,51). With rare exceptions, live viral vaccines are contraindicated in this population.

For patients on reversible immunosuppressive therapy, live viral vaccines are withheld for approximately 3 months after cessation of therapy. Patients receiving corticosteroids present an exception because the degree of immunosuppression is both dose and duration dependent. Children receiving high-dose systemic steroids (more than 20 mg or 2 mg/kg daily) for more than 14 days require a 1-month period after discontinuation before receiving live viral vaccines, whereas those on shorter courses can be immunized immediately after cessation. Lower doses and shorter durations generally are not immunosuppressive, and live-virus vaccines may be administered in many situations while the patient is on therapy (39).

Passive Immunization

An alternative form of protection to active immunization is passive immunization. Preformed antibodies are administered to the recipient, replacing or augmenting inadequate immunoglobulin levels in an attempt to prevent or minimize the severity of infectious diseases. Such preventive immunization strategy is considered for patients known to be deficient in antibody synthesis and for susceptible patients at high risk for complications of infection who are exposed or at high risk for exposure to specific pathogens.

Two basic types of products are available for passive immunization. These differ by the donor pool involved and the titer of specific antibodies transmitted. Processing is similar, with pooled donor plasma undergoing alcohol fractionation and the final products containing over 95% immunoglobulin G (IgG). Products are screened for blood-borne pathogens, including syphilis, hepatitis B, hepatitis C, HIV, and human T-cell leukemia viruses, and further processed to inactivate and remove viruses undetected in screening (39). Reactions are uncommon and similar to those experienced with any intramuscular (for immune globulin [IG]) or intravenous (for intravenous immune globulin [IVIG]) blood product.

Both IG and IVIG are derived from large plasma pools used to ensure a broad spectrum of antibodies. The U.S. Food and Drug Administration (FDA) guidelines specify the minimum concentrations of measles, diphtheria, polio, and hepatitis B antibodies. Antibody concentrations against common bacter-

ial pathogens vary widely. These products are indicated for prophylactic replacement therapy given on a regular basis (usually monthly) for antibody deficiency states such as primary immunodeficiencies (e.g., common variable immunodeficiency, X-linked agammaglobulinemia) and potentially offer protection to selected patients with pediatric HIV, chronic lymphocytic leukemia, after bone marrow transplantation, and perhaps very-low-birth-weight (39,52–54). Specific HIV patients in whom IGIV is recommended include those with documented hypogammaglobulinemia, recurrent serious bacterial infections, or inadequate antibodies to common antigens (e.g. measles, *S. pneumonia, H. influenza*) (55,56).

Hyperimmune globulins are immunoglobulin preparations with high levels of antibodies against specific pathogens. Plasma is obtained from selected donors with high antibody titers against the required antigens through immunization or natural disease. Products such as CMV immune globulin intravenous (CMV-IGIV) and respiratory syncytial virus immune globulin intravenous (RSV-IGIV) or monoclonal intramuscular are currently indicated for specific patients at high risk for exposure or severe disease if infected with these viruses. Varicella zoster immune globulin (VZIG), tetanus immune globulin (TIG), rabies immune globulin (RIG), hepatitis B immune globulin (HBIG), and IG for exposure to hepatitis A and measles are indicated for postexposure prophylaxis in potentially nonimmune persons after likely contact with contagion, often with simultaneous active immunization (39,57)

Immune Modulation and Hematopoietic Growth Factors

Augmentation of immunologic function may provide significant protection from infections for immunodeficient patients. As the role of cytokines in immune regulation and response continues to be defined, clinical research progresses in utilizing interferons, lymphokines, and monokines as therapeutic immunomodulators of disease. Some investigations suggested that antiinflammatory mediators, such as interleukin (IL)-4, IL-6, IL-10, and IL-13, may prevent some sequelae of infections and appear to have utility in the treatment of some malignancies. More significant for immunodeficient patients are the proinflammatory cytokines and interferons that may stimulate immunologic function, including IL-1, IL-2, IL-3, IL-5, IL-7, IL-8, IL-9, IL-11, IL-12, IL-14, IL-15, IL-16, IL-17, tumor necrosis factor, colony-stimulating factors, and interferons alpha, beta, and gamma (58,59). Placebo-controlled trials of the proinflammatory interferon-γ in 128 pediatric patients with chronic granulomatous disease resulted in a two-thirds reduction in serious infections, especially in younger patients (60). Subsequently, interferon-γ was licensed for prevention of infections in patients with chronic granulomatous disease in the early 1990s.

More attention has been directed toward colony-stimulating factors involved in the proliferation and maturation of hematopoietic stem cells. Granulocyte colony-stimulating factor (G-CSF) induces the formation and function of granulocytes, and granulocyte–macrophage colony-stimulating factor (GM-CSF) induces both granulocyte and monocyte proliferation and activation. Since the initial cloning and clinical trials in the late 1980s and eventual licensure, use has expanded to include stimulation of hematopoiesis and therapy for neutropenia in a variety of settings.

Although both agents have been used in settings of myelosuppressive chemotherapy, GM-CSF has been studied more extensively. Empiric use of both G-CSF and GM-CSF has been shown to reduce the severity of neutropenia, the duration of neutropenia, and episodes of fever during neutropenia, although administration does not necessarily decrease infection rates or the need for hospitalization (61–65). Given the expense of such agents, the cost-effectiveness of routine prophylactic use after chemotherapy is still questioned (1,64,66); however, when selectively administered after the onset of febrile

episodes in neutropenic patients, there may be some measurable overall cost savings (65). Many investigators suggested that the utility of CSFs after chemotherapy is dependent on the intensity of the chemotherapeutic regimen involved (1,20,63,66). Currently, routine use of such agents after cancer chemotherapy is not recommended, except in circumstances where prolonged marrow recovery is expected or documented or where clinical evidence suggests deterioration, focal infection, or sepsis (67).

Colony-stimulating factors may have a more substantial role in stem cell transplantation. Administration of either GM-CSF or G-CSF increases circulating peripheral hematopoietic stem cells in donors, offering an increased cellular yield for later infusion, whether for actual transplantation or rescue from febrile neutropenia (68–70). After autologous and allogeneic bone marrow transplantation, both CSFs effectively decrease the duration of neutropenia and enhance engraftment without increasing relapse rates or GVHD (71–74). Although such regimens do not necessarily reduce rates of infection, some studies have shown a significant decrease in days of empiric antibiotic therapy and hospitalization (72, 74). When used during graft failure after transplantation, survival rates have been greatly improved (75).

In the setting of HIV therapy, leukopenia is a relatively common toxicity of the chemotherapeutic agents used to treat HIV or prevent opportunistic infections. Zidovudine, ganciclovir, and trimethoprim–sulfamethoxazole (TMP-SMZ) are frequently prescribed medications that commonly inhibit bone marrow activity, resulting in neutropenia that may limit their utility in HIV-infected patients. Both GM-CSF and G-CSF have been studied in leukopenic HIV patients, resulting in dose-dependent increases in all leukocytes, including neutrophils (76). In addition, use of G-CSF in 71 neutropenic HIV-patients was associated with a significant decrease in the risk for bacteremia and prolonged survival compared with 81 untreated neutropenic HIV-patients, controlling for degree of immuno-suppression, medication regimens, and inter-current opportunistic infections (77). Al-though CSFs have become an accepted and useful adjunctive immunomodulator for se-lected HIV patients with neutropenia, there is still some concern regarding routine use be-cause *in vitro* macrophage activation pro-motes HIV replication (58,59,78); however, one small *in vivo* trial administered GM-CSF to 12 HIV-patients on zidovudine. Virologic analysis revealed no increase in HIV replica-tion, and CD4-lymphocyte counts remained stable, whereas absolute neutrophil counts increased (79).

Colony-stimulating factors have shown great potential in treating congenital and cyclic chronic neutropenias. In a small cohort of four children with congenital agranulocy-tosis (Kostmann's syndrome), in which neu-trophil production is impaired, treatment with G-CSF resulted in elevated peripheral neu-trophil counts, and reduced episodes of in-fection requiring antibiotics (80). Six children with cyclic neutropenia, an uncommon syn-drome thought to represent disregulation of stem cell proliferation, have been similarly re-sponsive to G-CSF, with improved neutrophil counts and a reduction in infections. This re-sponse is thought to be at least in part a result of improved neutrophil function because most patients continued to have some cycling of peripheral neutrophil counts despite regular administration of G-CSF (81). Interestingly, GM-CSF administered to three children with cyclic neutropenia resulted in more inhibition of neutropenic cycling but eosinophilia and less impressive neutrophil counts (82). Recent data also suggest a role for G-CSF in selected patients with autoimmune neutropenia. Al-though spontaneous remission was seen in 95% of a large cohort by age 24 months, a small subset with significant infections re-sponded to G-CSF with improved neutrophil counts (83). Neutropenias associated with Shwachman's syndrome, Fanconi's anemia, glycogen storage diseases, and prematurity have been reported to improve with both GM-CSF and G-CSF (84–88). Administration of

G-CSF in a randomized trial of 42 premature infants with presumed sepsis did show in-creased peripheral and marrow neutrophils but was clinically inconclusive because of a paucity of documented infections (85). Clini-cal research continues to determine what role these CSFs may have in the therapy and pre-vention of infection in other patients at risk, with and without neutropenia (58,59).

MEDICINAL INTERVENTIONS

Chemoprophylaxis

Because immunodeficient patients are pre-dictably at risk of infection by opportunistic pathogens, the administration of antibiotics with activity against select organisms is fre-quently used as a preventive measure. The po-tential benefits of such chemoprophylaxis measures are clear. Unfortunately, such strate-gies pose some hazards, including medication toxicities and the selection of resistant organ-isms, including fungi.

Bacterial infections are the most common cause of morbidity and mortality in neu-tropenic patients as well as in those with many other immunodeficiencies. Because infecting bacteria generally arise from the patient's en-dogenous flora, antibiotic regimens have fo-cused on decontamination of the gastrointesti-nal tract. Total decontamination utilizes broad-spectrum nonabsorbable antibiotics. Selective decontamination attempts to maintain benign anaerobic flora while eliminating pathogenic aerobes using absorbable agents.

Nonabsorbable Antibiotics

A variety of oral nonabsorbable antibiotics, including aminoglycosides, polymyxins, and vancomycin, have been examined as a means to eliminate potentially pathogenic organisms from the gastrointestinal tract. Few studies of such prophylactic regimens have shown any measurable decrease in rates of infection in immunodeficient recipients not residing in laminar flow units (89,90). A recent retro-spective evaluation of children with acute lymphoblastic and nonlymphoblastic leukemia who were receiving induction chemotherapy found no difference in infection rates during neutropenia between selective and total decontamination (91). Administration is further limited by the related cost and gastrointestinal side effects. Of more concern is antibiotic pressure on gastrointestinal microbial flora and the induction or selection of resistant organisms in these patients, as seen in four patients receiving total bowel decontamination with vancomycin who developed severe *Lactobacillus* sp. infections (92). Further evidence suggests that prolonged use of vancomycin in patients with fever and neutropenia is associated with the induction of resistance in enterococci (10). In this era of emerging antibiotic resistance, reserving aminoglycosides and vancomycin for treatment purposes rather than routine oral prophylaxis seems prudent.

Absorbable Antibiotics

Absorbable oral antibiotics that achieve systemic distribution appear to be better tolerated and more effective than nonabsorbable agents for chemoprophylaxis during neutropenia. Most studies have examined either the combination TMP-SMZ or a fluoroquinolone (generally ciprofloxacin, ofloxacin, or norfloxacin). Both regimens offer broadspectrum antibiotic activity against bacterial pathogens, are well absorbed, achieve adequate serum levels, and offer some intraluminal gut decontamination activity. TMP-SMZ is a sulfa-based combination with activity against both gram-positive and gram-negative bacterial organisms as well as some nonbacterial species (e.g., *T. gondii, P. carinii*). Most of the fluoroquinolones studied as chemoprophylactic agents offer broader activity against gram-negative organisms but are more limited against gram-positives than TMP-SMZ.

In pediatric patients, TMP-SMZ has been studied more extensively than the quinolones and is used more commonly for chemoprophylaxis. Studies evaluating TMP-SMZ for the prevention of infections in neutropenic patients of all ages are summarized in Table 23.4.

(93–133). In most of these studies, TMP-SMZ was considered effective at preventing infections, especially compared with no chemoprophylaxis or nonabsorbable antibiotic regiments. Infection rates were lowered most significantly in patients with neutropenia of greater than 2 weeks duration after chemotherapy for leukemia.

Adverse reactions related to TMP-SMZ administration are relatively few and include rash, decreased granulocyte counts, or prolongation of neutropenia (bone marrow suppression), fungal infections, and stomatitis. The highest rate of adverse reactions was reported by Verhoef et al. (127), who reported that 20% of patients experienced rashes attributed to TMP-SMZ. Rash was reported in another four of the 41 studies in Table 23.4, affecting fewer than 10% of patients in each (101,111, 113,128). Bone marrow suppression manifested by granulocytopenia was noted in seven of the 41 studies (98,107,108,112,113, 122,133). Side effects to TMP-SMZ were considered mild in all cases, were associated with higher doses, and were reversible on discontinuation of the medication (98,101,107, 108,111–113,122,127,128,133). Although adverse events were rare and considered insignificant in patients receiving such chemoprophylaxis, there is cause for concern regarding the rates of bacterial resistance and fungal colonization described in most studies. The routine use of such chemoprophylaxis remains controversial (1,20).

Recommendations differ for timing, dose, frequency, and duration of administration of TMP-SMZ, depending on the intent of the chemoprophylaxis. For preventing bacterial infections, TMP-SMZ can be used for uninfected afebrile patients with profound neutropenia that is likely to persist for 1 week or longer. Medication is administered orally by liquid suspension or tablet at a dosage of 150 mg of TMP and 750 mg of SMX/m^2 per day in two divided doses, which is approximately 5 mg/kg TMP and 25 mg/kg SMZ per day. The total daily dose should not exceed 320 mg TMP and 1.6 g SMZ. TMP-SMZ is also effective in preventing pneumocystis pneu-

TABLE 23.4. *Studies of prophylactic TMP/SMZ effectiveness in neutropenic patients*

Reference	Year	No. of Patients Studied	Control Agent(s)	Conclusion (comparative effectiveness)	Side effects
Enno et al. (93)	1978	30	NAA	Effective	None
Gurwith et al. (94)	1979	111	ND or NAA	Effective	None
Gaya et al. (95)	1980	186	Placebo	Partially Effective	None
Matarme et al. (96)	1980	63	NAA	Effective	None
Sleijfen et al. (97)	1980	105	NAA, Nalidixic acid	Effective	None
Dekker et al. (98)	1981	52	ND	Effective	BMS
Wade et al. (99)	1981	53	NAA	Same	None
Weiser et al. (100)	1981	29	ND	Same	None
Calvo et al. (101)	1981	20	NAA	Same	Rash
Preisler et al. (102)	1981	40	ND	Effective	None
Zinner et al. (103)	1981	248	NAA	Effective	None
Gurwith et al. (104)	1982	102	Placebo	Effective	Stomatitis
Watson et al. (105)	1982	88	NAA	Effective	None
Starke et al. (106)	1982	43	NAA + TMP-SMZ	Same	None
Scaglione et al. (107)	1982	139	ND	Effective	BMS
Pizzo et al. (108)	1983	150	Placebo	Effective	BMS
Gualtieri et al. (109)	1983	47	Placebo	Effective	None
Riben et al. (110)	1983	53	ND, TMP	Effective	None
Kauffman et al. (111)	1983	55	ND	Effective	Rash
Wade et al. (112)	1983	62	NAA	Effective	BMS, FI
Inoue et al. (113)	1983	64	TMP	Same	Rash, BMS
Rozenberg-Arska et al. (114)	1983	30	TMP/SMZ + NAA	Same	None
De Jongh et al. (115)	1983	61	Placebo	Effective	FI
Estey et al. (116)	1984	147	ND +/- Ketoconazole	Effective	FI
Hughes and Patterson (117)	1984	100	ND	Effective	None
Henry (118)	1984	43	ND	Effective	None
EORTC (119)	1984	342	Placebo	Effective	None
Lange et al. (120)	1984	67	ND	Effective	None
Kovatch et al. (121)	1985	74	Placebo	Effective	Thrush
Goorin et al. (122)	1985	60	Placebo	Effective	BMS
Van Eys et al. (123)	1987	126	ND	Same	None
Bow et al. (124)	1988	63	Norfloxacin	Same	None
Ward et al. (125)	1988	42	Placebo	Same	None
Cruciani et al. (126)	1989	44	Norfloxacin	Same	None
Verhoef et al. (127)	1989	164	+NAA, Ciprofloxacin	Less Effective	Rash
Liang et al. (128)	1990	102	Ofloxacin	Less Effective	Rash
Kern and Kurrla (129)	1991	128	Ofloxacin	Less Effective	None
Ward et al. (130)	1993	42	Placebo	Same	None
Murase (131)	1995	53	+/- Ciprofloxacin	+ciprofloxacin more effective	None
Lew et al. (132)	1995	146	Ciprofloxacin	Same	*Clostridium difficile*
Imrie et al. (133)	1995	40	Ciprofloxacin	Same	BMS

BMS, bone marrow suppression; FI, fungal infections, NAA, nonabsorbable antibiotics, ND, no drugs; SMZ, sulfamethoxazole; TMP, trimethoprim; TMP/SMZ, trimethoprim-sulfamethoxazole.

monia in patients at risk for such infection using different dosing schedules from those studied for prevention of bacterial infections during neutropenia (134). These regimens involve a similar dose given intermittently on three consecutive days per week, but this dosing has not been studied for preventing infections during neutropenia.

Pneumocystis carinii is an unusual ubiquitous primitive fungus or protozoal organism that infects susceptible patients and causes severe pneumonitis. Such infections have been well documented in patients with defects in cell-mediated immunity, including leukemia, HIV, and histiocytosis or who are undergoing bone marrow transplantation or receiving cancer chemotherapy, corticosteroids, or other immunosuppressive agents after organ transplantation (1,18,20,135). Decisions regarding the administration of chemoprophylaxis for *P. carinii* should be made based on the underlying disease, the degree of immunosuppression, and the prevalence of institutional *P. carinii* infections. For HIV-infected patients, lifelong prophylaxis is generally recommended after an episode of *P. carinii* pneumonia (PCP) regardless of CD4+ T-lymphocyte counts (17,135,136).

The most effective agent for preventing *P. carinii* infections is TMP-SMZ (17,20,134–136). In addition, TMP-SMZ provides prophylaxis against other opportunistic pathogens, most notably *T. gondii,* in HIV-infected patients (17,136). Unfortunately, patients with HIV have an adverse reaction rate to TMP-SMZ of nearly 50%. Successful desensitization with gradually escalating doses up to the final desired dose has been described and can be attempted in patients with minor rashes after the reaction has subsided (137). For patients intolerant of TMP-SMZ, alternative regimens include oral dapsone, pyrimethamine/sulfadoxine, aerosolized pentamidine for children over 5 years of age, atovoquone, and occasionally intravenous pentamidine (17,136, 138,139). In patients unable to receive any of these agents, limited data suggest that clin-damycin/primaquine and azithromycin may have a chemoprophylactic role (17). HIV patients not receiving TMP-SMZ or dapsone/pyrimethamine for PCP prophylaxis require serologic testing for *Toxoplasma* because alternative PCP drugs may not be effective (17).

With their limited side effect profile, the oral fluoroquinolones have become increasingly popular agents for both chemoprophylaxis against bacterial infections in neutropenic adult patients and as empiric therapy during febrile episodes. Table 23.5 summarizes a series of studies with various quinolones administered during episodes of neutropenia (124,126,128,129,132,140–146). As might be expected by the spectrum of fluoroquinolone antibacterial activity, there is a significant reduction in gram-negative infections during neutropenia compared with TMP-SMZ, placebo, or nonabsorbable antibiotic regimens (128,129,132,140–144). A metanalysis of quinolone efficacy was conducted by Cruciani et al. (147) in which 19 randomized trials including 2,112 subjects receiving chemoprophylactic antibiotics during neutropenia following chemotherapy were examined. Compared with other regimens, quinolone prophylaxis alone significantly reduced the rate of gram-negative infections, but it had no impact on gram-positive infec-

TABLE 23.5. *Studies of prophylactic fluoroquinolone effectiveness in neutropenic patients*

Reference	Year	No. of patients studied	Quinolone	Control agent(s)	Conclusion (comparative infection rates)
Winston et al. (140)	1986	66	Norfloxacin	NAA	Less gram-negative
Dekker et al. (141)	1987	56	Ciprofloxacin	TMP/SMZ + NAA	Less gram-negative
Karp et al. (142)	1987	68	Norfloxacin	Placebo	Less gram-negative
Bow et al. (124)	1988	63	Norfloxacin	TMP/SMZ	More gram-positive
Cruciani et al. (126)	1989	44	Norfloxacin	TMP/SMZ	Same
Liang et al. (128)	1990	102	Ofloxacin	TMP/SMZ	Less gram-negative
Winston et al. (143)	1990	62	Ofloxacin	NAA	Less gram-negative
Kern and Kurrla (129)	1991	128	Ofloxacin	TMP/SMZ	Less gram-negative
GIMEMA (144)	1991	619	Ciprofloxacin	Norfloxacin	Less gram-negative
Lew et al. (145)	1991	26	Ciprofloxacin	Placebo	Same
Lew et al. (132)	1995	146	Ciprofloxacin	TMP/SMZ	Less gram-negative
Patrick et al. (146)	1995	34	Ciprofloxacin	+/-NAA vs. Placebo +/– NAA	Same

NAA, nonabsorbable antibiotics; SMZ, sulfamethoxazole; TMP, trimethoprim, TMP/SMZ, trimethoprim-sulfamethoxazole.

tions, episodes of fever requiring empiric antibiotics, or infection-related mortality. A more recent metanalysis by Engel et al. (148) examined 18 randomized studies encompassing 1,408 patients receiving antibiotic prophylaxis during neutropenia. Here quinolone prophylaxis was found to have a significant effect in reducing episodes of gram-negative infections and febrile episodes, but it did not affect the incidence of gram-positive or fungal infections or mortality. Interestingly, in blinded studies, quinolones were less effective in decreasing episodes of fever than in unblinded trials and overall had minimal impact on empiric antibiotic use.

Of interest is the absence of an impact on episodes of gram-positive infections by quinolone chemoprophylaxis. Bow et al. (124) reported a significantly higher incidence of gram-positive infections in adult patients receiving norfloxacin compared with TMP-SMZ. Most other trials of quinolone prophylaxis found no significant difference in preventing episodes of gram-positive bacteremia compared with other chemoprophylaxis regimens (126,128,129,132,141–148); however many researchers continue to note increasing rates of gram-positive infections in adults receiving quinolone prophylaxis (2,3,8, 140,149). Krupova et al. (5) reported a statistically significant difference in the incidence of gram-positive bacteremias between neutropenic adults and children (65.7% versus 33.3%) and largely attributed the excess of gram-positive infections in adults to quinolone chemoprophylaxis compared with children receiving TMP-SMZ.

Several studies have examined augmenting quinolone prophylaxis with antibiotics that have better activity against gram-positive organisms, and results have been mixed. A large randomized, blinded European study of 551 patients demonstrated a reduction in episodes of fever and streptococcal bacteremia when penicillin was added to pefloxacin prophylaxis (150). A similar result was seen in one center after penicillin was added to the usual quinolone regimen, followed by a marked increase in penicillin-resistant organisms and associated mortality over a 7-year span (7). Another trial in a smaller group of 53 patients added amoxicillin to a ciprofloxacin regimen, but no difference in efficacy was found (151). The addition of rifampin to fluoroquinolone prophylaxis also had little impact. A small Spanish trial in 40 stem cell transplantation patients showed reduced incidents of gram-positive bacteremia, but adverse drug-related side effects were significant (152). A larger randomized multicenter Canadian trial studied 111 patients; whereas rifampin added to ofloxacin reduced the incidence of gram-positive infections, no effect on overall febrile episodes during neutropenia was noted (153). The meta-analysis by Cruciani et al. (147) similarly demonstrated a reduction in gram-positive bacteremia occurrences, with the addition of systemic penicillin, vancomycin, or macrolides but without any effect on episodes of fever or mortality.

In contrast to TMP-SMZ studies, most fluoroquinolone studies and use occurs in adult patients. Adverse reactions to fluoroquinolones are mild, with gastrointestinal upset (e.g., nausea, vomiting, diarrhea) affecting 5% to 10% and central nervous symptoms (e.g. dizziness, headache) seen in fewer than 4%. (154). Early reports of irreversible joint damage in juvenile animals raised concerns about the safety of these agents in pediatric patients. Surveillance during compassionate use of these drugs in selected pediatric populations failed to demonstrate significant adverse events. One large database of more than 1,700 patients aged under 17 years demonstrated no episodes of joint toxicity (155). A similar survey of more than 600 children with cystic fibrosis showed no arthropathies attributable to quinolones (156). Only two small studies examined fluoroquinolone prophylaxis in neutropenic children. Cruciani et al. (126) demonstrated no difference in documented bacterial infections of any type in 44 children given TMP-SMZ or norfloxacin. More recently, Patrick et al. (146) showed no significant difference in infections in 34 neutropenic children receiving either ciprofloxacin or placebo.

Organisms of the *Mycobacterium avium* complex (MAC) are ubiquitous in the environment. Patients with HIV infection and severely immunosuppressed (e.g., CD4+ T-lymphocyte counts <50/mm^3 if older than 6 years, <75/mm^3 for ages 2–6 years, <500/mm^3 for ages 1–2 years, <750/mm^3 for age <1 year) are at significant risk for disseminated infections and should receive chemoprophylaxis. The macrolide antibiotics clarithromycin twice daily or azithromycin once weekly or daily are the preferred agents (17). In a randomized, double-blind, placebo-controlled study of patients with acquired immunodeficiency syndrome (AIDS), Oldfield et al. (157) showed a 59% reduction in infections and a 68% survival benefit with azithromycin prophylaxis. A similar large multicenter trial of clarithromycin demonstrated a 69% reduction in MAC infections (158). Unfortunately, breakthrough infections are often macrolide resistant. Alternative regimens include rifabutin, which decreases infection incidence by about 50% but shows minimal survival benefits compared with the macrolides or rifabutin plus azithromycin (159).

The administration of broad-spectrum antibiotics for empiric or preventive therapy of infection in susceptible patients is an appealing concept. In selected settings, chemoprophylaxis or preemptive therapy may decrease the incidence rates of certain types of infection and perhaps some mortality and morbidity, such as episodes of fever and hospitalizations. With routine practice comes the risk of adverse drug reactions, including myelosuppression with some agents. Depending on the regimen selected, resistance among colonizing flora may be induced, and subsequent infections may become more difficult to treat. Indiscriminate use of these preventive strategies may accelerate this process, and caution should be exercised in selecting patients and regimens for consideration. Because of these concerns, no clear consensus has been reached concerning the use of prophylactic antibiotics in afebrile neutropenic children.

Antifungals

Fungal overgrowth and invasive infections are increasingly frequent complications of neutropenia. Such infections are closely associated with antibiotic prophylaxis and antibiotic therapy during febrile illnesses. To date, no single best method of prevention has been established. Candidiasis and aspergillosis are the most frequent fungal infections of concern in neutropenic patients, and fungemia has increased from 5% to 10% of nosocomial infections. In addition, endemic mycoses such as coccidioidomycosis, histoplasmosis, cryptococcosis, and penicilliosis may merit special attention in certain geographic areas. Agents that have been evaluated include nonabsorbable miconazole, clotrimazole, nystatin; oral, aerosolized, intranasal or systemic amphotericin B; and the azole agents fluconazole, ketoconazole, and itraconazole. Trials of antifungal prophylaxis are difficult to evaluate given the difficulty involved in diagnosing disease and the inconsistencies in disease definition.

Mucosal candida overgrowth in immunocompromised patients is of concern in terms of acute patient comfort and the theoretical risk of disseminated disease after damage to mucosal integrity. Nonabsorbable antifungal agents may reduce superficial colonization and local mucosal candidiasis. Trials of prophylaxis with nonabsorbable oral miconazole, clotrimazole, nystatin, and amphotericin B demonstrated inconsistent efficacy in preventing invasive candidiasis and until better data are available will be considered optional (17,160–166).

Systemic antifungal prophylactic strategies against invasive fungal infections in immunocompromised patients have been studied. Azole compounds offer some promise but are limited to some degree by their gastrointestinal side effects and impedement of the cytochrome p450 system, markedly affecting drug metabolism for many agents, including cyclosporine, some antihistamines, warfarin, and some anticonvulsants (167). The absorbable imidazole derivative ketoconazole has been demonstrated to have minimal effect in reducing invasive candidiasis (116,168,169). Newer orally available triazole agents appear to have some efficacy. The triazole fluconazole has been shown to reduce the incidence of mucosal and systemic candidal infections significantly in patients during and after bone marrow transplantation (170–173). Efficacy in neutropenic cancer chemotherapy patients is less convincing. Some trials demonstrated decreased colony counts of mucosal candida and episodes of oropharyngeal candidiasis and fever (173,174); however, these and other studies showed no effect on the incidence of systemic fungal infections or overall survival (164,173–175). One small study of 70 oncology patients by Yumac et al. (176) did show a decrease in systemic fungal infections patients receiving fluconazole 400 mg/day prophylaxis, but to date this result has not been replicated in a larger study.

With the increasing use of fluconazole, patient colonization with non-albicans *Candida* spp. such as *Torulopsis glabrata* and *Candida krusei* has increased (177). The prevalence of such non-albicans yeasts and *Aspergillus* spp. continues to increase as the infecting fungi of immunocompromised patients (1,14,15,16, 178). The newest oral triazole is itraconazole, which has activity against most yeasts, including *Candida, Torulopsis, Histoplasma,* and *Blastomyces* sp. as well as *Aspergillus* spp. Glasmacher et al. (179) performed a meta-analysis of itraconazole trials in patients with acute leukemia who were receiving chemotherapy; five of eight studies showed a reduction in invasive aspergillosis but in these studies historical controls received oral nonabsorbable antifungals or ketoconazole. The overall incidence of invasive fungal infections was decreased by 12%, although only three studies showed a statistically significant difference. A recent prospective study by Glasmacher et al. (180) showed a significant decrease in mortality from invasive fungal infections in leukemic patients receiving itraconazole compared with a nonprophylaxis control group. This study and others, including that by Lamy et al. (181), found that significant risk remains in patients with inadequate plasma intraconazole levels. The marked variations in plasma levels seen in all patients appear to be absorption dependent and are pronounced in bone marrow transplant patients, thus limiting the utility of this agent for chemoprophylaxis (182). Close monitoring of plasma levels in patients selected to receive itraconazole chemoprophylaxis is mandatory (183).

Amphotericin B was first introduced in the 1950s and remains the drug of choice for serious systemic fungal infections. This agent displays activity against a wide array of fungal organisms, including most *Candida, Torulopsis, Histoplasma, Blastomyces, Coccidioides,* and *Cryptococcus* yeast species as well as most *Aspergillus, Mucorales, Penicillium, Pseudoallescheria, Fusarium,* and *Malassezia* species (167). Because of concern over the increasing incidence of opportunistic infections by these previously unusual species, amphotericin B has been examined as a chemoprophylactic agent. Much of the limited efficacy data available are derived from trials of prophylaxis against invasive aspergillosis using a variety of low doses (0.1–0.25 mg/kg daily) compared with historical controls. Rousey et al. (184) demonstrated a significant reduction in incidence and mortality, from 14.5% to 5.5%, compared with historical controls, using a daily dose of 20 mg (0.15–0.25 mg/kg daily) for 186 patients during induction chemotherapy. Perfect et al. (185) randomized 182 neutropenic patients undergoing autologous bone marrow transplant to receive 0.1 mg/kg daily of amphotericin B or placebo. Although 6-week survival was greater using amphotericin B prophylaxis, the improved survival could not be attributed to prevention of fungal infections. In a retrospective review, O'Donnell et al. (186) found a reduction in invasive fungal infections in autologous transplant patients given extremely low-dose amphotericin B (5–10 mg/day) prior to high-dose corticosteroid prophylaxis for GVHD. Some studies suggested better efficacy in preventing mortality with the use of liposomal amphotericin B prophylaxis, but more investigation is required (187). Other modes of delivery, including intranasal and aerosol administration of amphotericin B to prevent inhalational aspergillus, showed no measurable reduction in disease (21,188). De Laurenzi et al. (166) reported a combination regimen that included intravenous, oral, and nebulized amphotericin B introduced in one institution after a dramatic increase in invasive fungal infections from 1.8% to greater than 20% was witnessed in high-risk patients. No cases of invasive fungal disease were seen in the subsequent 48 patients. Unfortunately, such limited data regarding safety and efficacy and a lack of extensive randomized controlled studies in high-risk immunocompromised hosts preclude an acceptable recommendation (1,189). Further investigation is required.

Antivirals

The most effective prevention of morbidity from viral pathogens in immunodeficient patients is to minimize contact with potential contagions and to maximize immunity to avoid primary infection. Many patients have been infected prior to their immunosuppressed state, however, with herpesviruses that may remain latent. Herpes simplex viruses (HSV) 1 and 2, varicella zoster virus (VZV), CMV, Epstein–Barr (EBV), and the human herpesviruses 6, 7, and 8 all may reactivate during periods of increased immunosuppression, causing significant mortality and morbidity. Antiviral agents may have some role in preventing reactivation by suppressing viral replication. All patients who can be anticipated to have periods of severe immunosuppression during intensive chemotherapy or transplantation should have serologic testing prior for CMV, EBV, HSV, and VZV.

Acyclovir has been demonstrated to have activity against many herpesviruses. A series of studies clearly demonstrated efficacy in reducing HSV reactivation and gingivostomatitis whether acyclovir is administered orally or intravenously (190–193). Patients with a history of recurrent herpes or seropositivity undergoing intensive immunosuppression should receive acyclovir until mucositis resolves or immunity improves. Acyclovir also displays activity against CMV and has been successfully administered in some centers for CMV suppression after autologous marrow transplantation or solid-organ transplants (194–196); however, some studies have suggested that acyclovir may not consistently prevent CMV reactivation after such transplants (197,198). Acyclovir also has been examined for the prophylaxis of varicella reactivation, but limited data suggest that zoster outbreaks are merely delayed rather than prevented; therefore, this agent is not routinely recommended (199,200).

Currently, intravenous ganciclovir is the only approved agent for prophylactic suppression of CMV. Randomized controlled trials demonstrated effective prevention from asymptomatic disease progression when CMV is cultured from body fluids (201,202). Ganciclovir has also been administered to CMV-seropositive stem cell transplant patients and appears to prevent reactivation of CMV (203). Currently, there are two accepted chemoprophylaxis strategies against CMV in transplant patients. Prophylaxis involves the administration of ganciclovir during the high-risk period of maximum immunosuppression and has been shown to be effective, although sometimes myelosuppression is a complication (197,203,204). Preemptive therapy requires highly sensitive laboratory monitoring techniques to diagnose active CMV and then initiate ganciclovir administration promptly (205). Both techniques have been shown to be effective, and trials and wider clinical use of each are now seen in patients receiving hematopoietic stem cell, liver, heart, lung, and kidney transplants (206).

Oral ganciclovir has been studied in HIV patients and may be considered for prophylaxis in seropositive patients with severe immunodeficiency (CD4+ T-lymphocytes <50/mm^3). Use is limited by myelosuppression, limited efficacy, and cost (17). In patients with CMV retinitis, suppression after primary therapy is recommended, and regimens include intravenous ganciclovir, foscarnet, and intraocular ganciclovir implants (17).

Although other antiviral agents are effective in treatment regimens for many of the herpesviruses, they are not commonly used in chemoprophylaxis regimens. Valacyclovir and famciclovir are oral acyclovir prodrugs with excellent absorption, bioavailability, and activity against HSV, but safety and efficacy data in immunosuppressed patients are limited. Oral ganciclovir is recommended for specific HIV patients who require lifelong prophylaxis, but it is not routinely used in other chemoprophylaxis settings. Foscarnet, cidofovir, and newer agents all may prove to have a role in viral chemoprophylaxis, but further investigation is needed.

Other Settings for Chemoprophylaxis

A different scenario evolves for the persistently immunocompromised patient after treatment for a documented opportunistic infection because the risk of recurrence is significantly increased. HIV patients and patients entering transplantation or continuing chemotherapy for oncologic disorders represent the largest groups of such patients. Specific infections of concern include documented PCP, *T. gondii* encephalitis, MAC, *Cryptococcus neoformans, Histoplasma capsulatum, Coccidioides immitis,* CMV end-organ disease, and *Salmonella* bacteremias. Chemoprophylactic agents are chosen based on specific organisms and antimicrobial susceptibilities whenever possible. For HIV-infected patients, such prophylaxis is generally continued for life (17). Individual decisions concerning the duration of prophylaxis must be made for other immunocompromised patients (1,136,207–209). Prophylaxis also can be considered after recurrent severe episodes of invasive bacterial infections, herpes simplex virus, and candidiasis.

Systemic antibiotic chemoprophylaxis is indicated for patients who are at risk for endocarditis or who are particularly susceptible to severe infection during procedures known to result in high rates of bacteremia. Guidelines for the prevention of bacterial endocarditis in patients with underlying cardiac conditions are reviewed and published periodically by the American Heart Association. Many complex congenital heart lesions, valvular defects, and postoperative shunts are associated with endocarditis. Prophylaxis is recommended based on the severity of the underlying lesion (high, moderate, or negligible risk), the potential for bacteremia, and the organisms involved from the particular procedure. For dental, oral, respiratory, or esophageal sites, oral prophylaxis for common colonizing organisms is sufficient when tolerated. Amoxicillin is considered standard, with alternatives including clindamycin, first-generation cephalosporins, and macrolides for penicillin-allergic patients.

For procedures involving the genitourinary and gastrointestinal tracts, the risk of enteric pathogens and bacteremia is significantly higher, with enterococci representing the most substantial risk for endocarditis. For this reason, moderate-risk patients can be administered amoxicillin alone, either parenterally or orally. High-risk patients should receive parenteral agents with broader coverage of enteric organisms, generally with ampicillin and gentamicin. Intravenous vancomycin is substituted in both groups for penicillin-allergic patients (210). The addition of parenteral metronidazole is recommended for neutropenic patients undergoing endoscopy because of the particular risks of anaerobic infection (211).

REFERENCES

1. Hughes WT, Armstrong D, Bodey GP, et al. 1997 Guidelines for the use of antimicrobial agents in neutropenic patients with fever. *Clin Infect Dis* 1997;25: 551–573.
2. Oppenheim BA. The changing pattern of infection in neutropenic patients. *J Antimicrob Chemother* 1998;41 (Suppl D):7–11.
3. Spanik S, Trupl J, Kunova A, et al. Risk factors, aetiology, therapy and outcome in 123 episodes of breakthrough bacteraemia and fungaemia during antimicrobial prophylaxis and therapy in cancer patients. *J Med Microbiol* 1997;46:517–523.
4. Pagano L, Tacconelli E, Tumbarello M, et al. Bacteremia in patients with hematological malignancies:

analysis of risk factors, etiological agents and prognostic indicators. *Haematologica* 1997;82:415–419.

5. Krupova I, Kaiserova E, Foltinova A, et al. Bacteremia and fungemia in pediatric versus adult cancer patients after chemotherapy: comparison of etiology, risk factors and outcome. *J Chemother* 1998;10:236–242.

6. Horvathova Z, Spanik S, Suflairsky J, et al. Bacteremia due to methicillin-resistant staphylcocci occurs more frequently in neutropenic patients who received antimicrobial prophylaxis and is associated with higher mortality in comparison to methicillin-sensitive bacteremia. *Int J Antimicrob Agents* 1998;10:55–58.

7. Spanik S, Trupl J, Kunova A, et al. Viridans streptococcal bacteraemia due to penicillin-resistant and penicillin-sensitive streptococci: analysis of risk factors and outcome in 60 patients from a single cancer centre before and after penicillin is used for prophylaxis. *Scand J Infect Dis* 1997;29:245–249.

8. Kukockova E, Spanik S, Ilavska I, et al. Staphylococcal bacteremia in cancer patients: risk factors and outcome in 134 episodes prior to and after introduction of quinolones into infection prevention in neutropenia. *Support Care Cancer* 1996;4:427–434.

9. Carratala J, Alcaide F, Fernandez-Sevilla A, et al. Bacteremia due to viridans streptococci that are highly resistant to penicillin: increase among neutropenic patients with cancer. *Clin Infect Dis* 1995;20:1169–1173.

10. Plessis P, Lamy T, Donnio PY, et al. Epidemiologic analysis of glycopeptide-resistant *Enterococcus* strains in neutropenic patients receiving prolonged vancomycin administration. *Eur J Clin Microbiol Infect Dis* 1995;14:959–963.

11. Cometta A, Calandra T, Bille J, et al. *Escherichia coli* resistant to fluoroquinolones in patients with cancer and neutropenia. *N Engl J Med* 1994;330:1240–1241.

12. Krcmery V Jr, Spanik S, Krupova I, et al. Bacteremia due to multiresistant gram-negative bacilli in neutropenic cancer patients: a case control study. *J Chemother* 1998;10:320–325.

13. Martina R, Subira M, Altes A, et al. Effect of discontinuing prophylaxis with norfloxacin in patients with hematologic malignancies and severe neutropenia: a matched case-control study of the effect on infectious morbidity. *Acta Haematol* 1998;99:206–211.

14. Orovcova E, Lacka J, Drgona L, et al. Funguria in cancer patients: analysis of risk factors, clinical presentation and outcome in 50 patients. *Infection* 1996;24: 319–323.

15. Hung CC, Chen YC, Chang SC, et al. Nosocomial candidemia in a university hospital in Taiwan. *J Formos Med Assoc* 1996;95:19–28.

16. Nucci M, Silveira MI, Spector N, et al. Fungemia in cancer patients in Brazil: predominance of non-albicans species. *Mycopathologia* 1998;141:65–68.

17. Centers for Disease Control and Prevention. 1997 USPHS/IDSA guidelines for the prevention of opportunistic infections in persons infected with human immunodeficiency virus. *MMWR Morb Mortal Wkly Rep* 1997;46(RR-12):1–46.

18. American Academy of Pediatrics. HIV Infection. In: Peter G, ed. *2000 Red book:* report of the Committee on Infectious Diseases, 25th ed. Elk Grove Village, IL: American Academy of Pediatrics, 2000:325–350.

19. Garner JS, Favero MS. CDC Guidelines for the prevention and control of nosocomial infections: guide-line for handwashing and hospital environmental control, 1985. *Am J Infect Control* 1986;14:110–129.

20. Pizzo PA, Rubin M, Freifeld A, et al. The child with cancer and infection. I. Empiric therapy for fever and neutropenia, and preventive strategies. *J Pediatr* 1991; 119:679–694.

21. Withington S, Chambers ST, Beard ME, et al. Invasive aspergillosis in severely neutropenic patients over 18 years: impact of intranasal amphotericin B and HEPA filtration. *J Hosp Infect* 1998;38:11–18.

22. Centers for Disease Control and Prevention. Guidelines for prevention of nosocomial pneumonia. *MMWR Morb Mortal Wkly Rep* 1997;46(RR-1):1–79.

23. Krasinski K, Holzman RS, Hanna B, et al. Nosocomial fungal infection during hospital renovation. *Infect Control Hosp Epidemiol* 1985;6:278–282.

24. Pearson ML, Hospital Infection Control Practices Advisory Committee. Guidelines for prevention of intravascular device related infections. *Am J Infect Control* 1996;24:262–293.

25. Garner JS. CDC Guidelines for the prevention and control of nosocomial infections: guidelines for the prevention of surgical wound infections, 1985. *Am J Infect Control* 1986;14:71–82.

26. Walsh TJ, Dison DM. Nosocomial aspergillosis: environmental microbiology, hospital epidemiology, diagnosis and treatment. *Eur J Epidemiol* 1989;5:131–142.

27. Centers for Disease Control and Prevention. Immunization of health care workers: Recommendations of the Advisory Committee on Immunization Practices (ACIP) and the Hospital Infection Control Practices Advisory Committee. *MMWR Morb Mortal Wkly Rep* 1997;46(RR-18):1–42.

28. Bolyard EA, Tablan OC, Williams WW, et al. Guideline for infection control in healthcare personnel, 1998. *Infect Control Hosp Epidemiol* 1998;19: 407–463.

29. Garner JS. Hospital Infection Control Practices Advisory Committee. Guidelines for isolation precautions in hospitals. *Infect Control Hosp Epidemiol* 1996;17: 53–80.

30. American Academy of Pediatrics. Infection control for hospitalized children. In: Peter G, ed. *2000 Red book:* report of the Committee on Infectious Diseases, 25th ed. Elk Grove Village, IL: American Academy of Pediatrics, 2000:127–137.

31. American Academy of Pediatrics. Sexually transmitted Diseases. In: Peter G, ed. *2000 Red book:* report of the committee on infectious diseases, 25th ed. Elk Grove Village, IL: American Academy of Pediatrics, 2000: 138–147.

32. Elliott DL, Tolle SW, Goldberg L, et al. Pet-associated illness. *N Engl J Med* 1985;313:985–994.

33. Centers for Disease Control and Prevention. Outbreak of Campylobacter enteritis associated with cross-contamination of food - Oklahoma, 1996. *MMWR Morb Mortal Wkly Rep* 1996;47:129–131.

34. Centers for Disease Control and Prevention. Poliomyelitis prevention in the United States: introduction of a sequential vaccination schedule of inactivated poliovirus vaccine followed by oral poliovirus vaccine. Recommendations of the Advisory Committee on Immunization Practices (ACIP). *MMWR Morb Mortal Wkly Rep* 1997;46(RR-3):1–25.

35. Centers for Disease Control and Prevention. Prevention

of varicella: recommendations of the Advisory Committee on Immunization Practices (ACIP). *MMWR Morb Mortal Wkly Rep* 1996;45(RR-11):1–36.

36. Perez-Schael I, Guntinas MJ, Perez M, et al. Efficacy of the rhesus rotavirus based quadrivalent vaccine in infants and young children in Venezuela. *N Engl J Med* 1997;337:1181–1187.

37. Centers for Disease Control and Prevention. Prevention and control of influenza: recommendations of the Advisory Committee on Immunization Practices (ACIP). *MMWR Morb Mortal Wkly Rep* 1998;47(RR-6):1–20.

38. Centers for Disease Control and Prevention. Use of vaccines and immune globulins in persons with altered immunocompetence: recommendations of the Advisory Committee on Immunization Practices (ACIP). *MMWR Morb Mortal Wkly Rep* 1993;42(RR-4):1–18.

39. American Academy of Pediatrics. Active and Passive Immunization. In: Peter G, ed. *2000 Red book:* report of the Committee on Infectious Diseases, 25th ed. Elk Grove Village, IL: American Academy of Pediatrics, 2000:1–81.

40. Centers for Disease Control and Prevention. Rotavirus vaccine for the prevention of rotavirus gastroenteritis among children: recommendations of the Advisory Committee on Immunization Practices (ACIP). *MMWR Morb Mortal Wkly Rep* 1999;48(RR-2):1–20.

41. American Academy of Pediatrics. Pneumococcal Infections. In: Peter G, ed. *2000 Red book:* report of the Committee on Infectious Diseases, 25th ed. Elk Grove Village, IL: American Academy of Pediatrics, 2000:452–460.

42. American Academy of Pediatrics. Meningococcal Infections. In: Peter G, ed. *2000 Red book:* report of the Committee on Infectious Diseases, 25th ed. Elk Grove Village, IL: American Academy of Pediatrics, 2000:396–401.

43. Centers for Disease Control and Prevention. Control and prevention of meningococcal disease: recommendations of the Advisory Committee on Immunization Practices (ACIP). *MMWR Morb Mortal Wkly Rep* 1997;46(RR-5):1–10.

44. Rennels MB, Edwards KM, Keyserling HL. Safety and immunogenicity of heptavalent pneumococcal vaccine conjugated to CRM197 in United States infants. *Pediatrics* 1998;101:604–611.

45. Gibb D, Spoulou V, Giacomelli A, et al. Antibody responses to *Haemophilus influenzae* type b and *Streptococcus pneumoniae* vaccines in children with human immunodeficiency virus infection. *Pediatr Infect Dis J* 1995;14:129–135.

46. Peters VB, Diamont EP, Hodes DS, et al. Impaired immunity to pneumococcal polysaccharide antigens in children with human immunodeficiency virus immunized with pneumococcal vaccine. *Pediatr Infect Dis J* 1994;13:933–934.

47. Kroon FP, van Dissel JT, de Jong JC, et al. Antibody response to influenza, tetanus and pneumococcal vaccines in HIV-seropositive individuals in relation to CD4+ lymphocytes. *AIDS* 1994;8:469–476.

48. O'Brien WA, Grovit-Ferbas K, Namazi A, et al. Human immunodeficiency virus-type 1 replication can be increased in peripheral blood of seropositive patients after influenza vaccination. *Blood* 1995;86:1082–1089.

49. Lum LG. The kinetics of immune reconstitution after human marrow transplantation. *Blood* 1987;69:369–380.

50. Somani J, Larson RA. Reimmunization after allogeneic bone marrow transplantation. *Am J Med* 1995;98:389–398.

51. Henning KJ, White MH, Sepkowitz KA, et al. A national survey of immunization practices following allogeneic bone marrow transplantation. *JAMA* 1997;277:1148–1151.

52. NIH Consensus Conference. Intravenous immunoglobulin: prevention and treatment of disease. *JAMA* 1990;264:3189–3193.

53. Sullivan KM, Kopecky KJ, Jocom J, et al. Immunomodulatory and antimicrobial efficacy of intravenous immunoglobulin in bone marrow transplantation. *N Engl J Med* 1990;323:705–712.

54. Wolff SN, Fay JW, Herzig RH, et al. High-dose weekly intravenous immunoglobulin to prevent infections in patients undergoing autologous bone marrow transplantation or severe myelosuppressive therapy. *Ann Intern Med* 1993;113:937–942.

55. Working Group on Antiretroviral Therapy: National Pediatric HIV Resource Center. Antiretroviral therapy and medical management of the human immunodeficiency virus-infected child. *Pediatr Infect Dis J* 1993;12:513–522.

56. The National Institute of Child Health and Human Development Intravenous Immunoglobulin Study Group. Intravenous immune globulin for the prevention of bacterial infections in children with symptomatic human immunodeficiency virus infection. *N Engl J Med* 1991;325:73–80.

57. Englund JAQ, Piedra PA, Whimbey E. Prevention and treatment of respiratory syncytial virus and parainfluenza viruses in immunocompromised patients. *Am J Med* 1996;102:61–70.

58. La Pine TR, Cates KL, Hill HR. Immunomodulating agents. In: Feigen RD, Cherry JD, eds. *Textbook of pediatric infectious diseases.* Philadelphia: WB Saunders, 1998:2719–2729.

59. Lau AS, Lehman D, Geertsma FR, et al. Biology and therapeutic uses of myeloid hematopoietic growth factors and interferons. *Pediatr Infect Dis J* 1996;15:563–575.

60. The International Chronic Granulomatous Disease Cooperative Study Group. A controlled trial of interferon gamma to prevent infection in chronic granulomatous disease. *N Engl J Med* 1991;324:509–516.

61. Furman WL, Fairclough DL, Huhn RD, et al. Therapeutic effects and pharmacokinetics of recombinant human granulocyte-macrophage colony-stimulating factor in childhood cancer patients receiving myelosuppressive chemotherapy. *J Clin Oncol* 1991;9:1022–1028.

62. Gutterman J, Vadhan-Raj S, Logothetis C, et al. Effects of granulocyte-macrophage colony-stimulating factor in iatrogenic myelosuppression, bone marrow failure, and regulation of host defense. *Semin Hematol* 1990;27:15–24.

63. Beveridge RA, Miler JA, Kales AN, et al. Randomized trial comparing the tolerability of sargramostim (yeast-derived RhuGM-CSF) and filgrastim (bacteria-derived RhuG-CSF) in cancer patients receiving myelosuppressive chemotherapy. *Support Care Cancer* 1997;5:289–298.

64. Wexler LH, Weaver-McClure L, Steinberg SM, et al.

Randomized trial of recombinant human granulocyte-macrophage colony stimulating factor in pediatric patients receiving intensive myelosuppressive chemotherapy. *J Clin Oncol* 1996;14:901–910.

65. Riikonen P, Saarinen UM, Makipernaa A, et al. Recombinant human granulocyte-macrophage colony-stimulating factor in the treatment of febrile neutropenia: a double blind placebo-controlled study in children. *Pediatr Infect Dis J* 1994;13:197–202.

66. Smith TJ. Economic analysis of the clinical uses of the colony-stimulating factors. *Curr Opin Hematol* 1996; 3:175–179.

67. American Society of Clinical Oncology. Update of recommendations for the use of hematopoietic colony-stimulating factors: evidence-based, clinical practice guidelines. *J Clin Oncol* 1996;14:1957–1960.

68. Socinski M, Elias A, Schnipper L, et al. Granulocyte-macrophage colony stimulating factor expands the circulating haemopoietic progenitor cell compartment in man. *Lancet* 1988;1:1194–1198.

69. Haas R, Ho A, Bredthauer U, et al. Successful autologous transplantation of blood stem cells mobilized with recombinant human granulocyte-macrophage colony-stimulating factor. *Exp Hematol* 1990;8:94–98.

70. Grigg A, Vecchi L, Bardy P, et al. G-CSF stimulated donor granulocyte collections for prophylaxis and therapy of neutropenic sepsis. *Aust N Z J Med* 1996; 16:813–818.

71. Kodo H, Tajika K, Takahashi S, et al. Acceleration of neutrophilic granulocyte recovery after bone-marrow transplantation by administration of recombinant human granulocyte colony-stimulating factor. *Lancet* 1988;2:38–39.

72. Nemunaitis J, Rabinowe SN, Singa JW, et al. Recombinant granulocyte-macrophage colony stimulating factor after autologous bone marrow transplantation for lymphoid cancer. *N Engl J Med* 1991;324:1773–1778.

73. Locatelli F, Pession A, Zecca M, et al. Use of recombinant human granulocyte colony-stimulating factor in children given allogeneic bone marrow transplantation for acute or chronic leukemia. *Bone Marrow Transplant* 1996;17:31–37.

74. Martin-Algarra S, Bishop MR, Tarantolo S, et al. Hematopoietic growth factors after HLA-identical allogeneic bone marrow transplantation in patients treated with methotrexate-containing graft-vs.-host disease prophylaxis. *Exp Hematol* 1995;23:1503–1508.

75. Nemunaitis J, Singer JW, Buckner CD, et al. Use of recombinant human granulocyte-macrophage colony-stimulating factor in graft failure after bone marrow transplantation. *Blood* 1990;76:245–253.

76. Groopman JE, Mitsuyasu RT, DeLeo MJ, et al. Effect of recombinant human granulocyte-macrophage colony-stimulating factor on myelopoiesis in the acquired immunodeficiency syndrome. *N Engl J Med* 1987;317:593–598.

77. Keiser R, Rademacher S, Smith JW, et al. Granulocyte colony-stimulating factor use is associated with decreased bacteremia and increased survival in neutropenic HIV-infected patients. *Am J Med* 1998;104:48–55.

78. Hammer SM, Gillis JM, Groopman JE, et al. *In vitro* modification of human immunodeficiency virus infection by granulocyte-macrophage colony-stimulating factor and gamma interferon. *Proc Natl Acad Sci USA* 1986;83:8734–8738.

79. Scadden DT, Pikus O, Hammer SH, et al. Lack of *in vivo* effect of granulocyte-macrophage colony-stimulating factor on human immunodeficiency virus type 1. *AIDS Res Hum Retroviruses* 1996;12:1151–1159.

80. Bonilla MA, Gillio AP, Ruggiero M, et al. Effects of recombinant human granulocyte-macrophage colony-stimulating factor on neutropenia in patients with congenital agranulocytosis. *N Engl J Med* 1989;320:1574–1580.

81. Hammond WP, Price TH, Souza LM, Dale DC. Treatment of cyclic neutropenia with granulocyte colony-stimulating factor. *N Engl J Med* 1989;320:1306–1311.

82. Wright DG, Kenny RF, Oette DH, et al. Contrasting effects of recombinant human granulocyte-macrophage colony-stimulating factor (CSF) and granulocyte CSF treatment of cycling blood elements in childhood-onset cyclic neutropenia. *Blood* 1994;84:1257–1267.

83. Bux J, Behrens G, Jaeger G, Welte K. Diagnosis and clinical course of autoimmune neutropenia in infancy: analysis of 240 cases. *Blood* 1998;91:181–186.

84. Roberts RL, Szelc CM, Scates SM, et al. Neutropenia in an extremely premature infant treated with recombinant human granulocyte colony-stimulating factor. *Am J Dis Child* 1991;145:808–812.

85. Gillan ER, Christensen RD, Suen Y, et al. A randomized placebo-controlled trial of recombinant human granulocyte colony-stimulating factor administration in newborn infants with presumed sepsis: significant induction of peripheral and bone marrow neutrophilia. *Blood* 1994;84:1427–1433.

86. Schroten H, Roesler J, Breidenbach T, et al. Granulocyte and granulocyte-macrophage colony-stimulating factors for treatment of neutropenia in glycogen storage disease type 1b. *J Pediatr* 1991;119:748–754.

87. Acachi N, Tsuchiya H, Nuoi H, et al. RhG-CSF for Shwachman's syndrome. *Lancet* 1990;336:1136–1137.

88. Guinan EC, Lopez KD, Huhn RD, et al. Evaluation of granulocyte-macrophage colony stimulating factor for treatment of pancytopenia in children with Fanconi anemia. *J Pediatr* 1994;124:144–150.

89. Storring RA, Jameson B, McElwain TJ, et al. Oral nonabsorbed antibiotics prevent infection in acute non-lymphoblastic leukemia. *Lancet* 1977;2:837–840.

90. Bender JF, Schimpff SC, Young VM, et al. A comparative trial of tobramycin vs. gentamicin in combination with vancomycin and nystatin for alimentary tract suppression in leukemia patients. *Eur J Cancer* 1979;15:35–44.

91. Muis N, Kamps WA, Dankert J. Prevention of infection in children with acute leukaemia: no major difference between total and selective bowel decontamination. *Support Care Cancer* 1996;4:200–206.

92. Fruchart C, Salah A, Gray C, et al. *Lactobacillus* species as emerging pathogens in neutropenic patients. *Eur J Clin Microbiol Infect Dis* 1997;16:681–684.

93. Enno A, Catovsky D, Darrel J, et al. Co-trimoxazole for prevention of infection in acute leukemia. *Lancet* 1978;2:395–397.

94. Gurwith MJ, Brunton JL, Lank BA, et al. A prospective controlled investigation of prophylactic trimethoprim/sulfamethoxazole in hospitalized granulocytopenic patients. *Am J Med* 1979;66:248–256.

95. Gaya H, Glauser M, Klastersky J, et al. Double-blind placebo-controlled trial of prophylactic trimethoprim and sulfamethoxazole for the prevention of infection in granulocytopenic patients. Presented at: *20th Interscience Conference on Antimicrobial Agents and Chemotherapy*; New Orleans; 1980(abst 331).

96. Malarme M, Meunier-Carpentier F, Klastersky J. Vancomycin plus gentamicin and cotrimoxazole for prevention of infection in neutropenic cancer patients. *Eur J Cancer Clin Oncol* 1981;17:1315–1322.

97. Sleijfer DT, Mulder NH, de Vries-Hospers HG, et al. Infection prevention in granulocytopenic patients by selective decontamination of the digestive tract. *Eur J Cancer* 1980;16:859–869.

98. Dekker AW, Rozenberg-Arska M, Sixma JJ, et al. Prevention of infection by trimethoprim-sulfamethoxazole plus amphotericin B in patients with acute non-lymphocytic leukemia. *Ann Intern Med* 1981;95:555–559.

99. Wade JC, Schimpff SC, Hargadon MT, et al. A comparison of trimethoprim-sulfamethoxazole plus nystatin with gentamicin plus nystatin in the prevention of infections in acute leukemia. *N Engl J Med* 1981;304:1057–1062.

100. Weiser B, Lange M, Fialk MA, et al. Prophylactic trimethoprim-sulfamethoxazole during consolidation chemotherapy for acute leukemia: a controlled trial. *Ann Intern Med* 1981;95:436–438.

101. Calvo F, Marty M, Lepors JS, et al. Antibiotic prophylaxis against infections in acute leukemia. *N Engl J Med* 1981;305:583–584.

102. Preisler HD, Early A, Hrymiuk W. Prevention of infection and bleeding in leukemia patients receiving intensive remission maintenance therapy. *Med Pediatr Oncol* 1981;9:511–521.

103. Zinner S, Gaya H, Glauser M, et al. Cotrimoxazole and reduction of risk of infection in neutropenic patients: a progress report. Presented at: *12th Interscience Conference on Antimicrobial Agents and Chemotherapy*; Chicago; 1981(abst 795).

104. Gurwith M, Truog K, Hinthorn E, et al. Trimethoprim-sulfamethoxazole and trimethoprim alone for prophylaxis of infection in granulocytopenic patients. *Rev Infect Dis* 1982;4:593–601.

105. Watson JG, Jameson B, Powles RL, et al. Cotrimoxazole versus nonabsorbable antibiotics in acute leukemia. *Lancet* 1982;1:6–9.

106. Starke ID, Donnelly P, Catovsky D, et al. Co-trimoxazole alone for prevention of bacterial infection in patients with acute leukemia. *Lancet* 1982;1:5–6.

107. Scaglione C, Tormena AM, Pavlovsky S. Estudios controlados de profilaxis con cotrimoxasol en pacientes neutropenicos afebriles con hemopatias malignas. *Sangre* 1982;27:912–918.

108. Pizzo PA, Robichaud KJ, Edwards BK, et al. Oral antibiotic prophylaxis in patients with cancer: a double blind randomized placebo-controlled trial. *J Pediatr* 1983;102:125–133.

109. Gualtieri RJ, Donowitz GR, Kaiser DL, et al. Double-blind randomized study of prophylactic trimethoprim/sulfamethoxazole in granulocytopenic patients with hematologic malignancies. *Am J Med* 1983;74:934–940.

110. Riben PD, Louie TJ, Lank BA, et al. Reduction in mortality from gram-negative sepsis in neutropenic patients receiving trimethoprim/sulfamethoxazole therapy. *Cancer* 1983;51:1587–1592.

111. Kauffman CA, Liepman MK, Bergman AG, et al. Trimethoprim/sulfamethoxazole prophylaxis in neutropenic patients. *Am J Med* 1983;74:599–607.

112. Wade JC, de Jongh CA, Newman KA, et al. Selective antimicrobial modulation as prophylaxis against infection during granulocytopenia: trimethoprim/sulfamethoxazole vs. nalidixic acid. *J Infect Dis* 1983;147:624–634.

113. Inoue M, Arai S, Kamiya H, et al. The prophylactic effect of trimethoprim-sulfamethoxazole against infection among children with acute leukemia. *Rinsho Ketsueki* 1983;24:26–33.

114. Rozenberg-Arska M, Dekker AW, Verhoef J. Colistin and trimethoprim-sulfamethoxazole for the prevention of infection in patients with acute non-lymphocytic leukemia: decrease in the emergence of resistant bacteria. *Infection* 1983;11:167–169.

115. de Jongh CA, Wade JC, Finley RS, et al. Trimethoprim-sulfamethoxazole versus placebo: a double-blind comparison of infection prophylaxis in patients with small cell carcinoma of the lung. *J Clin Oncol* 1983;1:302–307.

116. Estey E, Maksymiuk A, Smith T, et al. Infection prophylaxis in acute leukemia: comparative effectiveness of sulfamethoxazole and trimethoprim, ketoconazole and a combination of the two. *Arch Intern Med* 1984;144:1562–1568.

117. Hughes WT, Patterson G. Post-sepsis prophylaxis in cancer patients. *Cancer* 1984;53:137–141.

118. Henry S. Chemoprophylaxis of bacterial infections in granulocytopenic patients. *Am J Med* 1984;76:645–651.

119. EORTC International Antimicrobial Therapy Project Group. Trimethoprim-sulfamethoxazole in prevention of infection in neutropenic patients. *J Infect Dis* 1984;150:372–379.

120. Lange B, Halpern S, Gale G, et al. Trimethoprim-sulfamethoxazole and nystatin prophylaxis in children with acute lymphoblastic leukemia. *Eur Paediatr Hematol Oncol* 1984;1:231–238.

121. Kovatch AL, Wald ER, Albo VC, et al. Oral trimethoprim/sulfamethoxazole for prevention of bacterial infection during the induction phase of cancer chemotherapy in children. *Pediatrics* 1985;76:754–758.

122. Goorin AM, Hershey BJ, Levin MJ, et al. Use of trimethoprim-sulfamethoxazole to prevent bacterial infections in children with acute lymphoblastic leukemia. *Pediatr Infect Dis J* 1985;4:265–269.

123. Van Eys J, Berry DM, Crist W, et al. Effect of trimethoprim/sulfamethoxazole prophylaxis on outcome of childhood lymphocytic leukemia. *Cancer* 1987;59:15–23.

124. Bow EJ, Rayner E, Louie TJ. Comparison of norfloxacin with cotrimazole for infectious prophylaxis in acute leukemia. *Am J Med* 1988;84:847–854.

125. Ward TT, Ochi S, James K. Double-blind randomized trial of oral prophylactic TMP/SMZ for infection, in acute leukemia. Presented at: *28th Interscience Conference on Antimicrobial Agents and Chemotherapy*; Los Angeles; 1988(abst 1204)..

126. Cruciani M, Concia E, Navarra A, et al. Prophylactic cotrimazole versus norfloxacin in neutropenic chil-

dren: prospective randomized study. *Infection* 1989; 17:65–69.

127. Verhoef J, Rozenberg-Arska M, Dekker A. Prevention of infection in the neutropenic patient. *Rev Infect Dis* 1989;11:S1545–S1550.

128. Liang RH, Yung RW, Chan TK, et al. Ofloxacin versus co-trimazole for prevention of infection in neutropenic patients following cytotoxic chemotherapy. *Antimicrob Agents Chemother* 1990;34:215–218.

129. Kern W, Kurrle E. Ofloxacin versus trimethoprim-sulfamethoxazole for prevention of infection in patients with acute leukemia and granulocytopenia. *Infection* 1991;75:541–545.

130. Ward TT, Thomas RG, Fye CL, et al. Trimethoprim-sulfamethoxazole prophylaxis in granulocytopenic patients with acute leukemia: evaluation of serum antibiotic levels in a randomized, double-blind, placebo-controlled Department of Veteran Affairs Cooperative Study. *Clin Infect Dis* 1993;17:323–332.

131. Murase T. Chemoprophylaxis of bacterial infections in granulocytopenic patients with new quinolone: a comparison of trimethoprim-sulfamethoxazole (ST) alone with ST plus ciprofloxacin. *Kansenshogaku Zasshi* 1995;69:28–32.

132. Lew MA, Kehoe K, Ritz J, et al. Ciprofloxacin versus trimethoprim/sulfamethoxazole for prophylaxis of bacterial infections in bone marrow transplant recipients: a randomized, controlled trial. *J Clin Oncol* 1995; 13:239–250.

133. Imrie KR, Prince HM, Couture F, et al. Effect of antimicrobial prophylaxis on hematopoietic recovery following autologous bone marrow transplantation: ciprofloxacin versus co-trimazole. *Bone Marrow Transplant* 1995;15:267–270.

134. Hughes WT, Rivera GK, Schell MJ, et al. Successful intermittent chemoprophylaxis for *Pneumocystis carinii* pneumonitis. *N Engl J Med* 1987;316:1627–1632.

135. American Academy of Pediatrics. *Pneumocystis carinii* infection. In: Peter G, ed. *2000 Red book: report of the Committee on Infectious Diseases*, 25th ed. Elk Grove Village, IL: American Academy of Pediatrics, 2000:460–465.

136. Centers for Disease Control and Prevention. 1995 Revised guidelines for prophylaxis against *Pneumocystis carinii* pneumonia for children infected with or perinatally exposed to human immunodeficiency virus. *MMWR Morb Mortal Wkly Rep* 1995;44(RR-4):1–11.

137. Caumes E, Guermonprez G, Lecomte C, et al. Efficacy and safety of desensitization with sulfamethoxazole and trimethoprim in 48 previously hypersensitive patients infected with human immunodeficiency virus. *Arch Dermatol* 1997;133:465–469.

138. Yeung KT, Chan M, Chan CK. The safety of i.v. pentamidine administered in an ambulatory setting. *Chest* 1996;110:136–140.

139. Teira R, Virosta M, Monoz J, et al. The safety of pyremethamine and sulfadoxine for the prevention of *Pneumocystis carinii* pneumonia. *Scand J Infect Dis* 1997;29:595–596.

140. Winston DJ, Ho WG, Nakao SL, et al. Norfloxacin versus vancomycin/polymyxin for prevention of infections in granulocytopenic patients. *Am J Med* 1986; 80:884–890.

141. Dekker AW, Rozenberg-Arska M, Verhoef J. Infection prophylaxis in acute leukemia: a comparison of ciprofloxacin with trimethoprim-sulfamethoxazole and colistin. *Ann Intern Med* 1987;106:7–12.

142. Karp JE, Merz WG, Hendricksen C, et al. Oral norfloxacin for prevention of Gram negative bacterial infections in patients with acute leukemia and granulocytopenia: a randomized double-blind, placebo-controlled trial. *Ann Intern Med* 1987;106:1–7.

143. Winston DJ, Ho WG, Bruckner DA, et al. Ofloxacin versus vancomycin/polymyxin for prevention of infections in granulocytopenic patients. *Am J Med* 1990; 88:36–42.

144. The GIMEMA Infection Program. Prevention of bacterial infection in neutropenic patients with hematologic malignancies: a randomized, multicenter trial comparing norfloxacin with ciprofloxacin. *Ann Intern Med* 1991;115:7–12.

145. Lew MA, Kehoe K, Ritz J, et al. Prophylaxis of bacterial infections with ciprofloxacin in patients undergoing bone marrow transplantation. *Transplantation* 1991;51:630–636.

146. Patrick CC, Adair JR, Warner WC Jr, et al. Safety of ciprofloxacin as a prophylactic agent for prevention of bacterial infections in pediatric bone marrow transplant (BMT) patients. Presented at: *35th Interscience Conference on Antimicrobial Agents and Chemotherapy*, Washington DC, 1995 (abst LM17).

147. Cruciani M, Rampazzo R, Malena M, et al. Prophylaxis with fluoroquinolones for bacterial infections in neutropenic patients. *Clin Infect Dis* 1997;25:346–348.

148. Engels EA, Lau J, Barza M. Efficacy of quinolone prophylaxis in neutropenic cancer patients: a meta-analysis. *J Clin Oncol* 1998;16:1179–1187.

149. Spanik S, Trupl J, Ilavska I, et al. Bacteremia and fungemia occurring during antimicrobial prophylaxis with ofloxacin in cancer patients: risk factors, etiology and outcome. *J Chemother* 1996;8:387–93.

150. International Antimicrobial Therapy Cooperative Group of the European Organization for Research and Treatment of Cancer. Reduction of fever and streptococcal bacteremia in granulocytopenic patients with cancer: a trial of oral penicillin V or placebo combined with pefloxacin. *JAMA* 1994;272:1183–1189.

151. Fanci R, Leoni F, Bosi A, et al. Chemoprophylaxis of bacterial infections in granulocytopenic patients with ciprofloxacin vs. ciprofloxacin plus amoxicillin. *J Chemother* 1993;5:119–123.

152. Hidalgo M, Hornedo J, Lumbreras C, et al. Lack of ability of ciprofloxacin-rifampin prophylaxis to decrease infection-related morbidity in neutropenic patients given cytotoxic therapy and peripheral blood stem cell transplants. *Antimicrob Agents Chemother* 1997;41:1175–1177.

153. Bow EJ, Mandell LA, Louie TJ, et al. Quinolone-based antibacterial chemoprophylaxis in neutropenic patients: effect of augmented gram-positive activity on infectious morbidity. National Cancer Institute of Canada Clinical Trials Group. *Ann Intern Med* 1996; 125:183–190.

154. Patrick CC. Use of fluoroquinolones as prophylactic agents in patients with neutropenia. *Pediatr Infect Dis J* 1997;16:135–139.

155. Jick S. Ciprofloxacin safety in a pediatric population. *Pediatr Infect Dis J* 1997;16:130–134.

156. Chysky V, Kapila K, Hullmann R, et al. Safety of ciprofloxacin in children: worldwide clinical experi-

ence based on compassionate use-emphasis on joint evaluation. *Infection* 1991;19:3–10.

157. Oldfield EC, Fessel WJ, Dunne MW, et al. Once weekly azithromycin therapy for prevention of *Mycobacterium avium* complex infection in patients with AIDS: a randomized, double-blind placebo-controlled multicenter trial. *Clin Infect Dis* 1998;26:611–619.

158. Pierce M, Crampton S, Henry D, et al. A randomized trial of clarithromycin as prophylaxis against disseminated *Mycobacterium avium* complex infection in patients with advanced acquired immunodeficiency syndrome. *N Engl J Med* 1996;335:384–390.

159. Havlir DV, Dube MP, Sattler FR, et al. Prophylaxis against disseminated *Mycobacterium avium* complex with weekly azithromycin, daily rifabutin or both. *N Engl J Med* 1996;335:392–398.

160. Brincker H. Prophylactic treatment with miconazole in patients highly predisposed to fungal infection. *Acta Med Scand* 1978;204:123–128.

161. Cuttner J, Troy KM, Funaro L, et al. Clotrimazole treatment for prevention of oral candidiasis in patients with acute leukemia undergoing chemotherapy: results of a double-blind study. *Am J Med* 1986;81:771–774.

162. Owens NJ, Nightengale CH, Schweizer RT, et al. Prophylaxis of oral candidiasis with clotrimazole troches. *Arch Intern Med* 1984;144:290–293.

163. DeGregario MW, Lee WM, Ries CA. Candida infections in patients with acute leukemia: effectiveness of nystatin prophylaxis and relationship between oropharyngeal and systemic candidiasis. *Cancer* 1982;50: 2780–2784.

164. Egger T, Gratwohl A, Tichelli A, et al. Comparison of fluconazole with oral polyenes in the prevention of fungal infections in neutropenic patients: a prospective, randomized, single center study. *Support Care Cancer* 1995;3:139–146.

165. Edzinli EZ, O'Sullivan DD, Wasser LP, et al. Oral amphotericin for candidiasis in patients with hematologic neoplasms: an autopsy study. *JAMA* 1979;242: 258–260.

166. DeLaurenzi A, Matteocci A, Lanti A, et al. Amphotericin prophylaxis against invasive fungal infections in neutropenic patients: a single center experience from 1980 to 1995. *Infection* 1996;24:361–366.

167. Cross JT, Hickerson SL, Yamauchi T. Antifungal drugs. *Pediatr Rev* 1995;16:123–129.

168. Hughes WT, Bartley DK, Patterson GG, et al. Ketoconazole and candidiasis: a controlled study. *J Infect Dis* 1983;147:1060–1063.

169. Hansen RM, Reinero N, Sohnle PG, et al. Ketoconazole in the prevention of candidiasis in patients with cancer: a prospective, randomized, controlled, double-blind study. *Arch Intern Med* 1987;147:710–712.

170. Goodman JL, Winston DJ, Greenfield RA, et al. A controlled trial of fluconazole to prevent fungal infection in patients undergoing bone marrow transplantation. *N Engl J Med* 1992;326:845–851.

171. Ellis ME, Clink H, Ernst P, et al. Controlled study of fluconazole in the prevention of fungal infections in neutropenic patients with haematological malignancies and bone marrow transplant recipients. *Euro J Clin Microbiol Infect Dis* 1994;13:3–11.

172. Slavin MA, Osborne B, Adams R, et al. Efficacy and safety of fluconazole for fungal infections after marrow transplant—a prospective, randomized, double-blind study. *J Infect Dis* 1995;171:1545–1552.

173. Epstein JB, Ransier A, Lunn R, et al. Prophylaxis of candidiasis in patients with leukemia and bone marrow transplants. *Oral Surg Oral Med Oral Pathol Oral Radiol Endod* 1996;81:291–296.

174. Schaffner A, Schaffner M. Effect of prophylactic fluconazole on the frequency of fungal infections, amphotericin B use, and health care costs in patients undergoing intensive chemotherapy for hematologic neoplasias. *J Infect Dis* 1995;172:1035–1041.

175. Kern W, Behre G, Rudolf T, et al. Failure of fluconazole prophylaxis to reduce mortality or the requirement of systemic amphotericin B therapy during treatment for refractory acute myeloid leukemia: results of a prospective randomized phase III study. German AML Cooperative Group. *Cancer* 1998;83:291–301.

176. Yamac K, Senol E, Haznedar R. Prophylactic use of fluconazole in neutropenic cancer patients. *Postgrad Med J* 1995;71:284–286.

177. Wingard JR, Merz WG, Rinaldi MG, et al. Increase in *Candida krusei* infection among patients with bone marrow transplantation and neutropenia treated prophylactically with fluconazole. *N Engl J Med* 1991;325:1274–1277.

178. Bodey G, Bueltmann B, Duguid W, et al. Fungal infections in cancer patients: an international autopsy survey. *Euro J Clin Microbiol Infect Dis* 1992;11: 99–109.

179. Glasmacher A, Molitor E, Mezger J, et al. Antifungal prophylaxis with itraconazole in neutropenic patients: pharmacological, microbiological and clinical aspects. *Mycoses* 1996;39:249–258.

180. Glasmacher A, Molitor E, Hahn C, et al. Antifungal prophylaxis with itraconazole in neutropenic patients with acute leukemia. *Leukemia* 1998;12:1338–1343.

181. Lamy T, Bernard M, Courtois A, et al. Prophylactic use of itraconazole for the prevention of invasive pulmonary aspergillosis in high risk neutropenic patients. *Leuk Lymphoma* 1998;30:163–174.

182. Prentice AG, Warnock DW, Johnson SA, et al. Multiple dose pharmacokinetics of an oral solution of itraconazole in autologous bone marrow transplant recipients. *J Antimrob Chemother* 1994;34:247–252.

183. Poirier JM, Hardy S, Isnard F, et al. Plasma intraconazole concentrations in patients with neutropenia: advantages of a divided daily dosage regimen. *Ther Drug Monit* 1997;19:525–529.

184. Rousey SR, Ressler S, Gottlieb M, et al. Low-dose amphotericin B prophylaxis against invasive Aspergillus infections in allogeneic marrow transplantation. *Am J Med* 1991;91:484–492.

185. Perfect JR, Klotman ME, Gilbert CC, et al. Prophylactic intravenous amphotericin B in neutropenic autologous bone marrow transplant recipients. *J Infect Dis* 1992;165:891–897.

186. O'Donnell MR, Schmidt GM, Tegtmeier BR, et al. Prediction of systemic fungal infection in allogeneic marrow recipients: impact of amphotericin prophylaxis in high-risk patients. *J Clin Oncol* 1994;12: 827–834.

187. Tollemar J, Ringden O, Andersson S, et al. Prophylactic use of liposomal amphotericin B (AmBisome) against fungal infections: a randomized trial in bone

marrow transplant recipients. *Transplant Proc* 1993; 25:1495–1497.

188. Behre GF, Schwartz S, Lenz K, et al. Aerosol amphotericin B inhalations for prevention of invasive pulmonary aspergillosis in neutropenic cancer patients. *Ann Hematol* 1995;71:287–291.

189. Lortholary O, Dupont B. Antifungal prophylaxis during neutropenia and immunodeficiency. *Clin Microbial Rev* 1997;10:477–504.

190. Saral R, Burns WH, Laskin OL, et al. Acyclovir prophylaxis against herpes simplex infection in patients with leukemia. *Ann Intern Med* 1983;99:773–776.

191. Wade JC, Newton B, Fluornoy N, et al. Oral acyclovir for prevention of herpes simplex reactivation after marrow transplant. *Ann Intern Med* 1984;100: 823–838.

192. Wade JC, Newton B, MacLaren C, et al. Intravenous acyclovir to treat mucocutaneous herpes simplex virus infection after marrow transplantation. *Ann Intern Med* 1982;96:259–265.

193. Gluckman E, Lotsberg J, Devergie A, et al. Prophylaxis of herpes infections after bone-marrow transplantation by oral acyclovir. *Lancet* 1983;2706–2708.

194. Meyers JD, Reed EC, Shepp DH, et al. Acyclovir for prevention of cytomegalovirus infection and disease after allogeneic transplantation. *N Engl J Med* 1988; 318:12–18.

195. Gavalda J, de Otero J, Murio E, et al. Two grams daily of oral acyclovir reduces the incidence of cytomegalovirus disease in CMV-seropositive liver transplant recipients. *Transpl Int* 1997;10:462–465.

196. Prentice HG, Gluckman E, Powles RL, et al. Long-term survival in allogeneic bone marrow transplant recipients following acyclovir prophylaxis for CMV infection. The European Acyclovir for CMV Prophylaxis Study Group. *Bone Marrow Transplant* 1997;19:129–133.

197. Green M, Kaufmann M, Wilson J, et al. Comparison of intravenous ganciclovir followed by oral acyclovir with intravenous ganciclovir alone for prevention of cytomegalovirus and Epstein-Barr virus disease after liver transplantation in children. *Clin Infect Dis* 1997; 25:1344–1349.

198. Boeckh M, Gooley TA, Reusser P, et al. Failure of high-dose acyclovir to prevent cytomegalovirus disease after autologous marrow transplantation. *J Infect Dis* 1995;172:939–943.

199. Sempere A, Sanz GF, Senant L, et al. Long-term acyclovir prophylaxis for prevention of varicella zoster virus infection after autologous bone stem cell transplantation in patients with acute leukemia. *Bone Marrow Transplant* 1992;10:495–498.

200. Selby PJ, Powles RL, Easton D, et al. The prophylactic role of intravenous and long-term oral acyclovir after allogeneic bone marrow transplantation. *Br J Cancer* 1989;59:434–438.

201. Schmidt GM, Horak DA, Niland JC, et al. A randomized, controlled trial of prophylactic ganciclovir for cytomegalovirus pulmonary infection in recipients of allogeneic bone marrow transplants: the City of Hope-Stanford-Syntex CMV Study Group. *N Engl J Med* 1991;324:1005–1011.

202. Goodrich JM, Mori M, Gleaves CA, et al. Early treatment with ganciclovir to prevent cytomegalovirus disease after allogeneic bone marrow transplantation. *N Engl J Med* 1991;325:1601–1607.

203. Goodrich JM, Bowden RA, Fisher L, et al. Ganciclovir prophylaxis to prevent cytomegalovirus disease after allogeneic marrow transplant. *Ann Intern Med* 1993; 118:173–178.

204. Canpolat C, Culbert S, Gardner M, et al. Ganciclovir prophylaxis for cytomegalovirus infection in pediatric allogeneic bone marrow transplant recipients. *Bone Marrow Transplant* 1996;17:589–593.

205. Gotti E, Suter F, Baruzzo S, et al. Early ganciclovir therapy effectively controls viremia and avoids the need for cytomegalovirus (CMV) prophylaxis in renal transplant patients with cytomegalovirus antigenemia. *Clin Transplant* 1996;10:550–555.

206. Noble S, Faulds D. Ganciclovir. An update of its use in the prevention of cytomegalovirus infection and disease in transplant recipients. *Drugs* 1998;56:115–146.

207. Robertson MJ, Larson RA. Recurrent fungal pneumonias in patients with acute non-lymphocytic leukemia undergoing multiple courses of intensive chemotherapy. *Am J Med* 1988;84:233–239.

208. Bjerke J, Meyers JD, Bowden RA. Hepatosplenic candidiasis—a contraindication to marrow transplantation? *Blood* 1994;84:2811–2814.

209. Offner F, Cordonnier C, Llungman P, et al. Impact of previous aspergillosis on the outcome of bone marrow tranplantation. *Clin Infect Dis* 1998;26:1098–1103.

210. Dadjani AS, Taubert KA, Wilson W, et al. Prevention of bacterial endocarditis: recommendations by the American Heart Association. *JAMA* 1997;277:1794–1801.

211. Rey JR, Axon A, Budzynska A, et al. Guidelines of the European Society of Gastrointestinal Endoscopy: antibiotic prophylaxis for gastrointestinal endoscopy. *Endoscopy* 1998;30:318–324.

24

Antibiotic Therapy in the Immunocompromised Host

Stephen A. Chartrand

Department of Pediatrics, Creighton University School of Medicine, Omaha, Nebraska 68178

Broadly defined, an immunocompromised host has an alteration in phagocytic, cellular, or humoral immunity that increases the risk of an infectious complication or an opportunistic process such as lymphoproliferative disorder or cancer. Not only is the risk of ordinary infectious diseases significantly greater in the immunocompromised host, but the pattern and severity of infections vary markedly from that encountered in the immunocompetent host. Therapeutic interventions such as cytotoxic chemotherapy, bone marrow transplantation, corticosteroids, splenectomy, or irradiation compound the patient's immune susceptibility. Neutropenia, as a consequence of cytotoxic chemotherapy or bone marrow transplantation, is the most readily identifiable risk factor for severe bacterial infection. The suppression of T-cell defenses in patients undergoing allogeneic marrow transplantation is clearly associated with an increased susceptibility to invasive viral infections. Other therapy-induced alterations in host defenses include disruption of natural skin and mucosal barriers due to biopsies, placement of indwelling catheters, nasogastric and endotracheal tubes, chemotherapy-induced mucositis, and interference with adequate nutritional intake (1).

Initial therapy for the febrile immunocompromised child is complicated by the increased prevalence of antibiotic resistant pathogens in both the community and hospital environments. Like normal children, the immunocompromised child is at risk for community-acquired infection with multiple drug-resistant *Streptococcus pneumoniae* (DRSP), beta-lactamase producing *Haemophilus influenzae,* and, more recently, methicillin-resistant *Staphylococcus aureus* (MRSA). Overuse of antibiotics in the hospital has produced highly resistant gram-negative enteric bacilli that have acquired new, extended-spectrum beta-lactamases that shield them from the action of most currently available cephalosporins. Cephalosporin overuse has produced strains of *Pseudomonas aeruginosa* with derepressed chromosomal beta-lactamase or permeability changes that severely limit treatment options. Vancomycin-resistant enterococci (VRE) and highly resistant *Stenotrophomonas maltophilia,* among others, have emerged as nosocomial pathogens in many institutions. Infection resulting from these resistant gram-negative organisms is associated with a high morbidity and mortality because of ineffective antibiotic therapy.

To make an intelligent choice of effective antimicrobial agents, a brief review of important bacterial pathogens, important resistance mechanisms, and selected new antibiotics is warranted.

PATHOGENIC ORGANISMS

Most microbiologically documented infections that occur in immunocompromised hosts are caused by organisms that are part of the endogenous microflora of the gut or skin; however, the patient acquires approximately half of these pathogens after admission to the hospital (2). Within 24 hours of hospitalization, seriously ill patients undergo a change in their indigenous microflora toward one of aerobic gram-negative organisms (3). In the normal state, the endogenous microbial flora exists as a carefully balanced, synergistic microenvironment within the host. A unique feature of this balance is the capacity of intact anaerobic flora to resist overgrowth by more pathogenic aerobes, especially gram-negative organisms (4). When antibiotics, particularly the beta-lactam agents, suppress the anaerobic flora, this *colonization resistance* becomes impaired, and normal host flora may shift toward the more invasive aerobic species.

Providing antimicrobial coverage for all of the likely infecting organisms in a particular patient is usually impractical. The relative morbidity and mortality associated with the likely organisms can be used to guide antimicrobial selection (5). For example, in children with fever and neutropenia, coagulase-negative

TABLE 24.1. *Bacterial causes of febrile episodes in neutropenic patients*

Common	Intermediately frequent	Uncommon
Gram-positive cocci and bacilli		
Staphylococcus		*Bacillus* sp.
Coagulase positive (*S. aureus*)		*Listeria* monocytogenes
Coagulase negative		*Stomatococcus mucilagnosus*
(*S. epidermidis* and others)		
Streptococcus		
S. pneumoniae		
S. pyogenes		
Viridans group		
Enterococcus faecalis/faecium		
Corynebacterium sp.		
Gram-negative baccilli and cocci		
Escherichia coli	*Enterobacter* sp.	*Flavobacterium* sp.
Klebsiella sp.	*Proteus* sp.	*Chromobacterium* sp.
Pseudomonas aeruginosa	*Salmonella* sp.	*Pseudomonas* (other than *P. aeruginosa*)
	Haemophilus influenzae	*Legionella* sp.
	Acinetobacter sp.	*Neisseria* sp.
	Stenotrophomonas	*Moraxella* sp.
	Maltophilia	
	Citrobacter sp.	*Eikenella* sp.
		Kingella sp.
		Gardenerella sp.
		Shigella sp.
		Erwinia sp.
		Serratia marcescens
		Hafnia sp.
		Flavimonas oryzihabitans
		Achromobacter xylosoxidans
		Edwardsiella sp.
		Providencia sp.
		Morganella sp.
		Yersinia enterocolitica
		Capnocytophaga sp.
Anaerobic cocci and bacilli	*Bacteroides* sp.	*Peptococcus* sp.
	Colstridium sp.	*Veillonella* sp.
	Fusobacterium sp.	*Peptostreptococcus* sp.
	Propionibacterium sp.	

staphylococci are the most common blood iso-late in most studies, whereas *P. aeruginosa* infections are relatively less common. The morbidity and mortality associated with *P. aeruginosa* infection are high, whereas coagulase-negative staphylococcal infections rarely cause life-threatening injury in children. Consequently, empiric therapy regimens for fever and neutropenia are appropriately di-rected more toward *P. aeruginosa* and other gram-negative bacilli than toward coagulase-negative staphylococci. If coagulase-negative staphylococci subsequently are isolated, van-comycin can be added with little risk of a poor outcome. In institutions where the more viru-lent penicillin-resistant *Streptococcus viridans* group organisms are common, however, initial therapy should include vancomycin.

The spectrum of infecting organisms has changed over the past four decades. During the 1950s and early 1960s, *S. aureus* was the most frequent bacterial isolate in immunosup-pressed patients. When the beta-lacta-mase–resistant antistaphylococcal penicillins were introduced, gram-negative bacillary or-ganisms emerged as predominant bacterial pathogens (especially *Escherichia coli, Kleb-siella* sp., and *P. aeruginosa)* (2). The pre-dominant gram-negative isolates continue to be members of the Enterobacteriaceae (i.e., *E. coli, Klebsiella* sp., and *Enterobacter* sp.). In the 1990s, however, an increased prevalence of nonaeruginosa pseudomonas-like organ-isms (*Stenotrophomonas maltophilia, Burk-holderia cepacia, Pseudomonas stutzeri,* and others) has been observed in cancer patients as nosocomial infections or as a consequence of antibiotic resistance. An increase in mul-tiply resistant gram-negative bacteria also has been observed in many institutions, with antibiotic-resistant *Enterobacter, Klebsiella, Citrobacter,* and *Serratia* isolates being most commonly seen. Among gram-positive bac-teria, increased rates of infection resulting from MRSA, VRE, and penicillin-resistant *S. viridans* are now common in many insti-tutions. The bacterial causes of febrile episodes in neutropenic patients are listed in Table 24.1 (1).

ANTIBIOTIC RESISTANCE

The emergence of antibiotic resistant bac-teria in both inpatient and outpatient settings has profoundly affected the initial antibiotic management of potentially infected immuno-compromised children. A complete review of antibiotic resistance mechanisms and their clinical implications is beyond the scope of this chapter, but selected bacteria and mecha-nisms of resistance that impact the recom-mendations to follow are reviewed here. Readers are referred to the references (5,6) for more in-depth discussions.

Gram-Positive Organisms

As a result of the relatively simple cell wall in gram-positive bacteria, decreased perme-ability is not an option for significant antibi-otic resistance. Drug efflux is fairly uncom-mon in these bacteria, except for macrolide efflux pumps in *S. pneumoniae.* The TEM-1 family of beta-lactamases produced by gram-positive bacteria may be readily defeated by semisynthetic penicillins, penicillin/betalacta-mase inhibitor combinations, or cephalo-sporins. Clinically significant antibiotic resis-tance among these bacteria most commonly involves altered antibiotic targets.

Methicillin-Resistant S. aureus

Methicillin or "intrinsic" resistance is due to alteration of penicillin-binding proteins 2b or 2a. These proteins are enzymes that cat-alyze transpeptidation or carboxypeptidation reactions that are essential for cross-linking of the peptidoglycan backbone. They are the major targets of beta-lactam antibiotics. Synthesis of an altered penicillin-binding protein by the structural gene *mecA* confers methicillin resistance to *S. aureus* (7). This broad-based resistance encompasses all peni-cillins and cephalosporins. Although histori-cally viewed as a nosocomial pathogen, re-cent reports document an increasing rate of MRSA from community sources, including children. In general, community-acquired strains of MRSA have retained susceptibility to clindamycin, whereas hospital-acquired strains are resistant. Isolated strains of MRSA with intermediate resistance to vancomycin have been isolated recently, but clinical failure with vancomycin has not been reported.

Multiple Drug-Resistant S. pneumoniae

The prevalence of penicillin nonsusceptible *S. pneumoniae* increased dramatically during the 1990s. Once again, the mechanism involves alterations in the major penicillin-binding proteins, pbp2b for penicillins and pbp1a plus 2x for resistance to cephalosporins (8). Today, most penicillin-nonsusceptible strains are actually resistant to multiple drugs, including many cephalosporins, trimethoprim-sulfamethoxasole (TMP-SMX), macrolides, and even clindamycin, and are termed DRSP. Thus far, however, no strains resistant to vancomycin have appeared. The American Academy of Pediatrics recommends vancomycin as initial therapy for all children with life-threatening infections (9). Although pneumococci are not frequent causes of sepsis in immunocompromised children (except for those with sickle cell disease), vancomycin should be included as part of the initial regimen for most children.

Vancomycin-Resistant Enterococci

Strains of *Enterococcus faecium* resistant to vancomycin are now widespread in some institutions, especially among liver-transplant patients. Resistance is mediated by the *VanA* transposon gene, which encodes for an alteration of the D-alanine binding site in the bacterial cell wall. This resistance is both inducible and transferable, which raises concerns that this gene could be transferred to other streptococci and staphylococci (10). The overuse and misuse of both intravenous and oral vancomycin appear to be important factors in the development of resistance. Recent studies, including both adult and pediatric patients, found that 23% to 61% of institutions had evidence of VRE (11). Most pediatric isolates are nosocomial in origin. Contrary to popular belief, infections with VRE can be severe. In one pediatric study of enterococcal bacteremia, nearly 60% of deaths were attributed directly to the bloodstream infection (12).

Viridans Streptococci

Viridans streptococci have emerged as an important cause of overwhelming shock in neutropenic patients, especially those with severe oral ulcerations from chemotherapy-induced gingivostomatitis (13–16). Additional risk factors include prophylaxis with quinolones or TMP/SMX and treatment with antacids or H_2 antagonists. The most frequently isolated species are *Streptococcus mitis* and *Streptococcus sanguis*; up to 60% of the latter are resistant to penicillin. The mechanism of resistance again involves altered penicillin binding proteins, and many of these strains are also resistant to third-generation cephalosporins. The overall mortality in these patients seems to be higher in those not treated initially with vancomycin.

Gram-Negative Organisms

Because of their more complex cell-wall structure, gram-negative bacteria may possess additional mechanisms of resistance not available to gram-positive organisms. Decreased permeability through the outer membrane porin structures and drug efflux may act in concert with novel beta-lactamases or altered targets to produce a highly effective armamentarium against large numbers of antibiotics (6). This discussion is limited to recent developments in extended-spectrum beta-lactamases (ESBLs) and chromosomal beta-lactamase in those bacteria likely to cause infection in the immunocompromised host.

Extended-Spectrum Beta-Lactamases

The ESBLs are plasmid-mediated enzymes that confer resistance to the new oxyimino cephalosporins (e.g., ceftriaxone, cefotaxime, ceftazidime) and monobactams such as az-treonam, as well as narrow-spectrum cepha-losporins and anti-gram-negative penicillins (e.g., ticarcillin, piperacillin). Carbapenems such as meropenem and cephamycins (e.g., cefoxitin) are spared. Most of the organisms harboring these enzymes have been species of *Klebsiella,* especially *Klebsiella pneumoniae.* The predilection of *Klebsiella* sp. is explained partly by cross-infection, with clonal spread of producers, and this is facilitated by the fact that *Klebsiella* organisms survive longer than most other gram-negative rods on skin. Prior use of extended-spectrum cephalosporins or high-level use of such agents in a closed unit often is associated with outbreaks of ESBL-producing *K. pneumoniae.* ESBLs, however, also have been found in clinical isolates of *E. coli, Serratia marcescens, Enterobacter* sp., *Citrobacter* sp., *Salmonella* and *K. pneumo-niae,* all of which are frequent pathogens in im-munocompromised children. The prevalence of ESBL-mediated resistance among these bacteria varies widely, ranging from 10% to 40%; some hospitals report such strains rarely, if at all (17).

All ESBLs are not created equally, giving widely varying levels of resistance. Most hydrolyze ceftazidime and aztreonam more effectively than cefotaxime, although the op-posite is true for other ESBLs. Despite ap-parent *in vitro* susceptibility to third-genera-tion cephalosporins and cefepime, patients with ESBL producing gram-negative infec-tions have failed to respond to these oxyimino antibiotics (18). One explanation for this is the inoculum effect seen *in vitro* when such organisms are tested at 107 colony-forming units (CFU)/mL rather than at the usual 105 CFU/mL. The higher inoculum, a concentra-tion that could be attained easily in purulent secretions, typically increases the minimum inhibitory concentration (MIC) values beyond the susceptibility breakpoint. Beta-lactamase inhibitors, such as clavulanate, sulbactam, or tazobactam, are highly active against ESBLs and may be considered the drugs of choice. In fact, the susceptibility of ESBLs to beta-lactamase inhibitors provides a good labora-tory test for their presence. A disk containing clavulanate or sulbactam is placed 30 mm from disks containing oxyimino beta-lactams. Augmentation or distortion of the zone around an oxyimino disk indicates the pres-ence of ESBL (6).

Chromosomal (AmpC) Beta-Lactamase

Certain Enterobacteriaceae produce a chro-mosomal cephalosporinase that is not sensi-tive to beta-lactamase inhibitors and hy-drolyzes virtually every class of beta-lactam to some extent. Among clinical isolates, the most prevalent species producing this in-ducible AmpC enzyme are *Enterobacter cloa-cae, Enterobacter aerogenes, C. freundii, S. marcescens,* and *P. aeruginosa.* Most of these are common or frequent pathogens in im-munocompromised hosts (Table 24.1). Only trace amounts of the AmpC beta-lactamase are made in the absence of antibiotics, but transient high-level production can arise when the organism is exposed to certain antimicro-bials; this increased production is reversible

TABLE 24.2. *Inducers of chromosomal cephalosporinases*

Good	Variable	Poor
Cephamycins (e.g., cefoxitin)	Clavulanate	Sulbactam
Carbapenems (e.g., meropenem)	First- and second-generation cephalosporins	Third-generation cephalosporins[a]
Ampicillin	Desacetyl cefotaxime	Antipseudomonal penicillin Aztreonam[a] Cefepime

[a]Good selection of derepressed mutants.

when the antimicrobial is withdrawn. Many narrow-spectrum penicillins and older cephalosporins (e.g., cefoxitin) are strong inducers of the enzyme (Table 24.2) and may induce their own demise when used to treat infections caused by these strains. The carbapenems, such as imipenem and meropenem, are strong inducers of the enzyme, but they are relatively stable to AmpC and retain activity against both inducible strains and fully derepressed mutants.

Permanent hyperproduction (derepression) of AmpC can arise by mutation in the regulatory mechanism for the enzyme (6). In this case, extremely high levels of the chromosomal beta-lactamase are produced, and high-level resistance is seen. In *P. aeruginosa,* this mutation usually results in only partial derepression, and a second mutational event is required to complete the derepression. Derepressed mutants are highly stable and persist despite multiple *in vitro* passages. Prospective studies of emergence of resistance during therapy for infections due to gram-negative bacteria containing the AmpC enzyme reveal rates of 16% to 20% (19). Rates are highest for sequestered foci, such as peritoneal abscess and bone infections. Combination therapy does not prevent this emergence of resistance. Unfortunately, third-generation cephalosporins and aztreonam, which are poor inducers of the AmpC enzyme, are most likely to select for such derepressed mutants. Cefepime, by contrast, is both a poor inducer of the chromosomal enzyme and is less likely to select for derepressed mutants than third-generation cephalosporins.

Pseudomonas aeruginosa *Infection*

The prevalence of beta-lactam resistance among clinical isolates of *P. aeruginosa* is highest among children treated in tertiary care children's hospitals and transplant centers. Isolates of *P. aeruginosa* that produce plasmid-mediated beta-lactamases generally are resistant to all antipseudomonal penicillins. Although the enzymes themselves are susceptible to inhibition by clavulanate, this inhibitor usually does not reduce the MIC of ticarcillin for *P. aeruginosa* to clinically relevant levels. Thus, for most *P. aeruginosa* strains, the clinical effectiveness of ticarcillin–clavulanate is no greater than for ticarcillin alone. The chromosomal beta-lactamase is more often involved in clinically significant resistance than are plasmid-mediated enzymes. In large studies, emergence of derepressed mutants has occurred in 14% to 56% of those treated with third-generation cephalosporins, especially in neutropenic patients (19).

During therapy, *P. aeruginosa* also can develop resistance to carbapenems; however, the resistance is carbapenem specific and involves a selective permeability decrease to these drugs. Thus, isolates may remain susceptible to antipseudomonal cephalosporins even if they are resistant to the carbapenems.

Stenotrophomonas maltophilia *Infection*

Stenotrophomonas maltophilia is now emerging as an important clinical pathogen, especially in intensive care units, transplant units, and cystic fibrosis centers (20). This organism produces two inducible chromosomal enzymes: one primarily a cephalosporinase and the other a metallo–beta-lactamase capable of hydrolyzing penicillins and carbapenems. *S. maltophilia* usually is resistant to carbapenems, older penicillins, and most cephalosporins (21). Even when *in vitro* testing suggests beta-lactam susceptibility, clinical failures are common when cephalosporins or penicillin derivatives are used. Treatment always should be with TMP/SMX.

SELECTED NEW ANTIBIOTICS

Aztreonam

Although it is not a new agent, aztreonam is a widely underused antibiotic, primarily because of a lack of extensive studies in children. Aztreonam is a monocyclic beta-lactam antimicrobial that is active against strictly gram-negative aerobic bacilli (22). It has no activity against gram-positive or anaerobic organisms. Aztreonam's *in vitro* activity is almost identical to that of ceftazidime and should be considered an alternative to that drug. In fact, aztreonam's chemical structure is the left-hand side of ceftazidime. Parenteral aztreonam distributes widely, penetrates well into cerebrospinal fluid (CSF) and is excreted primarily unchanged in the urine. Dosage must be adjusted for patients with renal insufficiency. Adverse reactions are similar to those of parenteral cephalosporins. The main advantages of aztreonam include its narrow spectrum of activity, lack of cross-sensitization with other beta-lactam drugs, and lack of nephrotoxicity. Even patients with documented severe hypersensitivity to penicillins and cephalosporins may be safely treated with aztreonam. For patients with renal insufficiency, aztreonam delivers the same antibacterial activity as the aminoglycosides but is not nephrotoxic. The usual dose in children is 50 mg/kg every 6 to 8 hours. For adults, 1 or 2 g are administered every 6 hours.

Cefepime

Cefepime is a fourth-generation cephalosporin that is available as an intravenous or intramuscular preparation. Biochemically, cefepime is a zwitterion, which provides a high level of water solubility and consequently rapid penetration across the outer-membrane porin channels in gram-negative bacteria. Cefepime has fairly broad gram-positive and gram-negative activity, including highly penicillin-resistant *S. pneumoniae*. It is more active than cefotaxime against most Enterobacteriaceae, in particular *Enterobacter* sp. Cefepime's antipseudomonal activity is comparable to that of ceftazidime. Like all cephalosporins, cefepime in not active against enterococci (23). Cefepime is widely distributed within the body, and CSF levels are 20% of simultaneous serum concentrations. Adverse effects are similar to other cephalosporins. Compared with third-generation cephalosporins, cefepime is much less likely to induce resistance in bacteria that carry the *AmpC* chromosomal beta-lactamase gene

(Table 24.2). This is a major advantage for immunocompromised children, and in my opinion, cefepime should be the cephalosporin of choice for most patients. In a prospective study of febrile neutropenic patients, the combination of cefepime and amikacin was compared with ceftazidime and amikacin. Clinical and bacteriologic outcomes were comparable, but secondary infections were less with cefepime (24). Cefepime was safe and effective as monotherapy in 91 episodes of fever with neutropenia in 84 adult patients (25). The usual dose for children is 50 mg/kg administered every 8 hours (26).

Meropenem

Meropenem is a parenteral carbapenem antibiotic, which has excellent bactericidal activity against almost all clinically significant aerobes and anaerobes (27–29). A major difference compared with imipenem is the long, substituted pyrrolidine side chain present in the C-2 position in meropenem, which provides greater activity against penicillin-binding proteins in gram-negative bacilli such as *P. aeruginosa*. Meropenem is active against methicillin-susceptible *S. aureus,* penicillin-susceptible and resistant *S. pneumoniae,* and *E. faecalis* but not *E. faecium.* Meropenem is resistant to hydrolysis by the chromosomal *AmpC* beta-lactamase and is more active than ceftazidime against *P. aeruginosa* (27). Meropenem does select for derepressed *AmpC* mutants in *P. aeruginosa,* but it retains good activity against them (6). Resistance, although rare, has occurred with *P. aeruginosa* as a result of altered porin channel proteins that resulted in decreased antibiotic penetration into the periplasmic space. The drug is widely distributed within the body, and CSF levels are 16% of simultaneous serum concentrations. Meropenem is cleared by the kidney, with 70% of administered antibiotic being recovered unchanged in the urine. Dosage adjustments, therefore, are necessary with renal impairment (28). In a prospective study of fever and neutropenia in 154 children, meropenem monotherapy was as effective as the combination of ceftazidime plus amikacin (30). There are distinct clinical advantages to meropenem compared with imipenem. Meropenem is not degraded by the human renal tubular enzyme, dehydropeptidase, so there is no need to add cilastatin as in imipenem. Compared with imipenem, the incidence of central nervous system adverse effects, including seizures, is less with meropenem. Because of its broad spectrum, meropenem may be considered as monotherapy for fever in neutropenic children. The usual dose is 40 mg/kg every 6 to 8 hours (28,31).

UNEXPLAINED FEVER AND NEUTROPENIA

Because fever and neutropenia is the most common clinical condition facing the clinician, the recommendations that follow draw heavily on recent consensus guidelines published by The Infectious Disease Society of America and The National Comprehensive Cancer Network (1,32) for the use of antimicrobials in neutropenic patients with unexplained fever. The guidelines are general, and readers must take into consideration individual variations and types of infections, settings where patients are being treated, local antimicrobial susceptibility patterns, underlying causes of neutropenia or other immunosuppression, and expected time to recovery. Specific clinical syndromes that require more directed therapy are addressed individually.

Approximately 48% to 60% or more of neutropenic patients who become febrile have an established or occult infection and 10% to greater than 20% of patients with neutrophil counts of fewer than 100 cells/mm^3 will develop a bloodstream infection (32).

Definitions

Fever is defined as a single oral temperature greater than 38.3°C (101°F) in the absence of obvious environmental causes. A temperature of 38.0° or greater (100.4°F) over at least 1 hour indicates a febrile state. Some

physicians believe that, in the absence of a definable clinical focus of infection, a fever observed within 6 hours of the administration of a blood product is less likely to be of infectious origin. Although it occurs uncommonly, an immunocompromised patient who is afebrile but who has signs and symptoms compatible with infection (e.g., abdominal pain) should be considered at risk for infection (1).

When the neutrophil count decreases to below 1,000 cells/mm^3, increased susceptibility to infection can be expected, with the frequency and severity generally inversely proportional to the neutrophil count. Patients with neutrophil counts of 500/mm^3 or lower are at considerably greater risk for infection than those with counts of 1,000/mm^3, and patients with counts of 100/mm^3 or lower are at greater risk than those with counts of 500/mm^3. A rapid decrease in the neutrophil count and protracted neutropenia (<500 cells/mm^3 for 10 days) are major risk factors for impending infections (1).

Initial Evaluation

Empirical administration of broad-spectrum antibiotics is necessary for febrile neutropenic patients because the currently available diagnostic tests are not sufficiently rapid, sensitive, or specific for identifying or excluding the microbial cause of a febrile episode. If untreated, these infections may be rapidly fatal in the neutropenic host.

A thorough search should be undertaken for focal evidence of infection, remembering that the usual signs of inflammation may be absent in the neutropenic host. The sites most commonly infected include the periodontium and oropharynx; lower esophagus; lung; perineum, including the anus; skin lesions; bone marrow and skin biopsy sites; the eye (fundoscopic); vascular catheter access sites; and tissue around the nails. Two blood cultures should be performed in all patients.

If a central venous catheter (CVC) is in place, blood samples should be obtained from each lumen as well as from a peripheral vein.

Quantitative blood cultures may be helpful in distinguishing CVC infection versus from systemic sepsis, but they are rarely available and are not routinely recommended. If a catheter entry site is inflamed or draining, exuding fluid should be examined by Gram stain and culture for bacteria and fungi. If such lesions are persistent or chronic, stains and cultures for nontuberculous mycobacteria should be obtained. Little clinically useful information is obtained from routine cultures of the nasopharynx or rectum (1).

Diarrheal stools believed to be of infectious etiology should be tested for *Clostridium difficile* toxin and for bacteria (*Salmonella, Shigella, Campylobacter, Aeromomas/Plesiomonas,* and *Yersinia)*, viruses (rotavirus, adenovirus, or cytomegalovirus), or protozoa (*Cryptosporidium* sp.). All of these except *C. difficile* are uncommon as nosocomial pathogens. Pyuria may be absent in the presence of urinary tract infection in neutropenic patients. Therefore, urine cultures should be routinely obtained, especially if a urinary catheter is in place or if there are signs or symptoms of urinary tract infection. Examination of CSF is not routinely recommended unless central nervous system infection is suspected. Again, however, CSF pleocytosis may be absent in neutropenic hosts. Chest radiographs are recommended as part of the initial workup, even in patients with no overt signs or symptoms of pulmonary infection. Skin lesions suspected of being infectious should be aspirated or biopsied for cytology, Gram smear, and culture (33). A complete blood count and chemistry profile should be obtained at the onset and then frequently during therapy to monitor for possible drug toxicity.

Initial Antibiotic Therapy

All febrile patients with neutrophil counts below 500/mm³ and those with counts of 500 to 1,000/mm³ in whom further decrease can be anticipated should be promptly treated with intravenous broad-spectrum bactericidal antibiotics (1). Afebrile patients who are profoundly neutropenic but have signs or symp-

toms compatible with an infection also should receive empirical broad-spectrum therapy.

In selecting the initial antibiotic regimen, physicians should consider the type, frequency, and antibiotic susceptibilities of the bacterial isolates found in similar patients at the local hospital. For example, if penicillin and cephalosporin-resistant viridans streptococci is commonly found in febrile neutropenic patients at a particular institution, vancomycin should be included in the initial regimen (Fig. 24.1). If there is a high prevalence of cephalosporin-resistant *Enterobacter* or other gram-negative species, a carbapenem, a quinolone, or an aminoglycoside should be included in the initial regimen. Combinations of certain drugs, such as cisplatin, amphotericin B, cyclosporine, and aminoglycosides, however, should be avoided whenever possible. Plasma concentrations of the aminoglycosides and vancomycin should be monitored in patients with renal impairment or altered volumes of distribution (1).

In the 1990s and beyond, sites of infection are not often defined, especially in patients receiving prophylactic oral antibiotics. Grampositive organisms now account for 60% to 70% of microbiologically documented infections. Many of these (coagulase-negative staphylococci, *Corynebacterium jekeium*) are resistant to cephalosporins and penicillinase-resistant penicillins, but they are of relatively low virulence. Hence, a 24- to 48-hour period of delay in starting vancomycin is not detrimental. The increasing prevalence of multidrug-resistant *S. pneumoniae* and MRSA (7) now argue for adding vancomycin initially (34).

Some experts recommend administration of antibiotics through each lumen of the catheter, but there is only moderate evidence to support this approach. If initial cultures identify only one of the lumens as infected, antibiotics should be infused through that port.

Local antibiotic resistance patterns, a history of recent antibiotic use (including prophylaxis), and the potential for adverse effects all should be taken into account when choosing

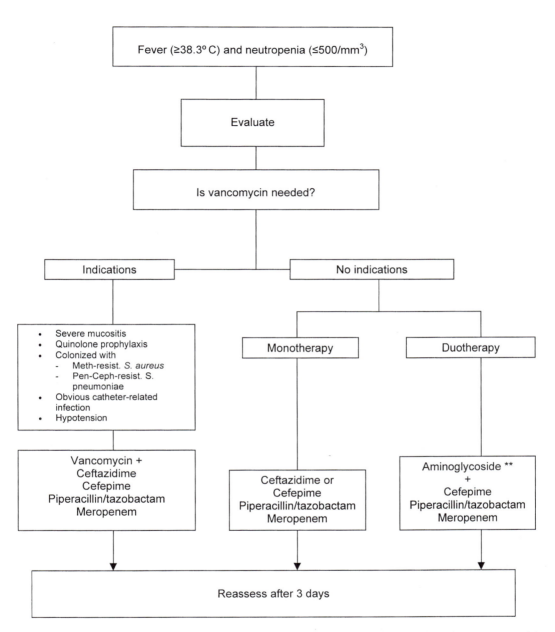

FIG. 24.1. Guide to the initial management of the febrile neutropenic patient. *Meth-resist.*, methicillin-resistant; *Pen-Ceph-resist.*, penicillin-cephalosporin resistant. (Modified from Hughes WT, Armstrong D, Bodey GP, et al. 1997 Guidelines for the use of antimicrobial agents in neutropenic patients with unexplained fever. *Clin Infect Dis* 1997;25:551, with permission.)

initial treatment regimens. Nevertheless, it is clear that not all antibiotics are equally effective (e.g., cefazolin versus ceftazidime for gram-negative bacillary infections) and that patients with true penicillin allergy should not be administered antipseudomonal penicillins. The recommendations that follow are consistent with the recent Infectious Disease Society of America (IDSA) and National Comprehensive Care Network (NCCN) guidelines, but they also take into consideration that resistance, especially among gram-negative organisms, is now widespread and that more rapidly bactericidal agents are preferred.

Monotherapy

Initial monotherapy directed against gram-negative organisms is comparable to multidrug combinations for most patients (35–37). The IDSA guidelines state that monotherapy with ceftazidime or imipenem/cilastatin can be considered a standard of therapy (1). Both drugs have broad-spectrum gram-negative coverage, including most strains of *P. aeruginosa*. Ceftazidime, however, is susceptible to hydrolysis by chromosomal *AmpC* beta-lactamase plus a number of ESBLs and selects for derepressed mutants. Cefepime, in my opinion, is preferable to ceftazidime (Fig. 24.1). Because meropenem is more potent than imipenem and better tolerated, it is now the preferred carbapenem agent. Meropenem is relatively resistant to both chromosomal and extended spectrum beta-lactamases, but it may select for permeability-mediated resistance in *P. aeruginosa*. If the local prevalence of carbapenem resistance is low, meropenem is also a reasonable initial choice. None of these drugs covers MRSA or coagulase-negative staphylococci. Meropenem is active *in vitro* against enterococci, penicillin-resistant viridans streptococci species, and highly penicillin and cephalosporin-resistant pneumococci, all of which are resistant to ceftazidime.

Many of the newer quinolones, such as levofloxacin, ofloxacin, and gatifloxacin demonstrate broad gram-positive and gram-negative coverage, including strains of methicillin-resistant staphylococci, viridans streptococci, and drug-resistant pneumococci. Previous studies in adults, however, showed both favorable and unfavorable results when these drugs are used as initial therapy in neutropenic patients. Because there are no prospective studies in children for this indication, they cannot be recommended at this time.

Combination Therapy without Vancomycin

Therapy with two beta-lactam agents is generally not recommended because of cost, a lack of improved efficacy over monotherapy, and the possibility of one agent inducing resistance to the other. The exception would be a combination of nafcillin (or oxacillin) plus an antipseudomonal cephalosporin, aztreonam, or antipseudomonal ureidopenicillin (e.g., piperacillin).

The most common dual therapy, excluding regimens with vancomycin, is an aminoglycoside (gentamicin, tobramycin, or amikacin) with an antipseudomonal ureidopenicillin or an antipseudomonal cephalosporin (Fig. 24.1). Piperacillin/tazobactam is the most potent of the ureidopenicillin/inhibitor combinations and is recommended. Advantages of the two-drug regimen include synergistic activity against gram-negative bacteria, anaerobe coverage, and possibly less emergence of resistant strains during treatment. The major disadvantage is the potential for nephrotoxicity, ototoxicity, and hypokalemia associated with aminoglycosides plus the added cost for toxicity-related drug monitoring.

Treatment with aminoglycosides alone is not recommended, even when the organism is susceptible *in vitro*. In my opinion, cefepime is now the preferred antipseudomonal cephalosporin because of its increased *in vitro* activity and decreased tendency to select for resistance (see later). Ceftazidime, however, remains an acceptable alternative. Ceftriaxone is not recommended because of its poor activity against *P. aeruginosa*.

Studies of quinolones in combination with other antibiotics are limited, especially in children, and no convincing evidence can be drawn for their superiority (38). Some of the newer fourth-generation agents such as gatifloxacin and gemifloxacin hold promise because of their activity against MRSA, VRE, and DRSP. Macrolide drugs such as erythromycin, azithromycin, and clarithromycin are bacteriostatic agents and should not be used as initial therapy unless infection from *Mycoplasma pneumoniae*, *Chlamydia pneumoniae*, or mycobacteria is suspected.

Vancomycin Plus One or Two Other Drugs

Although vancomycin has not been shown to influence the overall mortality associated with infections from gram-positive cocci as a group, the mortality associated with viridans streptococcal infections and the prevalence of DRSP in children argue for including vancomycin at least as initial therapy. Overuse of vancomycin, however, has led to the emergence of vancomycin-resistant organisms (e.g., enterococci) in many institutions. Readers are referred to the recent recommendations of the Hospital Infection Control Practices Advisory Committee of the Centers for Disease Control and Prevention for preventing the spread of vancomycin resistance (39). At least one study showed that vancomycin is not a necessary part of initial empirical antibiotic therapy (40); however, that study was carried out before the recent increase in multiple DRSP. I believe vancomycin should now be included in the initial regimen for all febrile neutropenic children, especially in institutions where fulminant infections caused by viridans streptococci are common. If initial blood cultures are negative after 72 hours or bacteria are isolated that are susceptible to other agents, vancomycin should be discontinued. The IDSA guidelines state that it is prudent to start vancomycin in selected patients with clinically obvious catheter-related infections, intensive chemotherapy that produces substantial mucosal damage, prophylaxis with quinolones, known colonization with DRSP or MRSA, a blood culture positive for gram-positive bacteria before final identification and susceptibility testing, and

hypotension or other evidence of cardiovascular impairment (1).

An initial approach to antibiotic therapy in the febrile neutropenic patient with unexplained fever is provided in Fig. 24.1. This approach is modified from the published IDSA guidelines and takes into consideration the increased prevalence of DRSP and beta-lactam resistant viridans streptococci plus the likelihood for cephalosporin-resistant gram-negative bacteria in this population.

A potentially interesting approach to initial empiric therapy is rotating antibiotic classes on a bimonthly or quarterly basis. For example, if ureidopenicillins are used in a particular unit during the first quarter, ceftazidime or cefepime might be used for the next 3 months, followed by meropenem before the cycle is restarted. If future studies of quinolones confirm their efficacy as initial therapy, this class could be included as a fourth rotation. Because the different classes of antibiotics tend to select different mechanisms of resistance in gram-negative strains, this approach has at least some microbiologic merit. Antipseudomonal cephalosporins and aztreonam tend to select for AmpC-mediated resistance or ESBLs, which do not generally affect meropenem. Meropenem tends to select resistance to itself attributable to permeability changes and decreases selective pressure for inducible AmpC and ESBL resistance.

Management during the First Week of Therapy

Usually, at least 3 days of antibiotic treatment are required to determine the efficacy of the initial regimen (1). At this point, further treatment is based on the fever response and whether the patient's condition has improved or deteriorated (Fig. 24.2). It should be stressed that the median time to defervescence with most initial antibiotic regimens is 5 days (range, 2–7 days).

Afebrile within 3 Days of Treatment

If an etiologic agent is isolated, the antibiotic regimen may be modified to enhance cov-

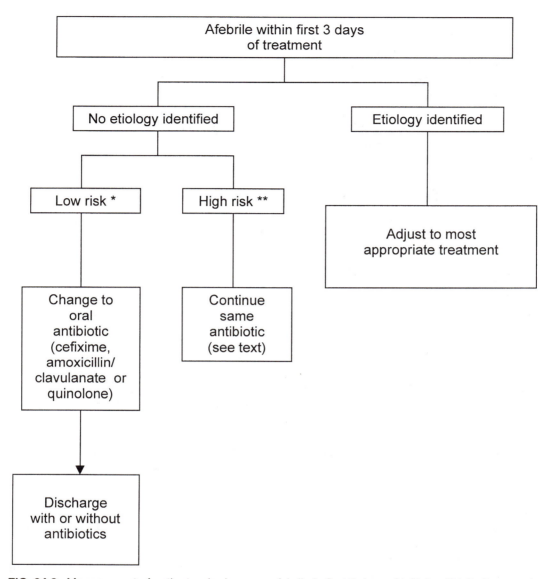

FIG. 24.2. Management of patients who become afebrile in first 3 days of initial antibiotic therapy. *, clinically *well;* **, absolute neutrophil count <100/mm³, mucositis, or clinically unstable. (Modified from Hughes WT, Armstrong D, Bodey GP, et al. 1997 Guidelines for the use of antimicrobial agents in neutropenic patients with unexplained fever. *Clin Infect Dis* 1997;25:551, with permission.)

erage for that organism, but broad-spectrum coverage should be maintained (36) (Fig. 24.2). Therapy should be continued for at least 7 days or until all sites of infection have resolved, and the patient is free of significant symptoms. In most cases, treatment should be continued until the absolute neutrophil count is greater than 500/mm³, but if the patient is afebrile and all signs and symptoms have resolved, antibiotics can be discontinued earlier. If no organism is isolated, treatment traditionally has been continued for a minimum of 7 days. Recent studies suggested that earlier discontinuance of treatment and discharge from the hospital may be feasible in some patients (see later).

For patients at low-risk for serious complications and no discernible focus of infection (Table 24.2), intravenous therapy can be changed after 2 or 3 days to any of several oral regimens. Such patients should be followed up closely as outpatients (41,42). With the ease and increasing use of CVCs, however, many pediatric oncologists prefer to continue intravenous therapy at home.

Persistent Fever after 3 Days of Treatment

If fever persists for longer than 3 days and no organism is identified, both the patient and the initial treatment regimen should be carefully reassessed, as shown in Fig. 24.3. This should include a meticulous physical examination, a thorough review of all cultures, a review of drug dosages, and consideration for additional radiographs. Additional studies should be considered to rule out viral, mycobacterial, chlamydial, and toxoplasmal infections.

If fever persists after 5 days of antibiotic therapy and reassessment does not yield a cause, one of three management choices should be made: (1) to continue treatment; (2) to change or add antibiotics; or (3) to add amphotericin B to the regimen, with or without changing the antibiotics. If no obvious changes in the patient's condition have occurred and the patient is clinically stable, the initial antibiotic

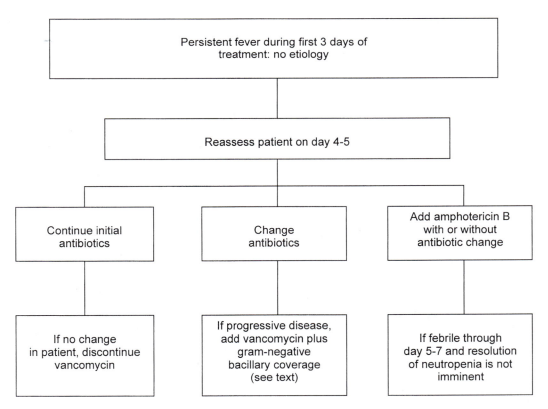

FIG. 24.3. Treatment of patients who have persistent fever after 3 days of treatment and for whom the etiology of the fever is not found. (From Hughes WT, Armstrong D, Bodey GP, et al. 1997 Guidelines for the use of antimicrobial agents in neutropenic patients with unexplained fever. *Clin Infect Dis* 1997;25:551, with permission.)

regimen can be continued. This option is most attractive if the neutropenia is expected to resolve within 5 days.

If the patient's condition has deteriorated or if focal infection becomes apparent, additional antibiotics should be added or the regimen changed. If the initial regimen did not include vancomycin and there is evidence of life-threatening sepsis, vancomycin should be added. Resistance to beta-lactam agents has become common among gram-negative organisms at many institutions, and persistent fever due to such organisms is becoming increasingly frequent. Widespread aminoglycoside resistance, however, remains relatively uncommon. Therefore, if aminoglycosides were not included in the initial regimen, gentamicin or tobramycin should be added despite the potential increased risk of toxicity.

If the initial treatment included vancomycin and cultures remain negative or organisms susceptible to less toxic agents are identified, vancomycin should be discontinued. If continued coverage for gram-positive organisms is deemed necessary, nafcillin (or oxacillin), a penicillin plus beta-lactamase inhibitor (ampicillin/sulbactam or piperacillin/tazobactam), or clindamycin can be added.

Most experts recommend adding amphotericin B to the treatment regimen if unexplained fever persists for more than 5 days in neutropenic patients (1,32,36). Every effort should be made to determine whether fungal infection exists (blood and urine cultures for fungus, skin biopsy, sinus radiographs, abdominal computed tomography [CT] scan) before amphotericin B is added. One prospective study found fewer breakthrough fungal infections and less toxicity with liposomal amphotericin B compared with amphotericin B (43). Liposomal amphotericin B is significantly more expensive, however, and generally is recommended only for *Aspergillus* spp. infections, unmanageable adverse effects with amphotericin B, and renal toxicity from amphotericin B.

Fluconazole is prescribed as an alternative to amphotericin B in some centers, but it is not active against *Aspergillus* species, *Candida krusei,* and some strains of *Candida glabrata* (44). Its efficacy as empiric therapy is unproven, however, and liposomal amphotericin B is preferred for patients who are unable to tolerate amphotericin B or who have renal dysfunction.

Duration of Antimicrobial Therapy

If the neutrophil count exceeds 500/mm³ by day 7 and the patient is afebrile, antibiotic therapy may be stopped (Fig. 24.4.). If the patient has been afebrile for 5 to 7 days but remains neutropenic, it is still reasonable to stop systemic therapy if the patient appears well with no discernible infectious focus and no laboratrory or radiographic evidence of infection. Antibiotic therapy should be continued for profoundly neutropenic (<100/mm³) patients, especially if there are mucous membrane lesions of the mouth or gastrointestinal tract and unstable vital signs.

If amphotericin B has been added and no focus of infection is subsequently identified, however, how long to continue amphotericin B becomes problematic. If a thorough clinical, laboratory, and radiographic workup fails to document a source of infection and amphotericin B has been administered for 2 weeks, treatment usually can be stopped.

For patients who remain febrile after the neutrophil counts have recovered to greater than 500/mm³, reassessment for undiagnosed infection should focus on fungal infections or undiagnosed viral infections (e.g., Epstein–Barr virus, cytomegalovirus, respiratory syncytial virus, adenovirus). Abdominal CT scans may be useful for identifying unrecognized hepatic or splenic fungal abscesses, especially as the absolute neutrophil count increases (45). Viral cultures of blood and respiratory tract, viral antigen detection tests, and polymerase chain reaction assays should be considered in the search for viruses. Antibiotics usually can be stopped 4 to 5 days after the neutrophil count reaches 500/mm³ or greater, despite persistent fever, if no infectious etiology is identified.

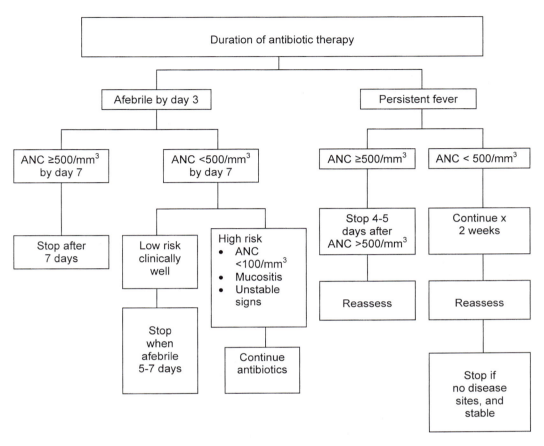

FIG. 24.4. Duration of antibiotic therapy. See section entitled "Early Discontinuation of Treatment" in text. ANC, absolute neutrophil count.

Discontinuation of Therapy

Recent studies from Texas, North Carolina, and Chile showed that low-risk febrile neutropenic children and adolescents can be safely discharged from the hospital without antibiotics before their absolute neutrophil count exceeds 500/mm³ (46–48). Criteria for early discharge included clinically well appearance, no fever for 24 hours, sterility of all blood cultures, control of local infection with antibiotic therapy, and evidence of bone marrow recovery (defined as any sustained increase in platelet count and absolute neutrophil count). Children or adolescents who were treated for bacteremia could be discharged before resolution of neu-

tropenia after a course of intravenous antibiotic therapy if repeated blood cultures were sterile and the patients otherwise met the low-risk criteria. Of 330 episodes, only 21 (6%) were associated with readmission for recurrent fever during the subsequent 7 days. None of the readmission blood cultures was positive, and all patients fared well during their second hospitalization. One confounding factor was that 25% of the patients received oral therapy after discharge for treatment of a specific source of infection.

Other investigators reported less favorable outcomes, although those studies were carried out more than 20 years ago (49). For older children and adolescents, it is arguable whether there is any real tangible benefit from discontinuing antibiotics altogether versus outpatient therapy with the new highly potent fluoroquinolones, for example. Nevertheless, any strategy to reduce excess antibiotic exposure in this population should be carefully pursued but closely monitored for any adverse outcomes.

Site-Specific Therapy

The NCCN recently published recommendations for the evaluation and therapy of site-specific infections in febrile neutropenic patients. The reader is referred to reference 32 for a more complete discussion, but those recommendations are modified and summarized here.

Mouth and Esophagus

The mouth and esophagus are common sites of infection in patients with fever and neutropenia. This is because of the propensity of the mouth and alimentary tract mucosa to be disrupted by cytotoxic therapy (*mucositis*). The clinical presentation of these infections is not etiology specific, and important bacterial, viral, and fungal pathogens often can be distinguished only by microbiologic culture.

When gingivitis or necrotizing ulcerations are noted in the mouth, viral and fungal cultures should be obtained. Empiric therapy for anaerobic bacteria should be started with clindamycin or metronidazole. Cultures for herpes simplex virus also should be obtained and consideration given to starting acyclovir. If vesicular lesions are noted, parenteral acyclovir should be started at once. Suspicious oral lesions should be swabbed and sent for fungal smear and culture, remembering that *Candida* spp. may be noninvasive colonizers of the oropharynx. Nevertheless, if yeast are seen or suspected, either topical antifungal treatment or fluconazole should be added. If there is no evidence of systemic fungal disease, amphotericin B may be withheld while a thorough laboratory and radiographic evaluation is pursued.

Retrosternal burning, dysphagia, and chronic nausea or vomiting should alert the physician to the possibility of esophageal infection with herpes simplex virus (HSV), cytomegalovirus (CMV), or *Candida* spp. Strong consideration should be given to early endoscopy for cytologic examination, Gram and fungal smears, fluorescent staining for HSV, and viral culture. If yeast infection is suspected or proven, treatment should be started with amphotericin B. Therapy with acyclovir or ganciclovir should be instituted for HSV or CMV, respectively.

Sinuses

The sinuses are a common site of bacterial and fungal infection in immunocompromised hosts (50). Cytotoxic therapy disrupts the natural ciliary cleansing mechanisms, and nasogastric tubes may lead to maxillary os obstruction. Sinus tenderness, periorbital swelling or cellulitis, nasal ulceration, or black patches on the roof of the mouth all strongly suggest sinus infection; however, signs and symptoms of sinus disease may be mild or even absent in neutropenic hosts until infection is far advanced. A limited sinus CT scan is usually more revealing than plain radiographs and no more expensive. Any suspicious lesion should be biopsied and sent for Gram and fungal smears plus aerobic/anaerobic and fungal cultures. Antibiotic therapy should be directed at *S. aureus* and anaerobes (clindamycin, ampicillin/sulbactam, piperacillin/tazobctam). If fungal infection is suspected, amphotericin B should be started. *Aspergillus* spp. sinusitis always requires surgical debridement.

Abdomen

Most infections in the abdomen are usually diagnosed and managed based on clinical presentation and radiologic findings. Symptoms may be obtuse and focal signs difficult to assess in a patient who is already chronically ill. Pain in the right upper quadrant suggests fungal or bacterial abscess in the liver. Evaluation should include ultrasound and enhanced CT scan. Initial therapy should include coverage for *S. aureus* as well as anaerobes and enterococci. A drug such as piperacillin/tazobactam plus gentamicin with or without metronidazole would be reasonable. If fungal infection is suspected, amphotericin B should be added. Infections in and around the rectum may also be polymicrobial, with anaerobes, enterococci, and gram-negative bacteria all potential pathogens. Stool cultures should include screening for *C. difficile* toxin. Broad-spectrum therapy should include anaerobes and enterococci (plus metronidazole if *C. difficile* screen is positive), accompanied by local care (sitz baths, stool softeners). Typhlitis (neutropenic enterocolitis) is a serious, life-threatening syndrome characterized by fever, diarrhea, and abdominal pain. Enhanced abdominal CT scans may be the only way to document the illness in many patients. Anaerobic bacteria predominate, but the same syndrome may result from *C. difficile,* CMV, and (in the allogenic transplant recipient) gut graft-versus-host disease. Polymicrobial bloodstream infection, bowel perforation, and hemorrhage may complicate typhlitis. Stool cultures for CMV and toxin screen for *C. difficile* should be obtained. Antibiotic coverage should include gram-negative bacteria and anaerobes. If CMV is proven or suspected, ganciclovir should be started.

Central Venous Catheter Infection

Catheter-related sepsis represents the most frequent life-threatening complication of CVCs (50–55). Unfortunately, there is as yet no consensus concerning either a useful definition of catheter-related sepsis or the optimal method of catheter management and prevention of infection. An extensive review of this subject was recently published by Greene (51).

It is useful to categorize CVC infections as shown in Table 24.3. CVC infections may occur anywhere along the length of the CVC from the exit site to the catheter tip. Infection may be intraluminal or extraluminal (or both), and it may or may not be associated with systemic symptoms. As part of the initial evaluation, an ultrasound study of the catheter tip should be obtained for all CVCs. If vegetations are found, catheter removal should be considered, regardless of the offending organism.

Exit site and tunnel infections usually are due to invasion by normal skin flora along the path of the catheter and usually are not accompanied by positive blood cultures drawn through the lumen. Intraluminal infections usually are due to contamination of the CVC hub by either the patient's skin flora or from organisms on the hands of medical personnel. Bacteria on the outer surface of the catheter may result from extension of an intraluminal

TABLE 24.3. *Central venous catheter (CVC) infections*

1. Exit (or insertion) site: Purulence from the catheter site or less than 2 cm of inflammation around the exit site
2. Tunnel infection: >2 cm of inflammation extending proximal from the catheter exit site of tunneled catheters
3. Pocket space abscess or cellulitis: Fluctuance around the subcutaneous implanted catheter hub or evidence of surrounding inflammation or cellulitis overlying the catheter hub
4. Central venous catheter-related bacteremia or fungemia:
   a. A positive blood culture drawn from the catheter with clinical symptoms and no apparent source for the infection
   b. A fivefold to tenfold or greater bacterial density per milliliter of blood obtained through the device compared with simultaneous peripheral blood cultures
   c. More than 1,000 CFUs or organisms obtained through the catheter in the absence of peripheral blood cultures
   d. A catheter tip culture of greater than 15 CFUs when the device is removed specifically for suspected catheter-related infection

CFU, colony-forming unit.

infection or may be due to seeding of the CVC during a bacteremic episode. The only definitive way to distinguish CVC infection from coincident bacteremia is to obtain semiquantitative peripheral and CVC blood cultures, a test that is rarely available in most hospitals (56). In clinical practice, a positive blood culture drawn through the catheter with clinical manifestations of sepsis and no apparent source for the infection is taken as a CVC infection. Pocket-space abscess or cellulitis of a subcutaneous infusion port is usually due to skin organisms introduced while accessing the port. In a study of pediatric oncology patients, subcutaneous ports resulted in fewer line-associated infections than percutaneous CVCs (57). Percutaneous CVCs are more likely to be used during intense chemotherapy and severe neutropenic episodes, whereas subcutaneous ports are used for long-term maintenance, which may explain in part the difference in infection rates.

Treatment

Most CVC infections can be treated with the catheter in place because most CVC infections are due to coagulase-negative staphylococci (50,54). For exit-site infections, a culture of any drainage should be obtained, along with local debridement and cleansing of the wound. The catheter may be left in place regardless of the organism. Local treatment with mupirocin plus an oral antistaphylococcal agent should be started unless fever or systemic symptoms are present. If fever is present, clinicians should consider adding vancomycin.

For tunnel-site infections, the catheter should be removed and sent for Gram smear and culture, including culture for *Mycobacterium* sp. (55). Empiric therapy with vancomycin should be initiated unless Gram smear of the drainage or catheter reveals gram-negative organisms. In that situation, ceftazidime or cefepime should be added.

The catheter may be left in place for infections from coagulase-negative staphylococci, non-*Corynebacterium jeikeium* diphtheroids

and some alpha-hemolytic streptococci. The catheter should be removed for infections with *S. aureus,* enterococci, *Bacillus* sp., *C. jeikeium,* all fungi, polymicrobial bacteremia, and nontuberculous mycobacteria. For any organism, if blood cultures remain positive for 72 hours despite appropriate antimicrobial therapy, the catheter should be removed. For gram-negative bacteremia in a clinically stable but neutropenic patient, the catheter may be left in place if (a) the organisms are presumed to have originated by transmigration from the gastrointestinal tract, (b) cultures sterilize within 48 hours, and (c) there is prompt defervescence. If *P. aeruginosa* or *S. maltophilia* is isolated, the CVC should be removed.

Treatment of pocket-space infections is rarely successful without removing the subcutaneous port, regardless of the organism. Cultures should be obtained through the port access site and from the pocket when the port is removed. Initial combined therapy with vancomycin plus ceftazidime or cefepime is recommended.

Replacement of infected catheters can be performed safely at a new site within the first 2 to 3 days after initial catheter removal if the blood is sterile for 48 hours. For uncomplicated CVC infection with coagulase-negative staphylococci, duration of treatment is 5 to 7 days after the blood becomes sterile. For *S. aureus* and gram-negative infections, antibiotics should be administered for at least 10 days from the first negative culture.

Prophylactic regimens to prevent CVC-associated infections include "antibiotic-lock" techniques, routine "changeout" of CVCs, vancomycin-added infusates, vancomycin flushes, and antimicrobial-impregnated catheters. Antibiotic locks are time consuming, expensive, and not always successful. Routine replacement of CVCs does not decrease the incidence of infections (58). Adding vancomycin to the infusate or line increases the risk for encouraging vancomycin resistance. Recent studies with catheters impregnated with rifampin–minocycline showed a significant reduction in CVC infection and hold some promise (50,59).

Outpatient Therapy

There is increasing acceptance that certain patients with neutropenia and fever can be managed safely and effectively as outpatients (60,61). The NCCN recommends that outpatient therapy be considered for low-risk patients who consent to home care, have a telephone, can access emergency facilities, have had at least two previous cycles of chemotherapy, have an adequate home environment, and are within 1 hour of a medical center or a physician's office. Risk factors to be considered in choosing outpatient therapy include the severity and duration of neutropenia; mucosal damage from cytotoxic chemotherapy or invasive procedures; nutritional status of the patient; cancer status (induction, remission, relapse); and comorbidities, such as hemodynamic instability, clinical bleeding, respiratory insufficiency, and mental status (60). Treatment may be administered at home or in the outpatient clinic. Outpatient regimens may include broad-spectrum intravenous therapy (similar to inpatient regimens) alone or with oral antibiotics such as ciprofloxacin or clindamycin. Alternatively, dual-agent oral therapy with a fluroquinolone (ciprofloxacin or levofloxacin) plus amoxicillin/clavulanate or clindamycin may be selected for older children and adolescents. Studies suggest that oral therapy is as effective as intravenous therapy for low-risk, febrile, neutropenic patients (62,63). Oral therapy has two distinct advantages in this patient population. First oral antibiotic administration does not require home health care teams and is therefore less expensive. Second, the risk of venous access, with the possibility of iatrogenic infection in the neutropenic host, is avoided (60).

SUMMARY

The immunocompromised patient is susceptible to a broad array of highly virulent and highly antibiotic-resistant bacterial pathogens. In selecting an antibiotic regimen, the clinician's initial goal is to provide broad-spectrum coverage with the most rapidly bactericidal, least toxic agents that are least likely to promote antibiotic resistance. Because of the increasing prevalence of penicillin and cephalosporin-resistant gram-positive pathogens, clinicians should consider including vancomycin in the initial therapy regimen. If no pathogen is isolated or the pathogen is susceptible to other agents, vancomycin should be discontinued as soon as possible. When specific bacteria are isolated, therapy may be modified to optimize coverage for that organism, but broad-spectrum coverage should be maintained during the patient's at-risk period. New strategies to improve therapy include oral therapy, outpatient therapy, and early discontinuation of antibiotics.

REFERENCES

1. Hughes WT, Armstrong D, Bodey GP, et al. 1997 Guidelines for the use of antimicrobial agents in neutropenic patients with unexplained fever. *Clin Infect Dis* 1997;25:551–573.
2. Freifeld AG, Walsh TJ, Pizzo PA. Infections in the cancer patient. In: DeVita VT Jr, Hellman S, Rosenberg SA, eds. *Cancer principles and practice of oncology*, 5th ed. Philadelphia: Lippincott–Raven, 1997:2659–2704.
3. Fainstain V, Rodriguez V, Turck M, et al. Patterns of oropharyngeal and fecal flora in patients with leukemia. *J Infect Dis* 1981;144:10–18.
4. Van der Waaj D. Gut resistance to colonization: clinical usefulness of selective use of orally administered antimicrobial drugs. In: Klastersky J, ed. *Infection in cancer patients*. New York: Raven Press, 1982:73–90.
5. Shenep JL. Antimicrobial therapy in the immunocompromised host. *Semin Pediatr Infect Dis* 1998;9:330–338.
6. Chartrand SA, Thompson KJ, Sanders CC. Antibiotic-resistant, gram negative bacillary infections. *Semin Pediatr Infect Dis* 1996;7:187–203.
7. Patrick C. Drug-resistant staphylococcal infections. *Semin Pediatr Infect Dis* 1996;7:182–186.
8. Coffey TJ, Dawson CG, Daniels M, et al. Genetics and molecular biology of beta-lactam-resistant pneumococci. *Microb Drug Res* 1995;1:29–34.
9. Committee on Infectious Disease. American Academy of Pediatrics. Therapy for children with invasive pneumococcal infections. *Pediatrics* 1997;99:289–299.
10. Cross JT, Jacobs R. Vancomycin-resistant enterococcal infections. *Semin Pediatr Infect Dis* 1996;7:162–169.
11. Jones RN, Sader HS, Erwin ME, et al. Emerging mutiply resistant enterococci among isolates. I. Prevalence data from 97 medical center surveillance study in the United States. *Diagn Microbiol Infect Dis* 1995;21:85–93.
12. Christie C, Hammond J, Reising S, et al. Clinical and molecular epidemiology of enterococcal bacteremia in a pediatric teaching hospital. *J Pediatr* 1994;125:392–399.
13. Elting LS, Bodey GP, Keefe BH. Septicemia and shock syndrome due to viridans streptococci: a case–control study of predisposing factors. *Clin Infect Dis* 1992; 14:1201–1207.

14. Bochud P-Y, Calandra T, Francioli P. Bacteremia due to viridans streptococci in neutropenic patients: a review. *Am J Med* 1994;97:256–264.

15. Richard P, Amador Del Valle G, Moreau P, et al. Viridans streptococcal bacteraemia in patients with neutropenia. *Lancet* 1995;345:1607–1609.

16. Reed EC, Arneson M, Vaughn W, et al. *Streptococcus viridans: a significant cause of neutropenic fever that caused death in some patients not treated for gram positive bacteria.* Proc Am Soc Clin *Oncol* 1990;9:321(abst 1239).

17. Jacoby GA. Extended-spectrum-lactamases and other enzymes providing resistance to oxyimino-lactams. *Infect Dis Clin North Am* 1997;11:875–887.

18. Rice LB, Willey SH, Papanicolaeu GA, et al. Outbreak of ceftazidime resistance caused by extended-spectrum beta-lactamases at a Massachusetts chronic-care facility. *Antimicrob Agents Chemother* 1990;34:2193–2199.

19. Sanders CC, Sanders WE. Emergence of resistance during therapy with the newer beta-lactam antibiotic: role of inducible beta-lactamases and implications for the future. *Rev Infect Dis* 1983;5:639–648.

20. Khardori N, Elting L, Wong E, et al. Nosocomial infections due to *Xanthomonas maltophilia: a case–controlled study of predisposing factors.* Infect Control Hosp Epidemiol 1990;11:134–138.

21. Neu HC, Saha G, Chin NX. Resistance of *Xanthomonas maltophilia* to antibiotics and the effect of beta-lactamase inhibitors. *Diagn Microbiol Infect Dis* 1989;12:283–285.

22. Orlicek SC. Aztreonam. *Semin Pediatr Infect Dis* 1999; 10:45–50.

23. Thornsberry C, Brown SD, Yee YC, et al. *In-vitro* activity of cefepime and other antimicrobials; survey of European isolates. *J Antimicrob Chemother* 1993;32(Suppl B):31–53.

24. Cordonnier C, Herbrecht R, Pico JL, et al. Cefepime/amikacin versus ceftazidime/amikacin as empirical therapy for febrile episodes in neutropenic patients: a comparative study. *Clin Infect Dis* 1997;24:41–51.

25. Eggimann P, Glauser MP, Aoun M, et al. Cefepime monotherapy for the empirical treatment of fever in granulocytopenic cancer patients. *J Antimicrob Chemother* 1993;32(Suppl B):151–163.

26. Reed MD, Yamashita TS, Knupp CK, et al. Pharmacokinetics of intravenously and intramuscularly administered cefepime in infants and children. *Antimicrob Agents Chemother* 1997;41:1783–1787.

27. Edwards JR. Meropenem: a microbiological review. *J Antimicrob Chemother* 1995;35(Suppl A):1–17.

28. Bradley JS. Meropenem: a new, extremely broad spectrum beta-lactam antibiotic for serious infections in pediatrics. *Pediatr Infect Dis J* 1997;16:263–268.

29. Bradley JS, Faulkner KL, Klugman KP. Efficacy and tolerability of meropenem as empiric antibiotic therapy in hospitalized pediatric patients. *Pediatr Infect Dis J* 1996;15:749–757.

30. Commetta A, Calandra T, Gaya H, et al. Monotherapy with meropenem versus combination therapy with ceftazidime plus amikacin as empiric therapy for fever in graulocytopenic patients with cancer. *Antimicrob Agents Chemother* 1996;40:1108–1115.

31. Blumer JL. Pharmocokinetic determinants of carbapenem therapy in neonates and children. *Pediatr Infect Dis J* 1996;15:733–737.

32. National Comprehensive Care Network: NCCN practice guidelines for fever and neutropenia. *Oncology* 1999; 13:197–257.

33. Allen U, Smith CR, Prober CG. The value of skin biopsies in febrile, neutropenic, immunocompromised children. *Am J Dis Child* 1986;140:459–461.

34. Committee on Infectious Disease. American Academy of Pediatric. *Pediatrics* 1997;99:289–299.

35. Freifeld AG, Walsh T, Marshall D, et al. Monotherapy for fever and neutropenia in cancer patients: a randomized comparison of ceftazidime versus imipenem. *J Clin Oncol* 1995;13:165–176.

36. Pizzo PA. Management of fever in patients with cancer and treatment-induced neutropenia. *N Engl J Med* 1993; 328:1323–1332.

37. Petrilli AS, Melaragno R, Barros KV, et al. Fever and neutropenia in children with cancer: a therapeutic approach related to the underlying disease. *Pediatr Infect Dis J* 1993;12:916–921.

38. Freifeld A, Pizzo P. Use of fluoroquinolones for empirical management of febrile neutropenia in pediatric cancer patients. *Pediatr Infect Dis J* 1997;16:140–146.

39. Hospital Infection Control Practices Advisory Committee (HICPAC). Recommendations for preventing the spread of vancomycin resistance. *MMWR Morb Mortal Wkly Rep* 1995;44:1–13.

40. European Organization for Research and Treatment of Cancer (EORTC) International Antimicrobial Therapy Cooperative Group and the National Cancer Institute of Canada—Clinical Trials Group. Vancomycin added to empirical combination antibiotic therapy for fever in granulocytopenic cancer patients. *J Infect Dis* 1991; 163:951–958.

41. Lucas KG, Brown AE, Armstrong D, et al. The identification of febrile, neutropenic children with neoplastic disease at low risk for bacteremia and complications of sepsis. *Cancer* 1996;77:791–798.

42. Finberg RW, Talcott JA. Fever and neutropenia—how to use a new treatment strategy. *N Engl J Med* 1999;341: 362–363.

43. Walsh TJ, Finberg RW, Arndt C, et al. Liposomal amphotericin B for empirical therapy in patients with persistent fever and neutropenia. *N Engl J Med* 1999;340:764–771.

44. Schaffner A, Schaffner M. Effect of prophylactic fluconazole on the frequency of fungal infections, amphotericin B use, and health care costs in patients undergoing intensive chemotherapy for hematologic neoplasias. *J Infect Dis* 1995;172:1035–1041.

45. Flynn PM, Shenep JL, Crawford R, et al. Use of abdominal computed tomography for identifying disseminated fungal infection in pediatric cancer patients. *Clin Infect Dis* 1995;20:964–970.

46. Aquino VM, Tkaczewski I, Buchanan GR. Early discharge of low-risk febrile neutropenic children and adolescents with cancer. *Clin Infect Dis* 1997;25:74–78.

47. Santolaya ME, Villarroel M, Avendano LF, et al. Discontinuation of antimicrobial therapy for febrile, neutropenic children with cancer: a prospective study. *Clin Infect Dis* 1997;25:92–97.

48. Jones GR, Konsler GK, Dunaway RP, et al. Risk factors for recurrent fever after the discontinuation of empiric antibiotic therapy for fever and neutropenia in pediatric patients with a malignancy for hematologic condition. *J Pediatr* 1994;124:703–708.

49. Pizzo PA, Robichaud KJ, Gill FA, et al. Duration of em-

pirical antibiotic therapy in granulocytopenic patients with cancer. *Am J Med* 1979;67:194–200.

50. Wald A, Leisenring W, van Burik J, et al. Epidemiology of Aspergillus infections in a large cohort of patients undergoing bone marrow transplantation. *J Infect Dis* 1997;175:1459–1466.

51. Greene JN. Catheter-related complications of cancer therapy. *Infect Dis Clin North Am* 1996;10:255–295.

52. Salzman MB, Rubin LG. Intravenous catheter-related infections. *Adv Ped Infect Dis* 1995;10:337–368.

53. Hiemenz J, Skelton J, Pizzo PA. Perspective on the management of catheter-related infections in cancer patients. *Pediatr Infect Dis* 1986;5:6–11.

54. Flynn PM, Shenep JL, Stokes DC, et al. In situ management of confirmed central catheter-related bacteremia. *Pediatr Infect Dis J* 1987;6:729–734.

55. Raad II, Vartivarian S, Klan A, et al. Catheter-related infections caused by the mycobacterium fortuitum complex: 15 cases and review. *Rev Infect Dis* 1991;13:1120–1125.

56. Siegman-Igra Y, Anglim AM, Shapiro DE, et al. Diagnosis of vascular catheter-related bloodstream infection: a meta-analysis. *J Clin Microbiol* 1997;35:928–936.

57. Ingram J, Weitzman S, Greenberg ML, et al. Complications of indwelling venous access lines in the pediatric hematology patient: a prospective comparison of external venous catheters and subcutaneous ports. *Am J Pediatr Hematol Oncol* 1991;13:130–136.

58. Cobb DK, High KP, Sawyer RG, et al. A controlled trial of scheduled replacement of central venous pulmonary artery catheters. *N Engl J Med* 1992;327:1062–1068.

59. Darouiche RO, Raad II, Heard SO, et al. A comparison of two antimicrobial-impregnated central venous catheters. *N Engl J Med* 1999;340:1–8.

60. Patrick CC, Shenep JL. Outpatient management of the febrile neutropenic child with cancer. *Adv Pediatr Infect Dis* 1999;14:29–47.

61. Mustafa MM, Aquino VM, Pappo Q, et al. A pilot study of outpatient management of febrile neutropenic children with cancer at low risk of bacteremia. *J Pediatr* 1996;128:847–849.

62. Freifeld A, Marchigiani D, Walsh T, et al. A double-blind comparison of empirical oral and intravenous antibiotic therapy for low-risk febrile patients with neutropenia during cancer chemotherapy. *N Engl J Med* 1999;341:305–311.

63. Kern WV, Cometta A, de Bock R et al. Oral versus intravenous empirical antimicrobial therapy for fever in patients with granulocytopenia who are receiving cancer chemotherapy. *N Engl J Med* 1999;341:312–318.

25

Immunomodulation

Uma H. Athale, R. Clark Brown, and Wayne L. Furman

Department of Hematology/Oncology, St. Jude Children's Research Hospital, Memphis, Tennessee 38105

As described in the preceding chapters, infectious complications are a chief cause of morbidity and mortality in immunocompromised children. The traditional approach to prevent and treat infections in these children has been to immunize, to administer aggressive antimicrobial therapy, or both. Although this approach led to remarkable improvements in the quality of life, far too many of these children still die of various infections. Advances in our basic understanding of the immune system enabled us to begin to explore how to manipulate the immune response (*immunomodulation*) in favor of these affected children. These efforts identified several small proteins, collectively termed *cytokines,* and elucidated

their vital biologic immunomodulatory functions. Table 25.1 describes the general biologic features common to most cytokines. Our understanding of the role of cytokines as immunomodulators in the treatment and prevention of infectious disease is still evolving. In general, the approaches to immunomodulation have been either to replace deficient states of effector cells by cytokine stimulation or to redirect the inflammatory cascade to prevent host injury.

This chapter reviews the role of cytokines in the development of an immune response and the uses of immunomodulators in preventing and managing infections in immunocompromised infants and children. These immunomodulators include anticytokine agents (e.g., monoclonal antibodies), hematopoietic growth factors or colony-stimulating factors (CSFs), interferons (IFNs), and interleukins (ILs). Although we focus on agents that have proven benefit in randomized clinical trials, we also introduce other immunomodulators with interesting results in preclinical and in early clinical studies and are likely to be evaluated further in future human trials.

TABLE 25.1. *General biologic features of cytokines*

Most cytokines are small to moderately sized (molecular weight ≤ 30 kDa), simple polypeptides or glycoproteins that occur most commonly as monomers or dimers.
Most cytokines are transiently expressed by variety of cells in response to wide range of stimuli.
Most exhibit autocrine or paracrine activity.
Most bind to specific high-affinity, saturable receptors on the surface of effector cells.
Most are bioactive at low concentrations.
Most mediate their action through transcriptional alteration of expression of the target gene.
Many are directly mitogenic.
Most act synergistically or antagonistically with other cytokines.
Most have overlapping functions and affect a wide variety of cell types.

CYTOKINES IN THE PATHOGENESIS OF INFECTION

Cytokines are central mediators of host responses to infection. Invasion of microorganisms leads to secretion of various cytokines, which initiate a complex interacting cycle of

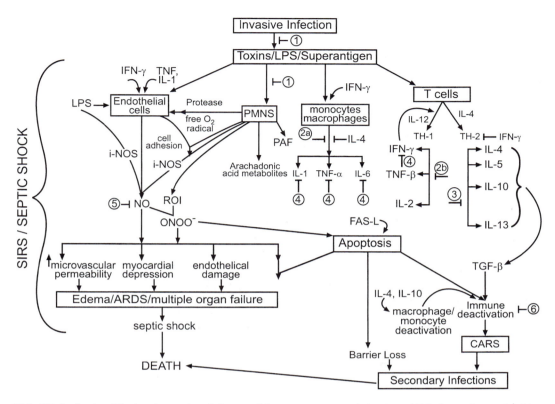

FIG. 25.1. A simplified schematic of the cytokine response to infection. *LPS,* lipopolysaccharide; *IFN,* interferon; *TNF,* tumor necrosis factor; *IL,* interleukin; *PMNs,* polymorphonuclear cells; *iNOS,* inducible nitric oxide synthase; *PAF,* platelet activating factor; *ROI,* reactive oxygen intermediates; *TH-,* T-helper; *TGF,* tumor growth factor; *FAS-L,* FAS ligand; *ONOO-,* perioxynitrite; *ARDS,* acute respiratory distress syndrome; *NO,* nitric oxide; *CARS,* compensatory antiinflammatory response syndrome; *SIRS,* septic inflammatory response syndrome; *TGF,* tumor growth factor; *1, 2, 3, 4, 5, 6* correspond to numbers in Table 25.4 and indicate potential targets for immune modulation of the inflammatory response to infection. (Adapted from Wheeler AP, Bernard GR. Treating patients with severe sepsis. *N Engl J Med* 1999;40;207–214; Weiss M, Moldawer LL, Schneider EM. Granulocyte colony-stimulating factor to prevent the progression of systemic nonresponsiveness in systemic inflammatory response syndrome and sepsis. *Blood* 1999;93:425–439; Glauser MP, Heumann D, Baumgartner JD, et al. Pathogenesis and potential strategies for prevention and treatment of septic shock: an update. *Clin Infect Dis* 1994;18[Suppl 2]:S205–S216; Anderson MR, Blumer JL. Advances in the therapy for sepsis in children. *Pediatr Clin North Am* 1997;44:179–205, with permission.)

events (Fig. 25.1). Cytokines modulate the responses of different kinds of effector cells, including neutrophils, monocytes/macrophages, and T- and B-lymphocytes and promote the secretion of various humoral factors. The aim of this critically balanced "cytokine cascade," in conjunction with other biologic response modifiers, is host protection by elimination of the invading pathogen. An inevitable by-product of this biologic event is modulation

of a wide array of inflammatory responses. Because of their important roles in upregulation or downregulation of inflammatory responses, the cytokines, despite their pleiotropism, are generally classified as either proinflammatory or antiinflammatory cytokines (Table 25.2). An imbalance in the production of these cytokines may lead to dysregulation of immune responses. An overstimulation leads to an exaggerated inflam-

TABLE 25.2. *Proinflammatory and antiinflammatory cytokines*

Type of cytokine	Proinflammatory cytokines	Antiinflammatory cytokines
Interleukins	IL-1, IL-2, IL-3, IL-5, IL-6, IL-7, IL-8, IL-9, IL-11, IL-12, IL-14, IL-15, IL-16, IL-17	IL-4, IL-10, IL-13
Hematopoietic growth factors	G-CSF, GM-CSF, M-CSF	—
Interferons	IFN-γ	—
Other	TNF-α, -β	TGF-β, IL-1ra

G-CSF, granulocyte-colony stimulating factor; GM-CSF, granulocyte-macrophage colony stimulating factor; IFN, interferon; IL, interleukin; IL-1ra, IL-1 receptor antagonist; M-CSF, macrophage-colony stimulating factor; TGF, tumor growth factor; TNF, tumor necrosis factor.

matory response with profound deleterious and unwanted systemic and pathologic consequences as seen in septic shock (to be discussed later). An inadequate immune response leads to the incomplete elimination of the pathogen and the subsequent persistence of infection (1–4). Thus, the nature of the cytokine response to a pathogen is crucial in determining disease resistance and susceptibility in humans.

FUNCTIONAL SUBSETS OF LYMPHOCYTES

The current concept of the complex cytokine cascade in infection depicts the T-cell component of the immune system as a central determinant of the host's inflammatory response. Therefore, to understand more fully cytokine regulation (or the role of cytokines in the pathogenesis of infection), one must understand the functional dichotomy of T-lymphocytes. Human CD4+ T-lymphocytes can be classified into two general populations: T-helper 1 (Th1) and T-helper 2 (Th2) (also known as type 1 or type 2, respectively). This classification is based on the pattern of cytokines released after T-cell stimulation. Invading pathogens along with natural killer (NK) cells and antigen-presenting cells will lead to differentiation of naive Th0 cells. Although most investigators refer to CD4+ cells as being Th1 or Th2 cells, CD8+ cells also are believed to exist as Th1- and Th2-type cells or to secrete cytokines in a polarized manner (5,6). Studies of mice indicate that the endogenous selection of Th1 versus Th2 cells is cytokine driven rather than antigen driven;

however, the origin of these cells and the initial process of selection are presently unclear. It is not known whether the subsets of Th1 and Th2 cells are terminally committed or whether their functions are interchangeable. Additional subsets of T cells have been described that cannot be completely accounted for by the Th1 and Th2 model. Nonetheless, the Th1 and Th2 model serves as an excellent framework for understanding the polarization of T-cell subsets in an immune response. A large percentage of lymphocytes do not secrete a specific pattern of cytokines (6). The characteristics of Th1 and Th2 cells are summarized in Table 25.3, and Fig. 25.1 depicts the developmental schema of Th1 and Th2 cells.

The Th1 cells, which secrete IFN-γ, IL-2, and tumor necrosis factor-α (TNF-α), are associated with macrophage stimulation and proinflammatory reactions. IFN-γ potentiates development of Th1 cells, which is primarily mediated by IL-12, and inhibits the proliferation of Th2 cells (Fig. 25.1). The Th1 cells trigger phagocyte-mediated hosts defenses and are the principal effectors of cell-mediated immunity (CMI) against intracellular pathogens and delayed type of hypersensitivity. They also stimulate production of IgG2a antibodies, which are effective in activating complement and opsonizing antigens for phagocytosis.

Because Th2 cells are thought to secrete antiinflammatory cytokines, they may ameliorate the effects of Th1 cells. The activated Th2 subset is involved mainly in phagocyte-independent host defense mechanisms. They secrete IL-4, IL-5, IL-6, IL-10, and IL-13 to

TABLE 25.3. *Characteristics of Th1 and Th2 cells*

	Type 1 (Th1)	Type 2 (Th2)
Stimulators	IL-12 IFN-γ	IL-4
Characteristic cytokines	IL-12, IFN-γ TNF-α/β	IL-4, -5, -6, -10 IL-13
Common cytokines	GM-CSF, IL-3	GM-CSF, IL-3
Major functions	CMI and DTH increased, macrophage activation with increased immunity, production of IL-1 and TNF, increased activity and number of CTLs, B-cell inhibition	B-cell help, humoral immunity, stimulation of mast cells and eosinophils, macrophage deactivation and decreased production of IL-1 and TNF, increased production of IL-1ra
Immunoglobulin isotypes	IgG2a	IgG1, IgE
Outcome	Augmentation of CMI	Augmentation of humoral immunity
Beneficial in	Leishmaniasis, leprosy, virus infection	Helminths
Detrimental in	Helminths	Leishmaniasis, leprosy, virus infection

CMI, cell-mediated immunity; CTL, cytotoxic T-cells; DTH, delayed type hypersensitivity; GM-CSF, granulocyte-macrophage colony stimulating factor; IFN, interferon; Ig, immunoglobulin; IL, interleukin; IL-1ra, interleukin-1 receptor antagonist; Th1, T-helper type 1; Th2, T-helper type 2; TNF, tumor necrosis factor.

promote B-cell activation and production of antibodies, especially IgE and IgG1. In addition, IL-3, IL-4, and IL-10 stimulate growth and activation of mast cells, IL-5 induces proliferation and activation of eosinophils, and IL-4 and IL-10 suppress monocyte/macrophage functions. IL-4 and IL-10 inhibit cytokine production by Th1 cells and can suppress the development of Th1 cells by down-regulating IL-12 production (5–8).

In summary, the Th1-mediated response, through promotion of CMI and inhibition of humoral immunity, results in a protective effect against pathogens and results in their elimination, primarily through CMI. The Th1-associated cytokine IFN-γ is necessary for controlling infection caused by intracellular organisms. In contrast, Th2 responses promote humoral immunity and inhibit CMI to confer protection against pathogens removed principally by humoral immunity.

CYTOKINES IN THE DEVELOPMENT AND PERPETUATION OF SEPSIS

Sepsis, which is defined as a clinical syndrome arising from a systemic hyperinflammatory response to infection, is a subset of a broader category called systemic inflammatory response syndrome (SIRS) (9). SIRS is a primary host response mounted to extreme clinical situations. In addition to sepsis, other insults, such as trauma, burns, pancreatitis, or major surgery, can result in SIRS.

Sepsis is a common cause of mortality and morbidity in immunocompromised patients. Cancer patients are at significant risk of developing sepsis, both as a consequence of their underlying malignancy and as a result of immunosuppressive therapy. Gram-negative bacteria are the most frequent cause of sepsis or septic shock, but infection by gram-positive bacteria as well as other organisms such as fungi, parasites, and viruses can result in septic shock (10). The pathogens or their products, especially the cell-wall components (e.g., lipopolysaccharide [LPS] from gram-negative bacteria and exotoxins or superantigens from gram-positive bacteria) are potent activators of various humoral pathways, endothelial cells, polymorphonuclear cells (PMNs), T cells, and macrophages (1,2,4, 10,11). This cascade of events is maintained and expanded by the host immune system reacting in response to the microbial toxins. Many different types of cytokines released in the process mediate the deleterious effects of sepsis.

The main proinflammatory cytokines involved in the septic cascade are TNF-α, IL-1,

IL-6, IL-8, IFN-γ, IL-12, and granulocyte macrophage (GM)-CSF. The production of IL-1 and TNF-α is triggered early in the cytokine cascade by microbial toxins. These two cytokines, whose actions are synergistic, promote endothelial cell–leukocyte adhesion, release of proteases and arachidonic acid metabolites (e.g., thromboxane A2, prostacycline, and prostaglandin E2), and activation of clotting factors (1–3,12). In addition to the proinflammatory cytokines, the immune system also produces endogenous antagonists to these cytokines. In the presence of LPS, the Th2 cells secrete the inhibitory cytokines (IL-4, IL-5, IL-10, and IL-13) that downregulate monocyte activation. Other agents involved in the antiinflammatory response include corticosteroids, prostaglandins, IL-11, TGF-β, soluble TNF receptors (sTNF-R), and IL-1 receptor antagonists (IL-1ra) (1,3,11). Th2 cells, in addition, stimulate B-cell activation and antibody production, which in turn may nullify the effects of Th1 cells. Fig. 25.1 summarizes a simplified working hypothesis of cytokine interactions in sepsis.

As shown in Fig. 25.1, the bacterial toxins and the cytokines stimulate the release of nitric oxide (NO) from the nitric-oxide synthase 2 (NOS-2) pathway in many cell types (1,3, 10,11). NO is thought to be a central mediator of the cardiovascular failure seen in many septic patients (3,11). Doughty et al. showed a strong correlation between NO production, organ failure, and an exaggerated proinflammatory response in children (13). NO reacts with the oxygen intermediates that are formed by the activated neutrophils to generate highly reactive perioxynitrite (3), which increases microvascular permeability, leading to edema and other clinical signs of septic shock and is thought to be an inducer of apoptosis (14).

Apoptosis of various cell types seems to play an important role in the development of multiple-organ failure associated with sepsis. In septic mice, apoptosis occurs primarily in hematopoietic cells (mainly T- and B-lymphocytes) and parenchymal cells of the bowel and lung and, to a lesser extent, in skeletal muscle and kidney (15). Systemic apoptosis of cells

of the immune system is a central feature in animals dying of multiple-organ failure as a result of septic shock (15,16). Apoptosis leads to lymphocytopenia, which is commonly observed in patients with sepsis. In addition, fas ligand-mediated apoptosis, known as activation-induced cell death, is shown to occur predominantly in Th1 cells (17,18). This maladaptive host response not only is ineffective in eliminating an infectious agent but also contributes to a state of immune deactivation known as *compensatory antiinflammatory response syndrome* (CARS) (2,3,12). The selective survival of Th2 cells may lead to the observed preponderance of Th2 cells after the proinflammatory response during sepsis and may contribute the development of CARS (1–3). In addition to the Th1 lymphocytopenia, patients with CARS have deactivated monocytes characterized by markedly reduced human leikocyte antigen DR locus (HLA-DR) expression, the loss of antigen-presenting cells, and a profound reduction in the *in vitro* production of LPS-induced TNF-α (19). Apoptosis of parenchymal cells and lymphocytes coupled with monocyte deactivation results in loss of a barrier defense and a decreased ability to eliminate pathogens. This immune deactivation increases the susceptibility to secondary infection and perpetuation of the sepsis/CARS cycle (2,3).

Relationship between Cytokine Levels and the Severity of Sepsis

Findings from several studies suggest that elevated levels of proinflammatory cytokines indicate a poor outcome for patients with sepsis. Significantly greater amounts of TNF-α and IL-6 were found in patients with septic shock than in patients with shock from other causes (20). TNF-α and IL-1β levels were significantly higher in children with sepsis than in healthy controls (21). In addition, TNF-α, IL-1β, and IL-6 levels were significantly higher in patients who died than those of survivors of sepsis who had comparable clinical Pediatric Risk of Mortality scores. Several patients who died, however, had low or absent levels of TNF-α and IL-1β, indicating that low levels of these cytokines do not always correlate with survival (21). Studies of adults indicated that the absolute value and persistent elevation of cytokine concentrations seem to correlate with the severity of sepsis and development of multiple-organ failure (20,22). Serum levels of IL-6 at presentation to the emergency department have been correlated with the risk for bacteremia and death (23); however, evaluation of cytokine levels remains a research tool.

TYPES OF IMMUNOMODULATORS

Anticytokine Agents

In 1985, Beutler et al. reported that the passive immunization of mice against TNF protects mice against the lethal effects of intravenously administered endotoxin (24). Since then, several strategies to interfere with excessive cytokine activity have been studied in animal models as well as in clinical trials. These approaches involve the use of a wide array of agents to try to induce a general anti-inflammatory state and modulate the end-organ damage of severe inflammation (11). Figure 25.1 and Table 25.4 describe some of these new agents and where they may be useful in inhibiting or modifying different steps in the inflammatory cascade.

In anticytokine therapy, antibodies, soluble cytokine receptors, naturally occurring inflammatory antagonists, or cytokine receptor antagonists are used to inhibit a particular proinflammatory cytokine. Because of the important role played by TNF-α and IL-1 in the development of sepsis, these cytokines have been a primary target in the development of immunomodulation therapy.

Anticytokine Antibodies

Several studies in animal models have shown that treatment with either purified anti-TNF-α antiserum or monoclonal antibody is highly protective against an intravenous infusion of a lethal dose of endotoxin or live bacteria (25–27). These studies also demonstrated that blocking TNF binding to its receptor significantly reduced IL-1β and IL-6 levels.

TABLE 25.4. *Investigational trials of immunomodulators in the prevention or treatment of sepsis*

Possible target	Intervention	Agent	References
Microbial toxins (*1*)	Antiendotoxin antibodies	E-5	(282–285)
		HA-1A	(286–290)
		EndoCAbs	(291)
	Endotoxin vaccine		(292, 293)
Inhibitors of proinflammatory cytokines (*2*)	Anti-inflammatory agents	Steroids	(294)
		Immunoglobulin	(295–297)
	Anti-inflammatory cytokines	IL-10[a]	(44, 298)
	Inhibition of TNF-α synthesis	Pentoxyphylline[a]	(299–301)
		Thalidomide[a]	(302)
Anti-inflammatory cytokines (*3*)	Stimulation of synthesis	G-CSF	(3)
Cytokine binding (*4*)	Soluble cytokine receptors	sTNF-α	(35)
	Anticytokine antibodies	anti-IL-6[a]	(303)
		anti-TNF-α	(28, 31, 304)
		anti-IFN-γ[a]	(305)
	Cytokine receptor antagonists	Il-1ra	(38, 41)
End organ effects of inflammation (*5*)	Modulation of NO synthesis	L-NAME	(306)
		L-NMMA	(11, 307)
		Methylene blue	(308)
Immune deactivation (*6*)	Monocyte stimulation, immune stimulation	IFN-τ	(19)

EndoCAbs, antiendotoxin core antibody; G-CSF, granulocyte-colony stimulating factor; HA-1A, human monoclonal antibody to lipid A; IFN, interferon; IL, interleukin; IL-1ra, IL-1 receptor antagonist; L-NAME, N^G-nitro-L-arginine methyl ester; L-NMMA, N^G-monomethyl-L-arginine; NO, nitric oxide; TNF, tumor necrosis factor; *1, 2, 3, 4, 5, 6* correspond to numbers in Fig. 25.1.
[a]Animal trials only.

Based on these results, several clinical trials of anti-TNF-α antibodies were undertaken to determine the efficacy of anti-TNF therapy in patients with sepsis (28–30). Although Fisher et al. demonstrated no survival benefit in the total study population of 80 patients with sepsis or septic shock, subset analysis of the 35 patients with TNF-α levels greather than 50 pg/mL at presentation suggested that patients who received the highest dosage of 10 mg/kg of antibody had a survival advantage (31). Abraham et al. stratified 971 evaluable patients with sepsis syndrome to "shock" or "nonshock" and then randomized them to receive a single infusion of either placebo (n = 326), 7.5 mg/kg (n = 322), or 15 mg/kg (n = 323) of a murine TNF-α monoclonal antibody (MoAb) (28). When all 971 patients were considered, there was no difference in all-cause mortality in those that received either dose of TNF-α MoAb versus placebo. In a subgroup of 478 septic patients with shock, however, there was a trend toward a reduction in all-cause mortality at 3 days (15 mg/kg TNF-α MoAb, n = 162, 25 deaths; 7.5 mg/kg TNF-α MoAb, n = 156, 22 deaths; placebo, n = 160, 44 deaths; p = 0.01, 0.004, respectively). Unfortunately, this difference was not significant at 28 days. In another study of a fusion protein consisting of the extracellular portion of the human TNF receptor and Fc portion of IgG1 (TNF:Fc), patients who received higher doses of TNF:Fc tended to have a higher mortality rate than did those in the placebo-treated group (30). Additional clinical trials with humanized anti-TNF-α antibody are under way (4).

The disappointing results of the anti-TNF trials may be explained by the fact that TNF is released early in the development of sepsis, even before many of these patients request medical attention. In almost all the animal studies, anti-TNF therapy was administered before, simultaneously, or immediately after intravenous infusion of the endotoxin or bacteria (25–27).

Soluble Cytokine Receptors

These naturally occurring truncated forms of membrane receptors that contain the ligand-binding domains compete with the membrane-associated receptors for binding of cytokines. Such soluble receptors have been identified for IL-1, IL-4, IL-6, IFN-γ, and TNF (4,10). Two types of soluble TNF receptors (sTNFr) have been identified: one corresponding to the type I transmembrane domain and another corresponding to the type II domain. The sTNFr is thought to be a host defense mechanism that inhibits circulating TNF; high levels of sTNFr circulate in patients with sepsis (32,33). Administration of recombinant type I sTNFr has been shown to be beneficial in baboons against lethal *Escherichia coli* sepsis (32). Because TNF-α has a low affinity for the monomeric TNF receptor ectodomains, a chimeric product with two sTNFrs coupled to a human IgG Fc region was created and shown to prevent endotoxin-induced death in mice (34); however, a recent clinical trial of the chimeric sTNFr resulted in an increased mortality rate for patients with sepsis, casting doubt on the utility of such soluble receptors as a treatment (35). In this randomized, double-blind, placebo-controlled multicenter trial, 141 patients were randomized to receive either placebo (n = 33) or 0.15 mg/kg (n = 30), 0.45 mg/kg (n = 29), 1.5 mg/kg (n = 49) of TNFR:Fc as a single dose by intravenous infusion. Ten deaths occurred in the placebo group (30% mortality), nine deaths in the 0.15 mg/kg group (30% mortality), 14 deaths in the 0.45 mg/kg group (48% mortality), and 26 deaths in the high-dose group of TNFR: Fc (53% mortality) (p = 0.02 for the dose–response relation). Baseline differences in the severity of illness did not account for the increased mortality in the groups receiving the higher doses of TNFR:Fc (35). It is possible that endogenous TNF-α is an essential component of the bactericidal network, making its removal harmful, as illustrated in this clinical trial. Other studies in humans have shown that the inflammatory response can be maintained even in the face of agents antagonistic to TNF-α. Thus, neutralization of TNF-α would not be beneficial in controlling the hyperinflammatory manifestations of sepsis (36).

Cytokine Receptor Antagonists

The IL-1ra is the only naturally occurring receptor antagonist identified so far (4,11,37). IL-1ra is produced by macrophages in response to endotoxin and is structurally related to IL-1α and IL-1β. IL-1ra binds to both IL-1 receptors and has no IL-1 agonist activity. Production of IL-1ra increases during various infections, especially in sepsis (38). This finding suggests that in the presence of endogenous IL-1ra, IL-1 cannot bind to its cellular receptors and thus cannot exert its proinflammatory activity. IL-1ra may help to limit the severity of infection and may be beneficial in the treatment of sepsis. In fact, several animal studies have shown that exogenously administered IL-1ra significantly decreased the number of deaths from septic shock (39,40). In one of these studies (40), IL-1ra also reduced the production of IL-6 (the elevated levels of which are associated with a poor outcome in humans) (37). Two large clinical trials of recombinant IL-1ra were performed after these encouraging animal studies (38,41). In the first trial, 99 patients with sepsis syndrome or septic shock were treated with standard supportive care, antimicrobial therapy, and, in addition, with escalating doses of IL-1ra or placebo. Patients received an intravenous loading dose of either 100 mg of recombinant human IL-1 receptor antagonist (rhIL-1ra) or placebo, followed by a 72-hour intravenous infusion of one of three doses of IL- 1ra (17, 67, or 133 mg/hour) or placebo.

All patients were evaluated at day 28 for all-cause mortality (38). There were 11 deaths among 25 patients who received placebo (44%), eight deaths among 25 patients receiving 17 mg/hour of IL-1ra (32%), six deaths among 24 patients treated with 67 mg/hr (25%), and four deaths among 25 patients receiving 133 mg/hour (16%). The IL-1ra was well tolerated. There was a dose-dependent, 28-day survival benefit associated with IL-1ra treatment ($p = 0.015$), and this same dose-related survival benefit was seen in patients with septic shock at study entry (n = 65; $p = 0.002$) and in patients with gram-negative infection (n = 45; $p = 0.04$).

These encouraging results led to a randomized, double-blind, placebo-controlled, multicenter, multinational trial in which 893 patients with sepsis syndrome were enrolled. Patients received an intravenous loading dose of 100 mg of rhIL-1ra or placebo followed by a continuous 72-hour intravenous infusion of rhIL-1ra (1.0 or 2.0 mg/kg per hour) or placebo (41). In contrast to the prior study, there was no significant increase in survival time for rhIL-1ra treatment compared with placebo among all patients who received the study medication (n = 893; generalized Wilcoxon statistic, $p = 0.22$) or among patients with shock at study entry (n = 713; generalized Wilcoxon statistic, $p = 0.23$), the two primary efficacy analyses specified *a priori* for this trial. Among patients with dysfunction of one or more organs (n = 563), however, there was a dose-dependent improvement in 28-day all-cause mortality (in the placebo group mortality was 43%, in the group who received 1.0 mg/kg/hour of IL-1ra, 40%, and in those treated with 2.0 mg/kg/hour of IL-1ra 33%; linear dose-response, $p = 0.009$). Similarly, in patients with a predicted risk of mortality of 24% or greater (n = 580), mortality in the placebo group was 45%, in the group who received 1.0 mg/kg/hour of IL-1ra it was 38%, and in those treated with 2.0 mg/kg/hour of IL-1ra it was 35% (linear dose response, $p = 0.005$). Those with both dysfunction of one or more organs and a predicted risk of mortality of 24% or greater (n = 411) also had a similar dose-related reduction in mortality (linear dose response, $p = 0.002$) (41). In a summary of these and other similar trials, Zeni and Freeman (42) concluded that IL-1ra probably results in less than a 10% decrease in mortality rate in sepsis syndrome patients and that further trials are likely not to be pursued because of the large numbers of patients that would be needed to demonstrate definitively such a small benefit.

Antiinflammatory Cytokines

The available data clearly indicate that the endogenous production of IL-10, a potent antiinflammatory cytokine, plays a physiologic role in dampening the immune response after a generalized inflammatory stimulus (6,43). Administration of IL-10 can prevent staphylococcal enterotoxin B-induced death and neonatal group B streptococcal sepsis in mice (44,45); however, endogenous IL-10 or exogenously administered IL-10 is detrimental to mice infected with *Streptococcus pneumoniae, Klebsiella pneumoniae, Listeria monocytogenes, Mycobacterium avium,* and *Brucella abortus.* Treatment with antibodies specific for IL-10 results in the clearance of bacteria from blood and lung of these mice and improves their outcome (43). This finding is not surprising because the clearance of intracellular pathogens requires an intact and competent CMI. Therefore, the anti-Th1-directed responses of IL-10 may be detrimental to mice with a systemic infection caused by intracellular bacteria or parasites.

Exceedingly high levels of IL-10 have been measured in plasma from patients with meningococcal septic shock. Moreover, high levels of IL-10 were correlated with monocyte-deactivating activities in patients recovering from meningococcal septic shock. Elevated levels of IL-10, which plays an important role in generating an immune refractory state after major surgery and SIRS, have been measured in patients experiencing a variety of infections or SIRS caused by various agents (43). In healthy human volunteers, increases in circulating neutrophils and monocytes and decreases in lymphocytes were seen in response to recombinant IL-10 (rIL-10). In this same study, pretreatment with rIL-10, in a time- and dose-dependent manner, suppressed the synthesis of the proinflammatory cytokines TNF-α and IL-1β by whole blood stimulated *ex vivo* with LPS (46).

Interleukin-10 offers the possibility of a new treatment modality for a variety of infections and inflammatory diseases in humans. It is under clinical evaluation for the treatment of ischemic-reperfusion injury at the time of surgery that disrupts blood flow to major vessels (43). IL-10 may directly diminish human immunodeficiency virus (HIV) replication by inhibiting transcriptional activation in infected cells or by limiting virus proliferation through its interactions with other cytokines. Preclinical studies showed evidence of significant reductions in the viral load of HIV-infected severe combined immune-deficient mice reconstituted with human fetal thymus and liver (SCID-hu). IL-10 is in clinical trials for the treatment of HIV-associated disorders (47). The results of recent pilot studies in patients with HIV infection appear promising (43).

In a rabbit model of bacterial meningitis with either *L. monocytogenes* or *Haemophilus influenzae* type B, intracisternal administration of rIL-10 significantly reduced TNF-β and lactate levels in cerebrospinal fluid. The effect was more pronounced when IL-10 was used with dexamethasone (48). These encouraging results suggest that a strategic and cautious use of IL-10 may be beneficial in limiting an excessive inflammatory response to sepsis caused by gram-positive and gram-negative bacteria or in other diseases in which systemic inflammatory responses are deleterious to the host. This approach, however, warrants great caution because inadequate protection of experimental animals from invasive infection in the presence of TNF and IL-1 blocking agents result in higher mortality rates as a result of overwhelming infection (49). Conversely, inhibition of IL-10 actions may have potential therapeutic utility in diseases such as lepromatous leprosy, disseminated tuberculosis, and visceral leishmaniasis, in which inadequate CMI contributes to disease progression or pathogenesis. Several clinical trials are in progress to define the role of IL-10 in the treatment of a number of inflammatory conditions including HIV infection, acute lung injury, thoracic–abdominal aortic surgery, inflammatory bowel disease, rheumatoid arthritis, multiple sclerosis, and psoriasis (43).

COLONY-STIMULATING FACTORS

Colony-stimulating factors are cytokines that control the proliferation, differentiation, viability, and activation of hemopoietic cells.

TABLE 25.5. *Colony-stimulating factors*

CSF	Effects	Approved indication	Pediatric dose	Investigational indications	Side effects
G-CSF	Stimulates growth and differentiation of granulocytes	Prophylaxis after chemotherapy for nonmyeloid malignancies to prevent serious infections; treatment of cyclic or idiopathic neutropenia, Kostmann's syndrome; enhancement of myeloid engraftment after BMT for nonmyeloid malignancies	5 µg/kg d i.v. or SC	Established infections, bone marrow failure syndromes	Bone pain; occasional splenomegaly, allergic reactions
GM-CSF	Promotes growth and differentiation of granulocytes and macrophages, stimulates, proliferation of hematopoietic progenitor cells	Enhancement of myeloid engraftment in patients with NHL, HD, or ALL after BMT; delayed engraftment after ABMT	250 µg/m² d i.v. (2-h) or SC; has been given up to 2,000 µg/m² d (309)		Fever, fluid retention, dyspnea, joint or bone pain, myalgias
M-CSF	Stimulates growth and differentiation of monocytes and macrophages	None	Unknown	Possible treatment of invasive fungal infections	Fever, rash, myalgia, headache, facial flushing, photophobia

ABMT, autologous bone marrow transplant; ALL, acute lymphoblastic leukemia; BMT, bone marrow transplant; CSF, colony-stimulating factor; G-CSF, granulocyte colony-stimulating factor; GM-CSF, granulocyte-macrophage colony-stimulating factor; HD, Hodgkin disease; i.v., intravenous; M-CSF, macrophage colony-stimulating factor; NHL, Non-Hodgkin lymphoma; SC, subcutaneous.

Adapted from Mueller BV, Pizzo PA. Cytokines and biological response modifiers in the treatment of infection. *Cancer Treat Res* 1998;96:201–222, with permission.

Many immunocompromised children have low numbers of neutrophils as a result of their primary disease (e.g., Kostmann's syndrome) or their treatment (e.g., cancer therapy, treatment of HIV infection, organ transplantation) and were logical places to begin to apply this new class of agents in attempts to replace these deficiencies. Here we summarize what is known about the biology and clinical utility of three of the CSFs (granulocyte colony-stimulating factor [G-CSF], granulocyte-macrophage colony-stimulating factor [GM-CSF] and macrophage colony-stimulating factor [M-CSF]) that have been shown to contribute to the prevention and treatment of infections in immunocompromised hosts (Table 25.5).

Granulocyte Colony-Stimulating Factor

Produced by several cell types, including monocytes, fibroblasts, endothelial and epithelial cells, G-CSF stimulates growth and differentiation of committed neutrophil progenitors and activates their function. The human gene encoding G-CSF is located on chromosome 17q11.2-21 and encodes a 174-amino-acid polypeptide that is minimally glycosylated (50). G-CSF interacts with specific receptors on neutrophils and their immediate precursors (and on some monocytes and leukemic myeloblasts) but not with receptors on eosinophils, lymphocytes, or erythroid cells (51,52). The number of G-CSF receptors increases during cell maturation (51): Mature granulocytes express 700 to 1,500 receptors per cell (53). Low levels of G-CSF (about 3 pM) preferentially stimulate neutrophil progenitors to proliferate and differentiate. Higher concentrations of G-CSF stimulate some macrophage progenitors to proliferate and differentiate (54) and can initiate, but not sustain, growth of multipotential and erythroid progenitor cells (51). Further, binding of the cytokine to its receptor activates mature PMNs, resulting in increased chemotaxis (55), expression of receptors for N-formyl-methionyl-leucyl-phenylalanine (fMet-Leu-Phe) (56,57), the release of arachidonic acid (58,59), membrane depolarization in response to stimuli, increased expression of Fc receptors for IgA (60), increased antibody-dependent cellular cytotoxicity (ADCC) (56), and the release of superoxide radicals (55).

Because G-CSF is a growth factor for neutrophils, it has been evaluated in a variety of clinical situations in which patients have reduced or defective neutrophil production. Recombinant human granulocyte-colony stimulating factor (rhG-CSF) was first approved for clinical use in the United States in 1991 for the primary prophylaxis of patients with cancer who were treated with chemotherapy (61). In addition to stimulating the proliferation and maturation of neutrophils, G-CSF can enhance phagocytic activity, respiratory burst activity, chemotaxis, and ADCC. Thus, G-CSF may be effective in treating critically ill patients with sepsis or SIRS (3).

Clinical Applications of G-CSF

Chemotherapy-Induced Neutropenia

The most common dose-limiting toxicity of conventional cytotoxic chemotherapy is neutropenia. The risk of serious infection is directly related to the severity and duration of neutropenia (62). Until recently, intensive supportive care with the early initiation of broad-spectrum antibiotics has been the only method of treatment available for children undergoing chemotherapy who developed fever. Delays in the onset of subsequent courses of chemotherapy, reductions in doses of potentially curative agents, or both were then necessary. Development and availability of the CSFs, particularly G-CSF, have greatly changed cancer therapy. Most children in the United States and North America with cancer are now treated on clinical research protocols in which CSF use is often specified.

The clinical investigation of G-CSF and other CSFs to ameliorate the infectious complications of cancer chemotherapy has been applied in three different ways: primary prophylaxis, secondary prophylaxis, and in the treatment of neutropenia. *Primary prophy-*

laxis is defined as the administration of a CSF in an attempt to prevent neutropenia or infection as a complication of neutropenia (63). Treatment with a CSF is usually begun 24 hours after the end of chemotherapy and continued through the expected neutrophil nadir, usually consisting of a 10- to 14-day course. *Secondary prophylaxis* is defined as the administration of CSFs to prevent new episodes of febrile neutropenia in subsequent cycles of treatment in a patient who has experienced febrile neutropenia in a previous cycle of chemotherapy but did not receive CSFs. This approach is usually in lieu of dosage reductions in chemotherapy (63). Secondary prophylaxis has been used in adults to try to direct CSF use to patients who are most likely to benefit while theoretically sparing those who may not need prophylaxis; however, secondary prophylaxis is rarely used in children because the dose intensity of most pediatric chemotherapy regimens produces a high likelihood of the development of febrile neutropenia. Thus, CSFs almost always are used as primary prophylaxis in children undergoing chemotherapy. CSF treatment of established *neutropenia* has been used to shorten the duration of neutropenia. Also, there is some evidence that CSFs may "activate" immune effector cells such as neutrophils and macrophages and make them more effective in clearing infections.

In several early clinical trials of recombinant human G-CSF (rhG-CSF), chemotherapy-induced neutropenia and its attendant febrile complications were improved significantly in adults (64,65). Twelve patients received rhG-CSF by continuous intravenous infusion in dosages of 1 to 40 µg/kg daily for 2 weeks after alternate cycles of chemotherapy. The use of rhG-CSF reduced the period of neutropenia by a median of 80%, and no infective episodes occurred during courses with rhG-CSF use compared with six episodes occuing during cycles of chemotherapy without rhG-CSF (64). In another trial, 27 adults with bladder carcinoma received 1 to 60 µg/kg of rhG-CSF by 30-minute intravenous infusion before the first cycle of chemotherapy after the first cycle or both (65). The use of rhG-CSF after chemotherapy reduced the number of days the ANC was below 1,000/µL ($p = 0.0039$) and reduced the use of empiric antibiotics for febrile neutropenia ($p = 0.0015$). Improvement in chemotherapy-induced mucositis also was demonstrated (11 vs. 44%; $p = 0.041$) (65). In a well-known trial, 211 adults with newly diagnosed small cell lung cancer were enrolled in a multicenter, randomized, double-blind placebo-controlled trial of rhG-CSF after they had received intensive multiagent chemotherapy (66). Administration of G-CSF or placebo was begun on day 4, approximately 24 hours after the last dose of chemotherapy, and continued through day 17 unless the postnadir neutrophil count exceeded 10,000/µL. Courses of treatment were repeated every 21 days for a maximum of six cycles. In the group treated with rhG-CSF, the incidence of fever with neutropenia (70% vs. 40%; $p < 0.001$), the duration of severe neutropenia (6 vs. 3 days; $p < 0.001$), and the total number of days of treatment with intravenous antibiotics (47% reduction in the mean number of days on intravenous antibiotics) were reduced.

Only a few randomized trials of G-CSF as primary prophylaxis have been performed in children (Tables 25.6 and 25.7) (67–71). Although rhG-CSF has been approved for the prevention of febrile neutropenia after chemotherapy (primary prophylaxis), the optimal schedule of rhG-CSF use after chemotherapy is still not known. In the best known trial, rhG-CSF was begun approximately 24 hours after the end of chemotherapy, and this is the primary schedule used for primary prophylaxis (66). In another trial of 33 adults with lung cancer, the schedule of rhG-CSF administration was randomly assigned to three groups: beginning 24 hours after completion of chemotherapy (*early treatment group*; n = 11), beginning 7 days after completion of chemotherapy (*late prophylaxis group*; n = 11), and on the first day of ANC below 1,000/µL (*therapeutic group*; n = 11). The results were also compared with those of ten patients who had received identi-

TABLE 25.6. Use of G-CSF in children as primary infection prophylaxis after chemotherapy

G-CSF regimen	Disease (no. of patients)	G-CSF vs. Control			Conclusions	Reference
		Incidence of fever and neutropenia	Median duration of antibiotic use	Median duration of hospitalization		
Randomized to chemotherapy ±G-CSF at a dose of 5 µg/kg given subcutaneously qd, beginning on day 7 and continuing for up to 14 d after chemotherapy	Metastic neuroblastoma	Not reported	Not reported	Not reported	78% of pts who received G-CSF and 5% who received chemotherapy without G-CSF were able to start next course of chemotherapy on time	(310) abstract
5 µg/kg, i.v. Randomized qd vs bid; begin day 1 vs. day 7 after chemotherapy	Nonhodgkin's lymphoma (10); neuroblastoma (11)	Not reported	Not reported	Not reported	Duration of neutropenia same for qd and bid; ANC reached > 500/µL more rapidly when G-CSF begun day 1 vs. day 7 (6.2 ± 3.5 vs. 10.4 ± 4.4 d $p < 0.01$)	(311)
Randomized to chemotherapy ±G-CSF; 10 µg/kg, SC	ALL (14 with G-CSF, 18 without G-CSF)	6 vs. 6	Not reported	5.8 ± 4 vs. 6.2 ± 5 d	G-CSF supportive therapy may be unnecessary in children with neutropenia of short duration	(67)
Randomized to chemotherapy ±G-CSF; 5 µg/kg, SC qd days 7 to 20 after each chemotherapy course	High-risk ALL (17 received G-CSF and 137 courses of chemotherapy; 17 received no G-CSF and 121 courses of CT)	17% vs. 40% ($p = 0.007$)	18.2 vs. 32.2 d ($p = 0.02$)	Not reported	G-CSF administered prophylactically in the interval between chemotherapy courses significantly reduced febrile neutropenia, culture-confirmed infections, and duration of i.v. antibiotic use	(68)
Randomized to chemotherapy ±G-CSF (or placebo); 10 µg/kg, SC qd until ANC > 1,000/µL for 2 consecutive days	ALL, beginning day 1 after induction CT (73 patients received G-CSF; 75 did not)	58% vs. 68%	6 vs. 9 d	6 vs. 10 d ($p = 0.011$)	G-CSF use did not reduce the rate of hospitalization for febrile neutropenia, prolong survival, or reduce the cost of supportive care	(69)
Randomized, CT ± G-CSF; 5 µg/kg SC qd	Nonhodgkin's lymphoma (149)	95% vs. 99%	13 vs. 16 d ($p = 0.07$)	31 vs. 33 d ($p = 0.15$)	Treatment with G-CSF after chemotherapy in children with NHL, previously shown to be of limited clinical benefit, also does not appear to reduce the costs of chemotherapy	(312)
Nonrandomized (20) courses of chemotherapy with G-CSF compared with 20 courses without in same children; 5 µg/kg, SC beginning day +1 after CT	Children with cancer receiving chemotherapy (16 patients)	2 vs. 10 ($p = 0.04$)	13 vs. 95 d ($p = 0.003$)	13 vs. 65 d ($p = 0.02$)	Use of G-CSF resulted in savings of $20,650 for 20 courses of chemotherapy or $1,033/course.	(125)

SC, subcutaneous; i.v., intravenous; ALL, acute lymphoblastic leukemia; CT, chemotherapy; qd, daily; pts, patients; ANC, absolute neutrophil count; bid, twice daily; G-CSF, granulocyte colony-stimulating factor; qd, daily.

TABLE 25.7. *Use of G-CSF to treat infections*

G-CSF regimen	Study design	Incidence of F/N	G-CSF vs. Control — Median duration of antibiotic use	G-CSF vs. Control — Median duration of hospitalization	Conclusions	Reference
Nonrandomized; 200 μg/m², SC; Three groups: Septicemia following CT for ALL (50 documented episodes of sepsis) Gr A: n = 25 Gr B: n = 16 Gr C: n = 9	Septicemia following CT for ALL (50 documented episodes of sepsis) Gr A: n = 25 Gr B: n = 16 Gr C: n = 9	NA	Same for 3 groups	Same for 3 groups	No significant differences seen between the groups in days of antibiotic use, hospital days, or mortality.	(126)
A, no G-CSF B, G-CSF begun as soon as sepsis documented C, Prophylactic G-CSF after CT						
Randomized, placebo-controlled; ±5 μg/kg G-CSF, SC upon hospitalization for fever/neutropenia	112 patients with cancer, 186 episodes of fever/neutropenia (112 first episode, 74 subsequent); 94 with G-CSF, 92 without	NA	Median 5 vs. 6 d (p = 0.02)	Median 5 vs. 7 d (p = 0.04)	The use of G-CSF produced a small but significant reduction in the duration of antibiotic use and hospitalization, with possible cost savings	(79)
Randomized, placebo-controlled trial; 1.0, 5.0 or 10 μg/kg (i.v. over 1 h) every 24 h × 3 days or 5 or 10 μg/kg every 12 h × 3 d	42 neonates (26 to 40 wk of age) with presumed sepsis for 3 d or less Placebo, n = 9; G-CSF at 1.0 μg/kg qd, n = 9; 5.0 μg/kg qd, n = 9; 10 μg/kg qd, n = 9; 5.0 μg/kg q 12 h, n = 3; 10 μg/kg q 12, n = 3	NA	Not reported	Not reported	G-CSF induced a significant increase in the peripheral blood and bone marrow ANC	(313)

ALL, acute lymphoblastic leukemia; ANC, absolute neutrophil count; CT, chemotherapy; F/N-fever with neutropenia; G-CSF, granulocyte colony-stimulating factor; Gr, group; i.v., intravenous; NA, not available; qd, daily; SC, subcutaneous.

cal chemotherapy without rhG-CSF support (72). The incidence of ANC less than 1,000/µL was significantly lower in the late prophylaxis group (8/18 courses, or 44%) than in either the early (16/20 courses, or 80%; $p < 0.05$) or the therapeutic group (17/18 courses, or 94%; $p < 0.01$). No differences were found, however, in the incidence of febrile neutropenia among the four groups (72). Although others evaluated the schedule for optimization of primary prophylaxis in various settings (73–76), no clear consensus has been achieved. The optimal timing of rhG-CSF for use as primary prophylaxis may also depend on the type of chemotherapy. Further clinical trials are needed to define the optimal schedule of rhG-CSF use for primary prophylaxis.

Another potential use of rhG-CSF is in the treatment of chemotherapy-induced febrile neutropenia. In the largest adult trial, (77), 218 patients with fever (>38.2°C) and an ANC less than 1,000/µL after treatment with chemotherapy were randomized to receive either rhG-CSF or placebo along with intravenous tobramycin and piperacillin. Patients treated with rhG-CSF experienced a decrease in the number of days of ANC less than 500/µL from 4 days to 3 days ($p = 0.005$) and an improvement in the resolution of febrile neutropenia from 6 days to 5 days ($p = 0.01$). Unfortunately, these did not result in a decreased duration of hospitalization (78).

In a similar randomized, placebo-controlled trial in children with established febrile neutropenia, 112 patients were studied during 186 febrile episodes. The use of rhG-CSF resulted in a small reduction in hospital stay (median 5 vs. 7 days; $p = 0.04$) and antibiotic use (median 5 vs. 6 days; $p = 0.04$) (79). A similar trial in 121 adults randomized patients to either rhG-CSF (n = 39), rhGM-CSF (n = 39), or placebo (n = 43) with "standard antibiotic treatments given to cancer patients for chemotherapy-induced neutropenic fever" (80). They found similar small reductions in days of hospitalization with CSF use (median, 5 days with either rhG- or rhGM-CSF vs. 7 days; $p < 0.001$).

These small clinical benefits warrant further trials to delineate the subset of patients who might benefit most.

Recommendations for rhG-CSF Use in Children

The available data suggest that G-CSF should be used as primary prophylaxis in children when the incidence of febrile neutropenia associated with a given course of chemotherapy is at least 40% (81–83). Treatment with G-CSF should be initiated at doses of 5 µg/kg daily given subcutaneously or intravenously, beginning 24 hours after the last dose of chemotherapy and continuing through the expected neutrophil nadir (usually 7 days or longer after most chemotherapy regimens) until normal levels of neutrophils have been restored (61,81,82,84).

Bone Marrow Transplantation

Randomized trials of G-CSF as primary prophylaxis after autologous bone marrow transplantation (85–89) also have generally shown similar benefits in fewer antibiotic days (85,88,89) but failed to show improvements in infectious mortality. The data after allogeneic transplantation are less compelling.

Myelodysplastic Syndrome

The myelodysplastic syndromes (MDSs) are a group of stem cell disorders characterized by a reduction in the number of neutrophils, impaired function of neutrophils, anemia, and hemorrhage. G-CSF, either alone or in combination with other cytokines, is being tested in a number of clinical trials, almost exclusively in adults, to determine whether G-CSF can be used to increase the neutrophil number and function and thus decrease the infectious complications of patients with MDS (90,91). Although the neutrophil counts and neutrophil function improved in most patients who received G-CSF, the clinical benefit of G-CSF in preventing infection in these patients is still unproven (61,90,91).

Aplastic Anemia

Although G-CSF has been tested in several small trials to determine its effectiveness in treating aplastic anemia (92), there are insufficient data to recommend routine use of G-CSF in children with aplastic anemia.

Congenital Neutropenia

Congenital neutropenia, also known as congenital agranulocytosis or Kostmann's syndrome, is a disorder that usually is detected in the first months of life and characterized by profound neutropenia (<500 neutrophils/µL) and by the absence of neutrophil precursors beyond the promyelocyte stage in bone marrow. This syndrome results in frequent bacterial infections that often progress to septicemia, meningitis, and death. G-CSF was given in doses of 3 to 60 µg/kg daily to five patients with this disorder (93). In all patients, the number of circulating neutrophils increased to 1,000/µL for 9 to 13 months during treatment, preexisting chronic infections resolved, and the number of new infections requiring intravenous antibiotics decreased. A larger, multicenter trial confirmed these findings (94). Similar benefits have been reported for some patients with idiopathic neutropenia (95).

Cyclic neutropenia is a rare disorder of myelopoiesis characterized by regular cyclic fluctuations (usually every 21 days) in the number of circulating hemopoietic cells. Children with this disease have recurring infections during periods of severe neutropenia. Six patients with cyclic neutropenia and histories of recurrent infections, aphthous stomatitis, and pharyngitis were treated daily with rhG-CSF for 3 to 15 months (96), all of which improved dramatically with treatment. In five patients, cycling of the blood counts continued, but the length of each cycle decreased from 21 to 14 days. Administration of rhG-CSF also increased the mean neutrophil counts, decreased the number of days of severe neutropenia, and reduced symptoms in most patients. Results from additional trials confirmed these findings (97). Use of G-CSF

essentially eliminated infectious complications in this group of children. Current investigations are focusing on reducing the number of injections of G-CSF per week needed to maintain clinical efficacy (98,99).

Acquired Immunodeficiency Syndrome

Neutropenia that results directly from infection or as a secondary effect of anti-HIV therapy is an important problem in children infected with HIV. Accumulating data suggest that the use of rhG-CSF in patients with acquired immunodeficiency sydrome (AIDS) increases neutrophil counts and can prevent neutropenic fever (61).

Other Disorders

Neutropenia from disorders such as glycogen storage diseases or dyskeratosis congenita can result in infectious morbidity. In one patient with neutropenia resulting from glycogen storage disease type Ib, this patient's clinical course of repeated infectious episodes improved greatly with the initiation of rhG-CSF treatment (100). This patient received rhG-CSF for 18 months and continues to show a marked reduction in infections. Similar results were seen in two other patients (101). Another patient with dyskeratosis congenita who received rhG-CSF treatment for a year had an excellent neutrophil response, from an ANC of less than 1,000/µL to greater than 1,500/µL by 2 weeks and greater than 10,000/µL by 6 weeks of treatment. Effects on complications resulting from infection were not reported (102).

Neutropenia is present at birth in 36% to 57% of newborns born to mothers with preeclampsia. About 6% of these infants will develop sepsis (103). In several small series, the effects of rhG-CSF on neutropenia in newborns have been evaluated (103–105). In the largest series, 15 neonates received rhG-CSF for 3 days by 1-hour intravenous infusion. The incidence of neonatal sepsis in the next 28 postnatal days was compared with that of 13 case-matched controls who also had prolonged preeclampsia-associated neutropenia (103). Sepsis was observed in 2 of 15 neonates treated with rhG-CSF; 7 of the 13 control infants experienced sepsis ($p < 0.05$) (103). Other potential uses of rhG-CSF are the treatment of diabetic foot infections (106), following liver transplantation (107), and as an aid to the treatment of fungal infections (108,109).

Prevention and Treatment of Sepsis

The role of rhG-CSF in preventing the progression of sepsis and reducing the incidence and severity of multiple organ dysfunction was reviewed by Weiss et al. (3). RhG-CSF administered prophylactically is thought to block the proinflammatory cytokine cascade before it culminates in severe tissue damage. G-CSF promotes the production of Th2-type cytokines (which produce IL-4 and IL-10) in mice and human T cells (110,111). These effects may help to restore immune dysfunction and imbalance in critically ill patients. Reduced expression of Th1-type cytokines and increased expression of Th2-type cytokines expression may downregulate NOS-2 activation and thus reduce NO synthesis. Through these direct and indirect effects, G-CSF may prevent the development of sepsis and reduce the risk of death in patients who have already developed sepsis.

Some experiments in animal models of infection or sepsis have produced encouraging results: increased survival rates of animals with sepsis (112–114), after severe burns (115,116), in models of neonatal sepsis (117), in models of soft tissue infection (118), in intraabdominal sepsis (113), and in a mouse model of pneumonia (115,119). For example, pretreatment of mice with rhG-CSF prevented death in two different models of septic shock (114). RhG-CSF (20 µg/kg/24 hours) given to rats 4 hours after intraabdominal sepsis was induced by a 4-mm cecal perforation reduced the mortality rate by more than half, from 96% to 42% (112).

Studies of humans have included evaluations of host immunity in postoperative and posttraumatic patients at risk of sepsis. In 16 of 20 patients at risk of sepsis, administration of exogenous G-CSF resulted in increased numbers of leukocytes and improved leukocyte function (120). In an additional clinical evaluation, 24 patients with granulocytopenia and sepsis who failed to respond to antibiotics (121) received 75 µg of rhG-CSF once daily for a mean of 5.2 days. Nineteen patients had increased leukocyte counts and survived. In contrast, the five patients whose leukocyte counts did not increase in response to rhG-CSF died (121). In another study, 214 adults with febrile neutropenia treated with tobramycin and flomoxef sodium were randomized to receive or not to receive rhG-CSF (122). No difference was found in the resolution of fever at day 4 or 7 of treatment in either group. Although administration of rhG-CSF had an observable effect on neutrophil recovery, it did not affect the response rate to empiric antibiotics (122). RhG-CSF also was evaluated as an adjunct to antibiotics in hospitalized patients with pneumonia (123). In this randomized, placebo-controlled trial, 756 adults who were receiving intravenous antibiotics for community-acquired pneumonia were randomized to receive rhG-CSF (n = 380) or placebo (n = 376). A 300-µg dose of rhG-CSF or placebo was given on the first day of randomization; additional doses were administered for a maximum of 10 days. Although the number of circulating neutrophils increased threefold in the rhG-CSF-treated group, no difference was found in the length of hospitalization or treatment-related mortality rates between the two groups (123); however, the use of rhG-CSF reduced the incidence of adult respiratory distress syndrome (4 vs. 14, $p = 0.017$), disseminated intravascular coagulopathy (2 vs. 7, $p = 0.007$), and empyema (1 vs. 6, $p = 0.068$) (123). All these data taken together suggest that rhG-CSF does have a role in the treatment of some patients with severe infections; however, additional trials are needed to identify the patients who will benefit most.

Toxicity

The toxicities of rhG-CSF in children have been mild and consisted of local hematomas at injection sites, occasional bone pain, and, rarely, asymptomatic splenomegaly associated with leukocytosis (79,124–126). In adults, the most commonly reported side effect, which occurs in about 20% to 30% of patients, is mild to moderate musculoskeletal and bone pain (50,127–129).

Granulocyte-Macrophage Colony-Stimulating Factor

A variety of cell types produce GM-CSF, many of which are present at sites of inflammation. These cells include T lymphocytes (130), macrophages, monocytes (131), endothelial cells (132), osteoblasts (133), smooth-muscle cells (134), trophoblasts (135), fibroblasts (136), and certain types of tumor cells (137). GM-CSF stimulates hemopoietic progenitor cells to proliferate and differentiate into granulocytes and macrophages and regulates some of their functions at maturity (138). In humans, the GM-CSF gene, located on chromosome bands 5q21-32 (139), encodes a 127 amino acid protein that can be glycosylated in different patterns, resulting in a native glycoprotein with a molecular weight ranging from 14 to 35 kDa (140).

Granulocyte macrophage-CSF exerts its biologic activity by binding to a specific cell-surface receptor that is widely expressed on hemopoietic cells, endothelial cells (141), and certain solid tumor cells (142). The GM-CSF receptor consists of two subunits: alpha and beta. The low–molecular weight α subunit binds ligand with low affinity, whereas the α and the β subunits together confer high-affinity binding (143). Low receptor occupancy appears to be adequate for maximal biologic activity (144), a property that confounds studies of the precise intracellular signaling cascade by which GM-CSF exerts its biologic effects.

Both GM-CSF and other CSFs may play a primary role in regulating the immune response by directly enhancing neutrophil function and by activating phagocytosis (145–147). GM-CSF enhances both chemotaxis to sites of injury (60,146,148) and cellular immobilization at inflammatory sites when neutrophils are exposed to GM-CSF for a prolonged time (60,146,149). The cytotoxicity of monocytes and eosinophils for both microbes (150) and tumor cells (151,152) also is enhanced by exposure to this cytokine.

All these effects, which are concentration and time dependent (146), involve coordinated interaction with other hemopoietins (60) and immune stimulants, including endotoxin, components of the complement system (C3b and C5a) (60), platelet-activating factor, leukotriene B4 (153), and formylpeptides such as fMet-Leu-Phe (a tripeptide released by bacteria that is chemotactic for inflammatory cells) (154).

Recombinant human GM-CSF (rhGM-CSF) was first approved for clinical use in the United States in 1991. Although three different recombinant human GM-CSFs have been produced, only Sargramostim, which is yeast derived, is clinically approved.

Clinical Applications of GM-CSF

Chemotherapy-Induced Neutropenia

Table 25.8 summarizes the use of rhGM-CSF as primary prophylaxis in children. Although several randomized trials of rhGM-CSF have been done in children (155–157) as primary prophylaxis, the findings have been less positive than those from trials of rhG-CSF. The reasons for this are unclear; however, the disappointing findings may be due to induction of cytokine fever by rhGM-CSF (63), weaker biologic activity of rhGM-CSF compared with that of rhG-CSF, or suboptimal protocol design.

Bone Marrow Transplantation

Brandt et al. (158) found that rhGM-CSF accelerated myeloid cell recovery in 19 adults

TABLE 25.8. *GM-CSF use in children as primary prophylaxis after chemotherapy*

GM-CSF regimen	Study group	GM-CSF vs. Control				Conclusions	Reference
		Incidence of fever and neutropenia	Median duration of i.v. antibiotic use	Median duration of hospitalization			
1,000 µg/m²/d; SC after ICE CT (12 patients with GM-CSF, 8 without) CT until ANC > 10,000/µL compared to historical controls	Solid tumors after ICE CT (12 patients with GM-CSF, 8 without)	100% vs. 79% (*p* = ns)	Not reported	8.25 vs. 6.75 d (*p* = ns)		GM-CSF did not reduce the proportion of courses associated with febrile neutropenia or the duration of hospitalization	(314)
Randomized to CT ± 5 to15 µg/kg/d (Leucomax), SC after each course of CT (began with course 3) until day 19 or ANC ≥ 500/µL × 2 d	ESFT (19 with GM-CSF and 167 courses; 18 without GM-CSF and 303 courses)	40.1% vs. 44.2%	8 vs. 7 d (total: 75 vs. 89 d)	0 vs. 0 d (Total: 165 vs. 226 d); (*p* = ns)		GM-CSF did not produce clinically meaningful reductions in the degree or duration of severe granulocytopenia, nor reduce the need for hospitalization or the incidence of fever and neutropenia.	(155)
Randomized to CT ± 250 µg/m²/d, CI 48 h after CT × 14 d on course 1 and 3 vs. 2 and 4	11 children with solid tumors; 42 courses with GM-CSF, 42 without	Not reported; 8 "infectious episodes" vs. 14 episodes	Not reported; (Total: 82 vs. 91 d)	Not reported		In children and adolescents undergoing intensive chemotherapy for solid tumors, GM-CSF reduces neutropenia and infectious episodes at the cost of mild thrombocytopenia	(157)
Randomized after autoBMT to placebo vs. 16 µg/kg/d (Leucomax) CI starting 3 h after marrow infusion × 14 d	21 children with metastatic NB; 16 pts part of double blind randomized cross over (arm A-6 after ABMT1, placebo after ABMT2; arm B-10 after ABMT2, placebo after ABMT1; 5 open label as arm A)	100%	ABMT1-19.6 vs. 26 d (*p* < 0.05); ABMT2-24 vs. 10 d (*p* < 0.02)	31 vs. 38 d (*p* < 0.02)		After the second ABMT, patients receiving GM-CSF have significantly longer episodes of febrile neutropenia	(315)

ABMT, autologous bone marrow transplantation; ABMT1, first ABMT; ABMT2, second ABMT; ANC, absolute neutrophil count; CI, continuous infusion; CT, chemotherapy; ESFT, Ewing sarcoma family of tumors; GM-CSF, granulocyte macrophage-colony stimulating factor; ICE, ifosfamide, carboplatin, etoposide; i.v., intravenous; NB, neuroblastoma; SC, subcutaneous.

treated with high-dose chemotherapy and autologous bone marrow transplantation (ABMT). This effect was not seen in 24 matched historical controls who did not receive this hemopoietin. Similar conclusions were reached by Nemunaitis et al. (159) in a study of 15 patients treated for lymphoid malignancies with autologous bone marrow transplantation and rhGM-CSF. Another study reported no difference in the time to hematologic recovery between a group of 25 patients with acute lymphoblastic leukemia who received autologous bone marrow transplants plus rhGM-CSF and historical controls who received only autologous bone marrow transplants (160); however, other studies demonstrated more rapid neutrophil (159, 161) and platelet (159) recovery in patients who received rhGM-CSF than in historical control groups. Because of these preliminary, encouraging findings, a randomized, double-blind, placebo-controlled trial in adults with lymphoid malignancies who were undergoing ABMT was performed (162). Preparative regimens differed, but the study design and the treatment schedule for patients receiving rhGM-CSF or placebo were identical. In this trial, 128 consecutive patients were enrolled at three participating medical centers. Sixty-five patients received daily 2-hour intravenous infusions of rhGM-CSF for 21 days, beginning within 4 hours of marrow infusion; 63 patients received placebo infusions. No particular type of toxicity was consistently ascribed to rhGM-CSF, suggesting that the toxic effects previously ascribed to this hemopoietin are associated with the effects of ABMT. Most importantly, the group treated with rhGM-CSF had more rapid recovery of neutrophils (ANC > $500/mm^3$ 19 vs. 26 days; $p = 0.01$) and needed three fewer days of IV antibiotics (24 vs. 27 days; $p = 0.01$). These improvements resulted in shorter initial hospital stays for the group treated with rhGM-CSF by 6 days (median duration, 27 vs. 33 days; $p = 0.01$) (162). No similar study of children has been reported. Our own experience suggests that rhGM-CSF will produce similar accelerated recovery of neutrophil counts in children who undergo a bone marrow transplant.

Myelodysplastic Syndrome (MDS)

Several phase 1/2 clinical trials have used RhGM-CSF in adults with MDS (90,91). Most demonstrated a dose-dependent increase in circulating neutrophils. Although a few also reported a reduced risk of bacterial infections, the routine use of GM-CSF in children with MDS cannot yet be recommended.

Aplastic Anemia

Several clinical trials using rhGM-CSF in patients with aplastic anemia (163–165), including one in children (166), have been reported. Again, dose-dependent increases in granulocytes, monocytes, and eosinophils were seen in most patients. Another study in seven children with Fanconi's anemia showed increases in neutrophil counts of 7- to 25-fold. RhGM-CSF was continued for up to 19 months (167). These studies were not designed to assess the impact of rhGM-CSF on the infectious morbidity of these patients, and therefore no recommendations can be made about its use in this group of children.

Congenital Neutropenia and Cyclic Neutropenia

There is very little published experience with the use of rhGM-CSF in either of these disorders (168,169). Furthermore, as discussed previously, because rhG-CSF is effective in these conditions, it is doubtful whether appropriate clinical trials will ever be done with rhGM-CSF to delineate its potential role in these diseases.

Acquired Immunodeficiency Syndrome

To enhance their immune function or to treat neutropenia, RhGM-CSF has been used in adults with AIDS (170,170–175). In most patients, it results in a dose-dependent increase in neutrophils, eosinophils, and monocytes (173). In this first trial, patients were treated with rhGM-CSF in doses ranging from 0.5 to 8.0 µg/kg. Dose-related increases in neutrophils were noted, with neutrophil counts as high as 35,000/µL at 8.0 µg/kg (173). Some patients received drug for up to 6 months without problems.

In other studies, rhGM-CSF was used in conjunction with antiretrovirals zidovudine (174) or azidothymidine (175). Its use resulted in continuation of antiretroviral therapy without interruption for neutropenia, a common problem with the use of these agents. Other potential uses of rhGM-CSF in patients with AIDS relate to its ability to activate and enhance neutrophil and macrophage phagocytosis of intracellular parasites, fungi, and bacteria (150,170,176). These properties make it of value in the prevention and treatment of opportunistic infections (170). A multicenter phase 3 randomized double-blind, placebo-controlled trial of rhGM-CSF is now under way to evaluate the incidence and time to first opportunistic infection (170).

Although there is some concern about rhGM-CSF increasing viral replication by stimulating macrophages (170,172), in a recent review of more than 270 AIDS patients treated with rhGM-CSF in 22 clinical trials, no increased risk of viral replication or clinical deterioration was found (171).

The potential benefits of rhGM-CSF use in patients with HIV infection are many, although no trial has yet demonstrated an improved survival. Currently, the routine use of rhGM-CSF in children with AIDS cannot be recommended.

Other Disorders

The use of RhGM-CSF in one patient with glycogen-storage disease has been reported (101). Dosages of 3 and 8 µg/kg daily resulted in increases in the average ANC to 1,200/µL from a baseline average of 300/µL. Therapy with rhGM-CSF had to be discontinued because of severe local side effects (101).

Very low birth weight (VLBW) infants have an increased risk of infectious complications. In a randomized, placebo-controlled trial, 264 VLBW infants aged 3 days or younger received a 2-hour intravenous infusion of rhGM-CSF (8 µg/kg/day; n = 134) or placebo (n = 130) daily for 7 days. Although

the ANC and eosinophil counts were significantly elevated on day 7 in the infants who received rhGM-CSF, there was no difference in the incidence of confirmed nosocomial infections in the two groups (40% in the rhGM-CSF group vs. 39% in placebo; p = not significant) (177). With these results in mind, the prophylactic use of rhGM-CSF in VLBW infants does not appear warranted.

Other potential uses of rhGM-CSF to treat or prevent infections include patients with congenital neutropenia (168) and drug-induced agranulocytosis (178), to enhance wound-healing (170,179,180), to treat severe refractory warts (181), as an adjunct in the treatment of severe fungal infections (182, 183), in the treatment of chemotherapy or radiation-induced mucositis (184,185), in children after orthotic liver transplantation (186), and as a vaccine adjuvant (170).

Additionally, GM-CSF is part of the "cytokine cascade" of SIRS and is involved in its pathogenesis (187). Although GM-CSF has a number of functional effects on neutrophils, monocytes, and macrophages related to their response to infection (188), it plays no obvious role as a systemic effector molecule in SIRS (3); however, its role as part of the supportive care of patients with sepsis is still being investigated. For example, in one study, 91 febrile neutropenic patients were randomized to receive ticarcillin–clavulanate plus netilmicin with (n = 45) or without (n = 46) rhGM-CSF (176). A significantly higher rate of cure occurred in the patients who received rhGM-CSF with antibiotics compared with those who received antibiotics alone (98% vs. 87%; p = 0.05). Although no mention is made of how many of these patients were considered to be clinically "septic," the use of rhGM-CSF in the group of patients with documented infections (33 episodes treated with antibiotics alone; 26 episodes treated with antibiotics and rhGM-CSF) also was associated with an improved cure rate (100% vs. 82%; p = 0.02) (176). The definitive role of rhGM-CSF in the treatment of sepsis awaits further clinical investigation. Table 25.9 summarizes the clinical trials of rhGM-CSF in children to treat presumed infections.

TABLE 25.9. *Use of GM-CSF to treat infections in children*

GM-CSF regimen	Study group	GM-CSF vs. Control			Conclusions	Reference
		Incidence of F/N	Duration of i.v. antibiotic use	Duration of hospitalization		
Randomized, placebo; ±5 µg/kg GM-CSF (Leucomax), SC on hospitalization for fever/neutropenia	40 children after CT/58 episodes of febrile neutropenia (28 with GM-CSF, 30 with placebo)	NA	Median 7 vs. 8.5 d ($p < 0.05$)	Median 9 vs 10 d ($p < 0.05$)	GM-CSF accelerated myeloid recovery and reduced the length of hospitalization for febrile neutropenia.	(316)
Randomized, placebo in VLBWN, GM-CSF 8 µg/kg d i.v. over 2 h × 7 days, then qod × 21 d	Neonates weighing 501 to 1000 g ≤72 h old (134 with GM-CSF, 130 placebo)	40% vs. 39% incidence of nosocomial infection	Mean, 15 vs. 14 d	Mean 28 vs. 28 d in NICU	Prophylactic administration of GM-CSF in VLBWN did not decrease the incidence of nosocomial infections.	(317)

NICU, neonatal intensive care unit; SC, subcutaneously; CT, chemotherapy; NA, not available; F/N, fever with neutropenia; GM-CSF, granulocyte macrophage-colony stimulating factor; i.v., intravenous; SC, subcutaneous; VLBWN, very low birth weight infants (50–1,000 g).

Toxicity

The dose-limiting toxicities of rhGM-CSF in both adults and children are mainly myalgias and fluid retention that is sometimes accompanied by pleural or pericardial effusions (159, 166,189). Rash and fever are frequent in children (166). A "first-dose effect" consisting of transient hypoxemia and hypotension has been reported (190). It is unclear whether this effect is unique to the nonglycosylated form of rhGM-CSF synthesized by bacteria. We have found that yeast-derived rhGM-CSF is tolerated well by children with cancer who have received myelosuppressive chemotherapy, even at doses more than three times higher (up to 2,000 μg/m^2) than those used in adult trials of the same product in which the maximum tolerated dose ranged from 250 to 500 μg/m^2 (160,191–193). The reasons for this are not clear. This finding could be explained by the possibility that the glycosylated products are better tolerated or that the toxicity profiles differ with underlying diseases or treatment histories. Another possible explanation is that children tolerate rhGM-CSF better than adults do (194). The findings of pharmacokinetic studies of rhGM-CSF in several children revealed no significant differences in drug disposition in children and adults (195).

Data on which to base a recommended dose of rhGM-CSF in children are few. The dose–response effect and toxicity profile we observed in children with cancer suggested that a daily dose of yeast-derived rhGM-CSF (750–1,500 μg/m^2) given by 2-hour intravenous infusion or subcutaneously may be appropriate. Few data are available from which to make firm recommendations for children with other illnesses, but the study reported by Guinan et al. (166) suggests that doses of 8 to 32 μg/kg daily (*E. coli*-derived rhGM-CSF) may be beneficial in children with aplastic anemia. Ongoing trials in a number of centers in the United States and Europe should provide more precise data in the future.

Macrophage Colony-Stimulating Factor

Also called CSF-1, M-CSF is produced by many different cell types (e.g., fibroblasts, bone marrow stromal cells, monocytes and macrophages, T lymphocytes, endothelial cells, uterine glandular epithelial cells) (196, 197). M-CSF binds to a high-affinity receptor on the surface of monocytes and macrophages and their precursors to promote the proliferation and differentiation of cells of monocyte/macrophage lineage and to maintain the functional integrity of these cells in the circulation. The human gene is located on chromosome bands 1p13-21 (197). Differential splicing of the M-CSF gene results in multiple mRNA species and subsequently polypeptide chains of variable length and carbohydrate composition (198). The native protein exists as a dimer of two identical subunits with a molecular weight of 70 to 90 kDa.

Although M-CSF has not yet been approved for commercial use, several trials of this cytokine have been conducted. Twenty-four adults who developed invasive fungal disease after bone marrow transplantation received standard antifungal therapy (199) and rhM-CSF given as a 2-hour intravenous infusion in doses ranging from 100 μg/m^2 to 2,000 μg/m^2. No toxicity directly attributable to rhM-CSF was observed. In six patients, their infections were resolved, and in another six, the infections did not respond to treatment. Twelve patients were not evaluable for response. No effects on monocyte, lymphocyte, or neutrophil counts were observed; however, patients who received the largest doses of rhM-CSF experienced a mean reduction in platelet count of 61,000/mm^3 during rhM-CSF treatment (199). Further evaluations of this cytokine in both adults and children with disseminated fungal infections resulting from cancer treatments are ongoing.

INTERFERONS

Interferons were discovered in 1957 by Isaccs and Lindenmann and were given their name because of their ability to interfere with viral replication (200). IFNs are divided into three classes—α, β, and γ on the basis of their antigenicity, amino acid sequence, and physiochemical properties. More recent guidelines for nomenclature, which are based

TABLE 25.10. *Biological characteristics and clinical applications of interferons*

	IFN-α	IFN-β	IFN-γ
Other names	Leukocyte IFN, acid-stable IFN	Fibroblast IFN, acid-stable IFN	Immune IFN, macrophage-activating factor
Chief cell source	Peripheral leukocytes	Fibroblasts	Lymphocytes, NK cells, alveolar macrophages
Effector cells	Neutrophils, macrophages	Neutrophils	Neutrophils, monocytes
Inducers	Viruses, dsRNA, LPS, bacteria	Microorganisms, dsRNA, cytokines	Microorganisms, superantigens, mitogens (augmented by IL-2), IL-12
Biological functions	Activates Ma, NK, T and B cells, modulates MHC class I expression, antiviral and antiparasitic activity, antiproliferative agent	Same as IFN-α	Acts as a weaker antiviral agent, is a strong activator of Ma, activates Ma, NK, T and B cells, modulates the expression of MHC class I and II antigens
Approved clinical applications	Antimicrobial effects condyloma accuminata, HCV infection, chronic HBV infection, laryngeal papillomatosis, HIV/AIDS Antiproliferative effects Kaposi sarcoma in AIDS, CML, gliomas, medulloblastomas, childhood hemangiomas, keloids and hypertrophic scars Immunomodulatory effects HIV infection when used in combination with antiretroviral agents	Condyloma accuminata, chronic HBV infection, laryngeal papillomatosis	Antimicrobial effects Mycobacterial infections: *M. leproe*, *M. tuberculosis*, MAC; Listeria monocytogenes infection, Immunomodulatory effect of interferon atopic dermatitis, rheumatoid arthritis, Job syndrome, congenital osteopetrosis, chronic granulomatous disease
Investigational uses	None	None	Prevention and therapy of neonatal infections: sepsis, pneumonia, septic shock, fungal infections

IFN, interferon; NK, natural killer cells; dsRNA, double stranded ribose nucleic acid; LPS, lipopolysaccharide; IL-12, interleukin-12; Ma, macrophage; MHC, major histocompatability complex; HCV, Hepatitis C virus; HBV, hepatitis B virus; AIDS, acquired immune deficiency syndrome; HIV, human immune deficiency virus; CML, chronic myeloid leukemia; MAC, *Mycobacterium avium intracellular complex*.

on the nucleotide sequences of IFNs, divide IFNs into two types: type I and type II (4,200). Although there is no structural homology between the two types, members of both groups share functional similarities. Table 25.10 summarizes the biologic properties and clinical applications of the human interferons.

Type I IFNs include IFN-α and IFN-β. The IFN-α family consists of three subclasses; IFN-α (subclass I), which consists of 14 closely related proteins encoded by distinct genes; IFN-ω (subclass II), and IFN-τ (subclass III), which is also known as trophoblast IFN (4,200). IFN-β, produced by fibroblasts, is a single-protein species that is homologous to IFN-α (201). This IFN αβ superfamily of genes is clustered on the short arm of chromosome 9 (9p21-22) (4,200–202).

Type II IFNs consist of IFN-γ. Mammals contain a single IFN-γ gene mapped to chromosome 12 (4,200,203,204). The mature form of human IFN-γ is a basic protein of 143 amino acids; the active IFN-γ molecule is a homodimer. (205)

Interferons induce the transcription of various genes. To date, approximately 30 IFN-inducible genes have been identified (203). The proteins encoded by these genes affect a wide variety of functions, which is the basis of the many and varied biologic effects of IFNs. These biologic effects include induction of an antiviral state, regulation of cell proliferation and differentiation, immunomodulation, regulation of cellular biosynthetic activities, and effects on cell membrane and cytoskeletal elements.

Interferons form the first line of defense against infections and are responsible for innate immunity against viral infection. The *in vivo* antiviral and antibacterial effects of IFNs are a combination of direct cellular effects and immunomodulation.

Early phases of viral infection stimulate type I IFN production and development of nonspecific immunity (e.g., immunity provided by increased NK cell activity). In addition, viral infection stimulates production of IL-12 by macrophages and NK cells. Later

phases of viral replication generate antigen-specific immune responses, which are dependent mainly on specific CD4+ cell subtypes (206,207). Type I IFNs usually are found at the site of viral infection; however, in certain types of viral infections (e.g. influenza, measles, and Dengue virus infections), type I IFNs can be found in the general circulation. Elevated circulating levels of type I IFNs usually are correlated with fever and general symptoms (e.g., chills, headaches, body aches, nausea) frequently associated with viral infections. Type I IFNs and IL-12, in presence of viral antigens, induce the differentiation of naive Th0 cells into Th1 cells. IFN-γ produced by these cells in the process of producing protective immune responses, along with other cytokines, may lead to fatal pathologic consequences (206,207). Several viruses are capable of producing proteins, termed *virokines,* which alter host cytokine networks. In addition, various viruses acquire and modify genes that modulate the host immune and inflammatory responses. Such genes include various cytokine genes that enable viruses to survive and replicate in different species in the presence of an active host immune response. The detailed mechanism of antiviral effects of IFNs against most viruses is not fully understood.

Interferons induce the differentiation of macrophages, granulocytes, and erythroid precursors and the maturation of B-lymphocytes to immunoglobulin-producing cells, but IFNs inhibit the differentiation of fibroblasts to adipocytes (208). IFN-γ, the best-known activator of macrophages and monocytes, greatly augments their tumoricidal and microbicidal activities (209). It improves antigen-presenting function (APC) and antibody-dependent cell-mediated cytotoxicity (ADCC) by upregulating the expression of IgG FcR; effects various cell surface antigens by inducing expression of both major histocompatability complex (MHC) class I and class II molecules, especially class II; and inducing de novo synthesis of MHC class II molecules (210). IFN-γ also enhances intracellular killing by augmenting respiratory bursts of macrophages and neutrophils in response to various cell surface stimuli. The generation of superoxide hydrogen peroxide radicals is important for the intracellular killing of microorganisms by macrophages and neutrophils. IFN-γ induces the cellular synthesis of nitric oxide synthase (iNOS), an enzyme involved in the synthesis of nitric oxide (NO). This is a major antibacterial mechanism and thought to be important for resistance to intracellular microorganisms (211,212). In addition, IFN-γ acts as a cofactor for proliferation of B- and T- lymphocytes and appears to be essential for the maturation of cytotoxic T-lymphocytes (CTLs).

Clinical Applications of Interferon-α and Interferon-β

In early trials, IFN-α was tested as a treatment for upper respiratory infections caused by rhinovirus, coronavirus, and influenza virus (213–216). IFN-α applied intranasally was able to prevent, but not cure, infections caused by these viruses (213,214,216). This treatment, however, was less effective against influenza virus infection (215). Nasal stuffiness and erosions resulting from daily intranasal sprays made the treatment unattractive for general use.

Hepatitis B and Hepatitis C infections

Hepatitis B virus (HBV) and hepatitis C virus (HCV) infection, either alone or in combination, in immunocompromised children can be acquired from the transfusions of blood products (217–219). IFN-α is an accepted form of therapy for chronic HBV infection. Long-term administration of recombinant IFN-α can cause virologic remission (i.e., clearance of viral DNA and eventual loss of hepatitis B core antigen [Hbe antigen]), normalization of aminotransferase levels, and even seroconversion in 25% to 40% of patients (4,200,220). Patients with high initial serum aminotransferase levels and low levels of HBV DNA are more likely to respond than those with high viral load or low serum amino-

transferase levels (221,222). Immunosuppressed patients usually belong to the latter category. The recommended dose of IFN-α, for adults, is 4 to 6 million international units (MIU) daily or 9 to 10 MIU thrice weekly, given either intravenously or subcutaneously for a prolonged period (220,222). Factors associated with poor response include high viral titers and cirrhosis before treatment.

The exact mechanism of action of IFN-α against HBV and HCV is not known (4,200,223). Endogenous IFN-α production and action is suppressed by viral replication; thus, supplementation of exogenous IFN-α may be a form replacement therapy (224). Alternatively, IFN-α therapy may lead to upregulation of viral antigens, making the virus-infected cells more susceptible to CTLs (4).

Currently, IFN therapy for HCV infection has not been approved for patients younger than 18 years of age (225). The aggressive nature of this infection and the poor outcome of infected immunocompromised patients may warrant exception to this general recommendation.

The recommended standard dose for adults of 3 MIU administered three times a week for 12 months leads to a biochemical response (normalization of serum alanine transaminase activity) in 50% and a virologic response (loss of detectable HCV RNA) in 33% of patients infected with HCV (225); however, disease in more than 50% of these patients recurs, and only 15% to 25% of patients have a sustained response when treatment is stopped. Longer duration of therapy (18–24 months), higher doses of IFN-α (up to 30 MIU per week), and treatment with other types of IFNs are neither effective nor practical (226). Recombinant IFN-β is currently indicated for HBV and HCV infections that are resistant to IFN-α. Recent clinical trials of combination therapy with IFN-α and ribavirin (a nucleoside analogue) have shown promising results for initial treatment and the treatment of relapse of chronic HCV infection (226–229). The role of interferon for postexposure prophylaxis to prevent HBV or HCV infection has not been determined.

HIV Infection and AIDS

Both IFN-α and IFN-β inhibit HIV-1 replication *in vitro* (230). Although IFN-α therapy is not beneficial in patients with advanced AIDS, IFN-α slows virus production and delays the development of AIDS in asymptomatic HIV-infected patients (231). Clinical trials are under way to evaluate the effectiveness of IFN-α in combination with other drugs (e.g., zidovudine) in the treatment of HIV infection and HIV-related diseases (4).

AIDS-Associated Kaposi's Sarcoma

Epidemic as well as endemic Kaposi's sarcoma (KS) is thought to have an infectious etiology. A large percentage of these tumors contain human herpesvirus 8 (232). KS is reported in young children and adolescents infected with HIV, especially those in Africa; however, the incidence of KS in children is extremely low compared with that in adults (233). Infection in approximately 30% to 50% of adult patients responds to high-dose (18–36 MIU daily) recombinant IFN-α therapy (234,235). Currently, IFN-α is recommended for the treatment of early or limited KS. It is speculated that IFN-α is effective because of its ability to activate CTLs and its profound antiangiogenic activity.

Papillomavirus Infection

Condyloma acuminata (genital warts), which is often associated with other sexually transmitted diseases, is a relatively common but recalcitrant condition caused by human papillomavirus infection. Approximately 5% to 38% of adolescents are reported to have asymptomatic infection (236,237). Intralesional application of IFN-α and IFN-β completely eliminated visible genital warts in approximately 60% to 70% of patients who were tested (238). IFN-α, 1 to 5 MIU three times week, administered parenterally, also has been effective (239). The combination of IFN therapy and cryosurgery is valuable in eradicating lesions and reducing recurrences (238, 239). IFN-α is also beneficial in reducing the number of lesions in patients with juvenile laryngeal papillomatosis (4,204,240). When used in combination with laser excision, IFN-α lengthens the remission period. For this purpose, the recommended dose is 3 to 6 MIU three times weekly for 3 or more months (240).

Clinical Applications of IFN-γ

Hyperimmunoglobulin E Syndrome

Recombinant IFN-γ has been proposed for the therapy of hyperimmunoglobulin E syndrome (Job syndrome) because of observations that IFN-γ can suppress the synthesis of immunoglobulin E (IgE) and also that IFN-γ production by mononuclear cells in these patients is extremely low or absent. *In vitro* studies have shown that incubation of neutrophils with IFN-γ leads to a threefold increase in their chemotactic response and inhibits IgE production of peripheral blood mononuclear cells by 67% to 93% (241,242). Preliminary trials of IFN-γ therapy suggested that clinical benefits include significant reductions in eczema, pulmonary symptoms, and secretions (242). The recommended dose is 50 μg/m² administered subcutaneously three times weekly.

Chronic Granulomatous Disease

Recombinant human IFN-γ was shown recently to be an effective and well-tolerated therapy for chronic granulomatous disease (CGD) (4,204,243). A possible explanation stems from the finding that IFN-γ can stimulate the respiratory burst in normal phagocytes (211,212) as well as in phagocytes from patients with certain variant forms of CGD (244). Similar but smaller responses were seen in patients with the autosomal recessive form of CGD (245). In a randomized, double-blind, placebo-controlled phase 3 trial, recombinant human IFN-γ significantly decreased the overall risk of infection, the relative risk of serious infection, and length of hospital stay of patients with CGD (246). These beneficial effects were independent of age, mode of inheritance of CGD, or concomitant prophylactic use of antibiotics. In most patients, IFN-γ improves the bactericidal activity of phagocytes without increasing the respiratory burst function. Thus, IFN-γ appears to augment other host defense mechanisms (243, 246). In addition, IFN-γ showed an additive effect with the prophylactic use of antibiotics, producing nearly a 20% increase in the infection-free rate compared with that of patients treated with IFN-γ alone (247). The recommended dose is 50 μg/m² subcutaneously three times weekly for up to 1 year.

Mycobacterial Diseases

Obligate or facultative intracellular microorganisms (e.g., *M. tuberculosis, M. leprae)* can cause granulomas. These nodular masses represent a cell-mediated, chronic inflammatory response to persistent infection and result from the continuous release of cytokines at the focus of infection. INF-γ, TNF-α and β, and other cytokines stimulate the accumulation of leukocytes and macrophage- and neutrophil-mediated destruction of intracellular pathogens mainly through generation of reactive oxygen intermediates and NO. If the intracellular pathogens cannot be cleared, the prolonged production of reactive oxygen intermediates may lead to tissue damage.

It appears that IFN-γ is crucial for the elimination of several intracellular pathogens known to infect macrophages. Mice with mutations either in the IFN-γ gene or in the gene for the IFN-γ receptor are much more susceptible to bacterial (e.g., *Listeria monocytogenes)* and mycobacterial (e.g., *Mycobacterium bovis*) infections (248,249). Induced NO production is believed to be a primary mechanism of macrophage cytotoxicity against intracellular pathogens such as bacteria, protozoa, helminths, and fungi (4,249). Because IFN-γ can induce NO production, it may be an effective treatment against diseases caused by such organisms.

Patients with lepromatous leprosy have selective anergy to the antigens of *M. leprae* (250). This anergy appears to be associated with deficient IFN-γ production and macrophage inactivation. Clinical trials have shown that intradermal or intramuscular IFN-γ may be helpful in patients with multibacillary leprosy (250,251). IFN-γ also may be a powerful adjunct to conventional therapy in treating nontuberculous mycobacterial infections (e.g., *M. avium)* that are frequently seen in patients with AIDS (252).

Visceral Leishmaniasis

High-dose recombinant IFN-γ (100–400 μg/m² daily) administered intramuscularly is effective in patients with visceral leishmaniasis resistant to pentavalent antimony treatment (253). A combination of these two agents is effective in treating seriously ill patients with refractory or previously untreated visceral leishmaniasis.

Neonatal Infections

Unlike adult cells, neonatal mononuclear cells and T cells are markedly deficient in the production of IFN-γ in response to various stimuli (254,255). Recombinant IFN-γ significantly enhances the chemotactic response of neutrophils from term neonates to levels comparable to that of adult neutrophils. These observations suggest that there is a potential role for the use of IFN-γ in preventing or treating sepsis or life-threatening infections common to this age group (204).

Sepsis

As stated, IFN-γ upregulates costimulatory and MHC molecules on the cell surface, increases the number of APCs, and primes monocytes and macrophages for the production of LPS-induced proinflammatory cytokines. Docke et al. showed that IFN-γ restores monocyte activation in a dose-dependent manner in patients whose monocytes have been deactivated during sepsis and in *in vitro* experiments by LPS desensitization or by IL-10 and TGF-β1 treatment (19). They further conducted a pilot trial to study the beneficial effects of IFN-γ therapy in nine patients with sepsis. These patients received IFN-γ in a dose of 100 μg daily administered subcutaneously if they had fewer than 30% HLA-DR+ monocytes on two consecutive days. The patients continued to receive the therapy until more than 50% of monocytes were HLA-DR+ for 3 consecutive days. IFN-γ therapy resulted in immediate restoration of the deficient HLA-DR expression in all patients and in LPS-induced TNF-α secretion *in vitro*. Recovery of monocyte function resulted in clearance of sepsis in eight of the nine patients. IFN-γ therapy was well tolerated without any adverse effects. Further evaluation of its role in the treatment of septic patients is warranted.

Toxicity

Adverse effects associated with and toxicity of interferons depend on the type of product used, the dose and route of administration, the treatment schedule, and the clinical status of the patients. In general, adverse effects are more common with IFN-α and IFN-β than with IFN-γ. These side effects tend to be more severe in initial treatments and with dose escalations. The primary dose-limiting effects of all IFNs include fatigue, leukopenia, elevated liver enzymes, and hypotension.

The side effects common to all IFNs include a flulike syndrome with fever, chills, tachycardia, headache, malaise, myalgia, fatigue, and sometimes nausea and vomiting. These effects occur in about 60% to 70% of patients (4,206,207). Headache, sleep disturbances, and hearing loss are experienced in 30% to 40% of patients (4). Nonsteroidal antiinflammatory agents can easily control these side effects. Frequently occurring dose-limiting hematologic toxicities include granulocytopenia and thrombocytopenia and occasionally anemia. Development of bone marrow suppression is dose related and is usually reversible. After high doses of IFNs, coagulopathy (with increased levels of prothrombin time and thromboplastin time) has been observed (206,207). Neurotoxicity, although uncommon, can be a dose-limiting consequence of IFN therapy. These neurotoxic effects include lethargy, altered mental states, disorientation, dysphasia, loss of sense of smell and taste, irritability, anxiety, panic attacks, emotional lability, depression, suicidal ideation, psychosis, and electroencephalogram changes. Other uncommon adverse events include elevation of liver enzymes (20%), hematuria, proteinuria, and cardiac disturbances (arrhythmias, ischemia, and hypotension). Patients with preexisting renal disease may develop nephrotic syndrome and rapid deterioration of renal function. Contraindications to treatment with IFNs include major depressive illness, cytopenias, hyperthyroidism, or renal transplantation (225).

Low levels of naturally occurring antibodies to IFNs are present in some persons who have not been previously exposed to exogenous IFNs. Neutralizing antibodies have been found in 10% to 20% of patients treated with IFN therapy; however, larger proportions of patients treated with recombinant IFNs (38% with rhIFN-α and 50% to 75% with rhIFN-β) reportedly developed antibodies (207). Antibody formation is associated with a decrease in the incidence of observed toxicities. Induction of autoantibodies to IFN-γ has not been reported.

INTERLEUKINS

The term *interleukin* was used originally to describe proteins that send signals between leukocytes. With further research, we now know that interleukins can be produced by and affect other cell types (256). The first interleukin to be discovered was IL-1, which was referred to as lymphocyte-activating factor. In 1986 the Sixth International Congress of Immunology decided that once the amino acid sequence of a new cytokine was known, it would be assigned an interleukin number (257); however, some cytokines such as the interferons and colony-stimulating factors have retained their original names (256). There are currently 18 interleukins that have been described (258,259). Of these 18 interleukins, only IL-2 is approved for clinical use. A complete review of their biologic properties and potential clinical applications is beyond the scope of this review. A brief synopsis of some of the approaches currently in clinical trials follows.

Clinical Application of Interleukins

Vaccine Adjuvants

Currently, vaccination is the most successful preventative immunotherapy against infectious diseases. In general, vaccines contain potent antigens that can serve as natural adjuvants to induce a prerequisite proinflammatory cytokine response. As described already, a level of proinflammatory cytokine release is needed to generate immune memory and can be tolerated by the host. Currently, the vaccines that are able to elicit such a response are predominately restricted to extracellular bacteria and some viruses. These vaccines generate predominately a humoral immune response in which antibodies neutralize pathogens or prevent subsequent infections. Vaccines to intracellular pathogens have been less successful in preventing infection because of their inability to elicit the appropriate cellular response required for clearance of infected host cells. To be effective, vaccines to intracellular pathogens must induce the appropriate balance of T-cell subsets (i.e., Th1 and Th2) and generate MHC class I-restricted effector cells (i.e., CTLs). Currently, the intracellular vaccines in clinical use are limited to the tuberculosis vaccine bacille Calmette-Guerin (BCG) and to a vaccine against invasive *Salmonella typhi*.

Several efforts are ongoing to overcome the inability of vaccines to generate the appropriate cellular immune memory needed for protection against intracellular pathogens. Some of these efforts focused on the use of immunoregulatory cytokines that influence cellular immune responses. This area of research has been predominately led by investigators who have used recombinant cytokines to develop antitumor vaccines. Several studies showed the combination of subunits of tumor antigens with immunoregulatory cytokines to be effective in eliciting immune responses against tumor cells. Unfortunately, the benefit of these vaccines is still unknown.

Additionally, preclinical studies have shown the combined administration of various cytokine adjuvants with microbial vaccines to be effective in preventing infections. These studies revealed an enhancement of both antibody- and cell-mediated immune responses. For example, the pioneering study by Xiang and Ertl (260) demonstrated that the murine immune response to rabies virus antigens was enhanced when DNA encoding murine GM-CSF was coinjected with DNA encoding the rabies virus glycoproteins. This approach has held up in other studies using a variety of antigens derived from pathogens such as *Plasmodium* sp., HIV, and HBV. In addition, other preclinical studies found that several cytokines may serve as effective adjuvants; these include many of the interleukins (IL-1, IL-2, IL-3, IL-4, IL-6, IL-7, IL-10, IL-12, and IL-15), growth factors (GM-CSF, G-CSF, M-CSF, and TGF-β), and IFN-γ; however, IL-2, IL-12, IFN-γ, and GM-CSF are currently the most promising cytokines, especially for eliciting a Th1-mediated response (261).

The use of GM-CSF and IL-2 in humans demonstrated that coadministration of either cytokine can lead to a potent, long-lasting, and specific immunity (262). Substantial data about the effects of GM-CSF in both neutropenic and nonneutropenic patients suggest that it acts as an immune regulator in addition to its role as a hemopoietic growth factor. Clinical trials are ongoing to examine the effects of coadministration of GM-CSF and microbial vaccines in both immunocompetent and immunocompromised patients. Clinical use of IL-2 in humans demonstrated that IL-2 can act as an immune regulatory agent. Several preclinical trials of IL-2 and microbial vaccines indicated that IL-2 enhances both antibody- and cellular-mediated immune response to viruses. IL-2 combined with an HIV vaccine strongly enhanced the activation of Th1 cells (263). Administration of IL-2 and herpes simplex virus type 1 antigens resulted in an enhanced mucosal immunity to the virus (264).

Interleukin-12 is also being evaluated as a vaccine adjuvant. IL-12 enhances the induction of Th-1 and CD8+ CTL-mediated immune responses (265). In a preclinical study, Kim et al. (266) showed that coadministration of DNA encoding IL-12 and HIV antigens resulted in augmentation of anti-HIV CTL function. Similar benefits were demonstrated with other microbial antigens, such as *Leishmania major* (267). In summary, the application of cytokines as adjuvants with vaccines is restricted to investigational use, predominately in cancer patients. Questions about the optimal dose, the optimal cytokine, the appropriate delivery method, and the optimal method of evaluating a beneficial immune response remain. The ongoing tumor vaccine trials should help to determine the risk of induced autoimmunity and generate some answers to the other questions. This knowledge and the rapid advancements in gene transfer technology ultimately should allow the rapid implementation of cytokine use in the development of improved vaccines against both intracellular and extracellular pathogens.

Anti-HIV Therapy

A recurring theme of cytokine and anticytokine therapy is to block active disease processes and restore immunocompetence. The successful use of recombinant IL-2 (rIL-2) in patients infected with HIV represents this type of therapeutic application. Patients infected with HIV have an increased risk of opportunistic infections because of progressive destruction of CD4+ lymphocytes. Depletion of CD4+ cells impairs the ability of the host to produce appropriate inflammatory and immune responses, in part because of impaired IL-2 production. IL-2 is expressed by activated T cells and generally functions as a

central proinflammatory and immunoregulatory cytokine (Table 25.2). IL-2 is necessary for expansion of effector cells, including NK cells, which are essential in clearance of viral and opportunistic infections. In addition, IL-2 triggers the release of other proinflammatory cytokines, including the secretion of INF-γ, GM-CSF, and TNF-α. These proinflammatory cytokines are potent stimulators of phagocyte effector cells. After incubation with IL-2 *in vitro,* T-lymphocytes from patients infected with HIV recover to some degree to proliferate in response to mitogen stimulation (268). Together, these observations led to clinical studies of exogenous IL-2 therapy to restore the IL-2-deficient state of patients.

In several phase 1 and 2 trials, rIL-2 therapy increased CD4+ lymphocyte counts and stimulated NK activity (269–271). Although no clear clinical benefit was demonstrated, probably because of the inability to quantify virus at that time and the limited number of patients in each study, these trials did establish some fundamental principles of rIL-2 administration. These studies suggested an increased benefit from combining rIL-2 with antiretroviral therapy and showed improved tolerance, better delivery, and a longer half-life of IL-2 when it was conjugated to polyethelene glycol (PEG-IL-2) (271,272). The adverse effects reported for these phase 1 and 2 studies included flulike symptoms (myalgia, arthralgia, fatigue, and malaise), fever, and asymptomatic hyperbilirubinemia. The most severe side effect reported was capillary leak syndrome, but this effect occurred infrequently at lower doses of IL-2.

Kovacs et al. (273) randomized 60 patients with an initial CD4+ cell count of more than 200 cells/mm³ to receive antiretroviral therapy with or without rIL-2. Patients who had follow-up for more than 50 months on combined therapy showed a mean increase in the number of CD4+ cells, whereas those on antiretroviral therapy alone had a decline in the number of CD4+ cells. Similar findings were observed in the study by Saraolatz et al. (274). In addition, this study suggested that the duration of rIL-2 therapy was more important than the total dose.

Another interleukin that may be effective in the treatment of patients with HIV infection is recombinant IL-12 (rIL-12). IL-12 is a central factor in the regulation of T-cell subset differentiation, especially in the regulation of Th1-type immune responses. *In vitro* evidence suggest that defects in Th1-type immune responses are present in patients infected with HIV (275,276), and a switch from a Th1-type to a Th2-type response may correlate with the progressive decline of patients with HIV infection (277). Findings from preclinical studies and preliminary Phase I trials suggest that rIl-12 therapy increases the number and function of phagocytic effector cells in patients (278). Further studies are ongoing.

LIMITATIONS OF CYTOKINE THERAPY

Despite identification of an increasing array of cytokines, their availability on an industrial scale, and advances in our understanding of their basic functions, with a few notable exceptions, they generally do not yet have proven clinical benefits. Although these agents still hold great promise, the multiple and often overlapping biologic effects of many cytokines are an important problem in their use as therapeutic agents. Furthermore, the timing of administration is critical, they are often active at small concentrations, their effectiveness is often short lived, or their effects may vary with concentration. Thus indepth investigations of the effects and determination of the optimal biologic dose to modulate a given deficiency is absolutely necessary. More precise laboratory predictors will be needed to identify the optimal biologic dose as well as the specific patient subgroups that will benefit most from a given intervention. The hemopoietic growth factors are relatively specific and thus have found several applications in children with various immune compromised states. Even with these agents, however, there is still significant controversy in how, in what dosage, and when to best use

these agents (84,279,280). A better understanding of the effects of cytokine interactions in the context of the immune response and inflammation should lead to more specific and effective therapies. In the future, it is likely that multiple combinations of cytokines will be used.

REFERENCES

1. Wheeler AP, Bernard GR. Treating patients with severe sepsis. *N Engl J Med* 1999;340:207–214.
2. Bone RC. Sir Isaac Newton, sepsis, SIRS, and CARS. *Crit Care Med* 1996;24:1125–1128.
3. Weiss M, Moldawer LL, Schneider EM. Granulocyte colony-stimulating factor to prevent the progression of systemic nonresponsiveness in systemic inflammatory response syndrome and sepsis. *Blood* 1999;93: 425–439.
4. Meager T. *The molecular biology of cytokines.* Chichester, England: John Wiley and Sons, Molecular Medical Sciences Series, 1998.
5. Carter LL, Dutton RW. Type 1 and type 2: a fundamental dichotomy for all T-cell subsets. *Curr Opin Immunol* 1996;8:336–342.
6. DiPiro JT. Cytokine networks with infection: mycobacterial infections, leishmaniasis, human immunodeficiency virus infection, and sepsis. *Pharmacotherapy* 1997;17:205–223.
7. Del Prete G, Maggi E, Romagnani S. Human Th1 and Th2 cells: functional properties, mechanisms of regulation, and role in disease. *Lab Invest* 1994;70:299–306.
8. Mosmann TR, Coffman RL. TH1 and TH2 cells: different patterns of lymphokine secretion lead to different functional properties. *Annu Rev Immunol* 1989;7:-145–173.
9. American College of Chest Physicians/Society of Critical Care Medicine Consensus Conference. Definitions for sepsis and organ failure and guidelines for the use of innovative therapies in sepsis. *Crit Care Med* 1992;20:864–874.
10. Glauser MP, Heumann D, Baumgartner JD, et al. Pathogenesis and potential strategies for prevention and treatment of septic shock: an update. *Clin Infect Dis* 1994;18(Suppl 2):S205–S216.
11. Anderson MR, Blumer JL. Advances in the therapy for sepsis in children. *Pediatr Clin North Am* 1997;44:-179–205.
12. Klosterhalfen B, Bhardwaj RS. Septic shock. *Gen Pharmacol* 1998;31:25–32.
13. Doughty LA, Kaplan SS, Carcillo JA. Inflammatory cytokine and nitric oxide responses in pediatric sepsis and organ failure. *Crit Care Med* 1996;24:1137–1143.
14. O'Connor M, Salzman AL, Szabo C. Role of peroxynitrite in the protein oxidation and apoptotic DNA fragmentation in vascular smooth muscle cells stimulated with bacterial lipopolysaccharide and interferon-gamma. *Shock* 1997;8:439–443.
15. Hotchkiss RS, Swanson PE, Cobb JP, et al. Apoptosis in lymphoid and parenchymal cells during sepsis: findings in normal and T- and B-cell-deficient mice. *Crit Care Med* 1997;25:1298–307.

16. Ayala A, Herdon CD, Lehman DL, et al. Differential induction of apoptosis in lymphoid tissues during sepsis: variation in onset, frequency, and the nature of the mediators. *Blood* 1996;87:4261–4275.

17. Lynch DH, Ramsdell F, Alderson MR. Fas and FasL in the homeostatic regulation of immune responses. *Immunol Today* 1995;16:569–574.

18. Suda T, Okazaki T, Naito Y, et al. Expression of the Fas ligand in cells of T cell lineage. *J Immunol* 1995;154: 3806–3813.

19. Docke WD, Randow F, Syrbe U, et al. Monocyte deactivation in septic patients: restoration by IFN-gamma treatment. *Nat Med* 1997;3:678–681.

20. Dofferhoff AS, Bom VJ, Vries-Hospers HG, et al. Patterns of cytokines, plasma endotoxin, plasminogen activator inhibitor, and acute-phase proteins during the treatment of severe sepsis in humans. *Crit Care Med* 1992;20:185–192.

21. Sullivan JS, Kilpatrick L, Costarino AT Jr, et al. Correlation of plasma cytokine elevations with mortality rate in children with sepsis. *J Pediatr* 1992;120: 510–515.

22. Pinsky MR, Vincent JL, Deviere J, et al. Serum cytokine levels in human septic shock: relation to multiple-system organ failure and mortality. *Chest* 1993; 103:565–575.

23. Moscovitz H, Shofer F, Mignott H, et al. Plasma cytokine determinations in emergency department patients as a predictor of bacteremia and infectious disease severity. *Crit Care Med* 1994;22:1102–1107.

24. Beutler B, Milsark IW, Cerami AC. Passive immunization against cachectin/tumor necrosis factor protects mice from lethal effect of endotoxin. *Science* 1985; 229:869–871.

25. Hinshaw LB, Tekamp-Olson P, Chang AC, et al. Survival of primates in LD100 septic shock following therapy with antibody to tumor necrosis factor (TNF alpha). *Circ Shock* 1990;30:279–292.

26. Silva AT, Bayston KF, Cohen J. Prophylactic and therapeutic effects of a monoclonal antibody to tumor necrosis factor-alpha in experimental gram-negative shock. *J Infect Dis* 1990;162:421–427.

27. Fong Y, Tracey KJ, Moldawer LL, et al. Antibodies to cachectin/tumor necrosis factor reduce interleukin 1 beta and interleukin 6 appearance during lethal bacteremia. *J Exp Med* 1989;170:1627–1633.

28. Abraham E, Wunderink R, Silverman H, et al. Efficacy and safety of monoclonal antibody to human tumor necrosis factor alpha in patients with sepsis syndrome: a randomized, controlled, double-blind, multicenter clinical trial. TNF-alpha MAb Sepsis Study Group. *JAMA* 1995;273:934–941.

29. Cohen J, Carlet J. INTERSEPT: an international, multicenter, placebo-controlled trial of monoclonal antibody to human tumor necrosis factor-alpha in patients with sepsis: International Sepsis Trial Study Group. *Crit Care Med* 1996;24:1431–1440.

30. Fisher CJJ, Agosti JM, Opal SM, et al. Treatment of septic shock with the tumor necrosis factor receptor:Fc fusion protein: the Soluble TNF Receptor Sepsis Study Group. *N Engl J Med* 1996;334:1697–1702.

31. Fisher CJ Jr, Opal SM, Dhainaut JF, et al. Influence of an anti-tumor necrosis factor monoclonal antibody on cytokine levels in patients with sepsis: the CB0006 Sepsis Syndrome Study Group. *Crit Care Med* 1993; 21:318–327.

32. Van Zee KJ, Kohno T, Fischer E, et al. Tumor necrosis factor soluble receptors circulate during experimental and clinical inflammation and can protect against excessive tumor necrosis factor alpha *in vitro* and *in vivo*. *Proc Natl Acad Sci USA* 1992;89:4845–4849.

33. Girardin E, Roux-Lombard P, Grau GE, et al. Imbalance between tumour necrosis factor-alpha and soluble TNF receptor concentrations in severe meningococcaemia: the J5 Study Group. *Immunology* 1992;76: 20–23.

34. Ashkenazi A, Marsters SA, Capon DJ, et al. Protection against endotoxic shock by a tumor necrosis factor receptor immunoadhesin. *Proc Natl Acad Sci USA* 1991; 88:10535–10539.

35. Fisher CJ Jr, Agosti JM, Opal SM, et al. Treatment of septic shock with the tumor necrosis factor receptor:Fc fusion protein: the Soluble TNF Receptor Sepsis Study Group. *N Engl J Med* 1996;334:1697–1702.

36. Suffredini AF, Reda D, Banks SM, et al. Effects of recombinant dimeric TNF receptor on human inflammatory responses following intravenous endotoxin administration. *J Immunol* 1995;155:5038–5045.

37. Dinarello CA. Interleukin-1 and interleukin-1 antagonism. *Blood* 1991;77:1627–1652.

38. Fisher CJ Jr, Slotman GJ, Opal SM, et al. Initial evaluation of human recombinant interleukin-1 receptor antagonist in the treatment of sepsis syndrome: a randomized, open-label, placebo-controlled multicenter trial. The IL-1RA Sepsis Syndrome Study Group. *Crit Care Med* 1994;22:12–21.

39. Ohlsson K, Bjork P, Bergenfeldt M, et al. Interleukin-1 receptor antagonist reduces mortality from endotoxin shock. *Nature* 1990;348:550–552.

40. Fischer E, Marano MA, Van Zee KJ, et al. Interleukin-1 receptor blockade improves survival and hemodynamic performance in *Escherichia coli* septic shock, but fails to alter host responses to sublethal endotoxemia. *J Clin Invest* 1992;89:1551–1557.

41. Fisher CJ Jr, Dhainaut JF, Opal SM, et al. Recombinant human interleukin 1 receptor antagonist in the treatment of patients with sepsis syndrome: results from a randomized, double-blind, placebo-controlled trial. Phase III rhIL-1ra Sepsis Syndrome Study Group. *JAMA* 1994;271:1836–1843.

42. Zeni F, Freeman B, Natanson C. Anti-inflammatory therapies to treat sepsis and septic shock: a reassessment [Editorial; Comment]. *Crit Care Med* 1997;25: 1095–1100.

43. Opal SM, Wherry JC, Grint P. Interleukin-10: potential benefits and possible risks in clinical infectious diseases. *Clin Infect Dis* 1998;27:1497–1507.

44. Howard M, Muchamuel T, Andrade S, et al. Interleukin 10 protects mice from lethal endotoxemia. *J Exp Med* 1993;177:1205–1208.

45. Cusumano V, Genovese F, Mancuso G, et al. Interleukin-10 protects neonatal mice from lethal group B streptococcal infection. *Infect Immun* 1996;64: 2850–2852.

46. Huhn RD, Radwanski E, O'Connell SM, et al. Pharmacokinetics and immunomodulatory properties of intravenously administered recombinant human interleukin-10 in healthy volunteers. *Blood* 1996;87: 699–705.

47. Kollmann TR, Pettoello-Mantovani M, Katopodis NF, et al. Inhibition of acute *in vivo* human immunodeficiency virus infection by human interleukin 10 treat-

ment of SCID mice implanted with human fetal thymus and liver. *Proc Natl Acad Sci USA* 1996;93:3126–3131.

48. Paris MM, Hickey SM, Trujillo M, et al. The effect of interleukin-10 on meningeal inflammation in experimental bacterial meningitis. *J Infect Dis* 1997;176:1239–1246.

49. Opal SM, Cross AS, Jhung JW, et al. Potential hazards of combination immunotherapy in the treatment of experimental septic shock. *J Infect Dis* 1996;173:1415–1421.

50. Demetri GD, Griffin JD. Granulocyte colony-stimulating factor and its receptor. *Blood* 1991;78:2791–2808.

51. Nicola NA, Metcalf D. Binding of ^{125}I-labeled granulocyte colony-stimulating factor to normal murine hemopoietic cells. *J Cell Physiol* 1985;124:313–321.

52. Begley CG, Metcalf D, Nicola NA. Binding characteristics and proliferative action of purified granulocyte colony-stimulating factor (G-CSF) on normal and leukemic human promyelocytes. *Exp Hematol* 1988;16:71–79.

53. Nicola NA, Vadas MA, Lopez AF. Down-modulation of receptors for granulocyte colony-stimulating factor on human neutrophils by granulocyte-activating agents. *J Cell Physiol* 1986;128:501–509.

54. Metcalf D, Nicola NA. Proliferative effects of purified granulocyte colony-stimulating factor (G-CSF) on normal mouse hemopoietic cells. *J Cell Physiol* 1983;116:198–206.

55. Wang JM, Chen ZG, Colella S, et al. Chemotactic activity of recombinant human granulocyte colony-stimulating factor. *Blood* 1988;72:1456–1460.

56. Welte K, Bonilla MA, Gabrilove JL, et al. Recombinant human granulocyte-colony stimulating factor: *in vitro* and *in vivo* effects on myelopoiesis. *Blood Cells* 1987;13:17–30.

57. Platzer E, Welte K, Gabrilove JL, et al. Biological activities of a human pluripotent hemopoietic colony stimulating factor on normal and leukemic cells. *J Exp Med* 1985;162:1788–801.

58. Steinbeck MJ, Roth JA. Neutrophil activation by recombinant cytokines. *Rev Infect Dis* 1989;11:549–568.

59. Sullivan R, Griffin JD, Simons ER, et al. Effects of recombinant human granulocyte and macrophage colony-stimulating factors on signal transduction pathways in human granulocytes. *J Immunol* 1987;139:3422–3430.

60. Weisbart RH, Golde DW. Physiology of granulocyte and macrophage colony-stimulating factors in host defense. *Hematol Oncol Clin North Am* 1989;3:401–409.

61. Welte K, Gabrilove J, Bronchud MH, et al. Filgrastim (r-metHuG-CSF): the first 10 years. *Blood* 1996;88:1907–1929.

62. Bodey GP, Buckley M, Sathe YS, et al. Quantitative relationships between circulating leukocytes and infection in patients with acute leukemia. *Ann Intern Med* 1966;64:328–340.

63. Miller LL, Smith MA, Nagler CH. The role of hematopoietic growth factors in supportive care. In: Pizzo PA, Poplack DG, eds. *Principles and practice of pediatric oncology.* Philadelphia: Lippincott–Raven, 1997:1115–1165.

64. Bronchud MH, Scarffe JH, Thatcher N, et al. Phase I/II study of recombinant human granulocyte colony-stimulating factor in patients receiving intensive

chemotherapy for small cell lung cancer. *Br J Cancer* 1987;56:809–813.

65. Gabrilove JL, Jakubowski A, Scher H, et al. Effect of granulocyte colony-stimulating factor on neutropenia and associated morbidity due to chemotherapy for transitional-cell carcinoma of the urothelium. *N Engl J Med* 1988;318:1414–1422.

66. Crawford J, Ozer H, Stoller R, et al. Reduction by granulocyte colony-stimulating Factor of fever and neutropenia induced by chemotherapy in patients with small-cell lung cancer. *N Engl J Med* 1991;325:164–170.

67. Dibenedetto SP, Ragusa R, Ippolito AM, et al. Assessment of the value of treatment with granulocyte colony-stimulating factor in children with acute lymphoblastic leukemia: a randomized clinical trial. *Eur J Haematol* 1995;55:93–96.

68. Welte K, Reiter A, Mempel K, et al. A randomized phase-III study of the efficacy of granulocyte colony-stimulating factor in children with high-risk acute lymphoblastic leukemia: Berlin-Frankfurt-Munster Study Group. *Blood* 1996;87:3143–3150.

69. Pui CH, Boyett JM, Hughes WT, et al. Human granulocyte colony-stimulating factor after induction chemotherapy in children with acute lymphoblastic leukemia. *N Engl J Med* 1997;336:1781–1787.

70. Weinthal J, Gillan E, Hodder F, et al. G-CSF significantly reduces the nadir of neutropenia, hospitalizations and costs during intensive chemotherapy in children with solid tumors. *Proceedings of the Annual Meeting of the American Society of Clinical Oncology* 1992;11:a1244(abst).

71. Okamura J, Yokoyama M, Tsukimoto I, et al. Treatment of chemotherapy-induced neutropenia in children with subcutaneously administered recombinant human granulocyte colony-stimulating factor. *Pediatr Hematol Oncol* 1992;9:199–207.

72. Soda H, Oka M, Fukuda M, et al. Optimal schedule for administering granulocyte colony-stimulating factor in chemotherapy-induced neutropenia in non-small-cell lung cancer. *Cancer Chemother Pharmacol* 1996;38:9–12.

73. Sawada KI, Sato N, Kohno M, et al. Efficacy of delayed granulocyte colony-stimulating factor after full dose CHOP therapy in non-Hodgkin's lymphoma: a pilot study for a leukocyte count oriented regimen. *Leuk Lymphoma* 1995;20:103–109.

74. Clark RE, Shlebak AA, Creagh MD. Delayed commencement of granulocyte colony-stimulating factor following autologous bone marrow transplantation accelerates neutrophil recovery and is cost-effective. *Leuk Lymphoma* 1994;16:141–146.

75. Cetkovsky P, Koza V, Jindra P, et al. Individual criteria could be optimal for starting G-CSF application after autologous stem cell transplantation. *Bone Marrow Transplant* 1997;20:639–641.

76. Morstyn G, Campbell L, Lieschke G, et al. Treatment of chemotherapy-induced neutropenia by subcutaneously administered granulocyte colony-stimulating factor with optimization of dose and duration of therapy. *J Clin Oncol* 1989;7:1554–1562.

77. Maher DW, Lieschke GJ, Green M, et al. Filgrastim in patients with chemotherapy-induced febrile neutropenia: a double-blind, placebo-controlled trial. *Ann Intern Med* 1994;121:492–501.

78. Maher DW, Lieschke GJ, Green M, et al. Filgrastim in

patients with chemotherapy-induced febrile neutropenia: a double-blind, placebo-controlled trial. *Ann Intern Med* 1994;121:492–501.

79. Mitchell PL, Morland B, Stevens MC, et al. Granulocyte colony-stimulating factor in established febrile neutropenia: a randomized study of pediatric patients. *J Clin Oncol* 1997;15:1163–1170.

80. Mayordomo JI, Rivera F, Diaz-Puente MT, et al. Improving treatment of chemotherapy-induced neutropenic fever by administration of colony-stimulating factors [see comments]. *J Natl Cancer Inst* 1995;87: 803–808.

81. Anonymous. 1997 update of recommendations for the use of hematopoietic colony-stimulating factors: evidence-based, clinical practice guidelines. American Society of Clinical Oncology. *J Clin Oncol* 1997; 15:3288.

82. Anonymous. Update of recommendations for the use of hematopoietic colony-stimulating factors: evidence-based clinical practice guidelines. American Society of Clinical Oncology. *J Clin Oncol* 1996;14:1957–1960.

83. Anonymous. American Society of Clinical Oncology. Recommendations for the use of hematopoietic colony-stimulating factors: evidence-based, clinical practice guidelines. *J Clin Oncol* 1994;12:2471–2508.

84. Anonymous. American Society of Clinical Oncology. Recommendations for the use of hematopoietic colony-stimulating factors: evidence-based, clinical practice guidelines. *J Clin Oncol* 1994;12:2471–508.

85. Gisselbrecht C, Prentice HG, Bacigalupo A, et al. Placebo-controlled phase III trial of lenograstim in bone-marrow transplantation. *Lancet* 1994;343: 696–700. [Published erratum appears in *Lancet* 1994; 343:804.]

86. Schmitz N, Dreger P, Zander AR, et al. Results of a randomised, controlled, multicentre study of recombinant human granulocyte colony-stimulating factor (filgrastim) in patients with Hodgkin's disease and non-Hodgkin's lymphoma undergoing autologous bone marrow transplantation. *Bone Marrow Transplant* 1995;15:261–266.

87. Linch DC, Scarffe H, Proctor S, et al. Randomised vehicle-controlled dose-finding study of glycosylated recombinant human granulocyte colony-stimulating factor after bone marrow transplantation. *Bone Marrow Transplant* 1993;11:307–311.

88. Stahel RA, Jost LM, Cerny T, et al. Randomized study of recombinant human granulocyte colony-stimulating factor after high-dose chemotherapy and autologous bone marrow transplantation for high-risk lymphoid malignancies. *J Clin Oncol* 1994;12:1931–1938.

89. Blaise D, Vernant JP, Fiere D, et al. A randomized, controlled, multicenter trial of recombinant human granulocyte colony stimulating factor (Filgrastim) in patients treated by bone marrow transplantation (BMT) with total body irradiation (TBI) for acute lymphoblastic leukemia (ALL) or lymphoblastic lymphoma (LL). *Blood* 1992;80:982a.(abst).

90. Geissler RG, Schulte P, Ganser A. Clinical use of hematopoietic growth factors in patients with myelodysplastic syndromes. *Int J Hematol* 1997;65: 339–354.

91. Hansen PB, Penkowa M, Johnsen HE. Hematopoietic growth factors for the treatment of myelodysplastic syndromes. *Leuk Lymphoma* 1998;28:491–500.

92. Kojima S. Use of hematopoietic growth factors for treatment of aplastic anemia. *Bone Marrow Transplant* 1996;18(Suppl 3):S36–S38.

93. Bonilla MA, Gillio AP, Ruggeiro M, et al. Effects of recombinant human granulocyte colony-stimulating factor on neutropenia in patients with congenital agranulocytosis. *N Engl J Med* 1989;320:1574–1580.

94. Dale DC, Hammond WP, Gabrilove J, et al. Long term treatment of severe chronic neutropenia with recombinant human granulocyte colony stimulating factor (r-meHuG-CSF). *Blood* 1990;76:139a(abst).

95. Jakubowski AA, Souza L, Kelly F, et al. Effects of human granulocyte colony-stimulating factor in a patient with idiopathic neutropenia. *N Engl J Med* 1989;320: 38–42.

96. Hammond WP, Price TH, Souza LM, et al. Treatment of cyclic neutropenia with granulocyte colony- stimulating factor. *N Engl J Med* 1989;320:1306–1311.

97. Dale DC, Bolyard AA, Hammond WP. Cyclic neutropenia: natural history and effects of long-term treatment with recombinant human granulocyte colony-stimulating factor. *Cancer Invest* 1993;11:219–223.

98. Jayabose S, Tugal O, Sandoval C, et al. Recombinant human granulocyte colony stimulating factor in cyclic neutropenia: use of a new 3-day-a-week regimen. *Am J Pediatr Hematol Oncol* 1994;16:338–340.

99. Boesen P. Cyclic neutropenia terminating in permanent agranulocytosis. *Acta Med Scand* 1988;223: 89–91.

100. Wang WC, Crist WM, Ihle JN, et al. Granulocyte colony-stimulating factor corrects the neutropenia associated with glycogen storage disease type Ib. *Leukemia* 1991;5:347–349.

101. Schroten H, Roesler J, Breidenbach T, et al. Granulocyte and granulocyte-macrophage colony-stimulating factors for treatment of neutropenia in glycogen storage disease type Ib. *J Pediatr* 1991;119:748–754.

102. Alter BP, Gardner FH, Hall RE. Treatment of dyskeratosis congenita with granulocyte colony-stimulating factor and erythropoietin. *Br J Haematol* 1997;97: 309–311.

103. Kocherlakota P, La Gamma EF. Preliminary report: rhG-CSF may reduce the incidence of neonatal sepsis in prolonged preeclampsia-associated neutropenia. *Pediatrics* 1998;102:1107–1111.

104. La Gamma EF, Alpan O, Kocherlakota P. Effect of granulocyte colony-stimulating factor on preeclampsia-associated neonatal neutropenia. *J Pediatr* 1995; 126:457–459.

105. Makhlouf RA, Doron MW, Bose CL, et al. Administration of granulocyte colony-stimulating factor to neutropenic low birth weight infants of mothers with preeclampsia. *J Pediatr* 1995;126:454–456.

106. Gough A, Clapperton M, Rolando N, et al. Randomised placebo-controlled trial of granulocyte-colony stimulating factor in diabetic foot infection. *Lancet* 1997;350:855–859.

107. Foster PF, Mital D, Sankary HN, et al. The use of granulocyte colony-stimulating factor after liver transplantation. *Transplantation* 1995;59:1557–1563.

108. Polak-Wyss A. Protective effect of human granulocyte colony stimulating factor (hG-CSF) on *Candida* infections in normal and immunosuppressed mice. *Mycoses* 1991;34:109–118.

109. Roilides E, Uhlig K, Venzon D, et al. Enhancement of

oxidative response and damage caused by human neutrophils to *Aspergillus fumigatus* hyphae by granulocyte colony-stimulating factor and gamma interferon. *Infect Immun* 1993;61:1185–1193.

110. Pan L, Delmonte J Jr, Jalonen CK, et al. Pretreatment of donor mice with granulocyte colony-stimulating factor polarizes donor T lymphocytes toward type-2 cytokine production and reduces severity of experimental graft-versus-host disease. *Blood* 1995;86: 4422–4429.

111. Hartung T, Docke WD, Gantner F, et al. Effect of granulocyte colony-stimulating factor treatment on *ex vivo* blood cytokine response in human volunteers. *Blood* 1995;85:2482–2489.

112. Lundblad R, Nesland JM, Giercksky KE. Granulocyte colony-stimulating factor improves survival rate and reduces concentrations of bacteria, endotoxin, tumor necrosis factor, and endothelin-1 in fulminant intra-abdominal sepsis in rats. *Crit Care Med* 1996;24: 820–826.

113. O'Reilly M, Silver GM, Greenhalgh DG, et al. Treatment of intra-abdominal infection with granulocyte colony-stimulating factor. *J Trauma* 1992;33:679–682.

114. Gorgen I, Hartung T, Leist M, et al. Granulocyte colony-stimulating factor treatment protects rodents against lipopolysaccharide-induced toxicity via suppression of systemic tumor necrosis factor-alpha. *J Immunol* 1992;149:918–924.

115. Nelson S. Role of granulocyte colony-stimulating factor in the immune response to acute bacterial infection in the nonneutropenic host: an overview. *Clin Infect Dis* 1994;18(Suppl 2):S197–S204.

116. Mooney DP, Gamelli RL, O'Reilly M, et al. Recombinant human granulocyte colony-stimulating factor and *Pseudomonas* burn wound sepsis. *Arch Surg* 1988; 123:1353–1537.

117. Cairo MS, Mauss D, Kommareddy S, et al. Prophylactic or simultaneous administration of recombinant human granulocyte colony stimulating factor in the treatment of group B streptococcal sepsis in neonatal rats. *Pediatr Res* 1990;27:612–616.

118. Yasuda H, Ajiki Y, Shimozato T, et al. Therapeutic efficacy of granulocyte colony-stimulating factor alone and in combination with antibiotics against *Pseudomonas aeruginosa* infections in mice. *Infect Immun* 1990;58:2502–2509.

119. Hebert JC, O'Reilly M, Gamelli RL. Protective effect of recombinant human granulocyte colony-stimulating factor against pneumococcal infections in splenectomized mice. *Arch Surg* 1990;125:1075–1078.

120. Weiss M, Gross-Weege W, Harms B, et al. Filgrastim (RHG-CSF) related modulation of the inflammatory response in patients at risk of sepsis or with sepsis. *Cytokine* 1996;8:260–265.

121. Endo S, Inada K, Inoue Y, et al. Evaluation of recombinant human granulocyte colony stimulating factor (rhG-CSF) therapy in granulopoetic patients complicated with sepsis. *Curr Med Res Opin* 1994;13:233–241.

122. Yoshida M, Karasawa M, Naruse T, et al. Effect of granulocyte-colony stimulating factor on empiric therapy with flomoxef sodium and tobramycin in febrile neutropenic patients with hematological malignancies. Kan-etsu Hematological Disease and\par Infection Study Group. *Int J Hematol* 1999;69:81–88.

123. Nelson S, Belknap SM, Carlson RW, et al. A randomized controlled trial of filgrastim as an adjunct to antibiotics for treatment of hospitalized patients with community-acquired pneumonia. CAP Study Group. *J Infect Dis* 1998;178:1075–1080.

124. Santana VM, Bowman LC, Furman WL, et al. Trial of chemotherapy plus recombinant human granulocyte colony stimulating factor in children with advanced neuroblastoma. *Med Pediatr Oncol* 1990;18:395(abst 116).

125. Riikonen P, Rahiala J, Salonvaara M, et al. Prophylactic administration of granulocyte colony-stimulating factor (filgrastim) after conventional chemotherapy in children with cancer. *Stem Cells* 1995;13:289–294.

126. Liang DC, Chen SH, Lean SF. Role of granulocyte colony-stimulating factor as adjunct therapy for septicemia in children with acute leukemia. *Am J Hematol* 1995;48:76–81.

127. Lieschke GJ, Burgess AW. Granulocyte colony-stimulating factor and granulocyte-macrophage colony-stimulating factor (2). *N Engl J Med* 1992;327: 99–106.

128. Lieschke GJ, Burgess AW. Granulocyte colony-stimulating factor and granulocyte-macrophage colony-stimulating factor (1). *N Engl J Med* 1992;327:28–35.

129. Root RK, Dale DC. Granulocyte colony-stimulating factor and granulocyte-macrophage colony-stimulating factor: comparisons and potential for use in the treatment of infections in nonneutropenic patients. *J Infect Dis* 1999;179:S342–S352.

130. Lusis AJ, Quon DH, Golde DW. Purification and characterization of a human T-lymphocyte-derived granulocyte-macrophage colony-stimulating factor. *Blood* 1981;57:13–21.

131. Thorens B, Mermod JJ, Vassalli P. Phagocytosis and inflammatory stimuli induce GM-CSF mRNA in macrophages through posttranscriptional regulation. *Cell* 1987;48:671–679.

132. Bagby GC Jr, Dinarello CA, Wallace P, et al. Interleukin 1 stimulates granulocyte macrophage colony-stimulating activity release by vascular endothelial cells. *J Clin Invest* 1986;78:1316–1323.

133. Horowitz MC, Coleman DL, Flood PM, et al. Parathyroid hormone and lipopolysaccharide induce murine osteoblast-like cells to secrete a cytokine indistinguishable from granulocyte-macrophage colony-stimulating factor. *J Clin Invest* 1989;83:149–157.

134. Munker R, Gasson J, Ogawa M, et al. Recombinant human TNF induces production of granulocyte-monocyte colony-stimulating factor. *Nature* 1986;323: 79–82.

135. Ruscetti FW, Chou JY, Gallo RC. Human trophoblasts: cellular source of colony-stimulating activity in placental tissue. *Blood* 1982;59:86–90.

136. Kaushansky K, Lin N, Adamson JW. Interleukin 1 stimulates fibroblasts to synthesize granulocyte-macrophage and granulocyte colony-stimulating factors: mechanism for the hematopoietic response to inflammation. *J Clin Invest* 1988;81:92–97.

137. Ruef C, Coleman D. Granulocyte-macrophage colony-stimulating factor: pleitropic cytokine with potential clinical usefulness. *Rev Infect Dis* 1990;12:41–62.

138. Coffey RG. Mechanism of GM-CSF stimulation of neutrophils. *Immunol Res* 1989;8:236–48.

139. Huebner K, Isobe M, Croce C, et al. The human gene encoding GM-CSF is at 5q21-q32, the chromosome

region deleted in the 5q-anomaly. *Science* 1985;230: 1282–1285.

140. Wong G, Witek J, Temple P, et al. Human GM-CSF: molecular cloning of the complementary DNA and purification of the natural and recombinant proteins. *Science* 1985;228:810–815.

141. Bussolino F, Wang JM, Defilippi P, et al. Granulocyte- and granulocyte-macrophage-colony stimulating factors induce human endothelial cells to migrate and proliferate. *Nature* 1989;337:471–473.

142. Baldwin GC, Gasson JC, Kaufman SE, et al. Non-hematopoietic tumor cells express functional GM-CSF receptors. *Blood* 1989;73:1033–1037.

143. Kwon EM, Sakamoto KM. The molecular mechanism of action of granulocyte-macrophage colony-stimulating factor. *J Invest Med* 1996;44:442–446.

144. Gearing DP, King JA, Gough N, et al. Expression cloning of a receptor for human granulocyte-macrophage colony-stimulating factor. *EMBO J* 1989; 8:3667–3676.

145. Klausmann M, Pfluger KH, Krumwieh D, et al. Influence of recombinant human granulocyte-macrophage colony-stimulating factor on granulocyte functions. *Behring Inst Mitt* 1988;83:265–269.

146. Weisbart R, Gasson JC, Golde DW. Colony-stimulating factors and host defense. *Ann Intern Med* 1989; 110:297–303.

147. Monroy RL, Davis TA, MacVittie TJ. Granulocyte-macrophage colony-stimulating factor: more than a hemopoietin. *Clin Immunol Immunopathol* 1990;54: 333–346.

148. Wang JM, Colella S, Allavena P, et al. Chemotactic activity of human recombinant granulocyte-macrophage colony-stimulating factor. *Immunology* 1987;60: 439–444.

149. Addison IE, Johnson B, Devereux S, et al. Granulocyte-macrophage colony-stimulating factor may inhibit neutrophil migration *in vivo. Clin Exp Immunol* 1989;76:149–153.

150. Fleischmann J, Golde DW, Weisbart RH, et al. Granulocyte-macrophage colony-stimulating factor enhances phagocytosis of bacteria by human neutrophils. *Blood* 1986;68:708–711.

151. Fabian I, Baldwin GC, Golde DW. Biosynthetic granulocyte-macrophage colony-stimulating factor enhances neutrophil cytotoxicity toward human leukemia cells. *Leukemia* 1987;1:613–617.

152. Grabstein KH, Urdal DL, Tushinski RJ, et al. Induction of macrophage tumoricidal activity by granulocyte-macrophage colony-stimulating factor. *Science* 1986; 232:506–508.

153. DiPersio JF, Billing P, Williams R, et al. Human granulocyte-macrophage colony-stimulating factor and other cytokines prime human neutrophils for enhanced arachidonic acid release and leukotriene B4 synthesis. *J Immunol* 1988;140:4315–4322.

154. Weisbart RH, Golde DW, Gasson JC. Biosynthetic human GM-CSF modulates the number and affinity of neutrophil f-Met-Leu-Phe receptors. *J Immunol* 1986; 137:3584–3587.

155. Wexler LH, Weaver-McClure L, Steinberg SM, et al. Randomized trial of recombinant human granulocyte-macrophage colony-stimulating factor in pediatric patients receiving intensive myelosuppressive chemotherapy. *J Clin Oncol* 1996;14:901–910.

156. Calderwood S, Romeyer F, Blanchette V, et al. Concurrent RhGM-CSF does not offset myelosuppression from intensive chemotherapy: randomized placebo-controlled study in childhood acute lymphoblastic leukemia. *Am J Hematol* 1994;47:27–32.

157. Burdach SE, Muschenich M, Josephs W, et al. Granulocyte-macrophage-colony stimulating factor for prevention of neutropenia and infections in children and adolescents with solid tumors: results of a prospective randomized study. *Cancer* 1995;76:510–516.

158. Brandt SJ, Peters WP, Atwater SK, et al. Effect of recombinant human granulocyte-macrophage colony-stimulating factor on hematopoietic reconstitution after high-dose chemotherapy and autologous bone marrow transplantation. *N Engl J Med* 1988;318:869–876.

159. Nemunaitis J, Singer JW, Buckner CD, et al. Use of recombinant human granulocyte-macrophage colony-stimulating factor in autologous marrow transplantation for lymphoid malignancies. *Blood* 1988;72:834–836.

160. Blazar BR, Kersey JH, McGlave PB, et al. *In vivo* administration of recombinant human granulocyte/macrophage colony-stimulating factor in acute lymphoblastic leukemia patients receiving purged autografts. *Blood* 1989;73:849–857.

161. Link H, Freund M, Kirchner H, et al. Recombinant human granulocyte-macrophage colony stimulating factor (rh GM-CSF) after bone marrow transplantation. *Behring Inst Mitt* 1988;83:313–319.

162. Nemunaitis J, Rabinowe SN, Singer JW, et al. Recombinant granulocyte-macrophage colony-stimulating factor after autologous bone marrow transplantation for lymphoid cancer. *N Engl J Med* 1991;324:1773–1778.

163. Antin JH, Smith BR, Holmes W, et al. Phase I/II study of recombinant human granulocyte-macrophage colony-stimulating factor in aplastic anemia and myelodysplastic syndrome. *Blood* 1988;72:705–713.

164. Champlin RE, Nimer SD, Ireland P, et al. Treatment of refractory aplastic anemia with recombinant human granulocyte-macrophage-colony-stimulating factor. *Blood* 1989;73:694–649.

165. Nissen C, Tichelli A, Gratwohl A, et al. Failure of recombinant human granulocyte-macrophage colony-stimulating factor therapy in aplastic anemia patients with very severe neutropenia. *Blood* 1988;72: 2045–2047.

166. Guinan EC, Sieff CA, Oette DH, et al. A Phase I/II trial of recombinant granulocyte-macrophage colony-stimulating factor for children with aplastic anemia. *Blood* 1990;76:1077–1082.

167. Guinan EC, Lopez KD, Huhn RD, et al. Evaluation of granulocyte-macrophage colony-stimulating factor for treatment of pancytopenia in children with Fanconi anemia. *J Pediatr* 1994;124:144–150.

168. Vadhan-Raj S, Jeha SS, Buescher S, et al. Stimulation of myelopoiesis in a patient with congenital neutropenia: biology and nature of response to recombinant human granulocyte-macrophage colony-stimulating factor. *Blood* 1990;75:858–864.

169. Guinan EC, Lopez KD, Huhn RD, et al. Evaluation of granulocyte-macrophage colony-stimulating factor for treatment of pancytopenia in children with fanconi anemia. *J Pediatr* 1994;124:144–150.

170. Armitage JO. Emerging applications of recombinant human granulocyte-macrophage colony-stimulating factor. *Blood* 1998;92:4491–4508.

171. Ross SD, DiGeorge A, Connelly JE, et al. Safety of GM-CSF in patients with AIDS: a review of the literature. *Pharmacotherapy* 1998;18:1290–1297.

172. Schaison G, Eden OB, Henze G, et al. Recommendations on the use of colony-stimulating factors in children: conclusions of a European panel. *Eur J Pediatr* 1998;157:955–966.

173. Groopman JE, Mitsuyasu RT, DeLeo MJ, et al. Effect of recombinant human granulocyte-macrophage colony-stimulating factor on myelopoiesis in the acquired immunodeficiency syndrome. *N Engl J Med* 1987;317:593–598.

174. Levine JD, Allan JD, Tessitore JH, et al. Recombinant human granulocyte-macrophage colony-stimulating factor ameliorates zidovudine-induced neutropenia in patients with acquired immunodeficiency syndrome (AIDS)/AIDS-related complex. *Blood* 1991;78: 3148–3154.

175. Pluda JM, Yarchoan R, Smith PD, et al. Subcutaneous recombinant granulocyte-macrophage colony-stimulating factor used as a single agent and in an alternating regimen with azidothymidine in leukopenic patients with severe human immunodeficiency virus infection. *Blood* 1990;76:463–472.

176. Bodey GP, Anaissie E, Gutterman J, et al. Role of granulocyte-macrophage colony-stimulating factor as adjuvant treatment in neutropenic patients with bacterial and fungal infection. *Eur J Clin Microbiol Infect Dis* 1994;13(Suppl 2):S18–S22.

177. Cairo MS, Agosti J, Ellis R, et al. A randomized, double-blind, placebo-controlled trial of prophylactic recombinant human granulocyte-macrophage colony-stimulating factor to reduce nosocomial infections in very low birth weight neonates. *J Pediatr* 1999; 134:64–70.

178. Sprikkelman A, de Wolf JT, Vellenga E. The application of hematopoietic growth factors in drug-induced agranulocytosis: a review of 70 cases. *Leukemia* 1994; 8:2031–2036.

179. Marques dC, Jesus FM, Aniceto C, et al. Double-blind randomized placebo-controlled trial of the use of granulocyte-macrophage colony-stimulating factor in chronic leg ulcers. *Am J Surg* 1997;173:165–168.

180. Arnold F, O'Brien J, Cherry G. Granulocyte monocyte-colony stimulating factor as an agent for wound healing: a study evaluating the use of local injections of a genetically engineered growth factor in the management of wounds with a poor healing prognosis. *J Wound Care* 1995;4:400–402.

181. Gaspari AA, Zalka AD, Payne D, et al. Successful treatment of a generalized human papillomavirus infection with granulocyte-macrophage colony-stimulating factor and interferon gamma immunotherapy in a patient with a primary immunodeficiency and cyclic neutropenia. *Arch Dermatol* 1997;133:491–496.

182. Peters BG, Adkins DR, Harrison BR, et al. Antifungal effects of yeast-derived rhu-GM-CSF in patients receiving high-dose chemotherapy given with or without autologous stem cell transplantation: a retrospective analysis. *Bone Marrow Transplant* 1996;18:93–102.

183. Mueller BU, Pizzo PA. Cytokines and biological response modifiers in the treatment of infection. *Cancer Treat Res* 1998;96:201–222.

184. Gordon B, Spadinger A, Hodges E, et al. Effect of granulocyte-macrophage colony-stimulating factor on oral mucositis after hematopoietic stem-cell transplantation. *J Clin Oncol* 1994;12:1917–1922.

185. Masucci G. New clinical applications of granulocyte-macrophage colony-stimulating factor. *Med Oncol* 1996;13:149–154.

186. Trindade E, Maton P, Reding R, et al. Use of granulocyte macrophage colony stimulating factor in children after orthotopic liver transplantation. *J Hepatol* 1998; 28:1054–1057.

187. Hack CE, Aarden LA, Thijs LG. Role of cytokines in sepsis. *Adv Immunol* 1997;66:101–195.

188. Root RK, Dale DC. Granulocyte colony-stimulating factor and granulocyte-macrophage colony-stimulating factor: comparisons and potential for use in the treatment of infections in nonneutropenic patients. *J Infect Dis* 1999;179(Suppl 2):S342–S352.

189. Antman KS, Griffin JD, Elias A, et al. Effect of recombinant human granulocyte-macrophage colony-stimulating factor on chemotherapy-induced myelosuppression. *N Engl J Med* 1988;319:593–598.

190. Lieschke GJ, Cebon J, Morstyn G. Characterization of the clinical effects after the first dose of bacterially synthesized recombinant human granulocyte-macrophage colony-stimulating factor. *Blood* 1989;74: 2634–2643.

191. Vadhan-Raj S, Buescher S, LeMaistre A, et al. Stimulation of hematopoiesis in patients with bone marrow failure and in patients with malignancy by recombinant human granulocyte-macrophage colony-stimulating factor. *Blood* 1988;72:134–141.

192. Phillips N, Jacobs S, Stoller R, et al. Effect of recombinant human granulocyte-macrophage colony- stimulating factor on myelopoiesis in patients with refractory metastatic carcinoma. *Blood* 1989;74:26–34.

193. Nemunaitis J, Singer JW, Buckner CD, et al. Use of recombinant human granulocyte-macrophage colony-stimulating factor in graft failure after bone marrow transplantation. *Blood* 1990;76:245–253.

194. Marsoni S, Ungerleider RS, Hurson SB, et al. Tolerance to antineoplastic agents in children and adults. *Cancer Treat Rep* 1985;69:1263–1269.

195. Furman WL, Fairclough DL, Huhn RD, et al. Therapeutic Effects and pharmacokinetics of recombinant human granulocyte-macrophage colony-stimulating factor in childhood cancer patients receiving myelosuppressive chemotherapy. *J Clin Oncol* 1991;9: 1022–1028.

196. Bajorin DF, Cheung N-KV, Houghton AN. Macrophage colony-stimulating factor: biological effects and potential applications for cancer therapy. *Semin Hematol* 1991;28:42–48.

197. Morris SW, Valentine MB, Shapiro DN, et al. Reassignment of the human *CSF1* Gene to chromosome 1p13-p21. *Blood* 1991;78:2013–2020.

198. Rettenmier CW, Sherr CJ. The mononuclear phagocyte colony-stimulating factor (CSF-1, M- CSF). *Hematol Oncol Clin North Am* 1989;3:479–493.

199. Nemunaitis J, Meyers JD, Buckner CD, et al. Phase I trial of recombinant human macrophage colony-stimulating factor in patients with invasive fungal infections. *Blood* 1991;78:907–913.

200. Vilcek J, Sen GC. Interferons and other cytokines. In: Fields BN, Knipe DM, Howley PM, eds. *Fields virology*, 3rd ed. Philadelphia: Lippincott–Raven, 1996: 375–399.

201. Taniguchi T, Mantei N, Schwarzstein M, et al. Human leukocyte and fibroblast interferons are structurally related. *Nature* 1980;285:547–549.

202. Sen GC, Lengyel P. The interferon system: a bird's eye view of its biochemistry. *J Biol Chem* 1992;267: 5017–5020.

203. Durum SK, Oppenheim JJ. Proinflammatory cytokines and immunity. In: Paul WE, ed. *Fundamental immunology,* 3rd ed. New York: Raven Press, 1993:801.

204. La Pine TR, Cates KL, Hill HR. Immunomodulating agents. In: Feigin RD, Cherry JD, eds. *Textbook of pediatric infectious diseases,* 4th ed. Philadelphia: WB Saunders, 1998:2719–2729.

205. Rinderknecht E, O'Connor BH, Rodriguez H. Natural human interferon-gamma: complete amino acid sequence and determination of sites of glycosylation. *J Biol Chem* 1984;259:6790–6797.

206. Mannering GJ, Deloria LB. The pharmacology and toxicology of the interferons: an overview. *Annu Rev Pharmacol Toxicol* 1986;26:455–515.

207. Fent K, Zbinden G. Toxicity of interferon and interleukin. *Trends Pharmacol Sci* 1987;8:100–105.

208. Affabris E, Federico M, Romeo G, et al. Opposite effects of murine interferons on erythroid differentiation of Friend cells. *Virology* 1988;167:185–193.

209. Howard MC, Miyajima A, Coffman R. T-cell-derived cytokines and their receptors. In: Paul WE, ed. *Fundamental immunology.* New York: Raven Press, 1993: 763–800.

210. Billiau A. Interferon-gamma: biology and role in pathogenesis. *Adv Immunol* 1996;62:61–130.

211. Nathan CF, Murray HW, Wiebe ME, et al. Identification of interferon-gamma as the lymphokine that activates human macrophage oxidative metabolism and antimicrobial activity. *J Exp Med* 1983;158:670–689.

212. Cassatella MA, Bazzoni F, Flynn RM, et al. Molecular basis of interferon-gamma and lipopolysaccharide enhancement of phagocyte respiratory burst capability: studies on the gene expression of several NADPH oxidase components. *J Biol Chem* 1990;265: 20241–20246.

213. Merigan TC, Reed SE, Hall TS, et al. Inhibition of respiratory virus infection by locally applied interferon. *Lancet* 1973;1:563–567.

214. Scott GM, Phillpotts RJ, Wallace J, et al. Prevention of rhinovirus colds by human interferon alpha-2 from *Escherichia coli. Lancet* 1982;2:186–188.

215. Treanor JJ, Betts RF, Erb SM, et al. Intranasally administered interferon as prophylaxis against experimentally induced influenza A virus infection in humans. *J Infect Dis* 1987;156:379–383.

216. Turner RB, Felton A, Kosak K, et al. Prevention of experimental coronavirus colds with intranasal alpha-2b interferon. *J Infect Dis* 1986;154:443–447.

217. Vergani D, Locasciulli A, Masera G, et al. Histological evidence of hepatitis-B-virus infection with negative serology in children with acute leukaemia who develop chronic liver disease. *Lancet* 1982;1:361–364.

218. Locasciulli A, Testa M, Valsecchi MG, et al. Morbidity and mortality due to liver disease in children undergoing allogeneic bone marrow transplantation: a 10-year prospective study. *Blood* 1997;90:3799–3805.

219. Locasciulli A, Testa M, Pontisso P, et al. Prevalence and natural history of hepatitis C infection in patients cured of childhood leukemia. *Blood* 1997;90: 4628–4633.

220. Perrillo RP, Schiff ER, Davis GL, et al. A randomized, controlled trial of interferon alfa-2b alone and after prednisone withdrawal for the treatment of chronic hepatitis B. The Hepatitis Interventional Therapy Group [see comments]. *N Engl J Med* 1990;323:295–301.

221. Freifeld AG, Walsh TJ, Pizzo PA. Infectious complications in the pediatric cancer patient. In: Pizzo PA, Poplack DG, eds. *Principles and practice of pediatric oncology.* Philadelphia: Lippincott–Raven, 1997: 1069–1114.

222. Brook MG, McDonald JA, Karayiannis P, et al. Randomised controlled trial of interferon alfa 2A (rbe) (Roferon-A) for the treatment of chronic hepatitis B virus (HBV) infection: factors that influence response. *Gut* 1989;30:1116–1122.

223. Peters M, Davis GL, Dooley JS, et al. The interferon system in acute and chronic viral hepatitis. *Prog Liver Dis* 1986;8:453–467.

224. Foster GR, Ackrill AM, Goldin RD, et al. Expression of the terminal protein region of hepatitis B virus inhibits cellular responses to interferons alpha and gamma and double-stranded RNA. *Proc Natl Acad Sci USA* 1991;88:2888–2892. [Published erratum appears in *Proc Natl Acad Sci USA* 1995;92:3632.]

225. Centers for Disease Control and Prevention. Recommendations for prevention and control of hepatitis C virus (HCV) infection and HCV-related chronic disease. *MMWR Morb Mortal Wkly Rep* 1998;47:1–39.

226. Liang TJ. Combination therapy for hepatitis C infection [Editorial; Comment]. *N Engl J Med* 1998;339: 1549–1550.

227. Poynard T, Marcellin P, Lee SS, et al. Randomised trial of interferon alpha2b plus ribavirin for 48 weeks or for 24 weeks versus interferon alpha2b plus placebo for 48 weeks for treatment of chronic infection with hepatitis C virus: International Hepatitis Interventional Therapy Group (IHIT). *Lancet* 1998;352:1426–1432.

228. McHutchison JG, Gordon SC, Schiff ER, et al. Interferon alfa-2b alone or in combination with ribavirin as initial treatment for chronic hepatitis C: Hepatitis Interventional Therapy Group. *N Engl J Med* 1998;339: 1485–1492.

229. Davis GL, Esteban-Mur R, Rustgi V, et al. Interferon alfa-2b alone or in combination with ribavirin for the treatment of relapse of chronic hepatitis C: International Hepatitis Interventional Therapy Group. *N Engl J Med* 1998;339:1493–1499.

230. Yamamoto JK, Barre-Sinoussi F, Bolton V, et al. Human alpha- and beta-interferon but not gamma- suppress the *in vitro* replication of LAV, HTLV-III, and ARV-2. *J Interferon Cytokine Res* 1986;6:143–152.

231. Lane HC, Davey V, Kovacs JA, et al. Interferon-alpha in patients with asymptomatic human immunodeficiency virus (HIV) infection: a randomized, placebo-controlled trial. *Ann Intern Med* 1990;112:805–811.

232. Schalling M, Ekman M, Kaaya EE, et al. A role for a new herpes virus (KSHV) in different forms of Kaposi's sarcoma. *Nat Med* 1995;1:707–708.

233. Athale UH, Patil PS, Chintu C, et al. Influence of HIV epidemic on the incidence of Kaposi's sarcoma in Zambian children. *J Acquir Immune Defic Syndr Hum Retrovirol* 1995;8:96–100.

234. Krown SE, Real FX, Cunningham-Rundles S, et al. Preliminary observations on the effect of recombinant leukocyte A interferon in homosexual men with Kaposi's sarcoma. *N Engl J Med* 1983;308:1071–1076.

235. de Wit R, Schattenkerk JK, Boucher CA, et al. Clinical and virological effects of high-dose recombinant interferon-alpha in disseminated AIDS-related Kaposi's sarcoma. *Lancet* 1988;2:1214–1217.

236. Martinez J, Smith R, Farmer M, et al. High prevalence of genital tract papillomavirus infection in female adolescents. *Pediatrics* 1988;82:604–608.

237. D'Angelo LJ. Sexually transmitted diseases in children and adolescents with HIV infection. In: Pizzo PA, Wilfert CM, eds. *Pediatric AIDS: the challenge of HIV infection in infants, children, and adolescents.* Baltimore: Williams & Wilkins, 1998:169–182.

238. Vance JC, Davis D. Interferon alpha-2b injections used as an adjuvant therapy to carbon dioxide laser vaporization of recalcitrant ano-genital condylomata acuminata. *J Invest Dermatol* 1990;95:146S–148S.

239. Bonnez W, Oakes D, Bailey-Farchione A, et al. A randomized, double-blind, placebo-controlled trial of systemically administered interferon-alpha, -beta, or -gamma in combination with cryotherapy for the treatment of condyloma acuminatum. *J Infect Dis* 1995;171:1081–1089.

240. Healy GB, Gelber RD, Trowbridge AL, et al. Treatment of recurrent respiratory papillomatosis with human leukocyte interferon: results of a multicenter randomized clinical trial. *N Engl J Med* 1988;319:401–407.

241. King CL, Gallin JI, Malech HL, et al. Regulation of immunoglobulin production in hyperimmunoglobulin E recurrent-infection syndrome by interferon gamma. *Proc Natl Acad Sci USA* 1989;86:10085–10089.

242. Jeppson JD, Jaffe HS, Hill HR. Use of recombinant human interferon gamma to enhance neutrophil chemotactic responses in Job syndrome of hyperimmunoglobulinemia E and recurrent infections. *J Pediatr* 1991;118:383–387.

243. Gallin JI. Interferon-gamma in the management of chronic granulomatous disease [see comments]. *Rev Infect Dis* 1991;13:973–978.

244. Ezekowitz RA, Orkin SH, Newburger PE. Recombinant interferon gamma augments phagocyte superoxide production and X-chronic granulomatous disease gene expression in X-linked variant chronic granulomatous disease. *J Clin Invest* 1987;80:1009–1016.

245. Sechler JM, Malech HL, White CJ, et al. Recombinant human interferon-gamma reconstitutes defective phagocyte function in patients with chronic granulomatous disease of childhood. *Proc Natl Acad Sci USA* 1988;85:4874–4888.

246. The International Chronic Granulomatous Disease Cooperative Study Group. A controlled trial of interferon gamma to prevent infection in chronic granulomatous disease. *N Engl J Med* 1991;324:509–516.

247. Hiscott J, Nguyen H, Lin R. Molecular mechanisms of interferon beta gene induction. *Semin Virol* 1995;6:161–173.

248. Dalton DK, Pitts-Meek S, Keshav S, et al. Multiple defects of immune cell function in mice with disrupted interferon-gamma genes. *Science* 1993;259:1739–1742.

249. Huang S, Hendriks W, Althage A, et al. Immune response in mice that lack the interferon-gamma receptor. *Science* 1993;259:1742–1745.

250. Nathan CF, Kaplan G, Levis WR, et al. Local and systemic effects of intradermal recombinant interferon-gamma in patients with lepromatous leprosy. *N Engl J Med* 1986;315:6–15.

251. Nathan C, Squires K, Griffo W, et al. Widespread intradermal accumulation of mononuclear leukocytes in lepromatous leprosy patients treated systemically with recombinant interferon gamma. *J Exp Med* 1990;172:-1509–1512.

252. Holland SM, Eisenstein EM, Kuhns DB, et al. Treatment of refractory disseminated nontuberculous mycobacterial infection with interferon gamma: a preliminary report. *N Engl J Med* 1994;330:1348–1355.

253. Badaro R, Falcoff E, Badaro FS, et al. Treatment of visceral leishmaniasis with pentavalent antimony and interferon gamma. *N Engl J Med* 1990;322:16–21.

254. Seki H, Taga K, Matsuda A, et al. Phenotypic and functional characteristics of active suppressor cells against IFN-gamma production in PHA-stimulated cord blood lymphocytes. *J Immunol* 1986;137:3158–3161.

255. Wilson CB, Westall J, Johnston L, et al. Decreased production of interferon-gamma by human neonatal cells: intrinsic and regulatory deficiencies. *J Clin Invest* 1986;77:860–867.

256. Balkwill FR. The other interleukins. In: *Cytokines in cancer therapy.* Oxford: Oxford University Press, 1989:150–181.

257. WHO-IUIS Nomenclature Subcommittee on Interleukin Designation. Nomenclature for secreted regulatory proteins of the immune system (interleukins). *Bull WHO* 1991;69:483–486.

258. Curfs JH, Meis JF, Hoogkamp-Korstanje JA. A primer on cytokines: sources, receptors, effects, and inducers. *Clin Microbiol Rev* 1997;10:742–780.

259. Dinarello CA, Novick D, Puren AJ, et al. Overview of interleukin-18: more than an interferon-gamma inducing factor. *J Leukoc Biol* 1998;63:658–664.

260. Xiang Z, Ertl HC. Manipulation of the immune response to a plasmid-encoded viral antigen by coinoculation with plasmids expressing cytokines. *Immunity* 1995;2:129–135.

261. Bermudez LE, Kaplan G. Recombinant cytokines for controlling mycobacterial infections. *Trends Microbiol* 1995;3:22–27.

262. Klausmann M, Pfluger KH, Krumwieh D, et al. Modulation of functions of granulocytes by recombinant human GM-CSF and possible complications of GM-CSF therapy. *Leukemia* 1988;2:63S–72S.

263. Xin KQ, Hamajima K, Sasaki S, et al. Intranasal administration of human immunodeficiency virus type-1 (HIV-1) DNA vaccine with interleukin-2 expression plasmid enhances cell-mediated immunity against HIV-1. *Immunology* 1998;94:438–444.

264. Hazama M, Mayumi-Aono A, Miyazaki T, et al. Intranasal immunization against herpes simplex virus infection by using a recombinant glycoprotein D fused with immunomodulating proteins, the B subunit of *Escherichia coli* heat-labile enterotoxin and interleukin-2. *Immunology* 1993;78:643–649.

265. Trinchieri G. Interleukin-12: a proinflammatory cytokine with immunoregulatory functions that bridge innate resistance and antigen-specific adaptive immunity. *Annu Rev Immunol* 1995;13:251–276.

266. Kim JH, Loveland JE, Sitz KV, et al. Expansion of restricted cellular immune responses to HIV-1 envelope by vaccination: IL-7 and IL-12 differentially augment cellular proliferative responses to HIV-1. *Clin Exp Immunol* 1997;108:243–250.

267. Afonso LC, Scharton TM, Vieira LQ, et al. The adju-

vant effect of interleukin-12 in a vaccine against Leishmania major. *Science* 1994;263:235–237.

268. Ciobanu N, Welte K, Kruger G, et al. Defective T-cell response to PHA and mitogenic monoclonal antibodies in male homosexuals with acquired immunodeficiency syndrome and its *in vitro* correction by interleukin 2. *J Clin Immunol* 1983;3:332–340.

269. McMahon DK, Armstrong JA, Huang XL, et al. A phase I study of subcutaneous recombinant interleukin-2 in patients with advanced HIV disease while on zidovudine. *AIDS* 1994;8:59–66.

270. Schwartz DH, Skowron G, Merigan TC. Safety and effects of interleukin-2 plus zidovudine in asymptomatic individuals infected with human immunodeficiency virus. *J Acquir Immune Defic Syndr Hum Retrovirol* 1991;4:11–23.

271. Teppler H, Kaplan G, Smith KA, et al. Prolonged immunostimulatory effect of low-dose polyethylene glycol interleukin 2 in patients with human immunodeficiency virus type 1 infection. *J Exp Med* 1993;177:483–492.

272. Wood R, Montoya JG, Kundu SK, et al. Safety and efficacy of polyethylene glycol-modified interleukin-2 and zidovudine in human immunodeficiency virus type 1 infection: a phase I/II study. *J Infect Dis* 1993;167:519–525.

273. Kovacs JA, Vogel S, Albert JM, et al. Controlled trial of interleukin-2 infusions in patients infected with the human immunodeficiency virus [see comments]. *N Engl J Med* 1996;335:1350–1356.

274. Saravolatz L, Mitsuyasu R, Sneller M, et al. Duration of proleukin IL-2 therapy is more important than total dose in achieving CD4 expansion. In: *Program and Abstracts of the Interscience Conference on Antimicrobial Agents and Chemotherapy* 1996:213(abst).

275. Clerici M, Yarchoan R, Blatt S, et al. Effect of a recombinant CD4-IgG on in vitro T helper cell function: data from a phase I/II study of patients with AIDS. *J Infect Dis* 1993;168:1012–1016.

276. Clerici M, Hakim FT, Venzon DJ, et al. Changes in interleukin-2 and interleukin-4 production in asymptomatic, human immunodeficiency virus-seropositive individuals. *J Clin Invest* 1993;91:759–765.

277. Clerici M, Shearer GM. A TH1—>TH2 switch is a critical step in the etiology of HIV infection. *Immunol Today* 1993;14:107–111.

278. Martelletti P, Stirparo G, Morrone S, et al. Inhibition of intercellular adhesion molecule-1 (ICAM-1), soluble ICAM-1 and interleukin-4 by nitric oxide expression in migraine patients. *J Mol Med* 1997;75:448–453.

279. Hoelzer D. Hematopoietic growth factors—not whether, but when and where [Editorial; Comment]. *N Engl J Med* 1997;336:1822–1824.

280. Croockewit AJ, Bronchud MH, Aapro MS, et al. A European perspective on haematopoietic growth factors in haemato-oncology: report of an expert meeting of the EORTC. *Eur J Cancer* 1997;33:1732–1746.

281. Anderson MR, Blumer JL. Advances in the therapy for sepsis in children. *Pediatr Clin North Am* 1997;44:179–205.

282. Ziegler EJ, McCutchan JA, Fierer J, et al. Treatment of gram-negative bacteremia and shock with human antiserum to a mutant *Escherichia coli*. *N Engl J Med* 1982;307:1225–1230.

283. Treatment of severe infectious purpura in children with human plasma from donors immunized with *Escherichia coli* J5: a prospective double- blind study. J5 study Group. *J Infect Dis* 1992;165:695–701.

284. Baumgartner JD, Glauser MP, McCutchan JA, et al. Prevention of gram-negative shock and death in surgical patients by antibody to endotoxin core glycolipid. *Lancet* 1985;2:59–63.

285. Calandra T, Glauser MP, Schellekens J, et al. Treatment of gram-negative septic shock with human IgG antibody to *Escherichia coli* J5: a prospective, double-blind, randomized trial. *J Infect Dis* 1988;158:312–319.

286. Greenman RL, Schein RM, Martin MA, et al. A controlled clinical trial of E5 murine monoclonal IgM antibody to endotoxin in the treatment of gram-negative sepsis: the XOMA Sepsis Study Group. *JAMA* 1991;266:1097–1102.

287. Romano MJ, Kearns GL, Kaplan SL, et al. Single-dose pharmacokinetics and safety of HA-1A, a human IgM anti-lipid-A monoclonal antibody, in pediatric patients with sepsis syndrome. *J Pediatr* 1993;122:974–981.

288. Warren HS, Danner RL, Munford RS. Anti-endotoxin monoclonal antibodies. *N Engl J Med* 1992;326:1153–1157.

289. Quezado ZM, Natanson C, Hoffman WD. Looking back on HA-1A [Editorial; Comment]. *Arch Intern Med* 1994;154:2393.

290. McCloskey RV, Straube RC, Sanders C, et al. Treatment of septic shock with human monoclonal antibody HA-1A: a randomized, double-blind, placebo-controlled trial. CHESS Trial Study Group. *Ann Intern Med* 1994;121:1–5.

291. Goldie AS, Fearon KC, Ross JA, et al. Natural cytokine antagonists and endogenous antiendotoxin core antibodies in sepsis syndrome: the Sepsis Intervention Group. *JAMA* 1995;274:172–177.

292. Madonna GS, Peterson JE, Ribi EE, et al. Early-phase endotoxin tolerance: induction by a detoxified lipid A derivative, monophosphoryl lipid A. *Infect Immun* 1986;52:6–11.

293. Astiz ME, Rackow EC, Still JG, et al. Pretreatment of normal humans with monophosphoryl lipid A induces tolerance to endotoxin: a prospective, double-blind, randomized, controlled trial. *Crit Care Med* 1995;23:9–17.

294. Lefering R, Neugebauer EA. Steroid controversy in sepsis and septic shock: a meta-analysis [see comments]. *Crit Care Med* 1995;23:1294–1303.

295. The Intravenous Immunoglobulin Collaborative Study Group. Prophylactic intravenous administration of standard immune globulin as compared with core-lipopolysaccharide immune globulin in patients at high risk of postsurgical infection. *N Engl J Med* 1992;327:234–240.

296. Fanaroff AA, Korones SB, Wright LL, et al. A controlled trial of intravenous immune globulin to reduce nosocomial infections in very-low-birth-weight infants: National Institute of Child Health and Human Development Neonatal Research Network [see comments]. *N Engl J Med* 1994;330:1107–1113.

297. Tracey KJ, Fong Y, Hesse DG, et al. Cerami A. Anti-cachectin/TNF monoclonal antibodies prevent septic shock during lethal bacteraemia. *Nature* 1987;330:662–664.

298. Gerard C, Bruyns C, Marchant A, et al. Interleukin 10 reduces the release of tumor necrosis factor and prevents lethality in experimental endotoxemia. *J Exp Med* 1993;177:547–550.

299. Zabel P, Schade FU, Schlaak M. Inhibition of endogenous TNF formation by pentoxifylline. *Immunobiology* 1993;187:447–463.

300. Strieter RM, Remick DG, Ward PA, et al. Cellular and molecular regulation of tumor necrosis factor-alpha production by pentoxifylline. *Biochem Biophys Res Commun* 1988;155:1230–1236.

301. Schade UF. Pentoxifylline increases survival in murine endotoxin shock and decreases formation of tumor necrosis factor. *Circ Shock* 1990;31:171–181.

302. Sampaio EP, Sarno EN, Galilly R, et al. Thalidomide selectively inhibits tumor necrosis factor alpha production by stimulated human monocytes. *J Exp Med* 1991;173:699–703.

303. Libert C, Vink A, Coulie P, et al. Limited involvement of interleukin-6 in the pathogenesis of lethal septic shock as revealed by the effect of monoclonal antibodies against interleukin-6 or its receptor in various murine models. *Eur J Immunol* 1992;22:2625–2630.

304. Quezado ZM, Banks SM, Natanson C. New strategies for combatting sepsis: the magic bullets missed the mark...but the search continues. *Trends Biotechnol* 1995;13:56–63.

305. Silva AT, Cohen J. Role of interferon-gamma in experimental gram-negative sepsis. *J Infect Dis* 1992;166:331–335.

306. Lorente JA, Landin L, De Pablo R, et al. L-arginine pathway in the sepsis syndrome [see comments]. *Crit Care Med* 1993;21:1287–1295.

307. Petros A, Lamb G, Leone A, et al. Effects of a nitric oxide synthase inhibitor in humans with septic shock. *Cardiovasc Res* 1994;28:34–39.

308. Daemen-Gubbels CR, Groeneveld PH, Groeneveld AB, et al. Methylene blue increases myocardial function in septic shock. *Crit Care Med* 1995;23:1363–1370.

309. Furman WL, Fairclough DL, Cain AM, et al. The use of GM-CSF in children after high-dose chemotherapy. *Med Ped Oncol* 1992;2(Suppl):26–30.

310. Michon J, Hartmann O, Bouffet E, et al. Preliminary analysis of the first open label randomized phase III study of recombinant granulocyte colony stimulating factor as an adjunct to combination induction chemotherapy in pediatric patients with metastatic neuroblastoma. *Blood* 1992;80:248(abst).

311. Kawa K, Yagi K. A multi-institutional randomized study on the effective schedule of G-CSF administration in pediatric cancer patients. Presented at: *18th International Congress of Chemotherapy*; June 27–July 2, 1993;173(abst).

312. Rubino C, Laplanche A, Patte C, et al. Cost-minimization analysis of prophylactic granulocyte colony-stimulating factor after induction chemotherapy in children with non-Hodgkin's lymphoma. *J Natl Cancer Inst* 1998;90:750–755.

313. Gillan ER, Christensen RD, Suen Y, et al. A randomized, placebo-controlled trial of recombinant human granulocyte colony-stimulating factor administration in newborn infants with presumed sepsis: significant induction of peripheral and bone marrow neutrophilia. *Blood* 1994;84:1427–1433.

314. Marina NM, Shema SJ, Bowman LC, et al. Failure of granulocyte-macrophage colony-stimulating factor to reduce febrile neutropenia in children with recurrent solid tumors treated with ifosfamide, carboplatin, and etoposide chemotherapy. *Med Pediatr Oncol* 1994;23:328–334.

315. Michon J, Bouffet E, Bernard JL, et al. Administration of recombinant human GM-CSF (RHUGM-CSF) after autologous bone marrow transplantation (ABMT): a study of 21 stage IV neuroblastoma patients undergoing a double intensification regimen. Presented at: *Annual Meeting of the American Society of Clinical Oncology* 1990;9:A712(abst).

316. Riikonen P, Saarinen UM, Makipernaa A, et al. Recombinant human granulocyte-macrophage colony-stimulating factor in the treatment of febrile neutropenia: a double blind placebo-controlled study in children. *Pediatr Infect Dis J* 1994;13:197–202.

317. Cairo MS, Agosti J, Ellis R, et al. A randomized, double-blind, placebo-controlled trial of prophylactic recombinant human granulocyte-macrophage colony-stimulating factor to reduce nosocomial infections in very low birth weight neonates. *J Pediatr* 1999;134:64–70.

Subject Index

Note: Page numbers in *italics* indicate figures; page numbers followed by t indicate tables.